D1294097

THE

PRINCIPLES AND PRACTICE

OF

OBSTETRICS

BY

JOSEPH B. De LEE, A.M., M.D.

PROFESSOR OF OBSTETRICS AND GYNECOLOGY AT THE UNIVERSITY OF
CHICAGO; CHIEF OF OBSTETRICS, CHICAGO LYING-IN HOSPITAL AND DIS-
PENSARY; CONSULTING OBSTETRICIAN TO PROVIDENT HOSPITAL, TO THE
CHICAGO MATERNITY CENTER, ETC.

*WITH 1221 ILLUSTRATIONS
ON 923 FIGURES, 265
OF THEM IN COLORS*

SIXTH EDITION, THOROUGHLY REVISED

PHILADELPHIA AND LONDON

W. B. SAUNDERS COMPANY

1933

Copyright, 1913, by W. B. Saunders Company. Reprinted May, 1913, October, 1913, and September, 1914. Revised, reprinted, and recopyrighted August, 1915. Reprinted August, 1916. Revised, reprinted, and recopyrighted November, 1918. Reprinted April, 1920, and August, 1921. Revised, reprinted, and recopyrighted August, 1924. Reprinted June, 1925, and January, 1927. Revised, reprinted, and recopyrighted April, 1928. Reprinted June, 1929, and June, 1930. Revised, reprinted, and recopyrighted January, 1933

Copyright, 1933, by W. B. Saunders Company

MADE IN U. S. A.

PRESS OF
W. B. SAUNDERS COMPANY
PHILADELPHIA

PREFACE TO THE SIXTH EDITION

GREATER difficulty than ever before was met in my attempt to keep the amount of material within the limits of one volume. Obstetric science and art are making rapid forward strides, and very little of the old is being disproved. This is true especially of the art, and therefore the reader will find few changes in the chapters devoted to the practical application of obstetric principles.

Owing to the undiminishing maternal mortality in the United States voices have been raised demanding a return to the midwife or, at least, a reactionary movement in obstetric practice. With the latter sentiment I agree—as it applies to the general surgeon, the occasional accoucheur, and to the family practitioner who has to do his work in the home, or in a small, usually understaffed, maternity ward of a general hospital. An expert obstetrician, working with the facilities of a well-equipped lying-in hospital, can and should seek to better the results obtainable by only natural obstetrics.

I have made an attempt to differentiate the two methods of practice and since the vast majority of births still occurs at home and in the hands of the family doctor, "the obstetrician to the people," very conservative advice, fitted to the milieu in which he works, has been given. Emphasis has been placed on intelligent expectancy, and I have shown how an efficient anti- and asepsis can be carried out in the most discouraging surroundings.

The text has been carefully revised and the illustrations too. A few obsolete ones were omitted, and many new ones added. I made a new set for the repair of perineal tears and episiotomy. Local anesthesia has been given the prominence it has come to deserve, and the newer narcotics, of the barbituric acid group, receive a proper evaluation.

A full description of the Aschheim-Zondek pregnancy test and a colored plate showing the reaction in the mouse are presented. The endocrinal changes in pregnancy are even less understood than in the normal woman, but after sifting an overwhelming mass of literature, the few kernels of probable truth have been shown in a colored diagram (dated).

It was not necessary to rewrite the chapters on the obstetric "diurnalia," hyperemesis, eclampsia, abruptio placentæ, placenta prævia, ruptura uteri, postpartum hemorrhage, breech—forceps—but they were carefully read, modern thoughts supplied and new illustrations inserted where necessary. The treatment of eclampsia always requires rewriting, and this was done.

The chapter on Contracted Pelvis seems too long in view of the great simplification of the treatment of this anomaly taking place of late. Most men do not trouble themselves with pelvic measurements and prepartal study of the probable mechanism of labor. All the fine nuances of the process in contracted pelvis are lost on them. They let the patient have a longer or shorter test, and perform cesarean section if difficulties arise. Such a course is degrading to our science and art, and results in a high maternal and fetal mortality. We have yet much to learn about contracted pelvis and nature's methods of overcoming mechanical difficulties. In this chapter only the treatment has been changed to harmonize with the latest scientific practice.

Much study is being given nowadays to the borderlands of gestation and internal medicine. Accordingly the subjects of tuberculosis, diabetes, heart disease, syphilis have been rewritten and brought up to date and the last one illustrated by a new colored plate showing the external manifestations of lues in a pregnant woman. Prof. v. Zumbusch of Munich, Germany, kindly provided the patients for the painting.

A great deal of time and effort were spent on the literature references. Since these take up much space and are useful only to the student and investigator, the authors are referred to tersely in the text and in the Bibliographies only the latest articles are mentioned. I took care to select such as possessed, themselves, the accumulated references to the literature. Thus the investigator is started out on his quest adequately directed.

My object always has been to supply the needs of the student and at the same time provide a wealth of instructive detail and illustrations for the practitioner—making the book an ever present help in time of trouble.

As in previous editions, the text reflects my teachings in Northwestern University Medical School and now at the University of Chicago. The principles of practice were developed in my service at the Chicago Lying-in Hospital and Dispensary. The obstetric technic is the result of my experience in many hospitals, in a large maternity out-department, and in private and consultation practice in the homes extending over a period of forty years. While formulating this system of obstetric thought and practice, the experiences and opinions of the best obstetric authorities as recorded in current literature have been duly respected. I have received much inspiration from the old volumes of Blundell and Ramsbotham of England, and Parvin of Philadelphia, and read with interest the works of Munro Kerr of Glasgow, and Eden of London; Schroeder, Bumm, Sellheim, and Stoeckel of Germany; Bar, Farabeuf, and Varnier of Paris, and our own Hirst and Williams. No book on obstetrics may now be written without a study of the monumental "Biologie und Pathologie des Weibes" by Halban-Seitz—an inexhaustible treasure house of information.

In the revision of the chapter on Embryology and the Physiology of the Fetus I had the benefit of the valued assistance of Dr. George W. Bartelmez, Professor of Anatomy, University of Chicago.

An appendix has been added giving a brief Chronology of Obstetrics. In a few minutes one can obtain a deep retrospect into the history of our art. This should be valuable for teachers.

Many physicians have written me, reporting unusual cases, or calling my attention to inaccuracies in the text, or expressing opinions of my work, and I offer them my appreciation. Mr. Felix Eisengräber, of Munich, and Miss Gladys McHugh, of Chicago, have continued to lend me their high artistic talents.

I wish to thank my Publishers who have gone to great expense in the preparation of this volume and whose consistent co-operation has enabled me to make the book just as I wanted it, and to keep it up to the very latest accomplishment in obstetrics.

JOSEPH B. DeLEE.

CHICAGO, ILLINOIS.
January, 1933.

PREFACE

THIS treatise is the outgrowth of a volume, by the author, entitled Notes on Obstetrics, and used for fourteen years as a text-book by the junior and senior classes at the Northwestern University Medical School.

Throughout its pages the author has constantly held in view the needs of the general practitioner and the student. Adequate space has been allowed the purely scientific subjects, and their direct bearing on daily practice has always been clearly emphasized.

Diagnosis has been made a particular feature, and the relations of obstetric conditions and accidents to general medicine, surgery, and the specialties have been fully brought out. Polemic discussion has been studiously avoided, at the risk, perhaps, of sometimes being too dogmatic.

In the preparation of the volume the works of the world's greatest authorities and the recent literature have been thoroughly studied, but the opinions expressed are mainly the result of the author's own experience in hospital, dispensary, consultation, and private practice. Twenty-one years' experience as a teacher of physicians, students, and nurses is reflected in these pages.

Lengthy bibliographies have been avoided, but sufficient recent references are given to enable the investigator to find all the literature.

For the student, owing to the crowded condition of the modern medical curriculum, brevity and system are essential, and the underlying principles of the art must be brought out. The practitioner needs a wealth of detail and of illustration to tell him what to do in a given case. To accomplish these purposes in a single volume two sizes of type have been used. Less important matter and details of treatment have been put in smaller type. For the same reasons lengthy descriptions of operations are omitted from the text, and put as full explanatory legends under the illustrations depicting the successive steps of the procedure. By studying the pictures serially, the reader will be better able to follow the operation than by referring to them from a distant text.

The subject matter is divided into four parts: The Physiology of Pregnancy, Labor, and the Puerperium; The Conduct of Pregnancy, Labor, and the Puerperium; The Pathology of Pregnancy, Labor, and the Puerperium; and Operative Obstetrics. Such an arrangement allows the easy division of the subject to fit the usual college curriculum, the Physiology and Conduct of Pregnancy, Labor, and the Puerperium being in the junior year, and the Pathology of Pregnancy, Labor, and the Puerperium, with Operative Obstetrics, in the senior year.

With very few exceptions the illustrations are original, having been drawn under the supervision of the author from fresh specimens, operations on the living and on the manikin, and from original photographs taken by himself. To Bumm's matchless work the author is indebted for many ideas, and for these, as well as for permission to copy some of his plates, the author is profoundly grateful.

James Kelly Parker drew most of the pictures; Grace Amidon did all the microscopic ones; and Hermann Becker, of Baltimore, those of the pelvic floor and the Porro operation. The tireless labor these artists put upon their work, which has extended over a period of eight years, is deeply appreciated.

The material for the illustrations came mainly from the Chicago Lying-in Hospital. The microscopic and wet preparations were generously furnished by

Professor F. Robert Zeit, of the Northwestern University Medical School. Professor H. Gideon Wells, of the University of Chicago, also placed specimens at the disposal of the author, for all of which he expresses his thanks.

To Dr. Heliodor Schiller the author is grateful for help in reading the proofs, and to the publishers, Messrs. W. B. Saunders Co., for most unusual generosity in the preparation of the volume.

JOSEPH B. DE LEE.

CONTENTS

PART II

THE PATHOLOGY OF PREGNANCY, LABOR, AND THE PUERPERIUM

SECTION VI

THE PATHOLOGY OF LABOR

SECTION VII

PATHOLOGY OF THE PUERPERIUM

PART III

OPERATIVE OBSTETRICS

INTRODUCTION

OBSTETRICS is that part of the science and art of medicine relating to the function of reproduction. The word obstetrics probably comes from the Latin *ob* and *stare*, "to stand before," "to protect." While, strictly, it should be applied to childbirth or parturition, usage justifies its application to all the phases of reproduction. "Midwifery" and "tocology" are synonyms for obstetrics. The function of reproduction is a closed cycle of events, interposed in the life of a woman, and comprises five periods—conception, pregnancy, labor, lactation, and involution.

The union of the male element of propagation, the spermatozoid, with the corresponding female element, the ovum, in the genital tract of the woman, results in the formation of a cell which is capable of attaching itself to the uterine wall and developing into a fully matured individual resembling its parents. The union of these two procreative elements is called conception. The production of a ripe human ovum requires about ten lunar months—*i. e.*, pregnancy lasts about two hundred and eighty days, and on the completion of this period the uterus expels its contents into the external world, the process being called labor, or parturition. The reproductive cycle is continued by the breasts taking up the further nourishment of the child,—lactation,—and is completed when the pelvic organs, concerned in the process, return to their former condition. This function is called involution. This cycle may be repeated more or less often during the period of reproductive activity of the woman, which extends from puberty to the menopause. One demands that it should not cause her death nor injure her health, and that the child be born alive, well, and capable of continued extra-uterine existence.

Unfortunately, this standard is seldom attained. The process of reproduction is disturbed by many pathogenic influences in all the periods of the cycle, and many permanent structural changes are inaugurated. The study of all these processes, both normal and pathologic, is the science of obstetrics; the application of this scientific knowledge and that derived from intelligent experience at the bedside of the patient comprises the art.

In the course of the study of obstetrics it will be seen that the function of gestation affects every organ in the woman's body, and, conversely, all conditions, medical or surgical, have a more or less direct influence on the process going on in the uterus. The child, too, has its own physiology and pathology, both medical and surgical. The obstetrician, therefore, must not alone be well versed in his particular science and art, but he must also be an internist, a psychologist, a surgeon, and a pediatrist. The borderlands of obstetrics, with medicine, surgery, and pediatrics, are narrow and intimate. In some universities the chairs of obstetrics and of gynecology are combined, it being held that the relations of the two branches of medicine are so interwoven that their separation is artificial and impractical. The obstetrician should not be a "midwife," caring only for actual births—his duty is to treat all the diseases and accidents that have to do with the reproductive function. Thus he must as skilfully repair an old perineal laceration as a new one, or treat sterility, as well as the surgical complications of puerperal infection. He must be able to remove a ruptured uterus, extirpate ovarian cysts complicating labor, as well as perform cesarean section.

While obstetrics is the most difficult and arduous of medical practice, it at the same time is the most satisfying. Nowhere can the physician accomplish so much, both in prevention of disease and accidents and in treatment and operation. The accoucheur very often has the positive conviction that without him either mother or child, or both, would have perished. With the erection of model maternity hospitals, the use of anesthetics, and the employment of sufficient assistants for the conduct of parturition the practice of obstetrics is being divested of most of its objectionable features, and with the public there is a growing sentiment toward the employment of obstetric specialists. These circumstances all tend to make the field of obstetrics more inviting to the ambitious physician, and will conduce to more rapid advance in both its science and art. The broader conception of the scope of obstetrics referred to above will also work to the same happy result.

Statistics show that there is need for this. It is generally conceded that the practice of obstetrics is on a low plane. Many reasons have been advanced to account for it, but in my opinion the basic cause is the prevalence of the notion that childbirth is a normal function.

Is labor in the woman of today a normal function? I say it should be, but is not. Imperfect as our statistics are, only four-fifths of the area of the United States being registered, and the returns from the registered portion being incomplete, we know that 16,000 women annually die in childbirth. We can form no conception of the late or postponed mortality from injury received during labor, and from diseases acquired during pregnancy and the puerperium, nor can any one tell how many women die from childbirth, but are buried under another diagnosis. I feel perfectly safe in stating that over 25,000 women die in the United States every year from the direct and indirect effects of pregnancy and labor.

The immense amount of invalidism resulting from childbirth is absolutely unmeasurable, but we know that annually hundreds of thousands of women flock to our hospitals for the repair of injuries and for relief from the effects of diseases contracted during labor. It is safe to say that 50 per cent. of women who have had children bear the marks of injury, and will, sooner or later, suffer from them. Laceration of the pelvic floor, of the supports of the uterus, bladder, and vagina occur in every labor. This fact, easily proved clinically by any accoucheur, has been demonstrated by Schultze and the anatomist Tandler. The late consequences of laceration of the pelvic floor, such as dislocation of the pelvic organs, especially uterus and bladder, infections of the genital tract, congestive conditions of the uterus, tubes, and ovaries, cystitis, ureteritis, pyelitis, etc., prolapse of the rectum, —indeed, a host of diseases, some fatal, and all inimical to the enjoyment of life,— all these conditions and others that could be named in considerable number that follow even natural delivery stamp the function of reproduction in women as pathologic. The symptoms of pregnancy often resemble those of sickness,—the nausea and vomiting, the psychic changes, the varicosities. Serologists tell us the blood changes are similar to those found in the reactions of immunity to infection or malignant growths. Between 3 and 5 per cent. of children die during delivery, and a great many are permanently crippled by the forces of labor.

Can a function so perilous that, in spite of the best care, it kills thousands of women every year, that leaves at least a quarter of the women more or less invalided, and a majority with permanent anatomic changes of structure, that is always attended by severe pain and tearing of tissues, and that kills 3 to 5 per cent. of children—can such a function be called normal? Much depends on what should be defined as "normal" for the human. Among insects it is the rule for the female to die soon after reproduction. The male bee is killed by the act of copulation. The salmon invariably dies after spawning. In domestic animals, laceration of the perineum and other birth injuries, endogenous sepsis, etc., are frequently met. Since these functions are considered natural and normal, the question arises, Are not a certain toll of mothers and a certain amount of damage to maternal structures natural to parturition, and therefore normal?   I know of no one who would take such a position.   All authors hold that the reproductive function should, normally, have no mortality, and it should not injure the woman nor the child.

Mauriceau epigrammatically called pregnancy a disease of nine months' duration.   Sir James Y. Simpson said that "parturition is always physiologic in its object, but not in some of the phenomena and peculiarities which attend upon it in civilized life."   Engelman, after comparing the labors of primitive and civilized peoples, says that a simple, natural labor is no longer possible, and, further, "the parturient suffers under the continuance of the old prejudice that labor is a physiological act."   Kehrer said that there was no sharp line between physiologic and pathologic pregnancy.   Kroenig says that modern conditions are such that child bearing has largely ceased to be a physiologic process.   J. O. Polak, in 1910, said that parturition is rapidly becoming a pathologic phenomenon.   F. S. Newell says that we must realize that "something has gone wrong with this normal physiologic process," or that the present methods are not efficacious.   E. P. Davis calls the statement that labor is a physiologic process a half truth.   Schwarz, of St. Louis, says, "tradition and ignorance are alike combined in spreading the fable that child bearing is a physiologic process."   Moran, of Washington (1915), asks for a "nation-wide propaganda to teach the laity that the long-cherished fallacy that pregnancy and labor are physiologic conditions should be abandoned."   Asa B. Davis, of New York (1923), believes 10 per cent. of pregnancies are pathologic and all of them potentially so.

J. Whitridge Williams (1923) says that 50 per cent. of women present evidences of toxemia, which he classifies as pathologic.   Sellheim in 1923, after comparing primitive woman and the animals, called attention to the incomplete adjustment of the modern, civilized woman to the demands of pregnancy, saying that she has reached her limit of power to meet the strain, and if she is not physically perfect she fails.   Eclampsia and other toxemias, therefore, are a failure of metabolism to adapt the organism to the new situation.   He emphasizes the diastasis recti abdominis, the striæ, pelvic floor injuries with prolapse, and comes "to the saddening conclusion, that through culture, i. e., in so far as it indicates estrangement from nature, pregnancy, labor, lactation, indeed, the whole function of reproduction, have become a load for woman which border on the pathologic or excessive, in part already must be appraised as a disease or as a pathogenic factor."

Later authorities also support my view of the matter.   Max Hirsch considering the damage done to the pelvic joints says that labor is a disease with anatomic foundation.   J. R. Goodall says that 80 per cent. of women are left with a pathogenic residuum from their labors—i. e., chronic endocervicitis.   Victor Bonney holds childbearing a physiologic phenomenon in the life of the race, but not in the life of the woman.

As was said before, 25,000 women die annually in the United States during childbirth; 6000 die from infection, 5000 from eclampsia, 4000 from hemorrhage. Of the immense number of wounded we can form no estimate.   That a large part of all this misery is preventable is the universal opinion of those who have studied the situation.   Why is it not prevented?   Because the standards of obstetric instruction and particularly of obstetric practice are very low.   Neither the schools, nor the hospitals, nor the profession itself, nor the public, hold the obstetrician and his art in very high esteem.   As a result the care of the child-bearing woman is left to the young, the inexperienced, the incompetent, or, indeed, even a non-medical person, the midwife.

It must be evident to anyone who will give the matter unbiased thought that, if we can invest obstetrics with the dignity it deserves, such regard will immediately place the practice on an elevated plane and more physicians will select this specialty for their life work; that the law-makers will hold the child-bearing woman with more respect and will protect her with proper legislation and will insist on sufficient obstetric instruction in the schools; prenatal care will come into its own, and that anachronism, the midwife, will spontaneously disappear. Finally, the public will properly evaluate the obstetrician's service and adequately remunerate him for his arduous labors. All these will inevitably reduce the deplorably high mortality and morbidity of childbirth.

But the present notorious disappreciation and disesteem of obstetrics will not be eliminated from the popular or from the professional mind until the pathologic dignity of the child-bearing function is recognized. No one need fear that the doctrine of the pathogenicity of parturition will invite undue interference with the natural powers. The contrary is to be expected. In medicine and surgery accurate knowledge of the nature of disease has often reduced the number of operations, and always has clarified and hardened the indications for interference. The best surgeons are the best pathologists. So in obstetrics, those men who know the dangers and possibilities besetting the child-bearing function will make the best accoucheurs, infinitely better than those who blindly call the function normal and lull themselves and their patients into a feeling of fancied security.

A text-book is not the place for an extended discussion of a subject of this kind, but the author must reiterate his conviction that not the majority, but the minority, of labor cases is normal, and that not until the pathologic dignity of obstetrics is fully recognized may we hope for any considerable reduction of the mortality and morbidity of childbirth.

LITERATURE

Ballantyne: "The Nature of Pregnancy," Brit. Med. Jour., February, 1914, p. 354.—*Bonney, Victor:* Newcastle Med. Jour., January, 1927.—*Davis, E. P.:* Jour. Amer. Med. Assoc., July 6, 1912.—*Engelman:* Amer. Sys. of Obst., vol. i, pp. 24 and 64.—*Goodall, J. R.:* Puerperal Infection, Montreal, 1932, p. 21.—*Halban and Tandler:* Anatomie und Ätiologie der Genital-Prolapse beim Weibe, Vienna, Braumüller, 1907.—*Hirsch, Max:* Zentrbl. für Gyn., April 23, 1932, p. 1064.—*Kehrer:* Volk. klin. Vort., 1905, Zur. Embr. Toxämia Grav.—*Kroenig:* Jour. Amer. Med. Assoc., February 12, 1910, p. 517.—*Moran, J. F.:* Jour. Amer. Med. Assoc., January 9, 1915, p. 126.—*Schultze:* Monatsschr. f. Geb. u. Gyn., December, 1913.—*Sellheim:* Mediz. Klinik., August, 1923, p. 1143.—*Simpson:* Collected Essays, vol. ii, p. 123.—*Williams:* Text-book, 1923.

PART I

THE PHYSIOLOGY OF PREGNANCY, LABOR, AND THE PUERPERIUM

SECTION I

PHYSIOLOGY OF PREGNANCY

CHAPTER I

PUBERTY, OVULATION, AND MENSTRUATION

Puberty.—At birth a girl and a boy baby are much alike. A close study will show small differences; the boy weighs, on the average, one-fourth of a pound more, the head is a little harder and larger, absolutely and also relatively to the body; a difference in the pelvis is also discernible: the female pelvis is larger and shallower than the male, and this is also true of the lower animals. More boys are born than girls—105 to 100, a proportion that prevails the world over, and for all the years, but since more boys die during labor—1 in 16—and during the first years of life, this proportion is reversed, so that later the females preponderate.

During the first years the characteristics of the sexes gradually become more marked, and as soon as the child walks the differentiation becomes apparent. The girl develops mentally and physically earlier than the boy, and one can sooner discover in her those traits of the female that distinguish it in later life. Sexually, the differences are less marked until the age of eight to ten years, when in the girl a change begins. In the boy it is noticed a few years later. The transformation becomes more apparent at the age of about fourteen years. It is called puberty, or in girls, menarche (from Greek μήν ἀρχή), and may be defined as that period in the life of the individual when it becomes capable of reproduction. The changes are more rapid and marked in the female—indeed, her sexual life is more intense and plays a greater rôle in her existence. Madame de Staël said: "L'amour n'est qu'une épisode de la vie de l'homme; c'est l'histoire tout entière de la femme."

The girl passing into womanhood changes physically and psychically. The pelvis enlarges, the limbs round out with fat, and the angularity of the body is replaced by graceful curves. The general carriage of the body is more womanly and dignified. The breasts enlarge, become more prominent, fuller, and firmer, the result of growth of the gland tissue and the addition of fat; the nipple becomes more prominent; the primary areola develops. Only very rarely may a droplet of secretion be squeezed from the nipple. The skin shows marked changes: its activity is increased, that of the sebaceous glands particularly, so that not infrequently comedones and acne result; in brunets the pigmentation deepens; the hair takes on more luxuriant growth, and it also develops on the mons pubis and axillæ; striæ—fine lines—sometimes appear on the thighs, and especially on the breasts. These striæ are due to stretching of the skin, the connective-tissue fibers arranging themselves in parallel lines, some of them tearing. They at first appear as purplish lines, but after several years turn a silvery white. The external genitalia grow larger, darker, more vascular, have more secretion, and emit a faint characteristic

1

odor. The thyroid enlarges, the larynx changes, especially in the male. In the female the voice also is altered, becoming fuller, lower in scale, and more melodious. In brunets the tendency is toward a contralto; in blondes, toward a soprano, range.

The mind undergoes alteration in its three parts—the will, the intellect, and the emotions. The will, especially during the change, becomes uncertain, and the girl loses to a good extent her control over it. Hysteric manifestations are quite common. The intellect broadens; new perceptions give a grander conception of life. The girl feels that a great transformation is taking place in her being, and the pride of womanhood and of anticipated wife- and motherhood swells in her. The emotions during the period of change also become unstable: the girl laughs and cries often without reason, is happy, gay, or sad and melancholy without cause. One must watch these manifestations—they may exceed the normal. The inclination toward the male increases, while at the same time a sense of modesty appears. Libido, unless artificially stimulated, usually does not fully develop until after marriage.

This transformation is the outward expression of the changes occurring in the internal organs of generation and in the ductless glands. The uterus is developing rapidly. The vagina lengthens and becomes rugous, the tubes grow longer, the ovaries take on a special activity, ova develop, the Graafian follicles ripen—in short, ovulation begins. With ovulation comes the ability to reproduce, but the girl at puberty is unfit to bring forth children. Cases are on record where girls of ten and even of nine years bore children, the one reported by Bodd weighing 3500 gm. (Literature, Dittrick). Plato set twenty years as the best age for the first child, and Wernich, from a study of the development of the children of young women, decided on the age of twenty-three as the best. At this time also the pelvis has achieved its full development; the bones are still somewhat elastic, the joints supple; the coccyx, particularly, can be pressed back, and the pelvic genital tract is soft and distensible. Hypertrophy of the thyroid and pituitary glands is constant during this period, and it is certain that the hypophysis has much to do with the changes above mentioned. Overfunctioning of the anterior lobe is associated with overactivity of the ovaries.

The most important sign of the advent of puberty is the appearance of the menses, or menstruation. This is a flow of blood of several days' duration, recurring every four weeks, attended by local symptoms referable to the genitalia and general symptoms. This phenomenon, again, is dependent upon or related to the changes going on in the ovaries, called ovulation. Therefore, puberty is marked by the inauguration of two new functions,—ovulation and menstruation,— each of which will now be considered.

OVULATION

Ovulation is that process by which an ovum ripens and is extruded from the ovary—that is, it is the maturation of the ovum or egg and expulsion of same from the ovary.

The ovary is a densely fibrous little organ, situated in the pelvis on the posterior surface of the broad ligament, in a shallow pouch—the "fossa ovarica." It averages 39 mm. long, 19 mm. wide, and 8 to 13 mm. thick, and weighs about 5 gm. The right is usually larger than the left, and is more liable to disease, because of the proximity of the appendix.

The organ is shaped like a large almond, being attached to the broad ligament by two layers of the peritoneum, between which the vessels and nerves enter its substance. The outer end is attached by one of the fimbriæ of the Fallopian tube to the tube. The ovary was first mentioned by Herophilus (Alexandria, 300 B. C.), and received its name from Steno, in the seventeenth century A. D. (Fasbender). The ovaries of different women vary much in size without apparently any relation to fertility. At birth the ovary is relatively quite large. Its growth up to maturity is caused by the formation of connective tissue, vessels, and the enlargement of existing primordial follicles. Corpora albicantia were found in the ovaries of new-born and very young children by Runge. Many ova are destroyed in all stages by the constriction of the fibrous tissue. After the menopause the ovary shrinks, and in old women may be as small as a navy bean. Accessory ovaries have been found on the broad ligaments, and are probably the result of faulty development, not of fetal inflammation. A third ovary and corresponding tube have been found, which is interesting from several clinical and medicolegal points of view. The ovary is covered by a layer of low columnar, lusterless epithelium, called the germinal epithelium, under which is the tough tunica albuginea. Beneath this are small unripe ova, while deeper down are larger ova

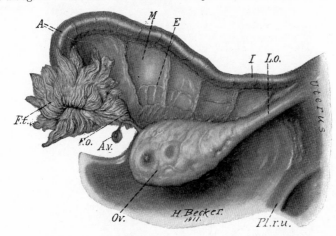

FIG. 1.—NORMAL OVARY AND FALLOPIAN TUBE.

F.t., Fimbria; *A*, ampulla; *M*, mesosalpinx; *E*, parovarium; *F.o.*, fimbria ovarica; *A.v.*, hydatid of Morgagni; *Pl.r.u.*, plica recto-uterina; *I*, isthmus tubæ.

in the process of ripening. These ova are surrounded by stroma, a characteristic, highly cellular, reticular connective tissue. The blood-supply is abundant, and numerous fine nerves form networks around the follicles.

The formation of ova begins early in fetal life. On the posterior wall of the abdomen of the embryo, to the inside of the Wolffian bodies, two light streaks of celom-peritoneal epithelium

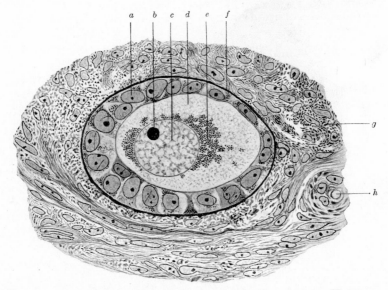

FIG. 2.—FOLLICLE IN THE FIRST STAGES OF GROWTH FROM OVARY OF ADULT WOMAN.

a, Follicular cells with mitochondria; *b*, nucleus of ovum; *c*, nucleolus of ovum; *d*, protoplasm of ovum; *e*, perinuclear accumulation of mitochondria (yolk nucleus); *f*, basement membrane; *g*, interstitial connective tissue; *h*, blood-vessel. Aniline acid fuchsin stain (× 780). From a preparation of C. M. Bensley (Maximow-Bloom, "Text-book of Histology").

appear. They are supported by connective tissue, and are the primary structures of the future ovary or testicle. In the somewhat proliferated peritoneal epithelium (germinal epithelium of Waldeyer) are seen many cells of greater size than the others, spheric in shape, and with a pale vesicular nucleus, the primordial eggs, or ova (Fig. 3). These may develop into primordial seminal cells if the fetus is a male.   The germinal epithelium proliferates actively, as do also the primordial ova, and is usually said to dip down into the stroma of the ovary, carrying with it the

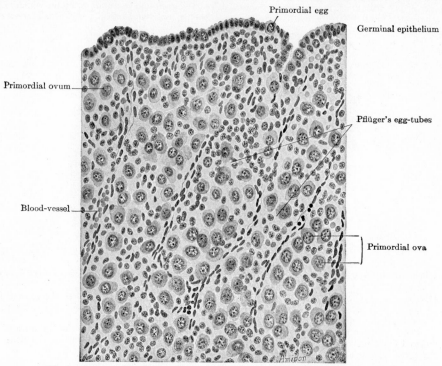

FIG. 3.—OVARY OF FIVE-MONTHS' FETUS, SHOWING EGG-TUBES AND PRIMORDIAL OVA.

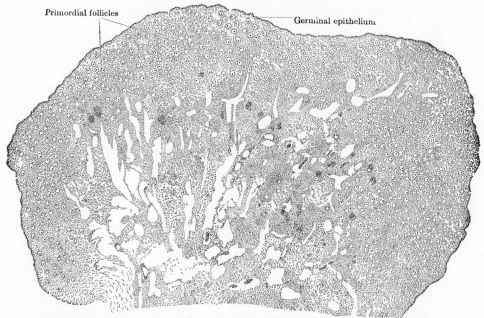

FIG. 4.—OVARY OF NEW-BORN, SHOWING PRIMORDIAL FOLLICLES. (From Dr. Zeit's specimen.)

ova. These groups of cells are called "egg balls," or the Pflüger "ovarian tubes." The connective tissue surrounding these columns of epithelial cells grows in such a manner that masses of germinal epithelium containing one or two primordial ova are split off, until finally the ovary is formed completely of such "primordial follicles" and connective-tissue stroma (Fig. 2). According to the recent work of Felix, Pflüger's tubes do not exist in the human ovary, but the follicles arise from a cellular mass just beneath the germinal epithelium. The primordial follicles develop into the larger structures, which de Graaf discovered in 1672 and have been named after him. The ova are nearly all completed during fetal life; perhaps some are formed during the first few years of life. The ovary of the new-born infant contains ovocytes of a number variously estimated at from 200,000 to 400,000. These are closely arranged in the periphery of the ovary, while toward the hilum are a few follicles in further advancement. The main function of the ovary is to mature and discharge the ova lying in the Graafian follicles. Other functions are ascribed to the ovary, but their discussion will be made later.

When a follicle begins to ripen,—and one lying near the hilum usually undergoes this change, —it sinks toward the center of the ovary. The follicle epithelium undergoes a rapid proliferation, a fluid appears in the center of the mass of cells, which are thus pressed against the wall of the follicle (Figs. 6 to 8). This layer of cells is called the stratum granulosum; the liquid, the liquor folliculi. The liquor folliculi is a clear, viscid, alkaline, albuminoid fluid, containing oil-globules and a few granules. At one part of the periphery of the follicle a small clump of cells of the stratum granulosum is seen, called the cumulus oöphorus or discus proligerus, and in this von

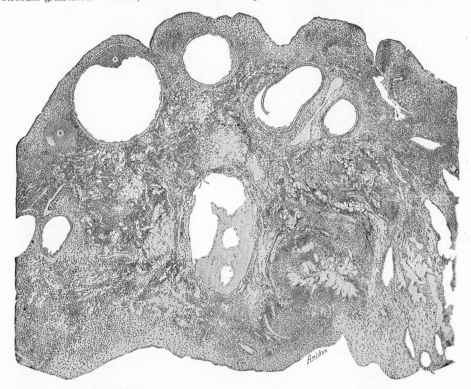

FIG. 5.—MATURE OVARY. TRANSVERSE SECTION. (Dr. Zeit's specimen.)

Baer, in 1827, found the dog ovum (Fig. 5). The stratum granulosum rests on a layer of loose connective tissue with characteristic large cells, the tunica interna, and this in turn on a layer of closely felted fibrous tissue, the tunica externa, both of the latter being derived from the stroma of the ovary, and called the theca folliculi (Fig. 6). The blood-supply of the ovary is increased, and there is a local congestion around the growing follicle. The cells of the follicle proliferate rapidly, the liquor folliculi increases, and the follicle nears the surface of the ovary. At the spot nearest the surface the theca folliculi atrophies, or its fibers separate, and the follicle bursts at this point (the stigma), the ovum, surrounded by cells from the cumulus oöphorus, escaping. Frequently the follicle does not burst, the ovum dies, and the follicle undergoes involution. This is not called ovulation. Coincident with the normal transformation in the follicle, changes destined to prepare it for the reception of the male element are going on in the ovum embedded in the cumulus oöphorus. The ovum is a typical cell, and consists of a cell wall, cytoplasm, deutoplasm, or yolk, which appear later in the development, and a nucleus, or germinal vesicle, with a nucleolus or germinal spot. During the later period of the ripening the nucleus nears the surface and undergoes karyokinesis. After the resolution of the chromatin into distinct chromosomes two successive cell divisions occur by which two small globules, or polar cells, are extruded and come to lie beneath the zona pellucida (Fig. 9). Through these divisions the chromosomes are reduced to one-half the original number. The polar globules were discovered

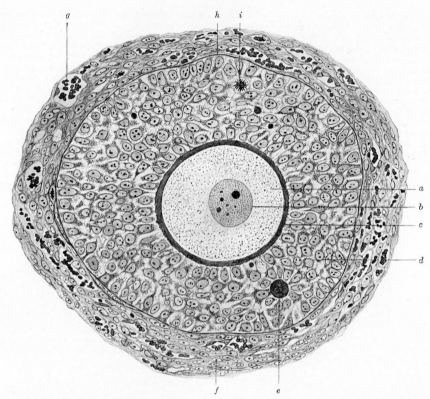

Fig. 6.—Growing Follicle from Human Ovary (Eighteenth Day of Menstrual Cycle).

a, Ovum; *b*, its nucleus; *c*, zona pellucida; *d*, follicular epithelium with mitochondria; *e*, vacuoles of Call-Exner; *f*, theca folliculi (outer and inner layer not differentiated as yet); *g*, blood-vessels with erythrocytes; *h*, basement membrane; *i*, mitosis of follicular cell (×375). From same section as Fig. 2 (Maximow-Bloom, "Text-book of Histology").

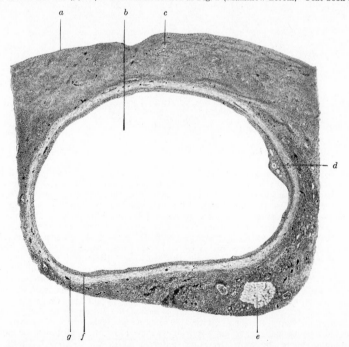

Fig. 7.—Large Follicle (5 mm. in Diameter) from Human Ovary (Eighteenth Day of Menstrual Cycle).

a, Surface of ovary with germinal epithelium; *b*, follicular liquid; *c*, primary follicle; *d*, cumulus oöphorus with ovum; *e*, corpus albicans; *f*, membrana granulosa; *g*, theca externa and interna (×20). From same ovary as Fig. 2 (Maximow-Bloom, "Text-book of Histology").

by Robin, a French histologist, in 1821–1825. The smaller germinal vesicle now rests, and is called the female pronucleus. The formation and extrusion of the polar globules are necessary to reduce the number of chromosomes of the female nucleus (Hertwig). A similar chromosome reduction takes place in the formation of the spermatozoid, except that the end-products are all of equal size and function. The halving of the number of chromosomes in both ovum and spermatozoid prior to their union at conception, when the normal number is restored, is believed to be important in maintaining the mechanism of inheritance.

The ovum as it is expelled from the Graafian follicle (Fig. 10) is just visible to the eye as a fine white point, measuring, naked, 0.2 millimeter in diameter. It

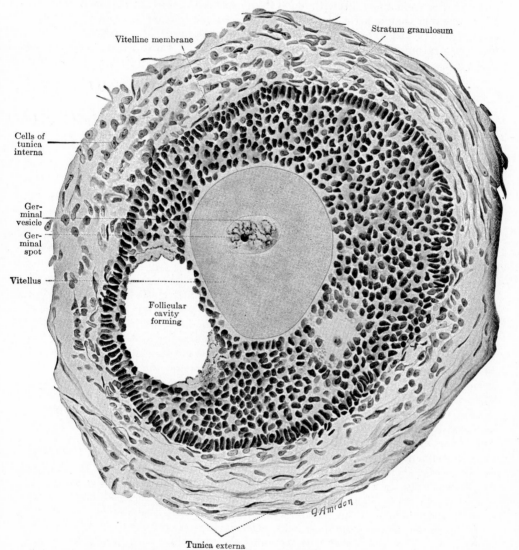

FIG. 8.—FURTHER DEVELOPMENT OF OVUM.

is surrounded by 100 or more epithelial cells derived from the stratum granulosum, arranged radially around the ovum, and called the corona radiata; inside this is the oölemma or zona pellucida, a thick membrane with radial fibrillations, not constant in all animals, and formed by the follicle cells; next comes a space, which also is not constant, the perivitelline space (Nagel), and may be only an optical effect, or it may occur after the extrusion of the polar globules; within the ovum itself is a broad peripheral zone of clear cytoplasm and a large central zone of

dark, coarsely granular deutoplasm; buried in the latter is the female pronucleus—
which was the germinal vesicle.

The expulsion of the ovum takes place when the Graafian follicle bursts, the
former having already been loosened from its bed in the cumulus oöphorus by
vacuolization of the cells of the stratum granulosum. The ovum finds its way
to the tube, there to await fertilization by the male element.

The Formation of the Corpus Luteum.—After the escape of the ovum and
part of the liquor folliculi out of the Graafian follicle the walls of the latter collapse,
and any space remaining fills with blood from ruptured vessels of the tunica propria.
It is probable that a little blood flows also into the peritoneal cavity. Rarely,
enough may be lost to be of clinical importance—even fatal. Many authors believe
that the stratum granulosum disappears, and the cavity is invaded by connective-
tissue cells from the theca, containing a yellow, refracting pigment—lutein or,

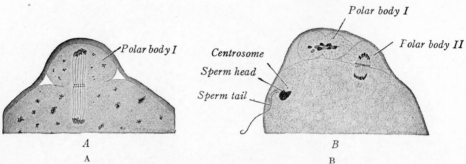

Fig. 9.—A, Formation of the First Polar Cell in the Mouse Ovum (Sobotta) × 1500. B, Separation of the
Second Polar Cell in the Bat Ovum (Arey, after Van der Stricht).

according to Escher, carotin, a substance identical with the coloring matter of
carrots. Bischoff believed the lutein cells are modified epithelial cells from the
stratum granulosum, and the latest work proves he was correct (Novak). There
is a very active production of luetin cells, which come to live in festoons around the
central blood-clot. The small collapsed follicle grows in the first two weeks to the
size of a bean, and shows the irregular yellow outline of lutein cells around the red
blood-clot. Fibrous tissue grows into the lutein mass and the blood-clot from the
periphery, giving the structure its irregular outline, and at the end of three weeks
the corpus luteum, as it is called, is 15 to 20 mm. in diameter. Now retrogression
occurs, the connective tissue replacing the lutein cells, whereby the yellow color is
changed to silvery white, the corpus albicans (Fig. 13); after several weeks more
the corpus luteum is represented only by a small retracted scar.

If pregnancy supervenes on this ovulation, the great vascularity of the parts,
or some other factor—late experiments of Aschheim, Zondek, Evans et al. seeming
to prove it to be the anterior lobe of the hypophysis—causes an excessive growth of
the corpus luteum. The histologic changes are the same as described, but they are
greater and prolonged (Figs. 11 and 14). Robert Meyer distinguishes four stages
—proliferation of the granulosa cells, vascularization, the stage of bloom, and
regression. The full growth is attained at the thirteenth week, when the
yellow body may take one-third the extent of the ovary, being the size of a
large hazelnut, sometimes palpable on bimanual examination. It continues
of this size until toward the end of pregnancy, when regressive changes begin
which are completed several months after delivery. The large corpus luteum of
pregnancy is sometimes called a true corpus luteum. The small corpus luteum of
menstruation is sometimes called a false corpus luteum. The French call these the
epithelial gland. Below suggests the term "glandula lutea." It is usually possible to
distinguish one from the other, but, as Hirst has shown, in the ovaries of two virgins

in which the corpus luteum of menstruation was almost exactly like a corpus luteum of pregnancy, one cannot always be certain. In cows they are not distinguishable. Some ripe Graafian follicles do not rupture, and a process of pseudocorpus luteum formation occurs also in them. Sometimes regression does not occur in the corpus luteum, but it enlarges into a cyst requiring operative removal.

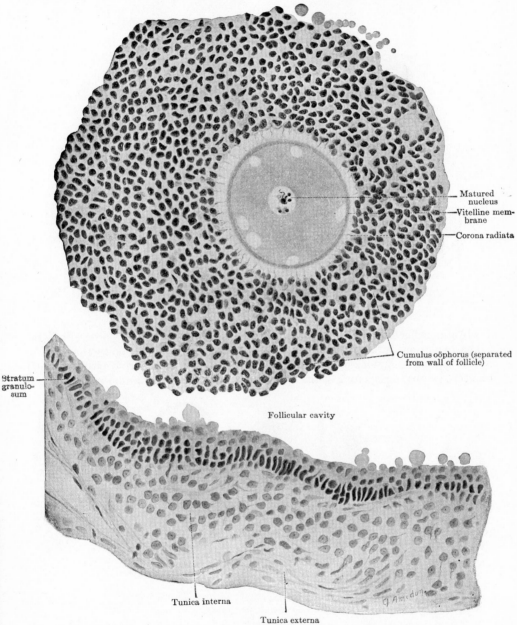

FIG. 10.—THE OVUM NEAR MATURITY.

The Functions of the Corpus Luteum.—It is more than probable that the glandula lutea has a vital relation to the function of gestation. G. Born and Prenant first suggested that it has an internal secretion, which circulating in the blood stimulates and regulates the changes of gestation. After castration the islands of

Langerhans and the hypophysis cerebri hypertrophy, showing an intimate inter-relation between these endocrinal glands. Leo Loeb found in guinea-pigs that the corpus luteum prepares an internal secretion, or hormone, which sensitizes the uterine mucosa so that it reacts to the stimulation of the ovum (or, indeed, any foreign body), with the production of exuberant decidua or maternal placenta.

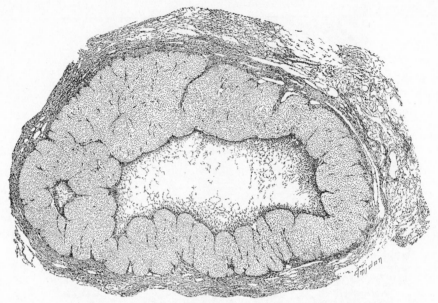

FIG. 11.—CORPUS LUTEUM VERUM.

Loeb also believes that the same hormone, which Allen called "progestin," in-hibits ovulation during pregnancy, though clinical experience shows that this is not invariable. Zondek describes two hormones in the anterior pituitary: (A) one that causes the ripening of the follicle; (B) one that causes luteinization. Both

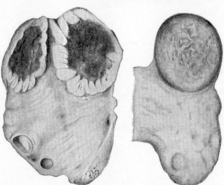

A   B
FIG. 12.—OVARY WITH CORPUS LUTEUM IN SITU.
A, Laid open; B, from outside.

are increased enormously by the presence of a pregnancy. Another hormone in the anterior pituitary is growth producing, especially effective on the genitals. The hypophysis is the motor of the sexual function. It seems that the nidation and stability of the pregnancy are dependent on the corpus luteum, because re-moval of the same in the early months usually causes abortion. Later, pregnancy is less likely to be interrupted—a point of practical importance. Some of the breast changes in pregnancy may also be due to this hormone in the blood.

The **ovary** has other functions. The mighty changes in the whole system of the female occurring at puberty are ascribable to influences emanating from the

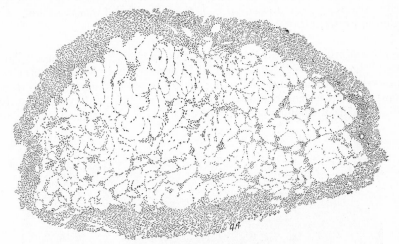

FIG. 13.—CORPUS ALBICANS. SEVEN WEEKS.

ovary. It is now generally believed that these changes are due to an internal secretion of the ovary prepared by the cells, easily demonstrated in lower animals, called the interstitial gland, which, experiments show, causes the sexual characters.

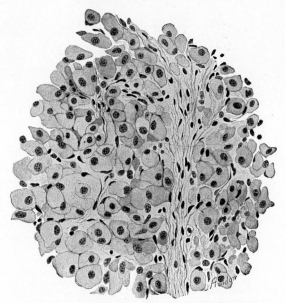

FIG. 14.—CORPUS LUTEUM VERUM. INDIVIDUAL CELLS.

Halban transplanted ovaries to distant parts of the body and proved the chemical theory of ovarian influence. Frank has found a substance in the follicular fluid of the ovary which he calls the female sex hormone, isolated by Doisy as "theelin," 1929. He can demonstrate it in the blood of menstruating women; it increases until the flow begins when it appears in the discharge. It also occurs in the blood of gravid women as early as the sixth week, and may be used in the diagnosis of pregnancy. The ovary is subject to the hormones elaborated by other glands of the endocrinal system, e. g., the hypophysis cerebri, the adrenals, the thyroid, the mamma, the pancreas (insulin), and, in turn, influences them. It also has a bearing on the formation of bone, e. g., osteomalacia. The most important function ascribed to the ovary, next to ovulation, is the induction of menstruation. (Literature: Chiriè, Frank, Graves.)

MENSTRUATION

Menstruation, also called the menses, the "periods," "catamenia," "monthly sickness," "the monthlies," "cleansing," "the flowers," may be defined as a periodic flow of blood from the genitals, recurring every four weeks, accompanied by general symptoms of malaise, nervous manifestations, etc., and local symptoms of pelvic congestion. This phenomenon occurs during the normal reproductive period of

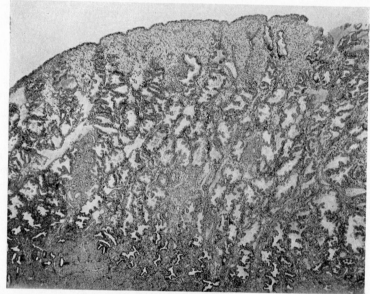

Fig. 15.—Mucous Membrane Removed Two Days Before Period Was Expected.   (Furnished by Professor G. W. Bartelmez, Culbertson Collection, University of Chicago.)

women, the *menacme* (Kisch), which begins with puberty, and continues up to about forty-five years. At this age, among other changes, the periods cease and the menopause, the climacteric, or the "change of life," takes place.

The menstrual flow begins as a whitish discharge, but soon becomes bloody, and contains red and white blood-corpuscles, degenerated, ciliated, and columnar epithelium, vaginal and uterine epithelium and secretions, and many micro-organisms, some of them pathogenic. Geist says we can differentiate menstrual blood from other bloody discharges microscopically.

The Anatomy.—For the first ten to fourteen days after beginning of the flow, the mucous membrane is thin (1 to 2 mm.), pale, and smooth, the glands are small, the secretion scant, the arteries and veins not prominent, but on the injected specimen they are seen to be numerous. Especially thick is the capillary network just under the epithelium and around the glands. The cylindric ciliated epithelium is continued into the glands. It is higher in the gland lumina. The connective tissue around the glands contains many large round-cells with large nuclei (Figs. 17 and 18). About ten days before the appearance of the menses the uterus becomes congested, enlarges, grows softer, the endometrium thickens to 5 or even 7 mm., the connective tissue is infiltrated with serum, the capillaries are filled to bursting, the epithelial cells enlarge, and the large round-cells in the connective tissue are seen to be proliferating rapidly, near the end of the cycle taking on the appearance of decidua cells. The glands increase in length, change form, become complex, and are filled with secretion. Viewing the surface with a lens, one sees many furrows with intense superficial hyperemia; it is shiny, but of a velvety appearance. The mouths of the glands are open, like minute

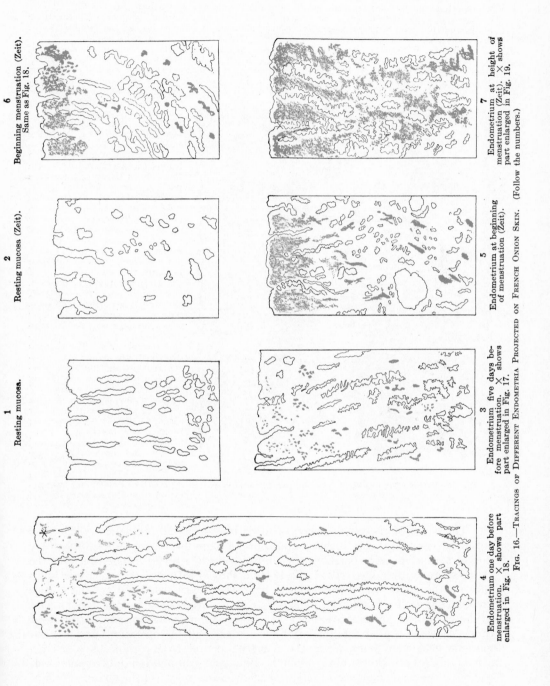

6
Beginning menstruation (Zeit).
Same as Fig. 18.

2
Resting mucosa (Zeit).

1
Resting mucosa.

7
Endometrium at height of menstruation (Zeit). X shows part enlarged in Fig. 19.

5
Endometrium at beginning of menstruation (Zeit).

3
Endometrium five days before menstruation. X shows part enlarged in Fig. 17.

4
Endometrium one day before menstruation. X shows part enlarged in Fig. 18.

FIG. 16.—TRACINGS OF DIFFERENT ENDOMETRIA PROJECTED ON FRENCH ONION SKIN. (Follow the numbers.)

funnels. This is the decidua menstrualis. The change is strictly limited to the mucosa of the corpus; the cervical mucous membrane does not take part. Until the researches of Hitschmann and Adler were published this normal state of the mucosa, a part of the physiologic menstrual cycle, was often called glandular endometritis.

At the height of the congestion the surface vessels are most strongly distended by blood, which often ruptures the thin capillaries and undermines the epithelium and superficial layers of the decidua menstrualis (Fig. 19). Small hematomata may form under the epithelium; these burst, and the blood appears externally. Some blood simply exudes through the capillary walls, and many leukocytes pass through by diapedesis. Menstruation is now at its height.

Sir John Williams believed that the whole mucosa down to the muscularis was exfoliated; Kundrat and Engelman, the superficial layers, the compacta; Schroeder, all the surface down to the basal layer; Lindner, 1921, showed that in most cases the compacta was lost, confirming Kundrat and Engelman's theory (Bohnen, 1927, Lit., Novak). These cells are dissolved by a tryptic ferment in the uterine secretion. In pathologic cases the deeper layers may exfoliate, and these women have dysmenorrhea and are sterile.

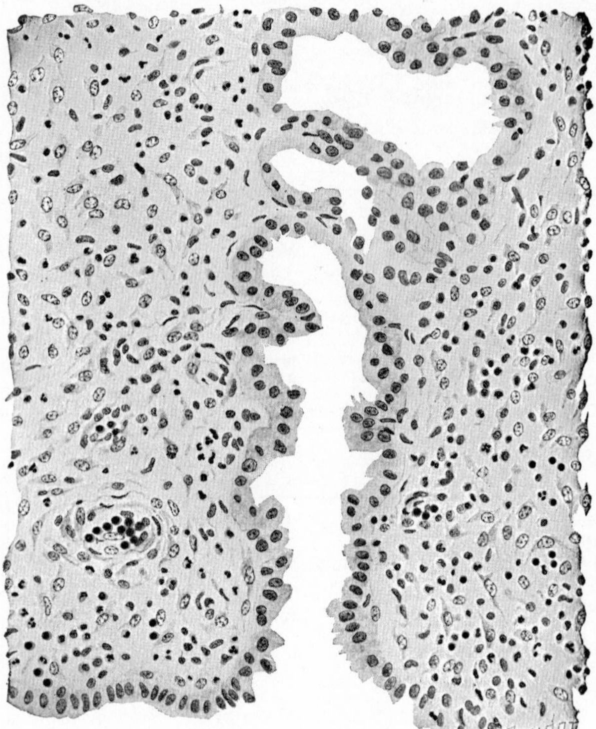

After a few days regression begins, the interglandular cells in the area of greatest congestion undergo a fatty degeneration, as do also a few of the epithelial cells. The remaining portions are gradually regenerated. The congestion subsides, the surface becomes anemic, the exuded serum and the small hematomata are absorbed, the endometrium becomes thinner, the cavity of the uterus gradually reduces in size, and the organ comes to rest, the process requiring about eight days. This period of rest lasts only a few days, because the preparation for the next menstruation begins again. The changes described are called the menstrual cycle, and this cycle is repeated every four weeks during the menacme, unless interrupted by pregnancy, lactation, or some pathologic condition. These four stages of the cycle—quiescence, premenstrual swelling or preparation, menstruation or period of flow, and regeneration—were accurately described by Engelman in 1875 and Hitschmann and Adler in 1908, and their relation to ovulation were studied by Schroeder et al.

Fig. 17.—Uterine Mucosa Five Days Before Menstruation (Progravid Stage).

The cause of the phenomenon of menstruation is still unknown. The most generally accepted theory is that an influence of some sort emanates from the ovary during ovulation, and, reaching the uterus, causes a severe congestion and the changes above described (Bischoff, 1844). Pflüger's theory of a nervous influence on the endometrium, emanating from the ovary distended by the corpus luteum, has been abandoned. There are many arguments for the theory that ovulation causes menstruation—(1) In some animals copulation during heat causes conception, therefore ovulation must occur. (2) At operations and at postmortems on women dying during the menstrual period, fresh corpora lutea or large atretic follicles are almost always found. Bimanual examination in favorable cases will often show an enlargement of the ovary, and one may feel the Graafian follicle burst under the pressure of the fingers. In an ovarian hernia the periodic swelling of the ovary has been observed. (3) Hyrtl describes the case of a girl who died after eight periods, where he found four corpora albicantia in each ovary. (4) Removal of the ovaries causes cessation of the menses, and in cases of congenital absence of the ovaries there are no menses. (5) There must be some dependence of the uterus on the ovary, because when the ovary is extirpated early in life, the uterus does not develop nor does the pelvis. (See Menopause.)

That the direct connnection between the two functions is not so clear is shown by these facts: (1) Ovulation may occur at any time, as is proved by laparotomies and autopsies. (2) It may occur before the birth of the child, during childhood, and after menstruation ceases. Pregnancies have occurred before puberty (see p. 2)—the child may have "fruit before flowers" (De la Motte). Conception has occurred during the prolonged absence of the menses, during the amenorrhea of lactation, and also after the menopause. (3) In some animals ovulation occurs long before heat. (4) Copulation has an influence on ovulation, as is proved by the fact that puberty occurs earlier when coitus is performed early, as in the countries of early marriages; (2) in rabbits it has been shown that copulation hastens the rupture of the Graafian follicle, and (3) certain tortoises cohabit two years before the eggs are fertile. Nevertheless, ovulation is by no means dependent on coitus, as virgins perform the function regularly.

Experiments on animals have been made by Fränkel, Bouin, Ancel, Loeb, and others to determine this relation. All that can reasonably be deduced from a study of the facts is that there is a strong connection between the functions of the ovary and of the uterus; that the impulses leave the ovary and affect the uterus; that the phenomenon of menstruation is probably the result of the stimulation of ovulation, and that, while

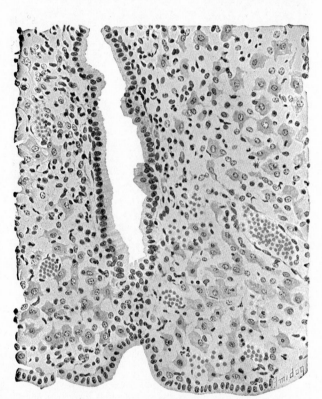

FIG. 18.—UTERINE MUCOSA ONE DAY BEFORE MENSTRUATION

ovulation may occur at any time, the monthly ovulation is the usual one, and affects the uterus, therefore, monthly also. Meyer, Ruge, Schroeder, and Fränkel have about proved that ovulation usually occurs fourteen to sixteen days after the beginning of menstruation, that the corpus luteum then begins to grow; the latter is at its height ten days later, the changes in the endometrium synchronizing with the changes in the corpus luteum. The changes in the uterus are designed to fit it for the reception of the fertilized ovum. Aveling called it "nest building." If conception occurs, the corpus luteum goes on growing (because of the increased vascularity perhaps, or because of the elaboration of a placental hormone) and continues throughout pregnancy, during which time it usually retards further ovulation and protects the security of the ovum. If implantation of the egg does not occur, the stimulus of pregnancy does not come to the corpus luteum, it degenerates, its secretion does not reach the uterus, which, therefore, shows regressive changes and later quiescence.   The woman menstruates because she does not conceive (Power).   The nest is not needed.

It is not necessary that the Graafian follicle rupture to produce menstruation. The development and regression alone suffice.   The influence of the ovary is transmitted to the uterus not via the nervous system, although Mandl has demonstrated nerves in the stratum granulosum, but through the blood, the process being similar to other internal secretory activities. Halban transplanted ovaries to distant parts of the body of monkeys, and a sort of menstruation continued.   Then he removed the ovaries and the menses disappeared.   Knauer transplanted the ovaries to another part of the abdomen in animals, and saw even pregnancy follow.   F. H. Martin, of Chicago, and Tuffier have successfully transplanted human ovaries.   Heterogeneous grafts are almost always absorbed within four months.   Tuffier also caused menstruation in the amenorrheic by injecting the blood of a normally menstruating woman. (See Bainbridge.)   A small piece of ovary will maintain the function of an endometrial transplant (Sampson).

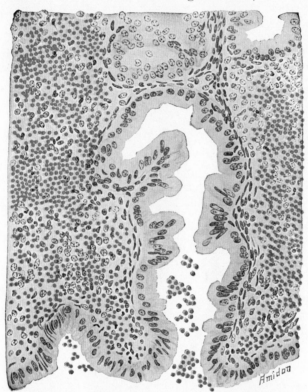

Fig. 19.—Endometrium During Early Menstruation (Zeit).

The object of menstruation has also given rise to much theorizing.   The oldest notion regarding the menstrual discharge is that it is the result of a general plethora.   The woman is endowed with greater blood-making powers, as she must nourish the fetus also.   If she remains sterile, there is no need for this extra blood, and it is thus gotten rid of.   While by no means accepting this theory, it is interesting to note that in poorly nourished girls, or those of a tuberculous type, nature withholds the menses for no other reason, obviously, than to save the organism this useless waste of blood.   Another theory, little less old, is that of a purification.   Even yet by some races women, while menstruating, are regarded as unclean.   The substances which were passed in the monthly discharges were supposed to be poisonous.   Macht has shown that the sweat of menstruating women will kill flowers held in the hand perhaps due to increase of cholin in the sweat.   Recently a southern writer said that cases of retention of the menses could result in headache, neuralgia, and rheumatic pains, even epilepsy.   In Germany the term "monatliche Reinigung," "monthly cleansing," is still used.   Schmoulker and Kieffer declared that the menstrual blood is an excretion relieving thus a toxemia.   Charrin proved that the woman's blood is more toxic before and during menstruation.   Turenne explained the toxemia of pregnancy as a menorrhemia, and administered ovarian extract as a remedy, but has no followers.   Aschner, 1922, reaffirmed the excretory theory.

Tubal Menstruation.—There are reasons for believing that the Fallopian tubes also take some part in menstruation—first, because tubes fastened in the abdominal wall often have periodic bloody discharges; second, cases of hematosalpinx point to this action; and third, a decidua menstrualis has been found in the tube (Arendt). One might argue against this supposition that the blood regurgitated from the uterus; that in all these cases the tube was diseased, which holds true for the first two cases, at all events. The mucous membrane of the tubes may undergo changes similar to those of the endometrium without the escape of blood, as one also observes a marked congestion of the cervix, vagina, and vulva, with increased secretion of the glands, during menstruation. Cyclical changes in the vagina analogous to those found in animals are also observed (Geist; Vinos).

THE CLINICAL ASPECTS OF MENSTRUATION

Time of Appearance.—In about 2 per cent. of new-born girls there appears a bloody, mucoid discharge from the vagina, which lasts one to four days. This is called pseudo-menses, usually indicates nothing pathologic, and requires no treatment unless prolonged and profuse. Bayer ascribed it to the ovarian influence of the mother transmitted as an internal secretion to the fetus by way of the placenta. It may be due to ovulation going on at the time of birth in the mother, or even in the child. Almost always this pseudo-menses does not recur, but precocious menstruation is on record. Plumb reports the case of a nine-pound girl with genitals like a fifteen-year-old, whose periods began six weeks after birth, and continued every six weeks thereafter. Cases of the menses beginning in the third and fifth month, with development of the genitalia and with hair on the pubis before the sixth year, are on record. This precocity is sometimes inherited. It may be due to abnormal action of the anterior lobe of the hypophysis, now known to have several hormones—one growth stimulating; one activates the follicle; one with luteinizing action. Often, however, it is the evidence of disease. The author saw very profuse pseudo-menses in two infants that died of cerebral hemorrhage. Several cases of precocious menstruation had hydrocephalus, sarcoma of the ovary, tuberculosis, or other disease.

The time of the advent of puberty and, with it, the menses, varies according to climate, environment, race, heredity, condition of life, and type of person. Warm climate seems to bring on early menstruation: the Hindus having the menses at twelve years, and English women living in India are affected likewise. In Greenland puberty begins from the seventeenth to the twenty-third year, and some of the Eskimos menstruate only in summer.

Races show marked variations. The Aryans and Slavs menstruate late, the Jews and most Orientals early. Brunets and red-haired girls menstruate early; blonds, late (Kisch). Environment exerts a strong influence. The highly strung city-bred girl has early periods, the country girl, later; the poor overworked factory girl, later; the girl reared in luxury, who dances, sees plays, reads novels, early. Chlorotic and tuberculous girls, by a wise conservatism of nature, do not menstruate or do so toward the twentieth year. Indeed, the late or scant appearance of the flow should call for a careful examination of the patient.

If the mother menstruated early, the daughter may also. The same is true of the cessation of the periods.

Symptoms.—At the onset of the menses the woman usually has symptoms referable to the genitalia and general symptoms, which are called menstrual molimina. Headache, throbbing in character, malaise, and a feeling of lassitude, neuralgias, especially of the face, chilliness, flashes of heat, all these occur and show the powerful effect of ovulation on the entire body. Sexual desire is sometimes exaggerated; there is increased sensibility, both of the skin and of the mind, and in those predisposed, hysteric outbreaks are common. The emunctories are more active, and the patient more likely to take cold at this time. The skin often emits a slight odor; attacks of urticaria, acne, and eczema have been noticed. The eyes often have dark circles; occasionally the lids darken as well; hordeolum, slight asthenopia, muscular and neural, have been often observed (Berger).

The bowels are disturbed, diarrhea and tympany occasionally occurring, and the appetite may be capricious. Senator and Chvostek believe they determined

2

a slight enlargement of the liver. Mild attacks of tonsillitis are not uncommon. There is pain in the back, in the groins (ovaries), sometimes exaggerated to pathologic dysmenorrhea, irritation of the bladder, and slight polyuria. The temperature is raised a degree, the pulse is faster and harder, the blood-pressure being raised 20 mm. until the bloody flow begins. Then it drops until the flow ceases, when a slow rise is observed. The erythrocytes increase before, and diminish during the flow. The amount of urea excreted is decreased, the CO_2 increased. In sick women, up to the start of the flow, there is an increase of the basal metabolic rate, little or none in the healthy (Lanz).

The external genitalia are somewhat engorged, darker, succulent; the discharges from the vulva, vagina, and cervix are augmented; the acid reaction reversed to alkaline and the flora changed—sometimes pathologically; indeed, the endometrium secretes freely only just before and during menstruation (Hitschmann). The cervix and vagina are more open; the uterus is larger and softer, the whole pelvis suffers from an acute vascular engorgement. The ovary containing the corpus luteum can often be felt. Normally no blood is spilled in the bursting of the Graafian follicle, but sometimes there are several drams (in pathologic cases up to 2 liters) which may produce peritoneal symptoms (Cornell). The acme of the changes is reached on the first day, after which regression occurs. The breasts also enlarge, become tender, and not seldom a few drops of colostrum may be squeezed from the nipple. The nipples are more erectile and darker, the findings thus resembling those of early pregnancy. The thyroid enlarges at puberty, and this may be permanent; it also swells during the period, but this engorgement rapidly subsides. A relation between the ovary and the thyroid gland is apparent in more than one condition.

The **character of the flow** varies in different women. It also changes from day to day. At first it is mucoserous, then bloody, then almost pure blood, which does not coagulate, a property it acquires from the secretions of the endometrium. The color is dark maroon, but in chlorotic girls it may be watery or even colorless. It is alkaline in reaction, slightly irritating, and has an odor like marigold. This depends on the constitution of the woman and the bacteria in the discharge. Some women have fetid menses. The menstrual blood is infectious for puerperæ. Clots normally are not present. The amount varies from four to six ounces, but this, as well as the duration of the flow, is not constant in the same woman nor the same in all women. Lahille holds that more than 80 grams is pathologic.

The **duration of the flow** varies within wide limits, but it usually lasts three to seven days. The English and American women flow three to five, the French five to seven days. At the beginning of puberty the flow is moderate; later more profuse and prolonged, especially after marriage, the result of the physiologic stimulation of intercourse or of endometritis, one of the late effects of gonorrhea or childbirth. Sexual stimulation increases the flow and sometimes its frequency. Brunets flow more than blonds; warm climates increase the discharge.

Periodicity.—At least 71 per cent. of women menstruate every twenty-eight days, and the majority during the new moon. If the flow starts a day earlier or later, it is of no importance. There are several types, as a twenty-eight-day type (71 per cent.), a twenty-one-day type (2 per cent.), a thirty-day type (14 per cent.), a twenty-seven-day type (1 per cent.), though some healthy women flow every six weeks. (Jessie L. King, Lit.) If one studies the life of woman carefully, clinically, and with the help of physical methods, one can determine an ebb and flow in her activities, mental and physical. It was described by Mary Jacobi in 1876. This cyclic movement, or "Wellenbewegung," or periodicity, reaches the highest point of its tide just before the appearance of the menses. Figure 20, from v. Ott, shows this graphically. The functions of the body, reflex excitability (King), the pulse, the blood-pressure, pulmonary capacity, heat radiation, temperature, excretion of urea, muscular power, the action of some of the endocrinal glands (Labhart and Hüssy), all increase according to the line in the figure, up to within a day of the menses; on this day there is an abrupt regression, then a gradual recovery, which rebounds and drops to normal about the seventh day after menstruation (Reinl). This periodicity is slightly manifest in the male, and recurs in five to six weeks' intervals. Perhaps it is the external evidence of the formation of spermatozoids.

During pregnancy the menses normally are absent. Occasionally a woman will have one, usually abortive period after conception, the "implantation sign" of Evans and Hartman. Cases where menstruation appeared throughout gestation are very rare, and the discharge of blood usually has a pathologic basis, *e. g.*, cervical polyp or erosion, double uterus, neoplasm. Wintz and Petty report instances. After delivery the menses reappear, according to Ehrenfest, in three months in 50 per cent. of the women, in 71 per cent. before six months, and in 81 per cent. before the women stopped nursing. The amenorrhea of lactation, therefore, is not so general as was formerly thought. Ed. Allen recently reported on the great variations of the periods in normal women.

The **menopause,** the "change of life," "the climacteric," "die Wechseljahre," "losing the periods," takes place between the fortieth and the fiftieth year. Thus the average length of the reproductive era of a woman's life is about thirty years.

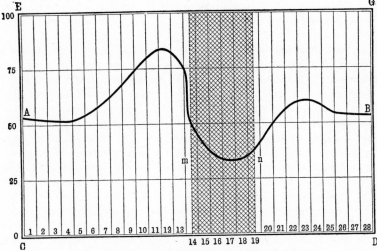

FIG. 20.—VON OTT'S TABLE OF PERIODICITY.

Statistics prove this for nearly all countries. The extremes are six to forty-six years. Krieger collected 2291 cases, and found the menses ceased in 12 per cent. of cases between the thirty-sixth and the fortieth year; in 26 per cent. between the forty-first and the forty-fifth years; in 41 per cent. of the cases between the forty-fifth and fiftieth years, and 15 per cent. of the cases from the fiftieth to the fifty-fifth years, the balance, 7 per cent., being distributed before the thirty-fifth and after the fifty-fifth years.

The climacteric occurs earlier in sterile women, in cold than in warm countries, in the poor than in the rich, in black than in white women. If puberty is early, menopause is late, the sexual function being strongly developed; but if the reproductive organs are overused or diseased, the menopause may be earlier. The menses may return after having ceased. Meissner (quoted by Krieger, *loc. cit.*) tells of this case: Menses at twenty; first child at forty-seven; up to sixty years, 7 children; cessation of the menses; seventy-five to ninety-eight years, regular periods; five years absent; one hundred and four years, menstruation again; end not known. Charpentier, quoted by Parvin, reports a case of menses ceasing at forty-eight, beginning again at sixty, then continuing for two years. In all such cases one should search carefully for pathologic conditions, as fibroid, cancer, atheroma, senile endometritis, etc. Pregnancy has occurred after the menopause. In addition to the above, Renaudin reports a case where, twelve years after the menses ceased, a living child was born. Kennedy reports the case of a woman who had five labors and one abortion after the fiftieth year.

Usually the advent of the menopause is announced by alteration, diminution, or irregularity of the flow. The amount of blood diminishes, mucus or serum replacing it. When the flow becomes more profuse than usual, attention should be directed more closely to the woman. The cessation of the menses, especially in nulliparæ, is often attended by nervous symptoms, such as loss of vasomotor control, flushings of the face and the body, flashes of heat and cold, trembling, hyperexcitability, cerebral and spinal irritability, indigestion, constipation, tympany, nosebleed, bleeding from hemorrhoids, profuse sweats, hysteric manifestations, and many of the symptoms that accompany the beginning of the function (Currier). The body puts on fat, which often hangs in ungainly masses on the back, thighs, buttocks, or abdomen; hair often appears on the face, and the habitus in general takes on a masculine type. All these symptoms are the result of the atrophy of the genitalia combined with changes in the ductless glands, thyroid, pituitary *et al.* The ovaries, tubes, uterus, vagina, and vulva undergo a process of senile involution and atrophy. For further information on the changes of the menopause the reader is referred to Kisch (*loc. cit.*), Aschner, Blair Bell, and A. F. Currier.

Vicarious menstruation is a periodic discharge of blood from some surface other than the uterus, which discharge is to represent the monthly flow, such flow being absent from the uterus. In the typical cases three conditions must be fulfilled—the uterine flow must be absent; the periodicity absolute, and the organ from which the vicarious discharge comes, normal. Such cases are rare, but authentic ones have been reported (Kisch, *loc. cit.*). Hemorrhages have been observed coming from the nose, stomach, lungs, breasts or nipples, mouth, gums, ear, arms, bladder, conjunctiva, named approximately in the order of frequency. Sometimes the organ from which the hemorrhage comes is diseased, as ulcer of the stomach, tuberculosis pulmonum, ulcer of the nasal septum, hemorrhoids, chronic otitis media, and in themselves would give rise to a bleeding surface, but when the periodicity of the flow corresponds to that of the menses, the latter being absent, we still speak of vicarious menstruation. Occasionally the usual flow is combined with a bloody discharge from another organ. After castration vicarious menstruation has been occasionally observed, and during pregnancy and the amenorrhea of lactation a vicarious flow may occur from another part of the body. The author had a case where, for nine months after delivery, the patient had a bloody discharge from the nipples lasting several days and recurring every twenty-eight days. The nipples were healthy and the patient amenorrheic. These hemorrhages are similar to the nosebleeds observed during pregnancy, the puerperium, and the menopause.

Occasionally one notices not a bloody flow, but an increased discharge from some organ, such as leukorrhea, diarrhea, otorrhea, salivation, recurring periodically at the time of the menses.

Midperiod Suppressed Menses.—Between the periods some women complain of menstrual molimina without the discharge of blood. The pain sometimes necessitates rest in bed or even an anodyne. Fasbender described the symptoms, and Martin named it "Mittelschmerz," or pain between the periods. There may be a slight increase of the leukorrhea at this time and microscopically one may find traces of blood, "the ovulatory bleeding" (Hartman). Since the height of the development of the Graafian follicle occurs at this time, it is probable that the pain is due to the distention of a tender ovary.

LITERATURE

Allen: See Smith and Smith, "Progestin in the Reproductive Cycle," Jour. Amer. Med. Assoc., 1931.—*Arendt:* "Über Decidua Menstrualis Tubarum," Verhandl. der Versammlung Deutscher Naturforscher, 1905.—*Aschner:* Die Blutdrüsenerkrank. des Weibes, 1918, Lit., also Zent. f. Gyn., July 29, 1927, p. 1596.—*Aveling:* Obstetrical Journal of Great Britain, July, 1874, p. 209.—*Bainbridge:* Amer. Jour. Obst. and Gyn., May, 1923.— *Berger and Loewy:* Diseases of the Eyes of Sexual Origin. Translated by Dr. Beatrice Rossbach, 1906.— *Bischoff:* Zeitschr. f. rationale Medizin. von Henle und Pfeiffer, 1855, vol. xiv.—*Bodd:* L'Abeille med., 1882, No. 4.—*Bohnen:* Archiv. für Gynaek., 1927, vol. 129, 3, p. 473.—*Charrin:* Arch. de Physiologie, October, 1898.—*Chiriè:* L'Obstetrique, May, 1911.—*Clark:* "The Origin, Growth, and Fate of the Corpus Luteum," Johns Hopkins Hospital Reports, 1898, vol. vii, p. 181.—*Currier, A. F.:* The Menopause, New York, 1896. —*Dittrick:* Jour. Amer. Med. Assoc., March 5, 1927, p. 722.—*Escher:* Zeitschr. für Phys. Chemie, 1913, lxxxiii, p. 198.—*Fasbender:* Geschichte der Geburtshilfe.—*Fraenkel:* Centralbl. f. Gyn., 1911, p. 1561.—*Frank:* Surg., Gyn., and Obstet., July, 1911; also November, 1914; also January 21, 1922, p. 182, Lit.—*Ibid.:* Jour. Amer. Med. Assoc., April 19, 1930.—*Geist, H. S.:* Surg., Gynec., and Obstet., 1930, 51, p. 848.—*Ibid.:* Amer. Jour. Obstet. and Gyn., October, 1931, p. 532.—*Goodman:* Amer. Jour. Obstet., 1878, vol. ii, p. 673. —*Gottschalk:* "Relation of Ovulation to Menstruation," Arch. f. Gyn., 1910, vol. xci.—*Graves, W. P.:* Hormonology, Saunders Co., 1931.—*Halban:* Arch. f. Gyn., vol. lxxv, H. 2.—*Hirst:* Text-book of Obstetrics, 1903.—*Hitschmann:* Zeitschr. f. Geb., 1907, and *Adler:* Monatsschr. f. Geb. u. Gyn., 1908, xxvii, I, S. 81.— *Keiffer:* L'Obstetrique, 1897.—*Kennedy:* Transactions of the Obstetrical Soc. of Edinburgh, 1882, vol. vii.— *King, Jessie L.:* Amer. Phys., 1917, 42, 607.—*Ibid.:* Publ. 363, Carnegie Instit., Washington, 1926.—*Kisch:* Das Geschlechtsleben des Weibes, 1904, 1906.—*Knauer:* Centralbl. f. Gyn., 1896, No. 20; 1897, No. 27.— *Krieger:* Die Menstruation, Berlin, 1869.—*Labhart and Hüssy:* Zeitschrift für Geb. u. Gyn., 1922, vol. lxxxiv, p. 713, Lit.—*Lahille:* Annales de Gyn., May, 1917, p. 535.—*Lanz:* Zeitschr. f. Geb. u. Gyn., 1925, vol. 89, p. 133.—*Leopold and Ravano:* Arch. f. Gyn., 1907, Bd. lxxxiii.—*Lindner:* Inaug. Diss., Breslau, 1921.—*Loeb:* Surg., Gyn., and Obstet., September, 1917.—*Ibid.:* Jour. Amer. Med. Assoc., February 25, 1911.—*Mandl:* "Anord. u. Endig. der Nerv. im Ovar.," Arch. f. Gyn., vol. xlviii, p. 276.—*Martin:* "Ovarian Transplantation," Surg., Gyn., and Obstet., September, 1917.—*Meyer:* Arch. f. Gyn., 1911, Bd. xciii, p. 354.—*Ibid.:* Internat. Abstract of Surgery, July, 1914, p. 13.—*Meyer, Robert:* Arch. für Gynaek., May, 1932, vol. 149, H. 2, p. 315.—*Nagel:* "Anatomie der weiblichen Genitalien," v. Bardeleben's Handbuch, 1896.—*Novak:* Jour. Amer. Med. Assoc., October 28, 1917; also vol. 83, p. 900, 1924.—*v. Ott:* Nouvelles Arch. d'Obstetrique et de Gynecologie, 1890.—*Pettey:* "Menstruation in Pregnancy," British Med. Jour., 1903.—*Pfister:* Beitrag. z. Geb. u. Gyn., vol. v, p. 421.—*Plumb:* New York Med. Jour., 1897.—*Reinl:* "Die Wellenbewegung, etc.," Volkmann's Sammlung klin. Vort., No. 243.—*Renaudin:* Compt. rend. de la Soc. de Med. de Nancy, 1861.— *Runge:* Arch. f. Gyn., 1907, Heft 1.—*Schmoulker:* Arch. de Gyn. et Tocologie, December, 1897.—*Stockard and Papanicolaou:* Amer. Jour. Anat., 1917, vol. xxii, p. 225.—*Tuffier:* Surg., Gyn., and Obstet., January, 1915.— *Turenne:* L'Obstetrique, December, 1904.—*Vinos:* Arch. für Gyn., 1932, vol. 148, H. 2, p. 351.—*Waldeyer:* Eierstock und Ei, Leipzig, 1870.—*Wintz:* Monatsschr. für Geb. u. Gyn., June, 1925.—*Zondek, B.-Aschheim:* Hormone, Berlin, Springer, 1931. Large monograph.

CONCEPTION

Conception, in its obstetric sense, means the union of the male and female elements of procreation, from which union a new being is developed. It is the means for the propagation of the species, and has variously been termed fecundation, impregnation, fertilization, incarnation.

The ovum is the female unit, or element, of procreation, and, as has been learned, is prepared in the ovary for the reception of the male unit, which is the spermatozoid, derived from the testicle. In the male the testicle is the important organ of reproduction; it is analogous to the ovary, and, like it, has many organs accessory to it. The testicle produces an internal secretion, the interstitial cells of Leydig probably making it.

The testicle and the ovary are developed in the fetus from identical structures— the germinal folds along the inside of the Wolffian bodies. The germinal epithelium in the one case develops into Graafian follicles; in the other it lines the tubuli contorti of the testicle. The genesis of the spermatozoids is very similar to that of the ovum. Whereas the spermatozoid is destined, in a sort of division of labor, to be the more active, aggressive agent in the function of impregnation and must seek the ovum, by a process of evolution it is given a shape which is capable of rapid locomotion. It is made very small, being among the smallest of cell elements, having been divested of all that is not needed for the performance of its function, which is to seek out the female pronucleus and fuse with it. The ovum, on the other hand, must possess the nourishment needed for the new life until the egg can derive nourishment from its parent. It is one of the largest cells in the body.

The spermatozoids were considered animalculæ by their discoverers, J. Ham and Leeuwenhoek (1677), but in 1840 Kölliker and Lallemand proved their origin from the epithelial cells. Spallanzani, in 1768, proved that they were the active fertilizing elements of the semen. The number of spermatozoids in a given ejaculation is sometimes enormous—227,500,000 in one discharge (Lode).

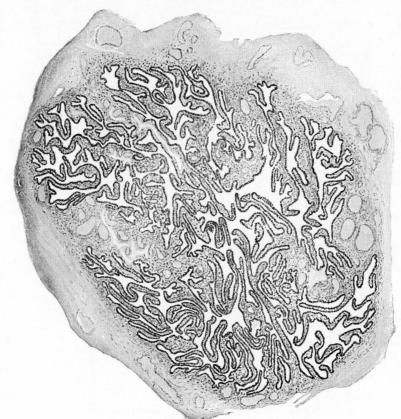

Fig. 21.—Cross-section of Tube at Ampulla (low power).

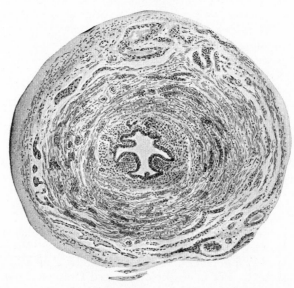

Fig. 22.—Cross-section of Tube Near Uterus.

Copulation.—Conception, impregnation, incarnation, and fecundation must be well distinguished from copulation, which means the sexual union of the male and the female.

The object of the voluntary act of copulation is solely to place the semen in such a location that its living elements, the spermatozoids, may reach the ovum. The rest of the function of reproduction is entirely involuntary. The act of copulation is not absolutely necessary; if the semen is injected into the vagina or even on the introitus vulvæ, conception may take place. The union of the spermatozoid with the ovum occurs, in all probability, in the outer end of the Fallopian tube —its ampulla. The frequency of tubal pregnancies indicates this. That the impregnation may occur in the ovary is proved by authentic ovarian pregnancies— indeed, several primary abdominal pregnancies, one attached to the omentum, have been reported.

How does the ovum reach the tube from the ovary? The ovary lies in a little depression—the fossa ovarica (Fig. 1)—and is covered in part by the mesentery of the tube, whose fimbriæ are in close proximity. The ampulla of the tube opens outward in numerous projections—the fimbriæ, the prolongations of the longitudinal foldings of the tube (Figs. 21 and 22). These are covered with ciliated epithelium. The waving of the cilia being toward the uterus, an efficient aspiratory current is produced in the peritoneal fluid of the neighborhood of the end of the tube. Experimentally in rabbits Lode saw tiny particles placed near the tubes gradually sucked into the fimbriated end. They appeared finally in the vagina. The ovum as it appears on the surface of the ovary, with its clump of cells from the cumulus oöphorus and a few drops of liquor folliculi, is caught in this current and led to the tube. Once in the tube, the peristaltic action of the wall of the latter will aid its progression toward the uterus, aided by the ciliary wave. Peristalsis of the tube is demonstrable by the x-ray and iodized oil. The length of time required for the passage from ovary to uterus in the dog is eight to ten days; the mouse, three days; the guinea-pig, three days; the opossum, one day; in the human, seven or more days—but of this one cannot be certain. The figures are for the fertilized ovum. Allen et al. from the washings of numerous tubes got more or less well preserved unfertilized eggs about the fifteenth day after the beginning of the menses.

The spermatozoids reach the ovum in the tube by means of their own locomotive power (Carleton). They sometimes overcome great obstacles, as occurs in impregnation when the semen is deposited on the vulva, in cases of rape, imperforate hymen, etc.

The vaginal mucus is acid, P_H 3.5, and kills the spermatozoids within a few hours, but that of the cervix is alkaline, P_H 9–9.6 (Miller and Kurzrok), wherefore the uterus would offer conditions much more favorable to their movement. The cilia of the tubes and uterus move in the direction of the internal os, and this serves to direct the course of the spermatozoids, for they swim always against feeble currents. The rate of travel of the spermatozoids has been variously estimated from 1 to 4 mm. a minute. Assuming the average rate to be 2 mm., the 70 mm. long trip through the uterine cavity would require thirty-five minutes, and the 120 mm. tube, sixty minutes more. It is not likely that the movement is aided by antiperistalsis of the tube; rather one would imagine the labyrinthine formation of the tubal passage would hinder progress. Spermatozoids are found in the tube, the pelvic peritoneum, on the ovary, within a few hours after cohabitation. They may live for at least three weeks (Dührssen and Nürnberger) in the favorable conditions supplied by the infundibulum of the Fallopian tube. Therefore, if there is no ovum ready to be fertilized on their arrival in the neighborhood of the ovary, they wait until one is ripened and expelled. If this is true it is very important in medicolegal cases, where the question of legitimacy arises, and for the exact computation of the length of pregnancy. Brodauf says they live only three days and Mall believes that while the sperms may be active they soon lose fertilizing power.

When the spermatozoid meets the ovum, its head is drawn into the ovum in a manner suggesting phagocytosis. It loses its tail, becomes round, is surrounded by a halo of radiating lines, and progresses toward the female pronucleus. Fusion takes place. The rest of the spermatozoids die—at least, they disappear. Kohlbrügge says that, in bats, the spermatozoids enter the blastula and affect the ovum, and that they also enter the mucosa uteri and unite with the cells. Waldstein demonstrated by means of Abderhalden's reaction that in rabbits the sperma is absorbed and Dittler showed that rabbits, immunized with homologous sperm, became sterile. If these things are proved for the human, they may explain several phenomena of conjugal life, e. g., sterility, monstrosities, serologic and endocrinal disturbances.

The woman is now pregnant, the fertilized ovum proceeds to the uterus, propelled by the cilia of the tube and aided by its peristalsis. The uterus has been prepared for the reception of the egg (see Anatomic Changes of Uterine Mucosa During Menstruation), the egg attaches itself to the decidua menstrualis, and the development of a new individual is begun. These processes do not always occur in the exact order described; observers have for a long time been aware that variations occur. The spermatozoids may pass out through one Fallopian tube and fertilize an ovum lying in the closed uterine horn of the opposite side. This is external wandering of the spermatozoid (Fig. 23). The ovum may wander from the ovary of one side into the tube of the other, as in a case of extirpation of the right tube and left ovary, the ovum crossed over and entered the healthy tube (Fig.

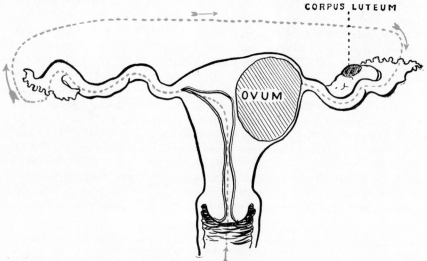

FIG. 23.—DIAGRAM TO SHOW THE EXTERNAL WANDERING OF THE SPERMATOZOID.
Red dotted line indicates course of spermatozoid.

24). In a case of extra-uterine pregnancy the corpus luteum was found on the right side, the ovum in the left tube (Fig. 25). In animals, too, one has found more fetuses in one horn of the uterus than there were corpora lutea in the corresponding ovary. It has been believed that the impregnated ovum could wander through the uterus up into the tube of the opposite side, because, if in certain mammals the ovary and part of the tube of one side be extirpated, ova are found in both horns of the uterus. All these experiments and clinical observations must be taken with a great deal of reservation, because the permeability of the stump of the tube comes into question. The operations to procure sterility by cutting and tying the tube have often been failures because the stump becomes pervious. The only sure method of permanently interrupting the connection between ovary and uterus is to exsect the uterine portion of the tube. In the above discussion accessory tubes or accessory ostia of the tubes must be considered.

It is easy enough to explain the occurrence of external wandering of the ovum. The ovaries are movable organs, and by certain positions of the parts, e. g., retroversion of the uterus with prolapse of the tubes into the culdesac of Douglas, are brought close together. One could also imagine the filling of the rectum and sigmoid as means of displacing the tubes. Pathologic adhesion of the tubes and ovaries may result in abnormal currents of serum created by the cilia of the tubes. For internal wandering of the human ovum there is no proof, though Andrews' case looks plausible.

The Time of Conception.—It is important to know the time pregnancy begins, but, unfortunately, we are in a position as yet only to guess at the exact date. The knowledge is wanted in order to determine the day of confinement and the actual

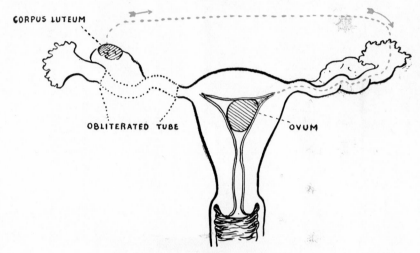

Fig. 24.—External Wandering of the Ovum.
Dotted red line indicates course of ovum.

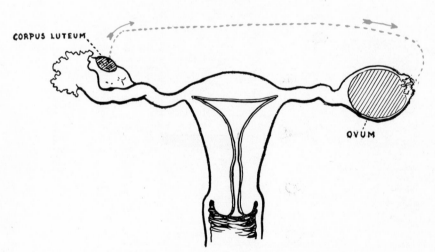

Fig. 25.—External Wandering of the Ovum (Oldham's case).

length of human gestation, for practical reasons, for the scientific study of the development of the ovum in the uterus, and for medicolegal processes in the question of legitimacy of a child or its paternity. All the points on which such a determination could rest are uncertain, as: (1) The date of the fruitful coitus (the woman's word must be accepted); (2) the date the ovum left the ovary, and whether it was fertilizable or not, and for how long (Mall says not more than one day); (3) how long it takes the ovum to reach the tube and uterus; (4) how long it takes the

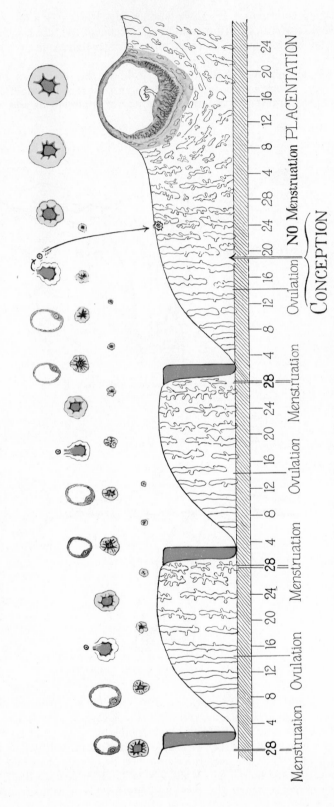

FIGS. 26, 27.—THE RELATIONS BETWEEN OVULATION, MENSTRUATION, AND CONCEPTION. (Modified from Schroeder.)

spermatozoids to reach the ovum; (5) how long the fertilized ovum rests before it begins to germinate—all unknown factors.

Halban, Ruge, and Meyer believe that ovulation occurs most often within sixteen days after the beginning of the menses and that the conception time lasts only a few days.

In all probability fertilization takes place soon after the ovum is discharged from the ovary. Hartman and Ball proved that in rats sperms are in the uterine cornua in about ninety seconds.

It is certain that rupture of the Graafian follicle and conception may occur at any time during the reproductive life of women. Kraus, Ogino et al. seek to prove that during the four to six days preceding menstruation conception cannot take place. Siegel, of Freiburg, from a study of statistics obtained from women whose husbands came home from the war on short furlough, concludes that most conceptions occur just after the menses cease and the incidence is least just before the next period. (See page 70.) No doubt the menses may occur after conception has taken place. It is customary to reckon the length of pregnancy as of nine calendar months, or ten lunar months, two hundred and eighty days' duration, dating from the first day of the last menstruation. Clinical experience shows that most labors occur at this time.

If further study shall prove, as Fränkel, Ruge, Meyer, Schroeder et al. claim, that ovulation occurs from fourteen to eighteen days after the beginning of the last menses, and if, as should be surmised, conception occurs also about this period, then we must conclude that human gestation is not two hundred and eighty days, but two hundred and sixty to two hundred and sixty-five days in duration.

The season of the year influences the number of conceptions. The months of May and June show the most, perhaps as an analogon to the mating of birds and animals. In many countries May, June, and October are favorite months for marriages. In country districts during the harvest-time there are fewer conceptions. The body is tired with hard work. After the harvest an increase is noticeable. In countries where conscriptions for soldiers take place, there are many conceptions before the time the men leave for the army. Illegitimate conceptions occur most often during the summer months. Climate exerts an influence, too; in the very cold regions the frequency of conception is less; in warm zones the contrary is true. Among the educated classes conception is voluntarily much interfered with, but there are those who believe that the number of impregnations falls off among them from natural causes.

LITERATURE

Andrews: Quoted by Corner, Johns Hopkins Bulletin, March, 1921.—*Benham:* Edin. Med. Jour., August, 1873, No. 19.—*Brodauf:* Zentralb. für Gyn., 1926, October 30, p. 2832.—*Carleton and Florey:* Jour. Obst. and Gyn. of Great Britain, Autumn, No. 1931, p. 550.—*Dittler:* Editorial Jour. Med. Amer. Assoc., 1921, p. 43.—*Fränkel:* Arch. für Gyn., 1910, xcl, S. 710.—*Graf Spee:* Doederlein's Handbuch d. Geb., 1915; complete literature.—*Halban:* Arch. für Gyn., 1914, ciii, S. 580.—*Hertwig, Oscar:* Lehrbuch der Entwickelungsgeschichte, eighth edition, pp. 21–24.—*Hoehne:* Centralbl. für Gyn., 1914, No. 1.—*Hyrtl:* "Beitrag zur Lehre von der Menst. und Befruchtung," Zeitschr. f. rat. Med., N. F., vol. iv, p. 156.—*Keibel and Mall:* Manual of Human Embryology, 1910, vol. i.—*Kohlbrügge:* Zeitschr. f. Morph. u. Anthrop., 1910, vol. xiii, H. 2.—*Kraus and Ogino:* Zentb. für Gyn., March 19, 1932, pp. 710, 721.—*Lode:* Arch. f. d. ges. Phys., Vienna, No. 50.—*Ibid.:* Arch. f. Gyn., vol. xlv, p. 292.—*Miller:* Arch. für Gyn., 1914, vol. ci, p. 600.—*Miller and Kurzrok:* Amer. Jour. Obstet. and Gyn., July, 1932, p. 19.—*Minot:* Text-book of Embryology.—*Newes:* Ergebnisse der Anat. und Entw., vol. xi, p. 197.—*Novak:* "Menstrual Reaction and Menstruation," Surg., Gyn., and Obstet., September, 1915, p. 343.—*Nürnberger:* Monatsschr. f. Geburtsh. u. Gynäk., July 5, 1920.—*Poehl:* Die physiol. Grundlagen d. Spermintheorie, St. Petersburg, 1898.—*Schreiner:* Annalen der Chemie und Pharm., 1878, vol. cxciv.—*Schroeder:* Surg., Gyn., and Obstet., June, 1914, p. 618; also Arch. für Gyn., 1915, civ, 27, S. 110.—*Tuffier:* Surg., Gyn., and Obstet., January, 1915, p. 34.—*Waldeyer:* Die Geschlechtzellen, Jena, Fischer, 1903.—*Waldstein and Ekler:* Wien. klin. Woch., 1913, p. 1689.—*Zondek, B.:* Die Hormone des Ovariums, etc., 1931, Berlin, Springer.

CHAPTER II

DEVELOPMENT OF THE OVUM

THE union of the spermatozoid and the ripened ovum has never been observed on the highest animals, but Sobotta has described the phenomenon as it occurs in the mouse, and Wilson and Matthews, in the sea-urchin. Barry, in 1838, first saw it, Hertwig, 1875, first explained it. The process in all is about the same, and

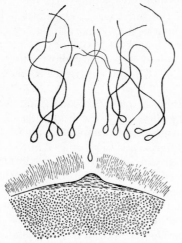

Fig. 28.—ENTRY OF SPERMATOZOID INTO OVUM (Fol).

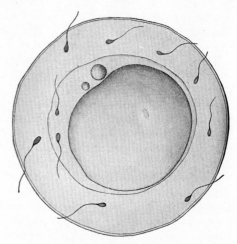

Fig. 29.—ENTRY OF SPERMATOZOID INTO OVUM (Kollman).

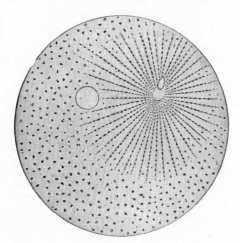

Fig. 30.

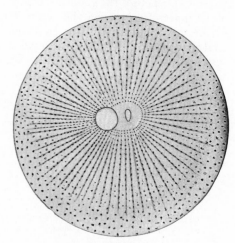

Fig. 31.

FIGS. 30 AND 31.—FUSION OF SPERMATOZOID AND OVUM (after Hertwig).

probably in the human varies little from what we observe in the lower forms of life. The spermatozoid—and only one—is probably received by the ovum through a process resembling phagocytosis. After the head has passed into the ovum, the

28

tail disappears and the cell-membrane thickens, which prevents other spermatozoids from entering the egg. The neck of the spermatozoid becomes the centrosome (not present in all species); the head swells up and becomes the male pronucleus. Both nuclei are made up almost wholly of chromatin (nuclein). The cytoplasm is arranged in radiating lines about the centrosome. The nuclei gradually approach each other and fuse (Figs. 30 and 31), the chromatin of the two forming one long convoluted thread. The nucleus is now capable of equal division; it is the primary "segmentation" or "cleavage nucleus."

When the first division of the embryonic nucleus has been completed (Figs. 32-35), each daughter nucleus receives an equal number of chromosomes; therefore

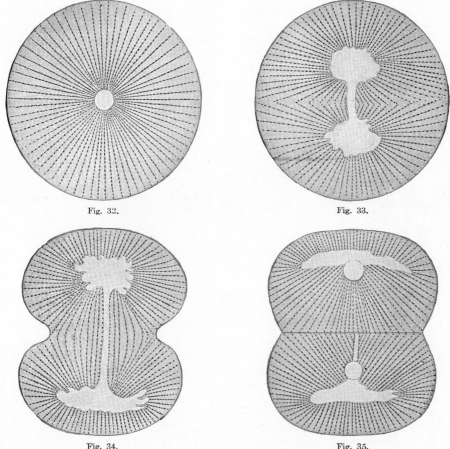

Fig. 32.   Fig. 33.

Fig. 34.   Fig. 35.

FIGS. 32-35.—FIRST CELL DIVISION. EGG OF SEA-URCHIN (Hertwig).

each cell is endowed with half paternal and half maternal qualities and attributes. The heredity of race, of external form, of family traits, of susceptibility to disease, and in rare instances of disease itself,—insanity,—is transmitted to the new individual through the chromatin of the male and female pronuclei. This must have chemic and structural qualities which are far beyond our physical powers of discovery, since within the microscopic mass of chromatin are contained the elements that develop into millions of cells, of the most diverse description, and carrying on most varied functions.

The segmentation nucleus forms a spindle with a centrosome at each end. Distinct chromosomes are arranged around the middle of the spindle at first, then each divides in two equal parts, which separate toward the ends. The achromatic fibers of the spindle dissolve in the middle, and, while this process goes on, the cytoplasm divides also. The process of karyokinesis is now complete. Two cells are formed, and thus the new individual is begun. Each daughter-cell divides again into two and again in geometric progression until a mass of cells results (Fig. 36). This mass, which resembles a blackberry in shape, is called the morula. In some animals all its cells have the same qualities as the parent cell, because broken pieces of the morula have been found to grow into a complete embryo (Driesch). These changes occur inside the zona pellucida, while the ovum is passing down the tube. The cells of the corona radiata are lost during the transit through the tube. When the morula has passed the uterine end of the tube, at which time it cannot be much more than 0.2 mm. in diameter, it attaches itself to the wall of the uterus.

The next step in the development of the egg is the blastula formation. The cells of the morula multiply with great rapidity, and a serum appears in their center which forces the cells to arrange themselves around the periphery of the egg, forming the blastodermic vesicle. The zona pellucida is stretched, persisting a varying length of time after the impregnation of the egg.

The blastodermic vesicle (Fig. 37) at first consists of a single layer of cells,

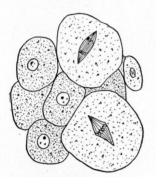

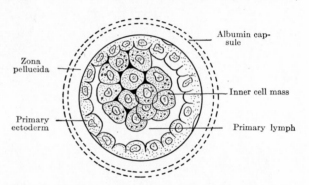

FIG. 36.—THE MORULA (MOUSE)
(Sobotta).

FIG. 37.—THE BLASTODERMIC VESICLE (RABBIT) (E. v. Beneden).

with, at one pole, an accumulation of cells—the later area embryonalis or inner cell mass. This mass divides into two—an outer, called ectoderm, epiblast, or ectoblast, and an inner, the entoderm or endoblast. The egg is now called a gastrula, and a third layer of cells develops between the other two, called the mesoderm, or mesoblast. This later divides into two—the splanchnic and the somatic layers; thus are we introduced to the study of embryology, which does not belong in the pages of this book. Only such points as are necessary for the consideration of the formation of the fetal envelopes will be presented.

The uterine mucosa has already been described. Under the influence of the corpus luteum it has been prepared for the reception of the fertilized egg. It is thicker, velvety, soft, spongy, vascularized, and the glands are full of clear secretion. The condition of the ovum as it enters the uterine cavity is unknown; probably it is in the blastula or gastrula formation. The zona pellucida has disappeared, and with it the cells of the cumulus oöphorus, the corona radiata.

One of the earliest human eggs ever described is that of Kretz Peters, and since the findings in this egg are supported, in the main, by those of other human ova (v. Spee) and of animals (Hubrecht and others), the conclusions drawn by Peters will be generally accepted in the following description. Bryce and Teacher published a description of a human ovum of about fourteen days. Herzog published, in 1909, a classic description of an early human ovum, and permits his plate to be here reproduced (Plate I). Miller's is the youngest human ovum discovered, ten or eleven days of age, described by Streeter.

PLATE I.

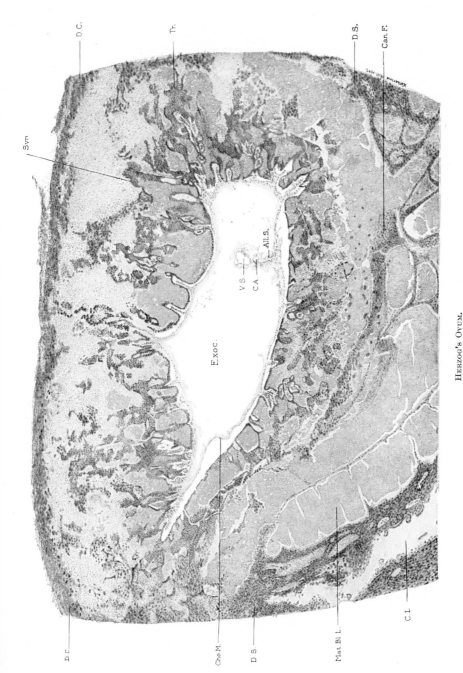

HERZOG'S OVUM.

All.S., Allantoic stalk. *C.A.*, Cavity of amnion. *Can.F.*, Canalized fibrin. *Cho.M.*, Chorion mesoderm. *D.C.*, Decidua capsularis.
Exoc., Exocoelom. *C.I.*, Gland-space. *Mat.Bl.L.*, Large cystic gland-spaces filled with blood; this is pathologic. *V.S.*, Vitelline sac. *Syn.*,
Syncytium. *Tr.*, Trophoblast.

Embedding of the Ovum in the Uterine Mucous Membrane.—When the ovum reaches a favorable spot in the uterus its ectodermal cells eat their way through the epithelium, probably in an area that happens to be without cilia, and the ovum thus

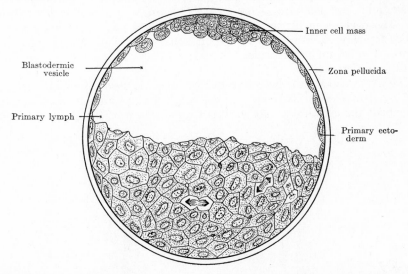

Blastodermic vesicle

Primary lymph

Inner cell mass

Zona pellucida

Primary ecto-derm

FIG. 38.—LATE BLASTULA (RABBIT) (E. von Beneden).

arrives in the edematous subepithelial connective-tissue stroma (Figs. 39 and 40). It is known that the epiblastic cells have tryptic power, and only a tiny surface, the space of a few epithelial cells, has to be denuded. The ovum does not enter the mouth of a uterine gland; it does not necessarily fall into one of the uterine

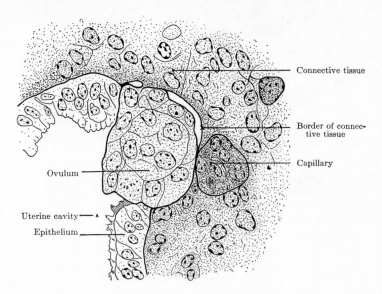

Connective tissue

Border of connec-tive tissue

Capillary

Ovulum

Uterine cavity

Epithelium

FIG. 39.—EMBEDDING OF OVUM IN MUCOSA (GUINEA-PIG) (v. Spee).

folds, though it is possible, but then the changes that would follow would not vary from the usual; it, by a process of arrosion, burrows into the endometrium. This reacts to the invasion by a local congestion, with edema, diapedesis of white and red blood-corpuscles, and a thickening of the outer layers of the stroma cells of the mucous membrane. The spindle-shaped cells under the epithelium and around the glands continue to enlarge into rounded or ovoid cells with a single nucleus, the decidual cells. These are much more numerous near the surface, forming a rather compact layer. The glands widen and undergo proliferation at the base, and are filled with secretion. In olden times this was called the uterine milk. The decidua menstrualis is being transformed into a decidua graviditatis, and the two layers, compacta and spongiosa, are already being differentiated. (See pp. 13 to 15, under Menstruation.) In the early stages the two may hardly, if at all, be differentiated.

The ovum sinks into the compacta; the opening through which it entered is closed by a mushroom-like cap. The changes in the human ovum up to this time—about the eighth day, not as Peters would have it, the third or fourth day

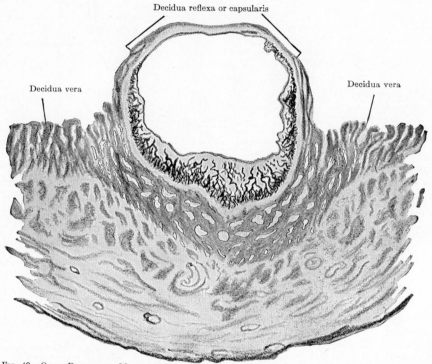

FIG. 40.—OVUM DISTENDING MUCOSA. SHOWS ARRANGEMENT OF UTERINE GLANDS (semidiagrammatic).

—are unknown. In the Kretz-Peters egg, the first fetal formation was already in progress, the amniotic cavity and chorion being completed. The epiblast or ectoderm—rather, that portion of the layer not concerned in the formation of the embryo—grows into the decidua, and provides for the nourishment of the egg. It is the epithelium of the chorion, and is called trophectoderm, because of its nutritive function. The cells are irregularly cubic, with a large, round or oval, slightly granular nucleus, and sometimes with a nucleolus. The trophectoderm grows into the compacta in all directions, but irregularly, and when it meets the dilated capillaries, it pushes into them, the endothelium of the latter being destroyed, thus allowing the blood to wash the surface of the trophectoderm. This causes the cell protoplasm to swell up, the cells to form a homogeneous mass, and the nuclei to alter and assume irregular forms—the syncytium. The trophectoderm forms a shell around the egg, which lies free in a cavity formed in the thickened mucosa. The area around the trophectoderm is called the trophosphere, and its dilated vessels, serous imbibition,

and hypertrophic and hyperplastic decidual cells provide the most favorable conditions for the nourishment and the growth of the ovum. In early fetation many uterine glands are filled with blood, and this occurs so regularly in all the latest specimens that it may be considered normal. The blood also flows in tunnels and lacunæ formed *in* the trophectoderm. We thus see the first act of the formation of the intervillous spaces.

The growth of the ovum is favored by the thickening or hyperplasia of the mucous membrane, which is soon bulged outward toward the cavum uteri in the form of a hemisphere. The glands are separated from each other (Fig. 40), and arrange themselves tangentially to the growing ovum. The layer of mucous membrane that is pushed up in the form of a cover is called the decidua capsularis; that portion on which the ovum rests, the decidua basalis, and all the rest of the lining of the uterus, the decidua vera. The term membrana decidua was applied to a supposed fibrinous exudation on the lining of the uterus during pregnancy, and named "decidua," or "caduca," because it is cast off during labor and the puerperium.

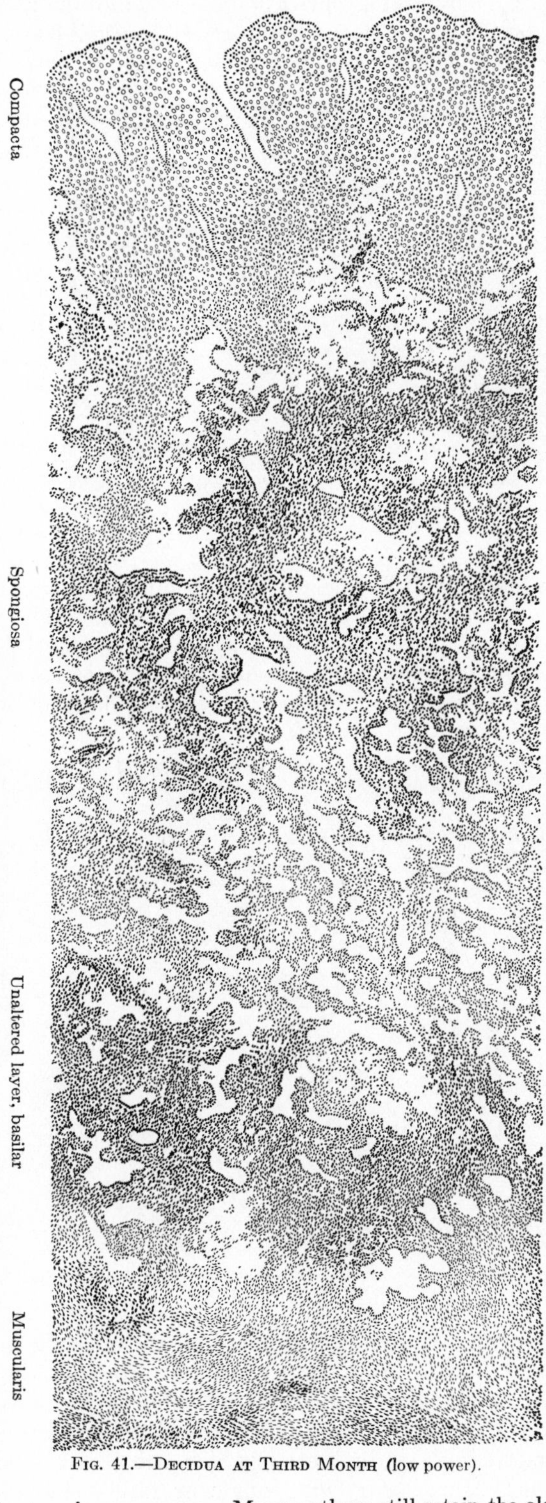

John Hunter taught that pregnancy caused an exudate to appear on the surface of the endometrium, and that the ovum coming down the tube pushed this membrane ahead of it, wherefore this latter portion was called decidua reflexa. Since the same kind of membrane was found under the ovum, it was thought that this was formed later, therefore, decidua serotina. Wm. Hunter (1774) used these names, but described a different mode of formation of the reflexa, according to which the ovum is surrounded by a reduplication of the decidua vera, is walled around, and covered over by the growth of the exuberant decidua. Another notion was that the ovum was caught between two folds of the thickened decidua menstrualis. This may be true in some cases. Many authors still retain the old names reflexa and serotina, but, according to modern ideas of the histology of the endometrium, the terms capsularis and basalis, proposed by His, are better.

FIG. 41.—DECIDUA AT THIRD MONTH (low power).

The endometrium undergoes many changes from the beginning to the end of pregnancy. The cervical mucous membrane normally takes no part in the formation of the decidua. It undergoes marked changes which will be considered later. Sometimes the ovum becomes attached in part to the cervix, but this is pathologic

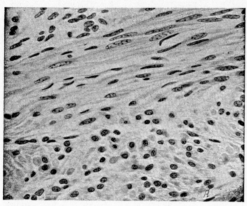

FIG. 42.—SECTION AT JUNCTION OF DECIDUA AND MUSCU-LARIS (high power).

(placenta prævia). In the first weeks the lining of the uterus is hardly distinguishable from the membrane of menstruation. The marked development of the glands, resulting even in a papillary formation with clumped epithelium, which Opitz declared characteristic for pregnancy, the vascularity, the beginning formation of decidual cells, the thickening, all these are similar, so that no one can positively identify a given bit of tissue as having come from one or the other condition. At the end of the third month the *decidua vera* has reached its greatest development (Fig. 41).

The membrane on the anterior and posterior walls is thickest, even as much as 1 cm., the areas at the sides of the uterus, and usually the fundus, are less thickened, and when the lining is cast off, as in abortion at this time, the edges present a sieve-like appearance from the openings of the uterine glands through the thinned portions (Fig 374, p. 460). The inner surface is rugous—that is, thrown into deep folds, but smooth; the outer, detached, is shaggy.

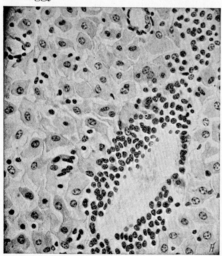

FIG. 43.—AREA COMPACTA. OBLIQUE SECTION OF GLAND. THIRD MONTH (high power).

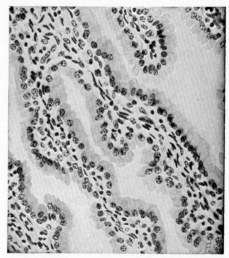

FIG. 44.—AREA SPONGIOSA (THIRD MONTH) (high power).

Microscopically, examination of an early decidua vera (Fig. 41) will show: (1) The epithelium, best preserved around the openings of the glands and in the deeper portions of the same; (2) the compact layer of the decidua, nearly one-half of the whole thickness, made up of the swollen and hyperplastic fibrillary stroma and many decidual cells, which are large, ovoid or spindle-shaped cells, with much protoplasm, with single or rarely several large vesicular nuclei, and derived from the stroma, not from epithelium, which they so much resemble (Fig. 43); (3) the glandular or ampullary layer, or spongiosa (Fig. 44), consisting of the enlarged, elongated, and convoluted uterine glands, often with papillary growths of the epithelium, which is low and cuboid without cilia, and containing fewer decidual cells; (4) a small, unaltered layer through which the glands' fundi pass to, and sometimes slightly into, the muscularis. The glands pursue a straighter course in the basilar portions of the compacta than in the spongiosa. The arteries rise in spirals around the glands, up to the surface, where they break into capillaries. Around the insertion of the ovum the blood-vessels are most numerous and the capillaries most dilated. The veins here are enlarged, and open into the inter-villous spaces. The glands are pushed aside by the growing ovum (Fig. 40).

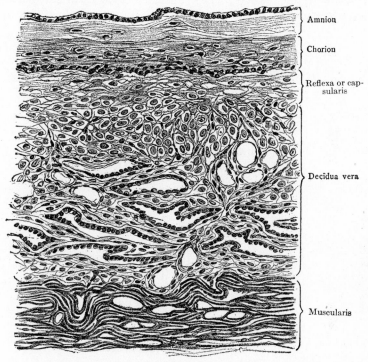

FIG. 45.—DECIDUA AT FIFTH MONTH (from Bumm).

The *decidua basalis* or *serotina* is a portion of the decidua vera altered only by the superimposed growing ovum. It has the compacta and spongiosa, but the glands and blood-vessels, which latter are enormously developed, are stretched to a plane parallel to the wall of the uterus, and, at the junction of the capsularis, curve in arches upward into it. (See Fig. 40.) The portion of the basalis next to the chorion or trophoblast is called the trophosphere, and will be again considered under the head of Placentation. The basalis, of course, must grow rapidly in the flat to keep up with the growing ovum, and this it does both by its own hyperplasia and by the splitting of the compacta of the neighboring vera. The glands of the basalis (or serotina) degenerate early, and, owing to the great and rapid growth of the area of insertion of the ovum (the site of the future placenta), are compressed into a low, lamellous layer of spongy tissue. The basalis shows progressive as well as degenerative changes, and they will also be considered under Placentation.

The *decidua capsularis*, or *reflexa*, is that portion of the vera which is stretched over the ovum (Fig. 40). It is thick at the equatorial portion and thin at the outer pole. This is the point where the egg buried itself in the mucosa. This point, which is microscopic, is soon covered in, so that in later stages it cannot be found. The portions near the base resemble the vera; the blood-vessels are more numerous; the veins larger, and the capillaries open into intervillous spaces. The glands are arranged tangentially around the ovum, and one finds glands opening obliquely on the surface (not into the cavity of the trophosphere), almost up to the vertex of the capsularis. The tissue is soft; the decidual cells numerous; also the so-called syncytial giant-cells. The uterine epithelium is flattened at the vertex, cuboid at the sides, usually without cilia, and disappears early. The portions of the decidua near the top of the capsularis early assume a fibrinous character, without glands, vessels, or epithelium, all these disappearing as the apex is reached.

As the ovum grows and fills out the cavity of the uterus the deciduæ undergo many and material changes. The capsularis at first is stretched over the ovum, and soon reaches the opposing wall of the uterus, on which it lies, but does not

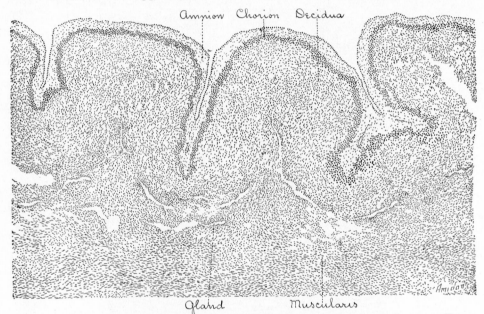

FIG. 46.—DECIDUA VERA AT TERM (low power). SHOWS WRINKLING DUE TO SHRINKING OF SURFACE OF UTERUS. (Specimen from cesarean section.)

adhere. The uterine cavity is completely obliterated by the fourth month. The capsularis undergoes coagulation necrosis, and is absorbed at the sixth month, though occasionally portions of it can be found on the membranes at term. The chorion adheres to the vera and on the delivered secundines large portions of the latter are found attached to the former. At the edges of the placenta one usually finds a thick layer of chorionic ectoderm in fibrinous degeneration, the site of the transition of vera and basalis into reflexa. This is the closing ring of Waldeyer-Winkler.

The decidua vera grows rapidly in thickness until the end of the third month; from then on it thins out until at term (Figs. 46, 47) it is only 1 mm. thick or in places even less. The epithelium is all gone except in the glands of the lowest layers of the spongiosa and those between the muscle-bundles. From these remnants the new uterine mucosa is reconstructed. The compacta is reduced to a narrow strip, and most of the decidual and stroma cells are in process of coagulation necrosis. The glands of the compacta are separated from each other, while in the spongiosa they form a thin, loose, flattened network, and since the stroma here too is beginning to degenerate, separation of the ovum from the uterine wall is easy. Nature is thus preparing the way for the release of the product of conception. The basalis undergoes the most marked transformation, because here the egg is inserted and the placenta is situated. Gentili has shown that the decidua possesses qualities similar to those of the glands with internal secretion. Its structure, therefore, is intimately associated with the placenta, and the description of the two will be combined.

PLACENTATION

We have learned how the ovum attaches itself to the uterine mucosa by burrowing through the epithelium into the stroma. At this time it is in the morula stage, and although it cannot be proved, probably there exists at this time an outer ectodermal layer with syncytial characteristics, *i. e.*, a trophoblast. At this time, also, and certainly within a few days, there exist the three layers of the ovum—the ectoderm, the entoderm, and the mesoderm. The amniotic cavity

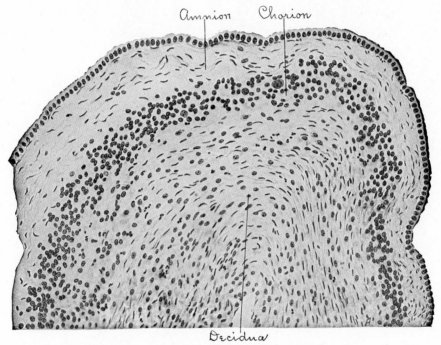

FIG. 47.—DECIDUA VERA AT TERM (high power).

also is formed, because one of the youngest human eggs, Peters', whose age is estimated at about sixteen days, shows this. The ectoderm is split by the amnion cavity (Fig. 61), the outer layer forming the trophectoderm, the inner layer sinking toward the center of the ovum, and, with the central mesoderm and entoderm, forming the embryo. While the trophoblast grows into the decidua in all directions, the mesoderm grows out underneath it, and blood-vessels with connective tissue spread out in the latter, coming from the body stalk of the embryo. Thus we have a condition represented in Figs. 63 and 64.

The trophoblast sends finger-like processes, called villi, into the decidua, the cells of which are dissolved and absorbed, as if by the action of an enzyme (Bryce and Teacher), and perhaps used in the nourishment of the ovum. These villi are at first solid masses of cells, and they break into the dilated and new-formed capillaries, pushing the endothelium before them, and destroying it. (See Plate opposite p. 30.) The maternal blood now bathes the outside of the trophoblast, and by its

action changes the superficial layers of epithelium into syncytial trophoblast
(Peters), and forms irregular blood-spaces or lacunæ in it. The lacunæ, therefore,
are both intravascular and extravascular, *i. e.*, are both dilated capillaries and
new spaces formed in the trophoblast, and they are the beginnings of the intervillous caverns soon to be described.

The solid trophoblastic processes or villi are invaded from the embryonal side
by mesoderm carrying the blood-vessels, and thus typical chorionic villi with an

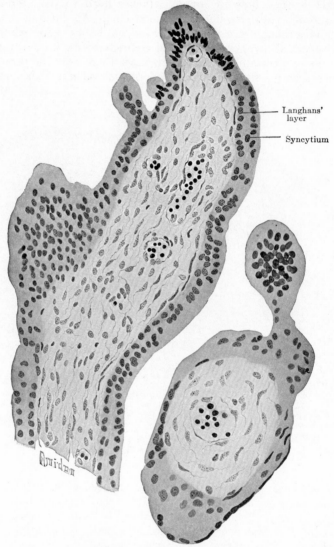

Fig. 48.—Chorionic Villi. Third Month.
Compare with hydatid mole, Figure 481.

inner core of mesodermal tissue, and a covering of trophoblast, in which two layers
can early be distinguished, are formed (Figs. 48–50). The outer layer is a strip of
protoplasm without cell-walls and with numerous large oval nuclei, the syncytium.
In places this syncytium is massed. Underneath is a layer of low cuboid mononucleated cells, which take the stain better—the Langhans layer. Langhans, in
1882, proved that there were two layers, and the lower one is named after him.

Preparations fixed in Flemming's mixture show the syncytium to be covered with stiff processes. The function of these processes is unknown. In the villi at term these are low, almost indistinguishable, and the layer of Langhans also has nearly all disappeared. The stroma of the early villus is made up of a reticulated substance, fibromucoid, spindle, or star-shaped cells, separated by spaces resembling lymph-spaces. There are also large vacuolated cells, often containing fat-globules distributed through the stroma (Hofbauer's cells). Possibly some of them are degenerated fibroblasts. In the later and more developed villi, and in the trunks of the villi, fibrous tissue preponderates in the stroma. In the stroma lies a mesh of capillaries, fed by an arteriole and emptied by a venule. From the start, the circulations of the mother and the fetus are distinct and do not intermingle. The blood of the child circulates inside the villus; the blood of the mother circulates

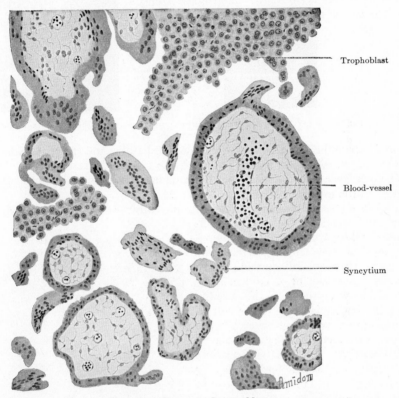

Trophoblast

Blood-vessel

Syncytium

Fig. 49.—Section of Placenta, Second Month.

outside, around the villus (Fig. 54). As the ovum grows the villi increase in number and complexity. They branch again and again, forming long tufts, and soon the whole surface of the chorion is covered by a thick fur of villi (Fig. 50). Those villi that grow toward the reflexa, or capsularis, find scant nourishment, and, too, a decidua that is being stretched and undergoing necrosis, wherefore they also soon atrophy and disappear. The process is started in the fourth week and is finished by the ninth, but sometimes villi persist in the capsularis, forming a reflexa placenta. The basalis is very richly supplied with blood; indeed, its structure is almost cavernous, and the villi here take on luxuriant growth (Figs. 50a and 51). This is the future placenta or chorion frondosum. The atrophied chorion is called the chorion læve. In the first weeks of life the ovum is firmly embedded in the uterine wall; then, owing to the rapid growth of the villi and their loose attachment (but still, attachment) to the dilated, newly formed blood-vessels, it is possible easily to lift the ovum out of its bed. Early abortions then give us specimens as in Figs. 50 and 50a. There are in such cases many villi and pieces of villi still remaining adherent to the basalis. These are called anchoring villi, because the syncytium on them has burrowed deeper into the decidua, and sometimes even has pierced into a dilated vein at the site of the placenta (Fig. 52). The villi continue to multiply, growing into the decidual base, which also grows outward among the tufts of the villi. These outgrowths of decidua carry the arteries and veins of the uterus, and in the ripe placenta are represented only by thin partitions between the large lobes or cotyledons of the placenta. The arteries pursue a

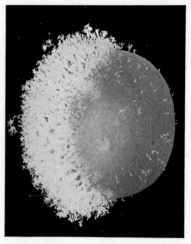

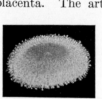

FIG. 50.—THREE WEEKS' OVUM (natural size).

FIG. 50a.—SIX WEEKS' OVUM.

spiral course through the uterine muscle, the basalis, and the septa, while the veins are straight. As these vessels approach the placental site they lose all their coats save one layer of endothelial cells, forming large sinuses, really not distinct vessels, between the muscular lamellæ and the decidua.

We have seen how the villi come to dip into the maternal blood, which flows in lacunæ formed by the dilated capillaries and cavernous spaces in the periphery of the trophosphere. The rapidly growing villi invade these blood-spaces, which, of course, communicate with those in the decidua basalis, and, finally, as the result of compression and absorption by the trophoblast, the compacta is nearly all destroyed, the villi lying against the spongiosa and a few (anchoring villi) dipping into it. The villi grow in the direction of the venous openings and away from the arteries, the blood-stream naturally swimming them in this direction. They stretch the venous sinuses, and by pressure necrosis destroy the decidua compacta between the veins until only the septa carrying the arteries are left (Fig. 54). The capillaries and veins of the compacta are developed, as the placenta grows large and heavy, into extensive caverns filled with the inextricably mingled branched trees of villi float-

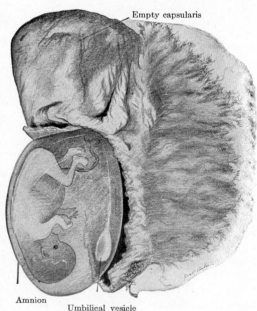

Empty capsularis

Amnion

Umbilical vesicle

FIG. 51.—NINE WEEKS' OVUM.

The amniotic sac with fetus has escaped from the capsularis.

ing in maternal blood (Fig. 53). These caverns are fed by the arteries which sometimes ascend the septa placentæ, and are emptied by the veins of the placental site. These vessels may be easily seen on the full-term placenta (Fig. 55).

The maternal blood in the intervillous spaces is in constant circulation. The arteries in the septa bring it, the veins on the surface of the cotyledons empty it, into the uterine sinuses. The circular sinus also collects the blood from all the

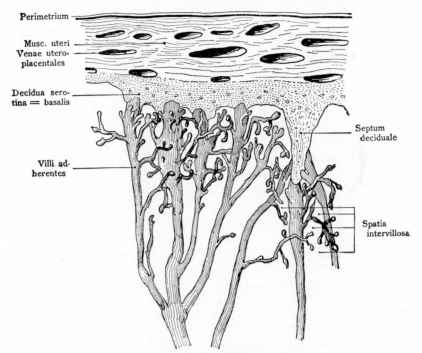

FIG. 52.—ANCHORING VILLI (Kollmann).

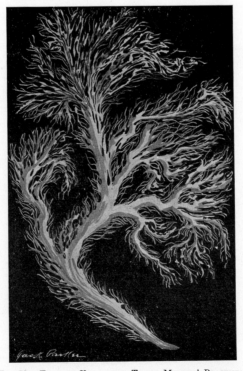

FIG. 53.—TREE OF VILLI FROM THREE MONTHS' PLACENTA.
Drawn floating in water.

cotyledons, serving as an anastomosis. The movement of the blood is aided by uterine contractions which occur at intervals throughout pregnancy.

The placenta grows laterally and in thickness, and about the fourth month

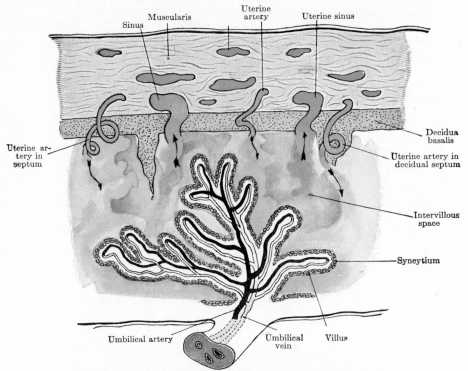

FIG. 54.—SCHEME OF PLACENTAL CIRCULATION (Kollmann, Hand Atlas). Arrows indicate supply and exhaust of blood in the intervillous spaces.

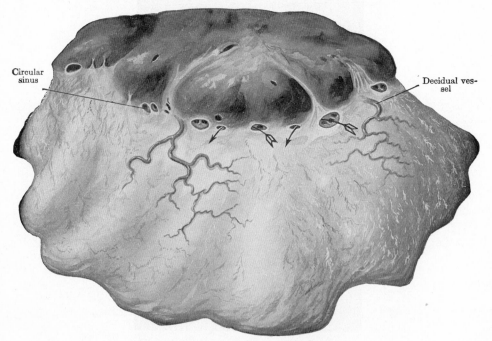

FIG. 55.—THE CIRCULAR SINUS OF THE PLACENTA.

takes up one-half of the area of the uterus; at the end of pregnancy the placenta occupies one-fourth to one-third of the uterine expanse. Its weight increases **at**

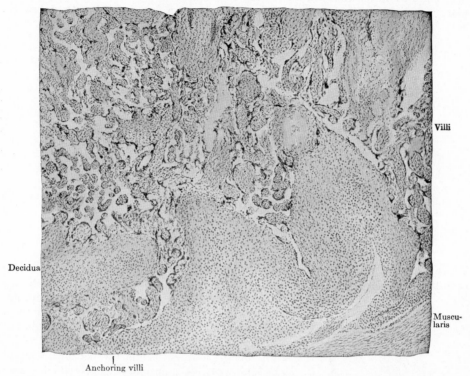

FIG. 56.—DECIDUA BASALIS (low power).

the rate of 60 gm. a month until the seventh month, then 50 gm., and, in the tenth month, less than 10 gm. The growth of the villi in the flat is permitted by a splitting of the decidua vera at the periphery of the placenta, and at the same time by an increase of the area of the placental base caused by the growth of the uterus. When the capsularis unites definitely with the vera, there remains a thickened ring of decidua at the junction of the basalis and capsularis, and the villi of the capsularis atrophying, while those of the basalis grow, the latter spread out under the attached ring of decidua for a short distance. This is exaggerated when there is a pathologically early adherence of the deciduæ, or if the natural splitting of the vera is interfered with. A placenta marginated and, in marked instances, placentæ circumvallatæ, are thus produced. The ring of decidua and chorionic ectoderm is called the decidua subchorialis.

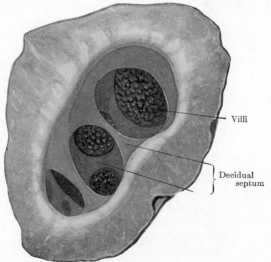

FIG. 57.—VENOUS OPENINGS IN THE PLACENTA (magnified). Author's specimen (idea from Kollmann, Hand Atlas).

By some it is referred to as the Waldeyer closing ring; by others, the edge of the closing plate of Winkler. The placenta is seen to be composed of two parts—one, very minute in quantity, derived from maternal tissues; the other from fetal, both inextricably intergrown.

The two umbilical arteries from the child spread out on the fetal surface of the placenta, divide and redivide, until each cotyledon is provided with a branch.

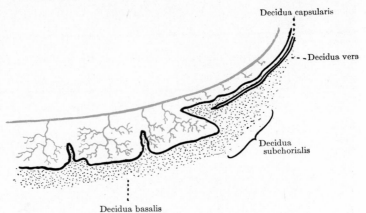

Fig. 58.—Diagram Showing Decidua Subchorialis (Pfannenstiel).

These branches, which have vasa nutrientia, split up into numerous twigs, and from each twig a bunch of villi hangs (Fig. 53). Each villus is provided with an arteriole

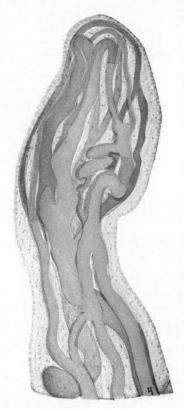

Fig. 59.—Circulation of a Villus (from an injected placenta).

which breaks into a convolution of intercommunicating capillaries. The blood is gathered by a venule to which the venules of the other villi are joined, until large venous trunks are formed which unite on the fetal surface of the placenta to form one large vein,—the umbilical vein,—which passes in the navel-string, the umbilical cord, to the child (Fig. 59). The circulation in the villi is, therefore, absolutely distinct from that of the intervillous spaces, as was proved by William Shippen in 1761, and the interchange of gases, water, and nourishment must take place through the villus-wall, by osmosis and by the vital action of the cells themselves, particularly the latter. The villus-wall consists of the following layers, naming them from within outward: endothelium of capillary, reticular mucoid stroma, Langhans' layer, and syncytium, both of the latter from the fetal ectoderm. Later in pregnancy Langhans' layer disappears or thins out; the syncytial band also grows narrower, until, at term, the villus has only a single layer of the stretched syncytium over it (Fig. 60).

The Development of the Amnion and Umbilical Cord.—According to the latest researches of Graf Spee, the amnion in the human is formed in a manner similar to that of many mammals. Very early a split appears in the ectoderm of the germinal area (Fig. 61); this fills with fluid and forces the embryonic plate toward the center of the egg. The mesoderm grows rapidly and separates this, the primary amniotic cavity, from the chorionic ectoderm everywhere except at the area of insertion of the body stalk, at the same time itself splitting into two layers—the somatic, external; the splanchnic, internal (Figs. 62 to 64).

A fluid appears in the space between these layers, which is called the exocelom, and takes in almost the entire content of the egg at this time. By the development of the exocelom the entoderm is separated from the periphery of the ovum and the yolk, or vitelline sac is formed (Figs. 64 and 65). The yolk sac is developed on the abdominal side of the embryo, while the amniotic sac is formed on its dorsal aspect. The vitelline sac, consisting of a layer of entoderm and one of mesoderm, and containing albuminoid matter, at first is much the larger; later the amniotic cavity is larger. The yolk sac communicates broadly with the primitive intestinal tube, and has blood-vessels, the vasa vitellinæ, which convey blood to the embryo. During the growth of the embryo and yolk sac, the neck of the sac, growing slower, appears to be constricted, the yolk stalk. (Fig. 81) These structures may often be found on the full-term placenta between the chorion and amnion, more or less distant from the insertion of the cord. The vesicle, which up to the fourth month measures 7 to 10 mm., is then the size of a split-pea, yellow and fibrous, and shows leading from it, lost in the cord, a fine white thread, the relics of the duct. Schultze's fold is a duplication of amnion (Fig. 67) at the point where the original vitelline duct left the body stalk.

The vitelline circulation ceases as the sac shrinks, and as the embryo receives its nourishment from the chorion frondosum, through the two veins and two arteries of the body stalk (Fig. 83). The amniotic cavity enlarges rapidly, and, coming around the embryo from all sides, causes

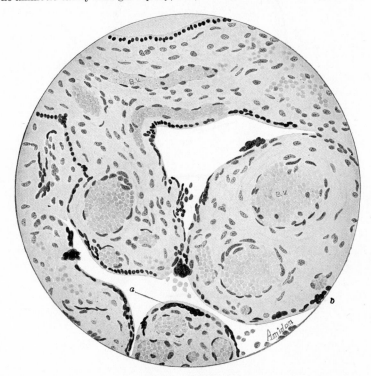

Fig. 60.—Ripe Placenta.
a, Intervillous space; *b*, syncytium.

the disappearance of the exocelom, and forces the body stalk, with its rudimentary blind allantoic stalk, and the four blood-vessels, and the vitelline duct together into a single short peduncle, the beginning of the umbilical cord (Fig. 66). This occurs in the fourth week, and the amnion completely fills the egg in the second month, coming to lie on the chorion throughout its extent. The embryo now floats freely in the cavity of the amnion, surrounded by the fluid there produced, the liquor amnii, and united to the chorion frondosum by the umbilical cord. It is nourished by the blood which circulates between it and the chorion frondosum. The nutritional organs are all formed as they will continue throughout pregnancy, requiring only further enlargement to accommodate the rapidly growing fetus. (For further details the reader is referred to text-books on embryology. The above description was necessary for the proper study of the clinical side of conditions met daily by the obstetric practitioner.) One of the best expositions of human embryology, placentation, etc., will be found in Grosser's portion of Halban-Seitz, Biologie und Pathologie des Weibes.

The **placenta at term** is a cake-like organ, and weighs about 500 gm., the proportion to the weight of the child being as one to six. Placentas vary in weight, size, thickness, form, and consistence (Fig. 69). Placentas from large children are heavier. In syphilitic cases the placenta is heavier than with normal children of the same size, and the proportion may be reduced to one to three.   A placenta may be small and thick or large and thin, the usual thickness being 1½ to 2 cm., and the breadth 15 to 18 cm.   The form is usually irregularly round, but the organ may assume any shape, depending on its direction of growth on the uterine wall.   Bilobate (the usual shape is apes), trilobate, and horseshoe shapes are observed, and

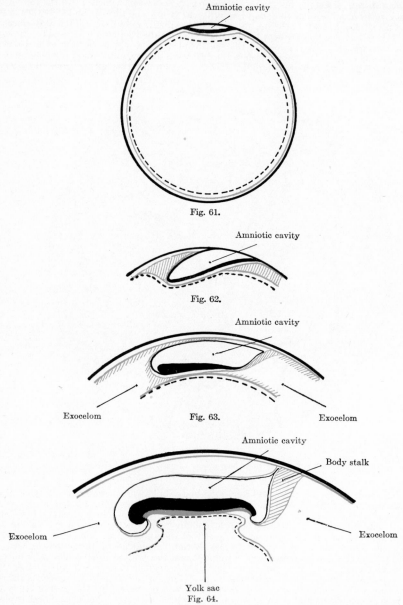

FIGS. 61, 62, 63, 64.—DIAGRAMS BY PFANNENSTIEL, TO SHOW FORMATION OF EMBRYO AND AMNIOTIC CAVITY.

the placenta may be spread out over a large area—placenta membranacea.   In addition to a main placenta, there may exist accessory portions connected to the former by an artery and vein; these are called placentæ succenturiatæ, or, if very small, placentulæ succenturiatæ.   If no blood-vessels can be seen. the piece is termed a placenta spuria.   These extra placentas are of immense clinical importance.   The shape of the placenta depends on the first location of the ovum after it enters the uterus. If the ovum attaches itself to the center of either the anterior or the posterior wall, the placenta probably will be round or oval. If it is embedded near one of the lateral angles of the uterus, the decidua, being thin at this point, offers poor nourishment to the villi, which then grow eccentrically,—either on to the fundus or on to the other wall of the uterus,—a bilobate or a trilobate placenta resulting. Such a division into lobes may also result from the pathologic formation of fibrinous masses in the placenta.

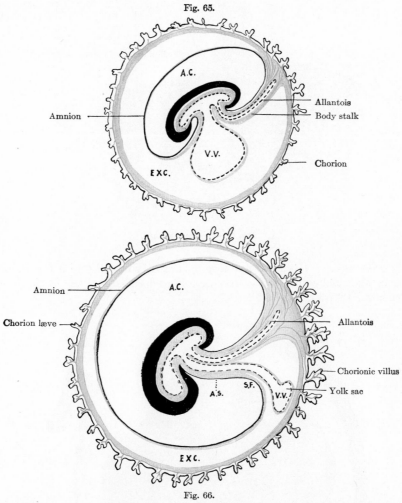

Figs. 65 and 66.—Diagrams by Pfannenstiel, Showing Formation of Abdominal Pedicle and Allantois. v.v., Vitelline vesicle; a.c., amniotic cavity; s.f., Schultze's fold; a.s., Amnion covering of umbilical cord.

Some placentas are soft and very vascular; others are harder and more fibrous, without being pathologic. The tissue of the organ is dark red, soft, friable, but interwoven with tough fibrous tissue and blood-vessels. The maternal surface— that surface which lies on the wall of the uterus—is covered with a thin, grayish, translucent, slightly roughened membrane, which cannot be peeled off, but tears away from the underlying soft pulp of the placenta. This is that part of the decidua basalis called the compacta, and which normally separates from the spongiosa and comes away with the placenta when it leaves the uterus. This gray membrane is broken here and there; small bits are absent, and in places it is thicker and opaque. At the rim of the placenta, and extending a little under the amnion, the chorionic ectoderm and decidua accumulate, the closing ring of

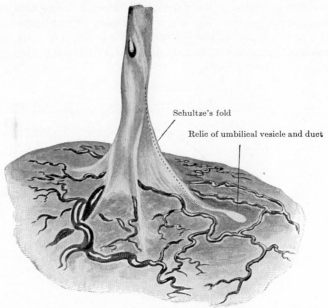

Fig. 67.—Schultze's Fold.

Waldeyer (Grosser). If you scrape into this area, you will find a large sinus, the circular or marginal sinus, and it may be followed all around the circumference of the placenta. (See Fig. 55, p. 42.)

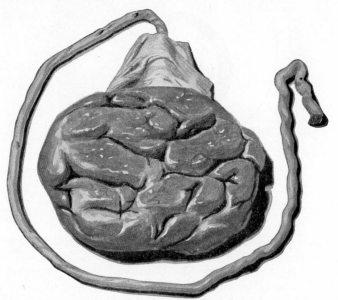

Fig. 68.—Normal Placenta (Maternal Surface).

The maternal surface of the organ is divided by decidual septa into numerous lobes called cotyledons. If one pushes the cytoledons asunder, the septum is split, and the venous sinuses which lead into the intervillous spaces are disclosed. (See Fig. 57, p. 43.) Occasionally a cotyledon will be sessile on the surface of the placenta, and may be left in the uterus. The most careful examination of the delivered placenta will fail to discover the absence of such a piece, and serious illness of the mother may result from its retention, such as hemorrhage or sepsis.

The fetal surface of the placenta is covered by the thin, glistening amnion, through which one sees the placental arteries and veins coming from the cord and branching in all directions until the smallest twigs disappear about one-fourth of an inch from the edge of the placenta. The surface is uneven, gray, and reddish, sometimes dotted with whitish and yellowish areas of fibrous tissue. These are

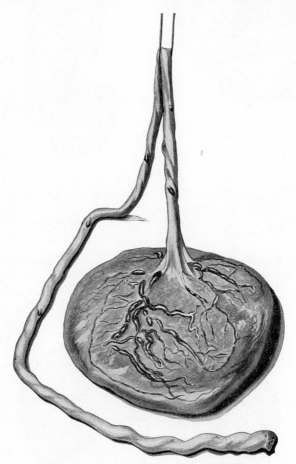

Fig. 69.—Normal Placenta (Fetal Surface).

called white infarcts, are very common, and will be considered under the pathology of the placenta (p. 602). The amnion may be stripped off the fetal surface except at the insertion of the cord. It is attached here only by the jelly of Wharton. In rare cases the amnion may be stripped off the cord also, the jelly of Wharton being present here too. The chorion læve, that portion of the periphery of the ovum which lay against the decidua capsularis, and in which the villi have atrophied, together with the amnion, forms a veil-like structure hanging from the placenta, and called the membranes. The chorion is the outer layer, thicker, cloudy, somewhat opaque, and easily torn. On its maternal surface are the remains of the decidua vera and capsularis, which can be scraped off with the finger-nail as débris. Early

4

in pregnancy and in pathologic cases it is a thicker membrane. Occasionally one sees blood-vessels running in the decidua, especially in the neighborhood of the placenta. The amnion is tougher and transparent.

The umbilical cord is inserted about the middle of the placenta, but it may be found at any point—at the edge (insertio marginalis) or even in the adjacent mem-

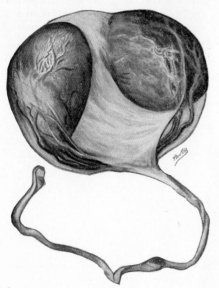

FIG. 70.—BILOBATE PLACENTA WITH VELAMENTOUS INSERTION OF CORD.

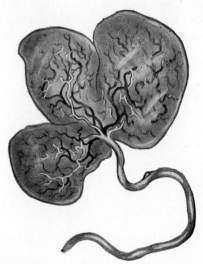

FIG. 71.—TREFOIL PLACENTA.

branes (insertio velamentosa). At its insertion are occasionally found small epithelial amniotic growths or caruncles, also the fold of amnion, carrying the ductus vitellinus, Schultze's fold. At some point in the membranes there is an opening through which the fetus passed. This lies usually 10 cm. from the edge

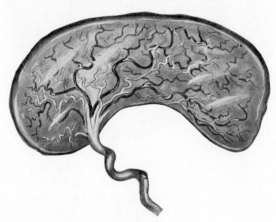

FIG. 72.—HORSESHOE PLACENTA.

of the placenta, showing that such was the distance from the internal os of the uterus to the edge of the placenta. The opening may be close to the edge, which shows that the placenta lay near the internal os, or even over it—placenta prævia. The placenta is situated usually on the anterior or the posterior wall of the uterus, seldom over the internal os (placenta prævia), and most rarely in the fundus. It may lap over from one side to the other. The causes of particular insertions of the placenta are unknown. Endometritis and subinvolution certainly have something to do with the location of the placenta low in the uterus.

The **umbilical cord** connects the fetus with the placenta, and is the means of conveyance of the fetal blood to and from the latter. It is formed by the abdominal pedicle of the embryo, as was described on p. 45. The amnion, as it develops, surrounds the cord, but is not attached to it. This occurs later. On cross-

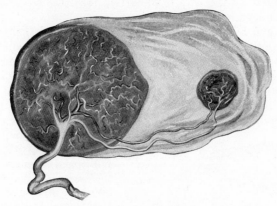

Fig. 73.—Placenta Succenturiata.

section the cord shows the covering of amnion epithelium, two arteries (sometimes one) and one vein (sometimes two), the relics of the vitelline duct (often lost), remains of the allantois, and the jelly of Wharton, which binds all together. If there is much jelly of Wharton, we speak of a fat cord; if little, of a lean cord. The amnion, with its pavement epithelium, passes over into the skin of the fetus at the navel, where there is a sharp line of demarcation between them. A plexus of capillaries ascends the amnion for $\frac{1}{8}$ inch, and Beckman and Zimmer found

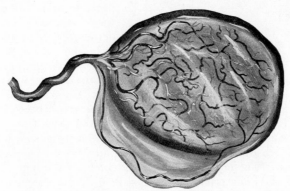

Fig. 74.—Battledore Placenta.

capillaries in the jelly of Wharton. Vasa propria do not exist here, but they do in the vessels of the placenta. Nerves were not found by Virchow and most searchers, but Kölliker and Valentine found them. At first the cord is very short, but as the child grows it lengthens until, at term, it measures about 50 cm. This varies from a few millimeters to 300 cm. A length of over 100 cm. is very rare. The spiral twists in the cord, of which there may be several hundred, are best explained by the movements of the child, but the direction of the growth of the arteries, and the effect of the pumping action of the fetal heart, may be partly causative. Stowe found that the tensile strength of the cord was from 8 to 15 pounds. Runge describes the anatomy of the vein.

The umbilical arteries are continuations of the hypogastric vessels; the vein comes from the umbilical vein. The arteries are twisted on themselves; they are twisted around the vein, and the vein is also twisted, and, as a result, there seem to be valves in the vessels, called valvulæ hobokenii. The arteries usually anastomose near the placenta. In 6 per cent. (Hyrtl) only one umbilical artery exists. They have a strong middle coat. The arteries and vein are sometimes curled into nodes which, covered by the jelly of Wharton, form the so-called false knots on the cord. True knots are also found.

The Amnion and Liquor Amnii.—The thin, transparent, silvery, tough membrane lining the chorion læve and frondosum (placenta) is the amnion. Its formation has already been considered. It is now being successfully used in skin-grafting. (See p. 44.) Occasionally a little of the jelly of Wharton exists between the two structures. The liquor amnii is produced by the amnion at the very earliest period of fetation, and at first it is crystal clear; later it becomes more opaque. The amount at full term varies from 500 to 2000 gm., depending on many conditions, one of which is the size of the child, another multiparity—more liquor in each instance. Quantities less than 300 gm. and more than 2000 are pathologic, the former being called oligohydramnion, the latter polyhydramnion. The amount of the fluid increases up to the seventh month; from then on it regularly decreases until, at term, there is usually but enough to fill out the spaces between the irregular contour of the fetus and the uterine wall. It is a clear fluid, more or less milky from suspended particles of vernix caseosa. This is the accumulated and exfoliated epidermis, sebaceous matter, and lanugo from the skin of the child and the cholesterids and glycerids secreted by the amniotic epithelium (Keiffer). There are also some leukocytes and unclassified cells. If the fetus dies, the liquor amnii becomes blood stained, and if the child is asphyxiated, one finds it green and thick from the admixture of meconium. It has a peculiar sperma-like odor, and a specific gravity varying from 1006 to 1015, which diminishes as pregnancy advances. The reaction is faintly alkaline or neutral. The cryoscopic (freezing) point of the liquor amnii is slightly higher than that of the maternal blood ($\Delta = 0.56$). Therefore, speaking generally, the liquor is destined to be absorbed (Keim). Clinically, one can observe fluctuations in the amount of liquor amnii. At the seventh month a sudden increase may often be noted.

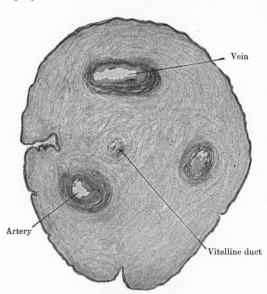

Fig. 75.—Section of Umbilical Cord at Term.

The chemic analyses of liquor amnii vary considerably. Prochownik found the following:

Reaction.	Specific Gravity.	Albumin.	Fats.	Inorganic.	Water.
1. Neutral	1081.5	6.81	0.20	6.27	986.62
2. Neutral	1006.2	7.70	0.10	5.50	986.09
3. Neutral	1007.1	8.20	1.22	5.68	985.30

Sandmeyer examined the liquor amnii with a view to determining its food value, and found it contains an average of 0.22 per cent. of albumin and a small amount of glucose. The salts are in about the same proportion as human blood-serum, i. e., 0.5 per cent., and are the chlorids, phosphates, sulphates, and carbonates of sodium and calcium, with very little potassium.

Dieckmann and Davis stained the liquor amnii with Congo red to measure its quantity during pregnancy. They find too that phenolsulphonphthalein is absorbed and appears in the mother's urine within five minutes.

An important finding is urea, which was found by Prochownik as early as the fourth week, and which increases toward the end of pregnancy and with the size of the fetus. The amount varies from 0.02 to 0.4 per cent. Ahlfeld, in a case where the bag of waters had ruptured thirty-one days before labor, could find so little urea in the collected liquor amnii that it could not be measured. Barnes says that since there is urea in the egg, the fetus must excrete it.

The albumins in the liquor are serum-albumin, globulin, and an ovovitellin-like substance (Goenner). The electrolyte concentration is less than that of the blood-serum.

Bondi found pepsin, a diastatic ferment, a fat-splitting ferment, and one like fibrin-ferment in the liquor amnii. These facts are important in connection with the maceration of fetuses after they die. In diabetes sugar is present in the liquor. Normally, bacteria are not present, but under pathologic conditions they may wander up the cervix and through the membranes, or through the musculature from adherent adjacent organs, e. g., inflamed bladder and appendix or decomposing fibroids.

The Sources of the Liquor Amnii.—Naturally, the liquor amnii comes ultimately from the mother, but much discussion has arisen as to whether the fetus excretes it, either as urine or through the cord and fetal placenta, or whether it passes directly into the cavity of the uterus from the maternal vessels. Probably both hypotheses are true. In favor of the first theory have been adduced—(1) Constant presence of urea in the liquor amnii (the fetus urinates into it); (2) the demonstration of urine in the bladder of new-born children; (3) the occurrence of polyhydramnion when the fetus has heart disease, in unioval twins, and in fetal monsters. In the latter, however, one must remember that monstrosities are frequently caused by amnionitis, which may also cause the polyhydramnion.

The theory that the liquor amnii is a transudate from the maternal vessels is most plausible. (1) When potassium iodid is given the mother, it will appear in the liquor amnii, but not in the fetal kidney (Haidlen). In diabetes sugar appears in the liquor amnii. (2) When the mother has heart disease or any affection attended by dropsies, one will often find an increase of the fluid. (3) Early in pregnancy, and when the fetus has been dead for some time, there is relatively too much fluid in the uterus. (4) Wohlgemuth and Massone experimentally showed that diastase in the maternal blood appears in the liquor amnii when the fetus is dead. Polano believes the liquor is a secretion of the amniotic epithelium, and since pathologic changes in the amnion have been found in cases of hydramnion, color is lent to this view. That the fetus urinates into the liquor amnii is improbable. If urea was excreted in this fashion, more of it should be found, and it is unreasonable to suppose that nature would have an individual floating in and drinking its own excreta. Cohnstein and Zuntz have proved that the arterial pressure in the kidney is too low even for the production of urine. Ahlfeld proves almost conclusively that the fetus does not, normally, urinate into the liquor amnii; that when this occurs, it is accidental, and probably due to some more or less serious circulatory disturbance but Minkowski and Makepeace are convinced the fetus does. (See Wagner, Kirstein, 1927.)

In a case where I administered methylene-blue to the mother before labor, it was excreted by the new-born child in the urine for several days after birth, but the liquor amnii was not blue.

The Uses of the Liquor Amnii.—The fluid around the child has most important functions: 1. First it is a food, which the fetus drinks. This is proved by— (a) The finding of lanugo in the meconium after birth, and real swallowing motions have been determined in the fetus during the latter months of pregnancy. (b) In a case of occlusion of the gullet the fetus was atrophied. (c) The liquor amnii contains albumin constantly, and if the fetus drinks enough, it will get a considerable amount of albumin.

2. It is a water-cushion taking up the shocks from external injury, and allowing free motion to the fetus; this prevents deformities, e. g., club-foot. In cases where the liquor is very scant the child is folded compactly together, and shortening of the muscles, wry-neck, and various distortions of the extremities result.

3. The young fetus is so delicate a structure that it can grow only in a liquid medium. It is possible the fluid prevents adherences of the amnion (Simonart bands). Later it preserves the cord from pressure and renders the movements of the child less painful to the mother. It stabilizes fetal temperature.

4. During labor it—(a) Helps dilate the passages by forming a fluid wedge with the membranes, and (b), surrounding the fetus completely, it distributes, as all fluids do, the compression exerted by the contracting uterus, equally in all directions, and thus saves any part of the fetus from injurious pressure. When the liquor amnii

has been discharged, the fetus is exposed to this pressure and may succumb to it. By the same action the placenta is held against the uterine wall. (*c*) It washes out the vagina for the passage of the child, and by its slightly bactericidal action, prevents infection of the child and the uterine cavity. Unfortunately, this germicidal action is weak.

THE FETUS AT DIFFERENT PERIODS OF DEVELOPMENT

At no time of life is the growth of the individual as rapid as it is during the period spent *in utero*. From the fifth week the fetus doubles its length five times, and its weight is 800 times greater at term than it is at two months. It is impossible to obtain these figures with scientific accuracy,

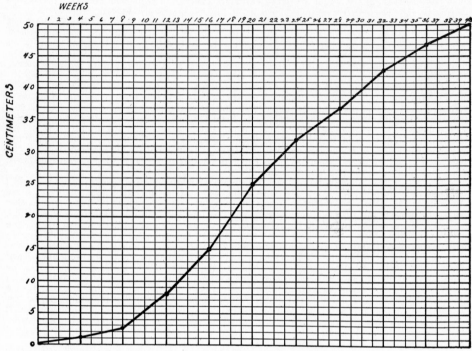

FIG. 76.—CHART SHOWING GROWTH IN LENGTH OF FETUS IN UTERO.

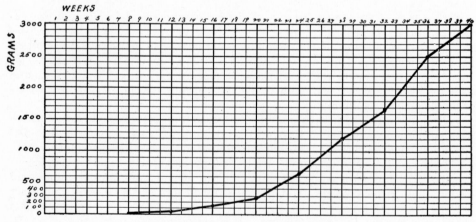

FIG. 77.—WEIGHT CHART OF FETUS IN UTERO.

first, because the exact date of conception cannot be determined in any of the cases, and, second, the individuals vary *in utero* as they do after birth. A good rule, which for practical purposes will suffice for the determination of the length of the fetus at a given period of pregnancy, is this: Square the number of the month, which will give the length of the fetus in centimeters until the fifth month.   After the fifth month add to this five each month; thus at four months a fetus should be about 16 cm. long; at six months, 30 cm. $(5 \times 5 + 5)$; at seven months $(5 \times 5 + 5 + 5)$, and so on. The length of the fetus is the safest guide in the determination of its age.   Children vary both in length and weight.   Some babies grow faster than others, and their growth, too, may be interrupted temporarily during pregnancy.   Frequent examinations during gestation will show this.

The Fetus at Various Periods.—Among the best works on the development of the early human ovum is that of His.   He distinguished three periods in the life of the child—the ovular, during the first two weeks; embryonal, the third, fourth, and fifth weeks; and fetal, from that on

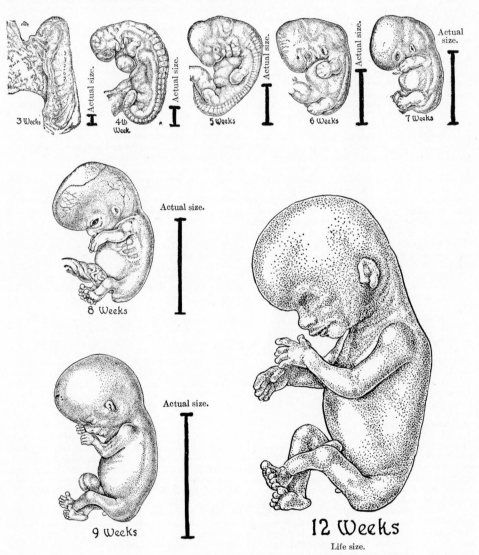

FIGS. 78, 79.—VERY EARLY EMBRYOS.   (Supplied by Prof. G. W. Bartelmez of the University of Chicago.)

until term.   The ovum in the first weeks interests the practical obstetrician little, because it can be studied only with a microscope.   It is almost impossible to judge the age of the little, shaggy, bladder-like ova that are expelled in early abortions, because they are often pathologic.   As a general rule, however, an ovum the size of a pigeon's egg is four weeks, and one the size of a hen's egg, six or seven weeks.   After this period the length of the fetus from nape of neck to sacrum, and still later the total length, or better the sitting height, give more certain conclusions.

End of the First Lunar Month.—An embryo of this period is 4 mm. long.   The yolk sac is still prominent and a distinct umbilical cord has not yet formed.   There are no external indications of the eye, ear, or nose, although a mouth and primitive jaws exist.   Buds representing the extremities appear during the following week. The visceral arches are distinct; the heart is a bulging, flexed tube lacking its characteristic chambers; the blind intestinal canal still opens rather broadly on the yolk sac; the first indication of the liver appears, but the kidney is undeveloped.

End of Second Month.—The fetus is 3 cm. total length; the branchial arches are prominent at the beginning of this period, but disappear at its end. The nose, ear, and eye are present, although the eyelids are still fused. The extremities, at first bud-like at the end, show the division into three parts: first, the arm, forearm, and hand; then the thigh, leg, and foot, and the digits are more marked. The tail-like process has disappeared. The navel begins to close; the liver develops, also the abdomen, which is not yet quite closed, and the external genitals appear, but it is impossible to determine the sex of the fetus, since the male and female genitalia are developed from identical organs and are differentiated later.

The villi in the decidua serotina grow luxuriantly, forming **the future placenta**, the permanent fetal maternal relations being now fully established.

End of Third Month.—The ovum is a little larger than a goose-egg, and the fetus 9 cm. long, weighing 5 gm. at the beginning and 20 gm. at the end of the month. The navel is closed, the internal genitals differentiated. The external genitals are alike in the two sexes. At the beginning of the eleventh week the scrotum closes, and the sex may be determined. The intestinal canal is formed and contains bile (Zweifel). The body resembles a human being, though the head is still proportionately extremely large. Centers of ossification are visible in many of the bones.

End of Fourth Month.—The fetus is 18 cm. long, and weighs 120 gm. at the end of this period. Meconium is present and is turning green (Charpentier). The muscles are active, fetal movements being occasionally felt by the mother. The heart-beat is strong and has been heard. The external organs of sex can easily be differentiated. The skin is bright red, transparent, so that all the vessels are visible. Lanugo—fine hair—appears on the skin.

Fifth Month.—The fetus is now 25 cm. long, and weighs 250 to 280 gm. (7 to 9 ounces). The head is still very large, being the size of a hen's egg, but the abdomen is less prominent. The fetus is lean. The skin is still red, but, owing to the deposition of fat, is less transparent. The lanugo is present all over the body, but on the head there are indications of hair. The nails can be distinguished. The eyelids are closed. Such a fetus may live for five to ten minutes with strong heart-beat and attempts at respiration.

Sixth Month.—The fetus, at the end of the sixth month, is 28 to 34 cm. long and weighs about 645 gm. (1¼ pounds). Its body is more in proportion, though still lean, the amount of fat in the skin being still small. The skin is wrinkled, and vernix caseosa begins to form. This is the accumulated, exfoliated epithelium and sebaceous secretion. The eyebrows and lashes are formed; the eyelids are separated, and such an infant born, may breathe, though superficially, and live for several hours under favorable conditions. Since its respiratory, digestive, and assimilative organs are physiologically undeveloped, no artificial means will preserve these fetuses from congelation and starvation. Reports of the rearing of such infants are to be discredited.

Seventh Month.—Length, 35 to 38 cm.; weight, 1000 to 1220 gm. (around 2½ pounds). The infant looks like a dried-up old person, with red, wrinkled skin. The wrinkles fill out with fat and disappear, but in later life or in illness they develop again in the same form and distribution. One can often trace family traits through these wrinkles. The eyes are opened; the testicles sometimes have entered the scrotum. The child cries with a weak whine or grunt, but, since the lungs are not adequately developed, it can seldom be kept alive. Rarely, an infant at seven months of gestation is as far advanced as another at eight months, and can, of course, survive. Those children of the early part of this period which the author has succeeded in raising have in later years not given him much satisfaction, having nearly all become hydrocephalic, dwarfed, or paralytic. From the twenty-seventh to the twenty-eighth week not a few have been saved and are growing promisingly.

Eighth Month.—The child is now 43 cm. long, and weighs around 1600 gm. (3¼ to 4 pounds). The pupillary membrane has disappeared. The skin, though still red, is not so much wrinkled, and the child is less lean. Vernix caseosa and lanugo are still present. The testicles are usually in the scrotum. The bones of the head are soft and flexible; ossification begins in the lower epiphysis of the femur. Meconium is passed with difficulty. Crying is stronger, but sometimes only a whimper. Such children may generally be reared with the aid of maternal milk, good nursing, and a proper incubator (Ahlfeld).

Ninth Month.—Weight, about 2500 gm. (around 5½ pounds); length, 46 to 48 cm. The lanugo begins to disappear from the face and abdomen, the redness fades, the wrinkles smooth out, the panniculus adiposus develops, the limbs become rounded. The nails are at the tips of the fingers. Circulatory, respiratory, and digestive organs are now well developed, though the child requires good care for a successful extra-uterine existence.

Tenth Month.—Weight, 3100 gm. (7 to 7½ pounds); length, 48 to 50 cm. Ahlfeld says the fetus may lose a little after the fortieth week. At the end of this period the child is prepared to cope with the factors of an extra-uterine existence. It is "ripe" or "at full term."

The Fetus at Term.—A fully developed, ripe fetus presents the following signs of maturity: length, 50 cm.; weight, 3400 gm. (7 to 7½ pounds); the skin is white or pink, a fleshy red denoting prematurity; vernix caseosa is thick in the creases and around the shoulders and back; the hair is several centimeters long; the lanugo mostly gone; the finger-nails are firm and protrude beyond the finger-tips and to the tips of the toes; the panniculus adiposus is well developed; the milia and comedones around the nose have usually disappeared; the chest is prominent; the mammary glands project; the navel is at the middle of the belly, and two or three centimeters below the middle of the body (higher in boys than in girls); the testicles are in the scrotum; in girls the labia majora cover the minora; the ear stands out from the head, its cartilage being well developed; the bones of the head are hard, the sutures narrow; the circumference of the head is equal to or less than that of the shoulders (Frank), the height of the head is one-fourth that of the body (Stratz), the voice is loud and strong; sucking movements are vigorous and sustained; meconium is passed early and often.

At autopsy one finds other signs of maturity in the advanced ossification of the bones, e. g., the ossification center in the lower end of the femur is 7 to 8 mm. broad, and the cerebral convolutions resemble those of the adult brain. x-Ray studies of fetuses to determine their age I have found unreliable because the appearance of the various ossification centers is not regular, but Hess and Adair have found that particular roentgenologic study of the upper extremities, the upper spine, and the head give data which are useful. von Winckel found the size of the liver and other organs a guide to the age of the fetus. The size and development of the placenta and cord are unreliable indices of maturity. Vascularity of the decidua at the border of the placenta is usually a sign of prematurity of the ovum, but endometritis must be excluded. Ahlfeld found scratch-marks on the amnion made by the fetus after its nails had grown beyond the finger-tips. This might be useful in medicolegal cases to determine, from the secundines, if the puerpera had delivered a viable infant. Szellö found that the presence of ossification centers in the metatarsal bones is a sign of postmaturity. (See Dr. J. H. Hess's book for an exhaustive consideration of this subject.)

Not any one of all these signs is absolutely reliable. The most certain is the length of the fetus, but even this varies from 48 to 52 cm., while children of 55 to 62 cm. have frequently been delivered. The weight of the fetus is especially uncertain, as a nine months' pregnancy may produce a child of only 1700 gm. ($3\frac{1}{2}$ pounds), while one of eight months may develop an infant of 3840 gm. ($8\frac{1}{2}$ pounds). Hodge (1850) taught that well-matured children are sometimes born before full term, and Parvin mentions a case of an infant weighing 7 pounds delivered after less than two hundred and twenty-six days of gestation.

Some children at term or over term are small and puny because of general debility of the mother or sickness during pregnancy. A prolonged febrile disease, for instance, typhoid, during pregnancy will compromise the growth of the fetus, as also will chronic diseases, diabetes, heart disease, tuberculosis, the various anemias, and syphilis. Bright's disease is particularly unfavorable, since the placenta is frequently infarcted (le placenta albuminurique) and its nutritional function interfered with. On the other hand, there is good reason for believing that the mother can become ill from toxins made by the child or placenta, or perhaps from abnormal fetal endocrinal gland actions. The influence of the endocrinal glands, both maternal and fetal, on the development of the child is now being studied; indeed, the relations of the fetus and host offer a promising field for investigation.

Diseases and abnormal location of the placenta restrict the growth of the child. The children in placenta prævia are usually undersized. Women with generally contracted pelves often have small babies, thus giving evidence of a hereditary tendency to arrest in development. La Torre finds no difference in size in the children from women with contracted pelves and those with normal pelves, but his observations were mainly on rachitic women. Large muscular women have large babies, and the same is true, to an extent, of the father. The head of the child bears a certain relation to that of the father and mother. Fat women usually have large babies. Women of the better classes have larger infants than the needy poor. Workers in factories have small children, and in some European countries pregnant women are not allowed to work in them during the latter months, many being sent to maternities to rest during the period. This restriction has been enforced even in the face of the demands for women's work by the necessities of war. Statistics have shown a distinct improvement in the general health of the mothers and a gain in the weight of their infants since this practice was instituted. Cigarmakers and workers in lead and phosphorus, if abortion and premature labor do not occur, have puny children. White children are larger than colored, American larger than European, boys larger than girls—3 to 5 ounces. Children born in wedlock are heavier than the illegitimate; this may be due to the attempts to produce abortion which many unmarried mothers make, to tight abdominal constriction practised to hide the evidence of pregnancy, and to the lack of nourishment and care they often suffer.

The children increase in size in successive pregnancies, which is due to the better development of the mother which comes with years, the more active circulation in the uterus, and the prolongation of the later pregnancies. The first child is likely to be small or thin, since it often comes a few weeks before term; the uterus is tense and allows little freedom of movement, and the health of women in their first pregnancy is usually not as good as in the subsequent ones. Statistics seem to show that the first children are less strong physically, and more often became tuberculous or insane. The children of later pregnancies, too, are better developed mentally than the first born. Many great men were later children in large families; for instance, Benjamin Franklin was the seventeenth; Napoleon, the eighth; Daniel Webster, the seventh; Wagner, the seventh; Irving, the eleventh; Coleridge, the thirteenth, child of their parents. After the eighth or ninth child a reduction in size is often apparent especially among the poor, due to a decline of the general health. Children from women after a long period of sterility are smaller than usual, and the infants of young girls are generally undersized.

If the child is carried over term, which is not seldom, it overgrows, the head hardens, and the muscles and fat become firmer. (See the chapter on Prolonged Pregnancy.)

The **evidences of life of the fetus in utero** form an interesting study. The fetal heart can be heard; heart and funic murmurs, too; one can feel the pulsation of the heart through the abdominal wall—all of which will be considered fully under the Diagnosis of Pregnancy. The fetus moves its limbs and body from the earliest months, and the movements are audible and palpable from the fifteenth week. Often one sees an extremity move under the abdominal wall, and sometimes the legs kick out with considerable force. These movements may be so active that they disturb the mother's sleep and require treatment, such as a tight abdominal binder and a dose of sodium bromid. The child has periods of sleep, of rest, and of activity. The mother may notice that the fetus stretches itself after a period of quiet. The author has felt the child flex or extend its head, withdraw its hand when the member was touched, and move out of a strained position into one more comfortable. The infant swallows the liquor amnii in large amounts, lanugo and vernix caseosa having been found in the meconium. These swallowing motions have never been diagnosed. The fetus also sucks its fingers in utero. Ahlfeld reports a case where the child's thumb was swollen at birth, and it immediately put the swollen member in its mouth and sucked it. In face presentation the child will suck the examining finger. One of the most interesting phenomena of intra-uterine life is fetal hiccup. Mermann first described it, but Ahlfeld has worked up the subject. The author has very frequently found it, and many intelligent women have remarked and correctly diagnosed the phenomenon. The movements are short, quick jerks of the shoulders and trunk, 15 to 30 a minute, regular, visible, audible, and palpable to the observer. They resemble hiccups perfectly except the absence of stridor. The author has heard them as early as the fifth month of gestation. They may continue fifteen to twenty minutes and become very annoying to the mother, recurring at more or less frequent intervals until delivery. In one case the author heard the sounds distinctly just before the child was born, and within a minute after the child was delivered it was hiccuping so loudly that it was heard in the next room. The contraction of the diaphragm has been felt by the hand in the uterus during the operations of version and extraction, but it was impossible to be sure that the infant was not suffering from asphyxia and was gasping for breath. The latter explanation of such a movement is the first one to be thought of in cases of this nature.

Another phenomenon, not so common, and more uncertain of diagnosis, is the respiratory action of the child in utero. If one carefully observes the umbilical region of a thin woman, pregnant near term, one may discover fine rising and falling movements of the abdominal wall. They occur 60 to 80 a minute, are intermittent, and are most pronounced in the region of the child's chest. Ahlfeld has studied these motions very thoroughly, and is convinced that they are due to minute excursions of the fetal chest, and he has succeeded in getting graphic tracings of them with the cardiograph, showing that when the chest expands, the abdomen contracts. As a support to this theory one may add the daily observations of the newborn child. Inspection of the chest will show, just before the gasp that precedes the first cry, tiny rapid inspirations and expirations. These are best observed on the apneic child delivered by cesarean section. The motion in utero serves to strengthen and prepare the diaphragm and chest muscles for the function of respiration, but it is not strong enough to suck liquor amnii further than the pharynx, whence it probably is swallowed (Schmidt, Lit.). Beclard saw them in animals in 1913.

The Mental State of the Fetus in Utero.—A child shows, very shortly after birth, a few evidences of mental action. It turns its face toward the light; it draws the foot or arm away from an obstructing object. The special senses are all present; even if only a few hours old it makes a wry face when a solution of quinin is placed on the tongue; a loud sound causes it to start; it feels pain, and it sees.

The mental condition of the fetus in utero has been the subject of much speculation. That the child lies in a continuous "dreamless sleep" (Parvin) is not probable. Intelligent mothers have said they could distinguish periods of sleep, of rest, and of activity. The child will assume a more comfortable attitude after it is disturbed by external manipulation with movements that are not all reflex. During labor it will wriggle its head away from the examining finger; it will draw its hand away from one's grasp. As Bailey said, it is probable that a vague and obscure will intervenes in the production of these movements.

Palpation of the fetus increases the rapidity of the heart. (For further information on this subject see Peterson and Rainey, Canestrini, and Pratt et al.)

LITERATURE

Adair: Amer. Jour. Obst. and Gyn., July, 1921, Lit.—*Ahlfeld:* Lehrbuch der Geb., 1903, p. 44.—*Ibid.:* Monatsschr. für Geb. u. Gyn., 1905, p. 144.—*Ibid.:* "Survival of Very Premature Children," Zeitschr. für Geb. u. Gyn., 1919, vol. lxxxi, Heft 2, p. 403.—*Allen, E., Pratt, J. P., Newell, Q. W.:* Amer. Jour. Anatomy, 1930, vol. 46, p. 1.—*Ibid.:* Publ. 414, Contrib. to Emb., Carnegie Institute of Washington, p. 44.—*Barnes:* Principles and Practice of Obstetrics.—*Barry:* "Researches in Embryology," Phil. Trans. Roy. Soc. of London, 1839.—*Beckman and Zimmer:* Zentb. für Gyn., August 15, 1931, p. 2518.—*Bondi:* Zentralbl. f. Gyn., 1903, p. 636.—*Ibid.:* Zent. für Gyn., 1905, p. 1075.—*Bryce, Teacher, and Kerr:* The Early Human Ovum, Glasgow, 1908, Maclehose and Sons.—*Canestrini:* Sinnesleben des Neugeborenen, Springer, Berlin, 1913.—*Cohnstein and Zuntz:* Pflüger's Arch., vol. xxxiv, p. 173.—*Driesch:* Zeitschr. f. wissensch. Zoölogie, vols. liii and lv, quoted by Nagel.—*Fetzer:* "Young Human Ovum," Zentralbl. f. Gyn., 1910, p 1413.—*Gentili:* Annal. di Ost. et Gin., August, 1913.—*Goenner:* Winckel's Handbuch der Geb., vol. i, p. 320.—*Grosser, Halban-Seitz:* Biologie u. Path. des Weibes, 1925, vol. vi, H. T., p. 119. Complete article.—*Heine and Hofbauer:* "Early Human Egg," Zeitschr. f. Geb. u. Gyn., 1911, vol. lxviii.—*Hertwig:* Lehrbuch der Entwickelungsgeschichte, eighth edition, p. 49 et seq.—*Herzog:* "Early Placentation, etc., in Man," Amer. Jour. Anat , July, 1909.—*Hess:* Amer. Jour. of Dis. of Children, December, 1917.—*Hess, J. H.:* Premature Infants, 1922.—*Keiffer:* Gynéc. et Obstét., Paris, July, 1926.—*Keim:* Paris Obstetric Soc., 1901.—*Kirstein:* Zentb. f. Gynæk., February 26, 1927, p. 522.—*La Torre:* Du Development du Fœtus ches les Femmes a Bassin Vicie, Paris, O. Doin, 1887.—*Makepeace et al.:* Surg., Gyn., and Obst., November, 1931, p. 635, Lit.—*Matthews:* "Maturation, etc., in the Echinoderm Egg," Jour. of Morph., 1895.—*Mermann:* Centralbl. f. Gyn., 1880, p. 377.—*Parvin:* Science and Art of Obstetrics, p. 211.— *Peters:* Ueber die Einbettung des menschl. Eies, Vienna, 1899.—*Peterson and Rainey:* Bull. New York Lying-in Hospital, December, 1910.—*Pfannenstiel:* Handbuch d. Geb., 1903, vol. i, p. 218.—*Pratt, Kraushaar and Sun:* Behavior of Newborn Infant, Ohio State Univ. Press, Columbus, 1930.—*Prochownik:* Arch. f. Gyn., vol. xi.—*Runge:* Zentb. für Gynæk., 1927, January 1, p. 49.—*Schmidt:* Zeitschr. für Geb. u. Gyn., 1927, vol. xc, H. 3, p. 559.—*Stratz:* Der Körper des Kindes, 1909, p. 69.—*Streeter:* The Miller Ovum, Carnegie Contributions to Embryology, No. 92.—*Szellö, F.:* Monatsschr. für Geb. u. Gyn., September, 1931, p. 41, Lit.— *Wagner:* Die Herkunft des Fruchtwassers, Vienna, Deuticke, 1913.—*Winckel:* Handbuch der Geb., vol. iii, p. 568.—*Wohlgemuth and Massone:* Arch. f. Gyn. u. Geb., July, 1911, vol. xciv, p. 381.

CHAPTER III

THE PHYSIOLOGY OF THE FETUS

THIS is a new science, and known facts are few, though many hypotheses have been advanced and supported by deduction from the study of the lower animals. The ovum is not a part of its mother, but simply a parasite, possessing all the functions of an organized being.

In the first days after fertilization the ovum probably is nourished by osmosis and imbibition of the fluids surrounding it in the tube. When it reaches the uterus, the trophoblast is already developed, and these cells eat into the uterine mucosa. The immense development of the decidual cells may be to serve as nutriment for the ovum, and the same is gotten and prepared by the trophoblast. The glands of the uterus enlarge enormously, and are filled with secretion, as is shown by Fig. 41. This secretion has fat from degenerated leukocytes, and was called uterine milk by the older writers, and their view that it furnished nourishment to the ovum may not be without foundation, though in the human placenta the villi do not dip into the glands. In earliest fetation the glands around the ovum contain blood. Until the placental circulation is established, the ovum very probably is nourished in the two ways indicated.

The Fetal Blood.—The blood at term has about the same appearance as maternal blood, but has less fibrin and hemoglobin and more salts (Preyer). It contains hemolysin, which has also been proved to pass through the placenta from the mother. Its blood may react, as does its mother's, to the introduction of foreign albuminoids, by the production of antibodies. It has less complement than the mother's blood. The Wassermann reaction is not determinable until the third week.

The nucleated red blood-corpuscles have all disappeared at the ninth month. The red blood-corpuscles are more easily decomposed than the mother's, but show increased resistance to hemolysis by cobra toxin. Boys have more than girls (8 per cent.). The fetus has a relative leukocythemia, and the number of leukocytes in the umbilical vein is greater than in the arteries; wherefore, since the white blood-corpuscles cannot pass over from the mother, one must conclude that they are made in the placenta. (For fetal blood chemistry see v. Oettingen.)

The hemorrhagic and icteric tendencies of the new-born and its weakness against infection show that it has a special blood pathology, but little is actually known about it. Its immunities are not yet developed, and, unless it receives antibodies from the mother via the milk, it succumbs easily to infections.

The Fetal Circulation.—The yolk sac has slight nutritive properties; it acquires a store of nutriment from the mother, and is concerned in blood formation. This is the first, or "vitelline," circulation; it is prominent for the first four weeks, and disappears later (Fig. 81). With the development of the chorionic villi and the umbilical vessels on the body stalk the fetus is provided with a new, rather a more direct, source of nourishment. The capillary system of the umbilical arteries and veins rapidly invades the growing villi, and thus the osmotic connection between the maternal and fetal blood is soon established. Figure 83 shows the vitelline and umbilical circulation existing side by side. The fetal blood now passes from the primitive heart through the primitive aorta, the umbilical arteries, to the capillaries lining the periphery of the ovum, and dipping into the chorionic villi, returning through the umbilical veins to the heart through the ducts of Cuvier. As the liver develops the blood returning from the chorionic area through the umbilical vein, traverses the liver, but soon, since the vessels of the liver cannot accommodate the rapidly growing demands of the developing placental circulation, a by-pass is formed from the umbilical vein through the liver to the inferior vena cava. Thus the returning blood from the now fully differentiated placenta passes, part through the liver with that from the portal vein, and part through the by-pass, the ductus venosus Arantii, into the inferior vena cava. The circulation of the blood

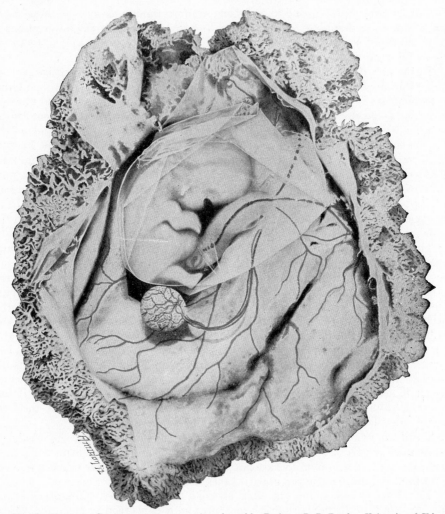

Fig. 81.—The Vitelline Circulation (from a specimen loaned by Professor R. R. Bensley, University of Chicago).

in the fetus before birth is different from that afterward, and at no part of the body is purely arterial blood supplied. This is easily seen in children delivered by cesarean section; they present a dull blue color, almost cyanotic.

The blood, oxygenated and cleansed in the placenta, provided with nutritive substances and water for the fetus, is collected by the branches of the umbilical vein and passes through the single vein of large caliber to the child, entering its body at the navel, then ascending behind the parietal peritoneum to the liver. Here the vein divides, several branches entering the liver directly, others anastomosing with the portal vein, while one large branch goes directly into the vena cava. This is the ductus venosus Arantii. The blood of the vena cava ascendens is, of course, venous, and mingles with that coming from the ductus venosus, both proceeding to the heart, which is entered through the right auricle. Here, already slightly venous, it meets the pure venous blood entering the auricle from the head and upper part of the trunk. In the right auricle a mingling of these bloods occurs, a fact brought out by Pohlman and confirmed by Kellogg in Arey's laboratory at Northwestern. This half arterial blood is now distributed as follows: Part goes through the foramen ovale into the left auricle, thence into the left ventricle and then up through the aorta as usual. Part goes into the right ventricle, whence, during systole, it passes into the trunk of the pulmonary artery, which has three branches, one for each lung and one that opens into the aorta. This by-pass into the aorta is called the ductus arteriosus Botalli, and serves to divert from the functionless lungs the excess of blood that the right ventricle throws out. One-half of the blood takes this shortcut to the aorta. Contrary to our old long-held notion, therefore, the heart distributes throughout the body blood of the same quality. The hypogastric—the former umbilical—arteries, leaving the internal iliacs in the pelvis,

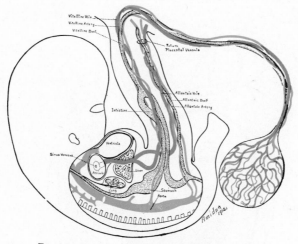

FIG. 82.—DIAGRAM OF THE VITELLINE CIRCULATION.

Embryo, 20 mm. long, seven weeks' growth. Vitelline circulation completed. Umbilical circulation increasing. Atrium dividing. Liver consisting of two equal lobes. Primitive aortæ partly united.

ascend alongside the bladder and urachus to the navel, then, winding spirally around the umbilical vein in the cord, reach the placenta. Here they split up into arterioles and capillaries in the villi. The fetal blood contained in the placenta is constantly undergoing the changes that in the adult occur in the lungs, the liver, the blood-making and other organs of the body. Late in pregnancy the opening of the vena cava inferior moves over to the right of the auricle, and the foramen ovale begins to diminish in caliber; thus the right auricle receives fresh blood, and more blood is forced into the lungs and through the ductus arteriosus into the lower portion of the body. A more equable distribution of nourishment is effected, and greater symmetry of the body results.

After the birth of the child important changes in the blood-currents occur. With the first inspiration the lungs expand. The pulmonary vessels are dilated, and blood rushes into them from the right ventricle. Since the lungs now take all the supply from the pulmonary artery, the by-pass to the aorta, the ductus arteriosus Botalli, collapses and shrinks up. It is solidly obliterated in a few weeks. The aspiration of the right auricle and ventricle draws the blood from the umbilical vein. This and the influence of cold air cause the vein to collapse. Tying the cord shuts off permanently the supply of blood from the vein. Its walls agglutinate, and in a few weeks the vein is obliterated, remaining as a cord-like ligament for the liver—the ligamentum teres. The ductus venosus Arantii also collapses and disappears. The pressure in the right auricle ceasing, that of the left auricle and ventricle increases, which results in the gradual closure of the foramen ovale. This opening sometimes persists for months, or may be the cause of permanent and fatal heart disease. Children with persistent patent foramen ovale are often cyanotic, especially when crying or on exertion, and are called "blue babies"—morbus cæruleus. The hypogastric arteries contract and thrombose, forming the obliterated

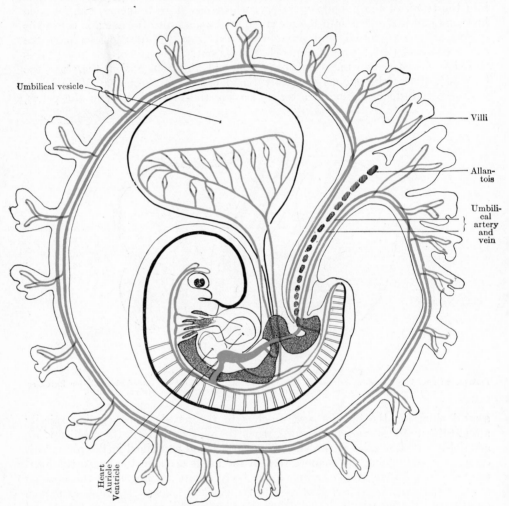

Umbilical vesicle

Villi

Allantois

Umbilical artery and vein

Heart
Auricle
Ventricle

FIG. 83.—SYNCHRONOUS VITELLINE AND CHORIONIC CIRCULATIONS (schematic).

hypogastrics of adult anatomy. This is due to the fact that the left ventricle, unassisted as formerly by the right ventricle via the ductus Botalli, cannot force the blood the long distance through the cord to the placenta. In addition, exposure to cold contracts the umbilical arteries. The pulsation in the cord ceases, and the adult circulation is established. Normally, no clots form in any of the temporary fetal vessels except the hypogastric arteries.

Special Physiology.—The fetus in utero has all the functions of the infant, respiration, digestion, assimilation, metabolism, heat-production and regulation, excretion, etc., but, owing to its particular environment, these are all much modified.

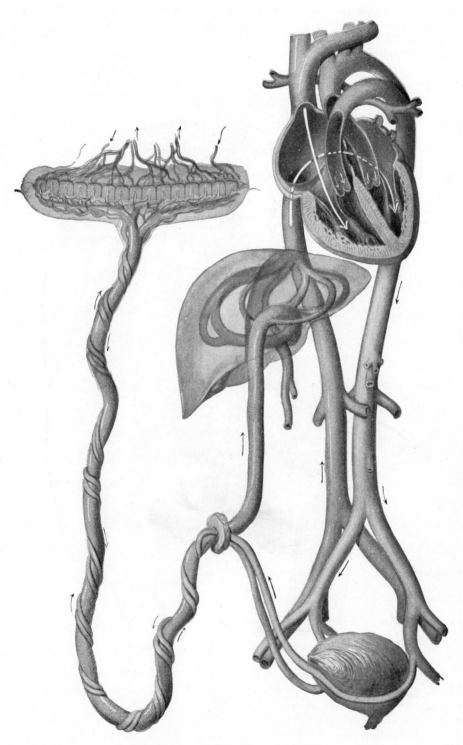

Fig. 84.—Diagram of Fetal Circulation—Diastole.

The placenta does several of the vital functions of the fetus almost entirely. It is the lungs of the child; it performs nearly all its digestion; it assimilates food; it stores up glycogen (Bernard), and it is the general excretory organ. The decidua seems to possess the glycogenic power—Zaretzsky. Its functions should be considered a little more in detail, though we will have to present much that is, at this time, unfinished or only partly proved.

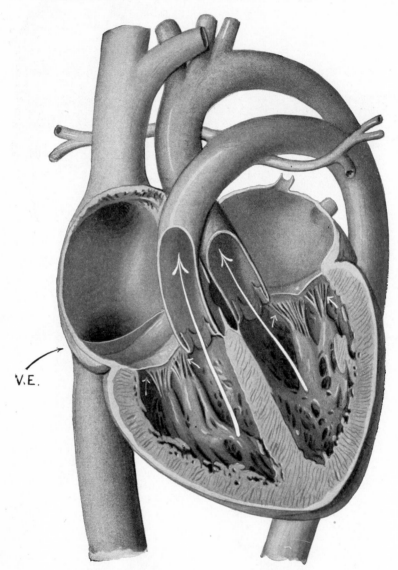

V.E.

FIG. 85.—DIAGRAM OF FETAL CIRCULATION—SYSTOLE.

Respiration.—Zweifel proved that the umbilical vein contains oxygenated blood, and the arteries venous blood. If the placenta becomes detached or the cord compressed, the child dies from asphyxia. These two facts prove that the fetal blood is supplied with oxygen in the placenta. The fetus needs little oxygen, as its combustion processes are slow; it moves little and meets with no resistance; it has no perspiration with evaporation from the skin. It loses no heat. Since this is so, the fetus tolerates withdrawal of its oxygen supply—asphyxia—very well for a time. As pregnancy goes on this toleration is lost. The fetus uses about 1.25 c.c. of O_2 per kilo per minute (Haselhorst). The process by which the fetal blood, carried to the placenta, becomes oxygenated is probably analogous to the process going on in the lungs. It is not by osmosis, because the oxygen is bound to the hemoglobin. The vital oxidizing power of the placental cells, perhaps through the medium of an enzyme, splits off the oxygen and carries it to the fetal red blood-corpuscles. The process is similar to internal or tissue respiration, and perhaps the fat in the villi facilitates the change (Hofbauer). Wolff has shown that in the Langhans cells granules exist which cause oxidative synthesis. Amyl nitrite given the mother quickens the baby's heart within forty seconds.

Digestion.—In many respects the villi of the placenta resemble the intestinal villi. In selective and vital action they exceed the latter in vigor and variety of function. The placenta is a large gland, and it probably assumes the functions which the adult glands later perform. The fetus needs albumin, fat, carbohydrates, water, and salts. Exactly how albumin is carried over from the mother's to the fetus' blood is not known. Albumose, but not peptone, is found in the placenta. Very probably the syncytial cells secrete an albumin-splitting enzyme, the protein going over into a compound of lower type, and the albumin is then re-formed inside the fetal vessels. Fat, according to Hofbauer, is found in the deeper parts of the syncytium and in the vacuolated cells in the form of fine droplets. It comes from the blood of the mother, and in small amounts from the glands of the uterus. In cows and dogs, for example, the connection of the villi with the glands is intimate, and the latter play an important part in fetal nutrition. Physiologists are not sure how fat exists in the blood, nor do they know how it passes over to the fetus. Emulsified fat does not pass the placenta. Probably here again a fat-splitting enzyme (lipase) is in action, fatty acids and glycerin being formed. The analogy between intestinal and placental villi is again strengthened (Guillemet).

Glycogen, demonstrated by Claude Bernard in the placenta in 1859, exists also in the decidua and syncytium (Langhans). How this and other organic compounds reach the fetus is not known. But we do know, thanks to the researches of Bergell, Liepman, and others, that many ferments exist in the placenta and probably the transfer is made in a way analogous to that of the intestinal digestion and absorption. Givens and Howe believe that the nutrient amino-acids and glucose pass to, and the catabolites, urea and uric acid, pass from, the fetus through the placenta by diffusion.

Water is readily absorbed by the villi, differences in the molecular concentration between the two bloods accomplishing the transfer. Of the metals, iron is one of the most important, and the fetus needs a great deal of it. There is no iron in the blood plasma of the mother, therefore the red corpuscles must be used by the trophoblast to provide the necessary amount. Probably the syncytium has a cytotoxic or hemolytic action on the erythrocytes, perhaps dependent on the transformation of the lipoid substances in the covering of the cells (Overton). The red blood-corpuscles are destroyed by the villi and the hemoglobin by complicated and not fully understood biochemical processes, is unmade and reformed in the fetal red blood-corpuscles. Perhaps this destruction of erythrocytes accounts for some of the anemia of women in the early months of pregnancy. Mayer, in 1827, proved that substances in solution in the maternal blood pass on to the fetus through the membrane separating fetal and maternal blood, *e. g.*, salts, potassium iodid, salicylic acid, atropin, etc., and in amount as they are dialyzable. We know that morphin, methylene-blue, the salts of mercury, lead, and arsenic pass over to the fetus. Gases pass over, as chloroform, ether, and carbon dioxid; therefore the danger of giving too much chloroform. Nicloux collected the literature on this subject up to 1909. Pregnant women should avoid large gatherings, or where large coal-stoves are used, as the carbon monoxid may injure the fetus.

As another source of nourishment mention must be made of the liquor amnii. It contains a slight amount of albumin, and the fetus drinks it in large quantities. This is proved by finding lanugo in the meconium, and the infant vomiting the liquor amnii after birth. The stomach of the fetus contains pepsin, and the intestines a tryptic enzyme; therefore the function of digestion could be carried on. Water is probably supplied the fetus in this manner. Until the second month the fetus is almost all water, has less solids even than milk. At the end of pregnancy the fetus is 74 per cent. water. The liver is active, demonstrated by its preponderating bulk and the presence of bile in the meconium. The meconium is a tarry, greenish-black substance, found in the colon of the fetus in considerable quantity even before the seventh month. It accumulates in the colon and, therefore, peristalsis must occur in the intestines. This has also been demonstrated experimentally. The meconium becomes thicker in the latter weeks, since the intestine is absorptive. It is composed of secretions of the intestinal canal,

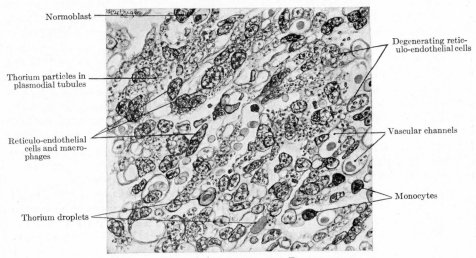

Fig. 85a.—Rabbit Placenta with Thorium.
Colloidal thorium (thorotrast) picked up by cells of rabbit placenta indicating a selective and protective function. (Department of Obstetrics and Gynecology, University of Chicago.)

the solid particles swallowed with the liquor amnii; lanugo, epithelium, vernix caseosa, and bile, and, chemically, cholesterin, bilirubin, fat, and mucin.

The placenta has protective and selective functions as recent tests with thorium show (Fig. 85a). Bacteria may pass the placental barrier (see page 526), and toxins, antitoxins, and immune bodies also, although proof is difficult. The fetus itself also makes small amounts of antitoxins, agglutinins, bacteriolysins, etc.

The Kidneys.—These are active from the early months, as Nagel has shown. Ahlfeld denies that the liquor amnii contains urine. He says the excrementitious matters which the kidney usually excretes are taken away through the placenta. Still, urea has been found in the liquor amnii; the bladder has been found distended, even so as to be a hindrance to labor; the kidneys are there, and, by analogy with other organs, must work. Urine is often found in the bladder of newborn children. They sometimes urinate freely during delivery. Probably the action of the kidneys before birth is not constant or considerable—rather, exceptional.

The child has its own general metabolism—internal respiration, anabolism, catabolism, heat production all go on as in the adult, but in varying degrees. The tissue changes are very active, since growth is so rapid, but the child needs to produce very little heat, being so well protected. Its temperature is one-half to three-fourths of a degree higher than that of the mother. The products of the fetal metabolism are carried to the placenta. Glands with internal secretion probably functionate.

Less is known of the excretory functions of the placenta, but such a function surely exists, since the fetus has very little other outlet for its waste matters. Some waste may accumulate as meconium in the intestinal canal, and a little more may be passed as urine or perspiration. That the mother can absorb materials from the child is proved by the injection of a salt, as iodid of potassium, into the child, and its demonstration in the saliva of the mother. That substances will pass from fetus to mother was suggested by Harvey and McGillivray and proved by Savory in 1858. Carbon dioxid passes from the fetus and is excreted by the mother.

The amount of actual waste furnished by the child cannot be large, because its nourishment is provided in a condition ready for immediate assimilation and conversion into living protoplasm.

The mother must, at whatever cost to herself, supply the building materials for the vitally active fetal growth, and since the fetus requires about 101 gm. of nitrogen, 32 of calcium, 18 of phosphorus, besides other important elements one need feel no astonishment if a weak, imperfect woman proves unequal to the task.

Relations of Fetus to Mother.—The symbiologic relations between the mother and fetus deserve intensive study. We know that a child may sicken, through the mother, of course, but independently, e. g., from bacteria normally present in her tonsils, carried via the blood to the placenta. Toxins absorbed from a diseased ovum may sicken the mother. See Adair.

The father may procreate a child which is symbiologically incompatible with its host, the mother. Congenital disease of the fetus, abnormalities of its endocrinal glands, improper chemism in the placenta may be due to paternal influences. The by-products of these perverted chemical changes may be destructive to the fetus, and, when absorbed, also to the mother. Clinically the author has reason for believing that hemorrhagic diathesis, hyperthyroidism, pregnancy nephrosis, "apoplexie uteroplacentaire," hyperemesis, and many other disturbances of pregnancy are due to incompatibility of the fetus with its mother. The author has not proved these theories experimentally. They are presented here in the hope they will stimulate some reader to adopt them as research problems. The child may belong to a blood-group differing from its mother.

The Determination of Sex.—It is felt that there must be a natural law governing the production of males and females, because the proportion between the two in live births in nearly all countries is as 105 or 106 is to 100. What this law is no one knows, but we have many theories, a review of which may be found in the literature indicated below (Cohn, Dawson, Lahms, Morgan, Rauber). The ratio of males to females in stillbirths is very high, at four months 357 to 100, at seven months 116 to 100, at nine months 137 to 100, and the high death rate during labor makes the proportion 150 to 100 (Greulich). Nature is prodigal with males.

Sex may be determined—(1) In the ovum itself (progamy); (2) at the time of fertilization by the spermatozoid (syngamy); (3) by the influence of external factors during the first formative period of the embryo (epigamy). All the theories proposed may be grouped under these headings.

Chromatic particles in the chromosomes of the germ cells are assumed to bear the hereditary qualities. During the course of development these particles are probably distributed to the various cells in a definite way, as are the chromosomes, by the process of mitosis. At maturation not only is the number of chromosomes halved (see p. 6), but it is assumed also that the number of hereditary qualities is reduced by half; in this manner a doubling of the number of hereditary qualities at the time of fertilization is prevented. The assumption that the chromosomes are the carriers of hereditary tendencies and determine sex is borne out by the observations of cytologists on the germ cells of invertebrates, especially insects, and of some vertebrates. According to Winiwarter after maturation all human ova possess 24 chromosomes, while half of the spermatozoids contain 24 chromosomes, the other half 23. There is thus one extra chromosome in each mature ovum and in each of half the spermatozoids. This chromosome, because of peculiarities of size or shape, can be identified easily in many animals, and is termed the *accessory chromosome*. McClung was the first to assume that the accessory chromosome is a sex determinant. It has since been shown by Wilson, Davis, and others that the accessory chromosome carries the female sexual characters. When, in the case under consideration, a spermatozoid with 24 chromosomes fertilizes an ovum, the resulting embryo is a female, its somatic nuclei containing 48 chromosomes. An ovum fertilized by a sperm cell containing only 23 chromosomes (without the accessory chromosome) produces a male with somatic nuclei containing only 47 chromosomes. (See monographs, Painter; Evans and Swezy.)

It seems pretty well settled that the male has the determining influence in the sex of the child—a fact that will bring practical solace to many wives, unable to present their husbands with sons.

J. Loeb, from a study of parthenogenetic frogs, concludes that all the ova are males, but that the spermatozoids are of two kinds, with and without a sex chromosome. If a spermatozoid with the chromosome fertilizes the egg, a female results. All his parthenogenetic frogs were males.

Regarding the influence of environment scientists differ. Ploss and Waldeyer claimed that in the lower forms of life, as melons, cucumbers, favorable conditions produce females, and Fürst claims that the larvæ of bees, when the nourishment is insufficient, result in hermaphrodites. On the other hand, Pflüger, Schultze, and Heapes (quoted by Ahlfeld, *loc. cit.*) have been unable to modify the sex of frogs, mice, and rabbits by altering their environment, but Trottet, by injecting epinephrin into rabbits during the first fifteen days of gestation, has produced a decided surplus of males.

Many conditions have been assumed as causative of sex distinction, and attempts have been made to influence nature, based on these, usually false, assumptions. Hippocrates and Galen believed that boys come from the right ovary, girls from the left, and Henke, in 1786, advised coition on the corresponding side when a child of that sex was desired. Hofacker and Sadler believed that the father, if older, would produce more males, while Janke claimed the weaker party of the sexual act produced his opposite, both theories are still to be proved (Alich).

Siegel utilized the unusual conditions of the Great War to determine the time of conception and the incidence of sex. He found that if the husband returned on his short furlough right after the wife's menstrual period the majority of the children were boys; if in the ten days before the period, more girls resulted. One of his tables of 115 cases shows of 56 conceptions occurring from the first day of the period to the ninth day, 48 boys and 8 girls; from the tenth to the fourteenth day, 10 boys and 14 girls; from the fifteenth to the twenty-third day, 5 boys and 26 girls; from the twenty-fourth to the twenty-sixth, no conceptions; from the twenty-seventh to the onset of the next menses, 4 boys and no girls. Siegel concludes the overripe ovum (two days before to nine days after the beginning of the flow) shows 86 per cent. boys; the young ovum (from the fifteenth day after the onset of the menses to the twenty-third day) shows 84 per cent. girls.

Düsing, from the study of 10,500,000 births, finds more boys are conceived in winter than in summer, and Ploss found that women in high altitudes give birth to more sons than those on the plains.

Nature still holds the secret of sex production, and it is a question if it is desirable, even if it were possible, for man to interfere in the matter.

Literature

Adair, F. L.: Jour. Amer. Med. Assoc., August 6, 1932.—*Alich:* Edit. Jour. Amer Med. Assoc., May 12, 1923, p. 1382.—*Bernard:* Ribemont, Dessaignes et Le Page, 1873, p. 103.—*Cohn:* Die willkürliche Bestimmung des Geschlechts, Würzburg, 1898.—*Dawson:* Causation of Sex, 1909.—*Driessen:* Arch. f. Gyn., 1907, 82, 279.— *Evans and Swezy:* Memoirs Univ. of Calif., 1929, vol. 1.—*Foster and Balfour:* Embryology, 1875.—*Givens and Howe:* Amer. Jour. Dis. of Children, January, 1923, p. 63.—*Greulich, W. W.:* Science, July 10, 1931, p. 53, Lit.—*Guillemet:* Passage de la Graisse a travers de la Placenta, Chantreau, Nantes, 1920, Lit.—*Guyer:* Journal of Morph., 1912, p. 52.—*Hartman and Ball:* Proc. Soc. Exp. Biology in Med., 1930, vol. 28.—*Haselhorst and Stromberger:* Zeitschr. für Geb. u. Gyn., 1932, Band 102, H. 1, p. 16.—*Hofbauer:* Biologie der menschl. Plazenta, Vienna, 1905.—*Lahms:* Zentb. für die Ges. Gyn., December 24, 1913.—*v. Lenhossek:* Das Problem der Geschlechts-Bestimmenden Ursachen, Jena, 1903.—*Liepman:* Zeitschr. f. Geb. u. Gyn., 1905.—*Loeb, J.:* Proceedings Nat'l Acad. Sci., 1916, ii, p. 313.—*Meyer and Overton:* Vierteljahresschr. der Naturforsherges. in Zürich, 1899.—*Morgan:* Heredity and Sex, 1913. Full literature on Causation of Sex.—*Nicloux:* L'Obstetrique, November, 1909, p. 840.—*v. Oettingen:* Arch. für Gynæk., 1926, Band 129, H. 1.—*Painter:* Jour. Exper. Zool., vol. 37, 1923.—*Preyer:* Specielle Phys. der Embryo, Leipzig, 1885. Complete literature.—*Rauber:* Der Überschuss von Knabengeburten und seine biologische Bedeutung, Leipzig, 1900.—*Riddle:* Bulletin Amer. Academy of Med., October, 1914.—*Savory:* Quoted by Strachan, Jour. Obstet. and Gyn., British Empire, 1925, vol. xxxii, No. 1, p. 89. Complete Review with Lit. of our Knowledge of Physiology of Placenta.—*Siegel:* Deutsche med. Woch., 1916, xlii, S. 1179.—*Stevens:* Publications of the Carnegie Institute, 1906.—*Strassman:* "Das Leben vor der Geburt," Volkmann's klin. Vort., N. F., No. 533.—*Trottet:* Jour. Amer. Med. Assoc., June, 1926, p. 1849.—*Wilson:* "Studies on Chromosomes," Jour. Exper. Zoölogy, 1906, vol. iii.—*Winiwater:* Arch. de Biol., T. xxvii.-*Wolff:* Monatsschrift für Geb. u. Gyn., February, 1913.—*Zaretsky:* L'Obstetrique, May, 1911. Gives full literature.

CHAPTER IV

CHANGES DUE TO PREGNANCY

LOCAL CHANGES

The rapidly growing ovum makes many demands on the maternal organism. It requires a great deal of room for its development, and a free blood-supply for its nourishment; then, too, the parturient canal must be prepared, and the means provided for the expulsion of the completed child. These are the local requirements: there are, in addition, demands on the organs of general metabolism—the liver, the kidneys, the ductless glands, the nervous system, etc., and, unless the proper balance is maintained, either mother or child or both will suffer. To meet these requirements of the growing fetus the whole body of the mother undergoes certain changes, which for the purpose of study are divided into local and general.

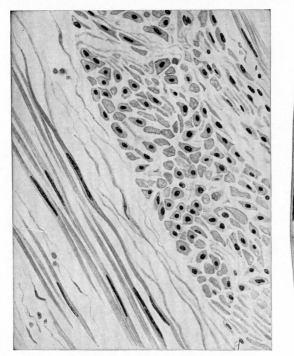

FIG. 86.—MUSCLE OF NON-PREGNANT UTERUS.

Local Changes.—Naturally the uterus is most markedly altered. The normal uterus of a nulligravida is a pear-shaped organ, 6½ cm. long, 2½ cm. thick, and 4 cm. wide, weighing 42 gm. In multiparæ the uterus is 7½ cm. long, 5 cm. wide, and 3 cm. thick, weighing 65 gm. It is made up of hard, unstriped muscle, covered in part by the peritoneum, moored to the pelvis by eight so-called ligaments, and attached to the pelvic floor by means of the vagina.

During the first half of pregnancy the uterus enlarges as the result of a hyperplasia of its muscular substance. This is a true eccentric growth, is much more rapid than is sufficient to accommodate the growing ovum, and is not due entirely to expansion by the growing ovum, as similar changes occur in the uterus with ectopic gestation.

There are hypertrophy and also hyperplasia of the cells. The wall of the uterus, which was 8 mm. before pregnancy, grows to be 25 mm. thick by the fourth month. After this, the decidua capsularis comes to lie on and fuse with the

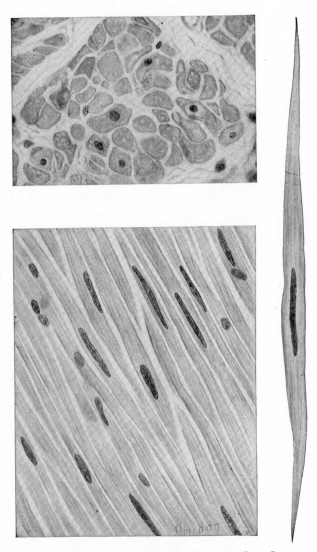

FIG. 87.—MUSCLE OF PREGNANT UTERUS. CROSS- AND LONG SECTIONS.
Removed at time of a cesarean section.

decidua vera, and the development of the uterus is co-equal with that of the ovum. At no time in pregnancy does the ovum actively distend the uterus. In cases of twins and polyhydramnion there may be pathologic distention of the uterus. At the end of pregnancy the uterine wall varies from 4 to 7 mm. in thickness, and it is remarkable what muscular power this thin-walled organ may develop. The muscle-fiber of the non-pregnant uterus is spindle shaped, and about 50μ

long. That of the full-term pregnant uterus is enormously enlarged (200 to 600μ) and presents fine longitudinal fibrillations (Figs. 86 and 87). The muscle-fibers of the cervix also undergo hypertrophy, but not as much as those of the fundus. Rarely cross-striated muscle-fibers have been found in the uterus, a phenomenon that may indicate metaplasia.

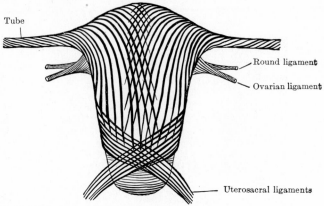

FIG. 88.—SCHEMA OF THE OUTER LAYER OF UTERINE MUSCLE-FIBERS.

The fibro-elastic tissue of the uterus is of great importance in view of the functions of the organ and its resistance to distention and the stress of labor. Dührssen and others have shown that the fundus is less rich in elastic tissue than the cervix, that the fibers are most numerous in the outer layers of the uterus and around the vessels, from which they probably arise.

The uterine connective tissue becomes augmented, softer, and slightly fibrillated, permitting free motion between the muscle-bundles and layers. How much hyperplasia exists is under question.

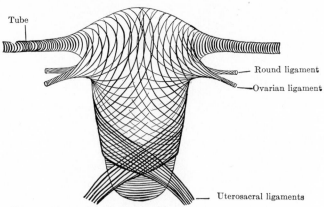

FIG. 89.—SCHEMA OF THE INNER LAYER OF UTERINE FIBERS.

The arrangement of the muscle-fibers has been the object of an immense amount of study, and it is not yet fully understood. Bayer gives a full history of the subject, and his description, with those of Helie and Chenantais, will be followed. In general three layers may be distinguished: an outer thin, an inner, also thin, and the middle, very thick and vascular. These layers are distinguishable only during pregnancy. At cesarean sections one observes them, and it is possible to unite them individually by suture. Since the uterus is the result of the fusion of the two Müllerian ducts, we would expect the tubes to play a rôle in the distribution of the

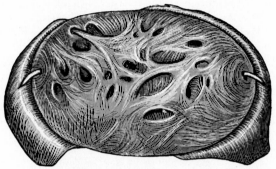

FIG. 90.—DISSECTION OF UTERINE MUSCLE. FUNDUS (from Helie and Chenantais).

uterine muscular fibers, and this is borne out by various dissections. The uterine ligaments also determine the direction of the muscular bundles (Ivanoff).

The outer layer of the uterus covers the fundus down to the point where the

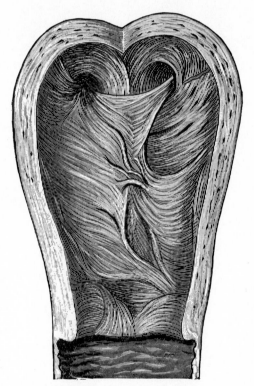

FIG. 91.—DISSECTION OF UTERINE MUSCLE. INNER LAYER (from Helie and Chenantais).

peritoneum is loosely attached, and is composed of the longitudinal fibers of the tubes (Fig. 88). It is hood-like, but does not cover the sides of the uterus, where the blood-vessels enter. The fibers are more or less longitudinal, and interlace in the middle, some crossing to the opposite side. The inner layer of the longitudinal fibers of the tube is continued under the endometrium, and forms the looped bundles of muscle around the tubal ostia and around the internal os. It also shows a thickening on both the anterior and posterior wall of the uterus and fibers run across the fundus to connect the two. Around the tubal ostia and the internal os there are also irregularly circular thickenings. The internal layer is more closely adherent to the middle portion than is the outer layer. The powerful middle layer is composed of the circular fibers of the tube and the radiating fibers from the sacro-uterine ligaments, the round and the ovarian ligaments (Fig. 89). These ligaments, during the development of the uterus in pregnancy, exert a marked effect on the direction of its growth, and during labor have a decided influence in

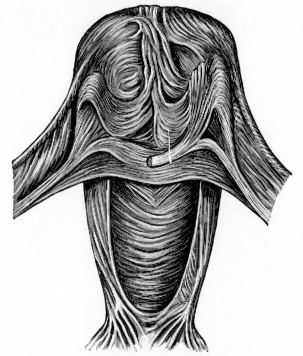

FIG. 92.—MIDDLE LAYER OF UTERINE FIBERS (from Helie and Chenantais).

the mechanism of the process. Many fibers run obliquely through the wall of the uterus binding all the layers firmly together, and they enable the uterine wall to be thickly felted together under the influence of the contractions.

As a result of the crossing and recrossing of the various muscular lamellæ and bundles, a most complicated network results, and through this network the blood-vessels of the uterus pursue their course. It is easily seen that when the muscle contracts, these vessels will be twisted, bent, and closed. This is what normally occurs in the third stage of labor after the child is expelled. The lamellar structure of the uterus is necessary to permit the distention of the uterus and its accommodation to the growing ovum.

The muscle-fibers of the cervix pursue simpler courses. At the isthmus the circular layers are prominent, especially at the insertion of the retractor fibers in the rear, i. e., the uterosacral ligaments. The plicæ palmatæ are made up of longitudinal fibers. Externally the cervix shows a layer of longitudinal and oblique fibers which spread out into the bladder through the vesico-uterine ligaments and into the bases of the broad ligaments. The portio vaginalis presents an inner, submucous, circular layer, derived from the vagina, an outer, longitudinal, from the same, and a middle layer, vascular and not pronounced, from the similar layer of the fundus compounded with the ligaments entering the cervix.

The cervix even at birth shows a tendency to the formation of two lips, an anterior and a posterior, the musculature at the sides being thinner. A virgin uterus may sometimes have what appears to be a bilateral laceration. During pregnancy the shallow lateral grooves are palpable, and during labor tears of the cervix usually occur at these places of less strength.

The **blood-supply of the uterus** must be very liberal to render possible the immense changes in the organ. The vessels undergo hypertrophy and probably

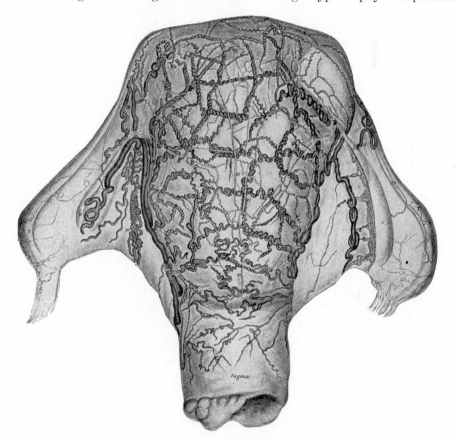

FIG. 93.—INJECTED ARTERIES OF PUERPERAL UTERUS (Nagel).

hyperplasia also. The arterial supply of the uterus is derived mainly from the uterine, a branch of the hypogastric, the ovarian or spermatic, a branch of the aorta, and the funicular, a branch of the vesical, which passes up the round ligament and joins the ovarian at the fundus uteri. The uterine artery, arriving at the side of the uterus at the level of the cervix, gives off several large branches which go down on the vagina (arteriæ cervicovaginales), the main trunk ascending in the broad ligament close at the side of the uterus. At the level of the internal os it begins to give off branches which cross through the substance of the uterus, to anastomose with those of the other side. The trunk, which is sometimes called the puerperal artery, rises, giving off branches all the way, and unites with the spermatic or ovarian artery. These vessels are wonderfully twisted, even to the smallest branches, and their anastomoses are frequent and full (Fig. 93). (See also Redlich for literature.)

The veins are much more developed than the arteries (Fig. 93a), and in general follow their course. They penetrate all the layers of the uterus, especially the middle, anastomose very freely, and empty into the plexuses at the sides of the uterus in the ovarian and broad ligaments. The former empties into the renal vein or the cava, the latter into the hypogastric vein, and thence into the internal iliac. The uterine veins have no valves.

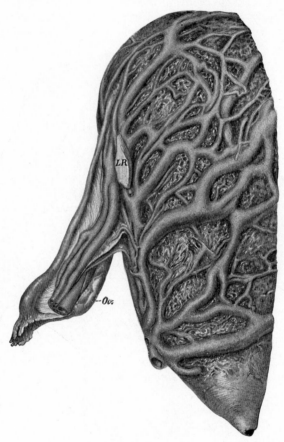

Fig. 93a.—Uterine Veins. Right Anterior Surface of Uterus, Seventh Month (adapted from A. Couvelaire). *LR*, Round ligament.

Microscopically, both arteries and veins, particularly the veins, undergo interesting changes in the uterine wall. They lose their outer coats, and come to lie on the muscle-bundles, with only an intima or with very little tunica media, really forming large blood-spaces called sinuses. The uterus thus seems to form part of the vascular system, and, as a matter of fact, it follows vasomotor impulses, for instance, the action of ergot and pituitrin and of nervous shocks.

The **lymphatics of the uterus** enlarge and multiply during pregnancy, so that the full-term organ is well honeycombed by them. They begin as large spaces under the endometrium and under the serosa, following the course of the muscle-bundles and blood-vessels; they anastomose freely under the serosa, communicating by stomata with the peritoneal cavity, and empty into the vessels of the broad ligament. The lymphatics of the corpus uteri empty into the lumbar glands; those of the cervix into the pelvic glands; those which accompany the round ligament into the upper set of deep inguinal glands; those of the lower vagina and vulva go to the deep and superficial inguinal glands, and through these to the glands around the external iliac arteries. The large size and great number of the

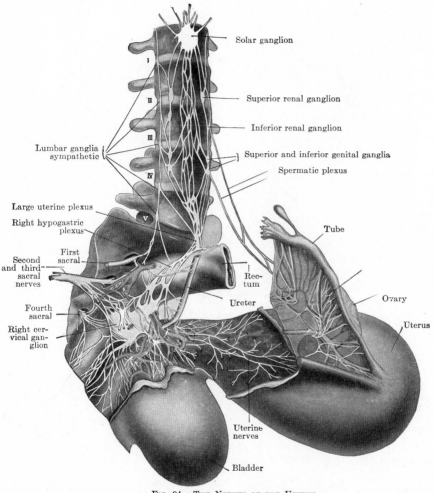

Solar ganglion

Superior renal ganglion

Inferior renal ganglion

Superior and inferior genital ganglia

Spermatic plexus

Lumbar ganglia sympathetic

Large uterine plexus

Right hypogastric plexus

Tube

First sacral

Second and third sacral nerves

Rec-tum

Fourth sacral

Ureter

Ovary

Right cervical ganglion

Uterus

Uterine nerves

Bladder

FIG. 94.—THE NERVES OF THE UTERUS.
Combined from Frankenhäuser and Bumm.

lymphatics in and around the uterus must be noted, also the distribution of the various streams of lymph, as this is important in the consideration of puerperal fever.

The **nervous supply of the uterus** is very rich, and comes from both sympathetic and cerebrospinal systems. Motor fibers are derived from the sympathetic, passing down from the aortic plexus; they are reinforced by fibers from the solar, renal, and genital ganglia, forming a large plexus above the promontory of the sacrum, near the bifurcation of the aorta, and called the great uterine plexus. From here the fibers pass on either side of the rectum through the hypogastric plexuses to the sides of the uterus, but mainly to the great cervical ganglion and thus into the uterus. Cerebrospinal fibers coming from the pneumogastric, phrenic, and splanchnic nerves follow the same course. Their function is unknown. The close nervous connection between the uterus and the stomach and heart may explain the reflex phenomena intercurrent between these organs. Sensory fibers come from the spinal cord through the sacral nerves, being also distributed via the great cervical

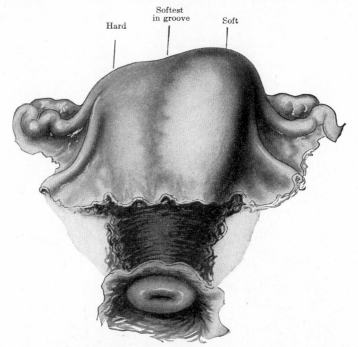

FIG. 95.—UTERUS AT EIGHT WEEKS.
Note enlargement of one half.

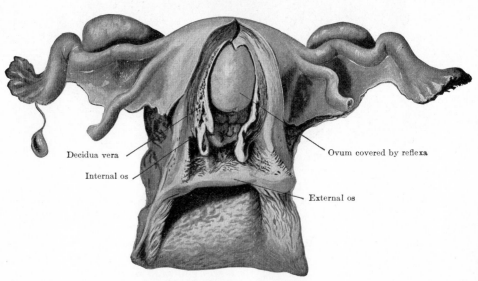

FIG. 96.—UTERUS AT FIVE WEEKS.
From Professor Jaggard's collection.

ganglion. That the sensory fibers come from the spinal cord in this way is shown by the clinical observation of painless labors in paraplegic women, and rendering the labor painless by the injection of procain into the spinal canal. The region supplied by the cauda is made anesthetic. The great cervical ganglion (Frankenhäuser) is a triangular mass of ganglion-cells and nerve-fibers lying at the side of the cervix and upper vagina, ½ inch wide and ¾ inch long. During pregnancy it grows to be 2 inches long and 1½ inches wide. Another ganglion exists on the posterior wall of the cervix.

The nerve-centers are less well known. Probably none exist (Ottow). There are independent nerve-centers in the uterus, because the organ acts even when removed from the body and perhaps there are nervous and muscular bundles similar to those in the heart. Cases of paraplegia are on record where labor was normal or even precipitate (Elkin). I delivered a paraplegic with forceps after the head was visible because of failure of the abdominal muscles to contract. This local center is supposed to be the great cervical ganglion, but there exist ganglionic

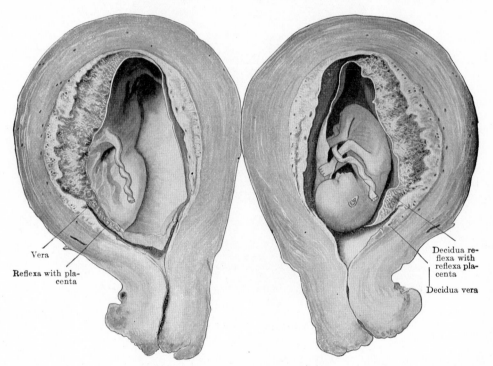

Vera

Reflexa with placenta

Decidua reflexa with reflexa placenta

Decidua vera

Fig. 97.—Uterus at Twelve Weeks.
Northwestern University Medical School Museum.

cells in the uterine muscle, and they form occasional small plexuses around the blood-vessels (Bar).

Changes in the Shape of the Uterus.—Within two weeks after conception the shape of the uterus begins to change. This is first appreciable in the anteroposterior diameter of the corpus. The ovum softens and distends that part of the uterus in which it is situated. As this is usually the anterior wall, we find a bulging here on one or the other side of the median line, making the affected side larger, thicker, and softer, while the other is smaller, thinner, and harder, there being a groove between (Fig. 95). These findings are useful in the diagnosis of pregnancy. The cervix softens, especially the supravaginal portion, its acquired compressibility giving Hegar's sign of pregnancy. The junction of the tubes with the uterus also softens. These conditions are brought about especially by imbibition of the uterine wall and the movability of the outer lamella of the uterine muscle on the middle

6

coat. After the second month one finds the uterus enlarged laterally, and in the third month the fundus has assumed nearly a spheric form. The consistence of the uterus at this time is spongy, elastic, and soft, like bread dough, and one often notices the organ harden under the examining hand—that is, it contracts.

After the fifth month the uterus enlarges in the direction of the fundus, the spheric form becoming ovoid or elliptic. The location of the tubal insertion and of the round ligaments shows this change, at the fifth month being near the vault of

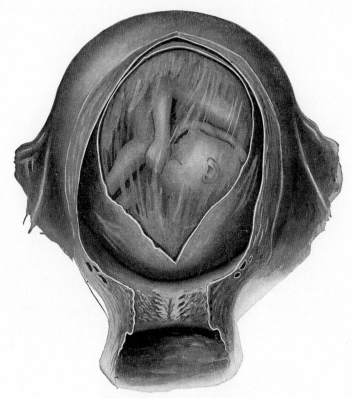

Fig. 98.—Uterus About Six Months.

the uterus, at the ninth month being 4 to 6 inches lower. During the last weeks of pregnancy the lower part of the uterus is developed to accommodate one pole of the infant, the so-called lower uterine segment being formed. This completes the ovoid or elliptic formation of the uterus (Figs. 98–102).

The virgin uterus is shaped like a flattened pear, and has a capacity of 2 c.c. or less; the full-term uterus resembles an immense gourd, and has a capacity of 4000 to 5000 c.c.

The configuration of the uterus is affected by the organs in the belly, the position and attitude of the fetus, the amount of liquor amnii, the location of the placenta, the attitude of the mother, uterine neoplasms, adhesions, etc. The spinal column presses into the uterus from behind; the intestines leave facets on its walls. Since the anterior wall is supported solely by the abdominal muscles, it bulges forward convexly. The fetus kicks out the non-resistant muscle, as may be observed during any abdominal examination. In shoulder presentation the uterine ovoid is transverse. A large quantity of liquor amnii makes the uterus spheric and tense.

The placenta develops that part of the uterus to which it is attached, and, from the location and course of the round ligaments, we make deductions as to the seat of the placenta (Palm). If the round ligaments run on the anterior surface of the uterus, the placenta is located on the posterior wall; if they are far to the side, the placenta is located anteriorly (Figs. 102 and 103).

We find, at term, uteri of various shapes—ovoid and elliptic, cordate and asymmetric (Figs. 104, 105, 106, 107, 108). Occasionally the fundus presents a shallow groove (Fig. 106), the uterus having an indication of horns—uterus arcuatus.

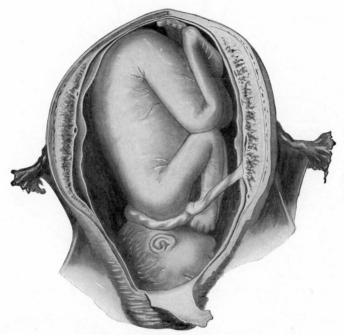

FIG. 99.—UTERUS NEAR TERM. Note primary brow presentation.

Sometimes one horn is developed more than the other (Fig. 107). The uterus at term, in 80 per cent. of cases, is deviated to the right side of the abdomen, and it is also twisted on itself from left to right. This dextroversion and torsion, which are also found in the virgin state, are due to the mode of formation of the uterus from the Müllerian ducts—in the embryo the left duct lies anterior to the right; second, the location of the mesenteric attachment of the sigmoid on the left side of the spinal column; third, congenital asymmetry of growth, which is noticeable even in vegetable life—for instance, trees and shrubs; fourth, the full rectum; fifth, the general habit of lying on the right side—the uterus falling over from the left. This dextroversion of the uterus is of considerable clinical importance. In abdominal examinations the left tube and ovary may be felt nearer the middle line, and the round ligament also is more prominent on the left side. During the operation of cesarean section it is necessary to bring the uterus to the middle line before making the incision for the delivery of the child.

For the first two months of pregnancy the uterus is below the pelvic brim. As it enlarges it becomes anteverted and anteflexed and lies on the bladder. The fundus is readily felt through the anterior fornix. The cervix is directed forward (Fig. 110). As the pregnancy develops the uterus rises up in the abdomen, coming to lie against its anterior wall. In primiparæ the uterus is molded against the spinal column more than in multiparæ, because in the latter the abdominal muscles are usually not so

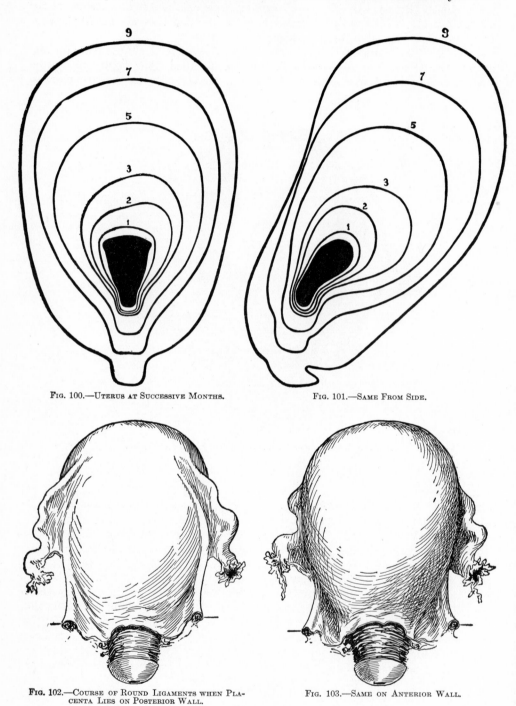

FIG. 100.—UTERUS AT SUCCESSIVE MONTHS.

FIG. 101.—SAME FROM SIDE.

FIG. 102.—COURSE OF ROUND LIGAMENTS WHEN PLA-CENTA LIES ON POSTERIOR WALL.

FIG. 103.—SAME ON ANTERIOR WALL.

The sign is usually but not invariably reliable.

strong and rigid. The intestines are forced upward and usually to the left. No intestine is normally found between the uterus and the abdominal wall. A hernia is sometimes emptied of gut during pregnancy. The cecum and appendix are forced upward and outward, but the colon is not displaced much. The fundus uteri at term is about the level of the second lumbar vertebra. It exerts no direct pressure on the kidneys, ureters, liver, or stomach, and is, therefore, not answer-

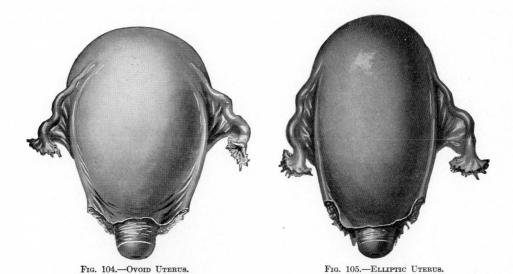

FIG. 104.—OVOID UTERUS.   FIG. 105.—ELLIPTIC UTERUS.

able for certain troubles of these organs ascribed to it, as nephritis, icterus, inter-costal neuralgia, hyperemesis, pyelitis.

The **bladder** during early pregnancy is a pelvic organ. In the last month, *pari passu* with the development of the lower uterine segment, the bladder is often

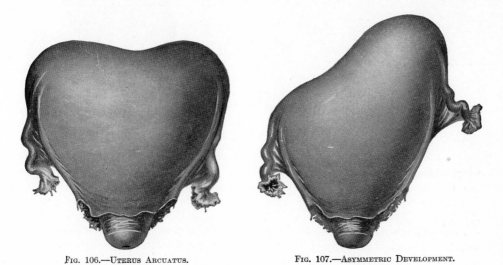

FIG. 106.—UTERUS ARCUATUS.   FIG. 107.—ASYMMETRIC DEVELOPMENT.

drawn up from behind the pubis into the abdomen, generally to the right. During labor the uterus draws away from the bladder, but the latter, when filled, may reach above the navel. The urethra is stretched only when the bladder is overfilled, or during labor when it is out of the true pelvis. Often the bladder is saddle shaped, extending on each side of the pelvis. It may also be asymmetric, and then the larger part is oftenest on the right.

The axis of the uterus varies in its relation to that of the axis of the pelvic inlet. In primiparæ, standing, the two axes sometimes correspond (Fig. 111). In multiparæ the lax abdominal wall allows the uterus to fall forward. If the recti abdominis are widely separated, the fundus falls between them, resulting in "pendulous abdomen," or "rupture," as the women term it (Fig. 113). When the woman lies in the horizontal position, the uterine axis sinks behind that of the inlet (Fig. 112).

Conclusions as to the duration of pregnancy based on the height of the fundus above the pubis must be carefully qualified. The author has found Bartholomew's "rule of fourths" to be nearer the normal than the old rule of thirds. If the fundus is one-quarter the way to the navel, the pregnancy is of two months; one-half the

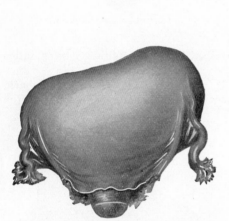

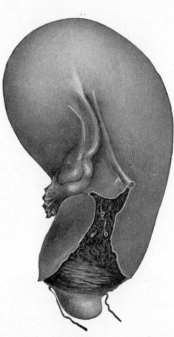

Fig. 108.—Uterus with Transverse Presentation of Fetus.

Fig. 109.—Ovoid Uterus from Side.
Shows flexion over spinal column.

way, of three months; three-fourths, at four months; at the navel at five months, and it rises one-fourth the way to the ensiform each month until the ninth. Now the uterus sinks down and forward, the process being called "lightening," and reaches the level it had at the eighth month. Naturally, the accuracy of these decisions is not great, being disturbed by the inconstancy of the location of the navel, the elasticity of the belly wall, and so many intra-abdominal conditions, the amount of liquor amnii, the size of the child, its position, etc. As Libow has shown the shape and size of the trunk alter the uterine relations. Toward the end of the last trimester the shape of the uterus alters. It becomes longer, which is due to the head passing into the newly formed lower uterine segment, a change less observable in pluriparæ until actual labor begins. The formation of the lower uterine segment is caused by several factors, and may be part of the process of lightening—the weight of the child, the intermittent uterine contractions, the action of the round ligaments, the tightness of the abdominal wall, and this is the reason that lightening is more likely to be found in primiparæ.

The uterus, owing to absorption of some of the liquor amnii, conforms a little more to the shape of the child and flattens at the fundus.

Lightening.—Two to three weeks before labor the uterus sinks downward and forward. The women call this "settling" or "dropping"; the technical term

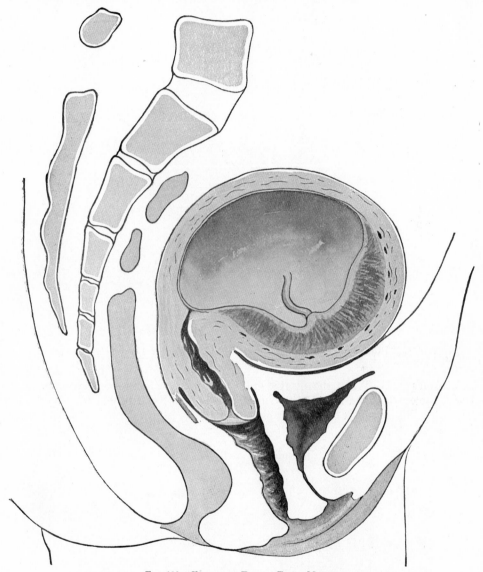

FIG. 110.—UTERUS AT END OF THIRD MONTH.
Shows long cervix, sharp anteflexion, and how the fundus sags heavily on bladder.

is "lightening." It occurs in about 75 per cent. of cases and is due to the gradual sinking of the child's head into the true pelvis, and is usual in primiparæ with normal pelves, or multiparæ with normal pelves and well-preserved abdominal muscles. Lightening may be simulated by the sudden weakening of the abdominal wall, which sometimes occurs late in pregnancy, and by the absorption of the liquor amnii. Both of these conditions produce the changes in the contour of the belly, relieve the distress in breathing, and show other symptoms attendant on true lightening.   The differential diagnosis is easily made by finding that the head has not engaged and that the changes in the cervix about to be described have

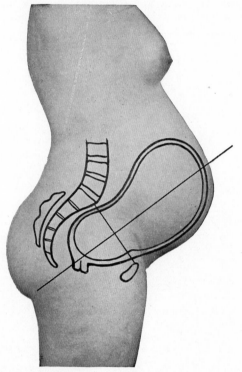

Fig. 111.—Shows Relation of Uterine Axis to Axis of Inlet in the Erect Posture (Primipara).

not taken place.   When the uterus sinks, the intestines and stomach have more room, the epigastrium is free, the diaphragm regains more nearly its usual level, the waist-line sinks so that the woman can fit her skirts better.   On the other

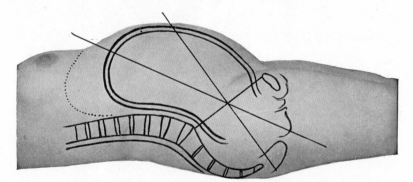

Fig. 112.—Same Primipara, Lying Flat.
Shows crossing of axes.

hand, the head presses upon the bladder and rectum, producing symptoms from these organs; walking is rendered more difficult, and many pains of a neuralgic nature and much distress referred to the pelvis are complained of.

On internal examination one finds the vault of the pelvis filled by the head, and the cervix, which before was a prominent protuberance on the lower uterine segment (Fig. 116), now has been flattened out against the head so that it can hardly be recognized as apart from the vagina.   Often too the vagina is folded on itself like a loose cuff, and this might be mistaken for the dilated os or a stricture (Fig. 118).

Sometimes lightening occurs suddenly, attended by more or less regular labor-pains. The patient summons the physician, but labor does not occur, and sometimes does not come on for two weeks.   These cases are not to be confounded with protracted gestation and postponed labor (*q. v.*).   Lightening may occur as early as the seventh month, and the head may recede and enter again, or later be prevented from engaging by having overgrown the size of the inlet in the meantime.   As a rule, however, the phenomenon indicates that that head is not too large to go through that particular pelvis, and, therefore, is always a welcome sign. If the head remains very low in the pelvis for several weeks, it may be molded to the pelvic floor, and be flattened on the posterior parietal bone, a deformity more or less permanent.

The Cervix and Lower Uterine Segment.— The unimpregnated uterus has three parts— the corpus, or body, the cervix, and the

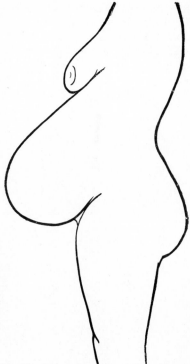

FIG. 113.—Multipara Standing. Pendulous Abdomen.

"isthmus," at the junction of the two.   The cervix is one-third as long as the body, and the insertion of the vagina makes three more or less sharp divisions (Fig.

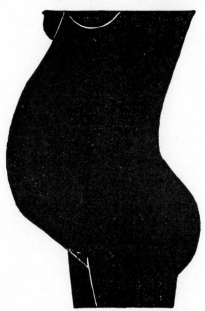

FIG. 114.—Silhouette of a Primipara before Lightening.

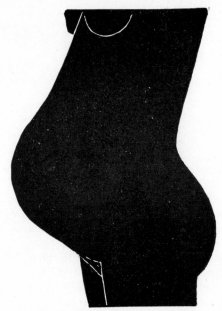

FIG. 115.—Same after Lightening.

119).   The anterior wall of the vagina is inserted 1 to 1½ cm. from the external os; the posterior wall about 3 cm. above the external os; and the cervix extends about 1 cm. above the latter point.   That portion of the cervix lying entirely in the vagina is called the vaginal portion—sometimes simply "portio"; that which lies behind in the vagina and in front against the bladder, the median portion ; and that which lies above the vaginal insertion, the supravaginal portion.   If one examines the cervix of a pregnant woman at successive weeks, marked changes in consistence, form, and position will be noticed.   Within a few weeks after conception the tip of the cervix begins

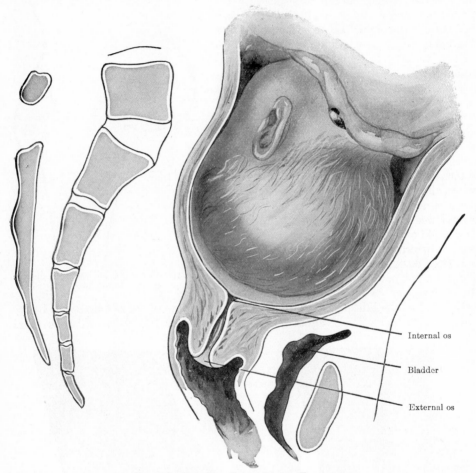

Internal os

Bladder

External os

FIG. 116.—HEAD AND CERVIX BEFORE ENGAGEMENT.

to soften, and this increases upward toward the corpus and from without inward. The softening is caused by imbibition of the tissues and increased vascularity, both hemic and lymphatic.   The anteflexion of the uterus being increased, the cervix points forward, and the uterus, as a whole, sinks lower in the pelvis.   This is especially noticeable if the woman wears tight corsets.   The cervical canal in the first three months runs from below and forward, behind and upward (Fig. 110). When the uterus rises up into the abdomen, the cervical canal takes a more vertical direction, the angle of the point of anteflexion becoming obtuse.   The softening now pervades the whole cervix and paracervical tissues.   The canal is closed by a tough mucous plug, which hinders the ascent of infection.   In multiparæ as early as the fifth month the external os is often patulous, and will admit the finger one-half inch. This is especially true if the cervix has been lacerated and not repaired.

In the seventh month the succulence which affected the cervix has pervaded the whole pelvis, and the outlines of the former are hard to distinguish. The cervix has taken a position higher and further back in the pelvic cavity. The external os always admits the finger in multiparæ, and occasionally in primiparæ. The cervical canal is directed backward, but exceptions are not uncommon. The author

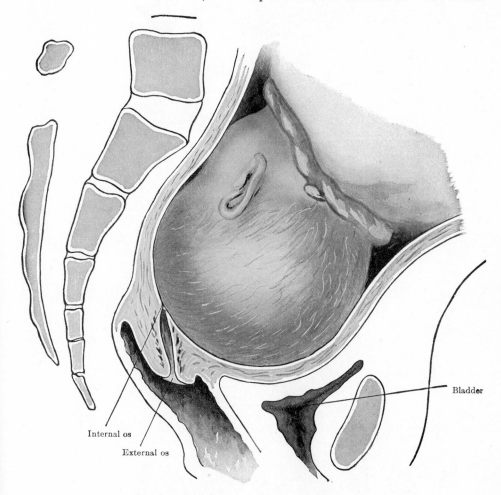

Internal os

External os

Bladder

FIG. 117.—EFFECT ON CERVIX OF ENGAGEMENT OF HEAD.
Sometimes the canal is directed backward.

has found it sometimes points forward and upward. The internal os is usually closed both in primiparæ and in multiparæ, though it occasionally admits the tip of the finger in the latter. The cervix begins now to flatten out against the fetal head, seemingly to be taken up and used as part of the uterine cavity. This is the impression one receives from the examining finger, but frozen sections prove that it is not always the case.

In the ninth month the softening and succulence of the cervix and neighboring tissues are greatest, since the venous congestion is at its height and the uterine contractions of pregnancy force a great deal of serum into the tissues. Sometimes even the educated finger experiences difficulty in outlining the structures. The imbibition of the epithelium often leads to erosions, and catarrhal affections of the

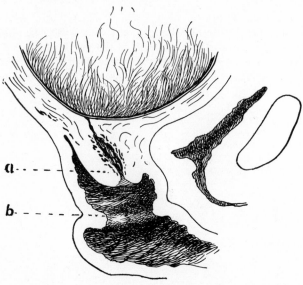

FIG. 118.—FOLDING OF THE VAGINA (*b*) DURING THE PROCESS OF LIGHTENING, SIMULATING THE EXTERNAL OS (*a*).

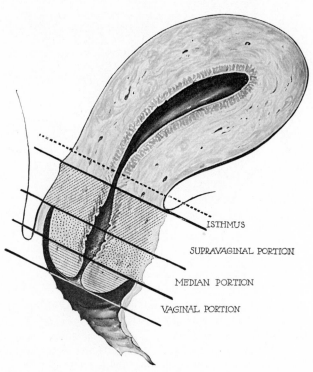

FIG. 119.—THE THREE CLINICAL DIVISIONS OF THE CERVIX. ABOVE THE CERVIX IS THE ISTHMUS.

cervix are much aggravated. Hence the gravidæ frequently have leukorrhea. If the patient previously had cervicitis with erosions, the condition may become so marked as to require treatment, because of hemorrhage, profuse and irritating discharge, etc. The mucosa does not have a decidua, although decidual islands are not infrequently found in the stroma, but its glands hypertrophy enormously,

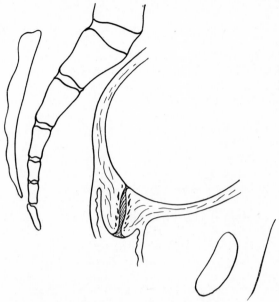

Fig. 120.—Cervix as Most Commonly Located.

forming a honeycomb-like structure. They secrete a tenacious mucus, constantly renewed which bars the upward march of infection. This "mucous plug" often with part of the superficial glands is expelled as the "show" at labor. Stieve also

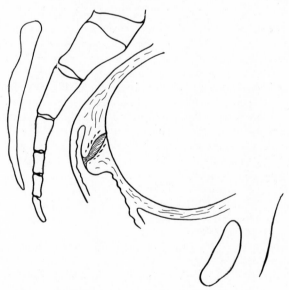

Fig. 121.—Cervix in Hollow of Sacrum.

proved that there is no increase of the connective tissue or muscle (both becoming softer) and that the veins multiply so markedly that the cervix almost resembles an erectile organ. The changes in the direction of the cervical canal have been described under the heading of Lightening (p. 87). The external os, even in primiparæ, now usually admits the index-finger, and in most of the cases the internal os will also allow the finger to pass. This is especially true of multiparæ in whom two or even three fingers may be inserted and the membranes may lie exposed to the vagina. The shape and size of the external os are much affected by previous laceration or scar formation. One will find many individual differences. The author has found the cervical canal in an old primipara enlarged at the thirty-third week so that the external os admitted the middle finger and the internal os was the size of a nickel. While the extreme softening and the enlargement of the cervical canal indicate that labor is near, still, in view of what has been said, absolute reliance may not be placed on these signs. In the last week or ten days the uterine contractions often bring about a true effacement of the cervix, and use it to form the lower portion of the uterine cavity, thus anticipating part of the first stage of labor. This is called "insensible labor" by the French, and is a welcome finding to the obstetrician, as it facilitates all operative manœuvers should hasty delivery be necessary. A cervix that remains long and tightly closed up until labor begins is not normal.

The location of the cervix at full term varies. Rarely one finds it anteriorly or at one side; most often it is in the middle of the pelvis (Fig. 120), and many times it is back in the hollow of the sacrum (Fig. 121). If it is high up near the sacrum and hard to reach with the finger, the condition is pathologic. In cases of antefixation of the uterus the cervix may be located above the promontory in the abdominal cavity.

The **relation of the cervix to the lower uterine segment** has been the subject of conflicting theories since 1746. Older writers taught that the cervix was un-folded, or effaced, drawn up and expanded to form part of the uterine cavity, until at term only a small part of the cervix was left. Modern investigators hold that it is the lower part of the uterine body which is developed to cover the inferior pole of the ovum, and that the cervix usually remains closed, at least not shortened, until labor begins.

The new cesarean section, in which the incision is made in the lower zone of the uterus, behind the bladder, enables us to study *in vivo* the anatomic conditions of the cervix and lower uterine segment, with an accuracy which vaginal examinations and even frozen sections do not permit and has thrown light in this polemic. Figure 123 shows the findings in a cervix at three months. At term the cervix is apparently slightly shortened, the external os hardly admits a finger to the internal os. From the internal os, extending toward the fundus uteri a variable distance, usually about 8 cm., the uterine wall is thin, the outer layer whiter and fibrous. A distinct layer of fascia, the continuation of the vesicovaginal fascia, can also be isolated, while the peritoneum over it is very loosely attached. The upper boundary of this part of the uterus is marked by three signs: first, the peritoneum becomes adherent to the muscle; second, a large transverse sinus is present; third, the muscle of the uterus suddenly becomes thicker, forming a sort of ridge or ring. This ring is demonstrable in pregnancy, but becomes more marked during labor, and it is called Braune's ring, because he first described it, or Bandl's, because he showed its immense clinical importance. It is more often and better called the contraction ring, because it marks the lower limit of the contracting or motor portion of the uterus.

The region from the contraction ring to the internal os is called the lower uterine segment and its origin has been much discussed. The old theory that it came entirely from the cervix is supported by Mauriceau, Braune, Bandl, Bayer, Bumm *et al.* A later view, that it comes in part from the uterus, that is, from the lower portion of the body, is supported by Stoltz, Schroeder, Barbour, Hofmeier *et al.*

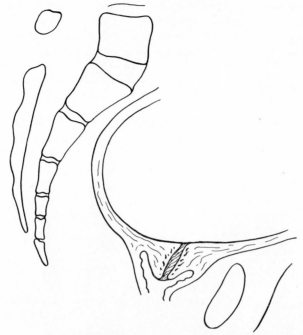

FIG. 122.—CERVIX NEAR PUBIS.

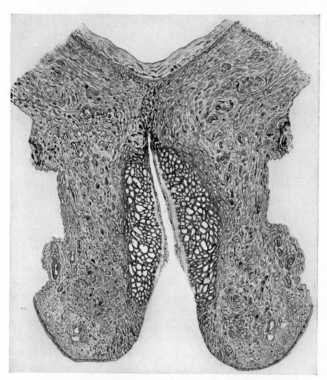

FIG. 123.—CERVIX AT THREE MONTHS.
Note immense development of the mucous glands and of the blood-vessels. Cervix seems almost like an erectile organ.

Aschoff, in 1906, showed that there exists between the internal os and the **proper** body of the uterus a slightly differentiated zone which he called the "isthmus." In it the musculature is not so well developed as in the corpus, but more so than in the cervix, the glands are fewer and less vertical, and there is less stroma. During pregnancy the isthmus develops greatly, but not as much as the corpus uteri. It stretches to accommodate the downward growing ovum and forms, with some of the outer fibers of the cervix, the lower uterine segment. This, in the fully formed structure, varies from 6 to 9 cm. in length, and one may deliver a fetus by an incision through it without encroaching on the contractile or motor portion of the uterus.

It is probable, in some cases, multiparæ notably, that the mucous membrane and a few layers of muscle—mostly circular—of the cervix remain unchanged until very near the advent of labor pains. This gives the sensation of a long canal and of a closed internal os, a condition well known to Bandl. It is just as probable that

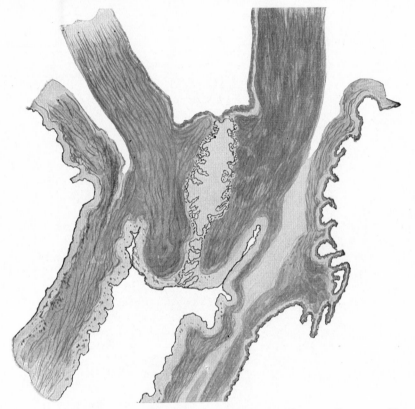

Fig. 124.—Closed Cervix in a Primipara After Pains had Begun. Condition Pathologic (Bayer).

the *outer layers* of cervical muscle are drawn up and expanded during the latter months of pregnancy, to form part of the uterine cavity—the so-called lower uterine segment. The upper boundary of this zone is the "contraction ring," or the lower edge of the contracting muscle of the corpus; the lower boundary is the so-called internal os of the cervix, the edge of the cervical mucous membrane. This zone is sometimes covered with decidua, but the membranes are loosely attached to it, showing its late formation. It has little, if any, contractile power. The movability of the muscular layers on each other permits the employment of cervical fibers for the formation of the lower uterine segment. It is probable, too, that sometimes, oftener in primiparæ, the cervical mucous membrane is also drawn up into the lower uterine segment. In this case one finds portions of the plica palmatæ spread out in the lower uterine segment, and one may even find the mucous membrane changed into decidua. It is certain that sometimes the cervix remains unchanged, except to soften and hypertrophy, and tightly closed until the advent of hard labor. These cases are, according to Bayer, pathologic, and the author agrees with him. A long closed cervix as in Fig. 124 is unusual.

That the changes in the cervix during pregnancy are not constant and typical will not surprise him who remembers the variously sized and shaped cervices he meets in the routine of gynecologic examinations, and one must agree with Bayer that sometimes the cervix unfolds in pregnancy and sometimes it does not.

During labor the differentiation in the uterus becomes marked and unquestionable. The corpus contracts strongly, the lower uterine segment feebly, the cervix not at all; thus two zones are formed—an upper, contracting, and a lower, dilating. In the consideration of the mechanism of labor this subject will again come up.

Changes in the Physiology of the Uterus.—During pregnancy the uterus acquires no new functions; those it has, however, are much developed. Menstruation normally ceases during pregnancy.

The sensibility varies in different women. Unless diseased, the organ is not tender. One may cut and sew the fundus uteri without causing pain. In neurotic patients the lightest palpation, even the fetal movements, evoke pain. In labor the uterus is more sensitive.

Irritability is that property which makes the uterus respond to external stimulation by contracting. Pregnancy develops this quality, but it also varies in different women. In some the ordinary abdominal examination evokes contractions; in others most powerful external and internal stimuli produce little, if any, effect. This is best observed when we try to bring on labor.

The dilatability of the uterus increases very much during pregnancy, and even when the uterus seems well filled by the ovum it can still stretch to hold a considerable amount of extra fluid. This is shown by the enormous acute distention in polyhydramnion and in the accumulation of large quantities of blood in cases of abruptio placentæ.

Contractility increases as pregnancy advances. Acting on impulses coming through the nervous system and the blood, the uterus contracts and relaxes. We note this power in the unimpregnated uterus when it expels clots, membranes, or fibroids. As early as the fifth week of gestation the contractions of the uterus are perceptible to the examining finger. These are painless, last twenty to thirty seconds, sometimes a few minutes, and may be observed to recur at irregular intervals up to the advent of labor, when they become regular, painful, and more powerful. The contractions are involuntary, but are sometimes affected by the nervous condition of the woman. They may continue postmortem for a brief period.

Retractility is a function of the uterine muscle not fully understood. It is that power which enables the uterine wall to close down on its diminishing cavity. This is brought about by a microscopic felting together of the muscle-fibers and a superimposition of the muscular lamellæ. This power is manifested most markedly in parturition. A retracted uterus cannot be completely re-expanded without danger to its structure. The property of retractility lies either in the muscle itself, or it is evoked through the nervous mechanism—probably the latter, since it seems to be affected by the same influences as contractility.

Elasticity is the ability of the uterine wall to return to a condition of rest after being distended. It must be sharply differentiated from retractility.

The **round ligaments** are part of the uterine muscle, and hypertrophy with it. Late in pregnancy they may be as thick as the little finger, and, owing to the high location of the fundus, they run vertically. When the placenta is situated on the posterior wall, the round ligaments are felt converging toward the fundus on the anterior wall of the uterus, and when the anterior wall is occupied by the placenta, the ligaments are pushed to the sides. The round ligaments contract synchronously with the uterus, and serve to moor the latter organ to the pelvis during labor. In pregnancy no such action is observable except in pathologic cases—as retroversion.

7

The **uterosacral ligaments** normally vary much in their development and in the place of insertion on the uterus. They too are part of the uterine musculature and hypertrophy in pregnancy. The part played by these ligaments as suspensors of the uterus has been much exaggerated. Normally, they are relaxed and are put on the stretch only when the uterus is drawn or forced down or up. If the displacement is kept up, they stretch and tear. During labor, however, they contract with the uterus, assisting to hold it in the proper axis of the pelvis, and they aid in the dilatation of the lower uterine segment and cervix.

The **broad ligaments** are also strengthened by the addition of muscular fibers, particularly around the arteries and veins. The two peritoneal layers are separated

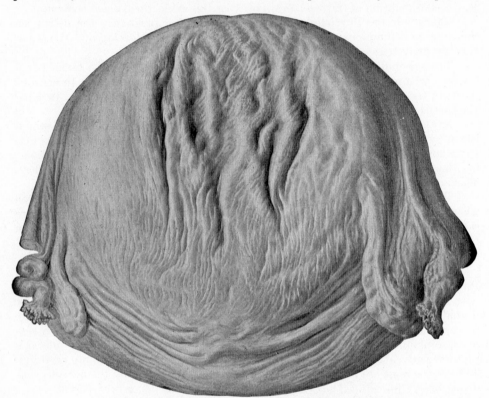

FIG. 125.—SHOWING WRINKLING OF UTERUS AT PLACENTAL SITE.
Specimen kindly loaned by Professor Piscaçek, of Vienna.

by the development of the uterus, so that a much larger portion of this organ is uncovered at the sides.

The pelvic connective tissue loses its fat; the unstriped muscle-fibers develop more abundantly in it; the lymph-spaces are larger; there is a serous imbibition of all the tissues, and the whole pelvis is congested and more succulent. Immense veins develop in and around the vagina and cervix, sometimes to a pathologic extent. The sides of the uterus may bulge with soft venous swellings. During labor these may burst, forming hematomata and hematoceles, and after labor they may thrombose and give rise to emboli and phleboliths.

Hofbauer has shown that, during pregnancy, a phagocytic tissue develops in the connective tissue around the cervix. It consists of monocytes and clasmatocytes, is increased by prolonged labor and especially by infection. The macrophages take part in the local immunity reactions.

The **peritoneum** grows with the uterus, a true hyperplasia occurring. Over the developing lower uterine segment the peritoneum becomes very loose and movable. In pathologic cases the peritoneum may not grow, and tears result. After delivery the peritoneum lies wrinkled in more or less typical directions on the contracted uterus, corresponding to the course of the muscle-fibers (Fig. 125). Walker, in 1887, and Schmorl called attention to decidua-like growths on the peritoneum of Douglas' culdesac, the posterior wall of the uterus, the tubes, ovaries, and omentum. The author has found them on the uterus and anterior abdominal wall in cases of cesarean section. They may be 2 to 3 mm. thick, are just under the endothelium, raising it up, resembling miliary tubercles, and may be pedunculated. They may be cystic or even calcareous. (See Fig. 126.) One finds these structures from the third to the tenth month, and the remains persist for several weeks after delivery. They are commoner after inflammations and irritations, and are due, according to Meyer, to ovarian hormones. Their microscopic structure resembles metastases of decidual cells, ectopic decidua (Geipel).

The **tubes,** which ordinarily vary in length from 5 to 19 cm., are stretched out in pregnancy, hanging almost perpendicularly at the sides of the uterus. There is no hypertrophy of the muscle-fibers, but much increased vascularity and succulence. A moderate decidual change of the mucous membrane has been observed even with intra-uterine pregnancy. The uterine end is usually closed, but the fimbriated end is open. The patulousness of the tubes is closely associated with the question of the possibility of superfecundation.

The **ovaries** are enlarged, especially the one containing the corpus luteum. In the early months the corpus luteum may be palpated—of course, only in favorable cases. In the later months one may feel the ovary through the abdominal wall hanging on the side of the uterus. The right one is less easily felt. They are always quite tender. The microscopic changes in the ovary are edema, vascularization, decidua-like formations under the tunica albuginea. Ovulation does not invariably cease during pregnancy, as was formerly taught.

The **vagina** increases in length and capacity by a real eccentric hypertrophy. It becomes more distensible, the elastic fibers increasing in amount, the muscle fibres hypertrophying and the tissues becoming infiltrated with serum. The rugæ deepen, the papillæ swell, so that sometimes they are palpable as small granules. The epithelium thickens like a true rejuvenation (Stieve). In pathologic cases a vaginitis granulosa may develop, and in cases of gonorrhea the surface may feel like a nutmeg-grater. The veins enlarge, the venules also, giving the surface a deep wine color (diagnostic of pregnancy), and this engorgement is attended by pronounced secretion or leukorrhea (Runge). Under bacterial or endocrinal action the glycogen changes to glucose and then to lactic acid which keeps the vagina relatively sterile (Adler).

The upper portion of the vagina enlarges as pregnancy advances, so that in the later months it is usually possible to touch the sides of the pelvis with the stretched fingers or a dilating pelvimeter. When the uterus ascends, the vagina is drawn up; when the head enters the pelvis in the last month of pregnancy, the vagina is pushed down and often thrown into the circular folds, which may simulate the dilating cervix (Fig. 118). The angulæ vaginæ become slightly movable. The anterior vaginal wall and thickened urethrovaginal septum may prolapse through the patulous vulva. Similar changes are seen on the vulva—softening, dark coloration, varices, pigmentation, thickening, enlargement, increased secretion of all its glands.

The **pelvic floor** takes part in the general imbibition of the pelvis. The levator ani becomes less rigid, more distensible. The fat in the ischiorectal fossa is partly absorbed by the end of pregnancy, but the infiltration with serum causes a pronounced swelling and sagging of the perineum. This sagging of the perineum below a line drawn from the under surface of the pubis to the tip of the sacrum is called *pelvic floor projection* (Fig. 127). Other conditions cause an increase of pelvic floor projection, such as pelvic tumors, marked intra-abdominal pressure, but in pregnancy it is most manifest, and in cases of incarceration of the gravid uterus one meets

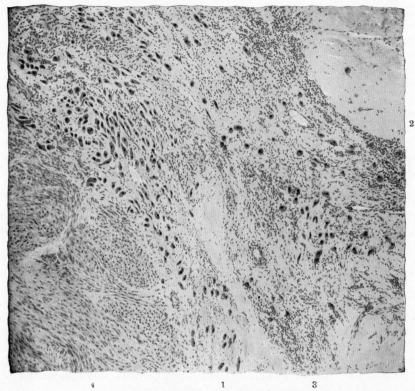

FIG. 126.—LOW-POWER SECTION OF UTERUS.
1, Invasion of decidual cells; 2, hyaline degeneration of muscle; 3, round-cell infiltration; 4, normal uterine muscle.

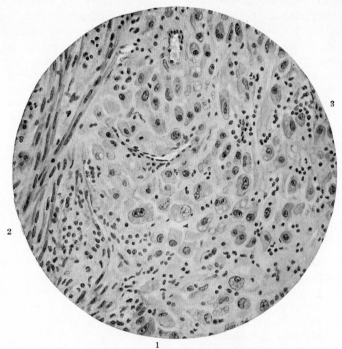

FIG. 126a.—HIGH-POWER SECTION.
1, Decidual cell invasion; 2, few strands of uterine muscle; 3, round cells.

Figures 126 and 126a are from a specimen removed from a normal uterus at cesarean section. They show how the uterine muscle is invaded by a mass of cells resembling decidual tissue. (See Figs. 483, 484.) The neighboring muscle is hyaline degenerated, and one can easily see how it might rupture. The significance of this specimen is much broader than in its bearing on ruptura uteri.

the greatest depression of the tissues. The pelvic floor projection during labor will be considered later.

The **bladder** is much concerned in the changes wrought by pregnancy. In the early months the fundus uteri lies upon it, but with no greater weight than the in-

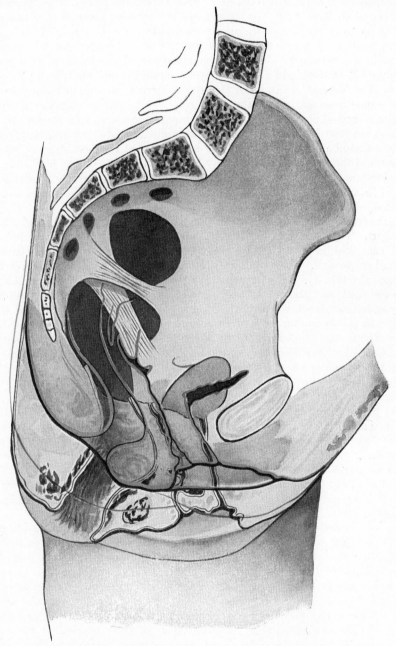

FIG. 127.—PELVIC FLOOR PROJECTION (adapted from Hart and Barbour).
Red indicates the parts before pregnancy.

testines. A certain amount of traction is exerted by the retroposed cervix on the neck of the bladder, and this, with the congestion of the parts, explains the frequent urination complained of by the women at this period. Cystoscopically, the indentation made by the fundus uteri is easily discovered; the color of the interior is darker, and one experienced in the use of the instrument may suspect the pregnancy from the appearance of the congested and newly vascularized bladder mucosa. Varicose veins in the base of the bladder are sometimes found. In the later months they may give rise to hemorrhage. Even after the uterus has risen into the abdomen the bladder remains a pelvic organ, unless distended, when it is flattened out against the abdominal wall. In these cases the bladder assumes a saddle shape, extending up to either side of the uterus—more toward the right. This is shown by the cystoscope, x-ray or by illuminating the filled bladder and observing the abdomen in a dark room. With the development of the lower uterine segment the attachment of the bladder to the uterus is loosened and the bladder is stripped off the wall of the latter. In labor the uterus retracts still further away from the bladder—sometimes so far that the latter comes to lie on the vagina. These facts were determined clinically in cases of extraperitoneal cesarean section at which operations we also learned that the bladder changes are not constant, varying much in different patients. During the latter part of the first stage of labor the peritoneum of the anterior culdesac may be partly stripped off the bladder. When the head enters the pelvis in the last month, it may press directly on the bladder or distort its base, thus giving rise to the frequent urination so often noted. Perhaps the diminished capacity of the organ is also causative.

The **ureters** are enlarged early in pregnancy. Thickening is one of the diagnostic signs. They are displaced to the side of the pelvis, and may be felt on bimanual examination as two cord-like, tender structures, coursing between the cervix and pelvic wall. Their walls are atomic, their lumen usually dilated, especially above the inlet (Hirst). Late in pregnancy they may be felt lying against the lower uterine segment and the fetal head. Halbertsma claimed that the ureters frequently suffer compression during the later months of pregnancy, and that eclampsia is due to the damming back of the urine. At no time can the uterus directly compress the ureters, and, further, the weight of the uterus is not greater than that of the intestinal mass. The entry of the fetal head into the pelvis in the last month distorts the course of the ureter or kinks or stretches it, and this may interfere with the passage of urine. Cystoscopically, the ureteral openings in the bladder appear elevated, thickened, and deeply congested.

The **pelvic girdle** is affected by the changes of pregnancy. The author has determined an actual increase of the size of the pelvic cavity. Measurements taken of contracted pelves before conception, and just before labor, will often show this, and women in whom labor was predicted as impossible may have spontaneous or easy operative deliveries. The constitution of the pelvic bones during pregnancy is altered similarly to the pathologic osteomalacia. Occasionally there is an irregular deposit of extra bone under the periosteum—the puerperal osteophytes of Rokitansky. The hypophysis is involved in these changes.

The pelvic articulations undergo marked changes. Hippocrates knew that they softened and became looser, and he believed that parturition was difficult if this relaxation did not occur. Perhaps part of the enlargement of the pelvic circle above mentioned is due to the thickening of the cartilages of the joints. Normally, and in man, there is a slight movability of the pelvic joints, but in pregnancy this is increased and during labor it is greatest. The tissues of the joint imbibe fluid, the capsule thickens, the vascularity is increased, and there is an augmentation of synovia. It is to be noted that these changes are most marked in women with varicose veins of the pelvis. The pubic, sacrococcygeal, and sacro-iliac joints are affected in the order named. In guinea-pigs these changes are part of the pregnancy and parturition, and may be so pronounced that the bones of the pubis may separate so far as to allow the animal's legs to lie alongside the body on the table. In cows the "sinking of the rump" informs the veterinarian that delivery is at hand. In women an actual enlargement of the pelvis in labor occurs only in very slight degree, but the softening of the joints allows freer motion of the bones and thus a certain configuration, which facilitates the delivery. After a certain point of stretching is reached the joint capsules tear, as Putschar has shown. It seems fairly well established that these joint changes are under endocrinal influences.

Many women in the later months of pregnancy complain of pain in the pelvic joints, a waddling gait, and difficulty in walking. Examination will usually show tenderness over the pubes, and riding of the two bones on each other when the pelvis is strongly rocked from side to side, or even a groove showing a larger degree of separation. (See Relaxation and Rupture of the Pelvic Joints.)

The **abdominal wall** distends as the pregnancy advances, and grows thinner, especially around the navel. Experiments by Kraus have shown that the tension is in the direction of radii from the navel. In primiparæ the abdominal walls are tenser and sag less than in women who have borne children. Sometimes the linea alba gives way to the strain, the recti muscles separate, and the pregnant uterus falls forward between them, covered only by a thin layer of skin and peritoneum. This is called "rupture" by the laity. The belly becomes pendulous,—"*ventre en besace*,"—and not seldom the condition gives rise to dystocia. Any tendency to hernia is aggravated by pregnancy, but during this period the uterus usually pushes the gut up and keeps it and the omentum from the hernial openings—that is, unless these are adherent to the sac.

In 90 per cent. (Credè), and in practically all cases of the author, the skin shows smooth, silvery, or pearly white or violet broad lines, called striæ or lineæ albicantes gravidarum. The lines are curved, irregular, sometimes confluent, and show a fine transverse fibrillation. They are arranged more or less concentrically, but sometimes radially around the navel, especially on the lower abdomen. Near Poupart's ligament they are always broader and deeper in color. One

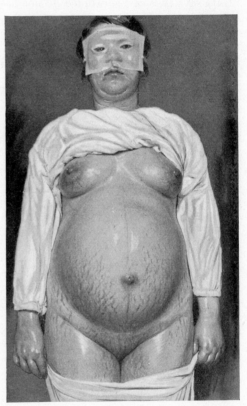

FIG. 128.—STRIÆ GRAVIDARUM.
Patient toxemic. Note swollen hands and face.

finds them on the nates, the thighs, more on the anterior aspect, but sometimes on the posterior too, and as far down as the knees. The breasts also show them, arranged radially to the nipple. Blonds are more affected than brunets, primiparæ more than multiparæ, fat women more than lean, large women more than small, young women more than those older than twenty-five. The number depends also on the degree of abdominal distention and the use of abdominal supporters, but there are other factors in the causation than mere abdominal distention, because in cases of immense abdominal enlargement due to ovarian tumors or ascites the striæ are not constant. Formerly they were considered positive proof of preëxisting pregnancy, but this is not true, since they occur in the following conditions: rapid accumulation of fat at any period, as at puberty; they are found in men (6 per cent.); dropsy and ascites; abdominal tumors; unusually rapid growth of the long bones may develop them at the epiphyses; after typhoid fever. If the lineæ are marked and with typical distribution, the presumption of previous pregnancy is strong, but never certain. The author has seen striæ on the breasts of a virgin. New striæ may appear among the old. The author has observed lineæ gravidarum in the sixth month. Histologically, one finds the connective tissue of the cutis and subcutis stretched, sometimes torn, and the former rhomboid arrangement of the fibers changed to a more parallel disposition of the strands across the striæ. The elastic fibers are always torn, and the retracted ends found at the edge of the striæ. The lymph-spaces are compressed and arranged parallel. Perhaps this explains the tendency of the lineæ to become dropsical. The papillæ are flattened, sometimes completely, and are also arranged in transerve rows. The epidermis is thinned. In brunets and colored women there is a tendency to pigmentation of the striæ. Stratz says that savage women do not have striæ, and advises massage with oil as a preventive. (See Taussig.)

The Physics of the Abdomen.—The pressure in the belly varies very little from that outside, and depends on the tonicity of the abdominal walls. In the relaxed horizontal position the abdominal walls support a pressure equal only to the weight of the viscera, which, being practically semifluid, seek the lowest portions of the cavity. In this position there is a slight increase of intra-abdominal pressure with inspiration, and a slight decrease during expiration.

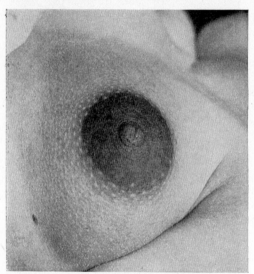

FIG. 129.—BRUNET'S BREAST. PREGNANCY, EIGHT MONTHS.
Shows primary and secondary areolæ.

In the erect position there is a slight increase of intra-abdominal pressure because the muscles are on tension, and this is augmented by inspiration, forced expiration, as by exercise, expulsive efforts, defecation, vomiting, parturition. The development of tumors in the belly, as fibroids, cysts, pregnancy, increases intra-abdominal pressure. In addition the lower portions of the abdomen, in the erect position, sustain the weight of the superimposed column of viscera. Therefore intra-abdominal pressure is not the same at all points. The changes in the pressure brought about by respiration are transmitted throughout the abdomen, and are evident on the perineum and organs resting on the pelvic floor, uterus, and bladder. The organs in the belly are not held in position by atmospheric pressure. They are fastened to the firm parietes by ligaments and floated on each other, getting indirect support from the abdominal muscles and pelvic floor. In the knee-chest position the weight of the liver and intestines falling toward the chest produces a negative pressure in the abdomen. If, now, the belly, vagina, rectum, and bladder are opened, air rushes in and distends them. We use this position therapeutically.

The Breasts.—In the embryo of six weeks there is found a line of cells running from the axilla to the groin, and called the linea or crista lactea. From the chest portion of this the breasts develop. Accessory breasts and supernumerary nipples are almost always found in this line on either side, and indicate a tendency to revert to a lower order in human development.

An ingrowth of epithelial cells, which later become tubulated, marks the site of the mamma. In the fetus at five months the gland consists simply of a collection of ducts which open at one spot—the future nipple. This spot is depressed; thus an inverted nipple in the adult is simply one retarded in development. Even at seven months the ducts are branched, and at term they divide two or three times. These primitive ducts represent the future lobules. Hardly any acinous structure exists at birth, but the tubules are capable of secreting milk and colostrum which do not differ in composition from those of the mother. The growth of the gland is very slow until puberty. Then acini develop in the primitive tubules, each of which becomes a tubuloracemose gland, and thus the breast comes to be made up of distinct lobules embedded in a fat cushion. Each lobe empties on the surface of the now prominent nipple by a duct. Before opening on the nipple each duct dilates a little—the sinus lactiferus. There are 15 to 20 ducts. The nipple is a muscular organ, and is covered by delicate pigmented skin, is quite vascular, and at the base is surrounded by unstriped muscle-fibers which unite with those of the

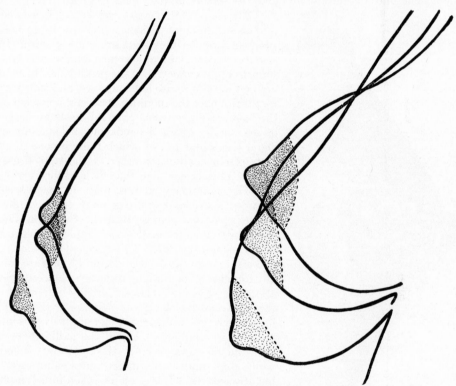

Fig. 130.—Variously Shaped Breasts (Primiparæ).

Fig. 130a.—Variously Shaped Breasts (Multiparæ).

nipple itself and thus produce the erection of the same. For a varying distance around the nipple the skin is very delicate, more or less pigmented, and raised from the fascia covering the mammary gland by soft connective tissue and fat. This is the areola. Embedded in this areola lie tiny milk-glands, Montgomery's tubercles, each opening on the surface by a microscopic duct. Sebaceous and sweat-glands are also found.

With the advent of pregnancy the glands take on renewed growth, and as early as the second month a change may be noted. The breasts increase in size and sensibility; the hard, tense feel of the virgin gland is lost; it softens and sags. The lobules become more marked, due to enlargement, development of acini in the periphery, and softening of the connective tissue and fat around them. The acinous formation on the tubules in the center of the gland is especially marked during pregnancy, there being both hyperplasia and hypertrophy. The veins enlarge and are seen as bluish streaks, especially at the periphery, and here striæ often (67 per cent.) develop. Hypertrophy of the lymph-system is also a feature. The nipple becomes more erectile, and, with the areola, becomes more deeply pigmented. The base of the areola becomes puffy, raising the surface above that of the rest of the gland, and the milk-glands of Montgomery enlarge prominently. Occasionally a droplet of secretion may be expressed from them. Around the primary areola, especially in brunets, a secondary areola, less pigmented, sometimes develops. It resembles "dusty paper sprinkled with drops of water." The clear spots are due to lack of pigment around the openings of sweat and sebaceous glands. From the early months—and the time varies—a little clear, sticky fluid may be expressed from the nipple. Later this is mixed with yellow material. It is called colostrum. Often it oozes out and dries into branny scales on the nipple. Unless cleaned off, these sometimes decompose and give rise to sore nipples, even in pregnancy.

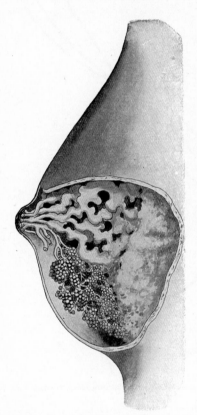

FIG. 131.—FUNCTIONATING BREAST, MOSTLY DIAGRAMMATIC.

The shape of the breast varies much in women, and also at different periods of life. In young, non-pregnant women they sometimes are hemispheric and prominent. In old women and in the later months of pregnancy they are pendulous. In some colored races they are like long sacs, and they may be thrown over the shoulder, for a child, carried on the back, to nurse from. Some breasts are large, others small, which depends on the amount of gland tissue and fat, of which there is sometimes more of one than of the other. The right breast is sometimes larger than the left, and vice versâ.

The mammary glands may be considered modified skin-glands, with a fetal origin similar to the sebaceous glands (Basch). Sometimes we find supernumerary glands and nipples above and below the normal one. This is called polymastia, and is rare. Accessory glands and nipples are usually found in a line running from the axilla onto the abdomen—the crista lactea already referred to; this and embryologic studies indicate that man had at one time a line of glands similarly to some of the lower animals. Up in the axilla there is often an aberrant piece of the mammary gland, which sometimes swells and becomes painful when lactation starts. It is often mistaken for a lymph-gland. It may enlarge outside of pregnancy. The sweat-glands in the axilla, too, are often enlarged and palpable, secreting freely. (See Knaebel.)

When the child is delivered and lactation begins, the breasts reach their highest development, but we will leave the consideration of this until we discuss the changes of the puerperium. Starling believes that the growth of the mammæ during pregnancy is due to the action of a "mamma hormone," developed in the growing ovum. Novak holds the placenta inhibits the formation of milk. Steinach believes the influence comes from the ovaries because he got the breasts to secrete in castrated male rats into which he had transplanted ovaries. Corner believes the impulse comes from the anterior pituitary. (See Fig. 131a, p. 110.) Hammond says it is the corpus luteum first stimulating the growth of the breast, then the secretion of milk follows in correlation to its involution. In the Blazek united twins, though only one was pregnant, in both the breasts were enlarged and secreted milk. The breasts possess an internal secretion which seems to inhibit ovarian activity, and, if produced in too large amounts, may cause atrophy of the uterus, the lactation amenorrhea. Extracts of the mamma have been employed therapeutically.

LITERATURE

Bandl: Über das Verhalten des Uterus und Cervix, Stuttgart, 1876.—*Ibid.:* Über Ruptura Uteri, Vienna, 1875.—*Bar:* La Pratique des Accouchements, 1907, p. 37.—*Bartholomew, Sale, and Calloway:* Jour. Amer. Med. Assoc., April 2, 1921.—*Basch:* Arch. f. Gynäk., vol. xliv. Gives literature.—*Bayer:* Freund's Gynäkol. Klinik, Stuttgart, 1885, p. 369.—*Ibid.:* Arch. f. Gynäk., vol. liv, p. 70.—*Bumm and Blumerich:* Ein neuer Gefrierdurchschnitt einer Gebärenden, Wiesbaden, 1907.—*Corner:* Quoted by Graves, Hormonology, 1931.—*Elkin:* Jour. Amer. Med. Assoc., January 7, 1922, p. 28.—*Geipel:* Arch. für Gyn., 1928, vol. 131, p. 650.—*Hirst, J. C.:* Amer. Jour. Obst. and Gyn., 1929, p. 528.—*Hofbauer:* Bull. Johns Hopkins University, April, 1926, p. 255.—*Ivanow:* Musculature de l'ute, Annales de Gyn., June, 1911, p. 327.—*Knaebel, A.:* "Mammae Accessoriae, Achselhöhlenbrüste," Monatschr. f. Geb. u. Gyn., 1910, vol. xxxi, p. 548.—*Krause and Felsenreich:* Arch. f. Gynäk., vol. xv.—*Libow:* Arch. für Gyn., 1931, vol. 147, H. 3, p. 773.—*Meyer:* Zeitschr. f. Geb. u. Gyn., 1913, vol. lxxiv, H. 2, p. 256.—*Ottow, B.:* Stöckel's Lehrbuch der Geb., 1930, p. 351.—*Palm:* Zeitschr. f. Geb. u. Gyn., vol. xxv, p. 317.—*Putschar:* Entwicklung, Wachstum u. Pathologie der Beckenverbindungen des Menschen, Jena, 1931. Excellent monograph with bibliography.—*Redlich:* Roentgen Atlas of Arteries of Uterus, Veit & Co., Leipzig, 1911.—*Retterer and Lalievre:* "Structur du muscle uterin," L'Obstetrique, October, 1909, p. 735; also March, 1911.—*Reynolds:* Surg., Gyn., and Obstet., July, 1911.—*Runge:* Arch. für Gynaek., 1924, Bd. 122, H. 3, p. 603.—*Sampson:* Surg., Gyn., and Obstet., May, 1914.—*Schill, L.:* Recherches sur la glande mammaire, Nancy, 1912.—*Schmorl:* Monatschr. f. Geb. u. Gyn., 1897, vol. v, p. 46.—*Schumacher and Hanlo:* Arch. für Gyn., 1931, vol. 147, Heft 3.—*Steinach:* Jour. Amer. Med. Assoc., February 26, 1916.—*Stieve:* Zentb. für Gynaek., 1925, No. 9, p. 484.—*Ibid.:* Der Halzteil der Menschlichen Gebärmutter, Leipzig, 1927.—*Taussig:* Surg., Gyn., and Obst., September, 1913.—*Walker:* Arch. f. path. Anat., vol. cxxvii.

GENERAL CHANGES IN THE MATERNAL ORGANS

Mauriceau called pregnancy a disease of nine months' duration, and there is much truth in the epigram. Generally, the pregnant state and labor are looked upon as physiologic, and in perfectly healthy women they may be so. No other function of the body is attended by such dangerous possibilities or is so easily deranged, so that one must always bear in mind how close to the borderland of pathology the obstetric case continuously runs. (See Introduction.)

Pregnant women ought to feel as well as during the non-pregnant state. In a percentage of the cases they do, or even feel better, but oftener this is not so. They are more irritable; their character changes; they are less trustworthy; they are less tidy; they have various aches and pains—neuralgia, toothache, headache— and innumerable symptoms, which the doctor is called upon to alleviate during the nine months. Sometimes severe mental disturbances arise. Every organ, every tissue of the body, feels the stimulus of pregnancy. The whole metabolism is changed to meet the new demands on the system, and it has been well said that "Gestation tests the integrity of every structure of the body" (R. Barnes). If there is any latent disease in the woman, pregnancy will bring it to the surface. This fact warns the accoucheur to study well the constitution of his patient and to watch carefully all weak points in the organism. The woman must provide a warm safe nest for the ovum and a mechanism by which it can be expelled when ripe. She must supply the fetus with water, oxygen, food, calcium, phosphates, iron, etc., and receive from the infant nearly all its waste, which must be converted so as to be easily eliminable by her emunctories. She must store up blood to replace that lost during labor, energy to furnish that needful for the physical strain of delivery, and fat and albumin to make milk.

It is the complicated processes of adjustment to these new necessities that we are about to study. Maladaptations, or insufficiencies, lead to the pathologic conditions to be considered later.

The Blood.—Investigators are not agreed on the changes which the blood undergoes during pregnancy, and it is because the blood reacts differently to the stimulus of pregnancy in different women. Kiwisch described the condition of the blood in early pregnancy as a "serous plethora," or hydremia. From external appearances many women, especially those generally ill nourished or living in poor circumstances, suffer from a condition of chloranemia. The fetus uses up a great deal of iron and calcium, but normally the blood lacks neither.

While in the first few months there may be a reduction in the reds and increase of the whites, the system soon reacts to the necessities imposed by pregnancy, and there is an increase of the reds, also of the whites, the latter out of proportion to the reds—the "physiologic leukocytosis of pregnancy" of Virchow. It is seldom more than 15,000. There is often an increase of the neutrophile polynuclears and also of the myelocytes, the latter indicating the part taken by the bone-marrow. Occasionally a few nucleated reds and poikilocytes appear. During labor there is a marked leukocytosis, especially of the polynuclear neutrophiles, values as high as 34,200 being obtained, average 18,000, and the eosinophiles disappear, which Adler ascribes to increased sympathicotonus. The leukocytosis is more marked in cases of obstructed labor and in primiparæ (Dietrich, Baer, 1916). Of the many theories as to its cause, that of Dietrich seems most plausible, that it is a reaction against the toxins of pregnancy; indeed, the blood in pregnancy resembles that in an acute infectious disease. The leukocytosis of labor is from muscular action.

Fahraeus found the precipitation rapidity of the reds, normally four times greater in women, increases with pregnancy, is greatest in labor, then quickly returns to normal. This is due to a difference between the electric charge of the corpuscles and that of the plasma (Hoeber).

The alkalinity of the blood is slightly diminished toward the end of pregnancy and in labor, as determined by the hydrogen-ion content, the alkali reserve, the CO_2 tension in the alveolar air, etc. The osmotic pressure is reduced, the freezing point being $-.533$, normal $-.55$. The ion and molecular concentration are also reduced. The amount of fibrin and fibrinogen increases from the sixth month of pregnancy, and may be one-third greater than usual. This increase of fibrin is probably a conservative act of nature to prevent dangerous loss of blood during labor. Perhaps the hyperinosis causes the thromboses sometimes observed in the veins of the leg and pelvis even before labor. Rebaudi says that the blood-platelets increase up to the time of labor, being 1,500,000 per c.mm., then rapidly decrease to 600,000. Their agglutinating properties increase with the number, therefore the coagulating power of blood is greatest just before labor.

The total quantity of blood is augmented, especially in the last months, a true plethora existing (Kaboth and Zuntz), a fact proved by Miller by means of the "vital red" method, the volume being between 6 and 9 per cent. of the body weight (Bohnen, 7–7.3 per cent.), the gain being 400 to 500 gm. The need for more blood must be admitted; the addition of the fetus and the fetal circulation, the development of the uterine arteries and veins, the enlargement of the veins of the lower extremities, which are sometimes so great that they appear to be veritable caverns. It would seem that they act as reservoirs and provide for the loss of blood at labor. The veins collapse afterward, but never completely or permanently. This surplusage of blood should not beguile the accoucheur to wastefulness of the vital fluid during delivery. The hemoglobin per kilo, fairly constant in pregnancy, decreases after delivery. Total hemoglobin is 6 per cent. + at term (Dieckmann).

Chauffard, in 1911, found an increase of the cholesterin in the blood, and at the seventh month a true lipoidemia. This and the lipemia are needed because the fetus uses much fat (Guillemet), and perhaps this increase has something to do with the augmented bactericidal power of the blood.

The blood-making organs show marked activity. The spleen grows from 140 to 180 gm. Barcroft found the spleen smaller in dogs. The lumbar glands enlarge, also the lymphoid structures of the endometrium. The lymph-glands all over the body are frequently enlarged in pregnancy (Meyer).

In the marrow of bone decided changes have been noted. Great congestion, and even a transformation of fat marrow to blood-forming marrow, have been found.

The Endocrine Glands.—An enormous literature has accumulated on this general subject, and not a little special work has been done on the relations of these glands to pregnancy, but the amount of proved knowledge is regretfully small. Here space permits only the barest outlines. For a fuller presentation of the theories and experimental work done, the reader is referred to Aschner, Bandler, Frank, Vignes, a review in 1926 by Capper, by Seitz in 1929, by Graves, 1931.

The *thyroid* becomes more vascular and almost always hypertrophies. The enlargement, sometimes a true hyperplasia, sometimes an increase of the colloid only, begins early in pregnancy and may not disappear completely after delivery. Lange claims that the thyroid has special bearing on toxemia and eclampsia. It has something to do with the growth of the fetus, the formation of monstrosities, and the stability of the pregnancy. The ovary (corpus luteum) activates the thyroid, sometimes to the point of producing symptoms of Basedow's disease (Frühinsholz, Lit.). Dysfunction of the thyroid, that is, maladaptation to the demands of the growing ovum, is not rare during pregnancy.

The *parathyroids* are also affected, though pathologic changes have not been seen, and if they do not supply sufficient secretion, symptoms of tetany appear during pregnancy, and in the child, too, after birth. Their action is bound up somehow with the calcium metabolism. Reduction of the calcium in the blood increases the irritability of the uterus, causing abortion, and upsets the sympathetic system, producing vasomotor symptoms.

The *hypophysis cerebri*, as first shown by Compte in 1899, hypertrophies during pregnancy. The chromophile cells are not affected, but the chromophobes are increased. The changes are most marked in the anterior lobe, which may become so large that it presses on the optic chiasm, causing hemianopsia and total blindness, or it may rupture its capsule. The changes in the chief cells are so pronounced that they are called "pregnancy cells." These cells persist and may be used for diagnosis of pre-existent pregnancy (Kolde).

The anterior lobe elaborates 5 (?) hormones more or less proven: (1) An ovarian follicle stimulating, prolan A; (2) a luteinizing, prolan B (Zondek), both of which increase so much during pregnancy that they appear in the urine, and when such urine is injected into immature mice, rats, rabbits, characteristic changes become visible in their ovaries (or testicles) which are used for the diagnosis of pregnancy (Zondek-Aschheim test); (3) a growth stimulating (Evans); (4) a metabolism regulating; (5) a breast activating hormone. (See Fig. 131a.)

Some of the symptoms and changes of pregnancy are acromegalic in nature, e. g., the large hands and feet, coarse features, the thick, coarse hair, the lowered voice pitch.

The posterior lobe, the part derived from the brain, possesses 3 hormones, one of which excites the uterus to powerful contraction, another raises the blood pressure, the third being antidiuretic.

The *adrenal glands* hypertrophy during menstruation and pregnancy, the change being more marked in the cortex. The secretion of the cortex is thought to be detoxicating, and tends to augment the lipoids in the body of gravida. Neu claims that a pregnancy adrenalinemia exists, but no one has been able to prove it, nor to show that the histology of the medulla (whence the adrenalin is supposed to originate) has undergone any change. Possibly the pigmentation of the skin, of the areolæ, and the mask of pregnancy are due to dysfunction of the adrenals.

The *pancreas* probably hypertrophies in pregnancy, and should this organ not adjust itself to the demands imposed on it, various symptoms might appear. Recurrent diabetes may be due to pancreatic inefficiency. Perhaps the vomiting of pregnancy may be related to the pancreas, at least it seems that the sugar metabolism is disturbed in hyperemesis. The kidney is very permeable to sugar even as early as the second and third months, and this fact is used as a basis of the sugar tests for pregnancy.

The *placenta* is one of the most important organs of internal secretion. Its hormones stimulate the development of the uterus and probably activate the thyroid, the hypophysis, parathyroids, adrenals, etc. Aschner ascribes the changes in the blood, in the liver, indeed, in the whole metabolism to the influence of the placenta. The placental hormone develops the breasts, but inhibits the formation of milk (Frankl).

Since one-half of the ovum is of paternal origin, its proteins are to an extent foreign to the mother, and one must be prepared to find reactions in her system similar to those which follow the introduction of other foreign proteins.

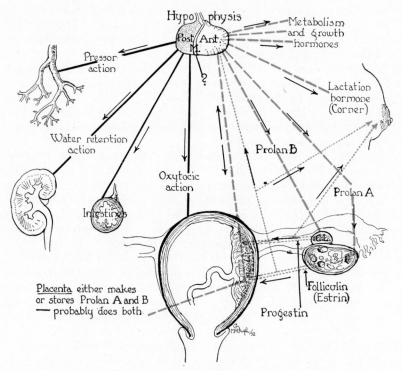

Fig. 131a.—Diagram Showing the Reciprocal Relations of the Hypophysis with Various Organs, as of August 1, 1932.

The functions of the ovary and the corpus luteum have been considered on page 9. After the placenta is fully developed it seems to take over the functions of the ovary and corpus luteum.

Of the other endocrines—the pineal, the thymus, the spleen—practically nothing is known. The endocrinal glands of the fetus functionate and probably affect those of the mother.

The Circulatory System.—The changes here are marked, the whole cardiovascular system being affected, though not in the same degree as was formerly believed. Larcher, in 1857, described an eccentric hypertrophy of the heart, especially of the left ventricle, Blot and other French authors agreeing with him. Later investigations (Müller and Dreysel), considering the weight of the body with that of the heart, have shown that there is only a slight if any enlargement, and that it is proportionate to the general increase of the body; and that Smith, aided by the electrocardiograph, found no hypertrophy. The arguments for accepting the theory of hypertrophy are: first, the physiologic need for more work by the heart; the increased amount of blood to be moved; the increased viscosity of the blood; the addition of the large area of blood-vessels of the placental circulation, and the dilated and new blood-vessels of the uterus; the increased abdominal tension; second, the results of postmortem measurements, the majority of authors finding some increase in weight; third, the clinical findings. There is an increase in the area of cardiac dulness due to the elevation of the diaphragm and leveling of the heart. Roentgen-ray examination of the chest in pregnancy (Kraus) shows two types— one with long thorax, a convex diaphragm, and undisturbed heart, another with short thorax, raised and flattened diaphragm, and heart placed horizontally. The heart in all cases is pressed against the anterior chest wall, displacing the lungs; thus the area of cardiac dulness is enlarged.

The cardiac output begins to rise in the fourth month, steadily grows to over 50 per cent. at term, is greater but undeterminable during labor, and returns to normal three weeks after delivery (Stander). Murmurs of various kinds are often heard over the heart, not transmitted far, and not always accompanied by accentuation of the second pulmonary sound. They are usually hemic in origin, but may be due to displacement of the heart, or kinking the pulmonary artery, and almost always disappear shortly after delivery. One must be slow to diagnose heart lesions in pregnancy, but it is generally admitted that the heart is peculiarly liable to disease during gestation, and that existing disorders are aggravated. Capillary angiospasm is found in 60 per cent. of normal gravidæ, and is one of the causes of edema (Hinselman).

The *blood-pressure* normally is 110 to 120, with 75 to 85 diastolic, subject to the usual fluctuations. The blood-pressure should not go above 140 mm., and even this advises caution, as indicating toxemia. During labor the blood-pressure is a little higher (130 to 140), especially during the pains (140 to 145). After the rupture of the membranes the pressure falls 40 to 50 points, but rises at once. It is highest during the expulsive efforts of the delivery, falls in the third stage (60 to 90 mm.), especially if there is hemorrhage, rises again after delivery, and slowly returns (in thirty-six hours) to normal during the puerperium (Slemons, Irving).

Pregnant women have a marked tendency to develop varicose veins of the lower half of the body. Nearly every one has at least one or more phlebectasiæ. In 20 per cent. of the cases the varicosities are marked. The usual sites are the legs, the vulva, the mons, the pelvis, the rectum, the anus, the vagina, the abdomen, the buttocks, in the order named. One or more or all the parts may be involved. One leg, usually the right, may exceed the other in the size and number of the varicosities. The surface veins are most affected. Of causes, several are given: increased venous congestion below the diaphragm, caused by the greater intra-abdominal tension of pregnancy; obstruction in the vena iliaca communis, due to the rush of blood from the enlarged vena hypogastrica; disturbed vasomotor conditions; increase in the total amount of blood, and enlargement of the veins to accommodate it; congenital anomaly of veins brought out by pregnancy; a toxic alteration of the blood and vein wall hypocalcemia. Predisposing causes are: Thin-walled veins, heart disease, tight girdles and garters, constipation, carrying heavy loads, frequent pregnancies. The state of pregnancy has mainly to do with the development of varices, because increased abdominal tension may exist without their occurrence, as in large ovarian tumors, ascites, etc. Parvin tells of a patient who knew she was pregnant as early as four weeks by the development of varicosities in the legs. Sometimes varicose veins shrink when the fetus dies. Compression of the cava by the uterus does not cause stasis in the veins below, because the specific gravity of the uterus is about the same as that of the intestinal mass. After the head has passed into the pelvis it may compress the internal iliac and hypogastric veins, but one does not often observe much difference from this unless there have been marked varicosities previously.

Edema is often associated with varices of the legs and has the same causes. It may occur alone, and may have other causes. The majority of gravidæ have some evidence of water retention, perhaps due to the incompetence of the kidney to excrete chlorids. Three kinds may be distinguished—the mechanical, due to the obstructed venous circulation in the abdomen, which disappears when the patient rests in the horizontal position; a general puffiness affecting the hands and face, as well as the legs, without urinary findings, commoner in hydremic patients, and which disappears rapidly after labor, perhaps due to wrong water balance;

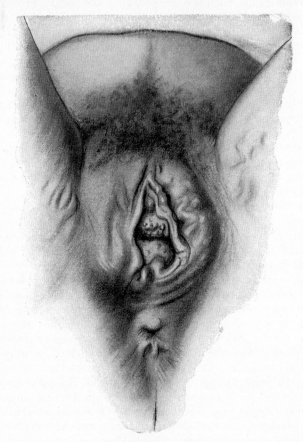

Fig. 132.—Varicose Veins of Vulva.
Drawn from a photograph.

a true anasarca, due to toxemia or nephritis, and always significant as a precursor of eclampsia. Possibly the latter two forms are allied. The edema of the legs may be enormous; the labia majora may be so infiltrated as to be translucent and as large as the fist; the sodden abdominal wall may hang down like a bag.

The **lungs** are displaced by the growing uterus. They retract to the sides, exposing more of the heart. The thorax is lifted up, is expanded laterally, and slightly diminished anteroposteriorly. Part of this change is permanent. The diaphragm is pushed up, but in fat subjects its upper curve is not convex, but flattened or even slightly depressed by the heart. These changes are more marked in primiparæ than in multiparæ, because of the lax abdominal wall in the latter. The respiration is more costal than abdominal because of the restricted excursion of the diaphragm, yet the lung capacity is increased, the breathing deeper and more frequent—cause, acidosis? More CO_2 is excreted. (See Alward and Klaften.) When lightening occurs at the end of pregnancy the chest is relieved. Changes which some rhinologists consider characteristic of pregnancy have been described as occurring in the nose and throat. The turbinates are turgid, even to closure of the nares or apposition against the septum. Perhaps these findings will explain the deafness and ringing in the ears some pregnant women have, or even some of the so-called neuroses (Freund). Brickner believes otosclerosis is peculiarly unfavorably affected by pregnancy. There seems to be an interrelation between the nasal cavities and the genitalia, cocainization of certain "genital" areas relieving dysmenorrhea and labor pains (Fliess). The larynx is somewhat congested, especially the false vocal cords, and there is some slight cellular infiltration of the tissues (Hofbauer), the changes being most evident in the interarytenoid fold. Sometimes symptoms result.

The Digestive Tract.—One of the first symptoms of pregnancy is the nausea and vomiting—the so-called "morning sickness." It may be present as early as the second week, but usually appears about the fifth, and persists until the twelfth week, though occasionally it continues until term. The patient is sick at the stomach on rising or after breakfast, and vomits the meal or only sour mucus, the overnight accumulation, being free from nausea the rest of the day. The feeling is similar to sea-sickness, and it is aggravated by sudden motion. The vomiting may recur at the end of pregnancy, after "lightening," due to the displacement of the stomach and intestines, but at this time the vomiting may also be due to toxemia, and mean that eclampsia threatens. Should the nausea and vomiting persist the greater part of the day, the case becomes pathologic. This will be considered under the subject Hyperemesis Gravidarum, p. 372. Morning sickness occurs in one-third of pregnant women. Its cause is obscure; perhaps it is a reflex from the uterus, or it may be toxemic, or due to disturbed relations of the ductless glands. Primiparæ are oftener affected than multiparæ. It occurs oftener in the higher classes of society and in the neurotic, perhaps from autosuggestion.

The salivary secretion is increased, and when the expectoration is frothy, it is called "cotton spitting." In some cases the patient is actually salivated; then the case is pathologic and needs treatment. The teeth easily decay due to the alteration of the secretions of the mouth, dentists say, probably not because of the demand of the fetus for more calcareous salts. Loosening of the teeth may occur. Gingivitis to a mild degree is also observed, but this borders on the pathologic. The taste is sometimes perverted, the gravida having a desire for unnatural things, as chalk, slate-pencils, sand, salt, etc. This symptom is called "pica," and may become morbid, as in the case of a woman who craved a bite of her husband's arm, and actually took it. It was considered dangerous to the fetus or mother to oppose these "cravings" of pregnant women, and all sorts of devices were employed to appease them. The appetite is usually increased unless nausea occurs; even then, after the vomiting, the patient is hungry. Some women have a voracious appetite in pregnancy, and often satisfy it to their detriment, in the belief, fostered by many, that they are eating for two. Again, anorexia is present or the appetite is fickle.

The *stomach* is displaced in the later months of gestation, being forced upward, backward, and to the left. The wall is congested, and pours out abundant watery secretion. Arzt found the hydrochloric acid decreased especially in the early months. Digestion is usually more active, and varies with the appetite.

The *liver* is forced upward, backward, and to the right in the late months. Liver dulness, therefore, must be corrected in this period. The liver is enlarged and hyperemic and Tarnier, in 1857, described a fatty infiltration around the intralobular veins, but this is not constant, and probably does not occur in normal pregnancy. There is more bile present, and dilatation of the bile-passages, also

8

ectasis of the central veins. The increased cholesterin content of the bile may explain the frequency of gall-stones in child-bearing women. Mechanical factors contribute also. Multinuclear cells, presumably from the placenta, even portions of villi, are sometimes found as emboii in the liver vessels. The integrity of the liver is severely tested by pregnancy and some of its functions do not always meet the demands. (See Couinard et Clogne.) (a) The need of the mother and fetus for iron causes much destruction of the erythrocytes which results in an excess of bile pigments—a cholemia occurring in at least 20 per cent. of cases. (b) The glycogenic function is often disturbed as evidenced by the hyperglycemia, the rapidity with which administered levulose appears in the urine, and the fact that a brief deprivation of carbohydrates results in acetonuria. (c) The ureogenic function is also subnormal and the liver is frequently unable to arrest all the unreduced albumin absorbed from the intestines. This is shown by Widal's test—leukopenia and hypercoagulability of the blood after ingestion of milk. (d) The complicated fat metabolism of the liver is often disturbed, and we therefore find a tendency to ketonemia because the fatty acids are not burned into CO_2 and water. The same is true of insufficiently aminized proteins and the alkali reserve is thus reduced. We find the alteration of the liver cells most marked in eclampsia, hyperemesis, and puerperal infection. (e) The requirements placed on the liver as a detoxicating organ are enhanced by pregnancy. (f) The excretion of bile pigments is reduced and we find urobilin in the urine and a high icteric index in the blood. (g) Finally, the internal secretion of the liver is of great influence in the genital sphere, especially during pregnancy and menstruation (Aschner).

The *intestines* are also affected by pregnancy. Constipation is almost the rule, being due to the displacement of the bowels, abnormal innervation, atony, general inactivity of the gravida, interference by the uterine tumor with bearing-down efforts in defecation. Hemorrhoids are common from the constipation and the increase of venous pressure below the diaphragm.

General Metabolism.—After a slight and inconstant initial loss the gravida puts on weight, rapidly up to the seventh month, then less rapidly until term, these changes corresponding to mutations of the general metabolism which Bar proved so clearly in dogs. The increase in weight is due to: (1) The fetus and secundines; (2) increased assimilation; (3) storing up of fat and albumin; (4) accumulation of water, especially in the lower extremities; (5) increase of the amount of blood. A store of potential energy is laid up for conversion into heat and force during labor, and milk during lactation. The hips round off and become broad; the breasts have more fat. If the fetus dies, this gain does not occur, or the patient may lose, and this fact may be used in the diagnosis of the death of the infant. The gain varies from 8 to 28 pounds, exceptionally less, and, pathologically, more, as much as 65 pounds. The rate of increase is 4 to 5 pounds up to the seventh month, then 4 to 3 pounds per lunar month until term (Hecker and Gassner, Kerwin, Toombs).

There is an increase of the basal metabolism rate sometimes reaching 35+ (Cornell, Baer). The thyroid incretion is increased (Eubinger). The nitrogen output is decreased, albumin being stored up amounting to 2000 gr. (about 300 gr. N.). Fat and iron are also stored up.

The eucolloidal state of the albumin and lipoids is dependent upon the presence of ions of sodium, calcium, potassium in proper proportion, *i. e.*, 100 : 2 : 2. In the last three months of pregnancy the amount of blood calcium is diminished (Rousseau, Lit.), which perhaps accounts for the increased irritability of muscles, nerves, heart, uterus, and possibly also for the high blood-pressure, edema and albuminuria. The action of other ions Mg, Fe, P, I, in varying concentration in the blood requires much study. (See Seitz, Macy, Adler et al.)

Most women feel better during pregnancy than at other times, but in some, especially the anemic and the neurotic, a condition of asthenia develops in the early months, the vegetative center in the brain not responding quickly enough to the call of pregnancy (Opitz, 1924). Later the nutrition is better, and the women may enjoy a permanent improvement in health from the stimulus of pregnancy. On the other hand, some women suffer a permanent neurasthenia from the strain of reproduction.

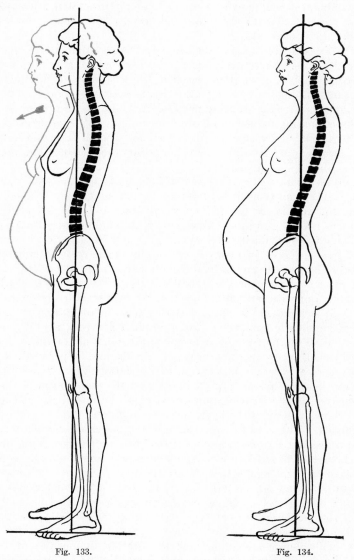

Fig. 133.   Fig. 134.

FIGS. 133 AND 134.—STATICS OF THE NON-PREGNANT AND PREGNANT WOMAN.
Arrow indicates direction of tendency to fall as abdominal tumor develops. Second figure shows effect of the adaptation.

The Urine.—The quantity is usually increased about one-fourth. This polyuria explains in part the frequent urination of pregnant women. The specific gravity is low, total solids and urea output being the same as or slightly less than in the non-pregnant state. The sulphates and phosphates do not change; the chlorids decrease, and water also is retained in the last months. Albumin is found in one-third to one-half of the cases of pregnancy, if one uses the finest tests. If one uses the hot and cold nitric acid tests, which, for practical purposes, are sufficient, one will find albumin in only 3 to 5 per cent. of gravidæ and 30 per cent. of parturients. The albuminura has been ascribed to lordosis, to latent bacterial influence, and to the abnormal permeability of the capillaries. Many times the albumin comes from the urinary tract or from the external genitals. Renal albuminuria, in the experience of the author, is rare in pregnancy, and should always be looked on with suspicion. Mild catarrhs of the bladder, pyelitis, and ureteritis are not uncommon in pregnant women. The highly congested, edematous bladder may permit the escape of albumin into the urine. The "kidney of pregnancy" is not normal. (See page 243).

Sugar is occasionally found in the urine during gestation, and is of two kinds— lactose and dextrose. Lactosuria occurs in 16 per cent. of gravidæ (Ney), is more pronounced near labor, most pronounced in the first week of the puerperium (77 per cent.), and disappears after lactation is discontinued, though it may be temporarily augmented by the weaning process. It is due to absorption of milk-sugar from the functionating breasts, and is not an unfavorable sign unless it is large in amount and attended by signs of disturbed nutrition. (See Literature.) True glycosuria, on the other hand, is more significant, though some authors describe a "physiologic diabetes of pregnancy."

The carbohydrate metabolism is not fully understood. The liver keeps the blood-sugar level from 0.09 to 0.18 per cent., but pregnancy is likely to disturb the mechanism and lower the kidney sugar threshold also, hyperglycemia and and glycosuria readily resulting. Alimentary, adrenalin and pituitary glycosuria are more likely to occur during gestation. One finds 0.01 per cent. of grape-sugar occasionally, as one does in men, but with the ordinary tests employed by the practitioner sugar is not regularly found in normal gravidæ. Its occurrence is always a matter of grave concern. (See Diabetes in Pregnancy, p. 552.) Acetone in the minute quantities usually found in women is also determinable during pregnancy. It is increased in amount during hard labor, during the first days of the puerperium, febrile conditions, toxemia and eclampsia, syphilis, ectopic gestation, and death of the fetus, but is not pathognomonic of this. Peptone, according to Fischel, occurs in 25 per cent. of gravidæ and 96 per cent. of puerperæ. It probably comes from the absorption of the fatty degenerative uterine tissue during involution and has no proved bearing on the metabolism of the fetus, the lochial discharge, or the fermentation processes of the intestine. It occurs in sepsis, acute yellow atrophy of the liver, toxemia, and eclampsia.

The Bones.—The bones in pregnancy show increased vascularity, especially the red marrow, and to a certain extent resemble the changes found in osteomalacia, but Loeschke has shown no demineralization exists; on the contrary, calcium, phosphorus, and magnesium are stored up. Fractures unite well in pregnancy, contrary to an old notion. In young women the author has observed a rapid growth of the pelvic bones during pregnancy, increasing materially the capacity of the pelvis due to osteogenesis around the pelvic joints under hypophyseal influence (Haslhofer).

The spinal column is straightened, the uterine tumor, prominent in front, changes the line of direction of the woman's person. This line of direction tends to fall anterior to her base of support. Therefore she throws her shoulders back and straightens her neck and head. The curve in the small of the back is exaggerated (Figs. 133 and 134), the pelvis being rotated slightly on the femora. These changes in the skeletal dynamics give the patient a peculiar attitude and gait or strut, which Shakespeare called the "pride of pregnancy." With marked softening of the pelvic joints, however, the patient has a waddling gait, because the innominates move on each other. These changes in the carriage require greater effort on the part of the gravida to maintain the erect position, which may cause weariness and backache. In cases of pendulous abdomen and with twins the changes in the attitude of the gravida are exaggerated. (See La Pointe; Putschar.)

The **skin** is much affected by pregnancy. Pigment is deposited in more or less typical regions—the nipples, the vulva, the linea alba, the navel, the face. The pigmentation of the linea alba changing it to a linea nigra, of the nipples already considered and of the face is most common. The forehead, cheek, and nose are covered with brown stains which cannot be wiped off. They, when marked, appear like a mask, and the condition has been called "the mask of pregnancy" (Fig. 135). This deposit of pigment in the rete cutis occurs oftener in nervous women or those suffering from uterine disease. Occurring outside of pregnancy, it is called chloasma uterinum. Brunets are more affected than blonds. Women of careless personal habits are more prone to manifest this sign, lack of attention to skin and

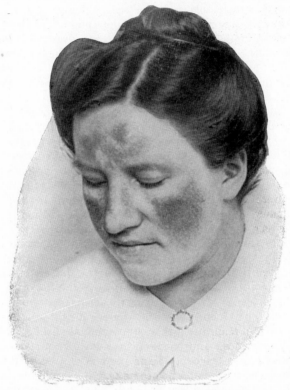

FIG. 135.—THE MASK OF PREGNANCY.
Photograph of case at the Chicago Lying-in Hospital.

bowels being a factor. The actual cause of the deposits is unknown—slow circulation in the capillaries, especially at the junction of the embryonal folds, hypertrophy of the suprarenals, active destruction of the red blood-corpuscles, abnormal iron metabolism, hepatic disturbances, and neurotic influences having all been invoked. According to Samuely, the pigmentation is due to the action of a ferment, tyrosinase, on the tyrosin in the blood during exposure to sunlight. Both the Blazek twins were pigmented, though only one was pregnant. A peculiar darkening of the eyelids has also been noted in pregnancy. It may be due to congestion or pigment. This pigmentation disappears mostly after labor, and especially when the menses are established, but some of it may persist for years. The vasomotor control of the cutaneous vessels is disturbed during pregnancy; thus one is able to produce red lines by simply drawing the finger over the surface. Sergent says that if a white line is thus produced the gravida has not enough epinephrin. The skin capillaries become more permeable to the serum, permitting the puffiness so frequently observed.

The sweat and sebaceous glands increase in activity, requiring more care of the patient to prevent odors. A delicate sense of smell may distinguish these odors as characteristic. In untidy women pityriasis versicolor is more likely to develop. The hair takes on increased growth, beginning about the third month of pregnancy; sometimes a fine lanugo appears on the face and chest (Apert). This excess of hair disappears two or three months postpartum—similarly to the effects of fevers. The nails are thinner. The subcutaneous fat becomes thicker, the finer features of the face coarser; the complexion in the early months is sallow, in the later months florid. Diseases of the skin are very common during pregnancy.

The Nervous System.—Pregnant women are more impressionable, subject to varying moods, are hyperexcitable, and sometimes a change in their character occurs, a quiet, sweet-tempered person becoming querulous and irritable, or vice versa. The author has only seldom observed such changes in any degree. In olden times pregnant women were considered morally irresponsible, and the condition was advanced in extenuation of crime. They are not reliable witnesses, perception being not so acute and interpretation false. Melancholia and real psychoses may develop, especially if there is a family taint. These symptoms may be the expression of a toxemia, as also may be neuralgias (especially facial, sciatic, and dental), the tingling and numbness in the extremities, headache, and disturbances of the special senses—hemeralopia, amaurosis, tinnitus. The exaggerated reflex excitability of the nervous system is manifested by marked skin and tendon reflexes, even ankle-clonus, occasionally Trousseau's and Chvostek's signs (tetany?), and by visceral reflexes, vomiting, indigestion. In the early months a tendency to sleep, especially after meals, is often noticed, and some women use this symptom to diagnose the pregnancy. Hysteric women suffer an exaggeration of their symptoms, and in them accesses of grand hysteria are more common.

The author has found many interesting mental phenomena by studying his cases psychologically. Pregnancy is the most momentous thing in the woman's life, and her mental adjustments, happy or unhappy, to the new condition will determine her health, spiritual as well as physical. In the majority of cases the patient rapidly adjusts herself to her new future even apparently overcoming the fear of death which all women admit they harbor more or less long. She may even be exalted in the realization that she is accomplishing the supreme purpose of a woman's existence. But to many the advent of pregnancy is undesirable or indeed a greater or less tragedy. Some become obsessed with the dread that they will die before the baby is born; others fear they will lose their beauty and, therefore, their attractiveness to the husband; some worry about having another mouth to feed, or because the child will interfere with their social pleasures; others, of masculine instincts, repudiate the responsibilities of motherhood because they hamper the "will to power." Deep undercurrents of feeling may be existent— such as antipathy to the family of the husband or to the personality of the husband or his religion; further, an undesire to bring more children into a contentious and chaotic world.

Many mental and nervous phenomena during pregnancy may be traced by psycho-analytic study to their hidden sources in the above-mentioned emotions— indeed, to deeper subconscious influences. Mental irritability, melancholia, psychoses, hyperemesis may be found to be a protest against the advent of pregnancy similar to the war psychoneuroses of soldiers.

A sort of fainting spell is a frequent complaint of pregnant women. It is accompanied by palpitation or fluttering of the heart, sometimes with pallor, and occasionally by slight loss of consciousness, resembling petit mal. Unless due to organic cardiac disease, the symptom, though annoying, is not dangerous.

LITERATURE

Adler, M.: Arch. für Gynaek., December, 1930, vol. 143, p. 236.—*Alward:* Amer. Jour. Obst. and Gyn., September, 1930, p. 373; also *Vejas:* vide infra.—*Apert, E.:* Jour. Amer. Med. Assoc., vol. 84, p. 925, 1925, Ref.—*Arzt:* Amer. Jour. Obstet. and Gyn., December, 1926, p. 879.—*Aschner:* Die Blutdrüsenerkrankungen des Weibes.—*Baer:* Surg., Gyn., and Obstet., November, 1916, p. 567.—*Bar, P.:* Leçons de Pathologie Obstetricale, Paris, 1907.—*Barcroft:* Jour. Amer. Med. Assoc., March 1, 1930. Current comment.—*Bohnen:* Arch. für Gynaek., 1925, Band 126, p. 144.—*Brickner:* Surg., Gyn., and Obstet., July, 1911.—*Capper:* Amer. Jour. Obstet. and Gyn., February, 1926.—*Chauffard:* L'Obstetrique, May, 1911.—*Couinaud et Clogne:* Gyn. et Obstetrique, 1923, vol. vii, No. 5, p. 372.—*Dietrich:* Arch. f. Gyn., 1911, vol. xciv, 2, p. 394. Gives literature.—*Evans:* See Novak, Jour. Amer. Med. Assoc., March 22, 1930.—*Fischel:* Arch. f. Gyn., vol. xxiv, p. 3.—*Fluhmann:* Collective Review, Amer. Jour. Obstet. and Gyn., November, 1926, p. 774.—*Frankl, O.:* Amer. Jour. Obst. and Gyn., October, 1923.—*Freund:* Monatsschr. f. Geb. u. Gyn., vol. xx, H. 3.—*Frühinsholz:* Rev. Mens. de Gyn. et d'Obst., 1921, p. 202.—*Guillemet:* Passage de la Graisse a travers de la placenta, Chantreau, Nantes, 1920.—*Hahl:* Arch. f. Gyn., vol. lxxv.—*Haslhofer:* Archiv. für Gyn., 1931, Band 147, H. 2, et seq.—*Hinselman:* Zentralblatt f. Gyn., 1921, No. 38, p. 1363.—*Hofbauer:* Zent. f. Gyn., 1908, p. 1196.—*Irving:* Jour. Amer. Med. Assoc., March 25, 1916.—*Kaboth:* Zentb. f. Gyn., 1923, March 31, p. 498, Lit.—*Kerwin:* Amer. Jour. Obst. and Gyn., April, 1926.—*Klaften:* Zentb. für Gynaek., April, 1925, p. 931.—*Kohn:* Münch. med. Woch., 1910, p. 1485.—*Kolde:* Arch. für Gyn., Bd. 98, 1912, p. 505.—*La Pointe and Thomas:* L'Obstetrique, December, 1911, p. 1148.—*Lange:* Zeitschr. f. Geb. u. Gyn., vol. xi, p. 34.—*Macy et al.:* Jour. Amer. Med. Assoc., June 14, 1930, p. 1920.—*Miller:* Jour. Amer. Med. Assoc., August 28, 1915.—*Miotti:* Annali di Ost. e Ginec., Milan, No. ix, p. 733.—*Müller and Dreysel:* Herzhypertrophie bei Schwangeren und Wochnerinnen, Munich, 1901.—*Ney, J.:* Arch. f. Gyn., vol. xxv, p. 239.—*Opitz:* Zentb. f. Gyn., 1924, p. 2.—*Putschar, W.:* Entwicklung, etc. der Beckenverbindungen des Menschen, Gustav Fischer, Jena, 1931.—*Rebaudi:* Amer. Jour. Obstet., October, 1907, p. 477.—*Rousseau, G.:* Dangers de la decalcification etc. au cours de la grossesse. Presses Universitaires, Paris, 1931.—*Seitz:* Monatsschr. für Geb., January, 1927, p. 323.—*Slemons:* Jour. Amer. Med. Assoc., September 8, 1917.—*Smith:* The Mother's and Newborn's Hearts in Pregnancy, Jour. Amer. Med. Assoc., July 1, 1922, p. 4.—*Stander, H. J., and Cadden, J. F.:* Amer. Jour. Obstet. and Gyn., July, 1932, p. 13.—*Toombs, P. W.:* Amer. Jour Obstet. and Gyn., December, 1931, p. 851.—*Vejas:* Volkmann's Sammlung klinische Vorträge, N. F. Gyn., 65.—*von Graff:* Arch. f. Gyn., 1912, vol. xcv.—*Zangemeister:* Zeitschr. für Geb. u. Gynaek., 1916, vol. 60, p. 325.—*Zuntz:* Zent. f. Gyn., October, 1911, No. 39; "Lactosuria," v. Noorden's Handb. der Path. des Stoffwechsels, vol. ii, p. 238; Hofmeister u. Kaltenbach, Zeitschr. f. physiol. Chem., vol. ii, p. 360; F. J. McCann, Lancet, April 24, 1897, p. 1174.

CHAPTER V

THE LENGTH OF PREGNANCY

WHILE it is important for many reasons to know the exact length of human gestation, we have to be satisfied with surmises and generalities. Ovulation may occur at any time. Authorities disagree as to the relation of the discharge of the ovum from the ovary to the time of menstruation. We do not know if an ovum is fertilizable when it leaves the Graafian follicle, or if it requires time, and if so, how much. We do not know how long it takes the spermatozoid to reach the ovum. Therefore it is impossible to determine the time of conception, even when the date of the fruitful coition is certain. Further, labor occurs often as the result of some trauma—physical or mental.

Since the beginning and the end of pregnancy are indeterminable, of course we cannot estimate the exact length of the period. As a datum for the reckoning the menses are absolutely unreliable, since a woman may menstruate during the first months of pregnancy, in which case it would seem that she bore a fully developed infant after a short gestation, and, on the other hand, a woman may conceive during a period of amenorrhea, thus giving the impression that pregnancy was prolonged to ten or even fourteen calendar months. This will explain those cases of pregnancy lasting three hundred and eighty to four hundred days (Parvin).

The most reliable datum from which to estimate the beginning is the date of fruitful coition, and, reckoning from this day, pregnancy has been found to vary from two hundred and twenty to three hundred and thirty days, the average being two hundred and seventy days. In cows the average length of pregnancy is two hundred and eighty-five days, but a fully developed calf may be delivered any time from two hundred and forty-one to three hundred and twenty-one days after the cow was covered (Ahlfeld, Schwarz). From time immemorial women have reckoned two hundred and eighty days, ten lunar months, or nine calendar months, from the first day of the last period as the length of normal gestation, and for practical purposes this may be accepted, because in the majority of cases it holds true, but one must remember and admit the exceptions. (See p. 25.) No doubt some children require a longer time in the uterus for full development than others. Some seeds in favorable soil grow faster than others. The writer has delivered children that were carried eight months that were as matured as full-term infants, and also in one case, he delivered a child weighing three and one-half pounds which was fully three weeks over term. Heyn had a case of two hundred and twenty-nine-day pregnancy, with child of 2980 gm. and 50 cm. length

The French law recognizes the legitimacy of a child born one hundred eighty days after marriage, and three hundred days after the death of the husband, the German law one hundred eighty-one and three hundred twenty-one days, respectively. In England, in 1921, the legitimacy of a child born three hundred thirty-one days after the husband went to war was allowed. (London Letter.) Fothergill reports a cesarean section three hundred and forty-four days after the last coitus. In America each case is decided on its merits.

The author delivered a viable child one hundred eighty-two days after the day of conception, Ronaldson one of one hundred eight-nine days. The reader desiring authorities in medicolegal cases of this kind should consult v. Winckel, Siegel, Eden, McCaffery, Engelman, (1927), and Peterson and Haines.

Without doubt pregnancy may be prolonged and an overgrown child delivered. Hannes found that in 50 per cent. of children weighing more than 4000 gm. (8¾ pounds) the pregnancy had lasted more than two hundred and eighty days. Ciulla

120

found that in 1 case of 200 the pregnancy lasted more than three hundred and twenty days. Children that are carried over term may be larger in all dimensions, or they may grow longer and harder (Bossi). The cranial bones ossify, the biparietal diameter increases, the body becomes firmer and less pliable; thus in both instances delivery is rendered difficult and more dangerous to mother and child Children that are being carried over time not seldom die before labor. A careful autopsy performed in a case of this kind showed no pathologic changes except granular degeneration of the epithelium of the kidneys. In some instances labor pains come on at the computed term of pregnancy, but they subside and a period of three or four weeks elapses until actual delivery occurs. The author considers it inadvisable to allow a woman to continue far beyond the normal date of term, and, in the interest of both child and mother, induces labor in such cases. "Missed labor" is a term introduced by Oldham to describe cases where pains come on when expected, but cease, the child dies, and is carried in the uterus a greater or shorter time, as, in one case, eleven months. A dead ovum carried in the uterus is not pregnancy. Various factors may influence the length of gestation, as the age of the woman, the sex of the child, etc. Young women are likely to have a shorter gestation; older women, longer. Women who have been sterile for years and old primiparæ are likely to go over term. Women who had delayed puberty, dysmenorrhea, who have long hard rigid cervices, are also likely to have delayed labor. Primiparæ, except old ones, not seldom fall into labor a few weeks before the date set, the tense abdominal wall forcing the head into the pelvis against the cervix, which evokes pains. Males are said to be carried longer than females. While this is true in animals, the author cannot confirm it from his own experience. Women who are active in the last months of pregnancy are less likely to go over term than the lazy ones, who take no exercise. One notices this in hospital practice. There is a popular notion that a gravida should exercise much during gestation or "the baby will be grown to her side," meaning that she will have a difficult labor from overgrowth of the infant. In summer women are likely to give birth earlier than in winter. Heredity seems to play a rôle. De la Motte reports the case of a woman who had two children at the seventh month. These girls grew up, married, and had children at seven months. Retzius describes an instance of a mother and her two daughters, in all of whom pregnancy was much prolonged.

Precocious and Late Pregnancy.—The earliest authentic pregnancy is reported by Bodd. The girl was eight years and ten months old, and delivered a child weighing 3500 gm. (about 7½ pounds), which had hair on the pubis. Pregnancy in girls of twelve to fifteen is not rare, and experience shows that most of the children live and that labor is seldom difficult. The pelvis develops rapidly during pregnancy, and the child is usually small, with a soft head, which accounts for the unexpected safety of these precocious labors. The latest pregnancy on record is the one reported by Kennedy. The woman was sixty-two years old, and this was her twenty-second labor. The author delivered a woman of fifty-two years safely of a living infant weighing over seven pounds. In some of the cases reported (Strassman) menstruation had been absent for years.

Literature

Ahlfeld: Lehrb. des Geb., 1903, p. 94.—*Bodd:* L'Abeille Medical, 1882.—*Bossi:* Gynäkologischer Rundschau, Vienna, vol. i, No. 1.—*Ciulla:* Zeitschr. f. Geb. u. Gyn., 1910, vol. lxvii, H. 2. Literature.—*Eden:* London Lancet, June 16, 1923, p. 1199.—*Engelman:* Zentb. für Gynaek., January 1, 1927, Lit.—*Fothergill:* Jour. Obst. and Gyn. of British Empire, vol. xxviii, No. 344.—*Hannes:* Zent. für Gyn., 1912, p. 1471.—*Heyn:* Ref. Zentb. für Gynaek., March 20, 1926.—*Kennedy:* Trans. Obstet. Soc., Edinburgh, 1882, vol. vii.—*London Letter:* A Ten Months' Child, Jour. Amer. Med. Assoc., August, 1921, p. 716.—*McCaffery:* Amer. Jour. Obstet. and Gyn., July, 1925, p. 107.—*Parvin:* Obstetrics, p. 210.—*Peterson and Haines:* Legal Medicine and Toxicology, I, 66.—*Retzius:* Ribemont, Dessaignes, and Le Page: Precis d'Obstetrique, p. 196.—*Ronaldson:* Edinb. Obs. Soc. Trans., vol. vi.—*Schwarz:* Zentb. für Gynaek., April, 1925, p. 905.—*Siegel:* Zentralbl. für Gyn., July 16, 1921, p. 994.—*Strassman:* Handb. d. Geb., vol. i, p. 95.—*v. Winckel:* Volkmann's klin. Vorträge, N. F., 1901, p. 293; Handb. d. Geb., vol. i, p. 652.

PHYSIOLOGY OF LABOR

CHAPTER VI

DEFINITION—CAUSES—CLINICAL COURSE

Labor is a function of the female organism by which the product of conception is expelled from the uterus through the vagina into the outside world, the regressive metamorphosis of the genitals started, and the secretion of milk inaugurated. There are three essential points in the definition, which excludes the extraction of the fetus by any other passage, as in cesarean section. Synonyms for labor are delivery, parturition, travail, childbirth, accouchement, confinement.

Abortion is the interruption of pregnancy before the fetus is viable, *i. e.*, capable of extra-uterine existence, which is after the twenty-sixth week.

Premature labor is the interruption of pregnancy after the fetus is viable, but before term, *i. e.*, the normal end of gestation.

Miscarriage is an expression used by the laity to signify the occurrence of a premature interruption of the pregnancy at any time.

Labor should be a normal function of the human female. It is so intricate, however, that a great many irregularities may mark its course. The unhygienic surroundings in which women live, prior diseases, the tendency to laziness, the evils of dress, of living, occupation, heredity, chronic endometritis, salpingitis, the evolution of the fetal head, *i. e.*, increased size of the child's cranium, due to the increased mental capacities of the race, all tend to produce conditions which influence the course of labor and may make it absolutely impossible in a given case, or fraught with great, even fatal, danger.

We must, therefore, divide cases into two groups:

1. Normal labor, or *eutocia*.
2. Abnormal (pathologic) labor, or *dystocia*.

As a matter of fact, a really normal labor without the slightest irregularity is rare; almost always there is some small point that is peculiar, although it may not affect the course of the labor, and the case may end favorably for mother and child. In general we call those cases normal where we do not have to interfere—where the woman expels the child and placenta herself, and she and the child live. Strictly speaking, however, unless the woman's condition is exactly as good as it was before conception and the child perfectly well and uninjured, the labor may not be called normal. Such cases as these are excessively rare. The boundaries between eutocia and dystocia are very narrow, and depend largely on the individual views of the obstetrician. Certain complications are classed by some under eutocia, while by others they are called distinctly pathologic. For example, I consider the vomiting of pregnancy, the kidney of pregnancy, breech and face presentation, rupture of the urogenital septum, to be pathologic conditions, while many authors hold them to be normal.

In the study of the phenomena of parturition four factors must be considered: (1) The *powers*, by which the expulsion of the ovum is accomplished; (2) the *pas-*

sages, which represent the road and the resistances met; (3) the *passengers*, the child and its adnexa (placenta, etc.); and (4) *external complications* which may disturb the course of the function. The last-named factor is the pathologic one, and will be omitted for the present. The other three factors make up the study of the mechanism of labor.

The Causes of Labor.—What brings on labor? Why should the uterus, which has carried the ovum for so many months, suddenly violently expel it? Nature certainly recognizes the right moment for the expulsion, since it is almost always accomplished at a time when the child is best able to carry on extra-uterine existence and before it has become too large to pass safely through the parturient canal. What the cause is that sets the uterus in action has been the subject of much speculation and investigation, but nature still hides the secret. It is probably hormonal. We wish to know because often it is necessary to bring on labor ourselves, and experience has shown that it is wise to follow nature's methods. The many theories can only be touched upon. (Lit. Jour. Obstet. and Gyn. of Brit. Empire, 1930, August.)

1. Through degeneration of the decidua the ovum becomes a foreign body. Untenable.
2. Increase of CO_2 in the maternal blood from thrombosis of the placental vessels, or of the fetal blood, irritates the uterus to contraction. Untenable.
3. Excessive distention of the uterine wall. True only of pathologic cases, twins, polyhydramnion.
4. That labor comes on through endocrinal influence is an attractive theory, but no proposition yet advanced has been proved. Dixon and Marshall believe that the decadence of the corpus luteum late in pregnancy removes the inhibitory influence which the folliculin of the ovary normally exerts on the hypophysis. The latter therefore secretes more pituitary hormone which evokes pains. Removal of the corpus luteum does not always bring on abortion or labor, and labor can occur without the ovaries. (See Bourne and Burn.)

The influence of menstruation continues during pregnancy as is evidenced by certain symptoms which occur, mostly in nervous women. Why labor should occur on the completion of ten menstrual cycles is unknown. Neuralgic pains, especially in the sacrolumbar region, insomnia, skin eruptions, increase of the varicosities, vomiting, nausea, diarrhea, constipation, decreased urine, sometimes albumin, uterine pain, sometimes small hemorrhages, and the tendency to abort are greater at these periods. G. de Paoli studied these changes in 30 women, and found: diminished lung capacity; lower blood-pressure; increased sensibility of the skin and of the reflexes; more rapid pulse. Aschner calls these symptoms of menorrhemia. Pathologic conditions are more common at these periods, for instance eclampsia, fainting, hysteria, pains in the bones. Labor is more likely to follow a slight trauma at this period.

V. der Heide and Sauerbruch in their experiments on rats (uniting one pregnant with a non-pregnant one in parabiosis) discovered that substances appeared in the blood which were poisonous to the non-pregnant animal, the reaction much resembling anaphylaxis. By injecting fetal serum into pregnant women pains were sometimes induced. The serum of a woman in labor rarely caused pains in a woman near term, but did sometimes cause anaphylactic collapse. In the Blazek twins (thoracopagi) when one was in labor the other was unaffected, probably being immunized during pregnancy by the first.

It does seem that something develops in the blood which either brings on labor or so sensitizes the uterus that an ordinary external irritant sets the process in motion. The uterus contracts throughout pregnancy and becomes increasingly irritable toward its end. Neu says this is due to the accumulation of suprarenin in the blood. Perhaps it is pituitary hormone. Blair Bell believes there is an increase of the pressor substances in the blood and tries to bring this into relation with the calcium content.

5. Pressure of the presenting part on the lower uterine segment, on the cervix, and the nerves of the great cervical and retrocervical ganglia, and other plexuses around the cervix and upper vagina, is an old (Galen. Power) and favorite theory, but it will not explain all cases, such as breech, and transverse presentation, and the uterine contractions of extra-uterine pregnancy. In some cases the head may be deep in the pelvis, and pressing hard on the cervix, without evoking pains. Still, clinical experience shows that when the child settles well into the lower uterine segment the dilatation of the cervix begins, and labor comes on. The methods employed in inducing labor nearly all operate by irritations applied to the nerves of this region, e. g.. the packing of the cervix with gauze, the application of colpeurynters, bougies, etc. One can often bring on labor by passing the finger around the internal os and stretching it a little.

6. The importance of accident, however, must not be overlooked. When everything is ready for labor, the parts softened, the cervix begun to unfold, the uterine muscle well developed and having attained a high degree of irritability, it is easy to see how some slight cause, mechanical or emotional, may suddenly start the uterine contractions. As soon as one contraction has occurred it seems to form the irritant for another, or forces the ovum against the cervix, stimulating the nerves, so abundant here, and thus labor is put in progress. Such exciting causes are: physical shocks—jolts, running up or down stairs, coitus, diarrhea, straining at stool; mental shocks—

sudden fright or joy—of which there are numerous illustrious examples. The Bible tells us that the wife of Phineas, upon hearing that her husband was killed in battle, went into labor. A patient of the author's, feeling that her labor was due, walked down and up the six flights of stairs to her hotel apartment. Pains came on within a few hours. She had a slight hemorrhage behind the placenta. A dose of castor oil or quinin will often bring on labor at term.

THE CLINICAL COURSE OF LABOR

It will be simpler to study the complicated problems of labor if, first, we get a clear picture of its clinical course; that is, what may be seen and felt while attending a woman in parturition.

In most primiparæ and many multiparæ there is a prodromal stage of labor, but in both the symptoms may be so slight that they may be unnoticed, and labor, therefore, seems to come suddenly. The prodromata are: (1) Lightening, with its symptoms, relief of pressure in the upper belly, and increase of pressure in the pelvis, together with a mucous discharge from the vagina. (2) False pains; in the latter weeks of pregnancy the patient is often annoyed by contractions of the uterus which are painful. They occur especially at night, subsiding toward morning. The uterus contracts at intervals throughout pregnancy, and shows greater irritability near the end. This sign is of value in determining that labor is at hand. Ordinarily, the contractions are not painful until actual labor sets in. False pains may be simulated by gas in the bowels, constipation, and appendiceal or gall-stone colic. Many women complain of drawing sensations in the pelvis similar to those experienced during menstruation, sometimes amounting to pain; these are called dolores præsagientes, and often accomplish effacement and dilatation of the cervix. (3) About twenty-four or forty-eight hours before labor there is a discharge of mucus, often mixed with blood. It is the plug which formerly filled the cervix, closing off the uterine cavity from the vagina. The blood comes from the surface left bare by the separation of the decidua. It is more or less profuse, is important, and is called the "show." If the placenta is situated low in the uterus, the show is likely to be quite bloody. Occasionally the show does not appear until labor has been in progress some time. (4) An examination in the last three weeks of pregnancy shows the cervix soft, shortened, perhaps completely effaced—in primiparæ the external os opened for one or perhaps two fingers. In multiparæ the cervix will admit two fingers to the membranes. Exceptionally, the external os, as well as the internal, remains tightly closed until labor begins, but this is abnormal, and is usually due to cervical disease. Occasionally the os is dilated to admit three or four fingers—the result of the "travail insensible" of the French. However, it is unsafe to predict with certainty the near approach of labor from the patulousness of the cervix, though it is quite probable. (5) The vulva is enlarged, succulent, and patulous, the pelvic floor projection very decided.

The painless contractions of the last weeks of pregnancy, the "insensible labor," force the head down into the pelvis and soften the structures—the lower pole of the fetus seems to slowly burrow its way into the pelvic excavation.

The transition into labor is usually very gradual, but we say that labor has begun when the contractions of the uterus become sensible to the patient—that is, painful; when they recur at regular intervals, and when they are effective in dilating the cervix and os.

The process of parturition naturally divides itself into three stages or periods:

The first stage extends from the beginning of regular uterine contractions until the os is completely dilated and flush with the vagina, thus completing the continuous channel called the "parturient canal." This is the stage or period of dilatation. The membranes usually rupture at the end of this stage—perhaps during it. The first stage does not include the rupture of the bag of waters, the time of which is very variable.

The second stage extends from the end of the first stage until the expulsion of the fetus is completed. It is the stage of expulsion.

The third stage extends from the delivery of the child until after the expulsion of the placenta and membranes and contraction and retraction of the uterus are completed. It is the period of the after-birth, or the placental stage.

In the first stage, recurring regularly about fifteen minutes apart, we notice the uterine contractions. These are appreciated by the patient as pain, and have been, therefore, designated by the various races from time immemorial as "pains," "dolores," "douleurs," "Wehen." No normal labor is painless, though quite a few such have been observed. Writers of all ages have described labor as painful

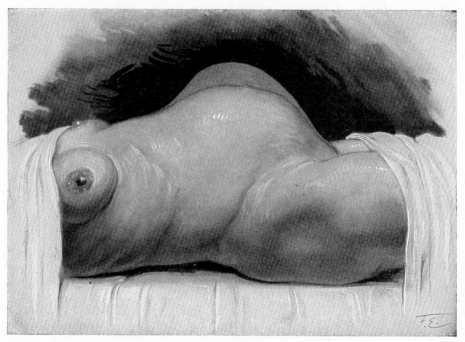

Fig. 136.—Composite Picture Showing the Uterus before and during Contraction.

The Bible mentions it in numerous places. Accounts of uncivilized races disprove the claim made by some that with them child-bearing is painless. (See Ploss, "Das Weib in der Natur und Völkerkunde"; Engelman, "Labor Among Primitive Peoples.")

Still, the severity of the pain varies. Some races, especially the uncivilized, have generally easy labors, whereas the highly cultured woman has hard, painful labors. This is true to a certain extent, in our civilized country, in the difference between the poor and the rich. The pain varies in different women, and the ability to stand pain varies in women, as it does in men.

As the labor progresses the pains gradually grow stronger. Whereas at first the patient just bends over a little, shows a change of countenance, after a few hours she may utter a cry. The cry is simply one of pain, similar to that of a severe toothache or intestinal colic. One observes much individual difference in women regarding the pain of labor. Those of quiet, even temperament and strong will-power bear their sufferings bravely and aid the physician and nurse, while the nervous, hysteric parturient cries out even early in the first stage, demanding an anesthetic or even delivery, and not seldom gives an otherwise normal labor a pathologic trend. The very first pains are usually felt in the small of the back, but soon they draw around to the front and are described as grinding, or like a severe general intestinal colic. They often seem to come in pairs—a mild one followed by a severe one. They last thirty to ninety seconds or longer. The character of the pain varies in different women, different labors, and different times of one labor. They may subside and recommence after hours or days (rare). The patient is cheerful between pains or may doze. As the pains grow stronger the intervals become shorter—ten, eight, five, four minutes. During the pain one observes the uterus contract. This begins before the pain is felt, and ends after the painfulness is over (Fig. 136). The uterus rises high in the abdomen, increases in diameter anteriorly and posteriorly, and decreases laterally, assuming a pear shape. At the same time it becomes

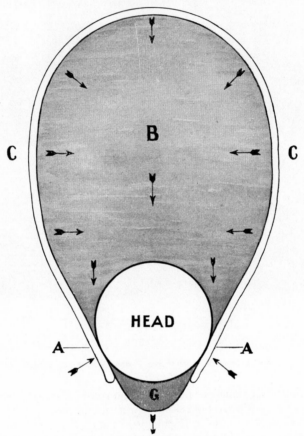

Fig. 137.—Ball-valve Action of Head.
Head at A–A divides uterus into two cavities. Pressure in G is much less than in B.

tender, tense, and the ligaments stand out sharply. There is a stage of accrement, acme, and decrement in each pain.

Under the influence of the uterine contractions—

1. A larger amount of the serum is forced into the lower uterine segment, cervix, and upper vagina.

2. The fibers of the lower uterine segment and cervix are drawn up into the body of the organ.

3. The liquor amnii is forced in the direction of the internal os.

4. The membranes are bulged out through the cervix.

5. The retraction of the fibers of the lower uterine segment and cervix, and the membranes being forced down into the cervix like a bladder, cause a dilatation of the cervix from above downward, and finally the full opening of the external os.

This dilatation of the cervix by the bag of waters is a very gentle and efficient one. The whole force of the uterus is not used, since the head resting against the lower uterine segment divides the cavity into two parts (Fig. 137). The resistance at A–A diminishes the power of C–C, therefore the tension in G is not so great as in B. Should the body not press fast to A–A, allowing the fluid in B to communicate with

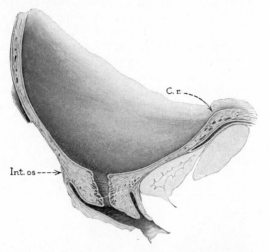

Fig. 138.—Cervix at Beginning of Labor. (From Schroeder's frozen section.)

the fluid in G, the tension in G would equal that of the space of B. This occurs often clinically. During a pain the tension in B rises; therefore also of G, but to a less degree; when the pain passes away the tension in both subsides. Thus it is seen how the head acts as a ball-valve, and becomes, with the membranes, the gentlest possible method to efface and dilate the cervix. Compare this to the rough dilata-

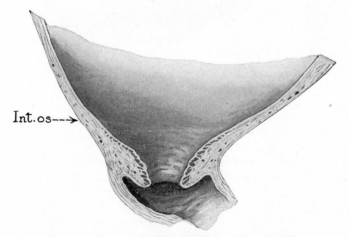

Fig. 139.—Effacement Half Completed. (From Leopold.)

tion which would occur were there no bag of waters, and if the head were driven through the cervix by uterine and abdominal forces. This happens when the bag of waters ruptures before labor, especially in primiparæ. These are called "dry labors," and are often long, tedious, and painful. Operative interference is oftener necessary in dry labors.

We have used two terms which need explanation—effacement and dilatation of the cervix. At the beginning of labor the cervix is shaped as in Fig. 138.

By the action of the uterus, which we will later study more minutely, the muscle-fibers are drawn up into the uterine body, the membranes are forced, pouch like, into the cervical canal, the two processes resulting in a dilatation of the cervix from above downward. The cervix is "taken up," it is "obliterated," it is "shortened," it is "effaced." The latter term is the one preferred by the author. When the cervix is so far taken up that only the external os remains, we say that effacement is complete. Dilatation now begins (Fig. 143). When the external os is opened so wide that it is flush, or nearly so, with the vagina, dilatation is complete, and the child is now able to pass through it (Fig. 144). Coincident with the dilatation the cervix is drawn up into the abdomen, so that, when the dilatation is complete, the external os is high—almost out of the reach of the finger. The bag of waters usually ruptures at this point.

The comparison of the parturient passage to two funnels, one placed above the other, is quite apt. The child has to pass first through the upper, the cervix, and, second, through the lower, the pelvic floor. Effacement of the cervix and dila--

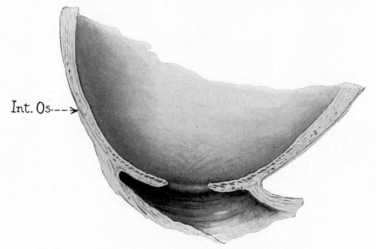

Int. Os--->

FIG. 140.—CERVICAL CANAL OBLITERATED
Effacement complete. Dilatation just beginning.

tation occasionally occur simultaneously, especially in multiparæ (Figs. 141 and 142). When the cervix is fully opened, the first stage of labor is ended, and the second stage begins.

The Bag of Waters.—Baudelocque defined the bag of waters as that portion of the membranes which pouched into the cervix during the uterine contraction. Later writers gave the name to that portion of the membranes which was uncovered by dilating the os. Others call the whole amniotic sac the bag of waters. The author prefers the latter view, though when speaking of the bag of waters the part presenting over the os is the part usually referred to. At the beginning of labor the membranes point into the cervix like a flat cone. As the dilatation progresses the bag of waters assumes the shape and appearance of a large watch-crystal, projecting through the os (Fig. 146). If the membranes are soft and exposed to the whole pressure in the uterus, they bulge out into the vagina or may rupture early. If the chorion ruptures, the amnion may project through the partly dilated os like a sac (Fig. 148). If the head fits closely on to the lower uterine segment and the membranes are firmly adherent, no bag of waters forms, and labor is usually delayed in such cases (Fig. 149).

The best time for the membranes to rupture is when the cervix is completely effaced and dilated, but they may break at any stage, even before the pains begin (dry labor). If the chorion ruptures alone, the amnion may be pushed out, cover-

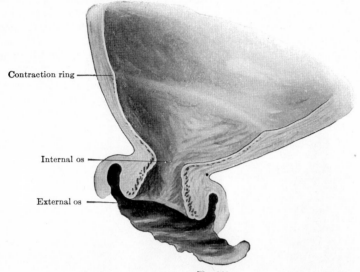

Contraction ring

Internal os

External os

Fig. 141.

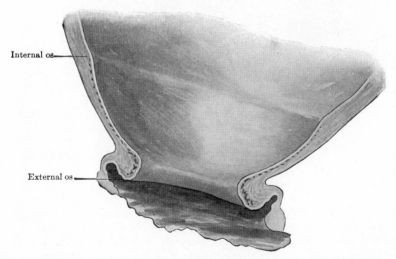

Internal os

External os

Fig. 142.

FIGS. 141 AND 142.—TWO STAGES OF THE COMBINED EFFACEMENT AND DILATATION OF A MULTIPAROUS CERVIX.

ing the head of the advancing child, and may be delivered with the latter. The child is said to be born with a "caul" and to be lucky. The caul must be removed as soon as the head is born, to allow the infant to breathe.

The rupture of the bag of waters usually takes place at the height of a strong pain, and is oftenest central, the waters coming with a gush. Or the rupture may take place high up, and the waters dribble away at each pain. Sometimes an ac-

9

cumulation of fluid between the two membranes occurs, and the chorion ruptures while the amnion remains intact.   Thus there seem to be two bags of water.

After the rupture of the bag of waters there is generally a short pause in the pains.   The uterus needs time to accommodate itself to the diminished size of its cavity and for the retraction of its muscular lamellæ.   A few drops of blood may now appear, coming from decidual separation.

Coincidentally with these changes in the cervix the fetal body has descended lower into the pelvis, the bag of waters or the head distends the vagina and may reach the pelvic floor.   It presses on the nerves of the rectum and outlet of the pelvis, and the parturient feels like bearing down as if at stool.

The Second Stage Has Begun.—The pains grow stronger, more frequent,— every three or two minutes,—and are changed in character, being expulsive.   The patient utters a peculiar cry.   She feels there is a body in the pelvis which she must force out; she closes the glottis, having fixed the chest in inspiration, braces the

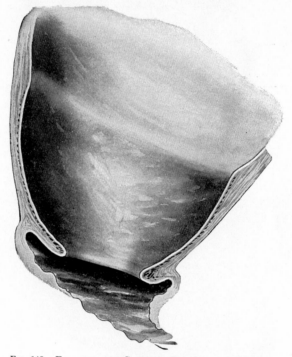

FIG. 143.—EFFACEMENT IS COMPLETE, DILATATION IS GOING ON.

feet against the bed, and, by a powerful action of the abdominal muscles, drives the head downward against the perineum.   During the contraction the uterus becomes board-like in hardness.   The parturient is working hard—indeed, the process is rightly called labor.   Her pulse is high, the veins of the neck stand out, the thyroid is swollen, a condition which Aëtius in 1567 said caused goiter, the face is turgid, the body bathed in sweat.

Owing to the pressure of the head on the sacral and obturator nerves as they go out of the pelvis, and to the distraction of the pelvic joints the patient complains of pains radiating into the legs and to the back.   In general she is more hopeful, since she can help and feels that there is progress in the labor, whereas in the first stage all she could do was to bear the suffering.

The perineum soon begins to flatten out and soften.   The glands pour out a glairy mucus which lubricates the passage.   The woman complains of pressure on the rectum, and may insist on having the bed-pan. Occasionally there are feces in the bowel which is being forced down by the advancing head, but more often the

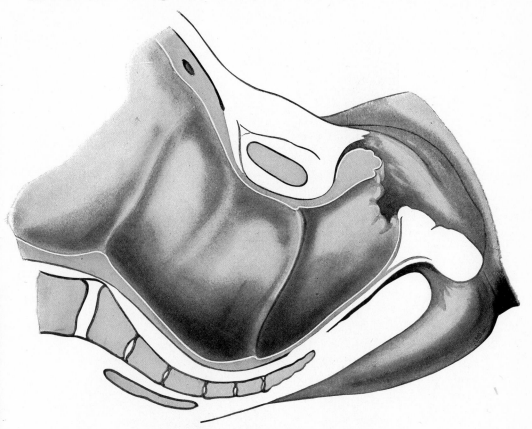

FIG. 144.—BOTH EFFACEMENT AND DILATATION ARE COMPLETE.

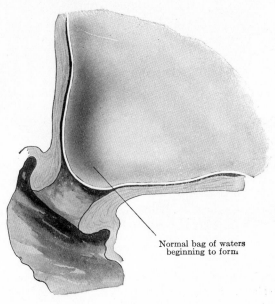

Normal bag of waters beginning to form

FIG. 145.

sensation is due to the head itself pressing on the rectum. After thirty to forty minutes the anus begins to open, and, if the woman has hemorrhoids, these swell up

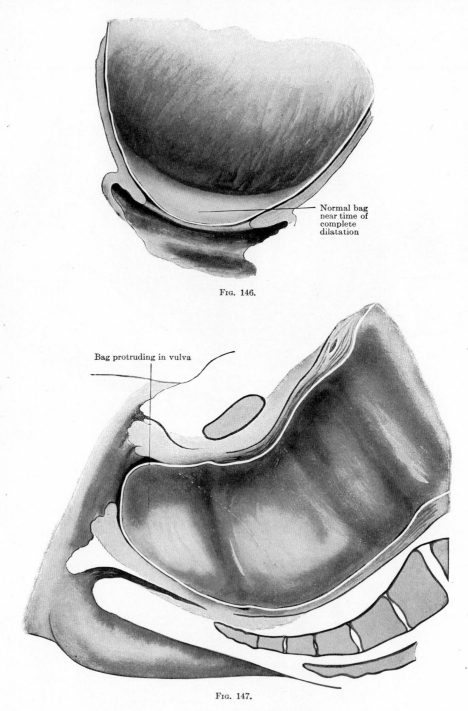

Normal bag
near time of
complete
dilatation

FIG. 146.

Bag protruding in vulva

FIG. 147.

almost to bursting. Soon the labia part during the height of a pain, allowing the wrinkled scalp to show. As the pain subsides the elastic pelvic floor forces the head back. With the next pain the perineum bulges more, the anus opens wider, so that one may see its anterior wall, the labia part further, and a larger segment of the scalp becomes visible. As the pain disappears the head recedes. In the interval between pains the woman lies back exhausted, or may have a few moments' re-

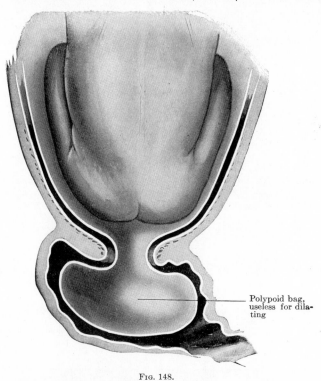

FIG. 148.

Figs. 145, 146, 147, and 148 represent the different shaped bags of waters.

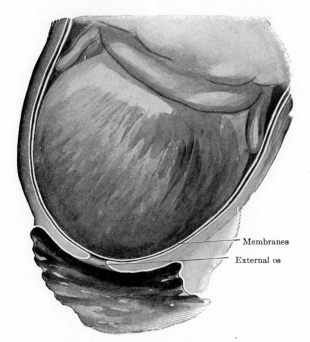

Polypoid bag, useless for dilating

Membranes

External os

FIG. 149.—BAG FITS FETAL HEAD LIKE A CAP. DOES NOT AID DILATATION, AND OFTEN OBSTRUCTS LABOR.

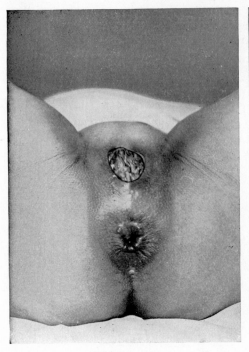

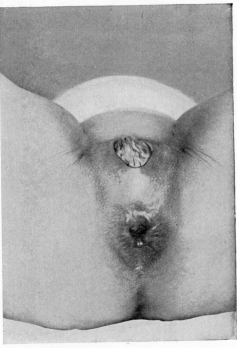

FIG. 150, *a*.—HEAD BEGINNING TO DISTEND PERINEUM.
Note anus is flattened.

FIG. 150, *b*.—PERINEUM MUCH DISTENDED AND THINNED.
Note glistening surface of the stretched skin.   Anus opened,
shows anterior wall of rectum.

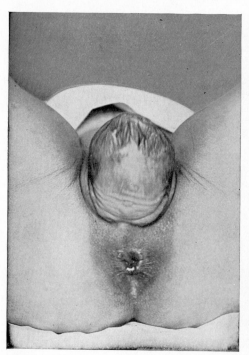

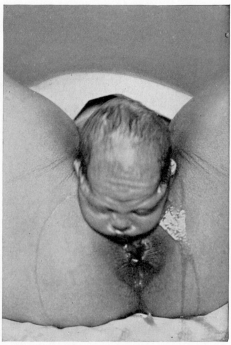

FIG. 151, *a*.—PERINEUM SLIPPING BACK OVER FACE.

FIG. 151, *b*.—HEAD DELIVERED.   PERINEUM RETRACTED
UNDER CHIN.   EXTERNAL RESTITUTION BEGINNING.

freshing sleep. When the resistance of the pelvic floor has been thus gradually overcome, the head comes to rest in the rima vulvæ, the nape of the neck stemming under the pubis. Now, by a crowning effort, under great nervous exaltation and powerful abdominal action, the head is forced out, the occiput coming from behind the pubis, the forehead, face, and chin rolling over the perineum. The woman feels as if she is being torn asunder. After this there is a pause of a few minutes, when the pains are renewed, the shoulders are delivered, and then generally the trunk, in one long, hard, expulsive effort. The child gasps, lying between the thighs of the mother, and soon cries vigorously. A little blood and the rest of the liquor amnii and the ends of the membrane are now discharged. The uterus contracts down into a ball. The patient feels much relieved. She may have a chill now, but this is considered physiologic. It may occur after the placenta is expelled and is not constant. The cause of this chill has been much discussed. The author has seen fewer

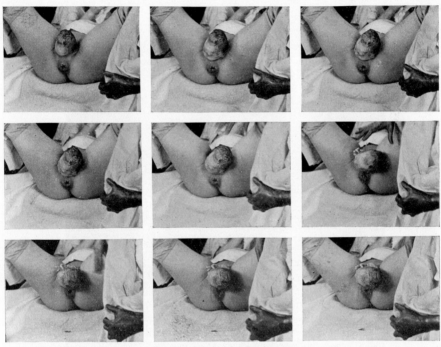

Fig. 152.—External Restitution.
From a motion picture. Note how baby's hand increases external rotation.

and fewer chills with the perfection of the aseptic technic of labor, and is inclined to believe they are due to absorption of toxins from the parturient canal, if not anaphylactic and due to the squeezing into the blood-stream (out of the uterine wall) of blood and lymph laden with products of the uterine activity, which occurs especially when the uterus contracts down on the placenta (Siedentopf). Abdominally, one finds the uterus contracted to a ball the size of a cocoanut. It still has the work of delivering the placenta. The second stage is ended.

The Third, or Placental Stage.—After from five to twenty minutes, devoted to rearrangement of its muscular lamellæ, the uterus begins to contract again. Some blood usually appears externally with the first pain. The uterus at first is somewhat relaxed, slightly flattened, but during a pain it becomes smaller, harder, and globular. The after-birth pains are usually not very painful; often the patient perceives only a slight drawing sensation, but the accoucheur can feel the regular (four to five minutes) contractions. After a period varying from a few minutes to an hour or more the fundus uteri rises high in the abdomen, generally under the liver, while below, over the pubis, the abdomen feels soft and boggy (Fig. 153). At the same time the cord advances a few inches from the vulva. These signs indicate that the placenta has loosened from the uterine wall and has descended into the lower uterine segment and upper part of the vagina. When the placenta is in the uterus the organ is large and globular. When the placenta has been forced from its bed into the lower uterine segment and upper vagina the uterus assumes a flattened pear shape. The flattening is from before backward and the fundus is sharp. On the anterior or posterior surface often a broad, shallow dimple is to be felt—the site of the placenta. The sharp fundus and the flat dimple are other evidences that the

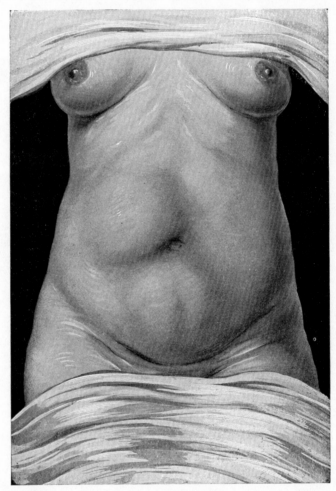

Fig. 153.—Uterus Risen in Abdomen Toward Liver. Placenta Makes a Soft Enlargement Above Pubis. Drawn from a photograph.

placenta has left the uterine cavity. After a few contractions the uterus again becomes more globular. If blood accumulates in the uterus it also becomes globular.

After a period, if the patient is let alone, varying from fifteen minutes to three hours or longer, the placenta is spontaneously expelled by the combined efforts of the abdominal muscles and the uterus. Generally, the attendant does not wait for this termination, but completes the process himself. The placenta is usually inverted like an umbrella, and draws the membranes after it, peeling them off the uterine wall (Schultze's method). Sometimes the placenta slides out without doubling up, the lower portion appearing first (Duncan's method). With the after-birth a lesser or greater quantity of blood is discharged. Now the uterus contracts down into a hard lump in the inlet of the pelvis, extending to the navel. It is the size of a fetal head. (See page 215.)

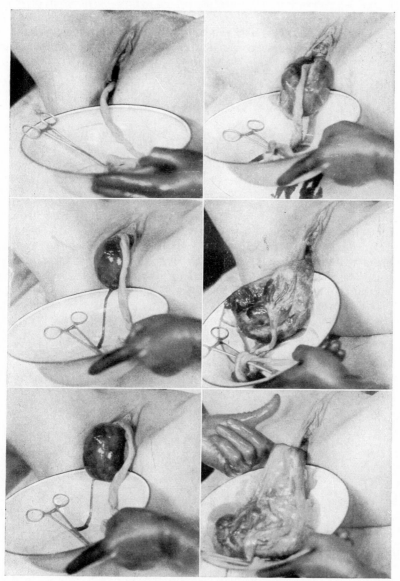

FIG. 154.—EXPRESSING PLACENTA.

When pituitary extract is administered, which is very frequently done now-adays, after the delivery of the child, the third stage is much altered. The effect of this hormone is to cause, in from two to five minutes, a powerful after-pain which usually loosens the placenta from its bed and expels it into the lower uterine segment and upper vagina. Another contraction soon follows and the placenta comes into sight. Thus the third stage is usually shortened to five or eight minutes.

Sometimes the uterus contracts unevenly and imprisons the placenta, requiring the intervention of art.

The third stage is ended. The *puerperium* has begun. The parturient has become a *puerpera*.

THE PAINS

The uterine contractions, the most prominent symptoms of labor, deserve more consideration.

1. They are involuntary. The woman has no control over them, but they are under the dominion of the cerebrospinal system. A mental shock may augment or

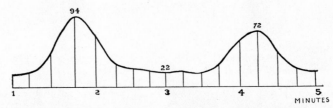

FIG. 155.—SCHATZ'S PAIN TRACING IN THE FIRST STAGE. THE FIGURES ON THE PEAKS INDICATE THE PRESSURE IN MILLIMETERS OF MERCURY. Ten mm. = 1 pound 1 ounce.

paralyze the uterine action. For instance, the abrupt entrance of a stranger may "drive the pains away." In one case of exceedingly slow labor the author expressed his intention to insert a colpeurynter. Strong pains came on at once and delivery was affected within an hour. It is known that fear produces an increase of epinephrin in the blood. Could it also flood the circulation with hypophyseal hormone and thus stimulate the uterus?

2. The action of the uterus is not peristaltic to the degree that exists in animals. The uterus may contract in one portion, the hardening extending quickly all over.

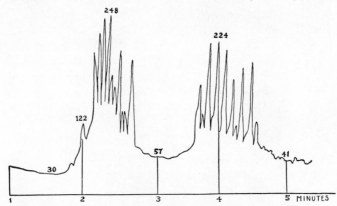

FIG. 156.—SCHATZ'S PAIN TRACING IN THE SECOND STAGE. THE FIGURES ON THE PEAKS INDICATE THE PRESSURE IN MILLIMETERS OF MERCURY. Ten mm. = 1 pound 1 ounce.

This the author has repeatedly observed after delivery of the child in cesarean sections. Portions of the uterus may contract while the rest remains in a state of retraction—for instance, "hour-glass" contraction; cornual contraction.

3. The action of the uterus is intermittent—that is, the pains recur at intervals. This intermittence aids the circulation in the parts. During uterine systole the blood in the veins is forced toward the broad ligaments; during diastole the uterus becomes turgid—to be observed at cesarean sections. Pelvic congestion is thus produced, and the resulting succulence of the cervix and vagina is a strong factor in their dilatation. By coördinated action the arteries dilate and more blood is brought

to the uterus (Werth). The blood in the uterine sinuses would be stagnant were it not for these intermittent uterine contractions, which much resemble the action of a local heart. The fetus is thus provided with sufficient oxygen. In cases of tetanus uteri the child may die of asphyxia because the hard, contracted uterus will not allow enough blood to flow through it.

The intermittence provides for the necessary rest of the muscle, the removal of waste, and the proper application of uterine force to the mechanical object of labor. The uterine action is a beautiful example of applied power.

4. The contractions are rhythmic, having three phases—increment, acme, and decrement. The increment is longer than the acme and decrement (Figs. 155 and 156). Schatz placed rubber bags in the functionating uterus and registered the pressure variations with a manometer, calling the apparatus a "tokodynamometer." His work is classic. The pain lasts from sixty to ninety seconds, the intervals from a few seconds to an hour, depending on the stage of labor and individual characteristics. Some pains are double. Sometimes a weak pain precedes a strong one. The first-stage pain differs from that of the second stage. The addition of the abdominal pressure alters the character of the curve. (See Figs. 155 and 156 and page 161.)

The contraction is well under way before the patient feels the pain, and continues a short time after the pain is gone. The pains grow stronger with the increased frequency. The educated hand, laid on the abdomen, can discover nearly all these points. The changes in the uterine form can also be seen.

5. The uterine contractions are painful. No other bodily function involving contraction of unstriped muscle is painful, and why these should be is incomprehensible if labor is to be considered a normal function.

Before labor has actively begun the pains are called dolores præsagientes. When the os is beginning to dilate, they become quite painful, and are called dolores præparantes. They seem to have their seat in different places—sometimes in the back, in the pelvis, again in the abdomen.

The first pains of labor are felt in the back, near the kidneys, and are called by the French women "pains of the kidneys." They may be felt only as a sensation of weakness, and the patient supports her back. Later the pains are felt more in the pelvis. In the first stage the pain is due to the pressure of the presenting part on the nerves of the cervix, to the stretching of the same during the dilatation of the os by the presenting part (Madame Boivin, who had personal experience), or to the compression of the nerves in the wall of the uterus. Perhaps all three causes are combined. The pains are described by the women as grinding, twisting, or resembling severe abdominal colic. Their power varies, see page 161.

The pain in the small of the back is due to radiation, such as is common in pelvic neuralgias and also to stretching of the pelvic joints. The nerves involved are the sacral and lumbar plexuses. The pain caused by the dilatation of the last fibers of the cervix is particularly acute, and sometimes a slight amount of blood may show itself, indicating a tear in the external os.

When the head passes down into the vagina and begins to press on the perineum, the pains are due to the stretching of these parts and are spoken of as tearing.

The patient now bears down and the pain cry is altered. She does not complain so much, but helps the labor along by pressing down with the abdominal muscles. When the head goes through the vulva, the greatest anguish is felt, the patient feeling as if she were torn open (dolores conquassantes). The pain may be so great that the patient faints or is temporarily insane, but both are rare.

These pains are called dolores ad partum. After the birth of the child the uterine contractions are called after-birth-pains, or dolores ad secundum partum. They usually are not so severe as the others, but in some patients they are very painful.

After delivery the pains are called dolores post partum, or "after-pains," and, especially in multiparæ, disturb the first days of the puerperium, often requiring treatment.

Painless labors do occur, but are very rare. If not due to disease of the spinal cord, it is hard to explain them. The women feel simply the desire to strain, as at stool, and delivery is usually quick. "Christian Scientists" claim to have no pain, but I have often observed they present positive evidences of suffering, reminding one of the stoical martyrs in Rome. Savage women have painful, though often quick labors, and they return to their work, not because they are well, but because their lot is labor under hardship. (Wright, Lit., Amer. Jour. of Obst. and Gyn., Aug., 1921, p. 208.)

CHAPTER VII

THE EFFECTS OF LABOR ON THE MATERNAL ORGANISM

It is not to be expected that a process requiring so much muscular exercise, such anxiety, and accompanied by such pain and traumatism, can be without a strong influence on the maternal organism. The patient eats little, sometimes vomits, is usually restless, and does not sleep much during labor. She may even have had pain at nights and very little sleep for a week, both of which exhaust her. A labor lasting a few days leaves the patient weak and completely tired out, with immunities against infection diminished, but this depends on the length of the labor and the strength of the woman in the first place.

The Duration of Labor.—The length of parturition is variable, which is true also of the same woman in different labors. In the uncivilized races labor is somewhat shorter. It is said that some Indian women, while the tribe is on the march, feeling the pains of labor coming on, go off to the side in the underbrush, bear the child, and, after expressing the after-birth, hurry to catch up with the rest of the train, but this is exceptional and true only of pure breeds. Later writers tell us that obstetric disease and mortality are large among the uncivilized women, particularly if crossed with whites. Labor is longer in the American negress.

In primiparæ labors are longer than in multiparæ; labor is shorter in warm climates, also during summer; in poor, hard-working women than in the rich and pampered; therefore shorter in the country than in the city.

The size of the fetus has a great deal to do with it—a large fetus, long labor. The same holds true if the fetal head is large and hard, and in contracted pelvis. In young, strong primiparæ labor is easier than in old primiparæ, the average in the latter being twenty-seven hours, but one is often surprised to see an easy labor in a primiparous patient over forty years old. Labor is longer in fat women, longer with boys than with girls, because they are larger. The lengths of the various stages of labor are about as follows: Primiparæ, first stage, sixteen hours; second stage, one and three-quarter to three hours; third stage, from a few minutes to several hours. Multiparæ, first stage, twelve hours; second stage, one-quarter to one-half hour; third stage, from a few minutes to several hours.

Extremes are not rare. We have had cases where labor was completed in even less than one hour. Again, there are labors which are slow from the start, requiring days for completion. Labor may intermit, an interval of hours or days occurring after the pains have begun and dilatation of the os has been effected. The difference in the length of labor in primiparæ and multiparæ is due to the slowness of dilatation of the cervix, perineum, and vulvar orifice in the former. In multiparæ, owing to stretching and tearing by previous deliveries, the resistances offered by the soft parts are less and much more readily overcome. If many years elapse between deliveries, some of the original resistance may have been regained. (See Calkins.)

In 1000 labors at the Chicago Lying-in Hospital the pains began and ended as follows:

Labor began.		Labor ended.
274 . . . . Between	6 P. M. and midnight	229
306 . . . . "	midnight and 6 A. M.	278
238 . . . . "	6 A. M. and noon	267
182 . . . . "	noon and 6 P. M.	226
1000		1000

The Temperature.—The muscular exertion during labor would raise the temperature if the loss of heat were not so great. Perspiration is increased, exposure of the body greater, respiration faster—all tend to keep the woman's temperature near normal. Accurate takings have shown, however, that there is a slight rise during labor, which is greatest right after delivery of the child, and varies with the usual daily variations, but does not normally exceed 1° F. During the pain the temperature rises a little. The temperature is likely to rise during a prolonged second stage. Overstrain and sleeplessness conduce to it (Adami). The author is convinced that fever of more than 0.5 degree during labor is toxinemic or septic in origin, and comes from the absorption of toxins or bacteria from the puerperal wounds. H. Müller came to the same conclusion. With the perfection of an aseptic technic slight fevers in labor are very rare, and the postpartum, so-called "physiologic" chill has become almost unknown. The chill formerly was ascribed to exhaustion of the mother, prolonged exposure of her person, loss of a source of heat, the child, readjustment of the abdominal circulatory conditions, nervousness, etc., but the author believes that the chill, too, is due to infection during labor. Proof of this is hard to bring, but if the other causes mentioned were real, the chill ought to follow nearly every labor, whereas statistics show that it occurs in only 20 to 30 per cent. In the author's practice it has almost disappeared with the perfection of asepsis, the use of rubber gloves, and the restriction of the internal examinations. If not due to infection, the possibility that it might be of an anaphylactic nature from absorption of fetal proteins during separation of the placenta is to be considered.

The Circulation.—The rate of the heart-beat increases somewhat during labor, reaching 100 or 110, but between the pains may be normal. The advent of a pain is heralded by a faster heart-beat. In the second stage, during the severe muscular exertion, the pulse-rate increases a good deal, but in the third stage, if no hemorrhage be present, it is usually normal. Any marked rapidity must put you on your guard against hemorrhage, external or internal. Arterial tension is increased until after the third stage unless there is hemorrhage or chloroform narcosis. During the pain the arterial tension is greater than in the intervals, 5 to 10 mm., and a moderately heightened blood-pressure continues a few days into the puerperium. The educated finger can determine these points, but the sphygmomanometer proves them scientifically (Slemons, Faught). In order to make a firm support for the action of the abdominal muscles in the second stage, the parturient fixes the chest in inspiration and holds her breath. If the bearing-down efforts are very hard and prolonged, the pulmonary circulation is interfered with, the right heart is congested, the blood cannot get into the chest, there is marked turgidity of the veins of the neck and head, and from this there sometimes result enlargement of the thyroid (which disappears postpartum), edema of the face, even tiny hemorrhages in the conjunctivæ. These evidences of venous congestion are, in bad cases, found also in the brain (Hodge). Paroxysmal tachycardia occasionally occurs.

The **respirations** are increased during the pains, but between pains are normal. Some nervous women hold the breath during the pains, even in the first stage. In the second stage breathing is more rapid, irregular, and altered by the bearing-down efforts and cries of pain. In the third stage they are again normal, unless there be hemorrhage, when an increase in number, or gasping, shortness of breath, persistent yawning, shows that there is something wrong.

More CO_2 is excreted during labor, and the rapid breathing helps to keep down the temperature. Too rapid breathing may produce acapnia, a condition which bears some relation to shock. Emphysema of the chest and head may result from too powerful bearing-down efforts. Usually harmless.

Turgidity and swelling of the turbinate bones are usually observed during labor. If the patient has a nasal catarrh, obstruction of the nares may result.

Fliess associates this condition with the uterine action, and claims that the latter may be influenced by treatment directed to the nose.

The Intestinal Tract.—Anorexia is the rule. Thirst is common. Many women vomit during labor. The old midwives say that sick labors are easy, but the author cannot confirm this. It was once the custom to give emetics on this theory to relax the cervix, but the practice is bad. When the head is passing through the os, the great distention may cause reflex vomiting, and some women vomit frequently during the second stage. Persistent vomiting at any stage of labor should always be suspected, and its cause sought for carefully. It may indicate threatened or actual rupture of the uterus, eclampsia, uremia, internal hemorrhage, peritonitis. In the third stage vomiting almost never occurs normally. Anesthesia, especially after operations, may cause it, but even then it is rarely so severe as in surgical cases. Persistent nausea and vomiting after a delivery are a significant symptom, and their cause must be discovered.

The bowels are often loose at the very beginning of labor, and borborygmus is often heard during its progress, but the head in the pelvis prevents defecation. In the second stage the advancing head forces feces from the rectum, an occurrence annoying to the mother, and dangerous, too, because, in the manipulations the doctor makes he may carry infectious matter into the parturient tract. A cathartic given in labor may stimulate the pains—an old remedy for inertia uteri.

The **mental condition** of the patient during the first stage of labor is what one would expect of a woman going through a mysterious ordeal full of fear and pain. In predisposed women it may be marked by hysteric manifestations. In the second stage, especially at the end, the parturient may become delirious or even maniacal from the suffering, but this is rare. Real fainting is also rare in normal labors. Whenever I have seen it, the cause has been hemorrhage or shock. That a woman may give birth during a faint is theoretically certain and medicolegally proved. This is important from a legal standpoint, as in cases of infanticide. (For full consideration of this subject see Moritz Freyer.)

The woman's demeanor is usually cheerful, but may be the opposite, she asserting her inability to bear the pain or that she will surely die. In the second stage, when the parturient feels the progress of the head, she complains less. Between pains the woman may doze or sleep soundly.

When the head enters the lower pelvis, it may compress the obturator or sacral nerves. Cramps in the leg are thus produced—in the anterior upper thigh in the former, on the posterior surface of the leg in the latter, instance.

After the child is delivered the parturient may fall asleep, which is especially common at the end of prolonged, exhausting labors.

The Urinary System.—The disposition of the bladder during labor varies in different women. Usually the lower uterine segment in its development pulls away from the viscus, leaving it behind the pubis, but in some cases, where the two organs are more intimately adherent, the bladder rises into the abdomen with the lower portion of the uterus. In either case the full bladder distends the lower hypogastrium, but there is a difference in the depth of the anterior culdesac.

The ureters are also drawn upward with the receding uterus. Early in labor they may be felt coursing around the cervix toward the brim of the pelvis. Later one cannot feel them. Frozen sections (Tandler) show that they cross the brim higher and more anteriorly than in the non-pregnant state. They are dilated, proved by pyelography, in three-fourths of normal pregnancies in the later months (Luchs). The ureters are obstructed by kinking, not pressure. The urethra is lengthened, compressed by the head, and much bruised during labor. If the head is too long impacted in the pelvis, the urethra and part of the bladder may slough out, leaving urinary fistulas.

In general the kidneys are more active during labor. The polyuria is due to the heightened arterial tension and stimulation of the kidneys through the sympathetic from the uterus. In nervous or hysteric women the general nervous system plays a part. Polyuria is usual, but not constant, some women having less than normal. The full bladder disturbs the course of labor, may prevent the engagement of the head, and in the third stage may delay the exit of the placenta and cause postpartum hemorrhage.

The specific gravity of the urine is reduced, urea, phosphate, and sulphate

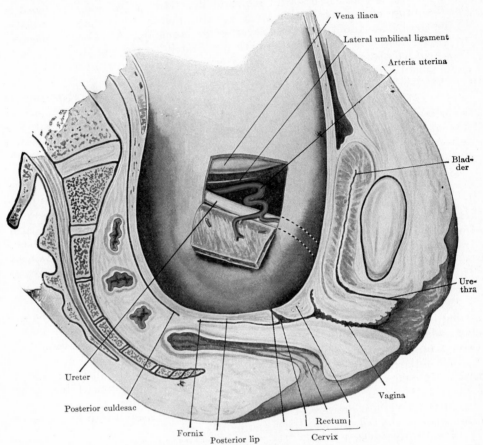

FIG. 157.—THE URETER AT TERM (from Tandler and Halban).

content also, while the sodium chlorid is increased (v. Winckel). Albumin is found in one-third of the cases, being three times commoner in primiparæ, more frequent in very young and very old parturients, in hard and prolonged labors, after the administration of anesthetics, with fever in labor, and in women who have had albuminuria during pregnancy. The amount in normal cases does not exceed 1/1000 Esbach. Larger quantities indicate pathogenic conditions. The cause of the albuminuria may be sought in the increased muscular exertion of labor, the high blood-pressure, and perhaps in the deportation of placental villi (Veit) under the force of the uterine contractions. (See Eclampsia.)

Formed elements, especially hyaline casts, are often found, even white and red blood-corpuscles, all three in proportion to the albuminuria. In general, it may be said that the urinary findings during labor bear only slightly less significance than at any other time during pregnancy.

General Metabolism.—The mother loses about one-tenth of her body weight (Baumm and Gassner). This is made up of the child, the placenta and membranes, the liquor amnii, blood, excretions from the skin, lungs, kidneys, etc.

A marked leukocytosis is found during labor, which, according to Hofbauer, is due to muscular work, but is more probably an antitoxic reaction. The whites

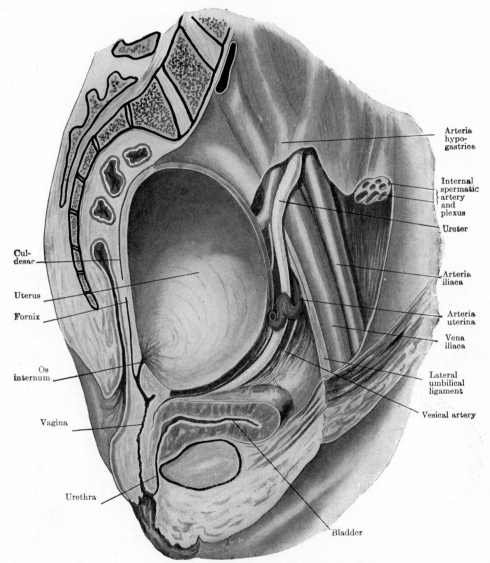

Fig. 158.—Topography of the Ureter (Tandler and Halban).

vary from 9 to 34,000. The polynuclear neutrophiles are increased, the eosinophiles much decreased (Cova).

Siedentopf found the non-protein nitrogen, acetone, diacetic acid are increased and the acid-base equilibrium disturbed, to the acid side, as labor advances, culminating at the end of the second stage, all due to muscular action.

Parturition is the only function normally attended by hemorrhage. Bloodless labors are rare, and are so usually because the fetus has been dead some weeks. The amount of blood lost varies in wide limits from a few ounces to several quarts. Where the normal limit lies depends on the individual patient. Authorities differ as to what should be considered normal. Ahlfeld says even 1000 gm. may be a normal loss, but that the average is 400 gm. The amount of blood lost is influenced by the size of the child, the area of the placenta, its location in the uterus, the rapidity of the separation of the placenta, the strength of the uterine contraction and retraction, the age of the parturient, and the number of children she has borne, being greater in multiparæ. The method of conduct of the labor by the medical attendant also influences the blood loss and pathologic conditions to be later considered.

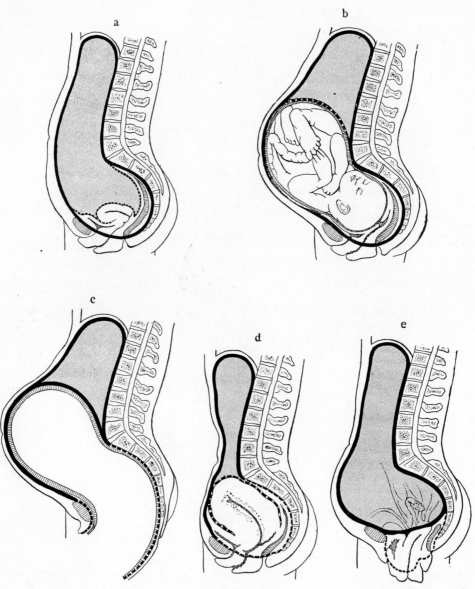

FIG. 158a.—Mutations in the Abdomen Caused by Pregnancy and Labor (Sellheim).

Pituitary extract given so frequently at present right after the baby is born, causes a powerful contraction of the uterus which diminishes the physiologic loss of blood. No exact figure may be given as to what is a normal loss of blood in labor. The author believes that 500 gm. should be the limit in ordinary cases, and that in small, anemic, or otherwise debilitated women the loss should not exceed 150 gm. Nearly all the blood comes during and after the third stage, either free or contained in the folded placenta as the retroplacental hematoma. A little blood appears in the "show" at the beginning of the first stage; a little more comes when the last fibers of the cervix are giving away; more may appear when the head bursts through the vulva, from tears of the clitoris and outlet. The bleeding now comes from the placental site and cervical and perineal lacerations, and when the placenta comes, the greatest discharge occurs. The oozing after the delivery of the placenta comes from the placental site and the puerperal wounds, and in the first two hours should not exceed 2 ounces. (See Calkins, Litzenberg, Plass.)

Figure 158a pictures schematically the astonishing mutations which occur in the female abdomen during pregnancy, labor and the puerperium. Following the normal, rather graceful, lines of the non-pregnant state (a) we see the great distortion produced by pregnancy, (b); this distortion is enormously exaggerated during labor, and that a woman should declare she feels as if she were being burst asunder by this mighty cataclysm ought not to surprise us at all, (c). After delivery the overstretched belly collapses and the pelvis is filled by the large uterus (d). If the pelvic diaphragm, which is the floor or bottom of the abdominal cavity, is overstretched or torn, the pelvic organs drop down and out. If the abdominal wall does not regain its tone, ventral hernia results (e).

It is very apparent, therefore, that the anatomy of the female is not constant. We must study it during a process of change and must recognize at least five stages: the non-pregnant state, the woman at term, at the end of labor, during the puerperium, and after involution is complete. The physics of the abdomen likewise must be studied at different periods and in transition, all of which makes the science of obstetrics very difficult and intriguing.

The results of the changes shown in Fig. 158a are more or less permanent and vary with the type of constitution of the pateint, e. g., women of the hypoplastic type are more prone to suffer as in (e).

LITERATURE

Adami: Gen. Pathology, 1909, p. 360.—*Ahlfeld:* Lehrbuch der Geb., 1903, p. 145.—*Calkins:* Amer. Jour. Obst. and Gyn., February, 1930, p. 274.—*Calkins, Litzenberg, and Plass:* Amer. Jour. Obst. and Gyn., 1931, February, p. 175.—*Cova:* Trans. Internat. Cong., Rome, 1902.—*Faught:* Blood-pressure, W. B. Saunders Co., 1913.—*Freyer:* Die Ohnmacht bei der Geburt, Springer, Berlin, 1887.—*Healy and Kastle:* Jour. Infect. Dis., 1912, vol. x, p. 244.—*von der Heide:* Jour. Amer. Med. Assoc., September 23, 1911, p. 1090.—*Koehler:* Zent. für Gyn., December 18, 1915, p. 891.—*Kolmer:* Jour. Med. Research, January, 1914, xxix, No. 3, p. 368.—*Luchs:* Zentb. für Gynaek., May 30, 1925, p. 1201.—*de Paoli:* Arch. di Ost. e Gin., January, 1903.—*Schatz:* Arch. f. Gyn., vol. iii.—*Sellheim:* Veit's Handbuch der Gynaek., 1926, vol. ii, p. 180.—*Siedentopf, H.:* Zentb. für Gyn., October 24, 1931.—*Ibid.:* Proc. Am. Gynec. Soc'y, June, 1932.—*Slemons and Goldsborough:* Zentralbl. f. Gyn., 1908, p. 700.—*Tandler and Halban:* Die Topographie des weiblichen Ureters, Vienna.

CHAPTER VIII

THE EFFECT OF LABOR ON THE CHILD'S ORGANISM

DURING the last weeks of pregnancy the child is quieter, due to the restriction of its movements from lack of room. The question, Does the child suffer pain during delivery? has been answered both ways. It probably does. The author has felt the infant withdraw its hand after being pinched, and it cries lustily immediately after birth, from the painful compression it suffered, and perhaps from the sudden decompression similar to that of men emerging from a caisson.

A not small percentage of children die, even in so-called normal labor—estimated by various authors from 2 to 5 per cent. The shock of labor to the infant must be reckoned with.

Careful examination of the fetal heart during labor shows that its rapidity is much affected by the pains. When the uterus begins to contract, the fetal pulse beats faster; during the height of the pain it is slow; as the pain wanes it beats fast again, gradually slowing down to normal. These findings are more pronounced after the membranes are ruptured and with strong pains. Sometimes the heart is accelerated by the pains. As labor progresses the fetal heart usually becomes

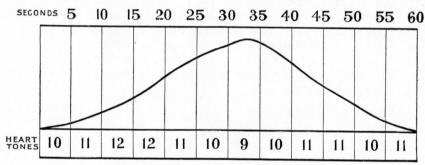

FIG. 159.—TRACING OF FETAL HEART-BEAT DURING A PAIN.
Lower figures are the numbers of beats per five seconds.

slower, and as the head passes through the inlet (Gauss) and the pelvic floor, the slowing may be so marked that the attendant becomes alarmed. The author has counted, during the pains, a beat as low as 60 while the head was being delivered. The cause of these variations is unknown. Schultze ascribed them to stimulation of the vagus by the insufficiently oxidized fetal blood, the uterine contraction forcing the maternal blood out of the placenta. Kehrer believed that the compression of the skull slowed the heart by direct vagus irritation, an opinion confirmed by Rech in 1931. The child is under the intra-uterine pressure—like a man working in a caisson—which slows the heart. Caisson workers sometimes become stuporous from over-pressure and perhaps the fetus does also. Guttner explains the bradycardia during the pain as a compensatory result of the fetal high blood-pressure. The slowing of the heart is not constant; the author has noticed that the pulse does not vary much, in some few labors, from the beginning to the end. When the child is in danger, its heart beats very fast, very slowly, or irregularly, yet occasionally we note these signs and the child does not suffer. The child may, in pathologic cases, make respiratory movements before its delivery. Even in normal deliveries close observation of the head as it lies in the vulva will discover little twitchings that indicate attempts to inspire, and the accoucheur will find that the infant has filled its mouth with blood or mucus from the vagina. It is wise to hasten the delivery when such action is discovered, because the infant may get foreign matter into the lungs or stomach and later develop pulmonary atelectasis or intestinal infection. Occasionally the infant will gasp and cry as soon as the head is out, but usually the first cry escapes after the body is delivered. At first the chest moves with tiny excursions; in a few moments a deep gasp fills the lungs, then comes a sneeze or a cough, which expels the mucus from the throat, following which is the lusty cry of the new-born.

The Cause of the First Respiration.—The theory of Preyer, that the irritation of the skin from the trauma of labor causes the respiration by stimulating the respiratory center reflexly, is very probable, although other conditions must be present.

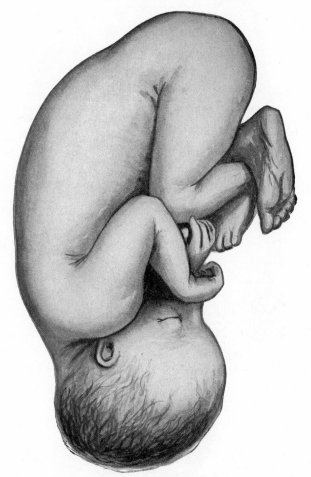

FIG. 160.—ATTITUDE OF CHILD IN UTERO AT BEGINNING OF LABOR.

Rough palpation, attempts at version, forceps, usually do not affect the child *in utero*. Should the child, however, be partly asphyxiated, the respiratory center will react to these stimuli and asphyxia alone will induce respiration. Ahlfeld delivered several children into warm saline solution and the respiration began as usual. While the fetal blood may become more venous toward the end of pregnancy, Haselhorst has shown that, during labor, there is no change in the O_2 content, in normal cases, at least in the cord blood. All students of this problem agree that the respiratory center grows more irritable as labor nears and becomes acutely so when the pains are strong. This is due to fluctuations of the circulation in the medulla and especially to the accumulation of CO_2 in the blood. As a result the fetus passes from a state of apnea to one of dyspnea and in this condition any physical shock can evoke a gasp or start breathing and crying. Such irritations are pain from the impacts of the forces of labor, touching the child, the cold air, the sudden release of the head and chest from compression, etc. If the child is rapidly delivered, as in cesarean section, or in multiparæ with a short second stage, it may come into the world with sufficient oxygen for a short time; it is in its intra-uterine condition of apnea, and a few minutes may elapse before the

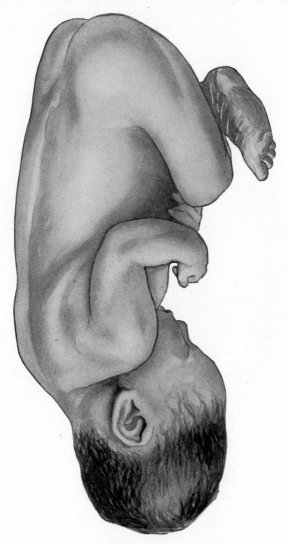

Fig. 161.—Attitude of Child During Period of Expulsion. Shows Marked Cephalic Molding.

respiratory center becomes sufficiently sensitized by the increasingly venous blood to evoke respiratory action. But we still need an explanation for the first respiration in cases of quick easy labor and in cervical cesarean where there can be no thought of asphyxia and yet the baby cries as soon as its face is exposed to the air. Perhaps this is it.

The trachea is collapsed, and the glottis partly filled with a bit of mucus (Barton). Its own muscle, aided by air rushing by the mucus, opens the lumen of the trachea.

The Changes in the Fetal Circulation.—With the first inspiration the lungs expand. The pulmonary vessels are dilated, and blood rushes into them from the right ventricle. There is no blood to pass through the ductus Botalli. It, therefore, collapses. This may be due to a valve-like formation at its junction with the aorta (Strassman) or to a twisting of the duct, due to the change of position of the heart, caused by the filling of the auricles and distention of the lungs. There is less blood coming from the ascending vena cava, the umbilical vein contracting; the pressure in the right auricle sinks. The result is an aspiration toward the heart of the blood in the vena cava and umbilical vein.

The distal ends of the hypogastric arteries contract and thrombose. This is due to the fact that the left ventricle cannot send the blood the long distance through them, since it is no longer assisted by the right ventricle through the ductus Botalli. Also, cold contracts the arteries, which have a powerful muscular coat. The pulsation in the cord ceases. Since the pressure in the right auricle is low and that in the left higher, the valve of the foramen ovale applies itself to the septum auriculorum, and thus the two sides of the heart become distinct.

The circulation is now just the same as in the adult. The ductus Arantii and ductus Botalli grow smaller by contraction of their muscular fibers, the latter

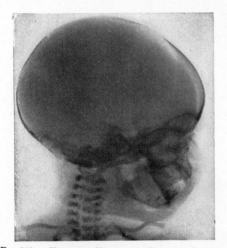

FIG. 162a.—UNMOLDED HEAD; FROM CESAREAN SECTION.

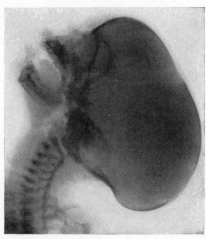

FIG. 162b.—EXTREME MOLDING—CASE OF FACE PRESENTATION.

through torsion of the vessel and the application of their walls to each other. No thrombosis occurs in them, nor in the vein of the umbilical cord—only in the arteries. They become obliterated in one or two weeks.

The Plastic Changes Wrought on the Fetus.—The conditions during labor are unlike those enjoyed by the child during pregnancy. The contracting uterus compresses the fetus into a definite shape, and gives it a certain attitude, both of which are to facilitate its passage through the parturient canal. The legs are flexed on the thighs and crossed over each other, the thighs on the abdomen; the arms are folded across the chest, the head flexed so that the chin rests on the sternum (Fig. 160). The pressure of the uterus on the crossed legs may bend the tibia and fibula, but the deformity lasts only a week or more.

The head undergoes marked changes, which vary with the presentation of the child for delivery, and are caused by pressure exerted by the maternal structures. In ordinary head presentations, with a moderately tight parturient passage, the face and the forehead are flattened, the occiput long drawn out (Fig. 161), the bones overlapped. Usually the occipital bone is pressed under the two parietals—the frontal also somewhat below them. One parietal overlaps the other, the one that lies against the promontory being the one that is depressed (Figs. 163 and 164). The head offers thus a long narrow cylinder to the birth-canal, instead of a round ball. These changes in shape, or "molding," are possible because of the softness of the

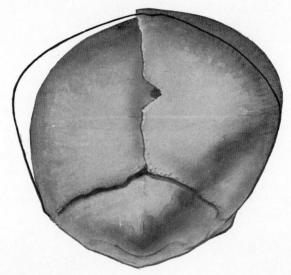

FIG. 163.—REAR VIEW OF SKULL MOLDED IN O.L.A.   Line-shape before molding.

bones and the loose connection they have with each other at the sutures. When this molding is absent, labor is more difficult. Some slight diminution in the size of the head occurs in labor, especially if the pelvis is contracted, and it is due to the

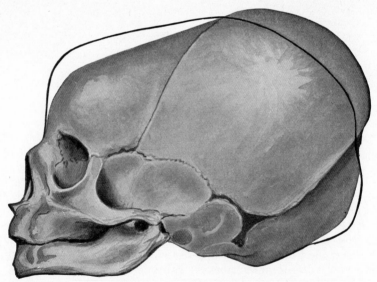

FIG. 164.—SIDE VIEW OF SKULL MOLDED IN O.D.A.   Line-shape before molding.

escape, under pressure, of the cerebrospinal fluid into the spinal canal. Necessarily, it is small and cuts little figure in the mechanism of delivery.

Along the sutures it is not uncommon to find numerous small hemorrhages in and under the dura mater and under the external periosteum. They are due to the overlapping of the bones, and are most marked in cases where the head has been forced through a narrow pelvis or compressed by the forceps (Fig. 165). On that part of the head least subjected to pressure there appears in long labors a soft, boggy, circumscribed tumor. In vertex presentations it is formed on one parietal bone. It is caused by the pressure of the uterus on the body of the child being greater than that on the portion which lies below the girdle of resistance—that is, through the opening in the cervix or the vagina, or even in the vulva (Fig. 166). The action is similar to that occurring in a limb tightly gartered—the blood cannot return; venous congestion with edema and extravasation of blood results, sometimes a blister. These small hemorrhages persist long after the edema is absorbed, and mark the site of the tumor on the head. The swelling is called caput succedaneum, and it occurs in and under the scalp, not under the periosteum, in ordinary cases. It is, therefore, movable on the skull. It may sag toward the side on which the child lies after delivery, but the blood extravasations will not change. If the pressure has been prolonged, the hemorrhagic infiltration affects the periosteum, the bone, and correspond-

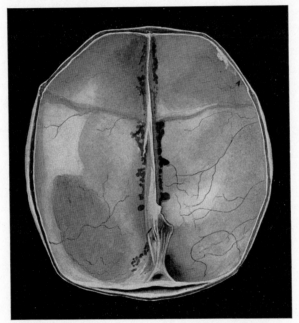

FIG. 165.—EPIDURAL HEMORRHAGES ALONG LONGITUDINAL SINUS.

ing regions of the meninges. A caput succedaneum can form before the bag of waters breaks because the pressure in the bag is less than that in the general uterine cavity, but it is rare. Most commonly we find the largest caput in a contracted pelvis with prolonged and powerful pains, and, second, when the head is arrested at the bony outlet. In either of these cases, but especially in the latter instance, the caput may be visible at the vulva. It may make the attendant believe that the labor is advancing, when, in reality, the growing caput indicates that the head has met an obstruction (Fig. 167). Thus it may give warning of the necessity to interfere in labor. One must distinguish between caput succedaneum and cephalhematoma, which is an accumulation of blood *under* the periosteum. (See Chapter LXII.)

The caput exaggerates the obliquity of the head produced by the depression of the parietal bone by the promontory of the sacrum or the pelvic floor. (See Figs. 163 and 164.) The caput is absorbed in twenty-four to thirty-six hours; the asymmetry of the head produced by the mechanical factors in labor disappears by the

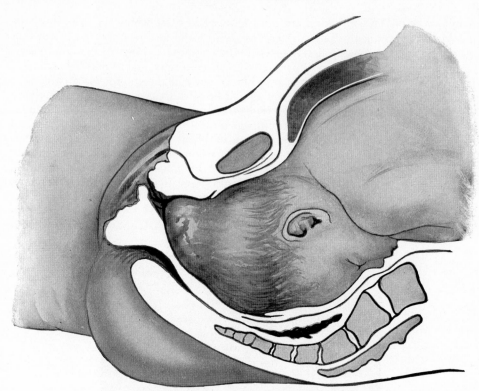

FIG. 166.—SHOWING HOW A CAPUT IS FORMED.

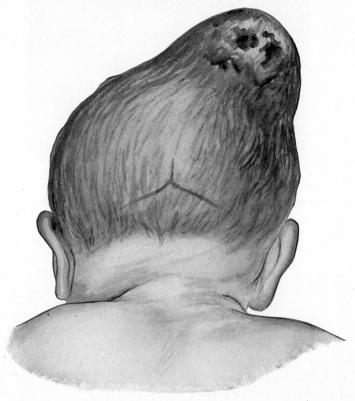

FIG. 167.—LARGE CAPUT SUCCEDANEUM SHOWING HEMORRHAGES INTO SKIN.

end of a week, but there often remains a permanent asymmetry of the skull, called that of Stadtfeld, who first described it. All forms of growth have a slightly spiral direction. This is true also of the fetus. There is a congenital scoliosis of the spinal column. The right parietal bone is pushed anteriorly in a horizontal plane, appearing flat, while the left is more convex. This asymmetry is permanent and has been demonstrated in the adult. The head tracings to be seen in any hat-shop show it. While the right side is usually affected, the twisting may be reversed. The asymmetry of Stadtfeld may be counteracted by the molding produced during labor. After the latter disappears, the true shape of the skull returns. In primiparæ long compression of the head by the lower uterine segment and pelvis results in dolichocephalus, which may be permanent. (Frommoltz, Lit.)

Sometimes the head occupies the pelvic cavity for the last three to five weeks of pregnancy, and is permanently deformed, flattened by the levator ani. The latero-flexion of the trunk shortens the sternocleidomastoid muscle, and during delivery the deformed muscle may rupture, causing hematoma, myositis, and wry-neck.

In breech presentations the head may be flattened by the pressure of the fundus against it for a long time. In a tightly built primipara the flattening may begin in the latter months of pregnancy and may be permanent. Sometimes corresponding shortening of the sternocleidomastoid muscle results from the strained attitude of the child, and wry-neck is produced in the same as above stated.

Without doubt labor affects the fetus in more ways than our present means of investigation disclose. Perhaps tiny hemorrhages in the brain may explain some of the so-called congenital deformities and diseases, for instance, strabismus, ptosis palpebrarum, epilepsy, persistent headache, idiocy. (See page 882.)

THE PROGNOSIS OF LABOR

In ideal labor there should be no mortality of either mother or child, but, unfortunately, we are far from this ideal.

In the United States of America, from a registration area comprising 94.7 per cent. of the total population of the country, over 15,000 women die annually in childbirth. (See following table.) The number seems to be growing all the time.

DEATHS IN CHILDBIRTH IN THE UNITED STATES

Cause of death.	1930	1929	1928	1927	1926	1925	1924	1923	1922	1921	1920	1919	1918*	1917
The puerperal state: Number	14,836	15,084	15,461	13,837	12,168	12,158	12,672	11,922	11,792	11,688	12,058	10,127	12,496	8,958
Rate per 1000 live births	6.73	6.95	6.02	6.47	6.55	6.47	6.56	6.65	6.64	6.81	7.99	7.37	9.16	6.61
Accidents of pregnancy: Number	1,332	1,530	1,576	1,259	1,282	1,093	1,165	1,229	1,145	975	1,732	1,470	3,034	733
Puerperal hemorrhage: Number	1,523	1,539	1,599	1,456	1,311	1,237	1,293	1,182	1,165	1,249	1,055	854	854	880
Other accidents of labor: Number	1,767	1,829	1,914	1,542	1,390	1,356	1,366	1,413	1,425	1,203	1,692	1,464	2,259	836
Puerperal septicemia: Number	5,385	5,718	5,590	5,353	4,484	4,569	4,704	4,495	4,249	4,639	4,036	3,366	3,473	3,710
Puerperal phlegmasia alba dolens, embolus, sudden death: Number	702	597	625	615	559	583	636	571	523	464	432	385	307	341
Puerperal albuminuria and convulsions: Number	4,082	3,821	4,098	3,556	3,091	3,256	3,441	2,966	3,211	3,081	3,050	2,527	2,496	2,405
Following childbirth (not otherwise defined): Number	45	45	48	48	48	57	59	53	70	72	54	52	62	43
Puerperal diseases of the breast: Number		5	11	8	3	7	8	13	4	5	7	9	11	10
Per cent of population of continental United States included in birth registration area	94.7	94.7	94.4	87.3	76.8	76.0	76.2	72.2	72.2	65.3	59.8	58.6	53.6	53.6

(The information for this table was kindly furnished by Dr. T. F. Murphy of the U. S. Census Bureau.)
* The highest rates were in the influenza years.

The increase year by year is explained by the increasing area of registration and the improvement in the statistical reports. Without doubt several thousand women die in childbirth every year and are buried under another diagnosis. Hundreds die months and even years after, but, nevertheless, from the direct results of labor, from their injuries, cancer, from infection, and from operations undertaken to cure them. W. Blair Bell estimates these to be more than those dying in labor.

During the agitation for the passage of the Sheppard Towner Maternity bill, the Children's Bureau published Maternal Mortality Statistics from various European nations and placed the United States sixteenth on the list. The author scrutinized these figures carefully, and agrees with Mongan that they are almost utterly worthless for purposes of comparison. The League of Nations, in 1925, published a chart showing the "International Incomparability of Mortality Statistics," and gave sixteen "Important Points to be considered when comparing statistics of causes of deaths for different countries." These were not considered by those who placed the United States low on the international list, and it would be just, therefore, not to quote that indefensible statement any more. The quality of obstetric work done in this country is certainly as good as that done abroad. A text-book is not the place to discuss such controversial matters; those especially interested may obtain the literature from the Children's Bureau at Washington, and the League of Nations, Geneva, Switzerland, and read Peller's article on European maternal mortality and Lowrie's on a new method of computing death rates.

Here suffice it to say that in Europe as well as in America of every 200 women who become pregnant at least one dies before the reproductive function is completed.

In speaking of these deaths we must distinguish between the preventable and the unavoidable. Without question the mortality of childbirth could be reduced to one per thousand if the public were properly instructed regarding the needful precautions, and if the physicians were all capable of meeting obstetric emergencies, and, most important, practised an aseptic technic. It will be noticed in all the statistics that nearly half the deaths were from infection.

There is an *unavoidable mortality* in childbirth, and it comes from disease of the uterus, adnexa, and pelvis, and from general affections aggravated by parturition, but it is small compared with the preventable mortality.

Labor shows a *high morbidity*, that is, the women are sickened or injured in the process of reproduction. The author has never seen a woman as anatomically perfect after delivery as she was before pregnancy occurred. Many women date life-long invalidism from a confinement. Overdistention of the abdomen often leaves weakness of the abdominal wall and visceroptosis; the urogenital septum is always torn, and prolapse of the urethra and anterior vaginal wall occurs, the patulous vulva opening the way for infectious catarrhs of the bladder and of the cervix and chronic metritis; laceration or overstretching of the pelvic floor is an almost invariable occurrence in greater or less degree, inviting prolapse of the uterus—these are some of the inevitable consequences of labor. If to these be added the frequent infections of the uterus and adnexa, the damage to the soft parts from operative deliveries, disease of the kidneys, of the liver, etc., one quickly appreciates the high morbidity of the reproductive function in the human female in our day. Naturally, it is impossible to compile statistics as to the frequency of these affections, but the records of the hospitals show a continual stream of women seeking relief from the bad effects of childbirth. Most of these diseases and accidents can, even with our present knowledge, be prevented, and no field in all preventive medicine promises greater results.

Prognosis for the Infant.—The highest mortality that befalls the human race in one day occurs on the day of birth. Schultze estimates that 5 per cent. of children are still-born, dying during labor, and 1.5 per cent. die shortly after birth, the result of the trauma of labor. In the United States in 1929 (excepting Texas and South Dakota) there were 85,678 still-births and 146,661 babies died during their first year, a large proportion from birth injuries. The statistics of the Chicago Lying-in Hospital, 1918–1931, are: 34,807 women had 35,179 babies after the period of viability, *i. e.*, twenty-eight weeks, and weighing more than 1500 grams. There were 356 twins and 8 sets of triplets. Of the 35,179 babies delivered there were 728 still-births, a gross mortality of 2.08 per cent. In 381 of these cases there were no fetal heart tones present on admission; 550 babies died during the first two weeks of life.

Total number of still-births and post-natal deaths, 728 plus 550 equals 1278. Therefore the *total fetal mortality was 3.6 per cent.*

Still-births...	728 or 2.7	per cent.
Still-births without fetal heart tones on admission...........	381 or 1.1	" "
Still-births with fetal heart tones on admission..............	347 or 0.9	" "
Died during the first two weeks of life.....................	550 or 1.6	" "
Still-births with heart tones on entrance plus post-natal deaths.	897 or 2.5	" "
Deducting 82 non-viable monstrosities, corrected fetal mortality is	815 or 2.3	" "

In Paris 9 per cent. die; in Glasgow, 13.6 per cent.; in Edinburgh, 11.5 per cent.; in England and Wales (1922), 7.7 per cent. (Bourne). These discrepancies show that we must use great caution in interpreting the data, and may never use them for comparison unless classified. At present there are no standards, *e. g.*, the term "still-birth" is not used in the same sense by the states and nations, some including abortions. Some statistics cover only the day of birth, some three days, some two weeks, etc. (See Bacon and Ferguson.) Asphyxia and injury during labor are frequent causes of fetal death, but a large part of the mortality is due to congenital defects, syphilis, alcoholism of the parents, and general diseases.

Besides this mortality, the children are frequently injured during delivery, either by the natural powers or, more often, by operative procedure. Hemorrhages into the brain, tentorium tears, fracture of the skull, dislocation and fracture of the vertebræ, joints, and extremities, often result from the brutal deliveries rendered necessary in cases of mechanical disproportion. Milder injuries of brain, nerves, and bones are very frequent, but are often overlooked until their later effects become prominent; for example, Little's disease from injury to the brain and spinal cord, chronic hydrocephalus, athetosis, idiocy, psychoses, etc.

One such brief glance into the subject will show the immensity of this field of preventive medicine, and prove to the reader that obstetrics is not one of the minor branches of medicine, but a specialty deserving the attention of the best minds in the profession.

LITERATURE

Bacon: Infant Mortality Due to Childbirth, Jour. Amer. Med. Assoc., June 19, 1915.—*Bell, W. Blair:* Maternal Disablement, London Lancet, May 30, 1931, p. 1171 and June 13, 1931, p. 1279.—*Bourne:* Recent Advances in Obstetrics and Gyn., Blakiston, 1926, p. 13.—*Cragin:* Practice of Obstetrics, 1916, p. 836.—*Dreyer:* Ref Zentralbl. f. Gyn., 1908, p. 1460.—*Dublin:* Mortality in Childbirth, Amer. Jour. Obstet., July, 1918.—*Ferguson:* Jour. Obst. and Gyn. British Empire, December, 1912, p. 334.—*Frommolt:* Zentb. für Gyn., January 1, 1927, p. 51.—*Gauss:* Zentralbl. für Gynaek., January 2, 1932, p. 1.—*Guttner:* Arch. für Gynaek., 1932, v. 149, H. 1, p. 70.—*Haselhorst and Stromberger:* Zeitschr. für Geb. u. Gyn., 1932, Band 102, H. 1, p. 16.—*Lowrie, R. J.:* New York State Med. Jour., October 1, 1931. See also Emerson, Amer. Jour. Obst. and Gyn., April, 1932, p. 605.—*Mongan:* Ill. State Med. Journal, July, 1922.—*Newsholme:* Jour. Amer. Med. Assoc., January, 1916, London Letter.—*Peller, S.:* Zentb. für Gyn., August 8, 1931, p. 2402.—*Rech:* Arch. für Gyn., 1930, vol. 144, p. 564.—*Schultze:* Handbuch d. Kinderkrankh., vol. ii, p. 15.

CHAPTER IX

THE MECHANISM OF LABOR

THE details of the wonderful process of parturition, whose clinical manifestations we have just considered, deserve separate study. The mode and manner by which the ovum is separated and extruded from the uterus comprise the mechanism of labor, and deserve the closest attention of the practising obstetrician. Indeed,

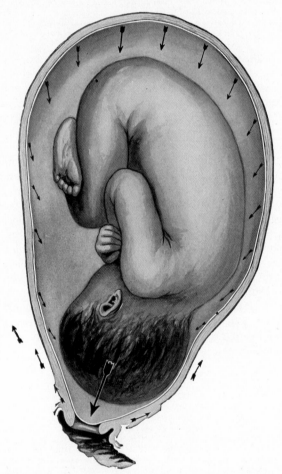

FIG. 168.—INTERNAL UTERINE PRESSURE (I.U.P.). SOMETIMES CALLED HYDRAULIC PRESSURE. EFFECT OF UTERINE CONTRACTION.

without accurate knowledge of this mechanism he ceases to be a scientific practitioner and becomes a midwife. The accoucheur who knows the science of the mechanism of labor will early recognize deviations from the normal, and, by some simple, harmless manipulation, may direct the course of labor into the normal again. He also will be able to deal with the pathologic mechanisms with the least possible danger of injury to the mother and child. The ignorant accoucheur, on the other hand, will allow the labor to go on until positive obstruction exists and the lives of parent and child are placed in jeopardy. Then he must use brute force to overcome mechanical difficulty, with the almost invariable result of severe maternal injury and frequent destruction of the child. Although a daily occurrence, and the object of a century of study by the most eminent accoucheurs, the intricate processes of parturition are not all understood, and many of them are not yet satisfactorily explained.

The subject falls naturally into the consideration of three factors: first, the *powers;* second, the *passages;* third, the *passengers.* After this the action of the

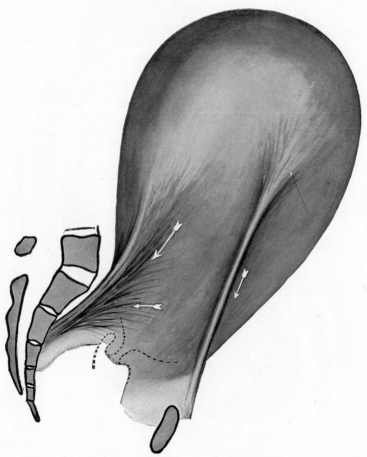

Fig. 169.—Action of the Uterine Ligaments.

powers on the passengers in forcing them through the prepared passages must be studied.

The Powers.—The uterus is the main driving engine, with the abdominal muscles as a powerful auxiliary. Gravity, that is, the weight of the child, is of small influence, while the elastic contraction of the vagina and perineal floor has hardly any effect on the propulsion of the ovum.

When the uterus contracts, it exerts equal pressure on its contents in all directions, obeying the law of pressure on fluids. If the pressure were met all over by equal resistances, it would return to the uterine wall nullified, but since there is a weak spot in the uterine wall, the lower uterine segment and internal os, the contents of the uterus will all be forced in this direction. The resultants of all the forces

applied to the bodies in the uterus will point toward the internal os (Fig. 168
Intra-uterine pressure (J.U.P.), as it has been called, is hydraulic pressure and
the most important factor in the work of the uterus, but other factors have be
invoked. Lahs and Schatz believed that the uterus, compressing the fetus fro
side to side, lengthened its spinal column, forcing the breech against the fund
and the head downward into the pelvis. This pressure is called the *fetal a*
pressure, and is absent in polyhydramnion, and with a small or macerated fet
Fetal axis pressure (F.A.P.) begins to act after the rupture of the bag of wate

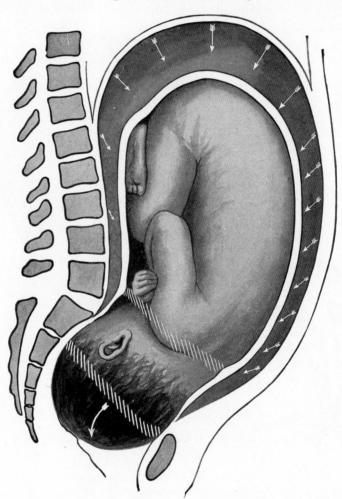

FIG. 170.—ACTION OF THE INTRA-ABDOMINAL PRESSURE IN AUGMENTING INTRA-UTERINE PRESSURE.
Girdles of resistance indicated by white lines.

Warnekros, with the x-ray, has shown that the spinal column is curved more by
uterine contractions in early labor, but later straightened after the bag of wat
is ruptured. The change of the C-formed spinal column to the straighter fo
results in a lengthening of the fetal cylinder of 10 cm. Radiographs show t
in some instances the uterus presses on the pelvic extremity of the fetal axis a
thus causes an advance of the child. While not constant F.A.P. may perform
function, which Liepmann denies.

Intra-uterine pressure accomplishes—(1) The protrusion of the bag of wate
(2) the dilatation of the lower uterine segment and cervix; (3) it causes edema a

succulence of the soft parts—the so-called "vital dilatation"; (4) the expulsion of the fetus and placenta.

The round, the uterosacral, and the broad ligaments have important functions. They are part of the uterus—mere extensions of its muscle-fibers—and contract when it contracts. These bands serve to moor the uterus to the pelvis and prevent too great retraction above the child. The round ligaments pull the fundus forward and bring its axis parallel with the axis of the inlet (Fig. 169). The uterosacral ligaments pull the cervix backward and downward and also help open up the lower uterine segment and upper cervix. All the ligaments, by the force exerted, increase the intra-uterine pressure and help expel the fetus.

The abdominal pressure is a powerful auxiliary in labor, and may substitute the uterine contraction more or less completely. During the first stage the abdominal muscles do not, and should not, take any part in the process of labor, but in the second stage they are called upon to assist and complete the work of the uterine contractions. During an expulsive pain the woman closes the glottis and makes a powerful bearing-down effort. She forces down the diaphragm and contracts the recti, the obliqui, and the muscles of the flanks. There is now a great increase of the intra-abdominal pressure, which, obeying the law, is transmitted equally in all directions, the uterus receiving its share. It is easy to see how the abdominal pressure is simply added to the intra-uterine pressure, resulting in increased general intra-uterine pressure—G.I.U.P. (Fig. 170).

After the dilatation of the cervix the abdominal muscles alone are able to expel the child, and usually do it, since the uterus by this time has retracted so high over the fetal cylinder and its muscle-fibers are so shortened that it has very little expulsive power.

In pathologic labor the abdominal muscles are particularly useful in overcoming the abnormal resistances, in preventing uterine rupture by restraining the upward displacement of the uterus, and in other ways. In the third stage of labor the placenta is expelled by the exertions of the abdominal wall, but only after the placenta is separated and lies in the lower uterine segment and vagina.

The **power** of the uterine contraction cannot be accurately measured. Duncan tried to do it by testing the resistance of the fetal membranes. The force necessary to rupture them varies from 4 to 37 pounds. Schatz, with his tokodynamometer, a rubber bag half-filled with water, lying in the uterus, connected with a manometer, found that the uterine contraction during the first stage showed a pressure of from 7 to 10 pounds, and during the second stage, when the force of the abdominal muscles was added, it was about trebled. Deffner, with Crodel's external tokometer, found about the same values. Joulin, with a dynamometer attached to his forceps, found a tractive effort of 80 to 100 pounds necessary to deliver some children—but these were pathologic cases and nature would have failed.

Clinically, the power of the uterine contraction may often be appreciated. It may crush the baby's head or fracture its bones. The accoucheur's hand in the uterus may be squeezed so hard that it becomes insensible and paralyzed. In rare cases tumultuous action of the uterus and abdominal muscles may eject the infant from the vulva with much force. Probably the ordinary amount of force exerted by the uterus and abdomen rarely exceeds 30 pounds.

Gravity plays but a small rôle in labor. The difference in specific gravity of the fetus and its liquor amnii is not great. The constant slight pressure exerted by the head on the lower uterine segment may soften this portion of the uterus, or it may elicit stronger pains. One often observes that a change of the parturient's position, which brings the weight of the fetus on to the cervix, such as walking or sitting up, will strengthen the uterine contractions.

11

CHAPTER X

THE PASSAGES

THE fetus has to traverse a bent passage, which is partly bony and partly fibrous and muscular. The bony portion is the pelvis, which is divided into two parts by a ridge called the linea terminalis. The upper, large, or false pelvis is of little obstetric interest. It is made up of the flaring iliac plates at the sides, the spine behind, and the gap in front over the pubis is filled in by strong abdominal

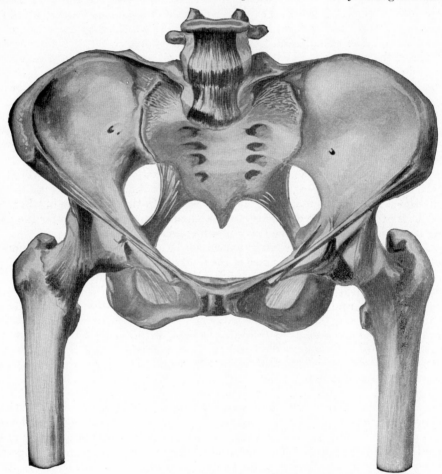

FIG. 171.—NORMAL FEMALE PELVIS.

muscles. The false or upper pelvis is shaped like a flat funnel, and forms a support for the uterus and child during pregnancy, directing the latter into the true pelvis at the proper time. The shape and size of the false pelvis, too, give the obstetrician some conception of the shape and size of the true pelvis. (See p. 252.) The true, lower, or small pelvis (pelvis minor) is of immense obstetric importance, since it supports the muscles of the pelvic floor and gives shape and direction to the par-

162

turient canal, itself forming part of same. A plaster cast of a true pelvis, as first made by Hodge, shows its cavity to have the shape of a cylinder with a bluntly pointed exaxial lower end. It is very slightly curved anteriorly. The entrance and outlet of the true pelvis are smaller than the middle portion, and have, therefore, been called straits—the superior and inferior. The region between, being large and roomy, is called the excavation. Anteriorly, the canal is short—4½ cm.; posteriorly, long, the length of the sacrum—12½ cm. Laterally, the pelvic canal is longer, and the sides narrow slightly from above downward, especially behind, near the spines of the ischia, but broadening out below at the tuberosities. The contour of the canal, therefore, varies much at different levels, and it is customary to describe these variations by means of planes drawn more or less arbitrarily through the pelvis. It must be clearly understood that the so-called planes about to be described are

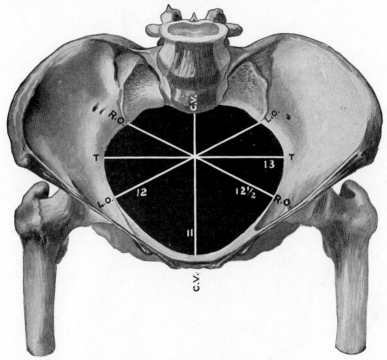

Fig. 172.—The Pelvic Inlet with Diameters.

really not such in a geometric sense, but represent regions or portions of the pelvis, and have three dimensions.

The **plane of the inlet,** brim, superior strait, isthmus, margin, or apertura pelvis superior, is bounded by the upper border of the pubis in front, the linea innominata or *linea terminalis* at the sides, and the sacral promontory behind (Fig. 172). This plane is heart-shaped—that is, a transverse ellipse on which the sacrum intrudes behind. The depth of the region of the inlet is about 2 cm., and represents the distance from a line drawn in the pubosacral diameter to a transverse line in the lowest level of the linea terminalis. (See Fig. 173.) It is deeper behind than near the pubis, and varies very much in all three dimensions—that is, in shape and depth. (For detailed description see chapter on Contracted Pelvis.) The inlet is a very important region of the pelvis, because contraction and distortion of the bones, due to disease, are likely to be marked here, and, further, it is an important factor in normal labor. Its diameters are, first, the anteroposterior, pubosacral, or *conjugata vera* (C. V.), named by von Roederer, extending from the top of the pubis to the

tip of the sacral promontory, measuring 11½ cm.   This is the true or anatomic
conjugate.   The shortest anteroposterior diameter is from a point 1 cm. lower on
the surface of the pubis to the promontory, and is called the obstetric conjugate
(Michaëlis), because intimately concerned in the mechanism of labor, especially in
contracted pelves.   It measures 11 cm. in the normal pelvis, but may be reduced to
a few centimeters in abnormal pelves.   When we speak of a pelvis of 8 cm. we
mean one with a C. V. of 8 cm.   It is impossible satisfactorily to measure the C. V.
on the living, though numerous instruments are vaunted for the purpose.   We can
gather an approximately correct idea of its length from the measurement of the
distance from the under margin of the pubis to the promontory.   This diameter is

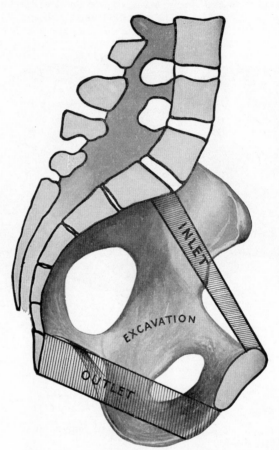

FIG. 173.—THE REGIONS OF THE PELVIS.

called the *conjugata diagonalis* (C. D.), and is, in normal pelves, about 1½ cm.
longer than the C. V. obstetrica, that is, about 12½ cm.   (See Pelvimetry, p. 252.)
Transversely, the inlet measures 13 cm., while the two obliques measure 12 and 12½
respectively.   The oblique diameters are named first and second or, better, right
and left, using the sacro-iliac joints as the denominator, according to the recommendation voted at the Congress at Washington in 1887 (Bar).   The right oblique extends from the right sacro-iliac joint to the left iliopubic tubercle; the left, between
corresponding points.   They are important diameters for the study of the mechanism
of labor at the bedside.   Since most individuals step harder on the right foot,
and since they also have a slight right scoliosis, the right half of the pelvis is a bit
flattened, and the left oblique, therefore, a trifle shorter than the right.   The inlet

is encroached upon by the iliopsoas muscles (Fig. 175), but probably not enough usually to disturb the mechanism of labor. If the child should be large and the muscle well developed, the muscle might delay the engagement of the head. Posture to relax the muscle would relieve the obstruction.

The **wide pelvic plane** is one passing from the middle of the pubis to the junction of the second and third sacral vertebræ (Fig. 176). It is about the center of the region called the "excavation" of the pelvis, and is, therefore, sometimes called the midplane, this latter term being much used in operative obstetrics. This plane

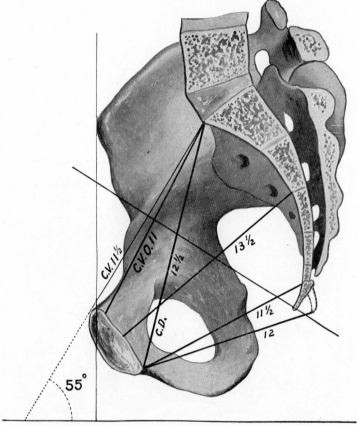

FIG. 174.—SAGITTAL SECTION OF PELVIS SHOWING DIAMETERS (Hodge).
C. V., Anatomic conjugate; C. V. O., obstetric conjugate; C. D., diagonal conjugate.

is irregularly ovoid, occupying the roomiest portion of the pelvis, and with an anteroposterior diameter of 13½ cm. and a transverse of 12½ cm.

The **narrow pelvic plane** passes through the apex of the pubic arch, the spines of the ischia, and the end of the sacrum (Fig. 177). This is the smallest strait of the pelvis, and is frequently the site of contracture, a fact which is only lately being adequately appreciated. This plane is ovoid, with the large end anteriorly and the smaller end behind, formed by the sacrosciatic ligaments. Owing to the incurvation of the spines of the ischia and the attachments of the levator ani muscle and fascia, the child, in its passage, is crowded into the anterior portion of this plane. Its most important diameter is that between the spines—10½ cm. An imaginary line drawn between the spines of the ischia is used to determine the descent of the head into the pelvis. The narrow pelvic plane is important also because it is the beginning of the bend of the cylindric birth-canal. In labor, the head descends straight into the pelvis until it reaches this plane, then begins to rotate and slide forward under the pubis.

The **plane of the outlet** passes through the arch of the pubis, the rami of the pubes, the tuberosities, and the tip of the coccyx. This plane is the lower boundary of the region of the bony outlet, and is not seldom the seat of contracture. There are really two planes, roughly resembling triangles bent at their applied bases on the tuberosities. During labor the head pushes the coccyx back (Fig. 174), bringing the two parts more into one plane, and at the same time increasing the antero-posterior diameter from 9½ to 12 cm. The transverse diameter of this plane is important—11 cm.

The above is a description of the classic pelvic planes dating from the time of

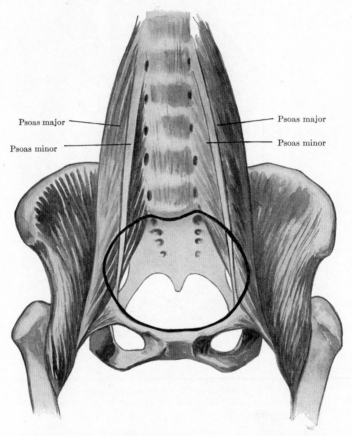

Psoas major

Psoas minor

Psoas major

Psoas minor

FIG. 175.—SHOWING INLET ENCROACHED ON BY ILIOPSOAS MUSCLES.

Levret (1770). Hodge, of Philadelphia, constructed a series of more arbitrary planes, all running parallel to the inlet (Fig. 179). The first parallel is in the inlet; the second parallel, called by Veit the "chief plane," touches the arch of the pubis and strikes the lower part of the second sacral vertebra; the third cuts the spines of the ischia, and the fourth goes through the tip of the coccyx and represents the pelvic floor. The Hodge system never obtained general recognition, and one modern author calls it obsolete, but Sellheim, to whom we owe much in the study of the mechanism of labor, as late as 1909 declared it the only scientific method for the study of the pelvis and the mechanism of labor, and recommended its general adoption by teachers and writers. It is a fact that the head enters the pelvis in the axis of the inlet, passing successively through these planes, and, too, since we can easily determine the location and direction of the inlet, it is a simple matter to orient one's self as to the location of the planes parallel to it. The author has used the Hodge system of planes in his studies of the mechanism of labor, and agrees with Sellheim as to their scientific worth. In the comparative study of contracted pelves (Hegar) and in gynecologic diagnosis they are equally valuable.

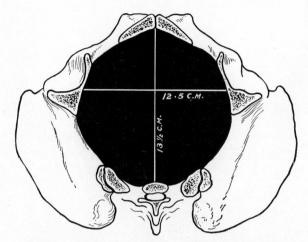

FIG. 176.—WIDE PELVIC PLANE.
Passes from the middle of the pubis to the junction of the second and third sacral vertebræ.

When the woman is in the erect position, the inlet makes an angle of about 55 degrees with the horizon, but this varies from 40 degrees to 100 degrees, depending on the rotation of the thighs and the carriage of the shoulders. This is called the *inclinatio pelvis*. A quick method to determine if this inclination of the pelvis is normal is to see if the anterior superior spine of the ilium and the pubis are in a vertical plane. In the lying position the inlet is 25 degrees below the horizontal.

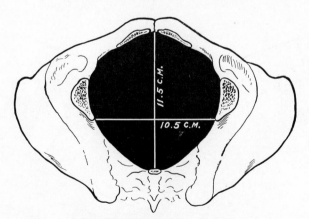

FIG. 177.—NARROW PELVIC PLANE.
Passes through the apex of the pubic arch, the spines of the ischia, and the tip of the sacrum.

The crests of the ilium run about parallel to the plane of the inlet. Formerly, great importance was attached to the pelvic inclination as affecting the mechanism of labor, lately not much.

Contrary to what would be expected, the pelvis is not a solid and fixed bony

structure. The coccyx is easily pressed back by the advancing head, enlarging the
outlet 2 to 2.5 cm. The pelvic joints are fixed by strong ligaments, but during

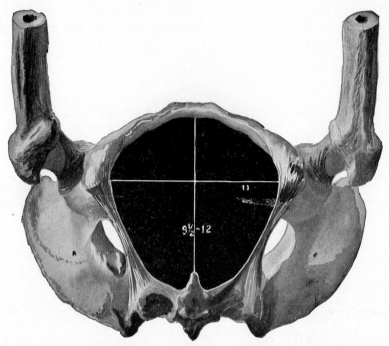

FIG. 178.—THE PELVIC OUTLET.
Passes through the arch of the pubis, the rami pubis, the tuberosities, and the tip of the coccyx.

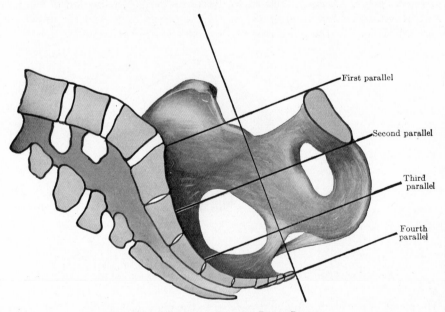

FIG. 179.—HODGE'S SYSTEM OF PARALLEL PELVIC PLANES.

pregnancy these soften and allow a certain degree of mobility to the bones. By
stretching and tearing as the head is driven, wedge-like, through the pelvis, they

allow a slight enlargement of the cavity. Also as occurs in many animals, the loosening of the joints allows the hip bones to rotate on the sacrum when the body is bent into forced extension and flexion. Thus, the sacrum being fixed, the pubis moves downward when forced extension of the thighs is made,—Walcher's position,—enlarging the inlet by 0.5 to 1 cm. (Fig. 180). In forced flexion, the knees being pressed against the abdomen, the pubis is forced up, the ossa innominata rotate upward and dip outward, enlarging the outlet of the pelvis. These changes in the shape of the pelvis are made use of in the conduct of labor. (See Chapter LVIII.)

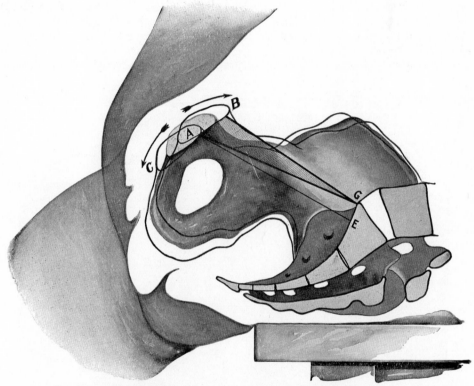

Fig. 180.—Showing the Mobility of the Pelvic Joints in Flexing and Extending the Thighs.

A represents the pubis when the patient lies flat on back; B, when the thighs are strongly flexed on the belly; C, when the legs are allowed to depend fully. A–E shows the available conjugate in the Walcher position, and the shaded area the gain in space in the region of the inlet.

LITERATURE

Bar, P.: Report sur l'unification de la nomenclature obstetricale au Congress à Rome, 1903.—Burns: Report of Committee on Obstetric Nomenclature to the American Medical Association, June, 1912.—Edgar: The Practice of Obstetrics.—Hodge: A System of Obstetrics, 1865.—L'Obstetrique, 1903, part 2.—Report of the Ninth International Medical Congress, Washington, 1887.—Liepmann: Zentb. für Gynaek., January 16, 1932, p. 136.—Sellheim: Die Geburt des Menschen, 1913.—Walcher: Zent. f. Gyn., 1889, p. 892.—Warnekros: Geburt im Roentgenbilde, Bergman, Berlin, 1925.

THE SOFT PARTS

Fig. 175 shows the relation of the psoas and iliacus muscles to the inlet. It will be seen that they give it a more quadrangular shape; that they encroach but little on its lumen; and that only in cases of transversely contracted pelves will they interfere in the mechanism of labor. The rectum lies on the left side behind, and projects into the cavity only when filled. It may thus cause dystocia. The midplane is encroached on by the obturator internus and behind by the pyriformis—very slightly, however. The nerves in the pelvis make no obstruction, and, owing to the projecting spines of the ischia and the forward dip of the pelvic floor, rarely are subject to pressure. When they do suffer pressure, the parturient has pains running down the legs and up the back. The peritoneum and fat count very little in the general configuration of the parturient canal, as was proved by Hodge with plaster casts.

The cervix and the lower uterine segment have already been considered. Of most obstetric interest is the pelvic floor. This consists of those soft tissues which fill out the irregularly shaped outlet of the pelvis. A great many structures enter into its formation—the pelvic fascia, the levator ani and coccygeus, the deep and superficial transverse perineal muscles, the constrictor cunni, the urogenital septum, fat and skin, and the organs—rectum, vagina, and urethra. Careful dissection and embryologic study enable us to distinguish two diaphragms in the pelvic floor (Holl) —an upper stronger, a muscular system, modified from that formerly used for the tail, and a lower, weaker, developed from the sphincter cloacæ, which closes the orifices in the pelvic floor.

The diaphragma pelvis rectale, or proprium, shortly referred to as the pelvic

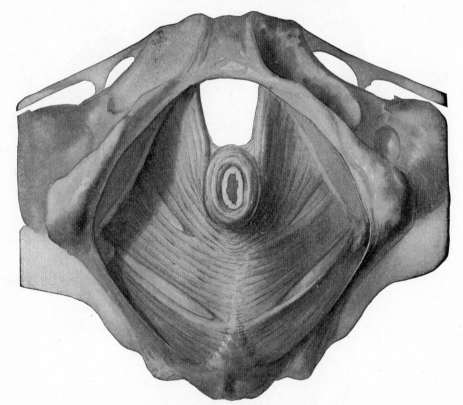

FIG. 181.—LEVATOR ANI FROM BELOW.
Drawn from a dissection made by E. Calhoun and E. Potter, N. W. Univ. Med. School.

floor or diaphragm, is made up of the levator ani and the coccygeus, together with the pelvic fascia above and below. Anteriorly, the muscle is attached to the back of the rami of the pubis, leaving an incomplete space, $2\frac{1}{2}$ cm. wide, behind the symphysis. It extends on either side across the opening of the obturator foramen, being attached to the fascia covering the obturator internus muscle underneath a tendinous duplication of the superior levator fascia (fascia diaphragma pelvis superiora), called the "white line," or arcus tendineus musculi levatoris ani. On vaginal examination this arcus tendineus can often be felt by the finger. The extent of the origin of the muscle varies. Usually it does not reach the spine of the ischium to which the ischiococcygeus is attached. Sometimes the two muscles fuse at their origins. The level of the "white line" also varies, sometimes it is higher, sometimes lower. In certain animals the levator ani takes origin from the linea innominata (Martin). Many divergent views of the anatomy of the pelvic floor exist, the reasons being that there are many individual differences even in normal women and, further, good subjects are hard to get, and dissecting artefacts easily lead to untrue conclusions.

From its area of origin the muscle-fibers pass downward and inward toward the median line. Posteriorly, they come together on the lower end of the sacrum and the coccyx; anterior to this they interlace in the median line behind the anus; next they fuse into a sling-like hammock under the perineal curve of the rectum, many of the medial fibers fusing with the upper border and sides of the sphincter ani and lower part of the rectum; finally, a very few fibers meet between the anus and vagina in the perineal body (Luschka's fibers). Holl gave different portions of

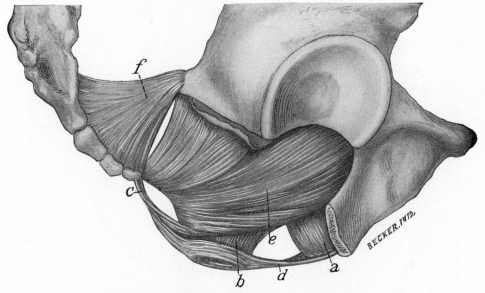

FIG. 182.—SHOWS LEVATOR ANI FROM SIDE—SLING-LIKE ACTION.

a, Vagina; *b*, rectum; *c*, posterior fibers of sphincter; *d*, anterior fibers of sphincter ani; *e*, levator ani, puborectal portion; *f*, musculus ischiococcygeus (somewhat modified from Luschka).

the broad muscle special names. That portion going from the spine of the ischium to the coccyx he called the ischiococcygeus; that from the arcus tendineus to the raphé, the iliococcygeus; that from the posterior surface of the pubis, passing alongside the urethra, vagina, and rectum, to meet its fellow in a tendinous raphé extending from the tip of the coccyx toward the rectum, the pubococcygeus; and, fourth, a strong band running from the pubis around the lower part of the rectum, sling-like, the puborectalis. The diaphragm thus resembles a concave broad horseshoe, incomplete in front, leaving an elliptic opening. Through this elliptic space pass the urethra, vagina, and rectum. The sides of the muscle slope together in the middle, forming a V-shaped gutter, leading down under the arch of the pubis. Figure 182 shows the distribution and action of the various portions of the levator ani and the opposing action of the sphincter ani. When the levator contracts it pulls the rectum and vagina up against the pubis; when the sphincter contracts it draws the anus and the lowest portion of the rectum backward, the result of the two forces being to bend the rectum, closing it most effectually.

On vaginal examination the puborectal portions of the levator can easily be felt as two roundish pillars at the sides of the vagina and when they contract the finger is raised up to the pubis. Beneath the pelvic diaphragm lie the ischiorectal fossæ, the perineal body, the diaphragma urogenitale, the vulva, and its glands. Of these we need consider only the diaphragma urogenitale (Fig. 184), which closes the hiatus genitalis. This is a three-cornered, musculo-fibrous septum, fitted into the pubic arch and extending backward to the anterior wall of the rectum. It is made up of the deep layer of the perineal fascia, inclosing the fibers of the musculus transversus perinei profundus and the compressor urethræ. A few of these fibers reach around the vagina and are called the sphincter urogenitalis (Kalischer). On this septum lie the musculi bulbocavernosi (sphincter cunni),

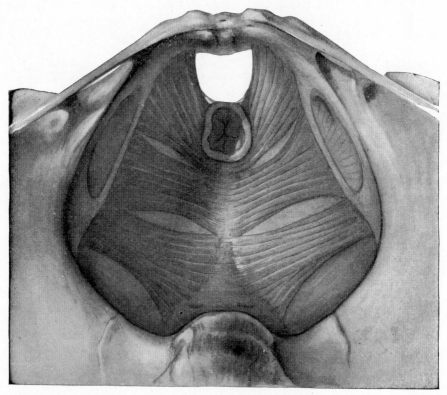

FIG. 183.—DIAPHRAGMA PELVIS.
Levator ani viewed from above. Same dissection as Fig. 181.

the ischiocavernosi, and the transversi perinei superficiales. These muscles, mostly rudimentary, center at a point between the rectum and the vagina called by Waldeyer the centrum perineale, or centrum tendineum perinei (Holl), or perineal body. The perineal body is a pyramidal structure, lying between the rectum and vagina, with its apex in the pelvic diaphragm. Its base is the skin between the anus and the vulva. Its anterior wall is the vagina and fossa navicularis, the posterior wall, the anus and rectum; at the sides it broadens out into the ischiorectal fossæ. It is composed of fat, fasciæ, the rear part of the urogenital septum, the fused ends of the transverse perineal muscles, the bulbocavernosi, the anterior fibers of the sphincter ani, and the skin. It has great obstetric importance, but not so much as that of the pelvic floor, a point frequently overlooked. During labor the perineal body is flattened out, its apex is pressed down and back, so that its structures come to lie on the distended pelvic diaphragm.

The sphincter ani externus lies between the skin and the pelvic diaphragm, surrounding the lower end of the rectum. It is attached posteriorly to the coccyx by the ligamentum anococcygeus, and anteriorly to the centrum tendineum. Most of its fibers go circularly around the anus, some continue into the bulbocavernosus, some circle in the skin near the anal margin. The puborectal portion of the levator ani fuses with the sphincter at the sides and behind. The sphincter ani varies

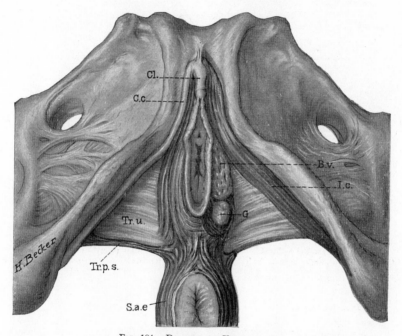

FIG. 184.—DIAPHRAGMA UROGENITALE.

Cl., Clitoris; C.c., crus clitoridis; Tr.u., trigonum urogenitale (triangular ligament); B.v., bulbus vestibuli; G., glandula vestibularis major (Bartholini); Tr. p.s., musculus transversus perinei superficialis; S.a.e., musculus sphincter ani externus; I.c., musculus ischiocavernosus.

much in size in different women: it may be as thick as the little finger and as broad as the thumb-nail, or only half the size. This is true of all the perineal muscles.

THE PELVIC FASCIÆ

The student is referred to books on anatomy for detailed descriptions of the fasciæ of the pelvis. Here only a brief résumé of those parts directly concerned in labor may be presented.

The endo-abdominal fascia passes down over the brim of the pelvis and soon splits into two layers. One covers the obturator internus muscle, one goes beneath it. About half-way down the inner surface of the obturator internus the fascia thickens into a ridge or seam, called the arcus tendineus musculi levatoris ani (commonly designated as the "white line"). Here the fascia splits, one layer passing downward on top of the levator ani and one layer continuing underneath it. A short distance below the white line the superior levator fascia thickens into another ridge or mass of fibrous tissue in which the hypogastric vessels, the ureters, and the fibers of the bases of the broad ligaments are found. This band of fibrous tissue is shown in Fig. 185 extending from the pubis around the pelvis to lose itself in the fascia over the pyriformis muscle. Martin called it the "retinaculum uteri." From its inner border four layers of fascia arise. One, very thin, goes anterior to the bladder, the second goes between the bladder and the vagina, the

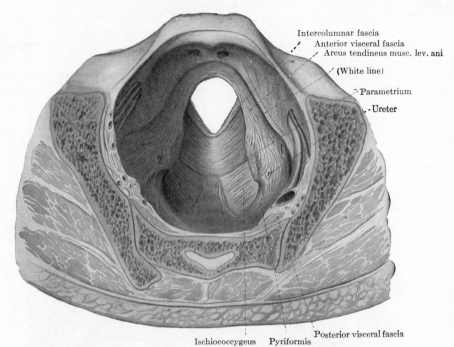

Intercolumnar fascia
Anterior visceral fascia
Arcus tendineus musc. lev. ani

(White line)

Parametrium

Ureter

Ischiococcygeus   Pyriformis   Posterior visceral fascia

FIG. 185.—THE CHIEF SUPPORTING FASCIAL SEAM (Wertheim).
All the pelvic organs are removed. The superior levator ani fascia, all except the portion between the pillars—the intercolumnar fascia—has been dissected away. The parametria have been cut off as they pass into the broad seam, which is part of the retinaculum uteri and is called the visceral fascia by Wertheim.

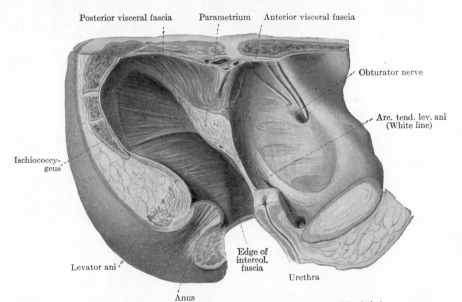

Posterior visceral fascia   Parametrium   Anterior visceral fascia

Obturator nerve

Arc. tend. lev. ani
(White line)

Ischiococcy-
geus

Levator ani

Edge of
intercol.
fascia

Urethra

Anus

FIG. 186.—THE SAME AS FIG. 185, SEEN FROM THE SIDE (Wertheim).
Shows the root of the visceral fascia. Incidentally, note the S-shaped conjunction of the levator ani stretching from the coccyx to the anus and forming a ledge on which the uterus rests.

third between the vagina and rectum, and the fourth is retrorectal (Fig. 187). The root stock of these four layers or leaves forms the base of the broad ligament.

It arises from the inner surface of the superior levator fascia and supports the pelvic viscera, hence, it should be called the visceral layer of this fascia. Anteriorly it is continued to the pubis to form the pubovesical ligaments, posteriorly to the sacrum to form the uterosacral ligaments, and laterally it makes the basis of the broad ligaments (called by Kocks ligamenta cardinalia.) One might liken this arrangement to a wire wheel—the cervix being the hub and the radiating ligaments the wire spokes. If any of the spokes are broken or stretched, the hub (cervix) will be displaced, resulting in disorganization of the whole system (Fig. 189).

The superior levator fascia now continues and covers the free edge of the levator ani muscle uniting with the deep layer of the fascia of the urogenital septum. Near the hiatus genitalis the fascia thickens into a ridge or strand of tough glistening fibers, called the arcus tendineus fasciæ pelvis. It can often be felt per vaginam

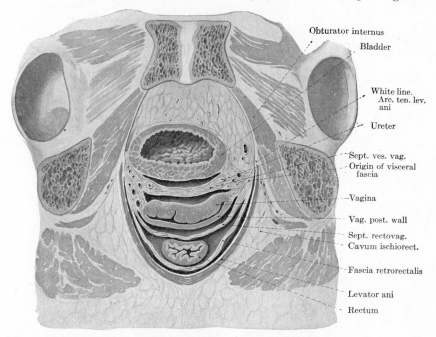

Obturator internus

Bladder

White line.
Arc. ten. lev.
ani

Ureter

Sept. ves. vag.
Origin of visceral
fascia

Vagina

Vag. post. wall

Sept. rectovag.
Cavum ischiorect.

Fascia retrorectalis

Levator ani

Rectum

Fig. 187.—Shows the Origin of the Visceral Fascia from the Endopelvic Fascia, and How the Broad Seam Splits Into Four Layers Enveloping the Pelvic Viscera (Wertheim).

on each side, as a sharp cord, coursing down the levator ani muscle. The fascia passes across from one pillar of the levator ani to the one on the opposite side between the rectum and the vagina, forming part of the centrum tendineum of the perineum and fusing with the third layer of the visceral fascia above described. It is somewhat thicker here, and holds the two pillars of the levator, while not in apposition—close together. I have given this portion, since it is so important in the mechanism of labor and in the repair of the pelvic floor lacerations, the name—"intercolumnar fascia" of the perineum.

These fascial planes and seams are of supreme importance in holding the cervix, bladder, vagina, and rectum in their proper relation to each other and to the pelvis. When they are torn or stretched in labor they allow the pelvic organs to descend *in toto*, or to be displaced one on the other. These fasciæ as shown by Goff in 1931 are more of the nature of areolar fascia and not the tough glistening structures usually so called.

The loose connective tissue and fat filling up the interstices of the pelvis are also of obstetric importance.

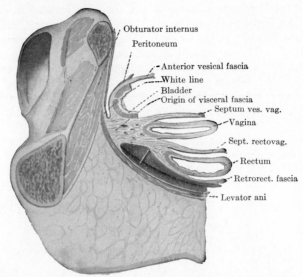

Obturator internus
Peritoneum

Anterior vesical fascia
White line
Bladder
Origin of visceral fascia
Septum ves. vag.
Vagina
Sept. rectovag.
Rectum
Retrorect. fascia
Levator ani

FIG. 188.—CORONAL SECTION OF THE SAME PELVIS AS LAST THREE (Wertheim).
Shows the root or origin of the visceral fascia from the superior levator fascia, and how it splits into four layers so as to ensheath the bladder, the vagina, and rectum.   Study with Fig. 187.

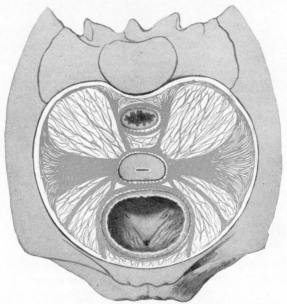

FIG. 189.—SEMIDIAGRAMMATIC (Tandler).
Shows how each pelvic organ has an individual sheath of fascia; the fibrous thickenings forming ligaments and fascial planes, supporting the organs and holding them in proper relation to each other and the pelvis; and the loose cellular tissue binding them all together.   Note the resemblance of the cervix to the hub of a wheel, the ligaments being the spokes.

THE FORMATION OF THE PARTURIENT CANAL

Before it can reach the external world the child has to pass through three rings—the cervix, the opening in the levator ani and the hiatus genitalis, the vulva, and perineum.   It is driven like a wedge against the resistance offered by these structures, and the overcoming of these structures is the main function of the powers of labor.   Normally, the head is forced through the cervix before it comes down on to the pelvic floor.   The dilatation of the diaphragma urogenitale occurs together with the diaphragma proprium, and together they are made to form a fibromuscular canal attached to the bony pelvic outlet. How the cervix is dilated until it is flush with the vagina has been described on p. 128. Figure 190 shows the condition of the parturient canal at the time when, dilatation being complete, the fetal head has passed through the cervix and come to rest on the pelvic floor. Now the levator ani begins to stretch. It is displaced downward and backward with all the soft parts of the pelvic outlet; thus these structures suffer a displacement in an axial direction, in addition to being dilated radially. This lengthening of the soft parts is greater on the posterior wall than on the anterior, being only 2 or 3 cm. here, while the posterior wall is stretched 10 cm. The bundles of the levator ani are separated and long drawn out (Figs. 191 and 192), so that they form, with the pubic arch, a canal whose circumference is equal to the head of the child—33 to 35 cm.

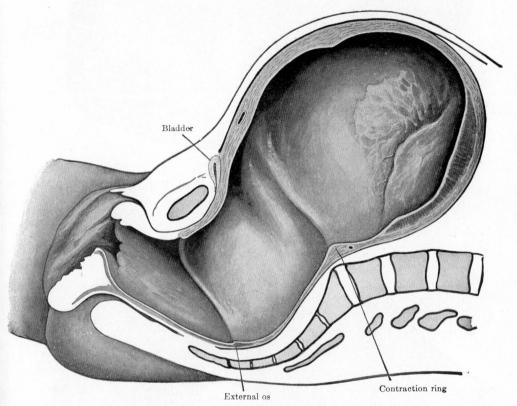

Fig. 190.—Braune's Frozen Section.
The head has passed through the cervix and come to rest on the pelvic floor.

The urogenital septum lies flat on the outside of the canal and dilates with it. Since the latter septum has little muscle, and connective tissue dilates poorly, it is the rule for tears to occur in this structure in all full-term labors. These tears allow a sagging of the anterior vaginal wall and urethra, producing the so-called "physiologic" prolapse of these structures. The sphincter ani is stretched from side to side as well as from before and backward. The anus, therefore, gapes widely as the head descends low, exposing the anterior wall of the rectum. The rectum is flattened out against the sacrum and levator ani. Owing to the attachment of the bladder to the lower part of the uterus it is drawn up into the abdominal cavity together with this portion of the retracting organ. Indeed, all the soft parts behind the pubis, the "pubic segment" (Barbour), have a tendency to retract upward, while those below, in front of the sacrum, the "sacral segment," are pushed

12

downward. Hart and Barbour have likened this action to that of folding doors, one being pulled, the other being pushed, to allow an object to pass through them.

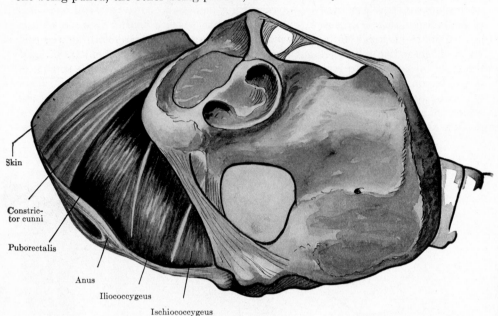

Skin

Constric-
tor cunni

Puborectalis

Anus

Iliococcygeus

Ischiococcygeus

FIG. 191.—PELVIC DIAPHRAGM RECONSTRUCTED AFTER DELIVERY (drawn from Sellheim's model. Outside view).

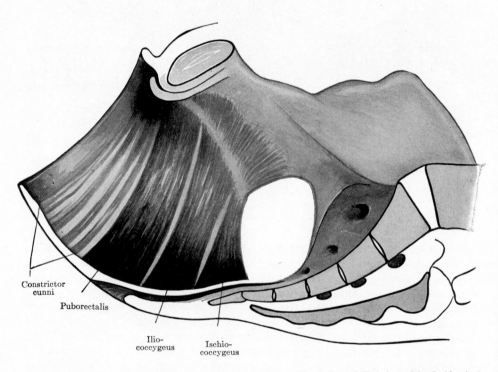

Constrictor
cunni

Puborectalis

Ilio-
coccygeus

Ischio-
coccygeus

FIG. 192.—PELVIC DIAPHRAGM RECONSTRUCTED AFTER DELIVERY (drawn from Sellheim's model. Inside view).

The vagina is dilated radially and axially, to form a lining membrane for the canal. When the pelvic floor tears, the vagina usually does also, but it may not. These submucous lacerations of the levator ani are difficult to recognize and hard to repair.

We have mentioned that the levator ani is stretched to form a muscular canal. Naturally the fascia above and below it take part in the dilatation. The retinaculum uteri, especially that portion around the cervix (the parametrium), is distended as the head is forced down, and the prolongations of the visceral fascia forward to the pubis (the pubovesical ligaments) are pulled down too. The same is true of the sacro-uterine ligaments.

The four leaves of the visceral fascia described on page 173 (Figs. 185–188) are distracted both radially and axially, *i. e.*, they are stretched circularly to the limit of the size of the fetal body, and at the same time they are forced down by

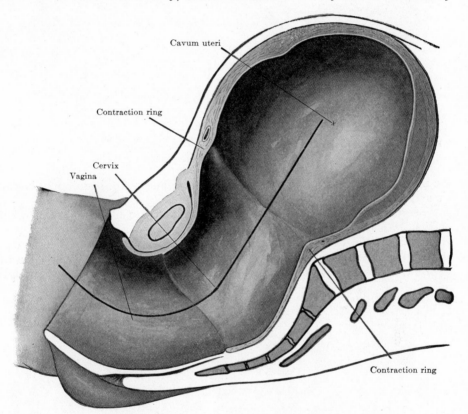

Fig. 193 —The Completed Parturient Canal.
Black line indicates the axis of canal. Note sharp bend at narrow pelvic plane.

the advancing head. As a result of this action these semi-elastic fascial seams and layers are thinned and destroyed in part. The vesicovaginal septum receives the first brunt of the attack, next the paracervical retinaculum, next the superior fascia levatoris ani, with the arcus tendineus fasciæ pelvis (Fig. 186); then the intercolumnar fascia gives way, which allows the levator ani pillars to separate (diastasis levator ani) and finally the urogenital septum.

In pathologic cases (*e. g.*, forceps operation before complete dilatation of the cervix, precipitate labor) the parametria and the root stock of the four leaves of the fascia visceralis are pushed off the superior layer of the levator ani fascia and prolapse of the pelvic organs follows. While overstretching and laceration during delivery are the determining causes of prolapse, the constitutional factor must always be borne in mind. Many women are of an asthenic nature, all their muscular and supportive structures being below par, either congenitally or acquired from bad habits of living. Easily 50 per cent. have enteroptosis. Infantilism of the genitalia is another basic factor. (See Sellheim.)

We may show the shape of the parturient canal, as in Fig. 193, but the reader will understand that it exists as such, in its entirety, at no time during labor. The advancing head produces such a disposition of the surrounding structures only at

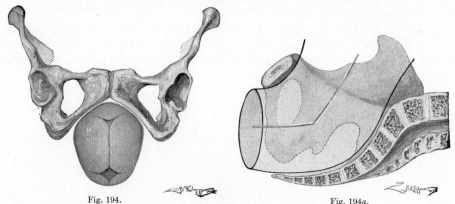

Fig. 194.   Fig. 194a.

FIGS. 194 AND 194a.—NORMAL SACRUM AND PELVIC OUTLET GIVING PROPER CURVE TO PARTURIENT CANAL. Note how head uses all available space under the pubis.

the moment it is passing through them. For the purpose of instruction, however, we may illustrate the completely dilated passages.

Schröder divided the uterovaginal canal into a contractile and a dilating portion. All under the contraction ring dilates; the uterine muscle above it contracts. Since the vagina is fastened to the pelvic floor, contraction of the uterus stretches the canal from this point upward, and the advancing head pushes the tissues from this point downward. This axial stretching of the canal, if carried

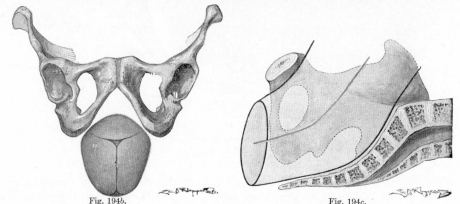

Fig. 194b.   Fig. 194c.

FIGS. 194b AND 194c.—OBTUSE ANGLE GIVEN TO PARTURIENT CANAL BY ABNORMAL PELVIC CONFIGURATION. ROTATION OF HEAD MAY BE DELAYED IN THIS PELVIS. Note how the head presses the perineum backward.

beyond the normal, may result in rupture of the uterus or vagina, and experience shows that this occurs most often in the zone extending from the contraction ring to the vagina. The radial stretching of the canal is greatest when the largest fetal plane is passing a given point. After this the elasticity of the walls of the canal adapts them to the reduced size of the fetal cylinder.

A study of the parturient canal will show that it runs straight down until it reaches the narrow pelvic plane or the third parallel of Hodge, then bends forward in

PLATE II.

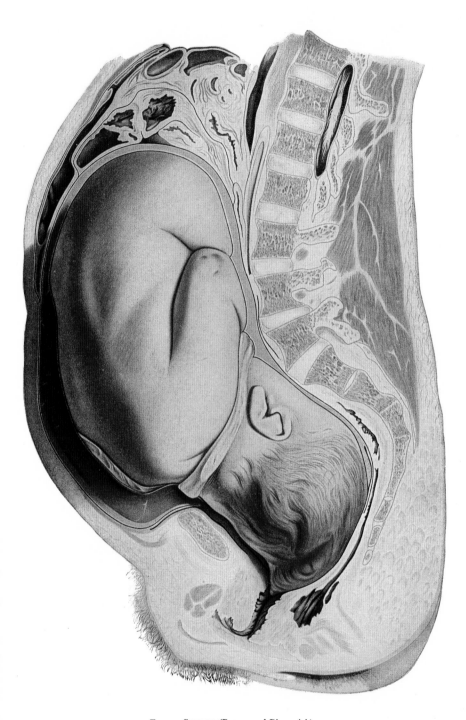

FROZEN SECTION (Bumm and Blumreich).

Cervix is completely dilated.   Note placenta on anterior wall and the formation of contraction rings to fit
depressions in fetal cylinder.

a sharp curve whose center is the symphysis pubis. If the passage uses the space under the arch of the pubis, the bend in it is quite sharp. If the arch of the pubis is narrow, or if the fetal head is very large, the occiput stems on the rami pubis, forcing the pelvic floor further back toward the sacrum, making a more obtuse angle in the parturient canal. The axis of the parturient canal is, therefore, not a curve (the curve of Carus), but a straight line with a bend at the pelvic floor and a curve (Plate II).

A great deal, in normal as well as pathologic labor, depends on the curve of the sacrum and the angularity of the pubic arch. If the sacrum is sharply curved and the pubic arch broad, as in Figs. 194 and 194a, the bend of the parturient canal will be more sudden. If the sacrum is not so deeply curved and the pubic arch narrow, as in Figs. 194b and 194c, the angle of the bend is very obtuse. Thus is created a factor in the mechanism of labor which affects the movement of the fetus along the birth-canal. (See p. 204.)

LITERATURE FOR CHAPTERS IX AND X

Deffner: Arch. für Gyn., 1932, vol. 148, H. 2, p. 502.—*Dickinson, R. L.:* "The Pelvic Floor," Amer. Jour. Obstet., May, 1902.—*Goff:* Surg., Gyn. and Obstet., January, 1931.—*Hart and Barbour:* Structural Anatomy of the Pelvic Floor, Edinburgh, 1880.—*Holl:* Handbuch der Anatomie des Menschen, v. Bardeleben, 1897, vol. vii, 2, Jena.—*Kalischer, O.:* Die urogenital Muskulatur des Dammes, Karger, Berlin, 1900.—*Martin:* Der Haftapparat der Weibl. Genitalien, Berlin, 1911, Lit.—*Schröder:* Lehrbuch der Geburtshilfe, 1899.—*Sellheim:* Veit-Stöckel, Handbuch der Gynaek., 1926, vol. ii, p. 179.—*Thomas:* "The Female Perineum," Amer. Jour. Obst., vol. xiii.—*Wertheim:* Operative Behandlung d. Prolapses, Springer, Berlin, 1919.

CHAPTER XI

THE PASSENGERS

FOR the study of the mechanism of labor a consideration of the fetus as a mechanical object is essential,—more so than has generally been allowed, —and we must consider its size, shape, compressibility, and pliability. The *head* is larger and more important, but the trunk takes no inconsiderable part in the normal mechanism of labor, and, when pathologically enlarged, may give rise to dystocia and even cause the death of mother or child or both. In the fetus at term the face is small, the vault of the cranium forming the major portion of the head. Four large squamous bones make up the cranial vault—the two parietal, the frontal, and the occipital. At the sides the temporal bones unite with the parietals. To provide for the molding necessary in the child's passage through the maternal parts,

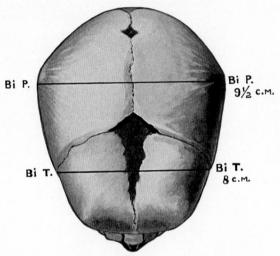

FIG. 195.—FETAL HEAD WITH DIAMETERS.

and for the rapid growth of the brain in the first year of life, these bones are not united, but the ossification halts at the lines of impingement, which later become the *sutures* of the skull. The bones are held together by the membrane in which ossification takes place—the chondrocranium. The lines of impingement are called *sutures*, and at the junctions of the sutures, owing to rounding of the bony corners of the separate bones, spaces filled by membrane are left, and these spaces are termed *fontanels* (fonticuli). Outside of the configurability conferred on the head by the sutures and fontanels, these spaces are of vital importance to the practising accoucheur, for by means of them he determines the relation of the head to the maternal pelvis, studies the mechanism of labor, and guides his application of the obstetric forceps.

Between the two parietal bones lies the sagittal suture (Fig. 195); between the parietals and occipital, the bent lambdoid suture; between the frontal bone and the parietals, the coronary suture, while between the two plates of the frontal bone lies the frontal suture, whose length varies. At the sides, where the parietal bones touch the temporals, lie the lateral or temporal sutures, of little obstetric importance.

At the junction of the sagittal, frontal, and coronal sutures lies a lozenge-shaped space, the anterior or large fontanel. Its size depends on the degree of ossification of the abutting bones, and its shape also, since with advanced ossification it becomes more square. Four sutures run into the large fontanel, which fact distinguishes it from the others, and, of its angles, three are acute and one obtuse, which points enable us to diagnose the position of the fetal head in the pelvis. The shortest, obtuse angle (Fig. 196) points toward the occiput, or posterior pole of the head, the long acute angle, toward the face.

Behind, at the junction of the sagittal suture with the lambdoid, a small triangular space exists, called the posterior or small fontanel. It is best to use the terms small and large fontanel to avoid confusion in the study of the mechanism of labor. Three sutures enter the small fontanel, which during labor is obliterated as

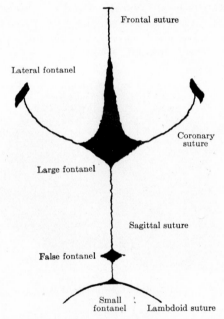

Frontal suture

Lateral fontanel

Coronary suture

Large fontanel

Sagittal suture

False fontanel

Small fontanel   Lambdoid suture

FIG. 196.—DIAGRAM OF THE SUTURES AND FONTANELS.

a space, the three lines coming together at a point like the letter **Y**. The stem of the **Y** is the sagittal suture and runs toward the face.

Where the lateral sutures meet the ends of the coronary and lambdoid, spaces exist which are called the lateral fontanels. They are important because they may impose as the other fontanels and lead to costly diagnostic errors. The ear is close to the posterior lateral fontanel, the bony orbit next to the anterior, and hereby mistakes are readily avoided. Wormian bones are accessory centers of ossification which sometimes occupy the spaces of the fontanels, but they have no obstetric importance. In the sagittal suture occasionally a quadrangular space is found (Fig. 195), which is most easily mistaken for the large fontanel, and may cause serious errors in diagnosis. It is a false fontanel. Confusion may be avoided by following the sagittal suture to its terminal fontanels.

We distinguish the regions of the skull by particular names. The occiput is that portion (Fig. 197) lying behind the small fontanel; the sinciput is that portion lying anterior to the large fontanel; the bregma, the region of the large fontanel; the vertex, the region between the two fontanels and extending to the parietal protuberances. In shape the fetal head is irregularly ovoid—narrow in front, broad behind. The frontal bone is quite square, the result of the angularity of the frontal protuberances, and the parietal bones have on each side a prominence which is more or less sharp—the parietal bosses (tubera parietalia). They mark the points where the head meets the greatest resistance in passing through the pelvis. No inference may be made regarding the shape of the child's head by considering those of its parents because it may resemble either one; usually, however, the mother makes the greater impress. Certain vagaries have been noted in the ossification of the sutures, which give the skull peculiar shapes. If the sagittal suture unites too early, a scaphocephalus results: the head is boat-shaped, being as broad in front as behind. If the frontal suture ossifies early, a three-cornered head results—trigonocephalus. In similar ways brachycephalus—short head—and dolichocephalus—long head—are produced. These various shapes modify the mechanism of labor and may produce dystocia.

The **fetal head diameters** vary quite a little within normal limits. The molding of the head by labor shortens some diameters and lengthens others. The measurements, therefore, should be taken a second time four or five days after birth, when the head has recovered its original shape. The measurements here given are the averages of a large number of children (Jaggard).

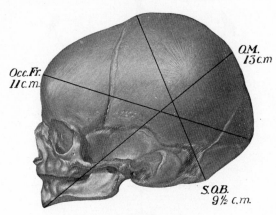

FIG. 197.—SIDE VIEW OF FETAL SKULL.

Diameter biparietalis—B.P., 9½ cm.
Diameter bitemporalis—Bi.T., 8 cm.
Diameter suboccipitobregmaticus—S.O.B., 9½ cm.
Diameter occipitofrontalis—O.F., 11 cm.
Diameter occipitomentalis—O.M., 13 cm.

There are many other diameters, but these are the only ones practically necessary. Two circumferences of the head should be taken, the large and the small, the first taken around the occipitofrontal diameter, the other around the suboccipitobregmatic. They measure 34 and 31 cm. respectively.

The **trunk,** while apparently larger, presents smaller diameters to the birth-canal, because it may be compressed to assume cylindric proportions. In some children the shoulders are very broad, in others relatively much smaller than the head. Boys usually have larger heads at birth, and this is also true of the first child, regardless of sex. The bisacromial diameter of the fetus is 11 cm.; the bisiliac, 9 cm. The circumference of the shoulders is 34 cm.; of the chest, 32 cm.

By "attitude" is meant the relation of the various parts of the fetal body to one another. The normal attitude of the child, when there is no scarcity of liquor amnii, is one of moderate flexion of all the joints, head slightly bent on the chest, the arms and legs free to move in all natural directions. The back of the child is curved.

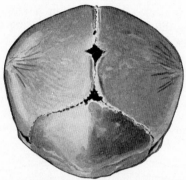

FIG. 198.—BACK VIEW OF FETAL SKULL.
Shows small fontanel and a "false" fontanel.

In addition, there is usually some lateral flexure of the head on one shoulder. (See Fig. 199.) When the amount of liquor amnii is small, so that the child has insuffi-

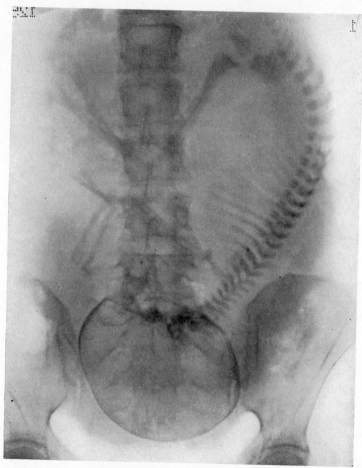

FIG. 199.—POSTURE OF CHILD IN UTERO.
Note that the child has much freedom of motion with the extremities.

cient space to stretch out, its attitude is one of cramped flexion. The extremities are pressed into the body, crossing each other, sometimes even with bending the long bones, and shortening of the muscles. Occasionally one finds decubitus over the bony prominences. Labor in such cases is harder and is often attended by irregular, anomalous uterine action. (See Labor in Oligohydramnion.)

Changes in the Fetus the Result of Labor.—Sellheim's x-ray plates and Barbour's frozen section, together with clinical studies, give us a clear idea of the molding of the child during labor. The child as a mechanical object for labor presents two ovoids joined by a flexible shaft, the neck. The trunk is flexible to a certain degree, and more flexible in certain directions than in others. Since this jointed object has to pass through a bent canal, one can readily perceive that this adaptability will come into play. The neck is most readily extended, and extension is its greatest movement, because the strong posterior neck muscles prevent any great

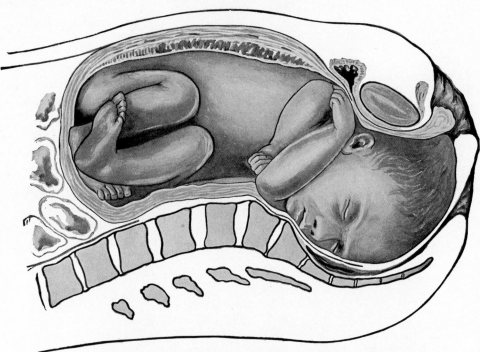

FIG. 200—FROZEN SECTION OF WOMAN WHO DIED IN SECOND STAGE (Barbour).

degree of flexion of the chin onto the sternum. The child can bend its dorsal spine best in a lateral direction, because the arms and thighs, by pressure against the trunk from the front, act like splints, stiffening it against flexion in this direction.

As the child is forced through the girdle of resistance its frankly ovoidal shape is squeezed into more cylindrical form, the better to pass the narrows and follow the line of least resistance or, as Sellheim says, the direction of least coercion. The uterus, by its contractions operating on its contents, forces open the lower uterine segment and cervix. Its cavity, therefore, lengthens, its walls apply themselves closer on the fetus, the extremities of the latter are pressed against the trunk, the latter is straightened out, the fetus is lengthened. This lengthening of the child is easily determined during every normal labor—one finds the fundus uteri rising higher toward the ensiform, while the head advances through the birth-canal and it is confirmed by x-ray pictures of a woman in labor.

By the same forces the head is flexed on the sternum, the shoulders sometimes thrown up under the ears, with the clavicles standing almost vertically, a condition found with normal pelvis and soft parts. This action fixes the head on the trunk, so that there is only one direction in which the head can bend readily, and that is extension. The effect of such a condition on the mechanism of labor will be studied shortly. In many cases the shoulder girdle is held back by the cervix or pelvis—then the shoulders are wedged through by hydraulic pressure aided by fetal axis pressure—or art helps with manipulation from below.

Fehling proved that the size of the head can be slightly reduced under the pressure of labor by the escape of cerebral fluid into the spinal canal. Perhaps, too, some of the blood in the brain may escape into the cervical veins. It is questionable, however, if such a small reduction as is thus possible is of any real influence in the mechanism of labor. The configurability of the skull, on the other hand, is of utmost importance. Figs. 162, 163, and 164 show how the head is molded in the most common delivery. When the child comes in face presentation, other cranial shapes are produced. The circular pressure of the uterus forces all the fetal tissues into conformation with the cylindric bore of the birth-canal, and one thus finds cross-sections of the fetal ellipsoid to show almost circular outlines. The reduction of the bisacromial diameter may be as much as 2 cm., depending on the hardness of the fetal tissues. If the child is overgrown, it is poor in water, and the flesh is tougher and less compressible. Dystocia is common in these cases.

PRESENTATIONS AND POSITIONS

Authors are not in accord in classifying the various ways in which the fetus may present itself for delivery. Baudelocque (1775) described 94 presentations. Almost any portion of the child's person can present itself first for delivery, and since the attitude and position of the child change during labor, the difficulties in the way of a universally acceptable classification are apparent. That accepted at the Ninth International Medical Congress at Washington, 1887, is generally recog-

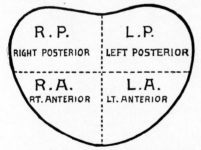

Fig. 201.—The Four Quadrants of the Pelvis. Looked at from above.

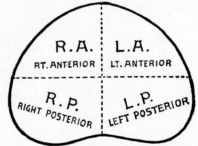

Fig. 201a.—The Four Quadrants of the Pelvis. Looked at from below.

nized as the best, but it is not complete enough. In the terminology, that adopted by the Basle Congress has been employed.

Definitions.—By "*presentation*" is meant that portion of the fetus which is touched by the examining finger through the cervix, or, during labor, is bounded by the girdle of resistance. According to Hodge, it is that part felt by the examining finger "toward the center of the pelvis." Much confusion will be avoided if the word *presentation* is adopted as here defined, and made synonymous with the much-used expression "presenting part."

"*Position*" is the situation of the child in the pelvis, and is determined by the relation of a given, arbitrary point in the presenting part to the periphery of the pelvic planes.

"*The point of direction*" is this arbitrary point in the presenting part, by which we determine the topographic relation of the presenting part to the periphery of the pelvic planes, *i. e.*, its position. In occipital presentation the occiput is the point of direction; in breech presentation, the sacrum; in shoulder presentation, the scapula; in face, the chin, etc. The Germans use the back as the point of direction.

"*Attitude*" is the relation of the fetal members to each other; it is habitus or posture. The attitude of the fetus has much to do with its presentation, but they are not identical. Attitude may be disturbed by the arms leaving the chest, the

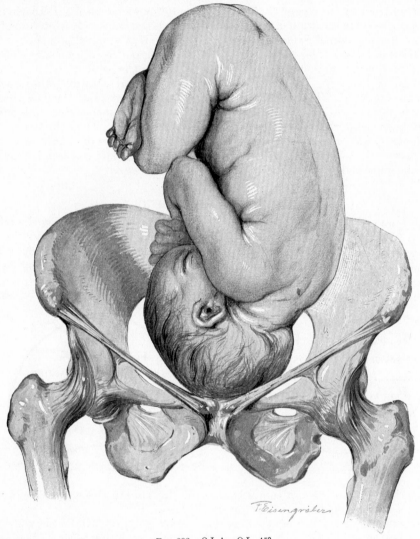

Fig. 202.—O.L.A.—O.L. 45°.

legs leaving the abdomen and prolapsing, or the cord prolapsing, the chin extending, making the various deflexion presentations, etc.

All terms as to direction are referred to the mother in the erect position. The term *upper* means the part in the direction of the fundus uteri; *lower*, the part nearer the vulva; *anterior*, means the direction to the front of the mother; *right*, the right side of the mother, etc.—these terms having no application to the child nor to the examiner nor are they changed in any position the mother may take. By keeping this rule in mind confusion will be avoided. These notions of direction have been taught by anatomists, physiologists, surgeons, and obstetricians for many centuries. In most of the illustrations the author has shown the conditions conformable to these ideas of direction, trusting the reader to transfer the images to the patient lying down.

For convenience of description the pelvis is divided into four quadrants— an anterior left, an anterior right, a posterior right and left (Fig. 201). The position of the presenting part is defined according to that quadrant in which the point of direction lies. Three grand divisions of presentation are recognized:

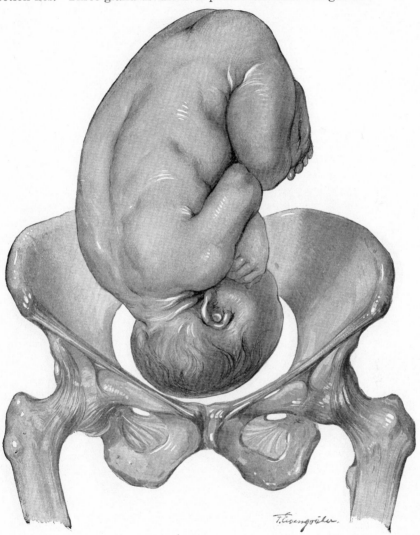

Fig. 203.—O.D.A.—O.D. 45°.

I. Cephalic presentation and its varieties—vertex, bregmatic, brow, and face. The vertex is the normal, the others are transitional, or pathologic, being due to deflexion of the head. They are sometimes called "deflexion attitudes."

II. Pelvic or breech presentation and its varieties—complete breech, footling, double footling, knee, double knee, and single breech.

III. Transverse presentation, including shoulder, arm, and any part of the trunk.

In the first two groups the axis of the fetus lies parallel with that of the uterus; in the last group it lies obliquely, more or less.

Presentation has to do with the part of the fetus which presents itself to the parturient passage first for delivery. It is determined by the attitude of the child and the relation of its axis to that of the birth-canal. Position, in its technical sense, means the topographic relation of the presenting part to the plane of the pelvis in which it lies; that is, to the four quadrants of the pelvis. Each presenting part

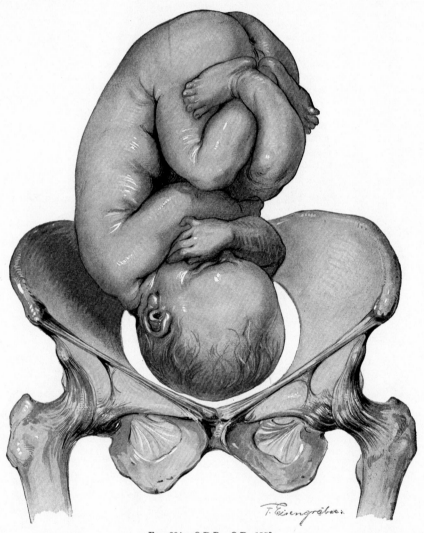

Fig. 204.—O.D.P.—O.D. 135°.
Radiography has shown that, before the actual labor, the child has much freedom of motion of its limbs and is folded together thus only in a dry uterus.

may so occupy the pelvis that its point of direction may lie in any pelvic diameter; for example, the occiput may be to the right, to the left, behind, in front, or at any intermediate point, when labor begins. The most common locations are used for teaching. The Committee at Washington adopted four main positions. Six are here given, and other writers (Williams, Farabeuf, and Varnier) also distinguish them. The Latin terms and abbreviations are to be preferred. In the following table the positions are named about in the order of frequency:

CEPHALIC PRESENTATIONS

1. Vertex—occiput, the point of direction.

Occipito-læva anterior ..........................O.L.A.
"   læva transversa .......................O.L.T.
"   dextra posterior ....................O.D.P.
"   dextra transversa ....................O.D.T.
"   dextra anterior.......................O.D.A.
"   læva posterior .......................O.L.P.

2. Face—chin, the point of direction.

Mento-dextra posterior.........................M.D.P.
"   læva anterior ........................M.L.A.
"   dextra transversa......................M.D.T.
"   dextra anterior........................M.D.A.
"   læva transversa .......................M.L.T.
"   læva posterior .......................M.L.P.

3. Brow—the brow the point of direction.

Fronto-dextra posterior.........................F.D.P.
"   læva anterior .........................F.L.A.
"   dextra transversa......................F.D.T.
"   dextra anterior........................F.D.A.
"   læva transversa .......................F.L.T.
"   læva posterior ........................F.L.P.

PELVIC OR BREECH PRESENTATIONS

1. Complete Breech—the sacrum the point of direction (feet crossed and thighs flexed on belly).

Sacro-læva anterior............................S.L.A.
"   læva transversa ........................S.L.T.
"   dextra posterior .......................S.D.P.
"   dextra anterior.........................S.D.A.
"   dextra transversa.......................S.D.T.
"   læva posterior .........................S.L.P.

When the breech is incomplete,—that is, when one or both feet have been prolapsed, or one or both knees are down, or when the feet are turned upward along the chest, so-called single breech,—the sacrum is still the point of direction, the designations remaining as above, and one simply adds the qualification, footling, knee, etc.

TRANSVERSE OR TORSO PRESENTATIONS

1. Shoulder—the scapula being the point of direction.

Scapulo-læva anterior ....Sc.L.A. ⎫ ⎧ Back,
                                              ⎪ ⎪ ante-
"   dextra anterior ....Sc.D.A. ⎬ ⎨ rior
                                              ⎪ ⎪ positions
"   dextra posterior ....Sc.D.P. ⎫ ⎧ Back,
                                              ⎬ ⎨ poste-
"   læva posterior..............Sc.L.P. ⎪ ⎪ rior
                                              ⎭ ⎩ positions

The back, side, or belly may present, but these are rare, and come readily under the above classification.

One important dimension is lacking in this presentment. How are we to determine the distance the fetus has advanced down the birth-canal toward the vulvar outlet? How shall we convey the idea of the location or degree of progression of the presenting part in the birth-canal? Müller suggested the word "station" or "statio," and used it thus, for example, "statio in aditu," presenting part in the inlet, "statio in exitu," at the outlet. Bacon is the only American teacher who has adopted this form. The term "degree of engagement" was used by Jaggard and is often employed, and the entry of the head into the pelvis he called "engagement." "Location" is another term, but "station" is better.

A head is "not engaged" when its greatest transverse diameter is still above the plane of the inlet. If freely movable, we call it "floating," or "caput ballitabile."

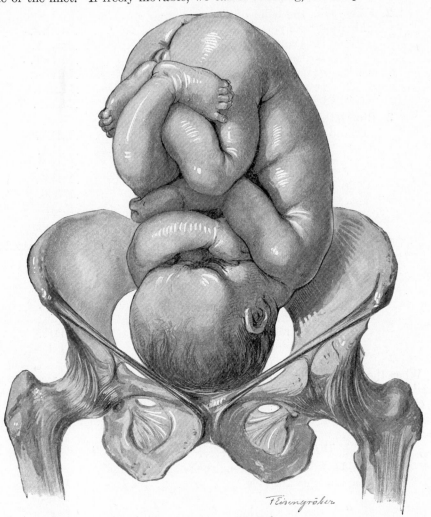

Fig. 205.—O.L.P.—O.L. 135°.

A head is "engaging" when the largest transverse diameter is just about to pass the inlet—"caput mobile." The term "engaging" should not be used in practice, as it expresses motion and conveys an indefinite idea of "station" (standing). A head is "engaged" when the largest transverse diameter has passed the plane of the inlet—"caput ponderosum." A head is "deeply engaged" when the largest diameter lies in the narrow pelvic plane. A head is "at the outlet" when the largest diameter is passing the bony outlet. The perineum is beginning to bulge at this time. A head is "on the perineum" when the largest diameter has passed the bony outlet and the head begins to show in the vulva. This might be called the period of *disengagement*.

A diagnosis of the mechanical conditions of a given labor, therefore, requires a statement of the presentation, the position of the presentation, and the station or degree of engagement of the presenting part. The last is of great importance, but much neglected, and often with fatal results to mother and child.

The author has devised plans for the designation of the different positions by "degrees," and the engagement, by centimeters. (See p. 310.)

FREQUENCY OF THE PRESENTATIONS AND POSITIONS

Karl Braun, in 48,449 cases, found vertex presentations in 95.9 per cent.; pelvic presentations, 2.7 per cent.; face, 0.6 per cent.; transverse, 0.7 per cent. Of the vertex presentations, 70 per cent. were O.L.A., 29 per cent. O.D.P., and 1 per cent. the other two positions. Schröder, from a clinical study of over 250,000 cases, finds the vertex in 95 per cent.; breech in 3.11 per cent.; the face, 0.6 per cent.; and transverse presentations in 0.56 per cent. At the Chicago Lying-in Hospital, in 35,179 births 94.95 per cent. were vertex, of which 12.1 per cent. were occiput posteriors and of these 52.7 per cent. were O.D.P. Breech occurred in 4.2 per cent., transverse in 0.45 per cent., brow in 0.068 per cent., and face 0.33 per cent. During the last few weeks of pregnancy both the presentation and the position of the fetus may change, most frequently from breech and shoulder, to head. Ordinarily the presentation is permanent after the presenting part has engaged in the pelvis, but this is not invariable. The author has observed a head which had sunk deep into the excavation rise up into the abdomen again before labor set in. Hippocrates believed that at the seventh month the child, which up to then presented by the breech, turned a somersault (variously named, Culbute, Inversio Fetus—Peristrophe) and the head came over the inlet.

While changes of the long axis of the child are not infrequent, changes in position are of almost daily occurrence. Examination of the woman on successive days, in the morning and evening, will show the back now on one side, now on the other. Multiparæ, because of the lax uterine and abdominal walls, show the most marked mobility of the fetus. During labor the fetus may also alter its presentation and position, particularly the latter. If the observer happens to examine the patient early in labor, he may find an O.L.P.; if a few hours later, an O.L.T., and again later an O.L.A., or even an O.D.A. Hospital statistics differ from those in private practice because pathologic labors are sent to hospitals. Figures from the one source show a large percentage of abnormal presentations; from the other, a necessarily smaller percentage. The effect of all these factors on the value of our statistical information is evident.

During pregnancy the child is more movable and accommodates itself to the varying position of the mother. When she is erect, its back falls forward; when on the side, it drops to the side on which she lies. This explains the frequency of O.L.T., O.D.T., O.D.P., and O.L.P. in our routine pregnancy examinations. One examiner may diagnose O.D.A., and his follower O.D.P., the change having resulted from the prolonged dorsal position of the mother and displacement by the palpating hand.

Causes of the Frequency of the Cephalic Presentations.—Hippocrates believed gravitation explained the predominance of head presentation. The heavier head sinks to the lowest part of the uterus, a fact which recent x-ray studies tend to prove. Dubois believed the fetus instinctively sought that position which was most comfortable; Simpson referred the head presentation to the reflex movements of the child when it was forced out of the position in which it could be most easily accommodated. Cohnstein gives the older theories in full.

The law of accommodation of Pajot explains it best. Where an ovoid body lies free in an ovoid container, the two long axes tend to become parallel, which is especially true if the container has contractile power, as has the uterus. The child, as it lies folded together, is ovoid; the uterus, at the end of pregnancy, likewise. The uterus is not a flaccid sac, but has some tonus and keeps its form, and further

it contracts frequently (the contractions of pregnancy). During these contractions
it assumes an exquisitely oval shape, and one can readily perceive how it would
gradually force the contained fetal ovoid to conform to the shape of its cavity
(Figs. 206–208). Even in early pregnancy the head lies in the lower segment of
the uterus, and this tendency is enhanced by the shape of the uterus growing more
ovoid all the time. After the head is once in the smaller end of the ovoid it is, to
an extent, anchored. This stability is favored by a normal pelvis and head (de
Snoo). The explanation of the occurrence of the various positions of the child
is easy. With the woman in the erect posture the back of the child will naturally
occupy the roomy anterior half of the uterus. Behind, the lumbar spine projects sharply into the uterine ovoid (Fig. 209), and, when the woman lies down,
the round heavy fetal back falls to one or the other side of it (Fig. 210). Since
the uterus has some dextrolateral torsion, and since the sigmoid and rectum
push forward the left side of the uterus, a cross-section of its cavity will appear
elliptic. A glance at the figures will show why the back is more likely to be found

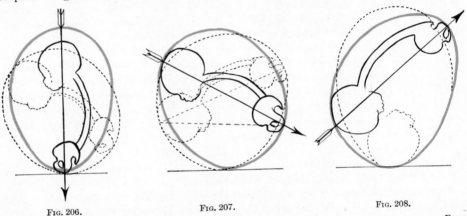

Fig. 206.   Fig. 207.   Fig. 208.

FIGS. 206, 207, AND 208.—DIAGRAMS TO ILLUSTRATE ACTION OF UTERUS IN ALTERING PRESENTATION OF FETUS
(modified from Kristeller).

in the left anterior portion of the uterus or in the right posterior. The back communicates its forward or backward tendency to the head, rotating it on an axial
diameter so as to bring the occiput to the front or rear. The left occipito-anterior
position is over twice as frequent as the right posterior, and this disproportion becomes greater until the end of pregnancy. During the twenty-four hours a woman
remains twice as long in the erect posture as lying down, and, therefore, the back is
more likely to fall to the front. This accounts for the predominance of O.L.A.
We use this knowledge to influence the mechanism of labor. Other reasons for the
frequency of O.L.A. have been advanced, as the flattening of the right half of
the pelvis and enlargement of the left half, the right oblique diameter of the inlet
being greater than the left; the inclination of the pelvis to the left side; the presence of the liver on the right side, but they have little influence. The location of the
placenta affects the location of the back, the latter usually lying opposite the former
(Figs. 209 and 210).

Abnormal and unusual presentations are caused by absence or inefficiency of
the above-mentioned factors. If the uterus is overdistended, as by polyhydramnion
or twins, its walls cannot grasp the fetal ovoid, which, therefore, is often found presenting wrongly. Multiparæ with flaccid uterus and lax abdominal walls (pendulous
belly) suffer often with malpresentations.

A small or premature fetus is more likely to present by the breech than an overgrown child. Hydrocephalic children predispose to breech presentation. Accident
is a factor, as when labor begins suddenly or the bag of waters ruptures when the
fetus is in an unfavorable presentation.

Abnormalties in the shape of the uterus cause malpresentations. Uterus arcuatus and bicornate uterus are often attended with breech or shoulder presentation. In one such case the author delivered two breech presentations, and in another the sixth successive footling.

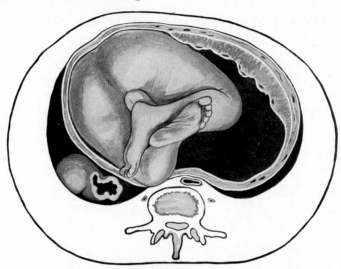

Fig. 209.—Showing Effect of Projection of Lumbar Spine, and also of the Location of Placenta on Anterior Uterine Wall. O.L.A.

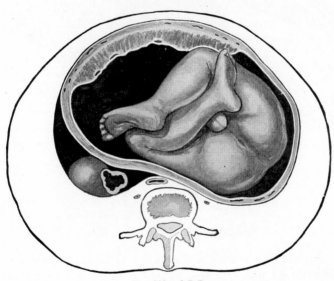

Fig. 210.—O.D.P.

Contracted pelvis, tumors of the lower uterus or pelvis, placenta prævia,—in short, all conditions which prevent the engagement of the head,—predispose to shoulder and breech presentations.

LITERATURE

Cohnstein: "Die Aetiologie der normalen Kindeslagen," Monatsschr. f. Geburtsh., 1868, vol. xxxi, p. 141.—*de Snoo, K.:* Arch. für Gynaek., 1931, 145, H. 3, p. 601.—*Müller:* Monatsschr. für Geb. u. Gyn., vol. xvi, p. 848.— *Schatz:* Arch. für Gyn., 1916, 105, T. 121.—*Schröder:* Lehrbuch d. Geburtshilfe, p. 139.—*Seitz:* Handbuch d. Geb., vol. i, 2, p. 1024.—*Sellheim:* Berl. klin. Woch., 1923, No. 36, p. 1684.

CHAPTER XII

THE MECHANISM OF LABOR IN OCCIPITAL PRESENTATION

ALTHOUGH the movements imparted to the child by the powers of labor were known to the older writers, Baudelocque, Smellie, and others, and Naegelè, in 1819, described them minutely, opinion is still divided as to their causes. If the student wishes to study these movements, a multipara will offer better advantages than a primipara, because, in the latter, the head is usually engaged when labor begins. The demands of asepsis restrict the frequent examination of the parturient which is necessary for a minute study of the mechanism. The use of sterile rubber gloves,

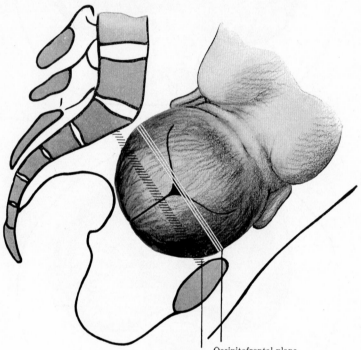

Plane of inlet Occipitofrontal plane

FIG. 211.—SYNCLITISM OR PARALLELISM.

rectal touch, and extreme asepsis will reduce the danger of infection, and a few thorough examinations will give the student a great deal of information. The radiologic study of the mechanism of labor, although a great deal of effort has been expended upon it, has not contributed much toward settling moot points, because of the technical difficulties in getting good pictures and the uncertainty of the readings made from them. Even slight distortion of the shadows will lead to erroneous deductions.

Broadly, the mechanism of delivery is as follows: An object consisting of two ovoids united by a hinge (i. e., the head and trunk united by the neck) is to be forced through a passage, straight at the beginning and sharply curved at its lower end. We must consider the manner of passage of the head and of the trunk. Each makes three movements—*engagement*, or entry into the pelvis; *rotation*, or adaptation to the shape of the pelvis, and *disengagement*, or exit from the pelvis.

Engagement of the Head.—*Multipara, O.L.A.*—At the beginning of labor the head lies over the inlet, inclined but little on either shoulder. The sagittal suture lies about midway between the promontory and the pubis—perhaps a little nearer the pubis if the promontory juts sharply forward. The head is then said to be synclitic or in synclitism (Fig. 211). The occipitofrontal plane lies parallel to the region of the inlet. If the woman has a pendulous belly, being a multipara, or if the pelvis is contracted, preventing a normal mechanism, the body of the fetus falls forward, the sagittal suture nears the promontory, the head presents its anterior parietal bone to the parturient canal, the parallelism between the occipitofrontal plane of the head and the plane of the inlet is destroyed, the head is asynclitic—it is in anterior asynclitism. This is often called Nägele's obliquity (Fig. 212). If the woman is a primipara, the abdominal walls holding the child firmly against the spine, the head may be inclined on the inlet with the posterior parietal

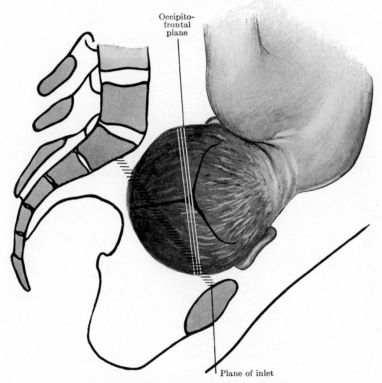

Occipito-
frontal
plane

Plane of inlet

FIG. 212.—ANTERIOR ASYNCLITISM (Nägele's obliquity).

bone more to the front, again disturbing the parallelism. This is posterior asynclitism (Fig. 213). Nägele believed the head usually entered the pelvis in anterior asynclitism, but extended investigation has disproved this view. The author has usually found the sagittal suture about midway between the promontory and the pubis. Marked asynclitism is pathologic. (See p. 750.) The sagittal suture also usually runs transversely across the pelvis, and, in a multipara, one finds the small and the large fontanels in the same plane of the pelvis.   The head, therefore, usually enters the inlet with its long diameter in the transverse of the pelvis; and since the two fontanels are about as easily reached by the examining finger, we conclude that the head is not strongly flexed on the chest. Many authors, including Williams, dispute the former of these statements, claiming that the head enters the pelvis in one of its oblique diameters, especially the right, but the author, after careful study of hundreds of labors, believes the head enters transversely in the majority of cases. Naegelè showed it entered either in the oblique or in the transverse. Sir Fielding Ould, of Dublin, corrected the ancient notion that the head entered the inlet with the occiput to the pubis. Pathologically it may do so.

Descent.—As soon as the uterine contractions begin, general intra-uterine pressure tends to force the fetus downward, and when the os is completely dilated, rapid *descent* begins. Descent of the head is also favored by the extension of the fetal body. (See p. 186.)

One result of descent is an increase of the *flexion* of the head. Mechanically the head acts like a two-armed lever, with the fulcrum at the junction of the spine with the occipital condyles. The sinciput and occiput meet equal resistances in the birth-canal, but the sincipital end of the head lever is longer than the occipital end, wherefore the sinciput is held back and the occiput descends. Any ellipsoid

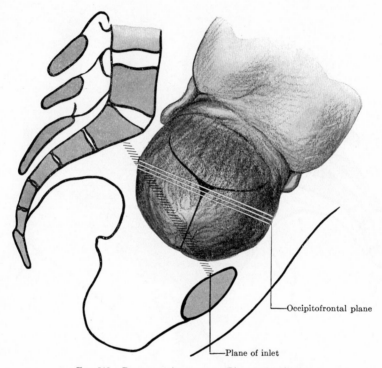

Fig. 213.—Posterior Asynclitism (Litzmann's obliquity).

body passing through a canal, in order to avoid resistance, will adapt its long axis to the long axis of the canal. The mechanical gain in flexion is that instead of an occipitofrontal diameter of 11 cm. and a circumference of 35 cm., there is presented to the birth-canal the suboccipitobregmatic plane with a diameter of 9 cm. and a circumference of 31 cm. Flexion may be marked, as occurs in generally contracted pelves. It may not occur until the head is well down on the pelvic floor, and thus labor may be delayed. Another result of descent and flexion is the disappearance of asynclitism, that is, the parallelism is restored, "leveling" occurs, the sagittal suture approaches the middle of the pelvis (Fig. 214).

In pathologic cases the asynclitism persists after engagement and may interfere with the next movement—rotation. Descent of the head into the pelvis, or engagement, is one of the most important phenomena of labor presented to the accoucheur for study, and clinically its importance is vital. A head is engaged in the pelvis when the biparietal diameter has passed the region of the inlet.

Internal Rotation.—The lowest part of the head now nears the pelvic floor and a new movement is imparted to it.   The occiput rotates from the transverse diameter into the oblique, and, finally, anteroposteriorly.   This movement is called *internal anterior rotation,* and many theories are advanced to explain it.   One of the oldest notions was that the pelvis presented a long transverse diameter in the inlet and a long sagittal diameter at the outlet, and that the head had to seek these diameters in its passage.   This is only partly true.   If one looks into a pelvis from above, one will see the spines of the ischia projecting sharply into its lumen.   The sides of the pelvis anterior to the spines curve gracefully downward, forward, and inward.   A finger following the curve glides gently forward under the pubis.   Without doubt this portion of the bone forming a part of the lateral inclined planes, so important to Hodge, has some slight function in anterior rotation.   Its action

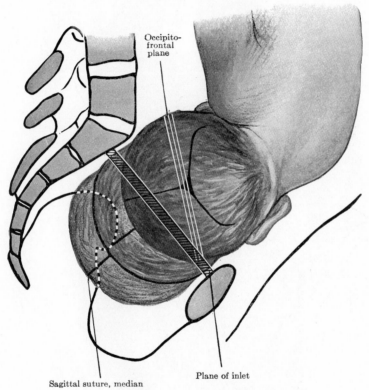

FIG. 214.—THE SYNCLITIC MOVEMENT, OR LEVELING.

with its opposite, together with the levator ani, may be likened to the ways of a ferry-boat.   The levator ani hangs like a sling, or trough or gutter, from the sides of the pubis and the ischia (which form the anterior lateral inclined planes), with the direction of its canal from behind forward.   The occiput, sliding down the side of the pelvis, is directed under the pubis, the long diameter of the head accommodating itself to the length of the trough, according to the law of inclined planes.   Since the occiput is almost always lower than the sinciput, it strikes the pelvic floor first, and, therefore, has the greater tendency to rotate anteriorly under the pubis (Fig. 215).   Examination at this period of labor will demonstrate the action of the pelvic floor in rotating the head forward.   Experiment—forcing the head through the pelvis of a female cadaver—shows that, as long as the integrity of the pelvic floor is preserved, its action is to direct the occiput forward, the head follow-

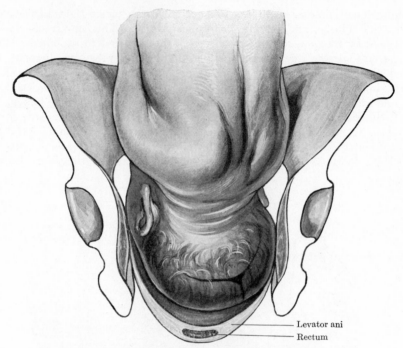

FIG. 215.—HEAD COMING DOWN ONTO THE LEVATOR ANI.
Note lateroflexion of head and twisting of body.

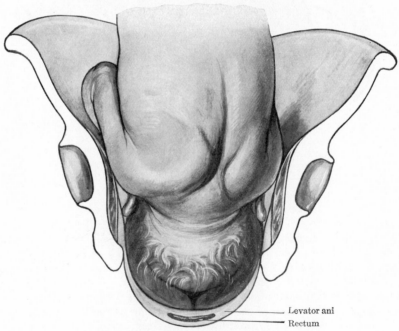

FIG. 216.—ANTERIOR ROTATION COMPLETED.
Head on the levator ani. Note lateroflexion is corrected.   Body still twisted.

ing the path of least resistance (Fig. 216).   In women with old lacerations of the
pelvic floor anterior rotation is often delayed or absent.   When the sacrum is
insufficiently curved, and the pubic arch very narrow, the trough or gutter is not

sufficiently sharply bent on the axis of the parturient canal to favor anterior rotation, which, therefore, is often arrested—a pathologic condition called "deep transverse arrest."

Schröder and Olshausen believed that the rotation of the back is communicated to the head. When the uterus contracts in the second stage it flattens from side to side, and the trunk of the child finds better lodgment in the anterior bellying of the uterus. That the back rotates to the front is easily demonstrable in most labors both by abdominal palpation and the x-ray picture. The flexion of the chin on the sternum and the raising of the shoulders against the head tend to fix the head and trunk, so that when the back turns, the head goes with it. One may easily convince himself of this by making the movement with a newborn infant. In cases where the back remains persistently behind, anterior rotation does not occur, and such conditions are pathologic. In manual correction of occipitoposterior positions the operator knows that unless he can get the back to the front, rotation of the head is incomplete or impossible or unstable.

Sellheim teaches that the body of the child possesses qualities which determine its movements in the birth-canal, and that during delivery, in order to

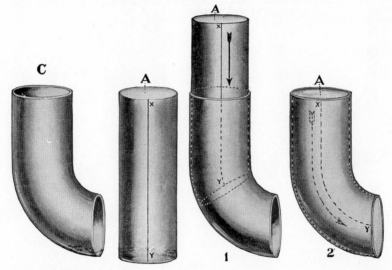

Fig. 217.—Action of an Evenly Flexible Cylinder when Forced through a Curved Passage. The cylinder A, uniformly flexible, in going through the canal C, will simply bend, the line x–y not changing its relation to C.

present the least resistance to the passage, it is compressed into the shape of a cylinder. This fetal cylinder bends with facility only in certain directions. The head bends backward, i. e., deflexes easily, and this deflexion is aided by the natural movements of the child. The head cannot be bent much on to the chest. Owing to the pressure of the arms and legs on to the body and the construction of the spinal column, the trunk cannot bend sagittally, but may bend easily toward one or the other side.

One may readily see that the fetal cylinder will be bent in its passage through the curved birth-canal, to correspond with the curve of the canal. If the child were flexible evenly in all directions, a bending of the cylinder in an anteroposterior diameter would be all that would be necessary. But the bending of the cylinder can occur only in certain ways—at the neck from before behind, in the trunk from one side to the other, and these two directions cross each other at a right angle. Therefore, in order for the fetal cylinder to pass through the curved canal, it must rotate on its long axis so as to bring the plane in which the bending can most easily occur to correspond with the axis of the birth-canal (Fig. 217). In other words, the child is forced to rotate until that part of its body which can be most easily bent, that is, the nape of the neck, comes to be adapted to the knee of the canal. The movement is similar to that of pushing the foot into a boot when the action is started wrongly—as the foot advances it rotates until the curve at the ankle corresponds to the curve of the boot (Fig. 218).

Anterior rotation of the child from all positions of the pelvis may be explained by this law of the accommodation of elastic resistance to the shape of the container (Sellheim).

While admitting the full power of Sellheim's arguments and proof, and agreeing with him that this law explains the rotation of the head and trunk, the other factors, especially the construction of the pelvic gutter and the action of the trunk on the head, must be also adequately evaluated. Further, the x-ray shows that the fetus is not always compressed to cylindrical form, but is sometimes more pyramidal, and the extremities are not flattened against the trunk except when they are passing through the girdle of resistance (Warnekros).

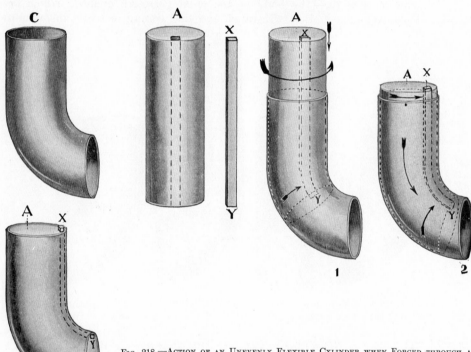

FIG. 218.—ACTION OF AN UNEVENLY FLEXIBLE CYLINDER WHEN FORCED THROUGH A CURVED PASSAGE.

The cylinder A has a flat steel rod at X Y. This rod cannot bend on the edge, only on the flat. Therefore, in order to accommodate itself to the curve of C, it must rotate the cylinder A. Note the direction of the arrows.

Disengagement.—Descent continues during anterior rotation, as also does flexion of the head. Indeed, flexion is exaggerated by the resistance of the pelvic floor, the forehead being pressed upward by the resistant sacrosciatic ligaments, the tip of the coccyx, and the levator ani (Fig. 219). After the forehead has passed the coccyx, and the nape of the neck has come to lie under the arch of the pubis, deflexion of the head begins. The chin leaves the chest, the occiput rises in front of the pubis, the forehead presses out the soft perineum, and the head is delivered in extension (Fig. 220). The causes of *extension* are generally agreed upon. The head meets an inclined plane—the perineum. The fetal axis pressure, or the general intra-uterine pressure, forces the trunk down upon the head, acting only on the sincipital arm of the head lever, since the occipital arm is under the pubis. The

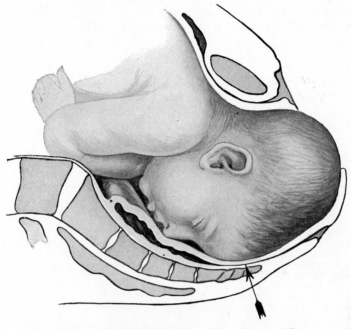

FIG. 219.—INCREASED FLEXION OF HEAD AT PERINEUM. ARROW INDICATES DIRECTION OF FORCE.

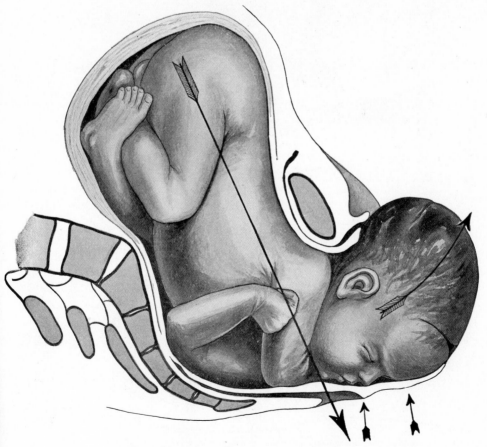

FIG. 221.—MOVEMENT OF EXTENSION AND DISENGAGEMENT.

parietal bosses strike the sides of the levator ani near the rami pubis, and are held firmly while the forehead is driven down and forward (Fig. 222). The perineum is

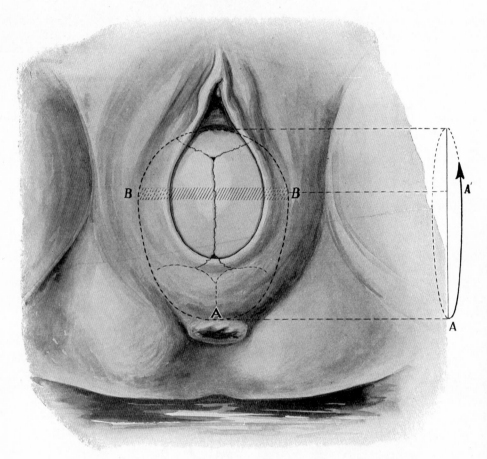

FIG. 222.—THE FACTORS IN EXTENSION OF FETAL HEAD WHEN ON PERINEUM.
Parietal bosses meet resistance at B B.   There is a tendency for A to come down, which is opposed by perineal floor, giving curve A A'.

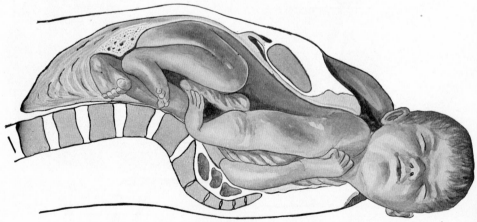

FIG. 223.—ZWEIFEL'S FROZEN SECTION OF A WOMAN WHO DIED AFTER DELIVERY OF HEAD.

thus displaced downward as well as backward, a point of importance in considering lacerations of the pelvic floor and their repair.

External Restitution.—After the head is delivered it slowly rotates in a direction opposite to that taken in internal anterior rotation; that is, in O.L. positions the occiput turns to the left, in O.D. positions it turns backward toward the right, side of the mother. The movement is called "external restitution," and is due to the untwisting of the neck and to the impulse imparted to the head by the internal rotation of the shoulders. External restitution or rotation does not invariably occur, and occasionally the occiput turns in a direction opposite to that which was expected. This is due to an unusual internal rotation of the shoulders.

When and where do these various movements take place? Descent or advancement, progression or translation (Sellheim), occurs throughout the whole process, even when the head is rotating—a point to bear in mind when imitating nature's method, as in a forceps delivery.

Flexion begins at the inlet of the pelvis, but may not until the head has reached the pelvic floor, when flexion and rotation occur almost simultaneously. It occurs toward the end of the first stage in primiparæ, and in all labors as the head is passing

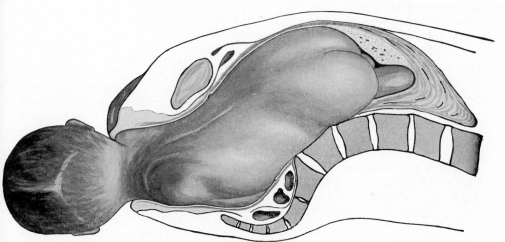

FIG. 224.—ZWEIFEL'S FROZEN SECTION OF A WOMAN WHO DIED AFTER DELIVERY OF HEAD.

through the cervix in the second stage. The flexion is exaggerated when the head is ready to disengage from the bony outlet of the pelvis, and this occurs about the middle of the second stage.

Internal anterior rotation takes place in the excavation of the pelvis, just as the head comes to rest on the pelvic floor, and is completed when the head has escaped the bony pelvis; though often, perfect rotation, bringing the small fontanel absolutely into the median line, may not occur at all, the head being delivered slightly oblique. Absence of rotation can occur only when the child is small and soft, or the pelvis very large, and is pathologic. Internal rotation usually begins in primiparæ when the first stage is ended and is completed before the second stage is half over. In multiparæ it occurs in the second stage.

Extension occurs after the forehead has passed the bony outlet, toward the end of the second stage of both primiparæ and multiparæ.

Mechanism of the Shoulders.—When the head becomes visible in the vulva, the shoulders engage in the inlet, the bisacromial diameter usually entering in the oblique opposite to that in which the head entered. In O.L.A. one finds the shoulders in the left oblique; in O.L.P. they enter in the right oblique. In O.L.A. the anterior shoulder rotates under the pubis from the right side of the pelvis, its direction of progression being opposed to that which the head underwent; while in O.L.P. the anterior shoulder follows the movement of the head from the left behind to the pubis in front.   The movements imparted to the shoulders are engagement, rotation, and disengagement.   General intra-uterine pressure forces the child down the parturient canal, and this action is reinforced by the direct pressure of the uterus on the fetal body.   The anterior shoulder slides down the lateral wall of the pelvis until it reaches the pelvic floor, then rotates under the pubis.   Anterior rotation of the shoulders is accomplished by the same factors which operate on the head— the shape of the pelvic floor, the direction of the opening in the pelvis, and the elastic resistances of the fetal body.   Flexion of the child's trunk is necessary to accommodate it to the concavity of the pelvic canal.   The child's body bends best laterally, and, therefore, according to Sellheim's law, the trunk will rotate until it corresponds to the direction of the curve of the canal through which it has to pass (Fig. 223). In rare cases no rotation of the back occurs, the shoulders appearing transversely, and sometimes the shoulders rotate to the opposite oblique, the back appearing on the other side to that in which it was expected.   Delivery of the shoulders is quite typical.   The anterior shoulder stems behind the pubis, the posterior rolls up over the perineum, after which the anterior shoulder comes from behind the pubis. If the perineum is much torn, a reverse mechanism occurs.   Often nature needs a little aid at this stage, and the accoucheur must imitate the natural modus of delivery.   Trouble with the shoulders is rare unless they are large, but laceration of the perineum frequently results from carelessness in their delivery, as also may fracture of the child's clavicle—even Erb's paralysis.   (See p. 884.)   After the chest is born, the rest of the child follows without any particular mechanism.

Over-rotation.—One is occasionally surprised to note that a labor starting out O.L.A. becomes, in its course, an O.D.A., and external rotation follows such a mechanism.   In these cases the internal rotation was excessive, carrying the occiput beyond the middle line to the opposite side, or the internal rotation of the shoulders was reversed or excessive.   The explanation of the phenomenon, after removing the question of error, is to be found in the laws governing the mechanisms, and one usually finds that the child was small or the parts large and yielding, the factors in the production of a perfect mechanism being weakened.

LITERATURE

Miller: Mechanik der Geburt, Zeitsch. f. Gyn., August 26, 1922, p. 1361.—*Ould:* "Positio Occipito-pubica."   Quoted
    in Jour. Obstetrics and Gyn. of Great Britain, October, 1909.—*Sellheim:* Die Beziehungen des Geburtskanales
    and Geburtsobjekts zur Mechanik, Leipsic, Thieme, 1906; also Handbuch der Geb. Doederlein, 1916, vol. i.
    —*Warnekros:* Roentgen Studies of the Mechanism of Labor, 1921; also 1926.

What One Observes of the Mechanism of Labor in O.L.A.—Careful observation of the course of labor enables us to closely follow the mechanism, to determine, at any time, its rate of progress, and to discover any variation from the normal. It is the knowledge of the mechanism of labor and the ability to recognize and correct abnormal variations that mainly distinguish the real accoucheur from the blind midwife, male or female.   It will simplify and clarify this study if the student will follow the described mechanisms on the manikin or with a pelvis and fetal skull.   Abdominal examination furnishes most valuable information, is less dangerous to the patient, less painful, and should always be practised first, though it is often necessary to supplement it by internal, rectal, or vaginal exploration.

At the beginning of uterine contractions the uterus is more globular than later, and slightly more pendulous.   The head is higher up, and movable above the inlet, especially in multiparæ, and the back is usually far to the side.   When the contractions attain regularity and severity, the uterus lengthens, the head becomes fixed over the inlet, and the back shows a tendency to come to the front, or go further back to the side, the latter movement depending on the position—whether an anterior or a posterior one. Fig. 225 shows the hands palpating the head before it engages in the pelvis; one sees how the fingers can move the head from side to side above the inlet. Fig. 226 shows the hands as they come to rest on the head, after it has engaged; one hand feels the occiput deep in the pelvis, to the left, behind the pubic ramus; the other hand finds the sharp forehead on the right and somewhat behind the median line. When flexion is marked, as in generally con-

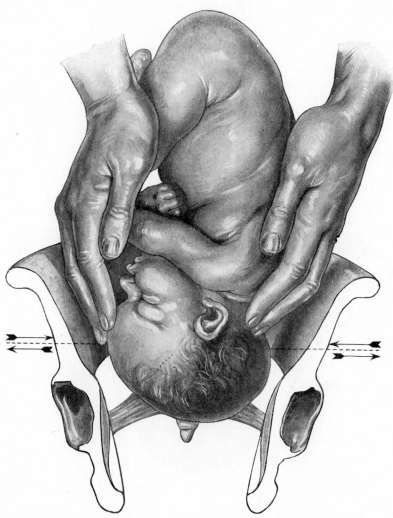

FIG. 225.—MOVING HEAD FROM SIDE TO SIDE ABOVE INLET. HEAD NOT ENGAGED.
Arrows show direction of movements. This manuever may also be carried out bimanually, with fingers in the vagina.

tracted pelves, one can hardly feel the occiput, it is so low in the pelvis, but the forehead is high up and easily palpated. If one now tries, with the two hands, to push the head from side to side, it will be found impossible: the head is fixed. As labor goes on and internal anterior rotation occurs, the occiput sinks behind the left pubic ramus out of reach of the external hand, and the forehead rises, then turns, disappearing in the right flank. When the occiput sinks beyond the reach of the fingers, the head is engaged.

The back at first is directed to the left side, but as labor advances it rotates to the front. One can follow the anterior shoulder as it goes from the left, behind, above, to the middle line just over the pubis. The movement of the back is also indicated by the course of the fetal heart-tones. At first the point of their greatest intensity is about the level of the navel, on the left; this point descends and comes to the median line until, when the head is on the perineum, the heart is best heard just above the pubic hair margin.

On vaginal exploration, early in labor, one finds the cervix closed or admitting only one or two fingers, which renders the diagnosis very difficult. In primi-

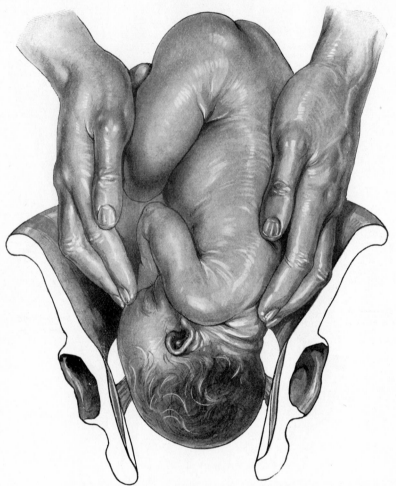

FIG. 226.—PALPATING THE ENGAGED AND STRONGLY FLEXED HEAD.

paræ the head is often engaged; in multiparæ it usually lies in the inlet, but freely movable, floating, or "caput ballitabile." The finger in the cervix comes upon the soft bag of waters, and through this feels the head. Lying across the os is the sagittal suture, running medially (synclitism) or nearer the promontory, or pubis (asynclitism), and at the end of the suture, in the left anterior pelvic quadrant, the finger finds the small fontanel. At the other end, in the right posterior quadrant, but nearly on a level with the small, lies the large fontanel. These findings indicate that flexion has not yet occurred. Flexion having taken place, one finds the small fontanel lower in the pelvis and nearer its center, the large fontanel higher and harder to reach, the sagittal suture more nearly paralleling the axis of the body, and lying almost in the right oblique. That fontanel which is nearer the center of the pelvis is the lower one. Internal anterior rotation occurring, the small fontanel de-

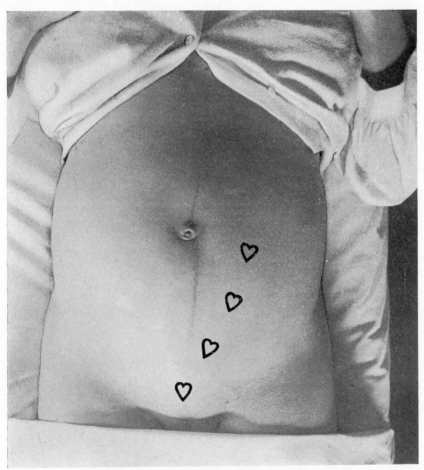

FIG. 227.—COURSE OF FETAL HEART-TONES AS DESCENT AND ROTATION OCCUR IN O.L.A.

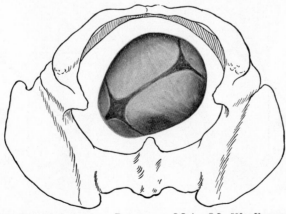

FIG. 228.—HEAD READY FOR ANTERIOR ROTATION IN O.L.A.—O.L. 50°. VIEWED FROM BELOW.

14

scends and sweeps around the left anterior quadrant of the pelvis until it lies directly behind the pubis, the sagittal suture now running exactly in the median line from before backward (Figs. 228, 228*a*, and 228*b*). Coincident with these movements the

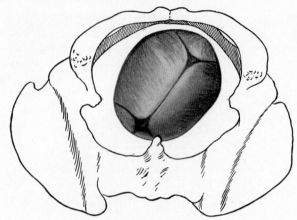

Fig. 228*a*.—O.L.A.—O.L. 40°. Flexion and Anterior Rotation Begun.

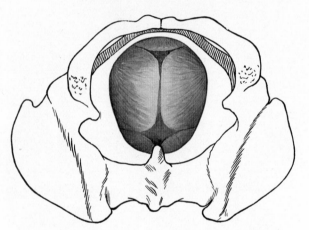

Fig. 228*b*.—O.L.A.—O.0°. Anterior Rotation Completed.

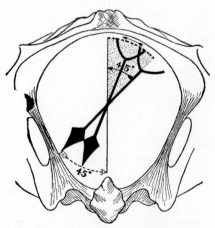

Fig. 228*c*.—Rotation in O.L.A.—O.L. 45°.
Occiput has an arc of only 45 degrees to travel.

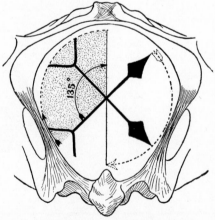

Fig. 228*d*.—Rotation in O.D.P.—O.D. 135°.
Occiput has an arc of 135 degrees to travel.

effacement and dilatation of the cervix have been taking place, and usually, by the time the head comes to rest in the perineal gutter, the os is completely dilated and retracted above the neck.   A caput succedaneum begins to form, and in long, tedious labors may grow so large that it makes the landmarks on the skull hard to find.   Firm pressure or massage will obviate the difficulty.   Of equal importance to the determination of the rotation is the recognition of the degree of engagement of the fetal head—the "station" (Müller).   It is not so easy to determine the degrees of advancement of the head along the birth-canal.   Older writers sought to decide this point by pushing the head up, and much use was made of the terms "caput

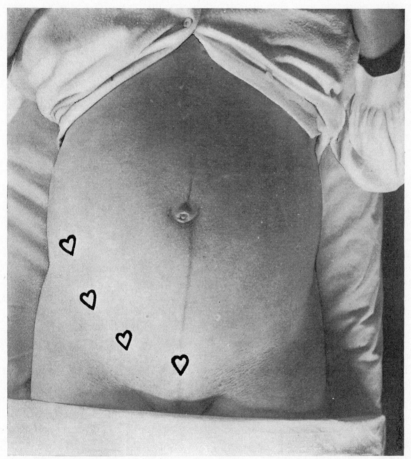

Fig. 229.—Course of Fetal Heart-tones as Descent and Rotation Occur in O.D.P.
One can also follow descent and rotation as they occur by observing the movement of the forehead and chin.

ballitabile, mobile, and ponderosum."   When the head floated above the inlet, it was called "caput ballitabile"; when it was fixed at the inlet, "caput mobile"; when deep in the pelvis, "caput ponderosum."   A head that is even visible at the outlet may be pushed up out of the pelvis, and a head that is not engaged may be fixed so that it cannot be moved; therefore, one may not be guided by the displaceability. The head is engaged when its largest plane—that is, the one through the parietal bosses—has passed the region of the inlet.   How may we determine that such has occurred?   We know that the head is engaged when, first, the most dependent portion of the skull (not the caput succedaneum) has passed a line drawn between the spines of the ischia; second, when two-thirds of the sacrum are covered by the cranial prominence, that is, the sacral hollow is occupied by the head; third, when the finger can feel only one-fourth of the pubis. Of these three criteria, the one measuring the distance of the head above or below the interspinous line is the most valuable and reliable. (See pages 310 and 766.)

Engagement varies with the different presentations of the head. It is prevented by highly contracted pelves, tumors blocking the inlet, and by pendulous abdomen. An abnormally large head engages with difficulty; the placenta may be in the way, or a large amount of liquor amnii (polyhydramnion) may confer great mobility on the fetus. Whenever the head does not engage, the cause must be sought out, and one may not attempt delivery until the degree of engagement is positively known.

In the occipitodextra anterior position, the mechanism of labor and the findings are the same as in occipitolæva anterior, but reversed.

MECHANISM OF LABOR IN OCCIPITODEXTRA POSTERIOR POSITION

One essential difference exists in the mechanism of O.D.P. as compared with O.D.A.—the occiput has to rotate through an arc of 135 degrees, three-quarters of a half-circle, while in O.D.A. it rotates through an arc of 45 degrees, only one-quarter of a half-circle (Figs. 228c and 228d).

Engagement of the head is slower because the broad part of the head is likely to impinge on the promontory of the sacrum, and for the same reason flexion is not so marked, and may not occur until the head is well down on the pelvic floor. Internal anterior rotation takes much more time—naturally, since the occiput has three times as far to travel. After it has occurred, the mechanisms of all positions are identical. The factors bringing about all the movements are the same in posterior positions as in anterior, and a new one is invoked. It is believed that the shoulder, striking on the promontory of the sacrum, prevents the back, and therefore the head, from rotating backward. Sellheim explains anterior rotation by his law of adaptability of a body, flexible best in one direction, being forced to accommodate itself to the curve of the container. Anterior rotation does not invariably occur—sometimes the occiput rotates backward to the hollow of the sacrum (3 per cent. of the cases), but then the labor is pathologic. This phase of the subject is considered on p. 632.

The Findings in Occipitodextra Posterior.—*Abdominally*, the back is felt to the right and posteriorly, and the heart-tones are deeper in the flank, further from the navel. During labor, both gradually come anteriorly, sinking at the same time (Fig. 229). The shoulder is on the right side of the median line, and turns to the front, then to the left side of the center, as labor progresses. The forehead, at first, is plainly felt above the left ramus of the pubis. It rises a little higher, due to flexion of the head, then it sinks lower as the head engages; finally, it sweeps backward, around the left half of the pelvis, disappearing at the side. The small parts, feet and arms, are felt anteriorly around the umbilicus. *Internally*, at the beginning of labor, the head is high up, the sagittal suture in the *right* oblique, the large fontanel in the left side anteriorly, the small fontanel high up, and at the right sacro-iliac joint. Flexion is less marked in these cases. After descent is started the flexion of the head throws the small fontanel nearer the center of the pelvis, the large fontanel recedes, and the sagittal suture becomes more vertical. Should flexion fail, the head reaches the perineum, the small and large fontanels descend in nearly the same plane, the sagittal suture running more or less transversely (Fig. 231). After rotation is complete the findings are the same as in O.D.A.

Labor is always longer, harder, and more painful, and effacement and dilatation of the cervix not so complete, in occipitoposterior positions. In pathologic cases

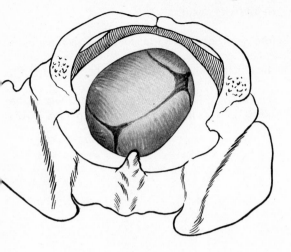

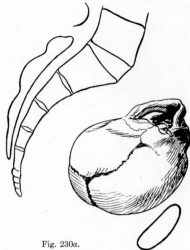

Fig. 230.

Fig. 230a.

FIGS. 230 AND 230a.—ROTATION IN O.D.P.—O.D. 135 DEGREES. (Seen from below and from the side.)

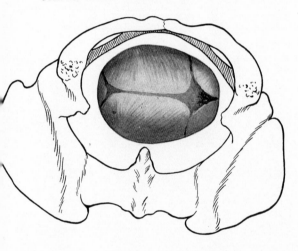

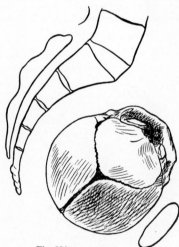

Fig. 231.

Fig. 231a.

FIGS. 231 AND 231a.—IT IS NOW CALLED O.D.T.—O.D. 90 DEGREES. (If rotation stops here, it is called transverse arrest or arrest at right 90°.)

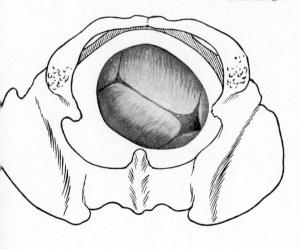

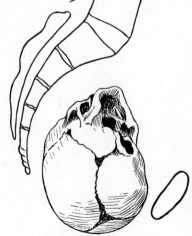

Fig. 232.

Fig. 233.

FIGS. 232 AND 233.—ROTATION IN O.D.P.—O.D. 135 DEGREES. (Now it has become O.D.A.—O.D. 45 Degrees.)

213

the powers of labor may give out before rotation is accomplished, and then we hav a condition known as "arrest," of which more later.

In O.L.P. the mechanism of labor and the findings are the same as in O.D.P but reversed.

The student should accustom himself to speaking of rotation in degrees of th circle. It will clarify his understanding of the mechanism and help him in hi operative obstetrics.

CHAPTER XIII

THE MECHANISM OF THE THIRD STAGE

Two acts make up the delivery of the placenta: separation or detachment of the organ and its expulsion.

It is not probable that the placenta always separates as the trunk of the child leaves the uterus. Observations at cesarean sections show that the placenta remains adherent to the uterus during the first moments of retraction of the muscle. The uterine wall is thick everywhere but at the placental site, which is somewhat thinner, though nearly as large as it was before delivery (Fig. 234). During the second stage of labor the placenta may shrink somewhat, to accommodate itself

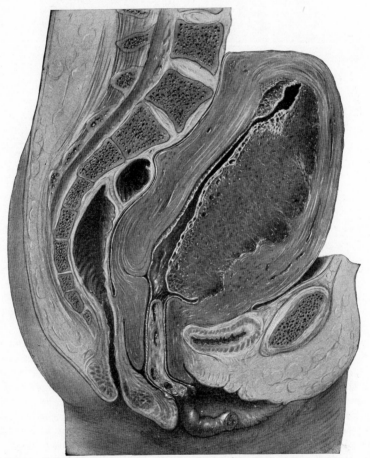

Fig. 234.—Placenta Still Attached to Uterus at Beginning of Third Stage.
Note thin uterine wall at placental site. V para, died in second stage, forceps, living child, frozen section (adapted from A. Couvelaire).

to the diminishing size of its area of attachment, but after the child is out, the first uterine contraction causes such a diminution of the surface area that separation is inevitable. Frankl has shown that when the child is born there is a rush of blood into the placental site, a *hyperemia ex vacuo*, which affecting particularly the thin walled vessels of the spongiosa causes rhexis, blood extravasations—in

215

brief, the retroplacental hematoma. He believes the placenta may be separated without uterine contractions. In either event the first break in continuity of the placental attachment allows a little blood to escape between the two organs, and the uterine contractions force this blood, like a fluid wedge, between the layers of the decidua serotina separating the placenta in the smoothest and most perfect manner from the wall of the uterus, the line of cleavage being in the spongiosa. Since the placenta is more adherent at the edges, the hemorrhage behind it will lift up the center, as is depicted in Fig. 235. This blood-clot is called the *retroplacental hematoma*, and varies much in size, depending on the method of extrusion of the placenta. When too brusque manipulations are made on the uterus, the edge of the placenta will separate at one place, allowing the retroplacental blood to escape externally, thus producing an abnormal mechanism of the third stage.

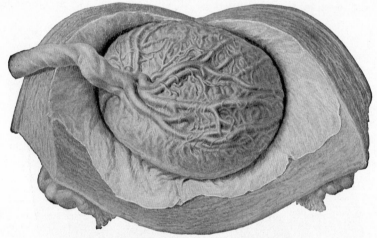

FIG. 235.—SHOWING HOW PLACENTA IS RAISED UP BY RETROPLACENTAL HEMORRHAGE.
Specimen kindly loaned by Prof. Piscaçek, of Vienna.

A third factor in the separation of the placenta, but a minor one, is the loss of the intra-uterine pressure. There is now nothing to hold the placenta against the wall of the uterus.

A fourth factor, traction on the placenta by a too short cord,—35 cm.,—or one coiled around the neck of the child, is pathologic.

Expulsion of the placenta begins when the separation is complete, or nearly so. The uterine contractions force the placenta against the internal os, and finally, through it, into the dilated cervix and upper vagina. From this point another force takes up the work—the abdominal muscles. Among the savages and ignorant people various methods of invoking the abdominal pressure are employed, as coughing, sneezing, blowing into a bottle or the fist, pushing on the belly, or squatting, as at stool. The accoucheur directs his patient to bear down, which failing, he expels the placenta by pressure on the uterus. Few authors commend pulling on the cord. In pathologic cases an accumulation of blood may force the placenta out of the uterus, and when pituitrin is given, the powerful uterine contraction which it usually evokes may detach the placenta and extrude it into the vagina simultaneously.

During the delivery of the after-birth one observes two mechanisms: First, the placenta turns inside out like an umbrella, the fetal surface comes out first, the cord leading the way, the membranes containing the retroplacental hematoma following after. This is called Schultze's method. Second, the lower edge of the placenta precedes, the whole organ sliding down the side of the uterus in the vagina. This is called Duncan's method. In the latter cases the retroplacental hematoma is small, or the edge of the placenta may have been inserted low, near the internal os, or the contractions of the uterus may have been unusually strong from the start, quickly separating the placenta and folding it together ready for extrusion. In opposite conditions we notice Schultze's method which is also more common when the placenta has a fundal insertion. Duncan's method is more likely to occur if the placenta is already near the internal os. Although Baudelocque described

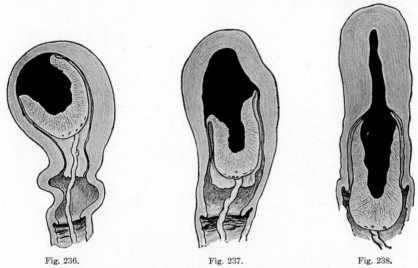

Fig. 236.   Fig. 237.   Fig. 238.

FIGS. 236, 237, AND 238.—SCHULTZE'S MECHANISM OF EXPULSION OF PLACENTA.

both mechnisms, they have been assigned the above names, and which is to be considered normal or more frequent for a time occupied the discussion of author- ities. My own observations, with the cervix exposed by broad retractors, prove that a pure Duncan method is rare, a combination of the two mechanisms being

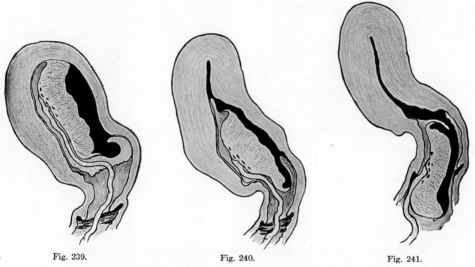

Fig. 239.   Fig. 240.   Fig. 241.

FIGS. 239, 240, AND 241.—DUNCAN'S MECHANISM OF EXPULSION OF PLACENTA.

the rule, but that the placenta emerges from the vulva most often like an inverted umbrella (see Figs. 242 and 245). The interesting x-ray studies of the placental stage by Weibel and Warnekros have not added much to our knowledge.

The membranes are mechanically drawn off the wall of the uterus by the de- scending placenta, but the firm contraction of the muscle also helps in their separa-

tion. They are also detached in part by the retroplacental hematoma, but when
this is extensive, the process is pathologic. After the placenta is outside of the
vulva, the membranes follow to gentle traction or by the weight of the placenta, or
by their own weight, if completely separated.   Normally, the membranes—consist-

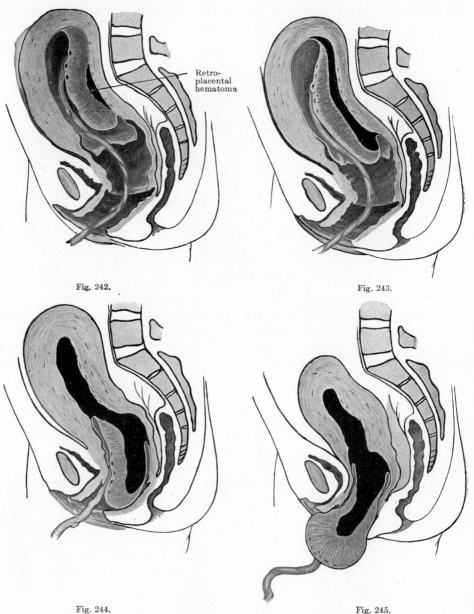

Retro-
placental
hematoma

Fig. 242.   Fig. 243.

Fig. 244.   Fig. 245.

FIGS. 242, 243, 244, AND 245.—USUAL MECHANISM OF EXPULSION OF PLACENTA.

ing of the amnion, the chorion, the decidua reflexa, with portions of the vera and part
of the decidua serotina—are expelled still adherent to each other.   Where the head
has been delivered covered with a "caul,"—the amnion,—a separation has occurred
between the chorion and amnion, and one finds the latter folded around the cord,
attached to the placenta only at the insertion of the latter.   In pathologic cases

(see p. 835). or where too brisk manipulations have been carried out in the third stage, the placenta is delivered, leaving more or less of the membranes still attached to the uterus.   These portions of the secundines undergo fatty degeneration and **are** cast off with the decidua during the puerperium; or, rarely, they become infected and cause puerperal fever.

Microscopically, one finds that the separation of the placenta and membranes occurs in the glandular or ampullary layer of the decidua—sometimes deeper, sometimes more superficially.   The soft. pink, incomplete layer of tissue to be found on the maternal surface of the chorion is decidua vera and reflexa, and one can often find blood-vessels in it.   The gray, translucent covering of the placenta is decidua serotina, and the broken-off veins and arteries of the placental site can always be demonstrated in it.   These thin-walled vessels, the glandular spaces, and the absence of fibrous tissue make the decidua a very soft structure, and, therefore, separation of the secundines is very easy.   One can rub the decidua off the uterus with a gauze sponge.   In pathologic cases the decidua serotina does not develop, or is absorbed early, and the chorionic villi burrow down into and between the muscle-fibers.   Dangerous adhesion of the placenta results, necessitating its operative removal.   (See Placenta Accreta.)

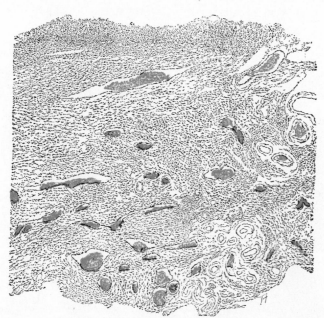

FIG. 246.—THROMBOSIS IN UTERUS AFTER ABORTION OF SIX WEEKS.   ABNORMAL, INSUFFICIENT RETRACTION. Woman twenty-six years old.

Hemorrhage from the large sinuses of the placental site is controlled by the contraction and retraction of the uterine muscular fibers and lamellæ. They act like "living ligatures" on the thin-walled vessels coursing through the uterus. The shifting of the layers of muscle and shortening of the bundles of fibers displace, compress, twist, and bend the thin-walled vessels, so that they are no longer pervious. Occasionally one finds, on the surface left bare by the placenta, a few thrombi occupying the open mouths of the vessels.   Thrombosis of the deeper placental site is pathogenic—it may lead to embolism and it invites sepsis.   Firm retraction of the uterus at the placental site, aided by strong contractions, guarantees the woman against postpartum hemorrhage and infection.

Pituitary disturbs the normal mechanism of the third stage.   Usually it hastens the processes, often it renders one pathologic.   (See p. 137.)

THE PHYSIOLOGY OF THE PUERPERIUM

CHAPTER XIV

LOCAL CHANGES

With the completion of the third stage, labor is ended; the puerperal state or puerperium has begun; the woman is a puerpera.

The puerperium may be defined as that period which extends from the delivery of the ovum until the return of the genitalia to the non-pregnant state is complete. Its length, therefore, is from six to eight weeks, though in common usage the

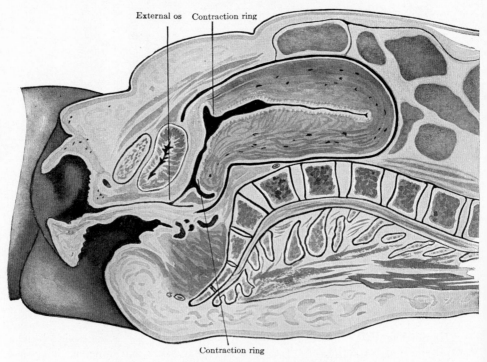

External os   Contraction ring

Contraction ring

Fig. 247.—Uterus Directly After Labor.
Frozen section of a primipara who died one hour after delivery, from hemorrhage and fatty heart (Stratz). Usually, there is no gut in front of the fundus.

puerperium means the time the woman is in bed after the labor. As has been repeatedly stated, a perfect restitutio ad integrum never occurs after labor. The woman carries the evidences of child-bearing all her life. The distinction between normal and pathologic conditions during the puerperium is not easy, even with the aid of the thermometer and of bacteriology. The rapid disintegration of the uterus, the changes in the endometrium, and in the open vessels at the placental site, are closely akin to the pathologic, and would be called such if they occurred at any other time or place. It is the same approach to the abnormal that renders permanent structural disease so prone to begin during the puerperal period.

In the physiology of pregnancy we learned of all the changes, local and general, which provided for the growth of the child and its expulsion from the mother. These were progressive changes. In the physiology of the puerperium we will study the retrogressive changes, local and general, which bring back the

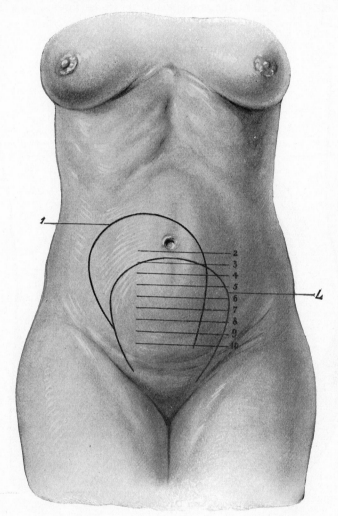

Fig. 248.—Height of Uterus Postpartum. The Bladder Empty.
L, After labor: 1, First day; 2, second day, etc.

organs of the mother to their original condition, and, second, those progressive changes in the breasts which enable them to carry further the function begun by the uterus—the nourishment of the child. The retrogressive changes of the genitalia are grouped under the general heading "Involution."

Changes in the Uterus.—Immediately after delivery of the placenta the uterus sinks below the level of the navel in strong anteversion and anteflexion, resting on the promontory behind and lying against the abdominal wall in front (Fig. 247). Owing to its previous displacement, its ligaments and vaginal attachments are so loose that the fundus may easily be moved to any part of the belly,—even as high as

the liver, or may be pushed down so that the cervix hangs out of the vulva.   The
uterus now resembles a flattened pear; it is 15 cm. long, 12 cm. broad, and 8 to 10
cm. thick, being about as large as a fetal head, and it weighs about two pounds.
The full bladder always displaces the uterus, and usually the latter rises toward the
right side.   On vaginal examination immediately after labor one can hardly outline
the cervix, it is so soft and succulent, hanging down from the hard contracted muscular fundus in folds, like a cuff.   It is about 1 cm. thick and 6 or 7 cm. long, but
may be stretched to 10 or 11 cm.   The internal os and contraction ring firmly close
the uterine cavity and mark the point where the thick fundus goes into the thin

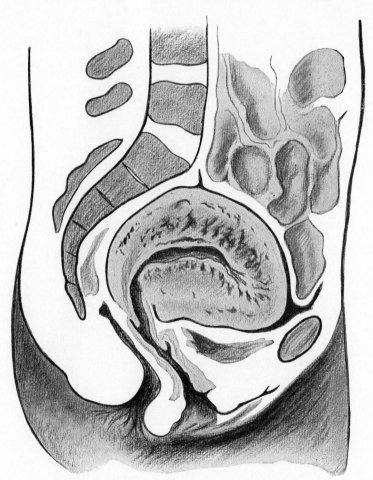

Fig. 249.—Uterus, Fifth Day Postpartum (from Bumm).

lower uterine segment and cervix.   Either a small blood-clot fills the cavity of the
uterus or the walls lie apposed.   At the placental site the uterine wall is thinner
than elsewhere until a few contractions have occurred; then it is thicker, and one
recognizes the location of the placenta by the roughened, raised surface.   This
roughened, raised surface is normal, and must not be mistaken for a piece of adherent placenta.   Measurements by Fehling show the thickness of the wall to
vary from 3½ to 5 cm.

Owing to the development of the elasticity of the vagina and pelvic floor, and
the filling of the rectum and bladder, the uterus rises in the abdomen on the first
day of the puerperium; but from then on one observes, from day to day, a steady

decrease in height above the pubis and in all its diameters (Fig. 248).   The table from Temesvary gives the measurements, which were taken when the bladder and rectum were empty and when the uterus was held up against the abdominal wall, *i. e.*, the anteflexion corrected.

Day	Height above Pubis	Breadth at Tubal Insertion
After delivery	10.91 cm.	11.05 cm.
First day	13.55 "	12.27 "
2d "	12.45 "	11.71 "
3d "	11.16 "	10.93 "
4th "	10.21 "	10.27 "
5th "	9.29 "	9.66 "
6th "	8.22 "	8.96 "
7th "	7.61 "	8.32 "
8th "	7.32 "	8.19 "

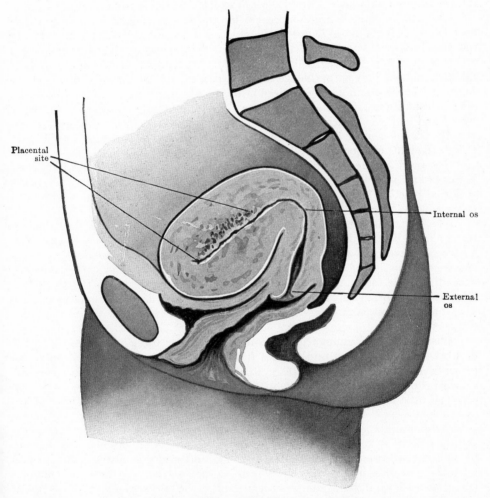

Placental site

Internal os

External os

Fig. 250.—Uterus, Twelfth Day Postpartum (Bumm).

While one may follow the descent of the uterus with the tape-measure, for practical purposes the rule of the fingers is sufficient.   On the first day the uterus is seven or eight fingerbreadths above the pubis; on the fifth day four or five, and correspondingly narrower across the fundus; while by the twelfth day it has sunk below the inlet so that it is not easily palpable from the abdomen (Figs. 249 and 250).

After delivery the uterus weighs $2\frac{1}{5}$ pounds, or 1000 gm.; by the end of the first week it has lost one-half—500 gm.; at the end of the second week it weighs 350 gm. (about 11 ounces); while in the eighth week it again is the small organ of two ounces, or 60 gm.

This rapid diminution of size is brought about by absorption of the tissue-juices and fatty degeneration of the muscle-fibers. Sänger showed that the fibers are not all nor fully destroyed, but the protoplasm undergoes cloudy swelling, hyaline and fatty degeneration. The fat is removed by the lymph-stream, by oxidation by the action of a fat-splitting ferment, and partly by the leukocytes. That fatty degeneration of the muscle protoplasm is not the only method nature has for reducing the uterus is indicated by the demonstration of glycogen (Broers) and peptone (Hofmeister) in the muscle. The connective-tissue fibers also undergo hyaline fatty degeneration and partial absorption. A multiparous uterus is usually thicker and more fibrous. Little is known of the changes in the nerves.

The uterine vessels are compressed by the contracting uterus, causing the anemia which is the basal factor of the changes described above, and obliterating the vessels themselves, with hyaline and fatty degeneration of their walls and occlusive growth of the endothelium (E. Ries). Thrombosis occurs in the walls of the deeper veins only in pathologic cases, but a superficial thrombosis is not abnormal. These thrombi are organized in the usual manner during the puerperium. The placental site, after the placenta has left it, contracts rapidly, presenting a raised and nodular surface about three inches in diameter; by the fourteenth day it is the size of a silver dollar, and in six weeks may still be recognized by its elevated, though not roughened, surface, which is the size of a quarter.

The uterine serosa, in spite of its elasticity, cannot follow the receding uterus. It lies in fine wrinkles which are well shown in Fig. 125, p. 98. They disappear within a week. Their distinctive grouping shows the direction of the contraction of the muscle-fibers.

The *cervix*, after labor, hangs down like a soft cuff, succulent, bruised, sometimes almost black with suffused blood, edematous, and more or less torn. The author has never failed to find more or less injury to this organ, even after natural and easy labors. The serous infiltration disappears rapidly, and within eighteen hours the cervix forms, quickly shortens, and becomes harder. On the third day two fingers still pass easily into the uterus; on the twelfth day one finger can attain the internal os, but cannot go through it; while in the fourth week the os is a small transverse slit.

Changes in the Endometrium.—During pregnancy the glandular layer of the decidua vera and serotina undergoes a fatty degeneration. The separation of the placenta and membranes takes place in this layer; therefore, when the uterus is emptied, its mucous surface is denuded, the connective-tissue spaces being exposed all over, and, at the placental site, almost to the muscle. The interior of the uterus is one large wound, with, at the placental site, immense veins, containing superficial thrombi, opening upon it. This condition explains the ease of infection and the severity of the disease if it once gains entrance. An invasion of the decidua by white blood-corpuscles takes place, forming a layer of granulation, which separates the necrosing parts of the decidua from the healthy. At first the endometrium varies from 2 to 5 mm. in thickness, the surface is rough, with shreds of degenerating decidua, blood-clots, and bits of fetal membrane. By the third day this, as the result of fatty degeneration, has softened so that it could be wiped off with the finger, but nature accomplishes it in a better way. The granulation wall separates the dead from the living tissues, the remaining decidua cells, in part, return to their original condition, the epithelium from the stumps of the glands which lay unaffected among the muscle-fibers and which now crowd closer together as the uterus shrinks, proliferates rapidly, grows out on the surface of the endometrium, and covers the new mucous membrane. Thus the larger part of the endometrium is cast off, regeneration taking place from the connective-tissue basis of the mucous membrane and from the epithelium of the deepest portions of the uterine glands (Fig. 251). It closely resembles the healing of a granulating surface on any mucous membrane.

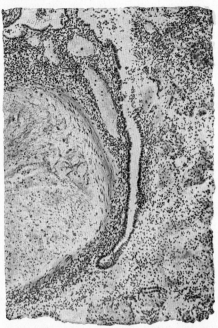

FIG. 251.—REGENERATION OF PLACENTAL SITE SHOWING NEW GLANDS FORMING NEAR BY NORMAL THROMBOSIS (specimen presented by Dr. Warthin).

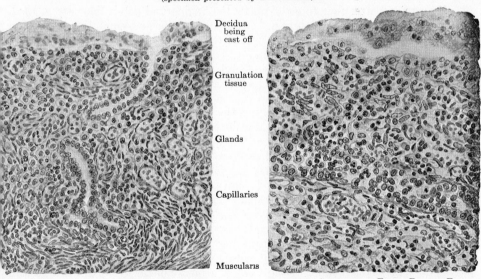

FIG. 251a.—REGENERATING ENDOMETRIUM ABOUT THE EIGHTH DAY OF PUERPERIUM, SHOWING NEW GLANDS FORMING.

FIG. 251b.—GRANULATION TISSUE FORMING ENDOMETRIUM DURING FOURTH DAY OF PUERPERIUM.

At the placental site similar processes occur, with, in addition, the thrombosis and organization of the open mouths of the vessels. The changes here are much slower than in the vera (Fig. 251). Williams, in his last work, published after his death, presented evidence tending to prove that the placental site is exfoliated, in six to seven weeks, by the growth of the endometrium which undermines it. The

15

decidua basalis, with the obliterated arteries and the thrombosed and organized veins—together with the tissue between them, much of which has been hyalinized are raised up and may touch the opposite, already regenerated, uterine wall New endometrial cells growing from the glands and deeper tissues break up and cast off this mass. This action is completed by the concentric ingrowth of cells which work their way in and under the mass from adjacent extra-placental areas. The necrotic, often hyalinized, tissue and vessels may be found, free in the uterus, for several weeks, being gradually discharged.

Changes in the Vagina and External Genitalia.—After labor the vagina may be found swollen, blue, bruised, pouting into the vulva; but it soon regains most of its tonicity, though only after years to a degree approaching normal. The extravasated blood is absorbed in a week, the prolapse of the walls becomes less, though the anterior wall of the vagina usually remains permanently lower. The elasticity of the perineum is reëstablished with surprising rapidity; perineal tears that looked large and deep are small the next day, but just as important, however. A peculiar consistence of the vagina and perineum remains for weeks after delivery. The tissues are distensible to only a certain degree, after which they break like card-board; the blood-vessels are friable, and operations performed during the puerperium are likely to be complicated by troublesome capillary oozing. Many cases of rupture of the vagina sub coitu have been reported as occurring in this period, and bleeding is always a prominent symptom. The vagina and mucous surface of the vulva have a deep-red, velvety appearance, by which the puerperal state can usually be diagnosed.

The pelvic floor, containing muscle, fat, and fascia, is infiltrated with bloody serum, full of small suggillations, even some larger blood extravasations. The muscle-fibers are often torn and overstretched. Absorption of the blood and serum quickly takes place, but many minute and larger scars are left, which result in atrophy and a weakened pelvic floor.

If examined after four to eight weeks the vagina and pelvic floor are relaxed presenting signs of hyperinvolution. Gradually the parts regain their tone and after four to eight months they are firmer, the closure is better, the vulva gaping very little, unless there has been an ununited laceration. It should be noticed that even after cesarean section, when the pelvic floor has not been dilated, there is considerable relaxation of the structures, occasionally the above-mentioned hyperinvolution.

The Puerperal Wounds.—A study of the healing process of the wounds made by labor forms an essential part of the duties of the accoucheur. The hymen tears in every labor, and its relics are found as a row of mucous membrane tags circling the vaginal orifice and called *carunculæ myrtiformes*. Around the clitoris, the labia minora, the introitus vaginæ, in the vagina, in the cervix—especially in primiparæ—occur larger or smaller lacerations, bruises, and scraped surfaces These may heal by apposition and primary union, or by granulation and suppuration. Lacerations of the perineum occasionally heal by primary union, but usually granulate up from the bottom. Sometimes the skin unites, but the body of the perineum, the physiologically important part, does not unite well. Lacerations of the vagina usually heal readily, but with scar formation, which, if marked, will distort the base of the bladder, producing incontinence of the urine, or dislocate the uterus, producing sterility and other noxious conditions. Cervix tears occasionally unite by primary union. If infected they do not, but may give rise to cellulitis in the adjacent broad ligaments, with resulting life-long invalidism.

In the absence of infection these wounds heal with very little inflammatory reaction. The surface is covered with a light-gray exudate. Underneath this pink, pointed granulations appear, the surface cleans off, epithelization rapidly occurs, and by the eighth day is usually nearly completed. Abnormal wound repair

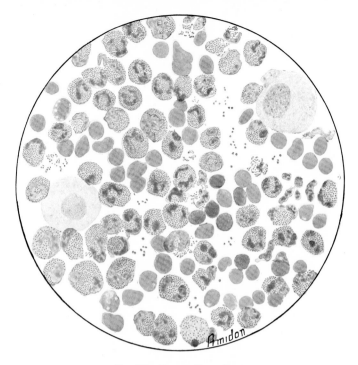

FIG. 252.—LOCHIA, THIRD DAY.
1. Blood-cells numerous.   2. Healthy leukocytes; nuclei contracted and normal.
3. Few bacteria.

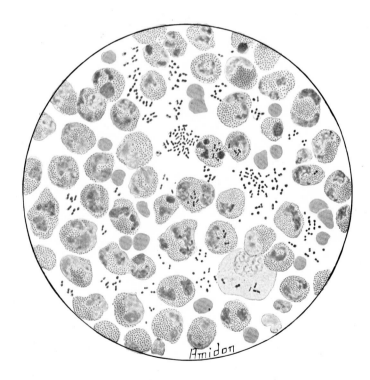

FIG. 253.—LOCHIA, FIFTH DAY.
1. Bacteria in abundance—one kind principally.   2. Leukocytes swollen, nuclei
swollen.   3. Phagocytes.   4. Blood-cells not so numerous.

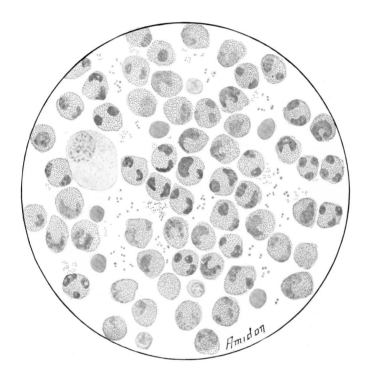

Fig. 254.—Lochia Alba, Eighth Day.

1. Bacteria less numerous and pale staining, probably dead. 2. Leukocytes more numerous and more normal in appearance. 3. Blood less.

indicates infection somewhere in the parturient canal. Swelling of the labia, edema around the wounds, which have a reddened, angry aspect, greenish, yellowish, even dark sloughing of the surface of the wounds, pain, fever, and illness, indicate that the normal process is being interfered with by infection.

The Lochia.—Another striking phenomenon of the puerperium is the appearance of the lochia, a discharge from the genitalia at first bloody, then sanguineous, then purulent, finally mucoserous, before ceasing entirely, in three to six weeks. On the first day the lochia are almost pure blood, normally not mixed with clots—*lochia cruenta* or *rubra*. Clots, unless large and numerous, are not insignificant. This flow is followed by one of blood-stained serum, which lasts a day or so, after which the discharge is thicker, of a maroon color and creamy consistence, with a characteristic odor—*lochia sanguinolenta*. Gradually the bloody admixture grows less, the white blood-corpuscles increase, the lochia resemble cream,—*lochia alba* or *purulenta*,—until at the end (thirteenth to the seventeenth day) there is only a slight mucoserous discharge.

The odor of the lochia varies from day to day, varies with the patient, some women naturally possessing a peculiar odor (even with the menses), and with the kind of bacteria present in the vagina. Normally, the odor is not very offensive, being faded or insipid, like old meat, or strong, like perspiration. If the lochia are fetid, or have a fruity, purulent odor, or sharp and biting, like sanious pus, the puerpera is more or less dangerously diseased. Decomposing clots or membranes, a forgotten piece of gauze, lend the lochia the foul odor of decomposition, even when the general condition of the puerpera is not disquieting. The other characteristics of the odor referred to indicate that the puerpera is suffering from one of the severer types of infection.

The lochia cruenta contain blood, shreds of membrane and decidua, and occasionally fetal remnants, vernix caseosa, lanugo, meconium, etc.

Lochia sanguinolenta contain blood in a state of solution, wound exudation, red and white blood-corpuscles, shreds of decidua in a state of fatty degeneration, mucus from the cervix and vagina, and microörganisms (Fig. 252).

Lochia alba are full of decidual cells—large mononucleated, irregular, round or spindle-shaped cells in process of degeneration, leukocytes, "lochiocytes," flat and cylindric epithelium, fat and débris from the uterus and the puerperal wounds, mucus, cholesterin crystals, and myriads of microörganisms (Fig. 254). In 34 per cent. of cases (Hoehne) the Trichomonas vaginalis is found.

The Bacteriology of the Lochia.—Even in normal puerperæ the lochia are infectious, as the frequent finger infections of nurses and the navel infections of children show. Kehrer vaccinated puerperæ on the thigh with their own lochia and produced abscesses. Likewise, inoculations of animals with normal lochia, in many cases, produced sepsis and death. Harris and Brown found the uterus sterile on the fifth day in 10 cases and in 20 it had diphtheroids. Döderlein found that the uterus, in the first few days after labor, was sterile in 83 per cent. of 250 cases examined. In the others were found the streptococcus, the staphylococcus, the gonococcus, and various saprophytes, aërobic and anaërobic. The uterus, from the fourth to the seventh day, shows a bacterial flora, including the Streptococcus pyogenes (Loeser). In the succeeding week the uterus gradually becomes aseptic. The vaginal lochia also contain these bacteria, and in greater frequency and number after the first day of the puerperium. (See p. 893.)

In spite of very extensive study and experimentation, it is yet impossible to distinguish the pathogenic from the non-pathogenic streptococcus. Therefore the streptococcus, found in the vagina of gravidæ and puerperæ, must be regarded as capable of developing destructive qualities if the conditions for it are ripe.

Since there is no doubt of the presence of these dangerous germs in the vagina, why is it that women do not all develop fever or infection during the puerperium?

First, because the bacteria do not wander upward into the uterus, where the most extensive wounded surface lies, until the third or fourth day, and by this time the protecting granulation wall is formed in the endometrium. The stream of lochia from above tends to wash them out. The thick, squamous epithelium of the vagina also acts protectingly against an invasion by bacteria. If a careless examiner, or indeed any manipulation, breaks through this protecting wall of granulations, the infection of the underlying blood- and lymph-vessels is inevitable. Clinical experience has taught us the danger of such interference.

Second, because the bacteria are of weak virulence, or—and this is probably a complement to such a statement—the puerpera possesses natural immunities against infection. When her general health is broken,—as by hemorrhage or eclampsia, shock from operation,—or if the local resistances are lowered from severe injury, the bacteria can develop their virulence and invade her organism. Analogously, the bacterium coli communis in the intestine and the bacillus diphtheriæ in the mouth, may live for years without producing disease. Perhaps part of this immunity lies in the presence of other bacteria in the vagina, and part in the acid reaction of the secretion (after the sixth day); but most of it, probably, is in the active immune bodies of the living tissues themselves (Stoltz, Walthard). Hofbauer proved that during pregnancy clasmatocytes and monocytes develop in the bases of the broad ligaments, forming a phagocytic tissue which acts as a defensive mechanism against invasion of bacteria and helps get rid of tear and tissue débris.

The Quantity of the Lochia.—Hippocrates estimated the amount of the lochia to be about 1300 gm.; later authors place it at about 500 gm., three-fourths of which is discharged in the first four days. Women who do not nurse their babies have more, nursing women less; indeed, in the latter, involution is faster and more perfect. These conditions are attended with increase of the lochia: Primiparity; young women; women who usually have profuse menses; twins; large placenta; severe operative deliveries, with bruising and injuries of the genitalia; retention of parts of placenta and membrane; too full meat diet; alcoholism; hemophilia; general atony. A strong, robust woman has more rapid reparative processes.

Source of the Lochia.—The lochia are very complex, containing the wound discharges, a serosanguineous exudate from all the puerperal wounds, from those of the endometrium, the lacerations of the cervix, indeed, of the whole parturient canal. A part of the flow comes from the uterine glands, the cervical glands, the vaginal and vulvar glandular organs.

The amount and quality of the lochia vary from day to day. If the patient sits up early, the lochia sanguinolenta continue longer or are more profuse. Sometimes the red lochia persist for several weeks, or they may reappear on the occasion of unusual exercise; or the lochia may cease as the result of disease (infection) or of obstruction to the flow. This almost always causes fever, which subsides when the drainage is reëstablished. The normal changes in the color and consistence of the lochia are interfered with by infection, and one of our best diagnostic means is the investigation of the puerperal discharges. The lochia contain a leukocyte proteolytic ferment (Jochman). Acidosis and hunger reduce lochia.

Involution.—All the foregoing changes are part of the function of involution, the most prominent of which is the reduction in size of the uterus. The reduction in size of the uterus is subject to many variations. In women who do not nurse, the reduction in size is slower. Sepsis stops involution or slows it—an important sign. On the other hand, involution offers a barrier to infection—the shedding of the decidua resembles the cleansing of a granulating surface; the lochia carry off the germs. The tightly contracted uterus does not absorb bacteria nor toxins.

Involution varies in different women and in the same woman after different confinements. The rate of decrease is not even, the greatest being during the first six days. Sometimes the process goes beyond the normal, the uterus at the tenth week being very small—superinvoluted. This superinvolution is sometimes called "lactation atrophy." It occurs only in women who nurse, and, in such cases, the periods do not reappear during lactation. The atrophy reaches its maximum about the fourth month. If nursing is stopped, the uterus is regenerated in six to eight weeks. This phenomenon is probably a conservative act of nature against too frequent pregnancies. If the nursing is continued too long, actual atrophy of the uterus may occur. When there are no general symptoms,—as pain in the back, nervous disturbances, anemia, weakness,—and if the uterus does not grow too small, the condition is not abnormal, and the uterus will regain its size after lactation ceases; sometimes, even before this. Occasionally (60 per cent.), about the third or fourth week, there is a slight return of bloody lochia. This is usually due to too much activity of the patient, and the blood comes from the placental site; perhaps a superficial clot is being exfoliated. A piece of placenta, thick membranes, sub-involution, infection of the endometrium, fibroids, and retroflexion are the commonest causes of profuse and abnormally long-continued lochia, or of a return of bloody discharge. An early return of the menses occurs in 43 per cent. of nursing women, but in only 26 per cent. are the periods regular. Intervals of weeks and months are noted, as are also great irregularities in amount and duration. If the women do not nurse, the menses usually return in six weeks and continue more or less regularly. The first menstruation after delivery is likely to be profuse.

The Abdominal Walls.—In many women the abdominal walls very slowly and imperfectly regain their previous elasticity. In but a few the tonus is well preserved. A great deal depends on the amount of distention of the abdomen during gestation, overstraining during labor, and the development of gas in the bowels after labor. Wearing tight corsets during pregnancy predisposes to weakness of the abdominal muscles. Attention to the bowels postpartum, and to the strengthening of the muscles, will aid in preventing what the women call "high stomach." Sometimes the belly is so weakened that the recti separate and the uterus comes to lie between them, a state which the women call "rupture," the scientific term being "diastasis recti."

Mathes calls attention to the influence of a congenital, inheritable, constitutional anomaly, manifested by a general laxity of the connective tissues and muscles. He calls this condition the status asthenico-ptoticus. The individual is hypoplastic in many ways, is predisposed to asthenic attacks on the occasion of a sudden mental or physical strain, or if a slow steady drain is made upon her reserve strength. She has ptosis of all her organs (Glénard's disease) and other signs of lack of tissue tonus (varices, hemorrhoids, edema, "poor circulation," vasomotor imbalance, dermographism, flat-foot, etc.). During pregnancy the abdominal walls readily give way to the distention. This is aggravated by the straining of labor and, to complete the picture of destruction, the hypoplastic and inelastic tissues of the pelvic floor are torn, overstretched, and dislocated, usually permanently, by the passage of the child, resulting in genital prolapse.

Changes in the Breasts.—These consist in the establishment of the function of lactation, whereby the woman is put in position to continue the nourishment of her offspring.

Nature has made woman an exception to the rule of other mammals. In her the secretion of milk does not begin until the second or third day, rarely on the first day after birth. In animals the milk is present in the glands the first few hours—even during labor. This delay is possibly an outgrowth of civilization, in that the function of reproduction is not allowed such full play as formerly, and lactation especially has been neglected for generations, resulting in hypoplasia of the glands.

The changes about to be described occur in the breasts after abortions from the fourth month on, as well as after labors at term. On the second day—or, as is usual in primiparæ, on the third day—the breasts grow harder, the veins become prominent, the whole organ fuller and heavier; the patient has the feeling that the secretion of milk is beginning and describes a prickling or burning sensation. Soon the swelling reaches a considerable degree, and the individual milk-ducts can be felt as hard strings—the lobes of the breasts as hard lumps. The gland is much fuller with blood and feels hot to the touch. Rarely, it becomes reddened and sometimes there is a bluish turgescence of the surface. The milk comes into the breasts much more stormily in primiparæ; they express it as "shooting in," and the distress caused is sometimes very severe.

The woman says the breasts feel like two hot weights on her chest, and if the little extension of the gland which sometimes lies in the axilla is involved, the patient keeps her arms outstretched in considerable discomfort, if not pain.

These phenomena are attended with a slight flow of milk from the breasts, even if the baby does not nurse. At each nursing the milk comes with greater force, but after twenty-four hours the process is not so active, though there may still be too much milk for a week, the binder being always more or less wet with it. Lesser degrees of activity of the breasts are common, even agalactia, absence of lactation, being observed. Even though the breasts show tumor, dolor, calor, and rubor, the phenomenon has nothing to do with inflammation; the patient has no temperature, or, at most, one-half degree F. There is nothing that could be called "milk fever."

In multiparæ the secretion begins earlier, sometimes even in the twelve hours after labor, and the breasts do not take on such sudden action, but lactation begins more gradually, and seldom do the breasts swell so that the skin is stretched over them tightly, as in primiparæ.

The enlargement of the breasts is not due wholly to milk. Only a small part of the milk is formed before the nursing, most being made while the child is sucking. The distention of the breasts is due to swelling of the gland-cells and lymphatic engorgement—both preparatory to the formation of milk. As soon as the child begins to nurse the gland-cells break down into fat-globules, the cells produce the milk plasma from the lymph in the distended lymphatics, and active secretion is established in a manner somewhat analogous to the action of the parotid gland. Completely established, the milk secretion becomes regular. The breasts fill up and are emptied in sequence, which is dependent largely upon training. If the child is put to the breast to nurse at regular intervals, the organ quickly accommodates itself to the hours, and one notices that, when the usual sequence is interrupted, the breast will begin to functionate at the proper time.

The first milk that comes resembles the secretion that may be pressed out of the nipple in the latter part of pregnancy; it is clear or only slightly cloudy, sticky, contains yellow streaks, and is called "colostrum."

The colostrum under the microscope is seen to be made up of fat-globules, a watery fluid, and the so-called colostrum corpuscles (Fig. 255). The fat-globules are often adherent by a thin substance which is visible after staining with certain reagents. The colostrum corpuscles are round, ovoid, or stellate cells which sometimes show ameboid movement and have one to three nuclei, which color with ammonia carmin. They contain numerous fine fat-globules. Where they come from has been disputed—they are believed to be changed gland epithelium or leukocytes, mast cells which have gathered up fat-globules. Since they are phagocytic they probably are not epithelial. They remain four to six days, and reappear if there is stasis or inflammation. In addition, lymphocytes are found, more or less full of fat drops; indeed, they may be balled together so that they can hardly be recognized as white blood-cells. Colostrum contains very little if any casein, but nearly 15 per cent. lactalbumin and lactoglobulin, with much fat. It, therefore, has a slightly cathartic action on the new-born babe. One sometimes finds colostrum in the breasts during menstruation, sexual excitement, always

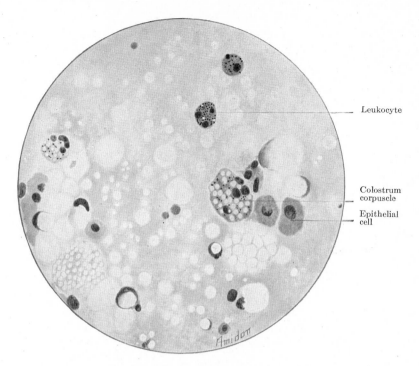

Leukocyte

Colostrum
corpuscle

Epithelial
cell

FIG. 255.—COLOSTRUM.

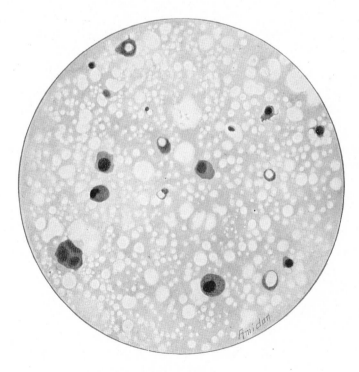

FIG. 256.—MILK.

during pregnancy, early lactation, and during the weaning process. The colostrum at this time helps the resorption of the milk. It has a proteolytic ferment (Jochman).

Human milk is an opaque, slightly yellowish or bluish-white liquid, with a characteristic odor and sweetish taste. Specific gravity varies from 1026 to 1036; it is neutral or alkaline; its freezing-point is $\triangle = -0.49$ to -0.63. Microscopically, one sees innumerable fine fat-droplets, alike in size if the milk is of good quality, and occasionally a glandular epithelial cell or a leukocyte.

It is still unsettled whether there is a membrane of casein around the fat-globules or not. The globules float in a thin, almost transparent, serum which contains albumin. Sometimes bacteria are present.

The composition of human milk varies from day to day and from hour to hour. It contains $87\frac{1}{2}$ per cent. water, $12\frac{1}{2}$ per cent. solids, of which 6.21 per cent. is milk-sugar, 3.78 per cent. fat, 2.29 per cent. proteins (lactoglobulin, 1.26 per cent., and casein, 1.03 per cent.), and 0.71 per cent. salts (König). Of these constituents, the fat is subject to the greatest variations, the proteids less, while most constant are the sugar and salts. In round figures, milk has 88 per cent. water, 2 per cent. proteids, 4 per cent. fat, and 6 per cent. sugar. Holt says the sugar is nearer $7\frac{1}{2}$ per cent., and he emphasizes the iron content, 1.7 mg. per liter. The fat of the milk comes from the epithelium lining the acini and alveoli. When the proper stimulus reaches these cells, which are low, cuboid, with one nucleus, they enlarge, the nucleus divides in a vertical direction, the cell becomes columnar, the protoplasm shows fat-globules, especially near the lumen of the acinus, and finally the cell membrane breaks, setting free the formed fat. After this process is repeated several times the cell itself is cast off, its place being taken by others made by lateral proliferation (Figs. 257 and 258). It is possible, but not proved, that the epithelia can select fat out of the circulating blood, or make it from the carbohydrates ever present in the gland. The casein, since it does not exist in the blood, must be made in the gland itself, as also must be milk-sugar or lactose. Bottazzi found a phosphoglycoproteid in the breast, and believes that through the splitting of this, casein and lactose result. If there is stasis of milk in the breasts, lactose appears in the urine.

The fluid parts of the blood do not reach the milk by filtration or exudation, but are separated from the blood by special secretive action of the glandular epithelium. One must accord the epithelium the most important function of making the milk.

Enzymes, or living ferments, are found in the milk and give it vital sustaining qualities, which are not to be discovered or imitated by the finest chemistry. Breast milk is a living secretion, and contains all the food requirements for the infant, ready for immediate absorption, vitamins and also the antibodies to infection. It is a clinically demonstrated fact that breast-fed children resist infection of all kinds infinitely better than those fed artificially. The author has seen such children, brought to the hospital in collapse, revive after a few breast-feedings as if a strong cordial had been administered. Wassermann has proved that the blood-serum of breast-fed children has stronger bactericidal power than that of those fed from the bottle. The quantity and quality of the milk vary:

First, with the individual—nervous women are not as good wet-nurses as the phlegmatic.

Second, with the race—Japanese, Jews, Swedes, Turks, gypsies, and negresses usually have abundant milk.

Third, with development of the body—a small, thin woman usually gives more milk than a large, muscular, or fat woman; the same rule holding good with cows. Nor does the size of the gland have much effect. The gland-lobes may be less in amount than the fat of the organ, though usually a well-developed breast and nipple presage a good milk supply.

Fourth, nutrition of the patient, to a certain degree—a woman in good health is more likely to give sufficient milk than a sickly mother, but, occasionally, one sees a tuberculous mother with a fat, healthy baby.

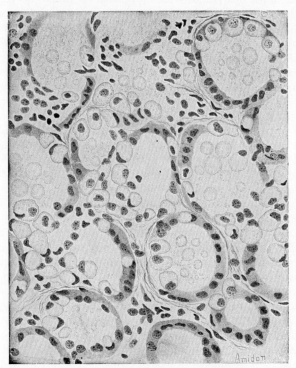

FIG. 257.—FUNCTIONATING HUMAN BREAST.

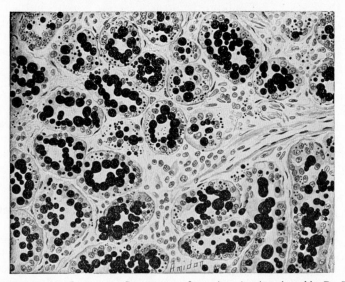

FIG. 258.—MAMMARY GLAND—LACTATING. STAINED WITH OSMIC ACID (specimen loaned by Dr. Gideon Wells).

Fifth, age of the patient. This has very little influence, though, before the age of eighteen and after forty, the milk is likely to suffer both in quality and in quantity.

Sixth, toward the end of lactation the milk gets poor in quality and less in quantity, though there are exceptions.

Seventh, the milk of the two breasts varies in quantity and quality, and from day to day, and at different times of the day, and during a single nursing. The proteids, fat, and sugar increase in amount with the emptying of the breasts.

Eighth, hunger decreases the amount of the milk; fat, casein, and sugar decrease, while the amount of albumin increases. These facts were found by Decaisne during the siege of Paris.

Ninth, emotions may alter quantity and quality—it is said that extreme emotional shock may so alter the milk that it will give the child colic, diarrhea, or even convulsions; that nervous shock may produce agalactia is well known.

Tenth, menstruation sometimes has a distinct effect on the nursing child—it may have colic, or cry a great deal, and may pass green stools, vomit, or have diarrhea; though, chemically, one can find no alteration in the milk. The changes last only a short time.

Eleventh, *pregnancy*—the milk gradually dries up, after becoming more watery. Very often the nursing mother observes a change in the nutrition of the infant and ascribes the same to the advent of a new pregnancy.

Twelfth, *drugs* often reappear in the milk. This has been known since Hippocrates, in connection with cathartics. One may, in order to purge the infant, give the mother the cathartic. Alcohol is said also to pass over, and cases are cited where the baby got drunk. Opium has caused narcosis of forty-three hours in the baby. Iron, arsenic, iodin, lead, and mercury are well known to pass over. Salvarsan may thus be used for the treatment of mother and babe.

Brieger has shown that immunizing doses of tetanus antitoxin pass over to the infant. The writer allowed a woman with diphtheria, who had large doses of antitoxin, to nurse her infant. The child did not take diphtheria, though Hofbauer claims that the diphtheria antitoxin is not transmitted to the child. Vaccinia is not believed to pass over. The only drug which has any effect on the amount of the milk secreted is iodid of potash. It limits the output.

Thirteenth, disease has an important effect on the milk. Diarrheas cause a diminution; in cholera, sometimes complete absence. In sepsis the milk sometimes dries up, which is a bad omen. Bacteria can pass into the milk in disease (Kehrer). Tuberculosis, anthrax, may pass over without any demonstrable change in the gland. In mastitis the milk may contain cocci and pus.

Fourteenth, irritation of the nipples causes an increase of the secretion. This is demonstrated clinically in many ways—e. g., by placing the baby to the breast early, the milk comes earlier, and by using the breast-pump too much to "relieve" the breasts, more milk is produced. It is possible to start lactation in a non-puerperal woman, even in young girls, by properly stimulating the breasts. Massage of the breasts and cold baths increase the milk supply.

Fifteenth, certain foods are said to increase the secretion, as tomatoes, oysters, and gruels. My experience with them is negative. Liquids, especially cows' milk, increase the amount of milk, and a rich supply of proteids in the diet seems to augment the fat content. Overfeeding, however, in the author's experience, only occasionally improves the nursing, and then, temporarily. Later, the mother puts on fat and the breasts dry up. If there is no gland tissue in the breast, no amount of stimulation will cause it to secrete.

Certain foods are said to alter the milk to the disturbance of the child—e. g., strawberries, tomatoes, beans, and acid fruits. It does seem that idiosyncracies, possessed by the mother, also become evident in her offspring.

Sixteenth, multiparæ usually have more milk than primiparæ, and women, after normal labor, are less likely to have disturbed lactation than those who have had difficult, operative deliveries, especially if attended with great loss of blood.

Seventeenth, the amount of milk varies with the demand. Ordinarily the breasts give 600 to 800 gm. per day, depending on the needs of the nursling, but Budin has recorded cases where a wet-nurse produced 2500 to 2800 gm. of milk per day, for a long period, without injury.

If the nursing is interrupted from any cause, it may be resumed, providing the interval is not too long. The author has seen the secretion of milk return after an absence of five weeks, and cases are recorded of its return after months.

Lactation has a not unimportant bearing on the general condition of the woman. A certain amount of blood and fat must be eliminated after pregnancy. Part of these go in the lochia, part in the excreta, and part in the milk. If the last is not excreted, the other organs must remove the excess and, according to Kehrer, congestion of the genitalia is likely to occur. It is a fact that, when the patient does not nurse, the lochia are increased, and the involution of the uterus is delayed, but this is generally explained by the absence of the reflex irritation which nursing causes on the uterus. The act of nursing causes uterine contractions in the early puerperium, which are a prominent symptom, as "after-pains," and these favor the rapid involution of the uterus. Positive observations are not on record, but, in general, it may be said that a woman recovers better from her labor if she nurses her offspring. Milk is also an excretion, containing amino-acids, urea, creatinin, creatin, and uric acid sometimes in the same proportion as exists in the blood. Taylor, of Aberdeen, has shown in goats that excess of protein in the food increases the non-protein nitrogen in the milk.

Literature

Budin: Le Nourisson, Paris, 1901.—*Duncan, M.:* Researches in Obstetrics.—*Fehling:* Die Physiologie und Path. des Wochenbettes, 2d ed., 1897.—*Harris and Brown:* Johns Hopkins Hosp. Bull.. 1928, 43, 190.—*Hoehne:* "Trichomonas Vaginalis," Zent. f. Gyn., 1916, No. 1, p. 10; Zentralblatt. f. Gyn., 1916, No. 6, p. 114.—*Hofbauer:* Bull. Johns Hopkins Hosp., vol. xxxviii, No. 4, p. 225, 1926.—*Holt:* Amer. Jour. Dis. of Children, October, 1915, p. 230.—*Jochman:* Arch. f. Gyn., vol. lxxxix, Bd. 3.—*Knapp:* Winckel's Handb. der Geb., vol. ii, 1.—*Loeser:* Zeitschr für Geb. u. Gyn., 1920, vol. lxxxii, H. 3, S. 648.—*Mathes:* Biologie u. Path. des Weibes, Halban & Seitz, 1924, Lief. 3, p. 42.—*Stoltz:* Die Bakteriologie des Genital-Kanales in der Schwangerschaft und in Wochenbett, Graz., 1903.—*Taylor:* Ref Jour. Amer. Med. Assoc , February 24, 1923, p. 557.—*Temesváry:* Arch. f. Gyn., vol. xxxiii.—*Walthard:* Stoeckel's Geburtshilfe, 1920, p. 90.—*Wassermann:* Deutsch. med. Wochenschr., 1903, No. 1.—*Williams, J. W.:* Amer. Jour. of Obst. and Gyn., 1931, November, p. 664.—*Wormser:* Arch. f. Gyn., vol. lxix, H. 3.—*Zangemeister:* Arch. f. Gyn., 1907.

CHAPTER XV

GENERAL CHANGES IN THE PUERPERIUM

It is surprising how little the general condition of the woman is affected by such a severe storm as is even a normal labor and, in the puerperium, by the absorption of the products of involution of the large uterus. In the absence of infection, most women feel quite well during the puerperal period. The soreness of the genitalia, due to the vulvar wounds, disappears in a few days, the soreness of the muscles likewise, and, even after a few hours, the patient feels rested from the severe exercise of delivery. Women unused to exertion recover less quickly from the strain. After a difficult operative delivery, however, and after a severe hemorrhage, we find the symptoms that would naturally go with such conditions, and the occurrence of surgical shock must also be mentioned. A multipara is likely to be annoyed by after-pains. These are painful uterine contractions which recur more or less regularly for one, two, three, or even six days. The contractions occur especially when the child nurses, a reflex or, perhaps, a mamma hormone going to the uterus from the breasts; also when the uterus is massaged, but most markedly when pieces of membrane, of placenta, or blood-clots have been left in the uterus. Women who have had endometritis, metritis, frequent abortion, rapidly successive labors, overdistention of the uterus by twins, polyhydramnion, or very quick labors, are likely to suffer more with after-pains. Primiparæ, because the uterus remains in a state of good tonus, are less likely to suffer with them. If these painful contractions reappear after they have once ceased, it is indicative of something wrong in the uterus—either infection or retained secundines, a fibroid, etc.

The Nervous System.—Puerperæ are more sensitive to irritations, a fact which was known to the Romans, and they placed a sign before her door, so that she was not disturbed—even by the tax collector. The reflex excitability is increased. Recent investigations of the knee-jerk show that in pregnancy this reflex is more active than usual, that it is most active in labor at the height of a pain, while during the puerperium the excitability gradually passes away. Puerperæ hear more acutely and are more sensitive to light and odors. Though many writers, and most nurses, believe that a nervous shock can cause fever, the author has never observed an unequivocal case where such a severe emotional storm has raised the patient's temperature. (See chapter on Puerperal Infection.)

The Temperature.—Variations in the temperature of puerperal women form a most important index of her health, and, together with the pulse, give us reliable information. Although attended by severe muscular exertion, labor does not, as a rule, raise the temperature more than one-half degree. If the labor terminates in the afternoon, the usual rise, at this time, may be exaggerated; but in normal cases, a parturient's temperature, should not go above 99° F. Even this makes one suspicious of infection. The so-called "physiologic chill" is, in the author's opinion, the result of the flooding of the system with toxins or bacteria from the puerperal wounds, or possibly alien proteids, as was told on p. 142. The temperature may rise one-half degree after labor, but falls to the normal within twelve hours, and then shows the physiologic diurnal variations, but these do not exceed 1° F. Many authorities assert that a puerperal woman may normally have fever. Fehling considers every rise above 101.1° F. pathologic; Winckel places the limit at 100.7° F.; Boxall, of London, at 100° F.; Williams, at 100.4° F. It is, to a great extent, arbitrary. My own experience is that, if the temperature rises above 99° F., almost always there is some cause for it—usually a mild infection. Goodall and Brindeau call all temperatures above 98.6° F. abnormal, in which I agree, but it is not meant that a woman showing a slightly higher fever must be very ill or in danger. In such cases one is warned to more careful asepsis in the daily technic of delivery and a painstaking study into the cause of the elevation in each individual case.

Primiparæ show higher temperatures and greater fluctuations than multiparæ, because in them there are more wounds and greater possibilities for the absorption of toxins. After hard operative deliveries, after many internal examinations, the temperature is often higher and more labile.

There is no such thing as "milk fever"! Formerly, in the non-antiseptic era, almost every puerpera had fever on the third day. Since at this time the breasts become large and hard, the fever was ascribed to the violent coming of the milk, and the real cause, the infection of the genitalia, was overlooked. With the advent of antisepsis there has been a great decrease in this so-called "milk fever," and large numbers of the best authorities deny its existence. Jaggard said he had never seen a case where there was fever and no other cause to be found than simply the coming of the milk. I have seen primiparæ with the breasts standing out hard and firm, the axillary lobe of the gland so swollen that the patient had to keep the arms from the sides, and yet the temperature was 98.6° F. Infection of the breasts is another thing. "Milk fever" is a misnomer that should be abolished from obstetrics. It too often forms the cover for severe puerperal infections, and many women have lost their lives because of neglect of the real disease.

The reason usually given that the puerperal woman should have some fever is this: The products of the regressive metamorphosis of the uterus and all the genitalia being absorbed, must be oxidized. This increased oxidation causes the increase in the body heat. But nature, by increasing the perspiration and other excretions, keeps the temperature nearly normal. The slight rise of temperature right after delivery is probably a mild infection. The older writers called it fibrin ferment fever.

On the third or fourth day the puerperal wounds are "cleaning themselves," the necrotic portions are being cast off, and the bacteria at this time often ascend into the uterine cavity, but nature protects the woman from invasion.

The temperature of the puerperal woman is subject to fluctuations on slighter causes as compared with the non-puerperal woman.

Constipation is said to give rise to temperature, which goes down when the bowels are emptied. This fever is probably due to obstruction to the flow of lochia, which is overcome when the rectum is emptied, but may be due to absorption from the intestine. It is safest, as soon as your puerperæ have fever, to think of infection first. A full bladder may act similarly, but it is wise to bear in mind the frequency of ureteropyelitis in puerperio. While fever may arise from the bowels, as from enteritis, I have never been fully convinced that constipation itself will cause it.

The Pulse.—In the second stage of labor the pulse is strong, rapid, perhaps irregular; but during the third stage it calms down and is normal throughout this time, unless there is a severe hemorrhage, when it becomes small and fast. Immediately after labor the pulse is soft; soon it has a high tension, especially in multiparæ, but the blood-pressure then sinks slowly to below normal or about normal.

A very high tension slow pulse must be regarded as a warning of eclampsia. In general, the pulse during the puerperium runs from 68 to 80, which is about normal, though higher rates are sometimes found, even in healthy women.

A peculiar phenomenon is sometimes observed in healthy puerperæ. The pulse-rate may be as low as 40 a minute, and some observers have found 30, but this is very rare. It occurs after labors at term more than after early abortions; in multiparæ more often than in primiparæ;

in lean oftener than fat women. The author has found a pulse of below 60 in only 10 per cent. of his cases. Other authors give 16.2 per cent. (Hemeys) and 63 per cent. (Olshausen). The cause is not known. Lynch gives the literature. There are many theories, of which the most plausible are: Fehling's—the sudden diminution of the intra-abdominal tension irritates the vagus reflexly; Schröder's—the heart, which hypertrophies during pregnancy, now need not work so hard; Olshausen's—the fat, which is absorbed from the uterus, slows the heart; that it is an evidence of vagotonia, as may be proved by pressure on the eyeball, which will make the pulse still slower. Further, the horizontal position, the quiet of the patient, the less amount of food, the great excretion of liquid in milk, lochia, sweat, etc., may combine to produce the bradycardia. It is of great prognostic significance. A slow pulse indicates that everything is going along nicely.

A very rapid pulse in the puerperium, in the absence of fever, points to hemorrhage, recovery from severe hemorrhage, or some heart disease. Not seldom a rapid pulse draws attention to the condition of the heart, but one must be careful in the diagnosis of heart disease during pregnancy and the puerperium, because murmurs are common (70 per cent.), and a displaced heart simulates hypertrophy. The pulse is more labile during the puerperium than the temperature. It warns much quicker of the advent of sepsis or other puerperal complication, but is less reliable. It fluctuates with the after-pains and with any little excitement—as visitors and nursing the baby. The usual relation between temperature and pulse obtains here as elsewhere.

The Blood.—There is a decrease in the amount of blood (Sengel), which had increased during pregnancy, an evidence of the loss during labor and especially if delivery was accompanied by much hemorrhage. The hemoglobin is disproportionately reduced. During labor, the leukocyte count varies from 9000 to 34,000, with an average of 18,000, the increase being in the polynuclear neutrophiles. The eosinophiles are often absent. The reds vary from 4,000,000 to 5,500,000. After labor the leukocytosis rapidly disappears, even within twenty-four hours, but usually it requires several days for the count to come down to the normal limits— 7500 to 15,000, which is somewhat higher than in the non-puerperal state. The normal proportion of the various whites is: Neutrophiles, 60 to 75 per cent.; lymphocytes, 25 per cent.; eosinophiles, 2 to 5 per cent. These proportions vary from day to day. About the fifth day one occasionally observes a slight eosinophilia, which is more marked after the birth of twins, of macerated fetuses, and in gonorrheal cases. Infection alters the blood-picture. (See p. 943.) The normal acidosis of pregnancy and labor continues during the puerperium (Burtscher), and may be increased by an acid base diet or hunger. Bardenheuer says it decreases the lochia and favors involution and wound healing.

The **respiration** is not much altered in frequency, but responds more readily to disturbances. The chest being free, expands more easily than during pregnancy, the type of breathing being costal and diaphragmatic. The vital capacity is increased after the third day. On percussion one finds a deeper resonance. The heart dulness sinks a little.

The Skin.—All the functions of the skin are more active, the sweat-glands particularly. After labor, when the patient is well covered up, she breaks out with a full, warm sweat, but this is rarely so profuse as to require a change of bed-linen. It is favored by the warm covers and the administration of warm drinks. That there is a sweating peculiar to puerpera is not true, but the perspiration has a peculiar odor, which varies in health and disease. During the lying-in there is a tendency to perspiration, especially in sleep, but it is less in the latter days, probably because of the establishment of the milk secretion and the free lochia.

The laity have great fear that the patient takes cold at this time. This is the outgrowth of the old belief that puerperal fever comes from catching cold, a view still held among the midwives, and in their practice it is not unusual to find the windows closed and the patient covered with heavy blankets, even in summer.

Ahlfeld says that there is some connection between the appearance of the sweat and the contraction and retraction of the uterus after labor.

The Kidneys and Urinary Tract.—Relieved suddenly from the increased intra-abdominal pressure by the delivery of the child, the kidneys become active. In the third stage it is not rare to find the bladder full and even overfilled, making an obstacle to the delivery of the placenta.

In the first twelve hours there is usually retention of urine, which sometimes may be enormous and cause ischuria paradoxa. This is due to the lack of elasticity of the bladder, inability to urinate in the horizontal position, the swelling of the vulva and urethra, kinking of the urethra (Olshausen), reflex spasm of the sphincter from stitches in the perineum, and injury to the bladder trigonum and urethral orifice, with edema. Still, quite a few puerperæ pass urine spontaneously. In many cases it is necessary to use the catheter. As a rule, patients pass urine three times daily, much less often than in the later months of pregnancy.

Cystoscopic examination of the bladder after labor shows the effect of the bruising sustained during the expulsion of the child. The trigonum and urethral orifice are edematous and strewn with minute blood extravasations. The epithelium desquamates and lies on the mucous membrane as a grayish film. After prolonged deliveries and hard operations, the bladder-wall is much crushed, and in the cystoscope we see the above effects much more marked (Fig. 259). The ureteral orifices are not easily found, but the ureters are very easily palpable, being usually somewhat enlarged. The laceration of the urogenital septum, and of the connective tissue around the base of the bladder, allows the anterior wall of the vagina to prolapse, carrying the urethra and neck of the bladder with it.

The urine collected just after delivery frequently (40 per cent.) contains a little albumin, white blood-corpuscles, a few reds, and scattered hyaline casts. In twelve hours the latter disappear. The amount of urine for the first eight days is 300 to 400 c.c. more than that of the non-pregnant woman, but is not much more than that of the pregnant woman in the latter months (Kehrer).

The specific gravity varies from 1010 to 1025, according to the amount of urine. The urea varies from 2.6 per cent. to 1.6 per cent., being highest on the third day, the excess being ascribable to the increased metabolism of lactation—the change of the albuminoids into fat. It is, therefore, less in women who do not nurse. The proportion of salts, phosphates, and sulphates does not vary much from the normal —perhaps the salt output is increased.

Milk-sugar occurs in 80 per cent. of puerperal urines (von Noorden). It is derived from the breasts. Blot first called attention to this physiologic lactosuria. It is greatest during the establishment of lactation, absent during its proper functionating, and appears again during the weaning process. The average is 0.2 per cent., but this may be increased to 1 per cent. by feeding with albuminoids and carbohydrates.

Peptone has been found in the urine by Fischel from the second to the tenth day, and is ascribed to the absorption of products of albuminoid degeneration going on in the uterus. Albuminuria occurs in 40 per cent. of the cases of labor, but this disappears before the third day. If it does not, or if albumin reappears, its cause must be sought out. Nephritis, pyelitis, ureteritis, cystitis, post-anesthetic effects, eclampsia, and sepsis must be considered. To avoid confusion from the admixture of lochia, only catheterized specimens may be used.

Lactic acid, acetone, pepsin, and toxins have been found in the urine of puerperæ. Creatin, discovered by Shaffer in the urine postpartum, is believed by Mellanby to be due to some unusual metabolism of nutrient material during the development of the fetus and the establishment of lactation.

The Intestinal Tract.—The puerperæ are very thirsty and drink much, but the appetite usually is poor for the first three days. Loss of fluids during labor, and in the lochia, urine, and sweat, explains the thirst. After labor, the belly is flat, even slightly concave, but soon a moderate tympany appears. In thin women the

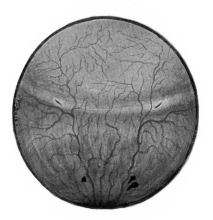

FIG. 259.—BLADDER THREE HOURS AFTER DELIVERY.
Note edema of trigonum and hemorrhages.

uterine tumor, the large and small intestines, with their peristalsis, the liver, spleen, and kidneys are very easily palpable, and one may use the opportunity for investigation of these organs.

A moderate tympany is normal in the puerperium; it is due to slight intestinal paresis, and accompanies the usual constipation. Rarely do the bowels move spontaneously in the first few days of the puerperium. The causes of the obstipation are: The bowels usually have been emptied by cathartics before labor; the woman eats little, and the excretion of fluids is so rapid that the intestinal contents dry up; the abdominal and perineal muscles, because of overstretching, cannot do their work; a patient usually has difficulty in defecating while lying on the back; and the pain in the parts may inhibit the action.

Older writers believed that constipation could cause puerperal infection. That constipation alone may cause fever I have some doubts, but in these cases the fever would come from the intestinal canal, not from the genitalia. A brisk purge may be followed by a fall of temperature in a case of real puerperal infection, and one may be misguided into ascribing the fever to the intestines, when, in reality, the purge simply stirred up the pelvic circulation, emptied the lower bowel, provided good drainage for the lochia, and perhaps increased the local and general leukocytosis so that the infection was taken care of. Errors of diet cannot cause puerperal infection.

The **weight** of the patient undergoes marked changes in the first months after labor. According to Gassner, the average weight of 238 women, on the day after labor, was 124 pounds. In the first two weeks they lost about 9 pounds, or 8 per cent. of their weight—Baumm, 6.58 per cent. The loss is greater in multiparæ, greater in large women, and after full term than premature labor, also greater after twins. This loss of weight is due to the moderate amount of food taken and the great amount of excreta—the sweat, the urine, but especially the lochia and the milk. The women look thin, pale, and washed out after getting up, and need a tonic diet. The weight is regained in four to six weeks, many women putting on excessive fat. Nowadays, since we do not starve the women so much in the puerperium, these losses are not so marked, but the custom of feeding puerperæ very lightly still exists in many places.

Literature

Bardenheuer, F. H.: Zentralb. für Gyn., December 19, 1931, p. 3636.—*Burtscher and Malfatti:* Klin. Woch., Berlin, April 18, 1931.—*Carton:* Annales de Gynecologie, 1903, vol. ii, p. 163.—*Goodall, J. R.:* Who quotes Brindeau, Puerperal Infection, Montreal, 1932, p. 20.—*Gräfenberg:* Arch. f. Gyn., 1908, vol. lxxxv, H. 2.—*Hahl:* Ibid., vol. xlvii, H. 3.—*Lynch:* "Bradycardia in Puerperio," Surg., Gyn., and Obstet., May, 1911. Literature.—*Mellanby:* Proc. Royal Soc., London, 1913, lxxxvi, p. 88.—*v. Noorden:* Path. des Stoffwechsels, 1906.—*Stengel:* "The Blood in Pregnancy, Parturition and Puerperium," N. Y. Med. Jour., 1903, vol. lxiii, p. 56.—*Wild:* Arch. f. Gyn., vol. liii, H. 2, p. 363.

THE HYGIENE AND CONDUCT OF PREGNANCY AND LABOR

CHAPTER XVI

THE CHILD

FEW women, in rearing a daughter, consider the possibility of her future pregnancy and labor, and make the attempt to prepare her for their successful accomplishment. Many women believe that while the child is in utero it can be influenced by the mental occupation of the mother; thus, for example, if she desires a musical child, she should study music assiduously during pregnancy. Then, too, most intelligent mothers try to live a hygienic life during gestation and do those things which seem to promise normal healthy offspring. Some few intelligent parents try to arrange the most auspicious circumstances at the time of procreation of their children, but, beyond such desultory efforts, very little attention is paid to the science of Eugenics. Indeed, to be well born one must go back many generations, but it is certainly demanded that a beginning should be made at once, to provide for posterity. Only in the human animal are the laws of successful procreation defied. The influences of heredity, of disease, of character, of environment, are all set at naught, and the propagation of the species left to chance, to lust, or to convenience.

Incontestable evidence exists to prove that the children of alcoholics are often weak, puny, imbecile, or epileptic. Insanity, the tendency to drug addictions, venereal disease, hemophilia, nephritis, and other affections, or a predisposition to the same, are undoubtedly transmitted, and their effects may be discovered even in the third generation. As far as the obstetrician is concerned, these facts carry weight as matter to be included in his history-taking in individual cases, for they will shed light on many complications occurring in the course of pregnancy and parturition, and indicate what measures to pursue in preventing and treating such complications (Ballantyne). Prenatal study and treatment of the child will do much to reduce infantile morbidity and mortality. After a girl is born much may be done to correct an evil ancestry and to prevent diseases which would affect her procreative ability. A well-developed child requires at least thirty-six weeks of uterogestation. Prematurely born girls not seldom show skeletal and genital infantilism, the latter causing dysmenorrhea and sterility and neuroses; the former, contracted pelvis with dystocia (abnormal labor). Another cause of infantilism, not generally recognized, is intestinal disturbances, especially infection, during the first two years of life. Atrophy of the intestinal glands leads to permanent hypoplastic changes in the whole system. Since bottle-fed children are most likely to suffer from such infections, the obstetrician will, all the more, seek to enforce breast-feeding with the future of the baby in view.

The new-born child is very easily infected, and vulvitis and vaginitis not seldom occur. That such may lead to subsequent pelvic disease is beyond question. Mastitis in the new-born girl may result in complete destruction of the mammary gland, with resulting agalactia in the puerperium. Rachitis in very early life is not uncommon, and it may distort the pelvic bones. While the resulting deformity only in severe cases produces an absolute disproportion between the child and the pelvis, milder degrees of pelvic distortion cause abnormalities in the mechanism of labor which not seldom cost the life of the mother or the babe, and often leave serious injury to both.

The acute infectious diseases—scarlatina, diphtheria, anterior poliomyelitis, etc.—not seldom leave permanent traces on the child, as nephritis, hepatitis, disease of the endocrine glands, and, in the last instance, paralysis, with shortening of the leg and consequent distortion of the pelvis. Psychic trauma in childhood may lay the foundation for later psychoses.

These few examples are given to indicate the scope of prophylaxis in early life, from an obstetric point of view, and much can be done by a wise hygiene to preserve the growing girl from the evils of disease, environment, and heredity.

PUBERTY

At this time, when mighty changes are going on in the internal and external genitalia, the foundation of permanent disease may be laid. It is beyond question that the crowding of the child's mind with studies and accomplishments, the premature social duties, together with inappropriate reading and company, and a lack of outdoor exercise and sports, tend to develop the mind at the expense of the body, particularly the sexual organs, which require so much of the girl's vitality at this period. Dysmenorrhea, hypoplasia of the uterus, later, chlorosis, are some of the results of these evils. Early womanhood also requires proper hygienic conduct if one wishes to develop a healthy nervous system and a normal reproductive function. Of transcendent importance is the proper instruction of the growing girl in the principles of sex and reproduction. Only in this way will it be possible to save the girl from ignorantly performing secret practices, e. g., masturbation, to restrict the spread of venereal disease, the number of illegitimate births and criminal abortions. It is impossible to go deeper into this important subject here, but that the obstetrician is concerned in this matter goes without saying, and by wise counsel, at this particular time, he may save the girl from permanent invalidism, even from death in childbirth (Surbled).

MENSTRUATION

Menstruation should not be regarded as an illness and the girl's mind should not dwell upon it. Her usual mode of life is to be continued, but excesses avoided. Immoderate dancing, exposure to cold with thin clothes, sexual excitement, hot baths taken to bring on the period, all cause catarrhal conditions of the uterus, which predispose to abortion, adherent placenta, and postpartum hemorrhage.

THE HUSBAND

The part played by the husband in obstetric complications has never been properly noticed. If he is unusually large and heavy boned, he may procreate children too large for his wife to bear. Venereal disease communicated to the wife is so common that obstetricians reckon with it all the time. Under this heading may be mentioned the local inflammations of the female urinary tract, cystitis, ureteritis, pyelitis, surgical kidney; vulvitis, endometritis, with adherent placenta, postpartum hemorrhage, subinvolution, etc.; pyosalpinx with gonorrheal and streptococcic (often fatal) peritonitis; syphilitic macerated fetus, with maternal hemophilic tendencies; gonorrheal ophthalmia of the new-born, and other fetal disease. These need only to be indicated to show that the husband is directly concerned in our discussion.

Too frequent intercourse during pregnancy often causes abortion, premature labor, and even abruptio placentæ. One important fact, and it will be again referred to, is that coitus in the latter weeks of pregnancy may cause infection of the uterus, which shows itself during and after delivery as a sometimes fatal puerperal fever.

16

CHAPTER XVII

HYGIENE OF PREGNANCY—PRENATAL CARE

WOMEN call the doctor and engage him for their confinement earlier now than formerly, earlier among the better classes than the poorer, earlier in the city than the country, earlier in the United States than in most other lands. Numerous advantages arise from this, in that it may enable the doctor to learn the traits or constitution of his patient, watch for any symptoms of disease, and prepare her properly for the labor. It, therefore, should be encouraged in practice.

Many and varied questions will be asked of the accoucheur, and it will be found convenient to supply each patient with a folder containing instructions for her to follow and other common information. The gravida should not change her usual mode of life unless the physician knows that some of her habits are bad and he must teach her the proper hygiene of living.

Dress.—The dress should be simple and warm. All the clothes should hang from the shoulders by suspenders or corset-waist, and heavy skirts not worn; better, warm drawers, closed, to prevent infection from street dust.

Low-heeled shoes with broad toes are best. The pregnant woman throws her head and shoulders back, in order to keep her balance. This makes an angle in the small of the back (see Fig. 133, p. 115) and gives the patient a peculiar gait, which did not escape the eye of Shakespeare, who called it the "pride of pregnancy." Elevation of the heels throws the body still more forward; the woman must throw head and shoulders further back, which causes pain in the loins and stretching of the abdomen. Gellhorn and Grossman call attention to the importance of caring for weak feet and fallen arches during pregnancy. These cause difficulty in locomotion, pains in the limbs and back. The usual orthopedic measures, good shoes, directed exercises and strapping of the feet are recommended.

There should be no circular constriction at any part of the body, which means that corsets, tight waistbands, round garters, may not be worn. The Latin term for the condition of pregnancy was "incincta," without a girdle, and had reference to the custom of laying off the girdle as soon as pregnancy was determined. Most multiparæ with a tendency to pendulous abdomen, and some primiparæ toward the end of pregnancy, like a light-weight, woven abdominal supporter or one of the maternity waists on the market. The corset is particularly injurious during pregnancy, because it forces the uterus and child down into the pelvis and against the lower abdominal wall, causing congestion of the pelvic veins and weakness of the abdominal muscles. Too tight corsets also, by restraining the expansion of the uterus, cause deformities of the child, for example, club-foot, wry-neck. Women who wish to conceal pregnancy by tight lacing may do themselves or the fetus even fatal damage.

The author advises all gravidæ to go without their corsets as much as possible, to sleep on alternate sides, and daily, after the seventh month, to gently knead the abdomen for a few minutes—all intended to move the child out of a cramped position, which, if too long held, may result in club-foot, wry-neck, etc.

Diet.—Simple, not strict, rules govern the diet. The amount of meat and broths should be small—not more than 4 ounces of meat or its equivalent in fish or eggs per day. Starches fried in fat and rich pastry should be avoided. Cereals, vegetables, and fruits should be eaten, especially fruit, to loosen the bowels. Water is taken freely, at least five full glasses daily—sterilized or filtered. Milk and, especially, buttermilk are commended. Alcohol is to be forbidden, first, because of the danger, exaggerated during pregnancy, of contracting the liquor habit; second, because of its demonstrable bad effect on the offspring, a fact which was known in Biblical times. Samson's mother abstained from wine during her pregnancy. A child begotten by a drunken father may be dull, stupid, or diseased, an observation made by Diogenes and confirmed by recent experiments on guinea-pigs.

Coffee in moderate amounts is not forbidden. Some popular books advise a special diet to reduce the bone salts of the fetus—a pernicious recommendation, because the mother's health will suffer before the infant is affected, and in all probability fetal rickets would result if an effect were possible.

It is absolutely essential for the growth of the fetus and for the woman in making the required adjustments of her metabolism that the food provide an abundance of all the vitamins, and plenty of calcium, phosphates, and iron. Milk, butter, fresh leafy vegetables, therefore, should not be missing from the dietary.

In general, a woman's ordinary habits need be little disturbed. She should not overeat, thinking she must feed two. (See Shukers.) Routine ultraviolet treatments and routine viosterol are not recommended. Cod and halibut liver oil may be given on indication.

The Bowels.—Constipation is the rule during pregnancy, and, if neglected, may lead to most serious consequences. A long-standing habit cannot be cured at this time, wherefore drugs must usually be resorted to. The following is the treatment pursued by the author:

First, the patient should make it an unfailing habit to go to stool at a certain hour each day. The best time is shortly after breakfast. Should no movement occur—and straining is not permitted—the action of the rectum may be provoked by a glycerin suppository or an enema. A desire to go to stool at any time must not be resisted. A sufficient amount of exercise must be taken. Abdominal massage is not permissible during gestation.

Second, every morning just after rising and every evening just before retiring the patient should drink a glass of cool water and eat some fruit—an apple or an orange. Between meals water is to be drunk freely.

Third, her diet should contain fruit and vegetables in abundance, especially spinach, peas, beans, barley, tomatoes, corn, bran bread, and foods of this kind. They give something for the bowels to act on, but one cannot use so much of them as in the non-pregnant state. Tea is forbidden, but coffee in moderate amount allowed. Prunes, figs, and dates are to be eaten, with care to chew them very fine, as they may cause indigestion. A little system in this helps a great deal, probably by suggestion. Let the patient begin with one prune a day, then one more each day up to ten or fifteen, gradually decreasing the number as the need disappears. Agar is being given lately, and certain foods which contain flaxseed, also psyllium.

Fourth, let the patient, every night before retiring, inject into the rectum 4 to 6 ounces of ordinary olive oil, leaving it there all night. In cases of spastic constipation this is a valuable remedy.

Fifth, drugs are withheld, as far as possible, and active cathartics entirely. Cascara, in bitter extract, administered in capsules, gives the best results, the dose being increased gradually and decreased as the desired effect is obtained. One may alternate, every month, with a saline aperient, and of the many on the market, the author has found Pluto water best. Liquid petrolatum is often used as an intestinal lubricant. Medicines are discontinued as soon as the patient is taught to do without them. A good prescription for atonic constipation attended with flatulence is the following:

R. Fluidext. cascaræ sagradæ 30
    Tr. rhei aromatici.. 30
    Tr. nucis vomicæ... 20
    Elixir taraxaci com., N. F..........................q. s. ad 120
    M. et S.—A half teaspoonful after meals, t.i.d.

If the patient has hemorrhoids, aloes may be substituted for the cascara.

The Kidneys.—It is generally conceded that the kidneys are the most vulnerable point in the body during pregnancy. One surely obtains very valuable information of the general metabolism from the urine, and its frequent examination is a duty of the accoucheur. The woman is directed to send him a four-ounce bottleful of the morning urine every three weeks until the seventh month; then, every two weeks, and if there is any suspicion of nephritis or toxemia, every day. She is also directed as often to measure the amount passed in twenty-four hours. This must be not less than 50 ounces. Tests are made for albumin, sugar, specific gravity, urea, and for casts. For practical purposes, finer examinations are not necessary. Albumin is significant if found by the usual tests.

Exercise.—Violent exercise, of course, is to be avoided. It is not possible to build up a strong muscular system during pregnancy. That should have been done before. To be avoided are jolts, running, sudden motions, lifting great weights, going up and down stairs quickly, horseback riding, cycling, golf, tennis, dancing, and swimming. Sea-bathing is adopted by some women to bring on abortion. To be encouraged are walks, up to two miles, in the sunlight, preferably not at night, and easy automobile rides. Housework is desirable, unless too strenuous.

Railway travel, the aeroplane, and ocean voyages had better be curtailed, and if travel is necessary, the most comfortable accommodations must be secured. Much depends on the individual, since many gravidæ do the most remarkable things and suffer nothing, while others miscarry from the slightest provocation. The author believes the automobile is responsible for many abortions and forbids touring entirely, and even short rides unless the roads are good. Much depends on the riding qualities of the automobile. If a woman has a known tendency to abort, she must be very careful, and had better even go to bed at the usual time of her menstrual periods. A general massage is often useful, care being taken to avoid the breasts, the abdomen, and varicose veins.

The patient may go to the theater, but must avoid crowds, for fear of getting into a crush. She must avoid gatherings in close rooms, especially with stove heat, because the fetus is very susceptible to coal-gas.

In practice among the well-to-do the children are larger and stronger than among the very poor, though the difference is not as great as one would expect. Studies of the factory workers in Europe, where the proportion of the operatives that are pregnant women is larger than with us, have proved that their children are more likely to be premature, puny, undersized, or weakly. Certain cities have arranged to give the pregnant woman a respite from work for six weeks before delivery and four weeks afterward, and France, Italy, and Switzerland are considering bills making such relief from toil obligatory. Austria, Germany, and Soviet Russia have passed such laws and have rendered their application possible by providing the financial aid such women need when they stop working. In Paris there are homes for women in the last weeks of pregnancy, and experience has shown their good effect upon the newborn children and the mothers.

Coitus During Pregnancy.—This is a subject on which much has been written, and deservedly, because it is of great importance. Many women have a distaste for intercourse during this time; in others the desire is increased, rarely to nymphomania. There are many reasons for forbidding coitus during gestation:

First, the danger of abortion, which is caused by the impact of the penis against the cervix, and the great congestion of the parts during the act. No doubt the frequency of miscarriage in the newly married is due to this cause.

Second, the nervous shock is not well borne by a woman whose nerve energy is already overtaxed. It aggravates the leukorrhea, and often increases the nausea and vomiting. In some cases the presence of the husband incites an attack of vomiting, and removal of the patient from home may be necessary.

Third, animals do not copulate when the female is pregnant, and, while the habits of other animals do not guide man, in many cases it would be wise for him to follow their instincts.

Fourth, the danger of infection. This is a real danger, the author knowing of two cases where fatal sepsis resulted from coitus just before labor, and several other cases where severe puerperal fever was in all likelihood the result of this pernicious practice.   The danger, of course, is greater in multiparæ in whom the cervix is patulous.

Other reasons that have been given are more or less fanciful—for example, that it makes the child sensual, that it weakens it, that the wife will lose respect for her husband.   The danger from coitus is greatest in the first three months, when usually the fact of pregnancy is not always sure, and in the last three months, when the abdominal tumor is large and the element of infection more prominent.   It is wise to restrict the practice to the intervening months, or, better, advise against it entirely.

Parvin devotes some space to this subject, and refers to the distaste of coitus in the wife as one of the signs of pregnancy mentioned by Susru-fa.   African tribes and other savages forbid it, the Chinese and Indians, likewise.   The Talmud forbids it conditionally.   Swift, in his terrible satire on the human race, in "Gulliver's Travels Among the Houyhnhnms," says that "this is such a degree of infamous brutality as no other sensitive creature arrives at," that is, "that the She-yahoo admits the male while she is pregnant."

The ancient Irans, Medes, and Persians punished the man heavily for such an act; he received 2000 lashes and was compelled to carry 3000 loads of heavy and light wood to the fire, sacrifice 1000 small animals, kill 1000 snakes, 1000 land lizards, 2000 water lizards, and 3000 ants, and build 30 bridges over flowing water (Ploss).

Bathing.—Cold and hot baths, Turkish and Russian, hot sitz-baths, and ocean bathing are to be avoided, because of the danger of exciting uterine contractions. Tepid baths, with cool spongings, may be taken freely.   They aid the kidneys in the work of excretion and preserve the person from odor.   During pregnancy the skin secretes more.   Sea-salt baths at home are good, but if the patient feels exhausted afterward, they are to be stopped.   A light general massage after the bath is very grateful to the patient.   For the profuse sweating which is sometimes an annoying symptom, a bath followed by a brisk rub with a "salt towel" is useful.   A "salt towel" is made by wringing a bath-towel out of a strong brine and drying it.

Among the poor there is a notion that bathing during pregnancy is dangerous. Is it possible that old experience discovered some harm in it?   We know that the full tub-bath, during or near labor, may cause infection, through the polluted water gaining entrance to the vagina.   Therefore the author advises his patients, in the latter weeks of pregnancy and in labor, to employ only the standing shower.

Vaginal douches, unless indicated are not used.   Only mild antiseptics may be employed, tepid, and given under low pressure, 12 to 18 inches.   One of the best medicaments is potassium permanganate, gr. v ad Oij.   Gonorrhea must be treated thoroughly to avoid conjunctivitis in the newborn and puerperal accidents in the mother.   After the eighth month no douches by the patient herself.

Mental Occupation.—Most women have sufficient to do in their household, and the question of an especial obstetric literature does not come up.   Occasionally the accoucheur will be asked to recommend a book on the subject of the care of the mother during pregnancy.   There are many on the market, some of the best being those by Brodhead and Slemons on Maternity.   The author questions the wisdom of giving gravidæ books which describe the anatomy and physiology of the function.   She should be advised to avoid them.

Some women believe that, by reading fine literature, the child will be intellectual, by studying music, musical, by practising the arts, artistic.   Since these enjoyments do no harm, but rather keep the mind away from injurious thoughts, the woman may be humored in the idea, though the physician may express a gentle disbelief in the notion.   This brings us to the subject of—

Maternal Impressions.—By this term is meant those impressions on the mind or body of the child in utero which result from a similar impression on the mind or body of the mother.   The belief that if a pregnant woman should see an ugly or terrifying object it would be reproduced in the offspring dates from remotest antiquity, and is spread all over the world, even in darkest Africa. The Biblical story of Jacob and the "speckled and spotted kine" proves its existence in the civilized, and the practices of the savages in many parts of the world show that the notion existed among the uncivilized, peoples for ages (Ploss). Novelists (Goethe, Scott, Dickens, O. W. Holmes, Shakespeare, Sterne, Hawthorne) have used the idea as a pet theme, and many names great in medicine and allied sciences could be quoted in its support. A few are Van Swieten, Boerhaeve, Morgagni, Rokitansky, Burdach, Stoltz, Liebrecht, Delassus, Monteggia, Montgomery, Tyler Smith, Fordyce Barker, Busey, Parvin, Goodell, Penrose, King, Davis, and Edgar. Nevertheless, most of the later writers, particularly the teratologists, call the belief a superstition, absurd and harmful. Blondel (London, 1727) fought against the theory. It must be admitted that the belief in the effect of the mother's mental state on the infant cannot be proved by appeal to physical laws, but we cannot always prove our medical beliefs in this way. We admit the influences of heredity, which we cannot as yet explain.

The arguments against the theory are, first, there is no nervous connection between the mother and the fetus. Virchow himself could find none. Kölliker found nerves in the umbilical cord, and Fedotoff in the placental vessels, but no connection was demonstrated. Second, the child is completely formed at the end of the sixth week, a time that pregnancy is usually not recognized, and in most of the cases reported the causative mental shock occurred much later in gestation. Third, all the monstrosities observed in the human are found in the lower animals, birds, fishes, even in plant life, and in much greater number. Many, many women see ugly or striking scenes during pregnancy and anxiously ask the doctor if the baby is "marked," but their fears are seldom realized. With our present scientific knowledge, the belief in the effect of the mother's mind on the *physical* well-being of the child is unfounded. How can we explain the innumerable cases, many reported by trustworthy physicians, where the deformity of the child resembled, in most striking manner, that of the alleged shocking experience of the mother? Very probably by coincidence, if pure invention be excluded.

That a violent emotion, experienced by a nursing mother, can so affect the milk that the nursling gets sick from it, even having convulsions, is a fact attested by honest observers. Bernheim claims that violent emotions can cause neuritis. That great mental excitement can produce abortion is a daily experience. A patient of the author, in her fifth month, was much frightened by fire in an adjoining dwelling and aborted. The fetus was tangled in its cord, the left leg being constricted in a hard knot. The author performed the autopsy on an otherwise healthy but macerated fetus weighing nine pounds. During a severe thunderstorm, a week previously, the mother had taken fright, the child's movements became excessively violent, and then ceased. The labor was normal. A hemorrhage in the placenta, due to circulatory disturbance in the uterus, will explain the first case, but there was no suspicion of abruptio placentæ in the second. These facts show that an impression on the mother's mind is transmitted to the uterus, but they do not explain how the destructive action on the fetus is produced. Experiments on animals have proved that fright can cause a sudden increase of the action of the suprarenal glands, the hyperepinephrinemia resulting in paralysis of peristalsis, stimulation of the heart, dilatation of the bronchioles, and stimulation of the uterus. (See Cannon.) Hemorrhages into the chorion may interfere with the nutrition of the embryo, even causing its death. Lesser degrees of interference may alter the growth of the embryo, producing a monster, since we know that the various cells of the morula are endowed with unequal resistance to external influence. Monstrosities have been produced by chemical action on segmenting eggs (see Teratology). If the emotions are not purely nervous, but partly chemical in action, would it be absurd to believe that toxins, produced by acute and chronic emotional conditions of the mother, passes through the placenta, as other chemicals do, and, exerting a selective action, as many toxins do, affected the delicate nerve-cells of the growing embryo? We know that physical, mental, temperamental, and emotional traits in either parent are transmitted to the offspring. How is the germ plasm affected in the first place, that it can carry these delicate but permanent impressions? The scope of this work does not permit going deeper into the subject, nor have our means of investigation been all tried on its solution. Perhaps modern biochemistry or serology will explain it.

The author has not seen, in the many cases of supposed maternal impression reported to him, even a plausible connection between the nervous shock and the deformity of the child, and has not the least ground for believing that such a teratogenic connection could exist. Nor have his ordinary observations discovered any relation between the mind of the mother and the babe that could not be explained by the laws of heredity as we at present understand them, but that such an influence may go from one to the other should not be ruled out as absurd and indiscussable.

When the gravida asks the question, "Could anything I have done or seen affect my baby?" a question that is so often put in great trepidation by the expectant mother, the physician can conscientiously answer, "No, in the present state of our scientific knowledge there is no basis for such fears." He can say, too, that a quiet, well-ordered mind conduces to a normal pregnancy and healthy offspring, which Plato, in the Seventh Book of Laws, recommended.

Care of the Breasts.—The breasts require care even from early infancy. The number of women unable to nurse their babies is enormous, and the evil effects are noticeable in our infant mortality tables. The number of women able but unwilling to nurse is small and growing smaller every year. It is a great misfortune if a woman cannot nurse her infant. The prevention of mastitis neonatorum has already been mentioned. Especially in the growing girl do the mammæ and nipples need care, and when they develop at puberty, provision for this growth by proper dress should be made. Pressure and injury must be avoided.

Some women, during pregnancy, require a form of bust supporter to hold up the large, heavy, pendent breasts. This supporter often forms a part of the "maternity waist." During her bath the patient exercises care not to hurt the glands. The fine, branny scales which accumulate on the nipple, if allowed to remain, form moist crusts and lead to cracks, fissures, blisters, and infection. The nipples should be washed frequently with a good soap, dried, and anointed with solid albolene, cocoa-butter, or any sterile fat. In blonds, red-haired women, and others with tender nipples a lotion that is very slightly astringent may be used:

R. Glycerite of tannin................................15
Spir. lavandulæ comp. 30
Aquæ destil.....................................80

After this has dried in, the nipples are to be anointed with the unguent. No strongly astringent washes or alcohol may be used. They harden the nipple, which then cracks under the sucking efforts of the child. The skin of the nipple must be made soft and pliable.

Inverted nipples (an atavistic reversion to an embryonal type) can seldom be improved by treatment. If the nipple is undeveloped, or pressed in by improper dress, gentle attempts may be made to draw it out with the fingers during the last six weeks of pregnancy.

Preservation of the Figure.—Naturally and properly, women are desirous that the function of child-bearing should not leave the person in an ungainly shape—for example, with protuberant abdomen. The most common complaint is that the patient develops a "high stomach" after labor.

It may be remembered that the Roman women had abortions performed so that they need not suffer the disfigurement produced by child-bearing. Certain changes in the body are the necessary consequences of childbirth, and beautify the figure, although some women do not look at it in this light. Such are the rounding of the hips, broadening of the bust, the more mature and matronly appearance. It is natural for some women to put on fat after delivery, and nothing done before, during, or after confinement will prevent it. An excessive accumulation is, however, amenable to the usual treatment for obesity.

For the prevention of "high stomach" or extreme prominence of the lower abdomen much may be done. The condition is caused by weakness of the abdominal muscles, or even by a separation of the recti muscles—when the woman is said to have a "rupture." As the result of either, the intestines fill with gas and fall forward; sometimes the kidneys become movable, or even the liver descends. The muscles give way under the stretching produced by the growing uterus, and, of course, will give away sooner if there are twins or an unusually large child, or if the walls are weak, as occurs in the "status hypoplasticus." If corsets are worn during pregnancy, they add to the strain on the lower abdomen, and thus favor muscular weakness. High-heeled shoes are another factor. Overstraining during labor and inattention to the bowels after labor are also causative. To prevent the muscular insufficiency, one must begin with the girl. She should develop herself as does the boy, with active sports—rowing, swimming, climbing, etc. The abdomen may need some support during the last three months of pregnancy, especially in multiparæ with already weakened walls or with twins, polyhydramnios, etc. After the birth of the child the nurse should see that the bowels are regularly emptied and that gas does not accumulate in the intestines. The binder, after labor, does not prevent "high stomach," and while the writer recommends it (see Treatment of the Puerperium), the most benefit obtained from it is when the patient first leaves the bed. To bring the abdominal walls back to their original tonus after delivery bed exercises are prescribed.

To prevent the overstretching of the skin and the formation of the lineæ or striæ gravidarum, our efforts are not very successful, but the writer recommends skin massage with albolene or fat. Several such remedies are much vaunted in newspaper advertisements.

General Instructions.—In general, the obstetric case is to be treated as a major surgical case. The woman is requested to report any symptom that annoys her, especially headache, disturbances of sight or sensation, edema of the extremities, bleeding from any part of the body, constipation, diminished urine, nausea, vomiting, excessive loss, or excessive gain in weight. Women complain that their accoucheurs do not take enough interest in them—a charge which is true.

PRENATAL CARE

The special attention given pregnant women has become a well-rounded system of treatment, to which has been given the title, Prenatal Care. While many physicians appreciate the importance of constant supervision of even the healthy pregnant woman, and, too, the public is slowly waking up to the necessity of such supervision, prenatal care has not yet become established practice with all doctors doing obstetrics. Yet there is no field in preventive medicine that offers the prospect of such glittering returns in saving human life and misery.

It is safe to say that 25,000 women die annually in the United States from the immediate and remote effects of childbirth. Statistics also show that 85,000 babies are born dead, and another 100,000 die within a few weeks after birth—these also, each and every year!

The invalidism and wretchedness of the mothers who are injured during labor, and the numbers of the babies who suffered damage, cerebral and other, during this process which should be normal, are alike indeterminable and uncountable, but every observant accoucheur knows both are enormous.

It is also safe to say that at least one-half of the mothers and babies could be saved by proper obstetric care before and during labor, and that the major part of the invalidism and wretchedness could likewise be prevented. That proper prenatal supervision helps to accomplish these purposes is a reasonable assumption and has been proved by the experience of every prenatal clinic.

Briefly, the objects of prenatal care are to so conduct the mother and baby through pregnancy that both are healthy and strong at the end, and ready for the ordeal of labor, with the assurance of a successful delivery, a living child, and a prompt recovery of the mother, while the new individual is given a good start toward healthy citizenship.

All that has been previously said in this chapter really has this object; but if one bends his mind to the matter, one will agree with Ballantyne that there exists here a scientific field still sparsely settled, very vast, and intensely alluring.

We first determine if the woman is fit for the ordeal of pregnancy and labor, searching particularly for heart and lung diseases and for factors which may influence the mechanism of labor, e. g., contracted pelvis, neoplasms, overgrowth of the fetus, etc. We seek to discover and counteract the effects on the fetus of syphilis, tuberculosis, hemophilia, alcoholism, and other chemical poisons, lead, arsenic, phosphorus, tobacco, etc. We seek to discern the causes of abortion and premature labor and to avoid them; also to learn to cure those diseases which necessitate the artificial interruption of pregnancy—for example, hyperemesis, chorea, placenta prævia, etc. We seek to trace the occurrence of fetal monstrosities, but have not advanced at all in this direction, even in the cases of those women who have such hereditary disposition.

We watch the woman carefully throughout gestation, early to discover those complications which, neglected, may cause her death or that of her child, especially eclampsia, nephritis, placenta prævia, and we treat the minor disturbances that so often make her life miserable.

We instruct the gravida in the hygiene of her state and regulate her mode of life so that her system can make proper adjustments to the new conditions, and we groom her for her approaching ordeal as a trainer does an athlete for a test of strength. We fortify her mind as well as her body. We decide what the course of the labor is likely to be and lay out the treatment in advance, e. g., we induce labor, arrange for an elective cesarean section, or determine upon watchful expectancy.

Finally, we prepare for the labor as we do for a surgical operation.

To do all this requires a great deal of time. A busy practitioner will delegate much of the routine to an assistant or to the office nurse, while the instructions may be conveyed by means of a booklet, which also contains answers to most of the questions a gravida is likely to ask.

The First Visit.—Upon the first visit of the prospective mother the diagnosis of pregnancy must be made, which is not always easy. When the physician is engaged for the delivery he starts the system of prenatal care by filling out the antepartum sheet.

The family history of obstetric accidents, eclampsia, hemorrhage, contracted pelvis, twins, may shed light on obscure possibilities, and Bright's disease, tuberculosis, or insanity in a parent may give some idea of what to expect in the daughter.

Next comes a recital of previous diseases, of the heart, lungs, or kidneys; of accidents or operations; of special predispositions—e. g., hemorrhage, infection, mental imbalance, adiposity, etc. Now follows the menstrual and the highly significant obstetric history. The nature of previous pregnancies, labors, and puerperiums should be elicited, searching carefully for the exact cause of the dystocia and its effects (lacerations, etc.), also recording the sex and weight of the babies, with, if they died, the reasons as fully as possible. By very tactful questioning venereal disease may be discovered.

Usually the vaginal examination precedes the general physical. Besides diagnosing the pregnancy the accoucheur determines the presence or absence of neoplasms, inflammatory masses, etc., and it is good to measure the pelvis also at this time. He must make sure that the woman is pregnant to spare himself mortifying surprises, and he may discover a contracted pelvis, an extra-uterine pregnancy, an ovarian tumor, or other condition which may be removed at this time safely for the patient, while if left for chance discovery, the favorable period may have passed by. In suspicious cases smears are taken of the vaginal and cervical mucus for microscopic study; gonorrhea, spirochetes, trichomonads.

The general physical examination (which the author often delegates to an internist) lays especial stress on the heart and lungs and includes the blood-pressure (usually slightly lowered during pregnancy), urinalysis, blood-count and hemoglobin estimation, the temperature, weight, and routinely a Wassermann.

The patient is now given general instructions regarding diet, exercise, future consultations, etc. (here the booklet serving its useful purpose), and special advice and medicines, if necessary for her particular case. The date of confinement is predicted and the domestic arrangements agreed upon, including the selection of a nurse.

The Routine Pregnancy Visit.—Every three weeks up to the seventh month and every two weeks thereafter the gravida appears for examination. It is best, though not always practicable, for her to send the urine midway between two visits and thus the accoucheur obtains knowledge of her condition twice as often. At each visit the blood-pressure, the temperature, pulse, and weight are taken, the urinalysis studied, the patient interrogated for symptoms of complications, and appropriate advice is given. The examiner is particularly alert to discover evidences of hyperemesis, eclampsia, anemia, nephritis, abortion, placenta prævia, and the beginning of heart and lung disease. All findings are conscientiously recorded.

In the long course of the pregnancy the general physical examination may be repeated and, toward the end, the condition of the child is given more attention, particular pains being taken to estimate its size and physical development. The breasts are also studied to learn of their fitness for lactation.

Every week, at a time set apart for the purpose, the physician looks over his records and gets in touch with the individual patients. If, for example, the chart shows that no urinalysis has been made for a long time, the patient should be reminded of such a necessity.

The Prepartal Visit.—It is not wise to allow the gravida to go into labor with an abnormal presentation. Shortly before the date set for confinement (see p. 25 for the determination of this date) the accoucheur should see the woman, inquire into her general condition, and make both an abdominal and rectal examination to determine the position and presentation of the child and the degree of engagement or the presence of twins. To avoid repetition, the methods of diagnosis of presentation and position will be considered in full in the conduct of labor. The author usually repeats the measurements of the pelvis at this time because it can be done more accurately and less painfully, the soft parts offering less resistance, and, too, the pelvis often enlarges during pregnancy. One may have to revise an opinion made in the early months regarding the probable course and treatment of the case. After these points are settled the heart of the infant should be auscultated. It is possible to diagnose fetal heart disease before delivery. A question usually put to the accoucheur is one regarding the sex of the child. This cannot be told before delivery. Frankenhäuser claimed that the girl's heart was more rapid than the boy's, and I have found that if the beat is persistently below 130, a boy, and above 150, a girl, is more likely to be born, but the patient is to be advised that any prediction thus made is a pure guess.

Other means of prediction of the sex have thus far failed. Injecting strontium iodide into the liquor amnii and x-raying the fetus is done by Menees to discover the sex. While instructive it is too dangerous. Dyroff, with an interferometric test, obtained 74 per cent. successes.

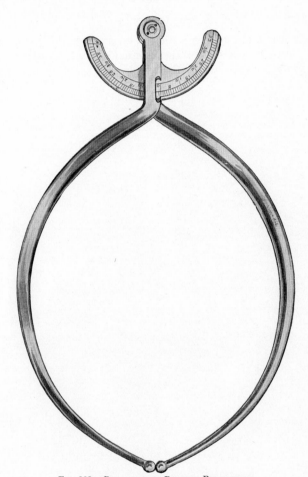

FIG. 260.—BAUDELOCQUE-BREISKY PELVIMETER.
Very slightly modified by the author.

The physician satisfies himself that the woman, as she stands on the threshold of labor, has been brought to the highest degree of mental and physical efficiency.

If the patient is to be confined at home the accoucheur selects the best room in the house for delivery, that is, the most commodious and lightest, and one that is close to the water-supply, provides for sufficient artificial light, a proper table for eventual operation, and satisfies himself that there are towels, sheets, cotton, basins, etc., all sterilized, ready for the event. (See page 265.)

At this visit the phenomena of beginning labor are explained to the patient and she is given explicit instructions as to how to call the doctor and the nurse and notify the hospital, and what physician to summon in the event of an emergency, if the regular attendant is not obtainable, also what to do should labor come on tempestuously. She is again advised not to take tub-baths, to keep the bowels very free, to limit the meat in her diet, and to drink a great deal of water. An important duty of the physician and nurse is to prepare the woman's mind for her approaching mental and physical ordeal, to which she looks forward with more anxiety than she will admit. She may be encouraged and assured that nowadays the science and art of obstetrics are so advanced that, with the prenatal care which she has enjoyed, women and babies do not die any more, and also that the suffering of labor has been largely eliminated.

PELVIMETRY

Of late years there has been a tendency to neglect pelvic mensuration. Most physicians are not skilful in taking the internal dimensions and the external ones are unreliable indices of the size of the pelvic cavity. Further, the practitioners

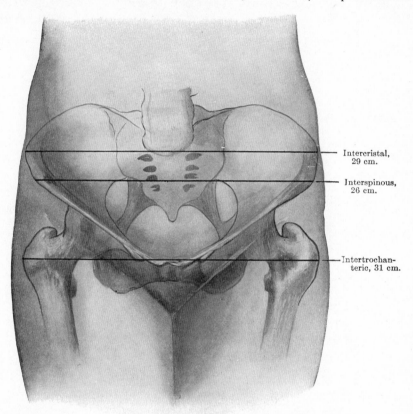

Intercristal, 29 cm.

Interspinous, 26 cm.

Intertrochanteric, 31 cm.

Fig. 261.—The External Measurements. Showing Where to Place Pelvimeter.

have got to rely on a test of labor—letting the patient have pains a certain length of time and, if the head fails to descend, they perform cesarean section. This is a blundering method of procedure, and, as we shall see later, is both unscientific and costly in human life. We should always strive to acquire as exact a knowledge as possible of the size and shape of the parturient passages.

In practice the *external measurements* are usually taken first.

1. The distance between the spines of the ilia, always taking the outer lip. The distantia spinarum iliorum, or **Sp. I. = 26 cm.**

2. The distance between the crests of the ilia, taking the outer lip, the distantia cristarum iliorum, or **Cr.I. = 29 cm.**

3. Between the great trochanters, distantia bitrochanterica, or **Bi.T.**=**31 cm.**

4. From the depression under the last lumbar spine to the anterior surface of the pubis—conjugata externa, diameter Baudelocquii, or **D.B.**=**20 cm.**

5. The circumference of the pelvis, **90 cm.**

6. The obliques, from the right posterior superior spine of the ilium to the left anterior superior, obliqua dextra, **Ob.D.** = **22 cm.**; and the corresponding oblique of the other side, **Ob.L.**=**21½ cm.**

The author takes the obliques only in cases where there is scoliosis and other evidence of pelvic asymmetry. Fig. 262 illustrates the manner of taking the external diameters. Baudelocque's diameter is best obtained when the patient is

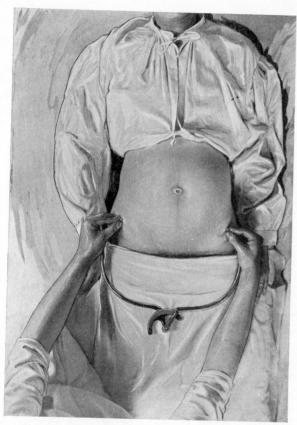

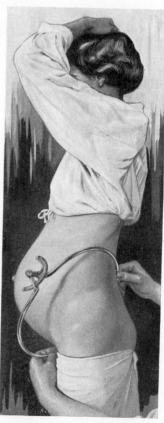

Fig. 262.—Taking Interspinous Diameter.

Fig. 263.—Taking Baudelocque's Diameter.

erect, as in Fig. 263, but one can get it with the patient lying on the side, with the upper leg straight, the lower drawn well up against the belly. The posterior branch of the pelvimeter is placed in the dimple under the last lumbar spine. This point is one inch above a line drawn between the two posterior superior spines. On the posterior aspect of the pelvis, in well-formed women, is a diamond-shaped depression formed by the dimples of the posterior superior spines of the ilia, the lines formed by the gluteal muscles and the groove at the end of the spine. It is called the rhomboid of Michaëlis, and is seen on beautiful statues—for example, the Capitoline Venus (Fig. 264). The point for the calipers is near the apex of the rhomboid. Variations in the shape and size of this landmark give us valuable information in deformed pelves. Anteriorly, the knob of the pelvimeter comes to rest on the most prominent portion of the bony pubis. It is wise to take Baudelocque's diameter three times and use the average of the three measurements.

The circumference is taken with the tape lying between the crests of the ilia and the trochanters on each side, and in a plane perpendicular to the long axis of the body. Naturally, in fat women the circumference does not give valuable information. Indeed, the value of the external measurements is but relative. Only marked deviations from the normal indicate a contraction of the pelvis, and one must rely on the internal examination for more positive information.

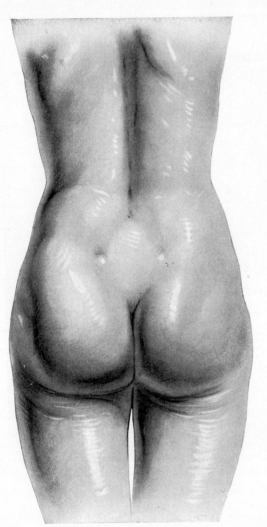

FIG. 264.—RHOMBOID OF MICHAËLIS.

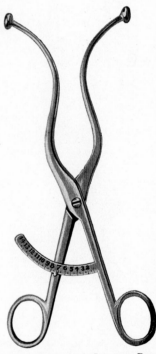

FIG. 265.—DELEE'S INTERNAL PELVIMETER.

Baudelocque believed that, by deducting 8 cm. from the external conjugate, the length of the vera could be obtained. This is not true, because the thickness of the bones and their conformation, produce differences of even $5\frac{1}{2}$ cm. (Skutsch and Goenner). The author possesses a pelvis with an external conjugate of 18 cm. and a C.V. of 14 cm., and another with an external conjugate of 21 cm. and a C.V. of $9\frac{1}{2}$ cm. If a woman has a conjugata externa of less than 18 cm., the probabilities are strong that the inlet is also narrowed.

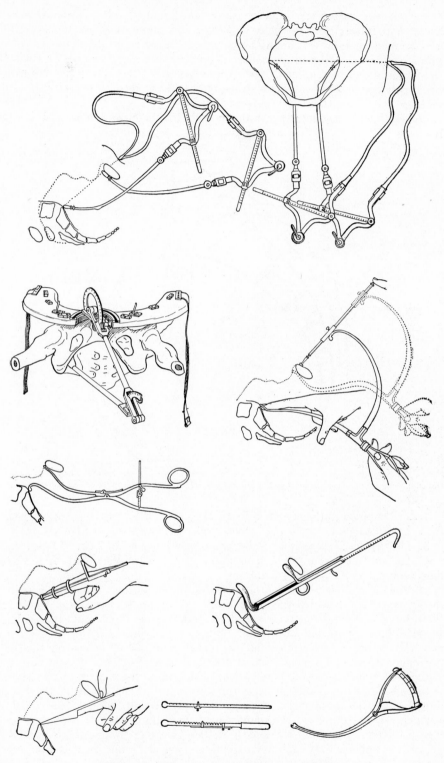

FIG. 266.—A FEW OF THE MANY INTERNAL PELVIMETERS.
Copied from Skutsch.

For the same reason the other measurements are unreliable.   The author has a
pelvis with an intercristous diameter of 21 cm. and an internal transverse of 13½
cm.   The relation between the interspinous and intercristous diameters is of more
importance, for when the interspinous diameter is equal to, or greater than, the
intercristous, we suspect a flat pelvis.   (See Chapter LIV.)   The author insists on
internal pelvimetry in all cases, excepting only those women who have had one or
more large children without the slightest difficulty.

The internal measurements are taken with the hand and a special internal
pelvimeter (Fig. 265).   These are essential:

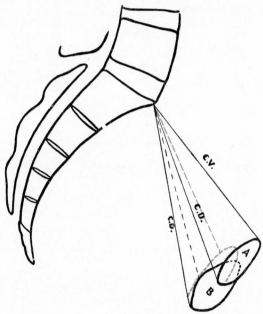

Fig. 267.—Diagram to Show the Effect of a High Pubis on the Length of the C.D.
Dotted line shows shortening due to a thick pubis or exostosis.   Red line shows effect of long pubic symphysis.

1. The conjugata diagonalis, **C.D.** = 12½ cm.   **C.V.** = 10¾ to 11¼ cm.
2. The distance between the spines of the ischia, bispinous, **Bi-sp.** = 11.
3. The distance between the tuberosities of the ischia, **Bi-isch.** = 11 cm.
4. The distance from the end of the sacrum to the ligamentum arcuatum
pubis; sacropubic, **S.P.** = 11½ cm.

Of the scores of instrumental methods of measuring the conjugata vera
directly, since the first by the elder Stein (1772) up to the latest by Biliçky
(1909), not one has proved practical (Fig. 266) because their application is painful and difficult, requiring anesthesia.   When used properly a few give accurate
results, but at present we still obtain our best information by measuring the conjugata diagonalis and deducing from it the length of the C.V.   Even though we
can measure the height of the pubis, and thus know the length of two sides of
the triangle, it is impossible to learn the arc of any of the angles of the triangle
subtended by the symphysis.   Trigonometry, therefore, cannot help here—we
must depend on estimates.   Examination of large numbers of pelves shows that
if one deducts 1½ cm. from the length of the C.D., one obtains the length of the
C.V.   If the pubis is very high, 6 cm. or more (Fig. 267), one must deduct 2 or 2½
cm.   If the upper border of the pubis inclines more than usual toward the sacrum
or is very thick, or if there is an exostosis of the posterior surface of the symphysis,

both of which last occur in rachitic pelves, 2 or even 3 cm. may have to be deducted from the length of the C.D. (Fig. 268).

The transverse diameter of the pelvis decreases from above downward. At the level of the inlet it measures 12 to 15 cm.; in the region of the spines, 11 cm.; anterior to the spines, 11½ to 12 cm.; at the outlet, between the tuberosities, 11 cm. In practice, it is only exceptionally possible to measure the transverse of the inlet directly. When labor has been in progress for a time, the vagina becomes so soft and distensible that one can spread the branches of the internal pelvimeter, pictured in Fig. 265, until they touch both sides of the pelvis, enabling one to read off the measurement on the scale with mathematical accuracy. Late in pregnancy it is easy with this instrument to measure the distance between the spines of the ischia. The distance between the tuberosities is not so easily gotten, because of the thick padding of fat over these bones. One must add 1 to 2 cm. to the measure-

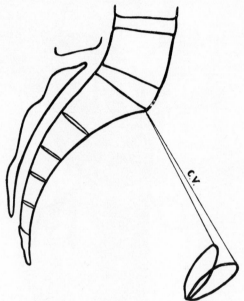

Fig. 268.—Diagram Showing Effect of Increased Inclination of Pubis on Length of C.V.

ment obtained with the pelvimeter. While the external measurements give only equivocal information, considerable dependence may be placed on internal mensuration, and this will increase with added experience.

Technic of the Internal Examination.—During the early part of the eighth month is the most favorable time for pelvic mensuration in general practice. During labor one may have the advantage of anesthesia. The patient must lie across the bed or on a table, with the hips hanging well over the edge, to enable the examiner to sink his elbow. Her person must be draped with a sheet, but the genitalia are to be exposed. For examination, at this period, the genitals need not be shaved, but they should be washed with water and soap, following this with a liberal use of antiseptic solution, 1 : 1500 bichlorid or 1 per cent. lysol. Sterile rubber gloves are to be worn. The internal pelvimeter is sterilized by boiling in a 1 per cent. soda or borax solution. On inspecting the vulva, one will note any suspicious discharge, abscess, varicose veins, the extent of previous lacerations, etc., after which two fingers are inserted between the widely separated labia, deeply into the vagina. It is well to study, in each case, the topography of the levator ani,

17

which can be easily done by pressing the fingers down on either side of the vagina. In a primipara the muscle is broad, sling-like, and on contraction powerfully crowds the fingers against the pubic arch. In a multipara the introitus is open, the levator ani is represented by two thick pillars at the sides of the vagina, which, upon contracting, do not crowd the fingers so tightly against the pubis. The condition of the vagina is noted. If there is a granular condition of the mucous membrane which might suggest gonorrhea, a smear should be taken with a view of

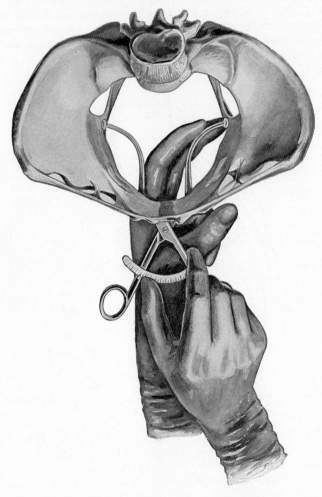

FIG. 269.—TAKING DISTANCE BETWEEN SPINES.

preventing ophthalmia neonatorum and sepsis postpartum. Next, the cervix is studied to learn whether it is long, tapir-nose-like, or short and broad; whether patulous, as in multiparæ, or closed; whether normal, smooth, and soft, or diseased, thick, knobby (ovula Nabothi), catarrhally inflamed, or eroded. Then the lower part of the uterus is palpated and the presence of the head determined, at the same time discovering any tumor which may block its entrance into the pelvis. The fingers now pass around the bony walls of the pelvis to obtain a mind picture of the capacity and configuration of the excavation. It requires years of practice for the accoucheur to be able to form correct mind pictures of these things, but they must be learned.   The height of the pubis, its inclination into the inlet, the presence of an exostosis on its posterior surface, the curve of the rami pubis, the height of the

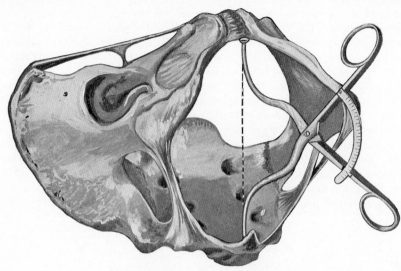

FIG. 270.—DIRECT MEASUREMENT OF ANTEROPOSTERIOR DIAMETER OF OUTLET.
Possible only at term.   Anesthetic usually necessary.

sacrum, the shape of the sacrum, the movability and shape of the coccyx are determined in the order mentioned.   Next the bispinous diameter is taken with the

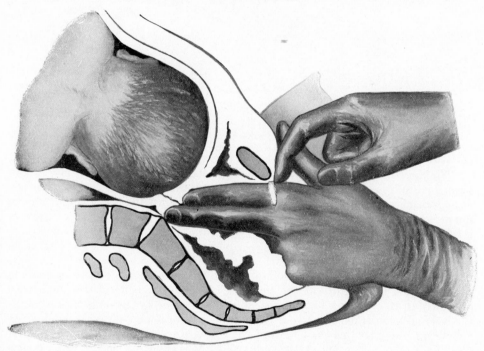

FIG. 271.—TAKING THE CONJUGATA DIAGONALIS.

pelvimeter.   The instrument is closed and passed, with the scale upward, along the finger until it has passed the grip of the levator ani, then the blades are spread until one knob comes to rest on, or just in front of, the spine of the ischium (Fig. 269).   Being assured that the patient's hips are horizontal, the blades are spread in the horizontal plane until they are arrested by the bony walls of the pelvis, and at this instant the amount of separation is read off the scale.   This measurement will cause little pain if the vagina is soft and dilatable (which is usual at this time), and if the examiner proceeds slowly and gently.   If the vagina is diseased, it is more tender.   Under no circumstances may force be used, as a tear of the vagina might occur.   If the blades easily spread to 10 cm. and there seems to be room beyond, it is not necessary to insist on the full measurement.   In a contracted pelvis it is easier to obtain the distance.   To take the sacropubic diameter from the inside is not always possible without anesthesia, and less often in primiparæ in whom the perineum rises high.   Fig. 270 shows how it is done.   One knob is steadied by the outside hand against the ligamentum arcuatum at the side of the clitoris, while the other knob is pressed against the end of the sacrum, being guided into place by the fingers in the vagina.   One may measure the sacropubic diameter with the fingers in the same manner as one obtains the diagonal conjugate.   Now the instrument is removed and the examiner takes the conjugata diagonalis (Figs. 271 and 272).

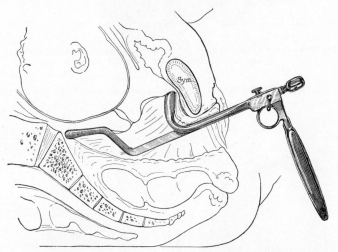

Fig. 272.—Measuring the Conjugata Vera with the Bilicky-Gauss Pelvimeter.

Sinking the elbow and resting it against the knee, the examiner gently, but with force, presses the middle finger-tip against the promontory of the sacrum. It may be necessary to keep up a steady pressure against the perineum for several minutes before the rigid muscles will relax.   As soon as the tip of the promontory is felt, the hand is raised against the ligamentum arcuatum.   A bit of cotton carried on the index of the other hand is now pushed along the index of the examining hand until it rests at the point where the examining hand is touched by the ligamentum arcuatum.   After making sure that the middle finger-tip was actually resting on the promontory at the time the bit of cotton reached the under edge of the pubis, the cotton is carefully steadied in its place by the outside hand while the internal hand is removed from the vagina.   With a tape-measure or any pelvimeter one now obtains the length of the conjugata diagonalis (Fig. 273).   After guessing at the inclination of the pubis and allowing for its height, one deducts $1\frac{1}{2}$ or 2 or more cm., and thus approximates the length of the C.V.   Numerous fallacies underlie this reading, the compression of the finger-tip, the bending of the joints, the slipping of the finger from the promontory, errors in estimating the height, thickness, and angle of the pubis, etc.

Several methods may be practised in obtaining the bituberal or biischiatic diameter. Schröder made marks on the skin of the buttocks to show the location of the inner surface of the tuberosities and measured the separation of the marks. An assistant may measure the distance between the two thumbs so placed on the tubers that the finger-nails represent their inner surfaces. Two, three, four, or five knuckles of the hand may be pressed in between the bones, and the distance across them later measured with a tape or, simply, an ordinary wooden tongue depressor

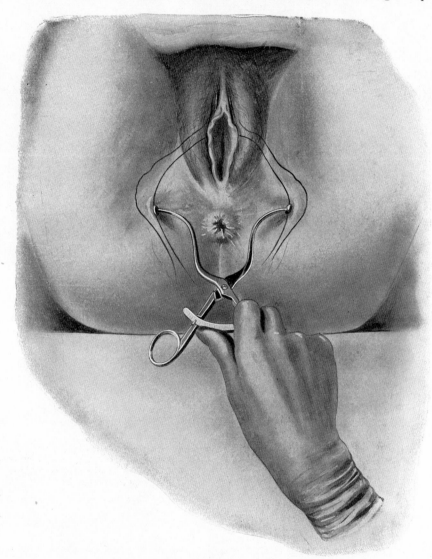

Fig. 274.—Taking Distance Between Tuberosities.

is whittled to fit between the tubers and measured (Fig. 280). Williams' pelvimeter may be used or the internal pelvimeter shown above. The closed knobs are inserted between the bones and separated until they are arrested (Fig. 274). It is necessary to press the tissues well against the bone and to add 1 to 1½ cm. to the reading for the thickness of the fat.

The posterior sagittal diameter of the outlet (see page 757) may be taken by holding the pelvimeter against a wooden tongue depressor cut to fit between the

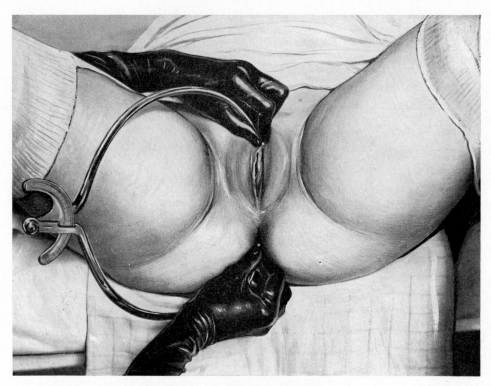

Fig. 275.—Measuring Sacropubic Diameter. Breisky's Method.
Photograph, Chicago Lying-in Hospital.

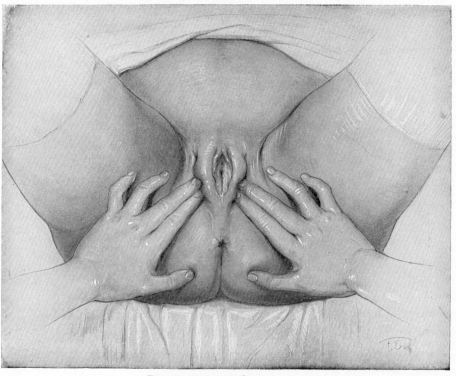

Fig. 276.—Palpating Pubic Arch.

tuberosities and subtending the distance between its middle and the tip of the sacrum (Fig. 280).

The sacropubic diameter may also be taken from the outside by Breisky's method (Fig. 275). One knob of the pelvimeter rests under the arch of the pubis,

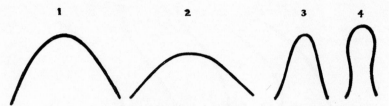

FIG. 277.—VARIOUSLY SHAPED ARCHES OBTAINED IN PRACTICE.
1, Normal. 2, Broad—as in flat pelves. 3, Narrow—as in male pelves. 4, Osteomalacic beaked pelvis.

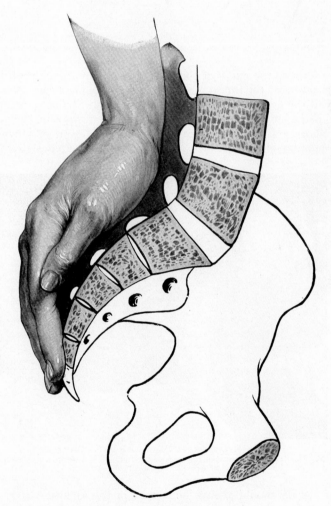

FIG. 278.—OUTLINING THE SACRUM.

the other is pressed against the sacrococcygeal joint, 1 cm. being deducted from the reading to obtain the result.

Finally, the examiner carefully palpates the accessible bony portions of the pelvis. The fingers of each hand are laid on the descending rami of the pubis and the acuteness of the angle of the arch thus easily determined (Fig. 276). Thickness of the bones, asymmetry of the two sides, a beak-shaped pubis (osteomalacia, rickets, see Chapter LIV) are thus discovered (Fig. 277). As the last maneuver, the hand is laid flat on the sacrum, the middle finger pressed firmly into the genital

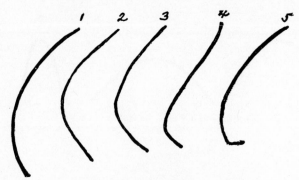

FIG. 279.—SACRAL OUTLINES.
1, Normal curve.   2, Rachitis.   3, Rachitis.   4, Rachitis.   5, Ankylosis of coccyx.

crease, to conform to the curve of the bone. On removing the fixed hand, the external configuration of the sacrum can be seen at a glance (Figs. 278 and 279).

A study of the general make-up of the gravida will tell us a great deal. Tall, muscular women seldom have contracted pelves, and, if they do, the type is usually masculine. Short, petite women may have generally contracted pelves. A woman that limps, or is hunchbacked, or has crooked legs, may have a distorted pelvis.

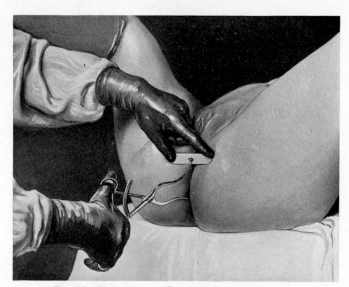

FIG. 280.—MEASURING THE POSTERIOR SAGITTAL DIAMETER.
A wooden tongue-depressor is cut to fit between the tuberosities, and the distance from its center to the end of the sacrum measured with any pelvimeter.

Evidences of rickets should always be sought in the rachitic rosary, the square, large head, enlargement of the epiphyses, bow-legs, curvature of the spine, etc.

All this information is to be carefully entered on the history sheet. If the physician conducts his examination systematically, he will not overlook any points and have the disagreeable necessity of putting the patient back on the table. On discovering anything unusual in the pelvis, soft parts, or child, the examination takes on extra interest, and special attention will have to be directed to the part. A discussion of these special subjects and the descriptions of deformed pelves will be found under the appropriate headings. A careful consideration of all the informaton obtained enables the accoucheur to make his diagnosis of the case, the prognosis of the labor, and any recommendation for treatment at this time, all of which are noted on the record. Too much emphasis cannot be laid on the importance of making a careful pelvic mensuration in pregnancy. It may discover a contracted pelvis and permit us to induce labor while the child is small, or prepare for cesarean section or other operative delivery at term. It will explain many anomalies in the mechanism of labor, and it will save many mothers' and children's lives.

Since the beginning of roentgenology attempts have been made to measure the pelvis and the fetus. Recently aided by the sitting posture and profile views and by the use of perforated plates and other devices fairly accurate results are being achieved. Bickenbach and v. Schubert in Germany, Thoms in the United States, and others have made the x-ray practical in pelvic mensuration, but the main factor in labor, the powers, only a labor itself can evaluate. An x-ray machine should form part of the equipment of every birthroom.

THE PREPARATION FOR THE ASEPTIC CONDUCT OF LABOR AT HOME

Unless the woman is to go to a maternity for delivery, the same preparations must be made at home as for a major surgical operation at home. Thousands of mothers and children die every year because of the lack of such preparation, and of the spirit that animates it. The principles of asepsis and antisepsis are not complicated nor hard to apply. They are only two: everything that is to come in contact with the puerperal wounds must be absolutely sterile; second, the external genitalia and introitus vaginæ must be thoroughly disinfected. If these two principles are deeply ingrained in the accoucheur's mind, the methods of carrying them out will suggest themselves. The ponderous and complicated system of asepsis practised in hospitals is not possible nor necessary in the home; but, on the other hand, the ideals of asepsis are not met by a basin of bichlorid solution and a roll of absorbent cotton.

LIST OF ARTICLES NEEDED FOR LABOR

3 basins (enameled).
1 pitcher (enameled), 4 quarts.
1 pitcher (enameled), 1 quart.
1 Perfection bed-pan.
1 fountain syringe (new), 2 quarts.
1 hot-water bag.
2 pieces rubber sheeting, 1 piece large enough to protect mattress, 1 piece 1 yard square.
1 medicine-dropper.
1 medicine glass.
2 bent glass drinking tubes.
8 ounces lysol.
1 bottle bichlorid of mercury tablets.
8 ounces tincture of green soap.
2 ounces castor oil.
1 tube white vaselin.
8 ounces alcohol.
1 ounce fluidextract of ergot.
4 ounces benzoinated lard or albolene.
1 rubber catheter, No. 14 French scale.

The following are used for making pads, sponges, applicators, etc.:
6 pounds absorbent cotton.
1 bolt of gauze.
10 yards unbleached muslin.
100 vulva pads.
1 accouchement pad, 1 yard square.
200 applicators.
18 cord dressings.
1 skein linen bobbin, ⅛ inch.
1 pair white stockings, long.
4 breast binders.
3 night gowns (short).
4 quilted pads, 2 feet square.
4 sheets.
18 towels (without fringe).
4 Mason jars, 4 jelly glasses (with covers).
Bundle of newspapers.
All the soft white rags the patient can gather.
Receiver for baby.

A list of the utensils (a copy of the author's being reproduced herewith)—dressings, cottons, brushes, etc.—needful for confinement is to be supplied each patient, with instructions how to prepare same, so that, when the time comes, everything is in readiness for an aseptic and correct accouchement. The nurse engaged for the case, three weeks before the day set for labor, goes to the patient's home and sterilizes a supply of towels, sheets, cotton sponges, gauze, umbilical pads, vulvar pads, and binders. The woman herself may be instructed in these matters. In the cities there are nurses who make a specialty of such preparations. Maternity outfits containing all the needed utensils, gauzes, dressings, pads, sheets, towels, etc., already sterilized, and neatly packed in sealed containers, are sold by surgical supply houses. Among the poorer classes the physician may have to carry everything necessary for an aseptic labor with him.

The basins, brushes, and douche-bag are carefully sterilized in dust-proof bags. One pound of the cotton is made into pledgets or sponges of convenient size, packed into glass jars, and sterilized. The other pound is made into large vulvar pads, covered with gauze. These are sterilized in packages of six. The newspapers are sterilized by steam with the pledgets and pads, or by baking in the oven, and serve many purposes—for example, to wrap up basins, towels, sheets, Mason jars, etc., that have been sterilized before labor, to place under the patient during labor, and to lay on tables and chairs to avoid marring them. A sterile newspaper wrapped in a sterile towel makes a good bed-pad during delivery. After everything has been sterilized, the packages are labeled and put away in a clean drawer or trunk. At the time of labor the accoucheur finds things all prepared and ready, a most comforting feeling. Well prepared is half the battle.

RULES FOR PREGNANT WOMEN

(This set of rules is printed on the reverse side of the slip giving the list of articles needed for labor.)

1. Consult your physician as soon as you believe pregnancy probable.
2. Dress warmly. Avoid circular constriction at any part of the body. As soon as the child's motion is felt lay off corsets; wear a maternity waist with breast supporter.
3. Take plenty of mild exercise in the open air and sunlight, especially walking, stopping short of fatigue. Avoid violent motions, golf, tennis, swimming, long trolley or automobile rides, etc. Traveling is permitted only when really necessary.
4. Take no hot nor cold baths, only tepid, with cool sponging. In the last three weeks before delivery, no tub baths; use the shower and sponging. Take no douches, unless ordered, and, especially in the last month, allow nothing to touch the internal genitalia.
5. Intercourse should be avoided if possible, always restricted, and absolutely forbidden during the last six weeks.
6. The bowels must move every day.
7. Eat your usual amount of food, restricting the meats or their equivalent, fish and eggs, to 4 ounces a day. Drink freely of water, milk, or buttermilk. No alcoholics. During the last six weeks reduce the diet generally, and especially the sweets and fats. Eat fresh vegetables.
8. Keep the breasts free from pressure. Bathe the nipples once a week with tincture of green soap, and anoint them daily with sterilized albolene.
9. Send a 4-ounce specimen of the morning urine for examination every three weeks; after the seventh month, every two weeks. Once every week measure the amount of urine passed in twenty-four hours. It should be 3 pints or more.
10. The blood-pressure should be taken every three weeks up to the seventh month, and every two weeks thereafter. Send the urine one week and appear for the blood-pressure reading the following week.
11. Report to your physician when you are troubled with nausea, vomiting, headache, swelling of the feet or eyelids, or other abnormal symptoms. Report also any marked reduction in the amount of urine and if there is hemorrhage from any part of the body.
12. Go without corsets as much as possible. Sleep on alternate sides. Daily, in the last two months, knead the abdomen very gently for a few minutes to relieve the baby from a cramped position.
13. If you are in need of advice during my absence, summon my Assistant, Dr.................................Telephone....................................... who will, if necessary, call my Associate, Dr.. Telephone..........................., or Dr.. Telephone..........................
14. At the first consultation a careful examination must be made, and near term, another.
15. When labor-pains begin, or if the waters break, or if the show of blood-stained mucus appears, go to the hospital, call your nurse, and notify the accoucheur.
16. Six to eight weeks after delivery come to the office for examination, to determine if the womb is in place and if there has been any excessive injury to the parts.
17. One year after the baby is born return with the baby for the "follow up" examination.
(The Author's "Booklet for Mothers," obtainable upon request, has supplanted this leaflet.)

The Engagement of the Nurse.—An accoucheur's success in obstetrics depends largely on the nurse. A careless nurse can undo his best work. After the diagnosis of the time of labor is made, the nurse is engaged and holds herself in readiness for a call at that time. The physician should select the nurse and, to avoid mistakes and meddlesome, though well-intentioned interference on her part, should provide a list of printed instructions regarding the care of the mother and babe during labor and puerperium. The author refers his nurses to a book written by him, "Obstetrics for Nurses," and thus avoids a great deal of detailed explanation.

INSTRUCTIONS FOR THE OBSTETRIC NURSE

Pregnancy.—Two to three weeks before the date of expected labor visit the patient and prepare the materials needed for confinement. See that everything on the list of articles needed (p. 265) is at hand.

Basins, bed-pan, brushes, douche-bag, and all utensils are carefully sterilized by steam; the Kelly pad, by soap and water and soaking in 1:1000 bichlorid for three hours; the douche-bag is to be boiled.

Prepare one dozen towels, three sheets, two pairs very long stockings, or special leggings, two pillow-cases, two night-gowns, two physician's gowns, two quart Mason jars of gauze sponges, two quart Mason jars of cotton sponges, two pads of cotton covered with gauze, one yard square, one receiver, and sufficient vulvar pads and umbilical cord dressings for the mother and babe during the puerperium. These are all packed in appropriately sized bundles, securely covered with towels or newspapers, distinctly labeled, then sterilized. All these things are carefully laid away, protected from dust, for the time of labor.

Instruct the patient how to determine when labor is at hand, and what to do until you or the doctor arrives.

During Labor.—When you are called, see that the accoucheur is at once notified.

See that there is a supply of hot and cold sterile water.

Prepare the patient as follows: Give colonic flushing of warm soapsuds; shave genitalia; full shower-bath; scrub torso with soap and water, paying special attention to the genitalia; rinse and wash thoroughly from ensiform to knees with 1 : 1500 bichlorid. Put on sterile night-gown.

Do not examine the patient internally nor give vaginal douches without permission.

Learn how to make rectal examinations and thus be able to report the progress of the labor.

Keep an accurate record of pulse, temperature, and all the occurrences during labor and the puerperium. Listen to fetal heart tones at least every thirty minutes and note.

See that the patient takes light nourishment during the first stage.

Provide quiet, cheer, and fresh air for the patient. Allow no gossip.

See that the bladder is emptied every four and the rectum every twelve hours, asking the accoucheur for orders regarding them.

When the second stage draws near, dress the bed and the patient with the sterile articles.

Be ready to assist the accoucheur in caring for the feces which may escape from the anus (basin of 1 : 1500 bichlorid and large cotton sponges).

Have sterile scissors, tape, and artery clamp ready for the cord, and gauze pledgets for wiping the eyelids and throat. Antiseptic for the eyes. Sterile catheter.

As soon as the child is severed, wrap it warmly in the receiver and put in a warm, safe place. Look at it occasionally for hemorrhage from the cord or choking.

Receive the placenta in a basin covered with a sterile towel, and be sure to present it to the accoucheur for his inspection.

During the Puerperium.—Treat the genitalia as an open surgical wound. Change the pads when soiled, douching the external genitals with 1 : 3000 bichlorid each time. Give no vaginal douches without orders. See that the patient urinates within eight hours after delivery.

Give her one ounce of castor oil on the morning of the second day after delivery. Get further instructions from the accoucheur.

Support the breasts and abdomen with light binders.

Report to the accoucheur sleeplessness, temperature above 99.5° F., pulse over 100, headache, hemorrhage, severe after-pains, abdominal distention or pain, dysuria, fetid or abnormal lochia, infected perineum, cracked nipples, engorged breasts, and anything unusual.

The diet is to be liquid for twelve hours, then light.

Take temperature, pulse, and respiration at 7 A. M., 4 and 9 P. M.

Consult the accoucheur regarding the time to get patient out of bed.

Care of Child.—See that the eyes are cared for according to the accoucheur's practice. Anoint the child with benzoinated lard, rub all off, then disinfect the cord with alcohol and dress with dry sterile gauze. Change only when soiled.

Wash eyelids and nostrils once daily with extreme gentleness. A half-bath daily or an oil rub until navel is cicatrized, then a full bath.

Take temperature and pulse A. M. and P. M. Weigh daily. Record everything.

Give 10 drops of castor oil on morning of second day.

Let infant nurse every four hours unless otherwise instructed, beginning at 7 A. M. Let nurse once after 10 P. M. until one week old, then train to sleep the night through.

Report to the accoucheur temperature above 99.5° F., absence of bowel movements or urine, convulsions or nervous symptoms, vomiting, redness of eyes or navel, hemorrhage from any place.

In general, the breasts, the genitalia, and the navel of the infant must be regarded as open wounds and treated invariably with extreme surgical cleanliness.

LITERATURE

Ballantyne: Antenatal Pathology, 1902.—*Barbaud-Le Fevre:* La Puberte, Paris, 1897.—*Cannon, W. B.:* Bodily Changes in Emotional Excitement, Appleton and Co., 1915.—*Chamberlain and Newell:* Amer. Jour. Roentgenology, May, 1921, p. 272.—*Dyroff:* Monatschr. f. Geb. u. Gyn., March and April, 1926.—*Fedotoff:* Ref. Jour. Amer. Med. Assoc., December 11, 1926.—*Forel:* The Sexual Question, 1908. What a Young Girl Should Know.—*Fry:* Maternity, 1907.—*Gellhorn:* Medical Record, August 25, 1917.—*Goenner:* Zeit. f. Geb. u. Gyn., vol. xliv.—*Parvin:* Obstetrics, 1895, pp. 219 and 225.—*Pinard:* Annales de Gyn., 1898; also June, 1915.—*Ploss:* Das Weib in der Natur and Völkerkunde, vol. i, p. 602; Das Weib, *loc. cit.*, p. 600 et seq.—*v. Mertz, v. Lüttge:* Zentb. für Gynaek., 1925, No. 9, p. 494, and idem, January 8, 1927, p. 76.—*v. Schubert:* Zentb. für Gyn., April 21, 1929.—*Sellheim:* Monatschr. f. Geb. u. Gyn., June, 1925, p. 290.—*Shukers, C. F.:* See Editorial Jour. Amer. Med. Assoc., July 2, 1932, p. 36.—*Skutsch:* Die Beckenmessung. Monograph. Gives history and illustrations of instruments, 1886.—*Surbled:* La Vie a Deux, Paris, 1901.—*Thoms:* Jour. Amer. Med. Assoc., July 5, 1930; Surg., Gyn., and Obstet., May, 1931.

CHAPTER XVIII

THE DIAGNOSIS OF PREGNANCY

CERTAINTY in the diagnosis of pregnancy cannot always be attained, but a high degree of probability can be reached. This most common condition, which any matron thinks she could diagnose with ease, may, after skilful application of all the means of investigation, assisted by long experience, and studied with a view to careful judgment, escape discovery or be mistaken for something entirely different. While we will admit that error may not always be avoided, it is also true that blunders are more often due to carelessness in making the examination, and lack of consideration of all the facts learned by it, than to ignorance. Socrates said that in studying ourselves, we should "lay aside prejudice, passion, and sloth," an axiom which could well apply to the diagnosis of pregnancy.

Sometimes the diagnosis may be made very quickly, but the accoucheur is warned to guard his statements, because the people believe the fact of pregnancy should be very patent and will discredit the physician if the event prove him wrong, and, further, much depends on his decision. The question of heritage of property, of prosecution at law of women accused of crime, of an illegitimate conception, whereby the fair name of a woman may be blasted, of legitimacy of offspring; the proper treatment of disease, as tuberculosis, cancer—all these depend on the correctness of his opinion, and mistakes are very disastrous to both mother and child.

The difficulties are greater in the first four months, before the fetus is large enough so that we can hear it or feel it, but sometimes the question of pregnancy is unsettled until the time for eventual delivery.

In uncomplicated cases, where only the question of pregnancy arises, the patient is more likely to be pronounced pregnant when really not so, but when it is to be determined whether pregnancy complicates some other pelvic condition or simulates something else, the pregnancy is more apt to be overlooked. Thus in operating for fibroids the surgeon is occasionally surprised by finding a pregnant uterus.

Sources of Error.—In the early months there is no absolute sign of pregnancy. The character of a gravid uterus can be perfectly mimicked by several other conditions. In the later months the positive signs, the fetal heart-tones and movements, may be absent, the child being dead or the perception of the movements being interfered with. The patient herself may render the examination nugatory; she may be too fat; have, in addition to pregnancy, a tumor, ascites, excessive tympany, etc., or she may hold the abdominal walls and perineum so rigid that the accoucheur can feel nothing in the pelvis. This may be due to nervousness or tenderness in the belly, or it may be practised with intention to deceive. Another source of error is deliberate falsifying by the patient. If she is pregnant, she may desire to conceal it, in order to get the accoucheur, unwittingly, to produce abortion, either with medicine given for amenorrhea or by passing a sound into the uterus for diagnostic purposes. When not gravid, she may desire a positive opinion of pregnancy in order to perform blackmail or institute bastardy proceedings, or to acquire an estate, as in the case of a widow being left property on the birth of a posthumous child. Under these circumstances she will declare all the symptoms of pregnancy to exist, and may even try to imitate the fetal movements by contractions of the abdominal walls. On the other hand, the accoucheur cannot always accept the statements of the patient as true, because she may even delude herself into believing she is pregnant. When approaching the menopause, especially if childless, women sometimes imagine themselves pregnant. The abdomen enlarges, the menses cease, they feel the movements of a child, and even go into labor, having pains. Pseudocyesis, spurious pregnancy, "grossesse nerveuse," as the disease is called, has even baffled the diagnostic ability of the ablest surgeons and accoucheurs. It is famous in history (see Montgomery), and exists in the animals—dogs, mares, and pigs.

For materials on which to build a diagnosis of pregnancy we must review those changes of the maternal organism wrought by conception which were considered in the Physiology of Gestation, for a minute study of which the reader is referred to that chapter. As in the discussion of a disease, we divide the findings into two groups—first, those which the patient tells of, called "symptoms," and those which the examiner himself discovers, called "signs." Symptoms are subjective or rational. Signs are objective or sensible. In general, in medicine, it is wise to adhere to objectivity, for then the chances of error are reduced, the suggestion element of the patient being removed. Subjective symptoms have, therefore, little value, and an opinion based on them, at best, is presumptive. Objective signs have greater value and may allow a probable or unequivocal opinion of pregnancy. Montgomery suggested such a division of the proofs of pregnancy—presumptive, probable, and unequivocal. It is wise to pursue a definite scheme in eliciting the proofs of pregnancy, then to assign to each one its proper valuation, and to compare it with the supposed time of conception. The order of appearance of the various phenomena of gestation, their mutual relations in time and severity, and the length of their existence—all these give valuable information for the determination of pregnancy, since irregularities from the typical course should lead to discovery of the causative anomaly. For purpose of study and practice the pregnancy is divided into three periods of three months each, that is, three trimesters.

FIRST TRIMESTER—SUBJECTIVE SYMPTOMS

Cessation of Menstruation.—This is one of the two really important symptoms of pregnancy, but to have value it must occur in a woman previously regular—it must persist until the time of examination. There may be no pathogenic cause for the amenorrhea and no disease may result from it. Three fallacies underlie this symptom:

A. Pregnancy may occur without menstruation: (a) As in a girl before puberty; (b) during the amenorrhea of lactation, or (c) amenorrhea from other causes, as heart disease, tuberculosis, the stress of war (Dietrich, Pok), and from no cause at all; (d) after curetage; (e) after the menopause. Several cases are on record where a woman conceived before the menses appeared, conceived again during the amenorrhea of lactation, and thus the reproductive cycle repeated itself several times without the appearance of the menses for years. Cases of conception occurring during lactation are so frequent that the popular idea of the preventive effect of nursing should be dropped. Pregnancies occurring two, even four, years after the climacteric have been reported.

B. Menstruation may continue after conception. It is not rare to learn of a woman having one or two periods after she is surely pregnant, but usually the amount of blood is small and the character of the flow otherwise abnormal. If the conception occurred just before the menses were due, there may be an abortive menstruation at the proper time. It is the rule in macacus monkeys and Hartmann calls it the "placental sign." That a true menstrual flow could occur is possible, because the two deciduæ do not fuse until the fifth month. A double uterus may menstruate from the unimpregnated half. Instances where a normal menstruation persisted during the nine months have been reported by Caruso and Pettey. The older writers cite cases where the periods appeared only during pregnancy. That the ovary sometimes continues to functionate during gestation is highly probable, as cases of superfetation and of menstrual molimina and autopsies on pregnant women prove. Rather than a menstruation a bloody discharge is more likely due to abortion, cervical erosions, disease of the endometrium, uterine polyp, fibroids, rupture of a varix at any point in the cervical, vaginal, vulvar canal, extra-uterine pregnancy, diseases of the ovum, as placenta prævia, myxomatous degeneration of the chorion, etc.

C. Other conditions may cause the amenorrhea: (a) Change of climate or environment, noticeable, for example, in girls coming from Europe. It seldom persists over three months. (b) Mental influence. Fear of conception, as occurs after illegitimate exposure, may cause the menses to cease. A strong emotion may do the same. (c) Pathologic conditions, tuberculosis, syphilis, anemia, hypopituitarism, other endocrinal anomalies, exposure to cold, and local disease, atresia of the hymen or the vagina. (d) Some women are habitually irregular, being amenorrheic for several months at a time, without apparent cause or any ill health. Occasionally a long interval will interrupt the regular periods, and the flow is likely to be uncertain during lactation and the approach of the menopause.

One is reasonably safe in regarding a woman who menstruates perfectly normally as not pregnant, and also one who can conceive and is otherwise well, and who suddenly ceases to flow, as presumably with child.

The value of this symptom is, therefore, only presumptive, but it is useful in fixing the date of conception and to determine the time of labor, and must always be noted for this purpose.

The Morning Sickness, or Nausea and Vomiting.—Among the so-called sympathetic symptoms, a tendency to nausea, often with vomiting, occurring in the early morning, must first be mentioned.

This usually begins after the fourth week, but may show itself earlier, as in a case quoted by Montgomery, where, at the end of the week after marriage, the patient felt squeamish. If the nausea is limited to a certain period of the day, mostly the morning, is not attended with symptoms of disease, comes on in a woman who can conceive and who previously was well, it is highly presumptive of the beginning of pregnancy.

About one-third of gravidæ have nausea and vomiting as a marked symptom; one-third complain of them occasionally or as being inconsiderable, and about one-third are free from them entirely. The nausea and vomiting occur earlier, more constantly, and more severely in primiparæ than in multiparæ. They recur in succeeding pregnancies, though usually in lighter form. Women of nervous, high-strung temperaments suffer more than those of the lower and hard-working classes. This symptom is further of value in that its continuance renders probable the life of the fetus, it having been observed that when the child dies the vomiting ceases. As we shall see when we come to discuss the pathology of pregnancy, the nausea and vomiting are probably of a toxemic nature. By the time of quickening the stomach is usually settled. The value of this symptom is only presumptive, because there are so many other causes for stomach disturbances. It seems that many irritations in the pelvis, tumors, pelvic peritonitis, salpingitis, and appendicitis, may cause them.

Salivation.—A slight increase of saliva is a not infrequent accompaniment of the nausea, and has the same cause, probably a toxemia. Dewees called it "cotton spitting," and, occurring in a healthy woman, unattended with fœtor ex ore or other sign of mercurialization, it has some slight value in the diagnosis of pregnancy, though it may occur in other uterine conditions and hysteria. There is a gingivitis which occurs at this period, with salivation, loosening of the teeth, bleeding from the gums, etc., which is distinctly pathologic, and will be considered in the Pathology of Pregnancy, as also will the profuse salivation, an exaggeration of the above symptom.

Change in disposition, the feeling of being pregnant, various neuralgias, and other subjective symptoms are unreliable in a serious diagnosis, because they can all be auto-suggested by the patient, especially if she is yearning for a child. However, when an intelligent multipara, having missed a period, believes she is pregnant, one must attach at least presumptive value to the symptom.

The tingling and even shooting pains in the breasts, with their enlargement, also serve to draw the physician's attention to the possibility of pregnancy.

Irritability of the Bladder and Symptoms of Pelvic Congestion.—The pregnant uterus does not weigh heavily on the bladder because its specific gravity is about the same as that of the intestines, but the anteversion of the fundus throws the cervix toward the hollow of the sacrum and stretches the base of the bladder, causing the frequency of urination so often mentioned by gravidæ in the first trimester. Later, when the fundus comes to be supported by the abdominal wall, the cause and the symptom disappear. The softening of the parts and the congestion of the pelvis lead to a leukorrhea of which the patient complains only if there was previously some catarrh of the organs, which catarrh is usually much aggravated by the pregnancy. The value of these two symptoms is obviously only presumptive.

OBJECTIVE SIGNS—FIRST TRIMESTER

The Breasts.—As early as the fourth week there may be some enlargement of the breasts, and often the patient notices a tingling or burning sensation in them. The enlargement progresses from periphery to center, and continues throughout pregnancy, though not evenly. Lineæ albicantes or striæ gravidarum appear on them, and blue veins may be seen coursing under the thin skin, especially near the nipple. The nipple darkens and becomes more sensitive and erectile; the primary areola darkens and becomes puffy, as if there were air under the skin. One may sometimes feel the sinuses lactiferi in the areola. The tubercles of Montgomery enlarge, and occasionally, even in the first trimester, on pressure, a fine stream of colostrum may be expressed from them. They may connect with the sinuses lactiferi. These tubercles not seldom become infected during pregnancy or the puerperium. Around the areola, especially in brunets, there often develops another pigmented area—the secondary areola. It is lighter in shade than the pigmentation of the primary areola, and resembles dusty paper on which water has been sprinkled, an effect due to the absence of coloring around the sweat-glands. The nipple and primary areola are often covered with branny scales, made up of dried sebaceous matter and epithelium. The epithelium of the areola sometimes exfoliates, carrying the pigment with it, showing that the latter is deposited in the deeper epidermal layers. Much of the coloring disappears after weaning of the baby, but, especially in brunets, more or less remains permanently.

Colostrum may be expressed from the nipple as early as the twelfth week, but it may not be present until after delivery. Of these findings, the most significant is the change in the areola, the deepened color, and the puffiness. All the signs are more marked in primiparæ, as in multiparæ traces often hold over from previous pregnancies. The breast signs have no value in an old multipara as the breasts are enlarged and often contain milk for years. Aside from these fallacies—(1) neurotic women may have tingling in the breasts, enlargement of the areola, and even colostrum during the menstrual periods. (2) Cases of pseudocyesis may show all the signs. (3) Prostitutes and masturbators not seldom show the signs, especially if they have pelvic disease. (4) The breast changes have been observed in cases of ovarian cyst, fibroids, hematometra. It must be admitted that under these circumstances the findings are not so typical, but their occurrence in other conditions than of pregnancy lowers the value of the sign. Especially is the presence of colostrum deceptive. It occurs in neurotic women, even if unmarried, and in men, and the lower animals not pregnant (Gärdlund). Cases are on record where girls have

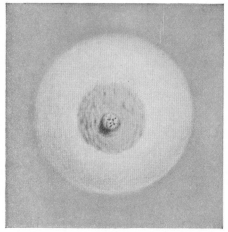

FIG. 281.—VIRGIN BLONDE, NINETEEN YEARS.

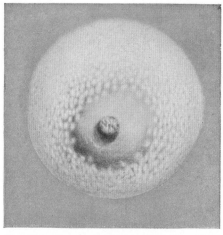

FIG. 281a.—PREGNANT BLONDE, PRIMIPARA, EIGHT AND ONE-HALF MONTHS.

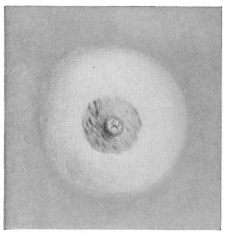

FIG. 282.—VIRGIN RED-HAIRED GIRL, SEVENTEEN YEARS.

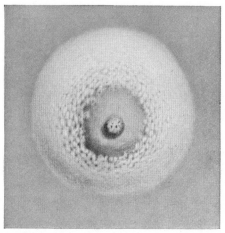

FIG. 282a.—PREGNANT RED-HAIRED WOMAN, PRIMIPARA, EIGHT MONTHS.

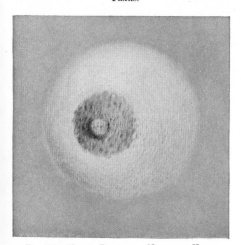

FIG 283.—VIRGIN BRUNETTE, NINETEEN YEARS.

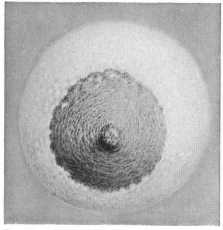

FIG. 283a.—PREGNANT BRUNETTE, PRIMIPARA, ABOUT FULL TERM.

suckled infants, the breast being stimulated by irritating poultices and suction, and men have nursed children (Tanner). The value of this sign, therefore, is presumptive, and, if the changes are all marked and typical, which usually occurs about the fifth month, the pregnancy might be said to be probable.

It serves to call attention to the necessity of a pelvic examination. During lactation a sudden diminution of the quantity and alteration of the quality of the milk, which usually produce effects on the nursling, are suggestive of the existence of a new pregnancy.

Bluish Discoloration of the Vulva, Vestibule, and Vagina.—Jacquemin, in 1836, discovered this bluish, dusky hue of the vestibule and anterior wall of the vagina, but Chadwick, in 1886, emphasized its importance. The sign is named after both these men. It is usually most marked around the meatus and in the vestibule, extending up the anterior vaginal wall, and is likened to the color of the lees of wine

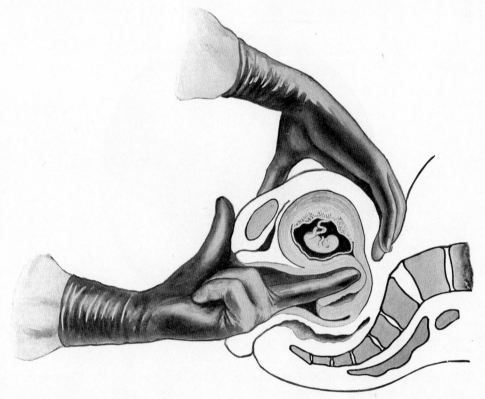

Fig. 284.—Hegar's Sign. Usual Method. Unless Performed with Utmost Gentleness the Pressure Used to Elicit this Sign May Cause Abortion.

—that is, an opaque, bluish tint with a tendency to violet. It appears about the eighth to the twelfth week, and becomes more marked as pregnancy advances. It is more marked in multiparæ than in primiparæ, in women with catarrhal or other disease of the genitalia, and in those with contracted pelvis, especially if they have had previous hard deliveries. It is almost always present, but may not appear until very late, and in rare cases not at all. It often disappears if abortion, with hemorrhage, begins and if the ovum is blighted. Since the discoloration is essentially a local venous congestion, it may be simulated by other conditions which may cause the latter—for example, menstruation, rapidly growing pelvic tumors of all kinds, displacements of the uterus, residua of previous pelvic inflammation which disturb

18

the pelvic circulatory conditions (parametritis, scars, plebitis, thrombosis), and in heart disease and obesity. All these circumstances detract from the value of the sign, leaving it only presumptive. Attempts have been made to diagnose pregnancy with the cystoscope, and when all the other pelvic organs show the non-inflammatory congestion of pregnancy, the bladder shows it also.

Softening of the Cervix and Vagina.—The congestive hyperemia of the pelvis is early manifested by a softening of the vagina and the cervix. These may be noted in primiparæ in the sixth week, and even earlier, by an acute observer, in multiparæ. The upper and lower portions of the cervix soften first, and at the same time one notes the succulence of the vagina, with an increase of the leukorrheal discharge. Goodell ascribed much diagnostic value to this sign, saying: "If the mucous membrane of the cervix feels as hard as the cartilage of the nose, no pregnancy exists; if it feels like the mucous membrane of the lip, pregnancy is possible." The same fallacies underlie this sign as the last, and its value, therefore, is only presumptive. Further, in cases of chronic cervicitis the cervix may soften but

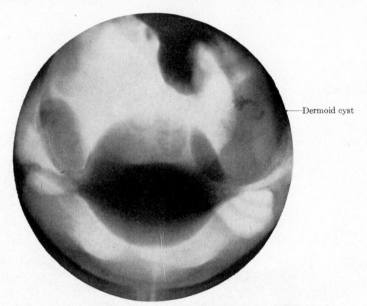

Dermoid cyst

FIG. 285.—x-RAY WITH PNEUMOPERITONEUM. PREGNANCY OF SIX WEEKS COMPLICATED WITH DERMOID CYST. NOTE TUBE, ROUND LIGAMENT, AND POSSIBLY CORPUS LUTEUM ON RIGHT SIDE. (Courtesy of Dr. I. S. Stein and Dr. R. Arens.)

little until the last months of pregnancy. Sometimes one of the earliest pelvic signs is the softening of the congenital thin areas at the sides of the cervix, felt as shallow grooves on its lateral walls.

Hegar's sign, or softening and compressibility of the isthmus uteri and lower uterine segment (Fig. 284). On bimanual examination the isthmus uteri is compressed between the two fingers in the anterior fornix and the abdominal hand. In typical cases one can bring the fingers together so that the uterine tissue between seems reduced to the thinness of paper. In fat women, or those in whom the abdominal muscles are held rigid, one may elicit the sign with one finger in the rectum and the thumb in the vagina. It may be necessary to give ether and to draw the uterus down with a vulsellum to get the information, but cases are rare where such a procedure is indispensable. This sign is only another evidence of the softening of the uterine muscle. The succulence of the tissues is most marked in the lower uterine segment and upper cervix (the isthmus), and permits the pressure, exerted by the fingers, to displace the ovum toward the fundus uteri and to slide the various muscular lamellæ away. In some favorable cases the muscle is so soft that it can be raised in a fold or ridge. Hegar's sign appears in multiparæ at the sixth week, and in primiparæ at the eighth week, but is seldom fully developed until the tenth week, disappearing when the uterus attains a size and height which make the part inaccessible.

When well marked and typical, the sign is highly presumptive and one of the most reliable of the first trimester, but that is all. The author has found the isthmus uteri soft and compressible in many cases months after an abortion or labor, in congested uteri, chronic pelvic peritonitis, and occasionally just before and during menstruation. The findings may be imitated by a retroflexed uterus, the angle of flexion being soft, and by a fibroid in the uterine wall. Indeed, the isthmus may be so softened and elongated that the cervix has been held for the whole non-pregnant uterus and the pregnant fundus has been diagnosed as a tumor of the uterus or adnexa. On the other hand, even in pregnancy, the sign may be absent or very slightly marked, or, owing to fat or rigidity of the parts, it cannot be elicited.

Changes in Form, Size, Consistence, and Position of the Uterus.—These have been described in the Physiology of Pregnancy and Local Changes (p. 72).

(a) *Form.*—The change from the thin pear shape of the virgin uterus to the rounded, plump, bulbous form, is very noticeable. If the ovum nests very near to

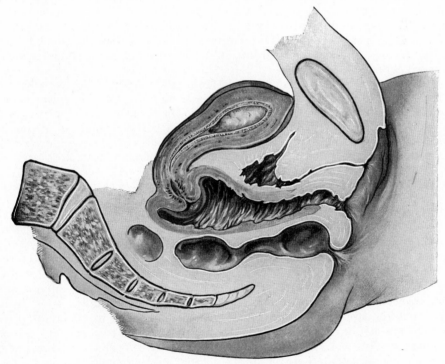

Fig. 286.—Flattening and Lengthening of Uterus in Early Pregnancy.

the entrance of one tube, that half of the uterus will develop first and give the fundus great asymmetry, and it might lead to a false diagnosis of extra-uterine or cornual pregnancy (Fig. 349). (See Ectopic Pregnancy.) It is called "grossesse angulaire" by the French. In the later development of the ovum the symmetry is reëstablished. Early in pregnancy one lateral half is thicker than the other, or either the anterior or the posterior wall of the uterus is bulged outward more, these variations being due to the location of the ovum (Fig. 286). Toward the end of this trimester the bulging of the fundus at the sides, above the relatively small cervix, may be appreciated by the finger placed in the lateral fornices.

(*b*) *Size.*—Every enlargement of the uterus gives rise to the suspicion of pregnancy, and steady characteristic increase in size is one of the most valuable signs we have, but at least two examinations four weeks apart are required. Hematometra and fibroids do not grow like this. The same rate of growth is found with no other uterine tumor. A phenomenon that has not been explained is a sudden softening and enlargement of the uterus, sometimes asymmetric, followed, after a short period, by a return to the original conditions. It easily leads to errors in diagnosis. If a uterus that has shown the usual gradual enlargement of pregnancy suddenly begins to grow too fast, one will suspect a polyhydramnion or hydatid mole; if the growth is interrupted and recession begins, a blighted ovum.

(*c*) *Consistence.*—An experienced hand can very often make a diagnosis of early pregnancy from this one sign. A pregnant uterus is elastic, spongy, and soft, resembling dough. At the site of the ovum the corpus is a little softer than the empty part of the uterus, sometimes feeling like fluid, while between lies a groove which is quite soft. This last phenomenon is not constant and hard to elicit, and the conditions must be unusually favorable (Fig. 95). Braxton Hicks called attention to the intermittent uterine contractions of later pregnancy. The author has felt the uterus contract as early as the eighth week, and it may even contract in spots. This sign may be used for diagnosis (Dickinson). A soft spot above the cervix in the early weeks, Ladinsky believes, is a valuable sign and Douglass noticed pitting of the uterine wall just above the cervix as early as ten days after a missed period.

(*d*) *Position.*—The strong anteversio-flexio of the uterus, lying like a lump of dough upon the bladder, serves to draw the attention to a possible pregnancy immediately on the introduction of the finger into the vagina. The uterus seems to be somewhat imbedded in the pelvis and does not partake readily of motion imparted to it.

These four signs, taken together, and by an experienced examiner, are sufficient to make a highly probable diagnosis of pregnancy. The changes in form, size, and position may be shown by the *x*-ray combined with pneumoperitoneum (Peterson). This procedure is not without danger and seldom necessary.

General Considerations.—The examination should be conducted systematically, all the points being elicited, not being satisfied with one or two. The bowels and bladder should be emptied, all constriction of the abdomen removed, with the patient lying, appropriately draped and at ease, on a table. If a definite order is followed, none of the signs will be overlooked, and the accoucheur will be spared the mortifying necessity of requesting the patient to go back on the table for reëxamination. It need not be reiterated that the usual antiseptic precautions are to be followed, but the advice to be gentle in all manipulations on or about the uterus must be repeatedly emphasized. Beside the unnecessary pain caused by rough pressure there is real danger of provoking abortion or damaging the tender ovum. Since a positive diagnosis in the first trimester may be made only under most favorable circumstances, the accoucheur should leave the answer doubtful, rather than to announce a probable condition as certain, and request the patient to return in four weeks. In cases where the reputation of the woman is concerned it is best to wait until the positive signs of the second trimester are present. If the examiner suspects that the woman desires a diagnosis with a view of going to an abortionist for criminal purposes, he should withhold it entirely for several months, as the public believes abortion is safe only in the earliest weeks. Under no circumstances may a physician prescribe a placebo to satisfy the woman's desire for an abortificient.

PLATE III.

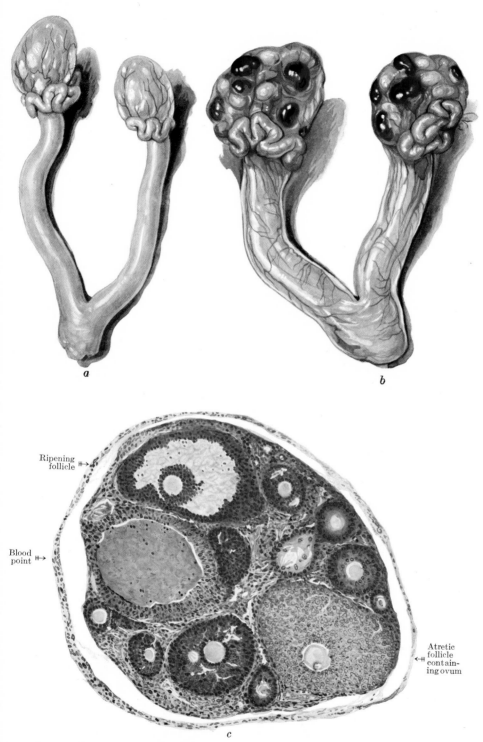

ASCHHEIM-ZONDEK REACTION IN THE MOUSE. (Preparations made by Dr. H. Stricker, Munich.)
a, The normal mouse; *b*, positive findings. Note blood points and atretic corpora lutea. *c*, Section of *b*.

THE LABORATORY DIAGNOSIS OF PREGNANCY

The numerous laboratory tests for pregnancy, Abderhalden's, Fahraeus', Rosenthal's, Ascoli's, et al., now have only historic value, but Zondek and Aschheim have developed one that is proving almost completely satisfactory.

Siddall in 1928 injected the serum of pregnant women into immature female mice and produced a remarkable growth of the genital organs. Zondek and Aschheim in 1928 published a test based on the fact that a peculiar hormone is excreted in the urine. Their experiments seem to prove that the anterior lobe of the hypophysis produces two hormones. One stimulates the ovarian follicles to hasty ripening, the other hurries the luteinization of the same. This double hormone is found in the blood, pregnancy colostrum, saliva, the placenta, decidua, and urine. Its origin is questioned. Zondek thought the hypophysis; Phillip, the placenta. Aschheim agrees with Phillip, as does Felz, which is confirmed by the fact that this element is much increased by pregnancy and is excreted by the kidneys. (See Fig. 131a, p. 110.) In a liter of normal urine there are 50 to 100 rat units of these hormones, but in pregnancy there are 12,000 units or more.

The urine of pregnant women therefore contains a new element, which injected into immature mice or rats produces such activity of development of the genital organs that it is striking to the naked eye—rarely needing a microscope. Concentrated early morning urine, 6 ounces, brought in a clean scalded bottle is used. Catheterization is not necessary if the patient will first cleanse the parts with soap and water and void into a scalded basin.

The urine is kept in the ice-box. A drop or two of toluol will preserve it for a week or longer.

Immature female rats, when they are twenty-five to thirty days old and weigh from 30 to 35 gm., are ideal for the pregnancy test. We prefer three rats which are litter mates, using two for the injection and keeping the largest for the control. The test rats are given two intraperitoneal injections each of 1 c. c. of urine (warmed) daily for two days. All three rats are anesthetized ninety-six hours after the first injection and the genital organs examined *in situ* and compared with those of the control.

The following changes may be noted in a positive test for pregnancy. The ovaries of the injected rats are grossly enlarged, irregular in outline, and hyperemic. On the surface one can note small hemorrhagic areas, the blood points. The accessories are also enlarged and congested in comparison with those of the control animal. Maturity of the entire genital tract is in evidence. However, only the findings of the ovary should be used to decide the pregnancy test. On microscopic section the ovary contains numerous large follicles in all stages of maturation. Massive hemorrhages are present in many of the follicles. The marked tendency towards luteinization is evidenced by numerous corpora lutea, the extensive replacement of theca and granulosa cells of many follicles by lutein cells, and the imprisonment of the ova within them, forming atretic follicles.

Immature male rats thirty-five to forty days old and weighing 40 to 50 gm. have proved in our experience to be excellent animals for this test. The test depends entirely upon the development and maturity of the secondaries, principally the seminal vesicles and prostate. The seminal vesicles are distended and filled with their secretions. The epididymis and Cowper's glands are only slightly hypertrophied. When the test is positive this change in the accessories is striking. On microscopic examination the cells of the seminal vesicles are all columnar in type and distended with secretion. Due to the size of the test animal the gross examination of the genitalia *in situ* is sufficient to make the diagnosis. Furthermore, they can tolerate injections of 2 c.c. of urine twice and three times daily so that five to six injections can be given over a forty-eight-hour period. The males can be examined forty-eight to seventy-two hours after the last injection (Davis and Ferrill).

Brouha uses male mice but Aschheim believes the reaction is not conclusive in male animals, though Neumann and Czyzak think it is. Friedman and Stricker inject the urine intravenously in rabbits—claiming quicker and more constant results (White), and Brown says the same of the gravida's blood serum.

A Word of Warning.—The simplicity of the test and its availability to the public through commercial laboratories might invite malingering, blackmail, etc. Already the women are getting an early diagnosis from the laboratory and then going to the abortionist. Legal precautions should be taken in collecting the specimen and throughout the examination. Further, a positive result is not pathognomonic—teratomata, hypophyseal tumors, etc., may also produce it. Corroborative evidence must always be sought. A negative Zondek-Aschheim is not proof of a dead fetus.

Literature

Aschheim and Zondek: Zentb. für Gynaek., 1931, July 11, p. 2200.—*Ascoli:* Münch. med. Woch., 1910, vol. lvii, p. 62. —*Bourne:* Recent Advances in Obst. and Gyn., Blakiston, 1926, p. 78.—*Brouha:* Bull. de l'Academie de Med. de Paris, 1930, 103, 150.—*Brown, T. K.:* Amer. Jour. Obst. and Gyn., 1932, March, p. 379.—*Davis, M. E., and Ferrill:* Amer. Jour. Obst. and Gyn., April, 1932, p. 567.—*Dietrich:* Zentb. f. Gyn., 1917, No. vi.—*Douglass:* Jour. Amer. Med. Assoc., 1929, vol. 93, No. 6, p. 453.—*Falls and Welcker:* Jour. Biol. Chem., 1918.— *Felz:* Zentb. für Gynaek., August 30, 1930, p. 2191; also Szarkoid.—*Fieux and Mauriac:* Ann. de Gyn. et d'Obstet., May, 1912.—*Flatow:* Münch. med. Woch., March 13, 1914.—*Gardlund:* Jour. Amer. Med. Assoc., April 21, 1917, p. 1221.—*Hirsch:* Zentb. für Gyn., May 2, 1925, p. 968.—*Jellinghaus and Losee:* Bulletin of the Lying-in Hospital of the City of New York, June, 1913. Full literature; also *Van Slyke:* Jour. Biol. Chem., 1915, xxiii, 337.—*King:* Jour. Obst. and Gyn., British Empire, December, 1913.—*Kraul:* Am. Jour. Obst. and Gyn., March, 1931.—*Neumann, Czyzak:* Zentralblatt für Gyn., June 29, 1931.—*Paine:* Boston Med. and Surg. Jour., February 20, 1914. Full literature.—*Peterson:* Jour. Obst. and Gyn., 1921, Pneumoperitoneum.— *Phillip:* Zentb. für Gynaek., 1930, p. 1858.—*Pok:* Zentb. f. Gyn., 1917, No. 20.—*Rosenthal:* Zeitschr. für Klin. Med., 1911, vol. lxxii, No. 6.—*Schwarz:* Amer. Jour. Obstet., January, 1914. Full literature.—*Seiffert:* Abnormal Lactation, Jour. Amer. Med. Assoc., June 12, 1920, Lit.—*Stricker, K.:* Münch. med. Woch., February 5, 1932, p. 213.—*Wells, H. G.:* See Editorial, Jour. Amer. Med. Assoc., December 25, 1920, p. 1786, Lit.— *White and Severance:* Jour. Amer. Med. Assoc., October 31, 1931.—*Widal:* Pregnancy Test, Zentralbl. für Gyn., June 2, 1923, p. 892.

CHAPTER XIX

SYMPTOMS AND SIGNS OF THE SECOND AND THIRD TRIMESTERS

During the second three months of pregnancy there is usually a subsidence of the symptoms called sympathetic,—the nausea and vomiting, salivation, neuralgias, and the irritability of the bladder,—with an increase of the mechanical symptoms. Menstruation is still absent, and a new subjective symptom develops—the patient feels the motion of the child.

Quickening.—About the sixteenth to the eighteenth week the woman begins to feel something in the abdomen, entirely unlike any previous sensation. It is said to resemble the fluttering of a tiny bird in the hand. It usually takes her a week to determine what it is, and finally she concludes it is the movement of the child within her. She is usually beset with various emotions, especially if this be her nature, and immediately feels the full glory of maternity. "Quickening" is the term applied to the first perception of the active fetal movements, and is a relic of the barbarous time when the ovum was considered inanimate until it was felt. The law reflected this belief and, until recently, a woman could be hanged for murder if she had not "felt life," or "quickened," and the innocent babe thus executed too.

Fetal movements are felt earlier by women who have felt them before, and thus have learned to recognize the faint impulses, and cases are recorded of " feeling life " at ten weeks after conception. The motions may not be sensible until the sixth or seventh month, and in rare instances not at all throughout pregnancy. The author had one such case where, in two pregnancies, the child was never felt and was born well at term. The movements, which are weak at first and later stronger, may be so vigorous that the patient's rest is disturbed, or they may be very sluggish throughout pregnancy. Rest, warmth, and narcotics diminish the motion; their opposites increase them. A shock, physical or mental, may abolish the movements for a time, even if the child is well. The motion may also cease, without cause, for periods of days or weeks. Hunger and fever at first stimulate the fetus; later, paralyze it. As a symptom of pregnancy, the quickening is of but presumptive value, because the mother, if she desires offspring, only too easily imagines the sensation. Fetal movements are declared in nearly every case of pseudocyesis. Montgomery refers to the famous case of Queen Mary, whose disappointment on learning that her fancied fetal movements were only the signs of a beginning dropsy, caused her to instigate terrible persecutions of the Protestants. Active intestinal peristalsis gives the patient the impression of the movements of a child, as also may contraction of the recti muscles, a tumor in the belly falling from side to side, and contractions of portions or all of the uterine wall when there is a fetus, but it is dead.

One may use the symptom for diagnosis in intelligent women who are without motive for deception. It may serve as a sort of check on the date of the last menses, in determining the length of pregnancy. In primiparæ, count twenty-two weeks ahead to find the probable date of confinement; in a multipara, twenty-four weeks.

OBJECTIVE SIGNS—SECOND TRIMESTER

Owing to the presence of positive signs, the diagnosis of pregnancy may be affirmed during this trimester. Although some authors assert that conditions exist where one must wait until the physiologic end of gestation arrives for a sure diagnosis, the writer has never met such a case.

The Intermittent Uterine Contractions.—Braxton Hicks first described them, and they are sometimes named after him. As early as the tenth week the whole uterus can be felt to contract, assuming more of a pear shape and then relaxing, without any perception by the mother. The contractions recur at very irregular intervals—minutes or hours and perhaps days. Parts of the uterine muscle may also contract and confuse the diagnosis. A cold hand, brusk manipulation, the active movements of the child (B. Hicks), bring on the contractions, and toward the end of pregnancy, or when premature labor is threatening, the irritability of the uterus is such that even ordinary palpation causes the uterus to harden. Normally not felt by the mother, they may be present in the latter weeks and disturb her rest seriously as "false pains." These usually produce no dilatation of the cervix, and thus are distinguished from true labor pains. A neurotic temperament explains the phenomenon. It is claimed that the virgin uterus contracts, and we know that a non-pregnant uterus can expel blood-clots, membranes, and fibroid tumors. The contractions of pregnancy, therefore, are only the evidence of an exaggerated normal function of the uterine unstriped muscular fibers. The intermittent uterine contractions have the action of a local heart, squeezing the blood out of the sinuses and allowing the influx of new blood in diastole; second, the pelvic tissues and cervix are softened by the local hyperemia produced, and the so-called "vital dilatation" is favored; third, the regular assumption of the uterus of its proper pear form causes the fetus to take, and keep, a position favorable to labor.

Soft fibroids and hematometra may cause the uterus to contract, but not in typical fashion, and the recti muscles sometimes imitate the sign; but with these eliminated, the intermittent uterine contractions become positive evidence of pregnancy, and are found irrespective of the life or death of the fetus.

Active fetal movements felt, seen, or heard by the obstetrician are a certain sign of pregnancy, and, in favorable cases, the observer being skilled, may be determined as early as the twelfth week (Pinard). One may see the slight shock of the abdominal wall, or the passage of a limb under it, and sometimes the motions are so vigorous that they are visible through the clothes, much to the embarrassment of the mother. With the stethoscope, one hears a light tap, like that of the finger against the back of the hand, held with its palm against the ear. With the hand laid on the belly, one perceives a weak knock, or stroke, but sometimes quite tumultuous actions of the extremities and back. Fetal hiccup has already been referred to. Active intestinal peristalsis bears some resemblance to this motion, as do also partial uterine contractions, and, remarkable as it may seem, these movements have been imitated by the abdominal muscles, so that even painstaking examiners have been misled. The famous case of Joanna Southcott, the false prophetess, who thus carried on an imposture for years, is one in point. Eliminating these sources of error,—and this is very easy,—the sign is a positive one of pregnancy and of the life of the child.

Passive Fetal Movements.—Owing to the flaccidity of the uterine wall and the amount of liquor amnii, we can give certain movements to the fetus which have been called "ballottement" or "repercussion." The sign is best elicited with the patient in position for the usual gynecologic examination. Two fingers in the vagina give the body, felt just above the cervix, a gentle push; the abdominal hand feels it strike the fundus of the uterus, and the fingers feel it come to rest again on the cervix (Fig. 287). This is typical ballottement and is very rarely thus obtained, one usually feeling the body leave and return to the fingers in the vagina. Repercussion is found from the sixteenth to the thirty-second week. Before this time the fetus is too small and after it too large, with too little liquor amnii, but one may obtain partial ballottement of the head by means of the abdominal examination, especially in breech cases. Another method of obtaining the sign is to place the woman at the edge of the bed on her side, allowing the uterine tumor to hang over.   A stroke on the uterus from below is now given—a very uncertain procedure.

Ballottement may be simulated by an anteverted uterus floating in ascitic fluid, a fibroid or ovarian tumor with long pedicle in the same, and a stone in the bladder. It, therefore, becomes a positive sign of pregnancy only when these three are excluded.

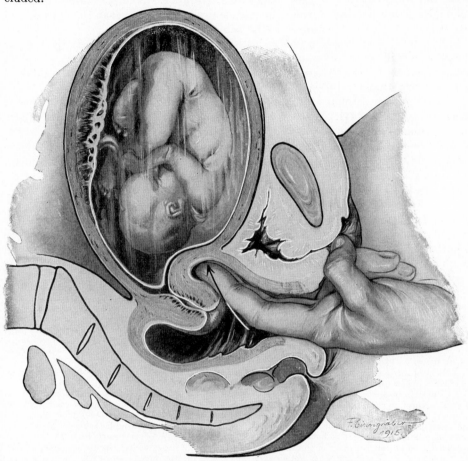

Fig 287.—Ballottement. Head Returning to Finger

Direct Palpation of the Fetal Body.—This sign depends entirely on the skill of the observer.   On palpating an enlarged uterus one will feel a hard body with parts which resemble the head or extremities of a fetus, but one must avoid hasty conclusions.

Fetal parts may be discovered as early as the fourth month, and as the child grows more and more, can be differentiated, so that later we can distinguish "large parts"—head and breech—and "small parts"—the extremities.   Lumps of feces in the sigmoid, carcinoma of the peritoneum, sarcoma of the ovaries, tumors of the omentum, fibroids of the uterus, can all assume shapes and positions which would mislead a careless observer.   The absence of fetal parts, in a case of pregnancy where they should be felt, will lead to the suspicion of a blighted ovum or polyhydramnion.

Auscultatory Signs.—*The Fetal Heart-tones.*—Mayor, of Geneva, in 1818, described the fetal heart-tones, but it is believed (Fasbender) that they were first heard by Philip le Goust, in 1650.   Lejumeau de Kergaradec, in 1822, published a monograph on the subject which is classic, and but little has been added to our knowledge since.   Both observers were listening to discover the sounds made by the fetus splashing in the liquor amnii.   Depaul heard the heart-tones as early as the eleventh week, but usually one finds them first in the fifth month of gestation, though it often requires close application and favorable external conditions, even at this time.   At first faint, the beat becomes stronger as the child grows larger. When nearer to the abdominal wall, the sound is heard better, also through a thin wall, and when the baby's back is directed anteriorly.   A large amount of liquor amnii, the placenta lying in front, the uterine bruit, rumbling gas in the bowels, and external noise all easily extinguish the sound.

The fetal heart-tones resemble the tick-tack of a watch heard by the ear through a pillow; tick—short pause, tack—long pause.   The first sound is isochronous with the systole of the heart and with the pulse in the umbilical arteries; the second sound is due to the closure of the semilunar valves.

The rapidity of the beat normally varies from 120 to 160 per minute, the usual range being 132 to 144.   Mention has been made of the supposed influence of sex, and experience does seem to show that girls' hearts beat faster than boys', but the knowledge is of little value in practice.   Marked variations in rapidity of the heart-beat occur without cause, the count running up to 180 even, and then subsiding. Fetal movements accelerate the beat; palpation of the fetal body does the same. Fever, fasting, asphyxia, and hemorrhage increase the rapidity of the heart. Uterine contraction, pressure on the fetal brain, slow it.

Pestalozza obtained a cardiogram of the fetal heart, and the writer has felt it beat through the abdominal wall in a case of face presentation, an experience reported by others also.   Falls has re-introduced the metroscope for listening to the fetal heart per vaginam.

Methods of Examination.—One will use the naked ear when without an instrument, and in places where rumbling exterior noises interfere, but it is disagreeable to patient and examiner.   A constrained position should be avoided, because this produces circulatory noises in the middle ear, and a smooth towel must always be laid between the ear and the skin.

During auscultation with the usual stethoscope, nothing may touch the instrument save the skin of the patient and the ear of the examiner.   Pressure with the fingers causes a faint hum, which often completely covers the sounds.   This may be obviated by holding the bell in place by means of a rubber band.

Best of all is the head stethoscope shown in Fig. 288.   One may hear the fetal heart with it when it is inaudible otherwise.   The author finds it indispensable in his practice.

The patient is comfortably arranged at the side of the bed or on a table, and appropriately draped, exposing the abdomen.   In doubtful cases the night-time should be selected, and all exterior noises rigidly excluded.   Up to the fifth month the stethoscope should be placed in the median line at the edge of the pubic hair.   When the child is palpable, one will be able to determine where the heart is located and listen there.   It may be necessary to push the child against the abdominal wall with the hand, so as to bring its heart nearer the stethoscope, and in the early months, if a diagnosis is imperative, one could lift the uterus up nearer the abdominal wall with the fingers or a colpeurynter in the vagina.   Experiments are now being carried on with telephonic amplification of the heart sounds.

The fetal heart-tones are the most reliable sign we have for the diagnosis of pregnancy.   Unless the mother's heart-beat is transmitted to the lower abdomen and has the same rapidity (fever, Basedow's disease), there is no question about the existence of a child in the belly.   By feeling the mother's pulse while listening over the uterus, and noting the difference, 72 and 140, and by following the line of increasing intensity of the sounds, the sign is easily proved.

The Fetal Souffle.—This is sometimes called the funic souffle, a name given to it by its discoverer, Evory Kennedy, in 1833.   It is due to the rush of blood through the umbilical arteries, and is heard when they are subject to pressure or torsion or tension, for example, coiling of the cord around the neck, cord too short, between the back of child and abdominal wall, and under compression by the stethoscope. Bumm believes the funic souffle arises in the fetal heart during pressure on the cord. In thin women the writer has felt the cord coursing over the fetal back.   In fetal heart disease one hears cardiac murmurs with the usual fetal heart-tones.   These murmurs may disappear after delivery, or, if the disease is organic, be permanent.

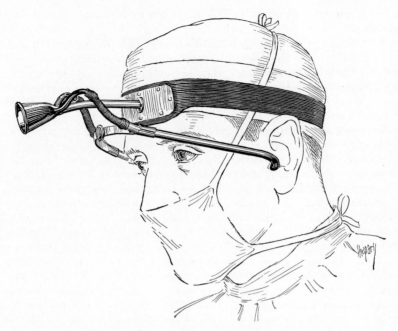

Fig. 288.—The DeLee-Hillis Obstetric Stethoscope.

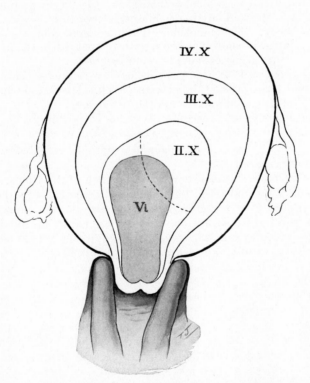

Fig. 289.—The Fingers Determine the Changes in the Shape of the Uterus.
The fornices are flattened and one feels the bulging uterus at the sides.

The fetal souffle is a soft, blowing murmur heard with the first sound, but it may be with both, or even diastolic. It occurs in about 15 per cent. of pregnant women, being more common during labor. When present, this sign is diagnostic of pregnancy.

The Uterine Souffle.—Kergaradec, in his paper (1822), described a sound which he heard while listening at the sides of the uterus, and he ascribed it to the rushing of blood through the placenta, calling it the "placental souffle." It is a soft, blowing sound, synchronous with the maternal heart, having a rushing character, similar to the bruit heard in an aneurysm or in the veins of the neck, or like the French "vous," pronounced in a low, blowing tone—"voo." During uterine contraction it is diminished or altered in quality; sometimes both.

It is heard best at the left side of the uterus, low down, but may be heard on the right side or anteriorly—occasionally all over the uterus, or on both sides.

It may be loud, drowning the fetal heart-tones, or soft, hardly audible—even absent in some (10 per cent.) cases. It may be heard at one time and be absent in the same place later. It may disappear during the examination.

In character it is humming, blowing, rushing, sibilant, or even musical. It may be continuous or intermittent or wavy. It is without shock, and is usually single, but may be both systolic and diastolic. Sometimes pressure with the stethoscope intensifies the sound and alters its character, and one may feel the rush of the blood at the side of the uterus with the fingers as a systolic, fine vibrant thrill. The origin of the sound is in the large vessels,—arteries and veins in the sides of the uterus,—and its similarity to the sound of a varicose aneurysm is striking. It is not in the placenta because it has been heard after the placenta is removed, and at locations far from the placental site. It seems loudest near the placental site. There is no sound by which we can locate the placenta, though in extra-uterine pregnancy a marked uterine souffle will serve to indicate the location of the ovum in the belly. The sound does not come from compression of the iliac arteries by the uterus, because it is heard with the patient in the knee-chest position and before the uterus has a chance to compress them.

Depaul has discovered the uterine souffle as early as the twelfth week, but most observers have not heard it until the sixteenth week. It is found whether the fetus is alive or dead, but usually diminished in the latter case.

As a diagnostic sign of pregnancy its value is only probable, because it is heard over all rapidly growing tumors—fibroids, ovarian cysts, even in enlarged spleen and liver, and in cases of anemia and maternal heart disease, the cardiac murmurs being transmitted.

Changes in Form, Size, Consistence, and Position of the Uterus.—These have already been considered under the Physiology of Pregnancy. In the diagnosis of pregnancy the shape of the uterine tumor, its size for the supposed length of gestation, the consistence and location—all these are hardly imitated by any other condition: the practised hand, with one grasp, can usually get enough information for a decision. Any doubt will be set at rest by determining the rate of growth of the uterus, when examined at intervals of three to four weeks. No other tumor grows so rapidly nor so typically. A peculiar phenomenon that is as yet unexplained, and which may confuse the diagnosis, is a sudden enlargement of the uterus to the size of one several months longer pregnant, and then, as sudden, a subsidence to the natural size. It is referred to by Buettner and Dickinson. In the author's case it very materially complicated the diagnosis. Should the uterus cease growing uniformly, or even get smaller, the ovum is probably blighted.

These signs, together, give us positive information of pregnancy.

O'Donnell, of Chicago, in 1911 demonstrated an x-ray picture of a woman six months pregnant. Since then much work has been done on the subject, and expert radiologists have discovered, in favorable cases, parts of the fetal skeleton as early as the eighteenth week. Peterson, of Ann Arbor, using the x-ray combined with pneumoperitoneum, can diagnose pregnancy as early as the sixth week, but now we have a safer early test, Aschheim-Zondek.

Changes in the Skin.—Pigmentation; the mask of pregnancy; the striæ gravidarum; the changes in the navel—at first retracted, then pouting, then drawn up; the varicose veins—all these are significant, but have little real diagnostic value. The secondary areola on the breasts is a useful but inconstant sign.

SYMPTOMS AND SIGNS OF THE THIRD TRIMESTER

The menses continue absent. Any bloody show now is either pathologic or means that labor is beginning. The morning sickness is usually absent. Its persistence or reappearance indicates the necessity for a careful examination of stomach, liver, and kidneys. Rarely, the vomiting is the result of cramping of the stomach by the high uterus. Active fetal movements are a more pronounced symptom, and may harass the mother, but the child usually quiets down as labor becomes imminent.

1. The painless uterine contractions become more and more noticeable as the months go by, until, toward the end of this trimester, the uterus often responds to very slight irritants. In this way the cervix and pelvic structures are prepared for the great dilatation they are about to undergo.

2. The examiner now has no trouble to feel the movements of the child.

3. Ballottement, or repercussion, is not obtainable, unless there is a great deal of liquor amnii (polyhydramnion), but partial repercussion is easily elicited, especially in breech presentations.

4. Direct palpation of the fetal body is plain, and toward the end of the trimester is the same as during labor. One may now diagnose the presentation and position.

5. The fetal heart-tones are louder and more constant, and one is more likely to hear the funic souffle and active fetal movements.

6. The uterine bruit is more intense and more distributed.

7. The changes in form, size, consistence, and position of the uterus are very marked. These have already been discussed. (See p. 84.)

8. The x-ray will always disclose the fetal skeleton.

Only gross carelessness will explain a mistake in the diagnosis of pregnancy during this trimester. Excessive fat in the abdominal wall, the presence of tumors, ascites, and general peritonitis, in the author's experience, have caused much difficulty, but have not rendered a working decision impossible.

SUMMARY OF THE DIAGNOSIS OF PREGNANCY

FIRST TRIMESTER

Cessation of menses....................................Presumptive
Morning sickness, salivation, etc.........................Presumptive
Changes in the breasts.................................Presumptive
Jacquemin's sign......................................Presumptive
Softening of cervix and vagina..........................Presumptive
Hegar's sign...Probable
Changes in form, size, consistence, and position of uterus....Probable
Aschheim-Zondek test.................................99 per cent. positive

Taken all together, with careful exclusion of conflicting conditions, a positive diagnosis may be made toward the end of the first three months.

SECOND TRIMESTER

Absence of menses....................................Presumptive
Quickening..Presumptive
Intermittent uterine contractions........................Probable
Active fetal movements discovered by the accoucheur.......Certain
Ballottement (with the three restrictions).................Certain
Direct palpation of fetal body..........................Certain
Fetal heart-tones and souffle............................Certain
Uterine souffle.......................................Probable
Changes in form, size, consistence, and position of uterus.....Certain
Skiagraph of fetal skeleton.............................Certain

Rarely it is impossible to make a positive diagnosis at the end of the sixth month of gestation. In the third trimester all the signs become more apparent and more convincing.

The Diagnosis of Lightening.—When the woman notes, toward the end of pregnancy, a subsidence of the symptoms referable to the upper abdomen and an increase of pelvic symptoms, and at the same time a change in the configuration of the belly, as is described on p. 89, it is fair to assume that lightening has occurred.

If, on examination, one finds the anteversion of the uterus increased,—the plateau-like fundus, the head deep in the inlet,—and on internal exploration the changes described and illustrated on p. 91, the diagnosis is positive. A real prognostic value attaches to this phenomenon. It means that the particular head can pass the particular pelvic inlet, and since the majority of serious pelvic deformities are at the inlet, it predicts a successful delivery. Lightening may be absent in the following conditions: Contracted pelvis and its equivalent—a large fetus; twin pregnancy; polyhydramnion; multiparity; occipitoposterior positions; presence of the placenta in the lower uterine segment; abnormal cervix; tumors blocking the inlet. In primiparæ lack of lightening is significant, and while labor may be prolonged, it mostly terminates favorably.

Diagnosis of the Life and Death of the Fetus.—Without positive evidence to the contrary, a fetus is considered alive. While we can easily assert that the child lives, we can less readily be sure that it is dead. The heart-tones, the fetal souffle, and active fetal movements determined by the accoucheur are convincing that the fetus lives. In a woman who is healthy and feels perfectly well it is usually safe to assume that the child is living.

Symptoms and Signs of Fetal Death.—1. Cessation of fetal movements after they have been felt. Presumptive.

2. Languor, malaise, light chilliness, foul taste in the mouth, symptoms which are due to the absorption of toxins from the dead fetus and are analogous to those arising from degenerating fibroids, are presumptive symptoms only. The same is to be said of the feeling of weight, or of a body lying heavily in the abdomen. Sudden cessation of the nausea and vomiting, in the early months, is suggestive of fetal death.

3. If a woman gives a history of losing several children at a certain month in pregnancy and now has identical symptoms, the information is suggestive. When a cause exists for anticipating fetal death, the diagnosis is rendered easier. Such conditions are syphilis, eclampsia, nephritis, high fever, cholera, etc.

4. Absence of heart-tones. This sign is of value only after repeated, prolonged examinations, under most favorable conditions (quiet room, proper position, etc.), have failed to find the heart-tones.

5. Cessation of growth of the uterus and abdominal tumor. A valuable sign if controlled by examinations repeated every three weeks. The uterus, instead of growing, gets smaller, harder, and usually more evenly resistant all over; though, occasionally, it becomes irregular, and then making the distinction from a fibroid is very difficult. The intermittent uterine contractions are more marked and there may be an occasional discharge of bloody or brownish mucus. Unless carefully considered, this sign may be fallacious, because, sometimes, the uterus apparently ceases to grow or even grows smaller for a time, even with a living child (one of the causes of placenta circumvallata), and, again, the uterus may enlarge after the death of the ovum, as in hydatidiform mole.

6. The only positive sign of fetal death is the palpation of the softened and macerated fetal head, with the bones freely movable on each other, the scalp hanging like a loose sac. This sign may be elicited through the vault of the vagina, through the cervical canal, or, rarely, through the abdominal wall. Maceration of

the fetus is usually so far advanced in a week to ten days that the softening of the skull may be discovered. On abdominal examination the uterus and fetus do not have the characteristic feeling of elasticity and firmness, but this sign is hard to elicit and is valuable only to an experienced accoucheur. Horner, in 1921, showed an *x*-ray picture of a macerated fetus *in utero* with overlapping of the skull bones, but this is not a positive sign as I have seen it on a living fetus. However, combined with marked curvature or angulation of the spine and general crowding together of the skeleton, it has much value (Kehrer, Hodges and Schnitker).

7. The discharge of bloody liquor amnii or milky fluid is suggestive, but one must eliminate hydrorrhæa gravidarum and early rupture of the amnion with subchorionic development of the ovum.

8. The breasts cease to grow, becoming flabby and pendent. Presumptive.

9. The patient loses weight, which is significant, because she ought to gain in the last four months.

10. The finding of acetone and peptone in the urine has no significance.

11. Absence of the usual basal metabolism increase in pregnancy (Baer).

12. Guirauden found that reduction of the clotting time of the blood to five minutes or less shows that the fetus is dead. The author's experience in 9 cases is confirmatory.

It is not absolutely necessary to make a positive diagnosis, since, if the fetus is dead, delivery will soon occur. (See Missed Abortion, Chap. XXXII.) It is usually not necessary to induce labor, because no harm results, except in the rarest instances. The woman is instructed not to have intercourse, to take no douches, etc., and to report any unusual symptoms.

Diagnosis of Multiparity.—It sometimes becomes necessary, especially in medicolegal cases, to determine if an existing pregnancy is the first one, or if a woman has previously borne a child. Such a diagnosis can usually be made if sufficient care be used, but if more than five years have elapsed since the birth of the last child, if it was small or prematurely born, if it was removed by a crushing operation or by a cesarean section, or if the genitalia be very large, it may be impossible to come to a positive decision, because the only signs we have are the relics of the traumatisms of labor.

1. The deep rupture of the hymen and perineum. If the perineum is torn and the patient avers that no operation on it had been performed and that she never suffered local injury or had an ulcerous disease, the sign is positive. If the patient wishes to hide the previous pregnancy, she may claim to have suffered injury in some way. Rupture of the hymen alone is not so certain a sign, since it almost always tears during coitus. Deep tears, forming later the carunculæ myrtiformes, occur only during labor or the delivery of a large body, as a fibroid. The hymen may be congenitally absent, or it may be so distensible that it does not rupture during delivery. The author saw only one such case, with a syphilitic fetus weighing three pounds.

2. Deep tears and scars in the cervix. In primiparæ the cervix is conic, with a round os. In multiparæ, owing to inevitable greater or less laceration, the portio vaginalis is more cylindric or knob-shaped, and the os is a transverse slit. Even if the laceration of the cervix is only moderate, one can distinguish two lips— an anterior and a posterior. Scars in the cervix may result from operation, ulceration, and disease, congenital or acquired. Prolapsus uteri and eversio cervicis have been found in infants; and chronic cervicitis, in virgins, may cause changes which imitate a parous cervix.

3. Vaginal scars are often the result of labor, but they may be due to operation, injury, or ulcerative process, which not infrequently complicates the acute infectious diseases, *e. g.*, measles and scarlatina. The vagina of a nullipara is

rugous, rough, and tight, the levator ani holding it well up against the pubic arch. In a multipara the reverse is true, but if many years have elapsed since childbirth, a great deal of the original condition is reëstablished. The laceration of the urogenital septum and of the anterior strands of the levator ani is one of the most constant of puerperal injuries.

4. The breasts are more pendulous, flabby, with deeply pigmented areolæ, and sometimes colostrum may be expressed from the nipples. The fallacies underlying this sign have already been mentioned.

5. Striæ gravidarum may be found on the breasts, abdomen, and thighs—old, white, crinkled, and silvery, mixed with the pinkish or purplish lines of a new pregnancy. Striæ are found in fat people, in girls as they round out at puberty, in some cases of abdominal tumors, after typhoid fever; and, further, they are absent in 5 per cent. to 10 per cent. of pregnancy cases.

6. The recti and abdominal muscles are usually relaxed and stretched after the woman has had a full-term child, but the author has seen several women in whom the abdominal figure was perfect after two or three full-term deliveries.

In medicolegal cases, therefore, one can seldom assert positively that pregnancy has, or has not, taken place. Abortions and premature labor leave still fewer traces behind them, and in such instances the medical witness must exercise still greater caution.

The Diagnosis of the Time of Pregnancy and the Prediction of the Day of Confinement.—Both physician and patient desire to know when labor will occur. One may wish to induce labor for contracted pelvis or to prevent overgrowth of the child; the other wishes to know so that she may arrange her household affairs, engage the nurse, and so forth, hence it is a matter of some moment to be able to discover the exact day, or come near it. Since the real duration of pregnancy is unknown, we can never be sure of the day when labor is to begin. The moment of conception varies, labor is more or less accidental, and, finally, the length of pregnancy varies in different women and in the same woman in her succeeding pregnancies. (See p. 25, The Duration of Pregnancy.)

Determination from Data Given by the Patient.—1. The date of the fruitful coition. No reliance is to be placed on the statement of the patient that the fruitful coition is distinguished by a peculiar sensation, and, therefore, may be used in the reckoning. The date of a single coitus is more reliable, and this may be known, as in cases of sudden death or absence of husband, rape, etc. If the monthly period, due within a few days of this date, remains absent, the probability that conception occurred about this time is very strong. One should count 273 days from the date of the single coitus to determine the date of confinement. In about one-half of the cases this date will be right within seven days.

2. The last menstruation. Naegelè's rule is to count back three months from, and add seven days to, the date of the first day of the last menstruation; for example, if the patient menstruated last beginning March 1st, December 8th will be the day of labor. In about 60 per cent. of cases this method is correct within eight days.

3. Quickening. It is customary to count ahead twenty-four weeks in multiparæ and twenty-two weeks in primiparæ; but in view of what was said regarding this symptom, it is plain that no reliance at all is to be placed on the data obtained.

Objective Signs.—1. Size of the uterine tumor, circumference of the abdomen, height of the fundus from the pubis or the navel—all these are valueless measurements, since so many conditions may disturb them; for example, the amount of fat in the abdominal wall, tumors and gas in the belly, the full bladder or rectum, polyhydramnion, twins, pendulous abdomen, contracted pelvis (Pendleton, Lit.).

2. The determination of the size of the fetus gives more certain information, as from this we may guess, with a fair amount of accuracy, its age. Direct mea-

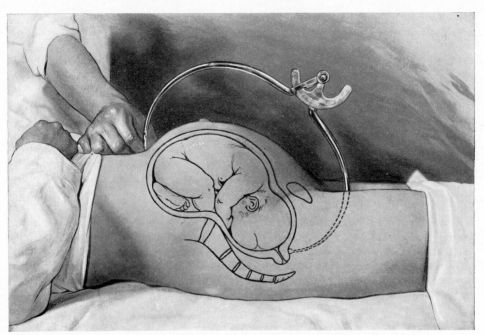

FIG. 291.—ASCERTAINING INTRA-UTERINE LENGTH OF FETUS.

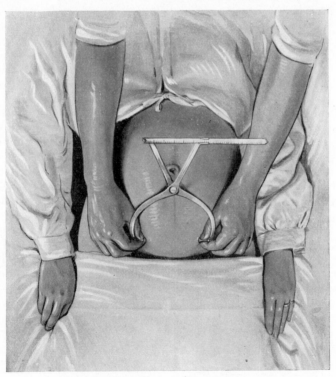

FIG. 292.—USING PERRET'S CEPHALOMETER.
Any pelvimeter may be used as well.

surement of the length of the fetus in the uterus, as practised by Ahlfeld (Fig. 291), is possible, and, since the length of the child is our best (but poor at that) guide to its

19

age, we frequently make use of this method. In primiparæ one branch of the pelvimeter (sterilized) is placed against the head from the vagina, the other branch resting on the breech. In multiparæ, since the head usually does not enter the pelvis until labor has begun, one puts the first branch of the pelvimeter over the upper border of the pubic symphysis. By doubling the figure obtained and subtracting 2 cm. for the thickness of the soft parts, one arrives at the length of the fetus and from this may deduce the period of the pregnancy. A ten months' child is 50 cm. long; one of nine months, 46 cm.; eight months, 42 cm.; seven months, 38 cm.

Direct measurement of the fetal head has been practised, using an ordinary pelvimeter (Fig. 292). One first carefully determines the position of the head with reference to the pelvis, and then places the branches of the pelvimeter as nearly as possible in the occipitofrontal diameter. One to 2 cm. must be deducted from an oblique measurement to obtain the biparietal diameter, and another centimeter for the thickness of the abdominal wall. Surprisingly accurate results are obtained, and the value of the procedure increases with experience. In breech and shoulder presentation the head is easily measured, unless labor has begun, but when the head has engaged, it can no longer be properly grasped; then, however, the measurement is not needed. A biparietal diameter of $7\frac{1}{2}$ cm. means that the child is of about thirty weeks' pregnancy, $8\frac{1}{2}$ cm., about thirty-four weeks, and $9\frac{1}{2}$ cm. about forty weeks.

The measurement of the fetal head is especially desirable in cases of contracted pelvis, where the question of the induction of premature labor arises, or of a radical operation at the time of full-term labor. Thoms claims good results by x-ray.

3. Direct palpation of the fetal body. Children may vary much in size even at identical periods of pregnancy. The author delivered, on the same day, a child at the eighth month of pregnancy which weighed eight pounds, and another, where the mother was three weeks beyond her reckoning, which weighed three and one-half pounds. It has also seemed that the child has periods of slower and quicker growth, similar to those of its extra-uterine existence. Again, the child may have a large head and a small trunk, or vice versâ. It is clear, therefore, that all estimations of the period of pregnancy and of the probable date of confinement, based on the size of the fetus, are unreliable, and even if we do guess accurately we have no way of being sure that the baby will live even if it turns out to be a large one. The large baby just referred to died, the small one lived. Viability and size do not go together.

4. Lightening before labor. It is quite safe to expect the delivery to occur within three weeks from the time the head settles into the pelvis. Often this occurrence is attended by regular uterine contractions which may simulate the real pains of delivery.

5. The changes in the lower uterine segment and cervix, as described in the physiology of pregnancy, give only relatively valuable information of the proximity of labor, because they have been observed three to six weeks before delivery, and may remain absent until actual pains have been in operation some time. The extreme sensitiveness of the uterus to external irritation which causes contractions may give a hint as to the nearness of labor.

LITERATURE

Baer: Basal Metabolism in Pregnancy, Am. Jour. Obst. and Gyn., October, 1921.—*Buettner:* Zent. f. Gyn., August, 1900.—*Caruso:* Arch. di Ost. e Gin., 1900.—*Depaul:* Traitè d'Auscultation Obstetricale, Paris, 1847.—*Dickinson:* Amer. Gyn. and Obst. Jour., 1892, vol. vii, p. 545; Trans. Amer. Gyn. Soc., 1901.—*Fasbender:* Geschichte der Geburtshilfe, p. 428.—*Guirauden:* Bull. Soc. d'Obst. et de Gyn. de Paris, September, 1924.—*Hegar:* Deutsche med. Woch., 1895, No. 35.—*Hodges and Schnitker:* x-Ray Diagnosis of Fetal Death. Lit.—*Horner:* Radiography in Obstetrics, Am. Jour. Obst. and Gyn., October, 1922.—*Kehrer:* Zentb. für Gyn., August 22, 1931.—*Montgomery:* Obstetrical Essays on Pregnancy, 1857, pp. 122, 128.—*Pendleton:* Am. Jour. Obst. and Gyn., September, 1926, p. 390.—*Pettey:* Brit. Med. Jour., 1903.—*Simpson:* Obstetrics and Gynecology, p. 101.—*Tanner:* The Signs and Diseases of Pregnancy, 1868.—*Thoms:* Amer. Jour. Obst. and Gyn., December, 1930.

CHAPTER XX

THE CONDUCT OF LABOR

It is a great satisfaction to the accoucheur to go to the home of the parturient knowing that everything for the proper conduct of labor has been provided and is in readiness. This sense of satisfaction is enhanced if he has with him a case or satchel containing all the instruments and apparatus, dressings, and medicines necessary for the usual case of labor and for the most common complications. What the accoucheur will carry in his obstetric satchel will depend on the conditions of his practice and individual preference. If his patients are on distant farms, he should take with him a complete obstetric armamentarium, which, though heavy

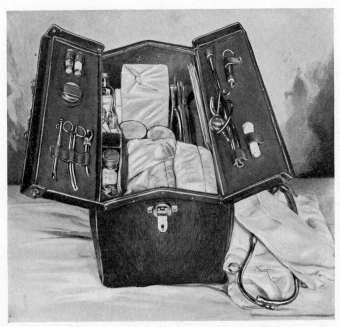

Fig. 293.—Author's Obstetric Satchel. White Suit and Stethoscope Taken Out.

and bulky, is necessary if he would give them all the benefits of his art. For a town or city practice, the instruments for the rarer operations—craniotomy, hebosteotomy, etc.—need not always be carried. It is absolutely essential that the physician be prepared for the operations of perineorrhaphy, forceps, and version, and for the complications, postpartum hemorrhage and asphyxia neonatorum. The author's satchel, for ordinary labor cases, contains the articles on the list subjoined. For complicated cases a separate bag, containing everything for operations from perineorrhaphy to cesarean section, is provided. It weighs 50 pounds and is very bulky, but when the parturient cannot be taken to the hospital operating-room, the operating-room must be taken to the parturient.

LIST OF ARTICLES IN OBSTETRIC SATCHEL (FIG. 293)

FOR ASEPSIS

Two sterile hand-brushes.
One surgeon's gown and cap (Fig. 780).
One white duck suit.
Four pairs sterile rubber gloves.
Four ounces lysol.
Three jars sterile gauze and cotton sponges.
Four ounces 70 per cent. alcohol.
One bottle bichlorid tablets.

MEDICINES

One quart of ether.
One ounce of fluidextract of ergot.
Six ampules "Gynergen."
Three of pituitary.
Two ampules 1 per cent. $AgNO_3$.
A working hypodermic syringe with tablets of morphin and scopolamin.
Sundry cardiac stimulants.
Two ampules Alpha Lobelin.
Four ampules magnesium sulphate, 50 per cent.
Three ampules of 1 per cent. novocain solution.

SUNDRIES

Linen bobbin (sterile) for cord.
Six tubes twenty-day catgut No. 2.
One wide-mouth jar with sterile silk gut.
C. P. sodium bicarbonate for boiling instruments.
One nickeled copper pan for same.
History sheets and cards for physician and nurse.

Birth-certificates.
Two sterile version slings.
Test-tube and reagents for testing albumin and sugar in the urine.
Blood-pressure apparatus.

INSTRUMENTS

One pair Simpson forceps.
Two scissors, long and short.
Four artery forceps, long and short.
Two tissue forceps.
Two vulsella.
Two special cervix holders.
One long uterine packing forceps.
Three broad retractors.
One box needles.
Two needle-holders.
One head stethoscope.
One silver catheter.
One rubber catheter.
Two tracheal catheters.
One baby scale and tape-measure.
One anesthetic mask.
One pelvimeter.
Syringes for local anesthesia.

FOR POSTPARTUM HEMORRHAGE

One douche-can and tube.
One 12-yard jar lysolized gauze.
One 8-yard jar of same.
One salt solution needle.
Three 2-dram bottles sterilized salt.
Two ampules 20 per cent. glucose sol.

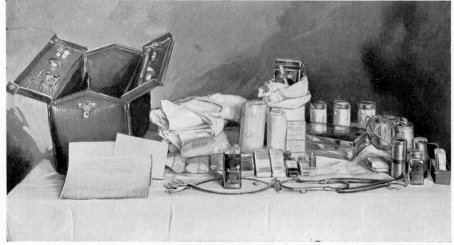

FIG. 294.—CONTENTS OF OBSTETRIC SATCHEL.

Basins and towels are to be found at the patient's house. If they are **not,** three one-quart cream pans and a package of six sterile towels must be added to the above outfit. All these things can be comfortably packed into a 17-inch "cabin" satchel. The instruments, all but the scissors and stethoscope, are packed in the pan, and are boiled in the same just before they are used. The medicine bottles are held in two bags made of ordinary white cotton duck, washable. Objection has been made to the leather satchel on the score of its becoming infected. This is possible if the physician is careless and allows it to become soiled with blood, etc. No contrivance can be invented to take the place of an aseptic conscience. By exercising care that the satchel is not soiled, by frequently cleaning it with a cloth dampened in alcohol, it may be kept in a safe condition. The instruments are boiled before using, and the aseptic articles are all in hermetically sealed bottles. When the satchel has been exposed to a known infected case, a half-ounce of formalin poured on a towel laid among the bottles, with the lids closed for a few hours, will sterilize it. A separate satchel should be used for infected cases.

The Question of Assistance.—The time has come to make a sharp distinction between hospital and home obstetric practice. Careful study of existing conditions will convince any one that the safest place for the parturient woman is the special, well-equipped lying-in hospital. Here are all the facilities for the aseptic conduct of labor and the puerperium, here is the danger of child-bed infection properly evaluated, here only are the refinements of an operative technic possible, because the operator has the help of trained assistants. The newer procedures—vaginal cesarean section, hebosteotomy, cesarean section and its modifications, the treatment of eclampsia, ruptured uterus, asphyxia neonatorum, the repair of lacerations, etc., all procedures which save life and reduce invalidism—can be carried out immeasurably so much better in the maternity than at home, that one could wish every woman would go to such a hospital for her confinement. That the obviously pathologic case belongs in the hospital cannot even be discussed. The maternity, while it relieves the physician of a great deal of the drudgery of obstetric practice, offers the temptation to undue operative interference in labor. Meddlesome midwifery is always deplorable but it is particularly dangerous in the small hospital where the prevalence of infections close to the maternity ward has, experience shows, increased the maternal mortality beyond all reason.

But the majority of births occur in the patients' homes and will continue so in our day, and it, therefore, becomes our duty to better the conditions we are forced to meet. The people must not expect such good results as are obtained by the accoucheur in his specially equipped maternity, but it is surprising how much may be accomplished, and with simple means. The preparations and the obstetric satchel have been described. It is essential that the accoucheur have sufficient assistants. Every labor case should have two physicians. The duties of the assistant are, first, to watch the fetal heart-tones so that if the child should show signs of exhaustion or asphyxia, it be recognized in time, and the frequency of still-births be thus diminished; second, to keep an accurate history of the labor; third, to care for the patient during the first stage while the accoucheur is attending to other work, or obtaining the rest he will need for the proper conduct of the second and third stages. In this way an impending convulsion, or rupture of the uterus, or internal hemorrhage or any other complications will be discovered early enough for successful treatment; fourth, to give the anesthetic, and assist at eventual operation; fifth, to care for the baby or for the third stage, if the accoucheur is busy with the baby; sixth, to stay in the house an hour or more after delivery to handle a possible postpartum hemorrhage.

If obstetrics is ever to attain the dignity of surgery,—and it should,—if the parturient woman is ever to enjoy the same benefits as the surgical patient, and she deserves them,—the accoucheur must be given sufficient help and the make-shift policies of obstetric practice must be abolished.

Response to the Call.—The pregnant woman is to be instructed to summon the physician immediately when she feels that labor has begun, or when she thinks that something—anything unusual—has taken place, and the physician should respond at once. If the call comes at a time when he cannot answer, the accoucheur sends his associate or assistant to care for the woman until his arrival. In this way a malpresentation of the child or other complication may be recognized early, at a time favorable for its correction, the preparations for labor may be made (if the patient has no trained nurse), the bowels and bladder properly cared for, and the nervousness of the parturient allayed.

Even before the accoucheur goes to the parturient he must have made up his mind exactly how he is going to conduct her labor. First of all, he must know how she stands at the threshold of her ordeal. Has she a good heart, good lungs, good kidneys, a good liver? Has she any hidden infection? Is her pelvis large enough? Is her baby too large? Does it lie in good position? Knowing all these things, he will have decided or will decide early in the first stage whether he will deliver the woman from below or perform elective abdominal section; he will have chosen the anesthetic best suited to the patient and will have prepared for all complications. Upon his arrival in the birth room he should refresh his mind by reading the antepartum record, and take the blood-pressure, examine the urine of his patient, and inquire into her present general health.

Asepsis and Antisepsis.—These have reference to, first, the physician; second, the patient; third, the environment, and the same minute attention to detail is required as for an abdominal section. It is a question if the uterus can care for more infection than the peritoneum.

Semmelweis, in 1847, called the attention of the world to *the physician as a carrier of infection*, and the latter's importance in this rôle has been recognized ever since—in fact it is exaggerated, for the public has held him responsible in cases of sepsis when he was not to blame. Cases of infection will occur under ideal conditions, and we must look for the cause elsewhere than in the accoucheur —probably in the woman herself, or even in the husband. The precautions the accoucheur is to take, as far as his work is concerned, are well recognized and ought to be the common property of the profession.

The accoucheur should be of clean personal habits, should not soil his clothes by contact with postmortem tables, pus-basins, contagious disease cases, etc., etc. The accoucheur should not attend contagious diseases, individual favorable experience to the contrary notwithstanding, AND HE MUST SCRUPULOUSLY AVOID GETTING INFECTIVE MATERIAL ON HIS HANDS.

This is the key-note of subjective asepsis and cannot be sufficiently emphasized. (Oliver Wendell Holmes first taught it.) All infected things—pus, dressings, etc.— should be handled with forceps and perfect rubber gloves. If the skin of the hands is once infected, it requires two days of frequent scrubbings, Zweifel says eight days, to obtain relative cleanliness again. No method of hand disinfection will do it at one operation.

Hand Sterilization.—*Fürbringer's Method.*—Pare the finger-nails and remove subungual dirt with a dull instrument. Scrub for five to ten minutes in very hot water with green soap. Soak hands in 65 per cent. alcohol one minute. Soak in bichlorid 1 : 1000 three minutes. Mercuric iodid is a newer mercury preparation said to injure the hands less than bichlorid and to be as strongly germicidal. The author uses bichlorid first and then alcohol.

Ahlfeld's Hot-Water-Alcohol Method.—Pare finger-nails and remove subungual dirt. Scrub with soap and hot water for three to five minutes; scrub in 95 per cent. alcohol three to five minutes, using a square of flannel in which the hands are wrapped until ready to examine or operate.

While, scientifically, it is impossible absolutely to sterilize the human skin, for practical purposes any one of the above methods, if conscientiously carried out, and providing the hands have not recently been soiled with virulent septic matter, will prove safe to the patient.

For absolute assurance against carrying infection the accoucheur should always wear rubber gloves in his practice, and these have the further real advantage that, to a great extent, they spare the skin of the hands from the corrosive action of antiseptics. The preservation of a smooth hand with well-groomed finger-nails is an essential item of an aseptic surgical technic. The frequent scrubbings and applications of corroding antiseptic solutions will ruin the skin of the hands, and make them harder and harder to sterilize. Other advantages of the gloves are: they prevent the finger-nails from scratching the softened and delicate mucous membrane; they render the examination less painful and distasteful to the woman —the gloves appeal to her sense of the esthetic; finally, besides preserving the hands, the gloves reduce the dangers of infection of the accoucheur by syphilis, pus, etc.

The possibility of injury to the gloves is the only real objection to their use, but this is reducible to a negligible minimum by proper technic. In the first place, the accoucheur must consider every puncture of the glove an error in technic, and throughout the operation must strive to avoid it. After each operation all concerned in it should publicly test the gloves and make note of the number of punctures. Then, too, the operator should dispense, as far as possible, with instruments that are sharp or have teeth—for example, fork retractors, bullet forceps, tenacula. The author, with this point in mind, has had dull instruments made to replace the rat-tooth tissue forceps, the vulsellum forceps, and the rat-tooth artery forceps. The ends of the scissors are blunt, and points, where necessary, are protected as much as possible. As a result of these and other precautions nearly every labor, and many operations—even craniotomy—are performed without injury to the gloves.

An important factor is the use of dry sterile gloves. If the gloves are drawn on over the wet hand, they macerate the skin, favor perspiration, and, if punctured, allow the accumulated secretions to escape readily. The dry glove has not these objections. The puncture of one finger does not communicate with the others, and the amount of secretion that escapes is negligible. In summer the author places a strand of gauze in the palm of the hand, leading it up to the sleeve of the gown at the wrist, as a capillary drain for the sweat. Further, *it is always understood that the hands are habitually kept free from infection and are carefully sterilized before putting on the gloves.* Without gloves, perspiration and scraped-off epithelium from two hands get into the wound; with intact gloves, neither escapes; with a few punctures, only a small portion escapes, and the chances of infection certainly are less than with the bare skin.

White duck trousers and a sterile gown are recommended for wear during normal delivery and obstetric operations. For the hours of waiting, the accoucheur is cleanly attired in a white duck coat. Street dirt and contagion are thus kept from the confinement bed. The head-piece shown in Fig. 780 is used by the author in all obstetrical operations and even normal deliveries. The author believes that spitting upon the puerperal wounds and the sterile instruments, etc., as unavoidably occurs during speaking, is a common cause of infection, and scales of dried mucus may fall out of the nose onto the sterile field.

Without doubt the physician carries the greatest danger of infection to the confinement room. The germs in the air, in the bed-clothes, in the patient's garments, even those of the vulva, may be the same in name as those he brings with him, but the former are not virulent, as they usually have been living a saprophytic existence. The physician comes in daily contact with infectious diseases, pus, and erysipelas cases, and his person, clothes, and especially his hands may carry highly virulent organisms. He or the nurse may have sinus or other infection and be an actual "carrier." MacGregor and Meleny have proved that a healthy person may disseminate puerperal and wound infections as throat carriers.

That everything introduced into the vagina should be absolutely sterile requires no mention. The author does not carry already sterilized instruments to the case because, to insure permanent sterility, the containers must be hermetically sealed, which is impractical. Gauze and sponges in glass jars can be thus carried. Instruments are boiled in 2 per cent. soda, borax, or lysol solution, in a tightly covered vessel, for twenty minutes just before they are to be used.

The Asepsis of the Patient.—Using culture-media very favorable to its growth Krönig and Pankow have shown that the Streptococcus pyogenes exists in 75 per cent. of the vaginas of pregnant women and in nearly all puerperæ. Walthard found pathogenic bacteria in 27 per cent. of the vaginas of pregnant women, and these bacteria could be made virulent by proper cultural methods. Logan found 35 per cent. streptococci. Albert in 1929 claims that even the uterus at term is

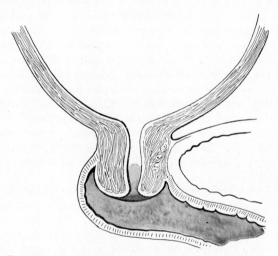

Fig. 295.—Diagram of Cervix Showing the Infected Zones.
The mucus is believed to be bactericidal. The worst infected area is the vestibule and vulva, the degree diminishing according to the red in the diagram.

infected in 50 per cent. of women. This is not proven but we know the cervix, the vagina, the vestibule, and the vulva are always infected with non-pathogenic and pathogenic bacteria. Why does not every woman in labor become infected? Why does not "auto-infection" occur more often? Auto-infection means the development of sepsis during the puerperium from germs which existed somewhere in the woman's person at the time of labor. Its existence was recognized by Semmelweis, later denied by many authorities, but recently admitted as possible, but of great rarity, by the majority of students of the subject. The reasons for the rare appearance of infection are: the parturient has developed local and general immunities against the germs which have made the vagina their habitat; the process of labor is a continual scouring out from above, the flow of the liquor amnii, the progress of the child and the placenta, the running of blood, all from above downward, all oppose the upward wandering of the vaginal bacteria; the vaginal mucus has slight bactericidal properties due partly to lactic acid the result of the action of the vaginal bacilli on the glycogen of the epithelium; the bacteria have a low virulence during labor, acquiring invasive properties only after the third day postpartum, but by this time the puerperal wounds are protected by granulations. (See p. 898.)

Let the natural immunities be broken down, as by severe hemorrhage, shock, eclampsia, etc., or let a new virulent bacterium be introduced; let the accoucheur in his manipulations carry too many of the vaginal bacteria up into the uterus (a procedure not entirely avoidable), or let him, by his operations, bruise and mutilate the parts too much, or let him break up the protective granulations above referred to, and the germs will rapidly invade the system, producing a disease known as "puerperal infection," termed by the older writers "child-bed fever."

The asepsis of the patient, therefore, consists mainly in the preservation of her immunities by sustaining her strength, procuring a normal course of labor, avoiding the necessity for operative interference, and conducting these with the least possible amount of damage. By restricting the vaginal examinations, and conducting the labor by external and rectal examination and observation of its course, we avoid carrying the infective material present in the vagina into the tissues. Rigid asepsis and antisepsis will prevent the access of bacteria from without.

In brief, the two main principles are: Limit the number of the puerperal wounds, and, second, prevent infection of the unavoidable puerperal wounds.

How to carry out these principles will occupy our attention throughout all the chapters devoted to the practical application of the science of obstetrics.

The Antepartum Bath.—As generally practised, the preparatory bath given in a tub is dangerous, because the wash-water, with the diluted soil from the body, gets into the vagina. Bacteriologic proof is not necessary to convince one of this fact. Any woman who has had children will know that the water of her bath frequently gains entrance to the vagina. Stroganoff has shown that the morbidity of the maternity in St. Petersburg has improved since the shower was substituted for the tub-bath, and the author recommends the shower in the antepartum preparation. First, the pubic region is carefully shaved, as for a gynecologic operation. A safety razor is best for this purpose. Then the whole body is scrubbed with soap and water. The person is then showered with lukewarm water, after which the pudendal region is again scrubbed with soap and hot water, using a wash-cloth (no stiff brush), and paying especial attention to the folds around the clitoris. Accumulated smegma is removed with olive oil, albolene, or soft soap. After the soap has been rinsed off, the region from the ensiform to the knees is liberally sponged with 1 : 1500 bichlorid of mercury, again paying especial attention to the pudenda. In preparing the genitalia for labor, extraordinary care must be observed not to allow soapy water, hair, or detritus to get into the vaginal orifice. This may be more dangerous than omitting all preparation.

At the Chicago Lying-in Hospital we made clinical experiments with 50 per cent. tinctura iodi and 4 per cent. mercurochrome preparation of the external genitals and compared them with bichlorid washings. The impression gained is that the essential part of the technic is to keep the vaginal orifice free from contamination. For details see author's Obstetrics for Nurses.

Before the bath is given, a colonic flushing of soapy water is administered, and the patient empties her bladder. After the bath, the patient is thoroughly dried with a sterile towel, dressed in sterile night-dress and stockings, with clean slippers and house dress, and conducted to the confinement room.

The Antepartum Douche.—Since germs with virulent possibilities are naturally present in the vaginas of parturients, it would seem wise to disinfect the vagina as we do before gynecologic operations. Theoretic consideration and practical experience, however, show that attempts to sterilize the vagina before labor invite the infections we seek to avoid. The scrubbing of the vagina and cervix robs the softened mucous membrane of its protective mucus and epithelium; the strong chemical antiseptics kill the delicate cells before they affect the bacteria. All that the treatment does is to remove some of the germs and the secretions, and within a few hours afterward the germs are as numerous as before. The tissues, however, have sustained permanent injury, and their natural immunities have been reduced. Experience in the Leipzig clinic under Menge, in parallel cases, treated with and without vaginal antisepsis, has shown a higher morbidity in the former class. Mayes of Brooklyn reduced his puerperal morbidity 40 per cent. by vaginal instillations of 4 per cent. mercurochrome. We tried these for two years at the Chicago Lying-in Hospital and our morbidity rose. Now we have discarded mercurochrome and returned to bichlorid and lysol solutions.

Further, it is as little possible to sterilize the vagina as it is to sterilize the skin. The author does not use antiseptic vaginal douches as a routine. Before opera-

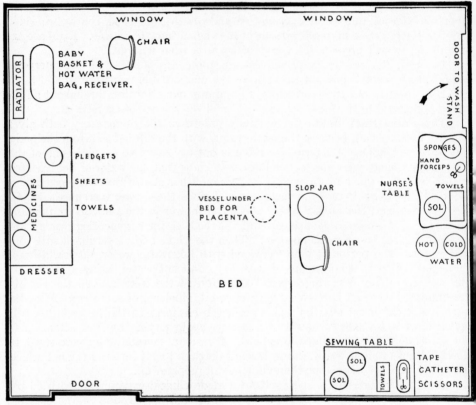

FIG. 296.—DIAGRAM OF ROOM PREPARED FOR CONFINEMENT.

tions, just before introducing the hand, the vagina is liberally flushed with 1 per cent. lysol solution squeezed from pledgets of cotton, the idea being to reduce the amount of infectious matter unavoidably carried into the puerperal wounds and up into the uterus by the manipulations. (See p. 947.)

Under Asepsis of the Patient may be mentioned abstinence from coitus during the last month of pregnancy. The danger of such a bestial practice is a real one. We have had four fatal cases. In one the procedure ruptured the membranes, the infant was born as the medical attendant entered the room. In another the patient acquired an acute gonorrhea ending in peritonitis.

Asepsis of the Environment.—The room selected for the confinement should be light, airy, with good plumbing, and may not have been recently used for a septic case. The air in the ordinary home does not contain any virulent bacteria, but this cannot be said of general hospitals admitting pus cases, pneumonia cases, and tonsillitis patients into the same wards with maternity patients. That under these circumstances puerperal infection may originate has been amply demonstrated to the author. The maternity case should be in a part of the general hospital absolutely isolated from the rest of the wards; best, in a detached pavilion of its own as the older obstetricians always taught and as new ones are learning.

The confinement room should be cleared of all unnecessary and of upholstered furniture. Heavy hangings, dust accumulators, and rugs should be removed before actual labor has commenced. Sufficient provision must also have been made for

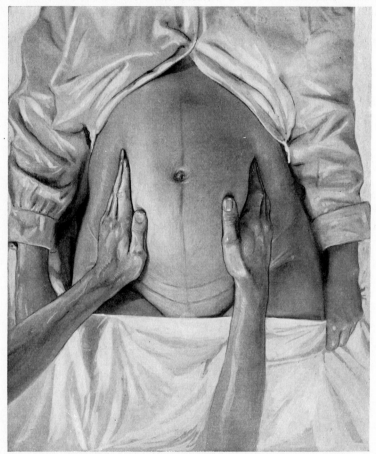

Fig. 297.—Is the Ovoid Longitudinal or Transverse?

light, especially for operations at night. The room should be conveniently arranged, some thought having been given to it. Figure 296 is an example.

The *bed*, preferably a narrow one, is moved away from the wall. Three table boards or shelves from a book-case are put under the mattress, on top of the spring, to give it a table-like character, and to prevent sagging in the center. The mattress is covered with a long rubber cloth; over this comes a sheet; at the middle of the bed is put a small rubber protector, and over this a sterile sheet, folded once, and all securely pinned with safety-pins. If the patient has no rubber sheeting, the mattress is covered with five layers of clean newspapers, and these also substitute the small rubber sheet under the buttocks. Sterile newspapers are easily procured, and they may be used in many places instead of sterile towels. A large bundle may be baked in the oven like a loaf of bread. The dresser, side-tables, and chairs on which the solution basins are laid are to be covered with newspapers.

To carry the solution basins, instrument tray, and pile of sterile towels, the ordinary sewing-table serves admirably, additional table room being obtained by means of the ever-present bridge table. The table from the kitchen or a strong library table is used for all operations. With a degree of effort and forethought the conditions of the lying-in hospital delivery room may be successfully imitated. The delivery has become an operation and the technic of the laparotomy has been adapted to it with but few alterations.

The First Examination.—On entering the lying-in chamber the accoucheur notices minutely the general appearance of the parturient, the frequency and strength of the pains; HE INQUIRES IF SHE HAS OTHER SUFFERING

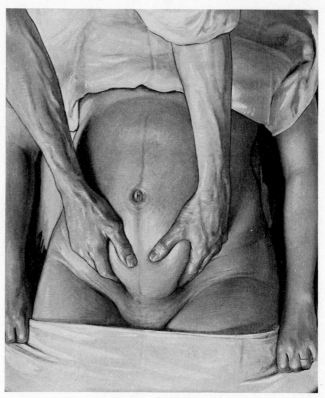

Fig. 298.—What is Over the Inlet?

THAN THE PAIN OF LABOR, takes the pulse, and later the temperature. It is not always necessary to proceed to the examination at once; the first few minutes may be devoted to general observations unless the indications point to a quick delivery. The accoucheur then takes off coat and cuffs, rolls sleeves above the elbow, washes the street-dirt off his hands, cleans his finger-nails carefully, scrubs his hands and forearms vigorously with soap and hot running or frequent changes of water for five minutes by the clock, then puts on a sterile gown. The nurse in the meantime prepares the patient for the external examination, bringing her near the side of the bed, uncovering the abdomen, but covering the limbs and chest with a sheet and a towel. The physician dries and warms his hands and proceeds with the abdominal exploration. Five questions must be answered: (1) Is the woman pregnant? (2) How many children has she had? (3) Is she at term? (4) Is she in labor? (5) Complete diagnosis of the case. The first three questions will have been answered by the pregnancy examinations unless the

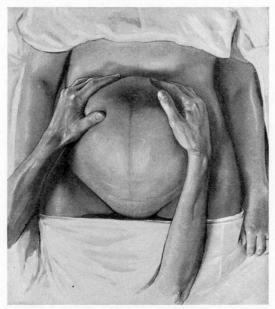

FIG. 299.—WHAT IS IN THE FUNDUS?

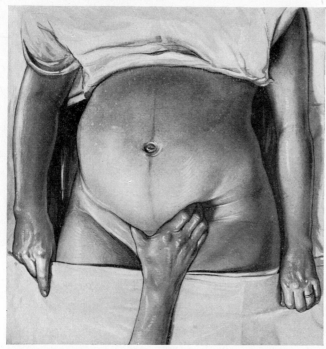

FIG. 300.—GRASPING HEAD WITH ONE HAND IN O.D.P. THUMB SINKS DEEP TO OCCIPUT. FINGERS STRIKE FOREHEAD (GREATER CEPHALIC PROMINENCE) OVER LEFT RAMUS PUBIS. OFTEN THE CHIN CAN BE DISTINCTLY FELT.

physician is first called during labor, but let a warning be sounded not to take too much for granted, but to proceed on the safe grounds of a careful physical objective examination. Is the woman in labor? The regular character of the pains, the hardening of the uterus, the show, the proved rupture of the membranes, and the findings on internal examination will determine this point; but labor may cease, even after partial or complete dilatation of the cervix, and pregnancy continue for days or weeks. The pains cease, the os closes, and the incident is called a "false alarm." False pains are painful uterine contractions occurring during the latter part of pregnancy, not followed by dilatation of the cervix or the appearance of a show. They often attend lightening, may occur at night, not seldom repeat, and may summon the physician and nurse on a fruitless errand. A warm bath and an enema or a dose of bromid will dispel them.

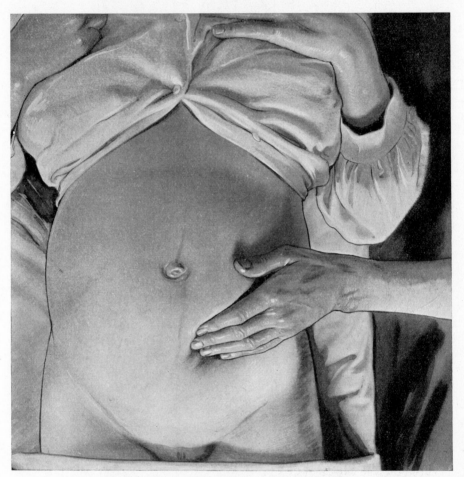

Fig. 301.—Palpating the Anterior Shoulder in O.L.T.

The **diagnosis of position and presentation** by abdominal examination was first developed by Pinard, and has since been amplified by many authors. One should have a certain plan, which, if followed, will lead to accurate results and prevent omissions. After noting the size and shape of the uterine tumor, the following four questions are answered: (1) Is the uterine ovoid longitudinal or transverse? (2) What is over the inlet? (3) What is in the fundus? (4) Where is the back?

1. *Ovoid, longitudinal, or transverse?* The hands are laid on either side of the belly, and the uterine tumor straightened between them, thus easily determining if the fetal and uterine ovoid lies parallel with the long axis of the mother or not.

If it is parallel, the presentation is either head or breech; if not, we are dealing with an oblique or a transverse presentation (Fig. 297).

2. *What is over the inlet?* The two hands are gently pressed into the inlet of the pelvis from the iliac fossæ. If they find a hard, ball-shaped body, it is the head. If they come almost together above the inlet, it means, first, that the head is very high, not having begun to engage; or, second, that the breech lies over the inlet and

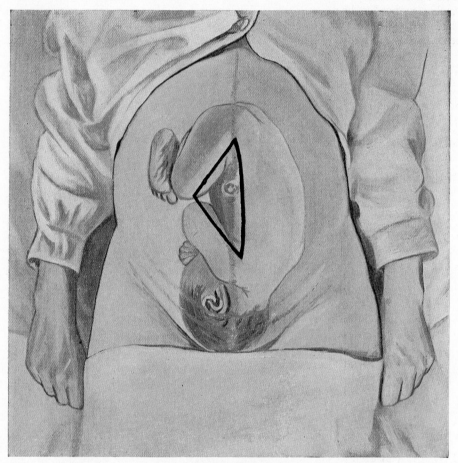

Fig. 302.—Fetal Triangle.

Four fingers of the right hand are laid in the broad base of the triangle and feel the side of the fetus. Pushing upward the thigh is felt, and downward, the arm.

is likewise pushed up; or, third, that there is no part over the inlet, the shoulder presenting and not being engaged. If the fingers come together on a soft, irregular body, it is the breech in the process of engagement (Fig. 298).

3. *What is in the fundus?* The two hands are laid on the fundus uteri, the examiner now facing the mother. In the other maneuvers his back was toward her face. Attempting to grasp the object in the fundus between his two hands, he determines its hardness and shape, and differentiates between the hard, round head and the softer, irregular breech. It is often easy to feel the genital crease, the crests of the ilia, and the small extremities of the child (Fig. 299). If he finds the fundus pushed to one side or full of small parts, he suspects transverse presentation or uterus unicornis.

4. *Where is the back?* The location of the back is determined by laying the

hands on the belly, as for the first maneuver, and pressing alternately inward toward the navel with them. The back offers more resistance, allows the hand to be pressed in less, and can usually be felt as such.

Having thus mapped out the child, one proceeds to the finer diagnosis of the position and attitude. The head is studied first. Two hands press downward toward the linea innominata. The occiput lies deeper in the pelvis; it is flatter than the forehead, nearer the middle line, and harder to outline. The forehead is reached sooner by the advancing hand, is angular, further from the middle line, and easier outlined. Having thus located these two points, the position of the head becomes clear. In case of flexion the forehead forms the greater cephalic promi-

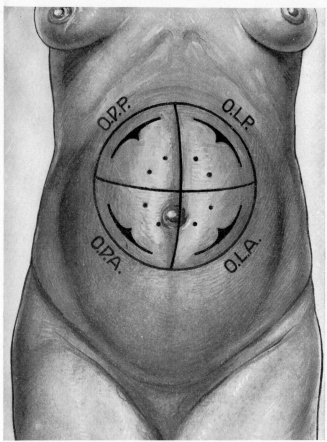

Fig. 303.—The Four Fundal Segments, Showing the Position of the Breech in the Four Positions of the Head.

nence. When the head is deflexed the occiput is more prominent. In partial deflexion the two portions of the head stand out equally. Another method, by a single grasp to palpate the head, is illustrated in Fig. 300. An expert diagnostician may often, with this one grasp, diagnose the presentation, position, and degree of engagement of the head. One determines the position of the head in the pelvis by the relation of the occiput and the forehead to the inlet. If the forehead is felt to the right side behind, and the hand, to reach the occiput, sinks deeply behind the left ramus of the pubis, the position is O.L.A. If the forehead or chin is over the left pubic ramus, it is O.D.P. Another method of determining position is by locating the shoulder. One hand passes upward from the rounding of the head and comes to rest on a soft prominence—the shoulder. If this is in the median line or to the right of it, when the back is on the left side, the position is O.L.A.; if to the left of the median line, the position is O.L.T. or O.L.P., and correspondingly when the back is on the right side. Passing upward the hand feels a triangular space (Fig. 302) made by the side of the baby's trunk—the thigh above and the arm below. Still another method of determining the position of the head in the pelvis is the study of the relation of the feet to the breech and the breech to the quadrants of the fundus (Fig. 303). Careful study of the subject has convinced the author that the breech and trunk very closely follow the movements of the head, so that, for example, if one finds the breech in a position which it would occupy in O.L.P., the head will lie in this position, and, by definitely outlining the breech, one may deduce the position of the head. The fundus is marked out with a circle and divided into four quadrants. If the breech, with the small parts, is found in the left anterior quadrant, the position is occipitolæva anterior, O.L.A.; if in the right posterior quadrant, the head is O.D.P. Gauss follows the mechanism of labor by palpating the chin above the pubis.

The Engagement of the Presenting Part.—What is the degree of engagement? Where does the head stand?—a most important question, which must be answered several times in every labor. (1) Place the two hands on the head, as in Fig. 298, and try to move the head—or breech—from side to side. If movable, the part is not engaged. (2) Note how much of the head can be felt above the inlet, using the pubis as a landmark. If only the forehead is palpable, and that on deep pressure, the head is well engaged. Other information is obtained on internal examination.

The Location of the Placenta.—In a few instances this may be discovered at this time, though, except in cases of placenta prævia and cesarean section, the information is of little value. The placental site has a boggy feel, the parts underneath are less sharp, and sometimes, if the abdominal wall is thin, one may see a somewhat circular groove on the uterus. When the placenta is on the anterior wall, the round ligaments are pushed to the sides, and when the organ occupies the posterior wall, the round ligaments converge on the front of the uterus (Figs. 102 and 103, p. 84) (Leopold and Bayer). There are no auscultatory signs which may be used in locating the placenta in the uterus. In cases of toxemia palpate especially gently to avoid abruptio placentæ.

The round ligaments, their course, thickness, tenseness, and tenderness, should be studied and noted.

Now the pelvis is measured, unless this has been done before labor (see p. 252), and an opinion is to be formed of the amount of resistance the child will meet. This comprehends the palpation of the child and the formation of a mental picture of its size, also fetal mensuration. It is a good plan to write down the probable weight of the child, to gain experience in estimating.

The presence of tumors in the uterus or abdomen, ascites, tympany, excessive or unusual tenderness, should all be noted. One may feel the umbilical cord coursing over the fetal back or around its neck; also feel unusual fetal movements, as hiccups and gasps; or may determine a fetal anomaly, as hydrocephalus, twins, etc.

Auscultation.—It is better to make the diagnosis of presentation and position by abdominal palpation, and confirm it by locating the fetal heart, than to rely on the location of the tones to give the former information, because there are vagaries in the transmission of the heart-sounds which may mislead. Fig. 227, p. 209, shows the location and course, during labor in O.L.A., of the fetal heart-tones, and Fig. 229 the same in O.D.P. As labor progresses, the child advancing and rotating, the point of greatest intensity of the heart-sounds comes anteriorly and sinks, until, when the head is distending the perineum, the sounds will be best heard just over the pubis. The auscultation of the fetal heart gives invaluable information as to the life and condition of the child. Normally, the rate is 120 to 150 a minute, and the beat is regular and rhythmic. Any slowing below 120, or increase above 160, is suspicious of danger threatening the infant, as also is irregularity of the beat or

20

lack of the normal rhythm. (See p. 869.) The fetal heart action should be studied every half-hour during the first stage of labor, and every three to five minutes, or even continuously, in the second stage, for the purpose of early discovering any danger which may beset the infant in utero. One may hear the funic souffle, especially if the cord lies over the fetal back or is coiled around the neck, and, if it is found, still greater caution is required.

Finally, the observer studies the uterine contractions, noting their character, frequency, and strength. The uterus is the engine of delivery, and the physician, as does the engineer, must know the power of the machine that does the work. Too little power, too much power, great power against great resistances—all such problems must be solved by the obstetrician during his observations.

Frey of Zürich judges the course of the labor and its normality by counting the labor pains, and Dodek and Crodel try to measure the strength of the pains with an external tokodynamometer, but practical results are not yet available. It is a step forward.

The main points in the abdominal examination are:

1. Accurate diagnosis of presentation and position.
2. Determination of the degree of engagement.
3. Condition of the child in utero.
4. Character of the uterine action. The power.
5. Consideration of the pelvic measurements and determination of the size of the child, and the kind and amount of resistance the latter will meet in its passage through the pelvis. The weight and resistance.

A large number of labors can be conducted by means of the information gained by abdominal examination alone, but often we need more, and this will be furnished by rectal exploration. In rare cases, and these are usually pathologic, one will have to resort to vaginal examination, but this method is restricted to a minimum because of the danger of infection, which is a real danger in spite of the employment of the most rigid aseptic technic.

For a complete obstetric diagnosis we wish to take the internal pelvic measurements, to confirm or correct the diagnosis of position and presentation, to determine the degree of effacement and dilatation of the cervix, the rupture of the bag of waters, the station of the head, etc., etc. Also, the accoucheur wishes to know if labor is so far advanced that he must stay at the bedside of the parturient.

All these points, except the pelvic measurements, can usually be obtained by rectal exploration and vaginal examinations are only exceptionally required. The author conducts all normal deliveries entirely without vaginal examination.

The Rectal Examination.—In 1893 Ries and Krönig recommended rectal instead of vaginal examinations in labor, but they obtained no recognition, and it was not until the employment of rubber gloves became general that it was possible to evoke any interest in the matter. The author has employed the rectal exploration for many years, mainly to determine the advancement of the head in the pelvis, but increasing experience is proving that it has a much wider field of usefulness. Smellie used rectal examination in 1750 (Krönig).

During pregnancy and especially in labor, the sphincter ani and levator ani soften and become more dilatable, both of which conditions permit one to insert the finger without causing pain. Indeed, after the head has engaged in the pelvis, the sphincter relaxes readily under pressure and later in labor the anus is patulous. The rectovaginal wall is so soft that it is easily compressed and the outlines of the cervix, the amount of its dilatation, and the presenting part are discernible. Furthermore, after the head has engaged, the examination gives more accurate results because the parts to be palpated may be steadied against the hard calvarium. In breech and face presentation the diagnosis is possible, but not so easy. After the cervix is thinned and dilated one can readily distinguish the cranial sutures or other landmarks on the presenting part, which enables us to diagnose its position.

The spines of the ischia are felt without difficulty, and thus the degree of engagement is determinable—this even better than by vaginal examination. Since the examination is practically painless and with a minimum of danger of infection, it may be repeated frequently, and thus the dilatation of the cervix, and the downward progress of the presenting part may be accurately followed.

With a little practice the pouting of the bag of waters can be felt, but if any doubt about the rupture of the membranes exists it cannot be settled by rectal

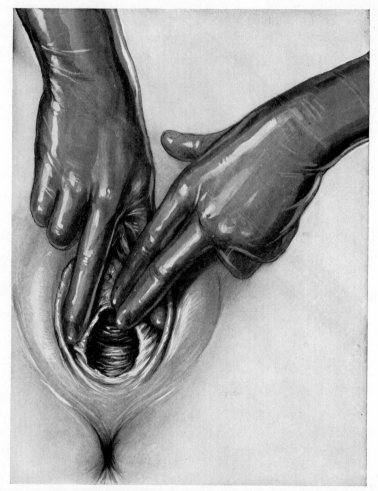

Fig. 304.—Fingers Entering Vagina from Above, to Avoid Contamination from Perineum and Anus.

touch alone. While one can form an idea of the size and shape of the pelvic cavity, the author does not trust the rectal examination for this purpose.

Breech, face, shoulder presentations, prolapse of the cord, of the extremities, placenta prævia, tumors blocking the pelvis, the advance of a colpeurynter through the cervix, abortion in progress—all these and more may be diagnosed by rectal examination. Indeed, the author has assisted labor by rotating the posterior occiput to the front, and by pushing up the forehead to aid flexion. Another advantage of the rectal method is, the finger cannot tear the cervix by premature attempts to dilate it, which injury results in chronic inflammation.

The hands should be washed and dried and *a sterile rubber glove* drawn on, the index-finger being coated with sterile vaselin or tragacanth jelly. Great gentleness is practised to avoid bruising the tender rectal mucosa. The presenting part may be pressed down on the examining finger by the hand from the outside. The examination should be conducted in the same manner as the vaginal, about to be described, and the points elicited in the same sequence.

Vaginal Examination.—The nurse is requested to drape the patient for the internal examination. This is always conducted by sight. The patient lies on her back, near the edge of the bed, but if she is very fat, and where the diagnosis promises to be difficult, she is best placed across the bed, or even on a table, in the lithotomy position. A sheet covers her person, the ends being twisted around the legs, leaving the genitalia exposed. Antiseptic solutions are prepared on a table near the bed—1 : 1500 bichlorid of mercury and 1 per cent. lysol, each basin

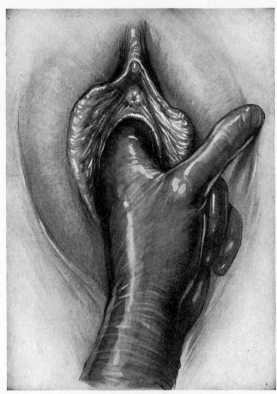

Fig. 305.—Fingers Inserted, Elbow Sunk, to Allow Finger-tips to Point Toward Umbilicus.

containing a good supply of cotton pledgets or gauze sponges. The hands are again scrubbed for five minutes in running water or frequent changes, soaked for a minute in 70 per cent. alcohol, and then for one minute in 1 : 1500 bichlorid. Since the genitalia have already been disinfected, in the primary preparation of the patient the physician needs only to liberally sponge the labia and introitus with lysol solution, then with the bichlorid, and again with the lysol solution, leaving a piece of cotton soaked in the latter lying in the vulvar canal. He now washes his hands again in the bichlorid solution, dries and powders them, and draws on his sterile rubber gloves. The talcum powder, which coats the gloves during sterilization, is washed off in the two antiseptic solutions, and then two fingers of the left hand— taking care to touch nothing on the way—are carried to the vulva, removing the bit of cotton left there. Then, separating the labia widely with the index and middle finger of the other hand, the two fingers enter the vagina, passing at once deeply into the canal, after which the labia are allowed to come together on the examining fingers (Fig. 304). Great care is to be employed to avoid the anal region, the fingers coming in contact only with the mucous membrane of the introitus vaginæ, and the inside of the two sterile fingers spreading the labia. These fine details are given because of the importance, as regards the dangers of infection, of the internal examination, and because it is so difficult to avoid carrying bacteria from the surface into the vagina and uterus.

Each and every examination is to be conducted with the same care. Six points are to be determined during vaginal exploration, and the laws of asepsis demand that they be made in a certain order:

1. *The Degree of Effacement and Dilatation of the Cervix.*—The fingers pass quickly to the cervix, noting its consistence and size, whether the external os is open, or the cervical canal shortened or effaced. The varying degrees of effacement and dilatation have been described and illustrated on pp. 127–132. One will speak of the cervix being effaced and the os admitting three or four fingers, or as being the

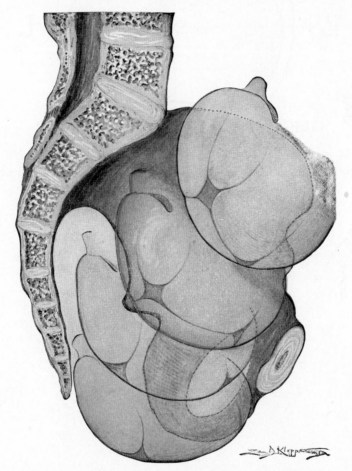

FIG. 306.—SHOWING THE HEAD IN FOUR DEGREES OF ENGAGEMENT.
The red shows the head just fully "engaged," the first "not engaged," the lowest "at the outlet."

size of a quarter, etc. The author prefers to use metric terms, saying the os is two, three, or more centimeters across, and sketches the shape of the cervix on the labor record.

Occasionally one will find the cervix partly effaced, much softened, or even somewhat dilated, without there having been many uterine contractions. This is called "insensible labor," and is very welcome in operative cases.

2. *Has the Bag of Waters Ruptured?*—The answer is usually easy, but may present great difficulty. If the membranes are of watch-crystal form, one feels a tense membrane, a short distance below the head, during a pain. In the interval this membrane is relaxed. If the membranes are pressed tightly against the head like a cap, it may be possible, by pushing the head up a little, to notice liquor amnii

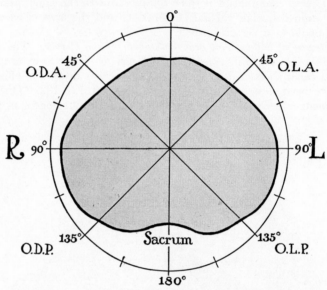

Fig. 307.—Diagram to Illustrate the Degrees of Rotation in Degrees of the Circle.

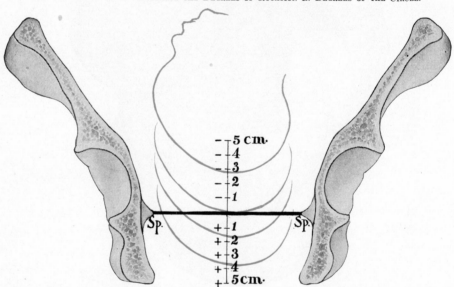

Fig. 308.—Designating the Station or Degree of Engagement of the Head by Centimeters Above or Below the Interspinous Line.

flowing down between the bag and the head, and no fluid will escape alongside the fingers. A practised touch will be able to distinguish between the smooth chorion or amnion, and the rough, hairy scalp. An attempt to wrinkle the scalp with the fingers, or catch a lock of hair between them, if successful, will show that the membranes are ruptured, and the head, when pushed up, will allow liquor amnii to flow into the hand. The discharge of liquor amnii, of vernix caseosa, or flakes of meconium will clinch the diagnosis. In doubtful cases the vagina may be opened by broad specula or the fingers, and the presence of the membranes over the head determined by sight. The bag of waters may rupture in two places— the first time high up, the second over the os; and there may be two bags, as in twins, or there may be an accumulation of liquid between the amnion and chorion.

3. *The Diagnosis of Presentation and Position.*—If the external and rectal examinations have been thorough, little more is to be learned from the vaginal, except to confirm or correct. (The findings on internal examination have been described on p. 206, to which the reader is referred.) It is usually impossible to outline the sutures and fontanels through the cervical wall, but the membranes do not hinder it except during the pains. After deciding that the hard, roundish body is the head, and the occipital part—not the face or brow—the finger seeks the sagittal suture. If it is near the promontory, the head is in Naegelè's obliquity, or anterior asynclytism; if near the pubis, in posterior asynclytism; if median, it is synclytic. Following the suture, the fontanels are felt—the lozenge-shaped one is the largest, and has four sutures running to it; the Y-shaped one is the smallest, having only three sutures running to it. The angle of the Y points to the face; the obtuse angle of the lozenge points back toward the occiput. (See Figs. 196 and 197.)

The lateral fontanels may impose as the large or small, but one always finds the ear close by, and the zygomatic process with the edge of the orbit. A false fontanel will confuse the diagnosis, and its presence should always be suspected when the findings are not typical. To distinguish the sagittal suture from the lambdoid or coronary, it is to be noted that the latter two lie in strongly curved planes, the sagittal lying in a less arched surface. Certainty in defining the position of the head can almost always be obtained by these means, but in cases of doubt it is well to *search for the ear*. The position of the ear will disclose the position of the head. In the second stage, after hard labor-pains have molded the head and developed on it a caput succedaneum, the landmarks are obscured, but still discoverable; and here also recourse may be had to the ear. The tragus points to the face.

The author has often, especially in teaching the mechanics of the forceps operation, felt the need of an accurate scientific method of conveying to others the exact position, or degree of rotation, of the presenting part. The usual method, O.L.A., O.L.T., etc., is good as far as it goes. To refine this part of our art he designed the plan shown in Fig. 307. The pelvis is laid on a circle with radii marking the degrees. The pubis is 0°, the sacrum 180°. With this plan O.L.A. would be O.L. 45°; O.D.P.=O.D. 135°; O.L.T.=O.L. 90°, etc. One can thus designate every stage of rotation, *e. g.*, O.L. 15°; O.D. 110°, and the figure stated represents the arc the occiput must travel to complete anterior rotation.

4. *The Advancement of the Head Along the Birth-canal.*—By means of external and rectal examination this point can always be determined and a vaginal would not be needed if this were all we wished to learn.

The head is "floating" when it is freely movable above the inlet. It is "fixed in the inlet" when moderate pressure will not dislodge it, but its parietal bosses have not yet passed the region of the inlet.

The head is "engaged" when its greatest horizontal plane has passed the region of the inlet. In occipital presentation this is the biparietal plane, and "engagement" is shown clinically, first, by the lowest part of the head having reached the interspinous line or passed it; second, by the covering of the sacrum, two-thirds *i. e.*, the lowest part of the head has reached the third parallel of Hodge and one can hardly insert two fingers between the head and the end of the sacrum; third, by the covering of the symphysis, three-fourths, by the advancing head. The head is in the "midplane" when the lowest part of the vault lies between the tuberosities, and "at the pelvic outlet" when the two parietal bosses are passing the tuberosities. After this the head comes well down "on the perineum" and lies in the distended vagina and vulva. In order to express in understandable scientific terms the exact station of the head the author has devised this plan. A vertical coronal plane is imagined passing through the spines of the ischium. This plane is divided in centimeters and numbered, as shown in Fig. 308. The interspinous line is zero, 0. The centimeters above are minus, those below plus. If the head has reached the spines, *i. e.*, just engaged, we say the head is "engaged at 0." If it is higher, we say "not engaged, —2, —3, —4," as the case may be. If it has passed zero we say "engaged +1, +2," etc.

By first touching the top of the head and then carrying the fingers to the bony wall of the pelvis, it is easy to determine the relation of one to the other, especially if the maneuver is combined with external palpation. Too great emphasis cannot be laid on the importance of accurately defining the location or "station" of the head in the birth-canal. Before operating this information is absolutely essential. (See p. 1048.)

5. *Abnormalities.*—The finger now notes any abnormality, the presence of the cord or fetal parts in the vagina, tumors, excessive rigidity of the perineum, etc.—points which will be touched upon later.

6. *Internal Pelvimetry and Diagnosis of Spacial Relations.*—Unless the pelvis has been carefully measured before, it is done now, or a previous examination complemented. Running the fingers slowly over the bony walls, the general size of the cavity is appreciated, the size and sharpness of the ischiatic spines determined, the sacrum, coccyx, and posterior wall of the pubis and as much as possible of the linea terminalis are palpated; then the relations of the head to the pelvis, as described on pp. 765, 766, are elicited and, finally, the fingers take the conjugata diagonalis, if the head is not too low. (See p. 259, Fig. 271.)

In the first examination all these six points are to be decided, and in the order named. By going slowly and gently the patient is not hurt, and all the required information will be gained. During a labor pain one must be careful not to rupture the membranes, but it is justifiable to pass the finger-tip lightly around the os to see how much it opens during a contraction, how well the bag of waters forms, and how tense the membrane becomes, thus forming some idea of the strength of the pains. After this the fingers rest at the side of the pelvis until the pain has passed away.

The accoucheur now fills out his history sheet or card.

The author wishes to emphasize the value of the rectal examination, and its superior guarantee, over the vaginal, in regard to safety from infection. Ninety per cent. of labors can be conducted without the latter, by abdominal and rectal exploration. Where the rectal touch gives doubtful information, a condition which is rapidly overcome by practice, if the fetal heart is unaccountably irregular and in operative cases, it is necessary to invade the vagina.

The Prognosis of the Mechanism of Labor.—After all the above information is obtained the various points are weighed and considered. The size and hardness of the child are balanced against the size of the pelvis, and both compared with the labor pains—*i. e.*, the power of the engine is compared with the work it has to do. An opinion is hazarded as to the probable mechanism, and possible abnormalities of the same studied in all their bearings.

The anxious patient will now put two questions to the accoucheur. One, "Is everything right?" should always be answered in the affirmative, with a word of encouragement. In the presence of an anomaly, the husband or near relative must be informed, for the doctor's own protection, but the parturient should be spared the alarm until it is needful to interfere, when the conditions are to be gently, kindly, and with great tact explained to her.

The second query, "How long will it last?" should be answered with consummate care. If a certain hour for the delivery of the child is stated, the clock will very often contradict the statement, and the parturient will lose faith and courage.

The writer usually replies that the length of the labor will depend on the strength and frequency of the pains, but that everything is in good order.

The Attendance of the Physician.—Ideally, every labor case should be continuously attended by a physician from beginning to end. The author enjoys this privilege, having a private assistant to stay with the parturient throughout the labor. How great the advantages of such a plan are and how comforting the practice is cannot be told. It undoubtedly saves the lives of many mothers and children, and it certainly prolongs the life and usefulness of the author. If the accoucheur must leave the house, he does so only after assuring himself that the presentation and position of the fetus are good, that the pelvis and child are normal, that the cervix is dilating naturally, that the mother is not threatened with eclampsia, that abruptio placentæ and placenta prævia do not exist, and that the infant is in perfect condition. The nurse is to be instructed to listen to the child's heart-tones every half-hour, and to report at once any unusual happening. Only accurate observation of many labors will give the accoucheur that knowledge which will enable him to determine if it is safe for him to leave the parturient—and when, and for how long—and even with such knowledge he will occasionally return to find the child delivered, the pains having suddenly become very strong. In a primipara it is best to remain in the house after the cervix admits three fingers; certainly with a multipara; and, also, if the pains are very strong and progress rapid, or if the woman's previous labors have been quick.

When the physician does leave the case, he must not visit infectious diseases or touch pus while absent. It is the physician's duty, in the absence of a trained nurse, to provide sufficient sterile water, towels, sheets, etc., as well as to have in readiness the materials for an aseptic reception of the infant. In the author's work "Obstetrics for Nurses" he has set down in great detail his obstetric technic.

LITERATURE

Albert: Arch. für Gyn., 1929, vol. 138, Heft 1.—*Dodek:* Surg., Gyn., and Obstet., July, 1932, p. 45.—*Gauss:* Zentb. für Gynaek., February 19, 1927, p. 449.—*Krönig:* Arch. für Gynaek., 1925, Bd. 123, p. 542.—*Logan, W. R.:* Jour. Obst. and Gyn., Brit. Empire, 1931, vol. 38, No. 4, p. 788.

CHAPTER XXI

THE TREATMENT OF THE FIRST AND SECOND STAGES

HAVING determined that everything is in order, that the parturient can deliver herself from below, and that there is no immediate or prospective danger threatening the mother or child, the obstetrician should remind himself that *the treatment of the first stage* is one of *watchful expectancy*. His duty is to observe the efforts of nature, not to aid, until she has proved herself unequal to the task or indicates that she will prove thus. Meddlesome midwifery has cost thousands of valuable lives. Attempts to hasten the dilatation of the cervix, either manually, by bags, or by having the woman bear down, may not be made. Premature bearing-down efforts of the mother aid very little in the first stage, and tire her so that she has no strength left for the expulsive work of the second stage; further, it is distinctly harmful, since the child is forced down before the os is dilated, overstretching the broad ligaments and laying the foundation for a future prolapsus uteri. Let the parturient walk around the room, the admission of dust into the vagina being guarded against by a large sterile pad and a T-binder. She may rest at intervals in a rocking chair, or on a couch, lying on her back or on the side to which the occiput is directed—for example, in O.L.T., on her left side, to favor rotation. Frequent external and occasional rectal examinations may be made to discover the progress of labor, and the fetal heart-tones should be listened to at least every half-hour. If this were more generally practised, intra-uterine asphyxia would be more often discovered early and more children saved by rapid delivery. Eclampsia, abruptio placentæ, rupture of the uterus, and the general condition of the mother must also be in the mind of the observant accoucheur, the possibility of the former, and the changes in the latter being constantly subject for thoughtful consideration. Temperature, pulse, and respiration should be taken and recorded every four hours. If labor is protracted, the accoucheur should try to procure some sleep for the parturient. Early in the first stage morphin and scopolamin may be given, but not near or during the second stage. Exhaustion is more common than most physicians think. They do not appreciate with what misgivings and dread the young mother approaches her trial. Add to these the sufferings of the first stage, the long sleepless vigil, with insufficient nourishment, a process terminated by an ordeal of racking pain which even anesthetics cannot entirely remove, and to these, furthermore, the loss of blood in the third stage, or eventual obstetric operation—and anyone will understand why some women suffer shock after delivery, are slow in regaining strength, and occasionally remain neurasthenics for years. Crile has shown that fear and worry produce microscopic changes in the brain and may lead to postoperative shock. One of the accoucheur's prime functions is to prepare the expectant mother's mind, as well as her body, for the severe test she is to undergo, and also to support both during the process. He must study each labor to learn "not how much a woman can endure, but what she can accomplish" (R. Barnes).

Diet.—During the labor the woman will refuse nourishment, but she should be pressed to take liquids in sugary drinks, in order to preserve her strength for the final ordeal of delivery and the third stage, and to forestall acidosis. Food is essential where labor is protracted. Postpartum hemorrhage is more formidable in a weakened patient. Nausea and vomiting are occasionally troublesome and medicines have little effect on them.

The Bowels.—Every twelve hours the lower bowel should be evacuated by a salt solution enema, but no enema should be given if the delivery seems very near, because of the danger of a flood of liquid feces accompanying the birth of the infant. If feces accumulate in the rectum, obstructing delivery, a milk and molasses enema may be given. During labor both physician and nurse take precautions against contaminating the vulva with fecal discharges.

The bladder should be emptied regularly every four hours, aided, if need be, by the catheter. If filled, it forms an obstacle of delivery, inhibits uterine action, delays rotation, and predisposes to incarceration of the placenta and postpartum hemorrhage (Fig. 309).

The Rupture of the Bag of Waters.—When the accoucheur judges this is imminent, the patient is put to bed, lying on her back. After it has occurred, a rectal examination is to be made to discover the size of the cervical opening and a possible prolapse of the cord. One can also learn if the head is ready to be delivered, in which event everything is prepared for this purpose. If labor is delayed long after the dilatation of the cervix, another rectal examination is made to discover the cause, and if the membranes have not ruptured, seeming to be an obstruction to labor, they may be opened vaginally, after proper aseptic preparation. Multiparæ often have very rapid deliveries after the membranes break, wherefore it is advisable to begin the sterilization of the hands and the general preparations for the delivery earlier than in primiparous labors.

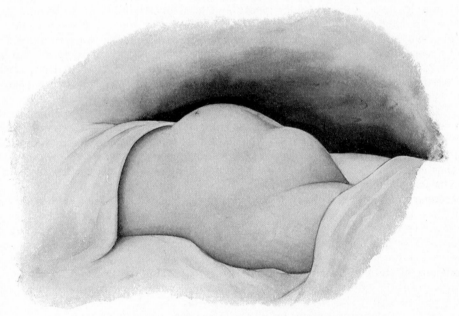

Fig. 309.—The Full Bladder During Labor.
From a photograph by Bar.

CONDUCT OF THE SECOND STAGE

Bearing-down pains do not always indicate that the second stage is begun, nor does the rupture of the bag of waters. The latter may occur before the pains start and, again, not even until after the head is visible. An experienced attendant, from the actions of the parturient, may usually decide that the cervix is fully dilated. A few particularly sharp pains, attended by a show of bright blood, usually indicate that the head is slipping through the cervix. The bed is prepared for delivery by being dressed with sterile sheets, the patient has a pair of sterile leggings or hose and a sterile night-gown put on; the table carrying the solution basins, sterile towels, sterile tape, and scissors for cord is drawn near to the bed, and the operator prepares his hands and puts on head-piece, mouth cover, and the sterile gown and gloves.

The patient often feels as if the bowels are to move, but she may not go to the closet; the movement, if any, being made on a sterile bed-pan. More often the sensation is due to pressure of the head against the rectum. Fecal particles that escape during the pressing efforts must be carefully gathered in sponges wrung out of 1 : 1500 bichlorid, and the anal region disinfected with the same solution. The bladder is emptied by catheter if necessary.

Four main points are to be considered during this stage: 1. Asepsis and antisepsis. 2. Anesthesia. 3. Protection of the life of the child. 4. Preservation of the perineum. 5. Complications, as abruptio placentæ, eclampsia, ruptura uteri. These should always be borne in mind, and will be treated under their respective headings.

Asepsis and **antisepsis** have been considered already, and will be touched upon in nearly every phase of the treatment here laid down.

Anesthesia.—It is our duty to mitigate the suffering of natural labor. We possess no drug which is without danger to either mother or child, but while striving to reduce these risks to a minimum we continually search for the perfect anesthetic. At present we are using several—ether, chloroform, nitrous oxid and oxygen, ethylene, narcylen (acetylene), morphin, scopolamin, magnesium sulphate, chloral hydrate, amytal, and regional and local anesthesia with novocain, etc. One or combinations of these drugs may be employed, and we give them in all three stages of labor, particularly the first and second, and also to varying degrees of unconsciousness. The "obstetric degree" is the use of the anesthetic to dull or relieve the pain without or with brief loss of consciousness; it is analgesia with forgetfulness of pain. The "surgical degree" is the abolition of consciousness attended by muscular relaxation.

It was formerly taught that parturient women enjoyed a certain degree of immunity against the bad effects of anesthetics, especially chloroform and ether. While this may be true to some extent as far as obstetric analgesia is concerned, it does not apply to surgical anesthesia with these drugs. Both may cause acidosis; ether causes ether bronchitis and pneumonia; choloroform affects the liver and kidneys, occasionally leading to acute yellow atrophy of the liver which resembles secondary chloroform death. It also hemolyses the red blood-corpuscles. Even nitrous oxid and ethylene produce similar changes in the blood which bear some resemblance to those of eclampsia (Stander). Sudden death from cardiac paralysis has also been reported. Littig collected 63 chloroform deaths, 5 obstetric, and condemns the drug unqualifiedly. Chloroform has another serious defect. In the presence of an open flame it is decomposed into carbonyl chlorid and hydrochloric acid, irritating gases which make the attendants cough, even poisoning them and the patient also. This may explain some deaths.

Ether is slower in action, bulkier to carry, less pleasant to take, causes more nausea and vomiting, and more is required for anesthesia, but it seems to be a little safer than chloroform for general use. It is inflammable, and one should avoid open flames.

Nitrous oxid and oxygen are giving way to ethylene when a gas anesthetic is required. This new gas, reintroduced by Luckhardt in 1922, has proved a valuable addition to our resources. One requires a skilful anesthetist, a good apparatus, a perfectly pure agent (free from CO), and extraordinary safeguards against ignition, because, when mixed with air, ethylene is highly explosive. Although Strauss has shown the coagulation and bleeding time of the blood is actually reduced under it, clinical experience is conclusive that ethylene causes increased parenchymatous oozing during cutting operations.

The uterine contractions are weakened by all anesthetics. Even under the obstetric degree the pains are weakened, are farther apart, and, contraction and retraction of the uterus in the third stage being delayed or insufficient, postpartum hemorrhage is favored. Ether acts thus to a much less degree than CHCl₃. Nitrous oxid and ethylene depress the pains very little, indeed, sometimes seem to strengthen the contractions as do the others occasionally in an indirect way. When the contractions are tumultuous or irregular, or too acutely painful, or when the woman will not bear down in the second stage because it hurts too much, an anesthetic will often calm and soothe, thereby actually hastening delivery. In pituitrin we now have a corrective for the paralysing action of all anesthetics, but only as far as the third stage is concerned.

Anesthetics affect the child. Ether and chloroform, if given for a long time, and morphin, pass over to the fetus which may be born deeply narcotised. The first two drugs also may produce an acute albumenoid degeneration of its vital organs, especially liver and heart, from which the child may die. Morphin must be given at such a time that the fetus has recovered from its effects before it is born, or at a moment when we are certain the drug will not have passed over to the child in any considerable quantity by the time it is delivered. In our experience morphin may be given up to four hours before birth, but not from then on until thirty minutes before delivery.

Ethylene and nitrous oxid and oxygen do not affect the baby very much. Asphyxiation is much less with ethylene, but it sometimes causes a bleeding tendency in the child.

Choice of Anesthetic, First Stage.—In a multipara with rapid labor it is seldom necessary to give any narcotic until the end of the first stage, when I usually give ether to the obstetric degree with a short period of complete unconsciousness as the baby's head is being delivered. Ethylene may be substituted for the ether.

With primiparæ and slow multiparæ I nearly always administer morphin (1/6 to 1/4) and scopolamin (1/200 to 1/150), or morphin and magnesium sulphate as soon as the pains are well established in regularity and strength, and the cervix 3 to 4 cm. dilated. This medication with kindly encouragement and a little suggestion (dark room, plugging the ears, etc.), a sort of medicinal hypnosis, will usually make the parturient fairly comfortable until the time has arrived to give ether or ethylene. If it does not, or if one sees the woman is suffering, Gwathmey's rectal instillation is added (Vide infra). Other drugs occasionally exhibited to alleviate the pain of the first stage are: heroin, chloral, bromid, amytal.

I have given sodium amytal by mouth and per rectum. It often fails to relieve pain, occasionally the parturient gets excited, the contractions may weaken, the babies are endangered; generally I found it inferior to morphine. Pernocton another barbituric acid derivative, used much in Germany, is said to have the same objections (Schmidt, Keller). It is not acceptable for N. N. R. of the American Medical Association, 1931. Avertin-tri-brom-ethanol, rectally, is too dangerous for routine use in obstetrics; it decomposes readily into the cauterizing dibromacetaldehyde, the placental stage may be abnormal and the margin of safety is so narrow that even the surgeons are restricting it to basal or preparatory anesthesia in combination with the inhalants. Nembutal, luminal, etc., have the same actions as amytal.

During the Second Stage.—Chloroform still enjoys some vogue, but most accoucheurs prefer ether. Nitrous oxid was gaining friends until ethylene came, and this new gas is even displacing ether for obstetric analgesia or operations where deep relaxation is not required. I use ether and ethylene, the latter more and more, especially if the patient has a cold, or is toxemic, or has goiter, nephritis, or sepsis. Ether is used when it is necessary to operate in heart disease or shock, or when uterine relaxation is required as for version or other intra-uterine manipulation. Many deliveries can be finished under local anesthesia.

Indications.—(1) Great pain at the end of the first stage or in the second stage. (2) Great excitability at these periods. (3) Tumultuous pains at any period of labor, especially if the cervix is not dilated or if the head is on the perineum, the idea being to moderate the power of the uterus and to save it, the cervix, or the perineum from rupture and the baby from injurious pressure and asphyxia. (4) To preserve the perineum when the bearing-down efforts are too strong. (5) To eliminate the inhibition of bearing down due to pain.

Conditions.—(1) Labor must be sufficiently advanced; ether is very rarely given in the first stage, best in the second. (2) The pains must be strong and regular, so as to offset the weakening effect of the drug. (3) When given simply for the relief of pain, special consideration must be given to toxemia, hepatic disease, goiter, hemophilia, and sepsis. (4) In cases of severe hemorrhage special rules apply. (See p. 853.)

Ether.—*Obstetric Degree.*—Any simple inhaler, or even a handkerchief held in the hand, will suffice. The open method is preferred, because in obstetrics the carbonization of the blood, so common in general anesthesia, must be avoided in the interests of the child. When the pain begins, 45 drops of ether are poured on the mask, and the patient takes deep breaths of the vapor; as the pain increases a few drops more are given; as the pain subsides, the mask is removed. The patient obtains relief from pain, but consciousness is not abolished. This procedure is repeated until the head is just about to escape from the vulva, when the ether is poured on frequently, and the first stage of surgical anesthesia is reached, consciousness being abolished for a few minutes, during which time the infant is delivered. Administration begins at the end of the first stage.

Surgical Degree.—Deep anesthesia is needed in obstetric practice under the same conditions as in surgery, to produce unconsciousness to pain and complete relaxation. The method of administration does not differ from that practiced in general surgery.

Ethylene Administration.—We start the inhalations toward the end of the first stage, rarely when the cervix is 7 cm. in diameter, and then only if the pains are severe. At the very beginning of the pain, diagnosed by the hand feeling the uterus harden, or from the parturient squirming a little, a few deep breaths of 50 per cent ethylene and 50 per cent. oxygen are given, and the mask is removed as the height of the pain passes. The patient does not go to sleep and does not change color. As the second stage pains grow stronger the percentages of the two gases are changed—60–40, 80–20, 90–10, but never pure ethylene. If a deeper anesthesia is necessary, a little ether vapor is added to the mixture. As soon as the head is born the administration is stopped, to be resumed when sutures are inserted. The baby is not asphyxiated unless the analgesia has been continued several hours, but experience shows one must be prepared for this complication.

Nitrous Oxid and Oxygen.—In 1800 Sir Humphrey Davy recommended N_2O for surgical operations not attended with much hemorrhage. In 1868 Edmund Andrews of Chicago suggested that oxygen be given with it. In 1880 Klikowitch of St. Petersburg recommended an 80 and 20 per cent. mixture for obstetric cases, and in 1881 v. Winckel reported favorable results in 50 deliveries. Guedel of Indianapolis in 1911, Lynch and Hoag in 1913 used this form of analgesia in normal labor. Capillary oozing is a fault common to both N_2O and ethylene, but the latter does not require partial asphyxiation to produce anesthesia.

N_2O may be given earlier than ether or chloroform, near the end of the first stage, and throughout the second. In toxemic conditions, for short, bloodless operations, like curettage, application of colpeurynters, minor perineorrhaphies, we use gas or, preferably, local anesthesia, with gas to assist. In major operations local anesthesia where possible, otherwise ether. The prolonged, deep anesthesia with gas is not safer than ether. For version, forceps, extensive perineorrhaphy, vaginal cesarean section ether is the agent of choice.

Method of Administration.—For surgical or deep narcosis the method of giving N_2O and oxygen does not differ from that employed by surgeons, and the reader is referred to appropriate text-books. Obstetric analgesia requires skill and attention to detail.

At the beginning of the second stage, and, in rare cases, toward the end of the first, the gas is started. The large inhaler is used, and at the very beginning of the pain, perceived by the hand laid on the belly, or felt by the patient, two deep breaths of pure N_2O are allowed, the next two inhalations are of a mixture of 90 per cent. N₂O and 10 per cent. oxygen, the next two of 50 and 50, then pure oxygen for three breaths—inhaler removed. At the proper time the parturient may be allowed to bear down and labor is conducted in the usual manner.

The patient must not become cyanotic, must not lose consciousness, must not complain of headache, which mean that too much N₂O has been given. Thirst is often marked, water should be allowed freely. The amount of N₂O needed varies with every patient, and this must be determined with care. The gas is given only during the pains, but more must be given as the second stage nears its end, and during the actual birth of the head deep anesthesia is produced for a few minutes. When the child is delivered the N₂O is turned off and pure oxygen given to prevent cyanosis in the baby, but how effectual this is cannot be proved scientifically. Occasionally it is necessary to change to ether for the actual delivery. Cases are recorded where this intermittent administration of the gases was kept up for ten and twelve hours, but the author is certain this is dangerous because of degeneration of the liver, maternal as well as fetal. In one case the author used gas for five hours and the patient suffered marked hemolysis, and nearly died from postpartum hemorrhage. Two to three hours are the usual requirements, but one should not continue over three hours. Contrary to experience with chloroform and ether, the uterine contractions are not weakened by gas, indeed, labor is shortened, the pains seem more effectual. Delivery may be very rapid and the patient make little or no outcry. Lacerations are not less frequent than with other narcotics. The puerperium is not affected, the child thrives as usual.

Other Anesthetics.—Anesthesia of the spinal cord, invented by Corning and elaborated by Bier and Tuffier, has recently been gaining vogue. Its dangers—respiratory paralysis, headache, vomiting, hyperpyrexia, tachycardia, muscular spasms, drug intoxication, meningitis, and peripheral necroses—are being gradually eliminated by improvement in the technic. Krönig said spinal anesthesia is dangerous in pregnancy and labor and present experience with all the drugs—stovain, spinocain, tutocain, procain—sadly confirms him. Stoeckel advised the injection of the novocain into the sacral canal, and Sellheim, blocking the pudic nerves, reaching them through vaginal puncture. Bonar and Meeker, in 1923, recommended sacral nerve block, and it seems practical for cases where general anesthesia is dangerous.

Procain is a very valuable local anesthetic, and the author uses it for obstetric and gynecologic operations wherever possible. For cesarean section it is ideal. To each ounce of ½ per cent. procain solution 3 drops of 1 : 1000 adrenalin are added. Ten ounces of this solution may be used with safety, but so much is seldom required. Local anesthesia should be used more extensively. It may be complemented by morphin and scopolamin. (See page 320.)

Hypnotism has been used in hysteric subjects, with reported good effects. Apollo was born of Latona under such influence. The writer frequently uses suggestion during labor to aid the parturient to bear the pain, and after labor gentle suggestion will aid in obtaining the quiet and restful sleep so conducive to rapid restoration of the patient's nerve equilibrium (Siemerling).

Women vary very much in their ability to stand pain and in their demands for anesthetics. One may often clean out a uterus, or repair a torn perineum without any narcotic, or just a ¼ of morphin and 1/100 of scopolamin.

Gwathmey's Synergistic Analgesia.—Dr. J. T. Gwathmey has developed at the New York Lying-in Hospital a method of analgesia to which he gave the name synergistic, because it combines the narcotic and analgesic action of several drugs—morphin, magnesium sulphate, ether, and alcohol. A small amount of quinin is added to counteract the paralysant action of the drugs upon the uterine contractions. Part of the medication is given hypodermically and part by rectal instillation. We have used this technic with some satisfaction, and have varied it to suit each case. While it is not uniformly successful in abolishing the pain of labor, and such is not the intention, most patients are much relieved and few harmful effects have as yet been reported. Occasionally the pains die down, and labor is delayed; laceration of the cervix may occur if the pains are too strong (quinin), and the narcotized patient gives no warning; rarely is the child too narcotized for easy resuscitation. Contraindications to its use are colitis, diabetes, and diseases of the ear. We do not use the rectal instillations unless the hypodermics are insufficient, *and we often omit the quinin when the uterine contractions are good and no stimulation of the pains is required.* For this reason, each case must be carefully individualized and only those drugs exhibited which are needful for the particular patient. Dr. Gwathmey has kindly permitted me to reprint his own description.

Ampules containing morphin and magnesium sulphate, magnesium sulphate plain, and the drugs for rectal instillation, already mixed, are now obtainable, but any nurse can prepare the medicines herself from the medicine closet. The rectal instillation requires care to make a smooth mixture; dissolve the quinin in the alcohol, add the ether, then the olive oil—shake well and filter through cotton. Cork tightly, keep at room temperature. Prepare two doses for each labor, the second one containing only 10 grains of quinin or none at all.

"When cervix is two fingers (1 inch) dilated, with pains three to five minutes apart, and lasting thirty or more seconds, give (1) intramuscular injection of 2 c.c. sterile 50 per cent. solution of magnesium sulphate and ¼ grain morphin sulphate. If sedation, wait until effect begins to wear off, or, if no relief within twenty minutes, repeat (2) intramuscular injection without morphin, and give by rectum the following instillation:

Quinin alkaloid	20	grains
Alcohol	45	minins
Ether	2½	ounces
Petrolatum liq. heavy (or olive oil) q. s. ad	4	"

"Twenty minutes after rectal instillation, give (3) intramuscular injection of 2 c.c. sterile 50 per cent. solution magnesium sulphate (no morphin). *The Standard Treatment is three (3) intramuscular injections and one (1) instillation.* If labor is prolonged beyond four hours from first injection, the entire technic can be repeated with safety, except that the morphin is omitted when delivery is expected within one hour.

"Apparatus: Five-ounce funnel; 20 inches rubber tubing, glass connection; French catheter, size 20 or 22; hypodermic needle, long (1½ inches); a container for 2 extra ounces petrolatum liq.

"*Details of Technic.*—1. When labor begins, give one soapsuds enema, then tap-water enemas until bowel is clean. Patient should walk to toilet when possible. Repeat tap-water enemas every eight hours. If practical, a rest of at least four hours should intervene before treatment. Catheterize if necessary.

"2. Practice perfect asepsis in injecting the morphine and magnesium sulphate. State to patient that object of injection is to relieve pain.

"*Give the intramuscular injection during a contraction.* Insert a *long* needle deep into the gluteal, deltoid, or subscapular region and inject solution *as needle is gradually withdrawn.* Avoid injecting solution into skin and subcutaneous tissues.

"Keep patient as quiet as possible. Place cotton in ears and cover eyes with some dark colored material, or with towel. If in a ward, the bed should be screened; if in a room, lower the shade, exclude light, and close door. Give only necessary attention, talking in a quiet voice and making all manipulations as gently as possible. Note time of intramuscular injection and fill out analgesic chart as labor progresses.

"3. Just before giving rectal instillation, state that object is to relieve pain. Place patient on left side, Sims' position. Apply vaselin (or oil) liberally around anus so that the ether, if expelled, will not burn. *Fill catheter and rubber tubing to funnel with warm oil in order to exclude air.* Insert gloved finger into rectum and direct catheter about 8 inches, *i. e.,* beyond fetal head (or buttocks). Lower funnel below level of anus and allow oil to return to funnel together with any gas that may be left. If unusual amount of fecal matter or water is present, allow it to drain away and refill with 1 ounce of oil, care being taken to exclude air. Now elevate funnel. As last of oil is leaving funnel, add mixture (which has been allowed to stand in warm water for a few minutes) care being taken not to admit air between oil in tube and mixture in funnel. *Finally add a sufficient amount of oil at 100° F. to make a 5- or 6-ounce mixture.* Between contractions, under gentle pressure, pass the fluid by 'milking' the rubber tube. Give the whole amount between three to five contractions. Clamp the catheter below glass connection so that no air can follow and then withdraw catheter. Make pressure on perineum with a towel for ten to fifteen minutes during contractions. Instruct the patient to breathe deeply with mouth open during contractions and to 'squeeze up' in order to induce reverse peristalsis. State that if contents are retained, there will be no pain, and thus secure co-operation. From now on the patient may be allowed to lie in the position most comfortable to her. Do not make a rectal or vaginal examination within one hour after instillation.

"4. Twenty minutes after instillation give third intramuscular injection of magnesium sulphate.

"5. A second or even a third instillation may be given at two-and-a-half-hour intervals, using only 10 grains of quinin, however. (I have found it possible to use too much quinin, endangering the child and the integrity of the cervix [author].)

"6. If an anesthetic is required when head is passing over perineum, use sparingly. No chloroform. To superimpose an anesthetic upon a partially analgetized patient is dangerous for the child (Harrar).

"7. Make full notes on Analgesic Chart."

Scopolamin-morphin Amnesia (Twilight Sleep).—Schneiderlin, a neurologist, in 1899 recommended the employment of morphin combined with scopolamin for the production of surgical anesthesia. In 1902 v. Steinbüchel recommended its use in labor. Naturally, the profession eagerly grasped this opportunity to relieve women of the pain of childbirth, and the drugs soon were extensively employed here and abroad.

The Freiburg method is as follows: After labor is well on its way, when the pains are four or five minutes apart and lasting thirty or more seconds, the first injection is made. This consists of $\frac{1}{6}$ grain of morphin and $\frac{1}{150}$ grain of scopolamin. Krönig and Gauss insist on the use of narcophin—a proprietary narcotin-morphin-meconate, and Straub's "Scopolamin Haltbar." The latter is a permanent solution of this delicate drug, purchasable in sterile ampules. Forty-five minutes after the first injection another is given, but only $\frac{1}{200}$ grain of scopolamin is used. After this the hypodermics are given every hour, using $\frac{1}{300}$ to $\frac{1}{150}$ grain of scopolamin, and, in prolonged labors, an occasional dose of morphin, $\frac{1}{8}$ grain—all depending on the individual case. The object is to maintain the patient in a state of amnesia, and this is determined by testing her memory. The room need not be fully darkened, only the patient's face should be well shaded. Quiet must be kept, and only necessary attentions permitted. Shortly after the second injection, the patient is asked if she remembers what has gone before, has she seen the nurse or intern? If she remembers, another dose is given. If not, nothing is done for an hour, when, if the mind seems to be clearer, $\frac{1}{300}$ grain of scopolamin is given. Care must be exercised that the woman does not attain full consciousness. Sleep, forgetfulness, and absence of pain are suggested to her by the environment, the actions of all the attendants, and by constant reiteration. Usually, after one and a half hours she drops off to slumber, the face reddened, the throat dry, the pupils contracted, the conjunctivæ congested, the pulse 90 to 120, the skin a little warm and dry. Food is not given, but water freely; the patient asks for attention to her wants. During the pains she moves about restlessly, or turns from one side to the other, or grunts a little, and occasionally opens her eyes —to drop off to sleep again when the pain passes. She will respond to questions, but incoherently, and often forgets to finish a sentence begun, dropping off to sleep. As the second stage draws near its end she bears down and becomes very restless. Occasionally this becomes extreme, and several nurses are required to hold her to prevent too rapid exit of the head, also to prevent her from clutching the pudenda with her hands. Her continual jactitation also disturbs the asepsis. A few whiffs of ether are often needed as the head passes through the vulva.

An acute observer will always know when the head has reached the perineum, though it requires greater watchfulness than usual. Throughout the labor, but especially in the second stage, the fetal heart-tones must be auscultated. I have found they often fluctuate decidedly, ranging from 100 to 180, but there is little cause for alarm unless they remain below or above these figures. In the second stage the irregular and slow or fast heart-beat is very much more significant and often indicates forceps. The passing of meconium is still more ominous. After delivery the child usually cries vigorously at once, but may be born in a state of apnea as one sees at cesarean sections. Mild means of resuscitation suffice, but the child may be asphyxiated or narcotized to a serious degree, requiring prolonged efforts to start respiration.

The woman wakes up from an hour to six after the birth, and has none or faint recollections of the parturition. If, however, she bends her mind to it she will recall more and more of the labor. It is best to keep up the amnesic effect by suggestion, with which much can be accomplished. Women that were noisy and intractable while under the influence of the drugs may remember nothing, while those that were quiet and apparently unconscious may remember nearly everything.

Contraindications.—Contracted pelvis of all types; inertia uteri from any cause; advanced pulmonary and heart disease; where there exists an immediate or prospective indication for the operative termination of labor, as placenta prævia, eclampsia, asphyxia in utero; where there is a known idiosyncrasy to atropin, or the first dose shows this; advanced labor (the best time is to begin from eight to four hours before actual delivery). A certain number of women will prove refractory and it would require too much of both drugs to produce amnesia. Again, the drugs may stop labor completely and must be discontinued on this account. The first stage may not be slowed but the second usually is, requiring more frequent use of forceps. It is also hard to maintain the aseptic technic as the parturient may become delirious and ungovernable.

In 1921 a revival of interest developed the fact that the fetal mortality of 2 per cent. had not been eliminated (Meyer). The danger to the child lies in the fact that morphin and scopolamin are not antagonistic in their action on the respiratory center, but cumulative and sometimes potentized, the latter especially in highly alkaline blood (Strube), and paralysis results.

In general, it may be said that the scopolamin-morphin method requires a high degree of obstetric skill aside from the ability to properly observe and conduct the seminarcosis. Therefore, (1) The drugs may not be used to produce anesthesia or insensibility to pain, only amnesia, forgetfulness or, rather, lack of appreciation of pain and slight analgesia. (2) The method is not adapted for general usage in the home, only in maternities with a sufficient and efficient staff of physicians and nurses. (3) The fetal heart-tones must be noted every five to ten minutes, during the second stage every two minutes, likewise the condition of the mother, and a capable accoucheur must always be at hand to interfere at once if need be. (4) While the life dangers to the mother can be eliminated, the patient must be willing to pay the price of possible lacerations and hemorrhage, and an occasional loss or injury of the child as the cost of her relief from suffering.

History.—Narcotic potions were administered by the ancients in labor. Theocritus mentions them as given to Antigone. Other examples are cited by Simpson. Sir James Y. Simpson was the first to use ether in obstetric practice on January 19, 1847, when he did a version and an extraction. In November of the same year he discovered the anesthetic properties of chloroform, and used it in labor cases to the exclusion of ether, and widely advocated the practice. A storm of adverse criticism against both anesthetics broke loose at home and abroad, and, to our minds, a curious and ridiculous polemic was waged between Simpson and his opponents. (See Obstetric Memoirs, Simpson, vol. ii, Anesthetics.) N. C. Keep, of Boston, was the first, according to Channing, to use ether in labor in America—April 7, 1847. The use of an anesthetic in labor spread quickly, particularly after Victoria, Queen of England, in 1853 and 1857 had enjoyed its benefits. It was called the Queen's chloroform, or *anesthesia à la reine.*

Preservation of the Life of the Fetus.

Preservation of the Life of the Fetus.—An effort should be made to reduce the infant mortality during childbirth. Even normal labor prepares dangers for the fetus and when complications occur, such as prolapse of the cord, abruptio placentæ, placenta prævia, eclampsia, breech presentation, they always compromise its life. We cannot discuss the subject in full here.

Asphyxia from interference with the placental or cord circulation is the commonest danger, and cerebral edema and hemorrhage from prolonged compression are next in frequency. Both are more likely to occur in the second stage, but our watchfulness for them, and for the other complications, must be unremitting until the baby is born.

Our only means of discovering the peril of the fetus is auscultation of its heart sounds and, therefore, it is best to deliver all women on the back so that the stethoscope may be frequently and easily employed. The head stethoscope (Fig. 288) is indispensable in obstetric practice and with it one should listen to

21

the child every thirty minutes in the first stage, and every two or three minutes in the second, and oftener if the heart tones are not of ringing quality and of proper frequency and regularity.

During normal labor the fetal heart beats 120 to 160 per minute, slowing up a little during the uterine contractions. Rates below and above these figures, irregularity or weakening should always excite suspicion and command discovery of the cause.

In general labor is to be conducted so as to prevent the natural powers injuring the child. Too strong pains should be moderated by narcotics; the bag of waters should be preserved until the second stage is well under way; and prolonged compression of the fetal brain is to be avoided.

Preservation of the Perineum.—Anatomic study of the pelvic floor after delivery always shows evidences of injury to all its structures. The connective tissue is torn in many places, the layers of fascia are loosened, the levator ani muscle lacerated more or less; the urogenital septum is always ruptured, the perineal body frequently, and all the tissues are bruised, showing larger or smaller hemorrhages and suggillations. The later results of these macroscopic and microscopic injuries are shrinking and atrophy of the pelvic diaphragm, relaxation of same, prolapse of the urethra, vagina, bladder, uterus—all depending on the extent of the traumatism. In importance these lacerations vary very much. Worst in their effects are the tears of the levator ani, the perineal ones being less harmful, and yet it is the prevention of perineal lacerations that occupies so much of the accoucheur's attention. Our best efforts are to be directed to preserve the levator ani, but some attention should be given to the perineum itself, because it has physiologic and pathologic dignity; extensive rupture of this body may cause sterility, vaginitis, cervicitis, endometritis from infection ascending through the patulous introitus; a perineal tear once started may go through the anus into the rectum, causing that great affliction—fecal incontinence; fresh tears may form the atria of bacterial invasion; the structures once torn can never be perfectly restored; finally, the injury may often be prevented, and, if not entirely, it may be limited to a safe degree. The author has found the hymen tears in all cases; 70 per cent. of primiparæ have tears of the fourchet—the so-called first-degree laceration; 25 per cent. of primiparæ and 10 per cent. of multiparæ have lacerations extending well into the perineal body, and in 10 per cent. the injury exposes the sphincter ani—the so-called second degree. Only in operative cases has a complete laceration—that is, through the sphincter ani—occurred. These percentages are larger than those given in most text-books, the reason being that the author, after the levator ani is well stretched, allows the head to issue rapidly, with a view to sparing the child's brain the traumatism of a prolonged perineal "protection." Without doubt children suffer brain injuries because of the accoucheur's anxiety to avoid perineal lacerations. The excessively slow delivery, too, has been responsible for cases of still-birth from asphyxia. (See Sellheim, 1931.)

Causation.—Rupture of the perineum may not always be prevented, even in the best hands and under the most favorable conditions. The pelvic outlet may be diseased, as by edema, excessive deposition of fat, a white-cell infiltration from syphilis, condylomata lata and acuminata, varicosities, or through lack of elasticity from scars, from previous operation, age, or constitution. In some women otherwise well the perineum tears like wet blotting-paper. A narrow pubic arch, by forcing the head back into the perineum and not allowing the occiput to crowd up close to the ligamentum arcuatum, favors rupture. A vulva situated high on the pubis is subject to injury. Necessity for rapid delivery often makes us disregard the perineum, as in breech cases and when the child is threatened with asphyxia. Delivery effected early in labor finds the perineum unprepared for the rapid dilatation. Exit of the head in unfavorable attitudes—face, brow, forehead, and in posterior rotation of the occiput—frequently causes lacerations, because the most favorable circumferences are not presented to the canal. A large child acts in the same way by overstretching the outlet.

Treatment.—Prevention of perineal lacerations naturally will proceed along lines indicated above. Here only those precautions needful in spontaneous labor will be described. How to care for the levator ani and perineum during forceps and other operative deliveries will be given in full in the proper chapters.

The levator ani and the fascia above and below it, making up the pelvic diaphragm, can be spared serious injury only by slow dilatation. While carefully watching the fetal heart-tones, the patient is not allowed to bear down overmuch during the first part of the second stage. The author does not hurry this period of labor without indication. If the pains and the bearing-down efforts are tumultuous, the woman is given ether as a moderator. While more frequent in operative deliveries, the tear in the levator sometimes occurs at the point of its attachment to the pubic rami, under the arch of the pubis. This accident may rarely be recognized before it has occurred, but if it is feared, one should incise the muscle in the right vaginal sulcus, because the high hidden tear may be impossible to sew up afterward, but the lower incision is accessible to the needle.

The principles of the protection of the perineum are two: (1) Deliver slowly, developing to the ultimate the elasticity of the pelvic floor; (2) deliver the head in forced flexion, to present to the parturient passage the smallest circumferences of the head. The first principle needs no elucidation. A hard body which has to overcome the resistance offered by an elastic cylinder will be less likely to tear the cylinder if forced through it very slowly. A brief study of the mechanism of labor will show the advantages of keeping the head well flexed until the larger part of it has escaped from the vulva. If the head were to come out in partial extension, there would be presented to the girdle of resistance, made up of the pubic arch and the pelvic floor, the occipitobregmatic, occipitofrontal, and occipitomental diameters and circumferences. If the chin is forced down on the sternum, and flexion thus maintained until the nape of the neck comes to fit closely into the pubic arch, the diameters and circumferences which have to pass the ring of the outlet are the suboccipitobregmatic, suboccipitofrontal, and suboccipitomental, which are less by 1½ to 3 cm.

Mode of Procedure.—The author has given up the practice of delivering women on the side because of the difficulty of preserving asepsis, and the inability of listening constantly to the fetal heart-tones. The illustrations of this method have been preserved because the reader can see the field better than if the patient were photographed lying on her back. The principles of the protection of the perineum, of course, are identical with the two operations.

The accoucheur, having put on head and mouth cover, and stethoscope, sterilized his hands, and donned his gown and gloves, stands on the right side of the patient, who lies on her back, the head supported by a low pillow, with her knees raised and abducted, the vulva being toward the best light. Every two or three minutes he lifts the sterile towel from the abdomen, bends his head down and listens to the fetal heart-tones. Unless the patient is bearing down too much and the head advancing too rapidly, he does not interfere by word or act until the scalp is visible to the size of an egg. The rapidity of the descent of the head may easily and safely be determined by pressing the fingers upward and inward along the ramus of the pubis (Fig. 311). One can feel the hard resistance of the presenting part if the part is low in the pelvis. The location of the anus also indicates the degree of dilatation and downward displacement of the levator ani. When the accoucheur decides that the head is coming through too fast, he asks the woman to cease bearing down, to open her mouth and breathe through it until the force of the effort is expended.

With each pain the head is allowed to come down to distend the perineum a little more.   If the pain is too strong, the head may be gently held back by evenly

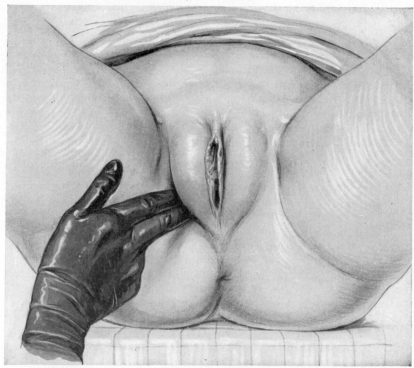

FIG. 311.—DETERMINING THE RATE OF ADVANCE OF THE HEAD BY PRESSING IN THE PERINEUM.

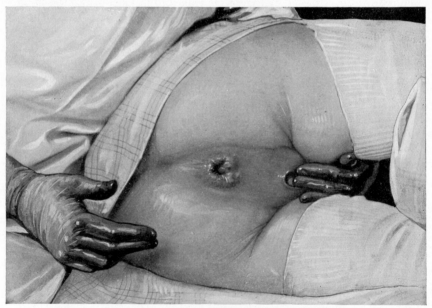

FIG. 312.—DELIVERY ON SIDE.   RESTRAINING TOO RAPID DESCENT BY GENTLE PRESSURE.
I do not recommend side position deliveries.   It is used here because it best shows the maneuvers photographically.

distributed pressure of both hands.   A word of warning against overzeal must here be given.   Many an infant has lost its life because the attendant was overanxious to deliver the woman "without stitches." The protracted second stage resulted in its loss by asphyxiation. Again, the infant may be injured by pressing on the head too forcibly, causing skull fracture, and, finally, if the uterine and abdominal efforts are violent and the child not allowed to come out, the uterus may rupture,

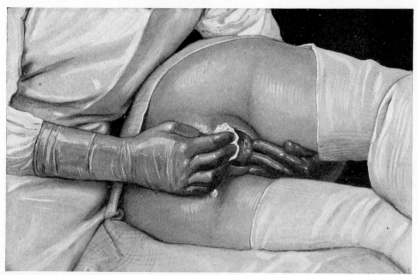

Fig. 313.—Directing the Occiput Under the Pubis by Pressure on the Head at Edge of Frenulum.

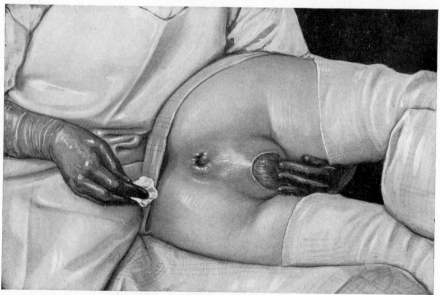

Fig. 314.—Restraining Advance, Yet, at the Same Time, Favoring Flexion. Sponge Ready to Catch Feces.

as it does under other circumstances of opposition to its powerful action. The author has seen all these injuries.

Not seldom feces and mucus are forced from the anal opening during the woman's bearing-down efforts. Since there is real danger of infection from this source, the accoucheur must collect such discharges in large cotton sponges soaked in 1 : 1500 bichlorid, using care not to soil his glove nor the region around the anus.

This region, as an additional precaution, is resterilized with both antiseptic solutions. The author has never seen any harm from the very liberal use of these antiseptics on the vulva and perineum.

In gentle fashion the head is permitted to descend until its greatest periphery stands in the distended vulva. It is now *delivered in the interval between pains.*

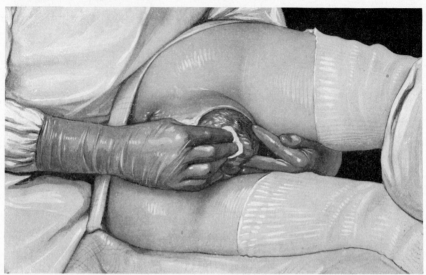

Fig. 315.—Tucking Labia Minora Behind Occiput.

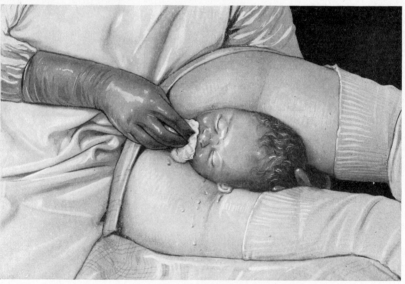

Fig. 316.—Cleansing Mouth.

The head is restrained at the height of the bearing-down effort, the woman is asked to breathe through her mouth or to cry out, while the accoucheur tucks the clitoris and labia minora behind the occiput under the pubis. By the proper administration of an anesthetic the pain of this stage is alleviated, and too violent bearing-down efforts, endangering both perineum and child, are moderated. After the pain has ceased the woman is asked to bear down, and during this effort the distended perineum is slipped back over the forehead and face under the chin, taking care that neither the hand nor the baby's face is soiled by feces issuing from the rectum.

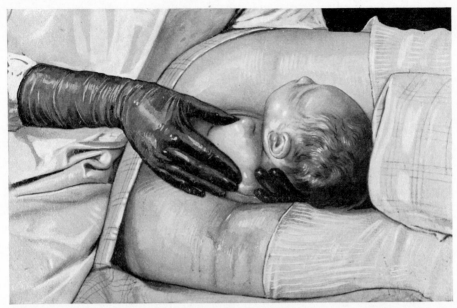

FIG. 317.—DELIVERY OF POSTERIOR SHOULDER.
Crowding the child gently upward into the pubic arch, to forestall injury by the broad chest.   The elbow of the left arm follows down the receding uterus.   The author prefers to turn the patient on her back, as in Fig. 319.

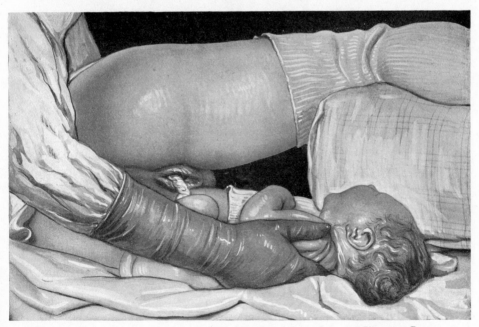

FIG. 318.—THE LEFT HAND NOW GRASPS THE UTERUS, THE RIGHT LAYS THE INFANT IN POSITION.

During this maneuver the head is maintained in a state of flexion, *not by pressure on the forehead through the perineum,* but by manipulation of the part that is accessible to the fingers. A gentle attempt to lead the suboccipital region under the pubis is first made by pressing the head back onto the perineum with the finger on the occipital protuberance, during two or three pains. When the head has descended far enough to give hold to the fingers, these applied right at the edge of the frenulum are used to press it up under the arch of the pubis, and, as the head finally rolls up onto the pubis, the flexion is maintained, as far as possible, by making pressure on the part delivered against the bone (Figs. 313 and 316). Some-

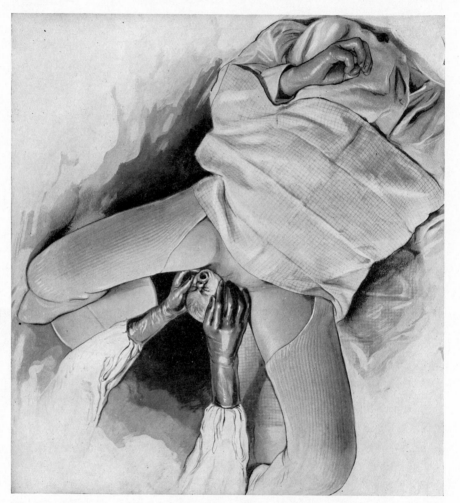

Fig. 319.—Patient on Back, with One Foot on Bed and One on a Stool, for the Delivery of the Shoulders, if Difficult.

With sufficient help, one puts patient across the bed.

times the head sticks in the vulva, here Ritgen's maneuver (Fig. 497, p. 624) may be used, but this is the only manipulation advised at this stage, excepting cleansing the parts with antiseptic solutions.

As soon as the face is delivered the forehead and eyelids are wiped with a gauze sponge wrung dry out of 1 : 1500 bichlorid solution, the mucus is squeezed out of the nostrils and wiped out of the mouth with the finger, covered, if need be, with a piece of soft linen or lintine. These details are important. Removal of the vaginal secretions from the neighborhood of the eyes is to prevent ophthalmia neonatorum; the removal of mucus from the nose and mouth, to prevent aspiration of the foreign matter, with subsequent intestinal sepsis, atelectasis, and broncho-pneumonia.

The accoucheur now feels for the cord and notes if it is around the neck, and if it is tight, making an obstacle to delivery. If it does this, and cannot be slipped over the shoulder, it should be clamped and cut. A cord that is too short, or rela-tively too short, may, unless cut, pull on the placenta and cause anomalies in the third stage, or even inversion of the uterus.

Delivery of the Shoulders.—A tendency to hurry this part of labor should be resisted. If the child's face is normally blue and reacts to stimuli, *e. g.*, rubbing,

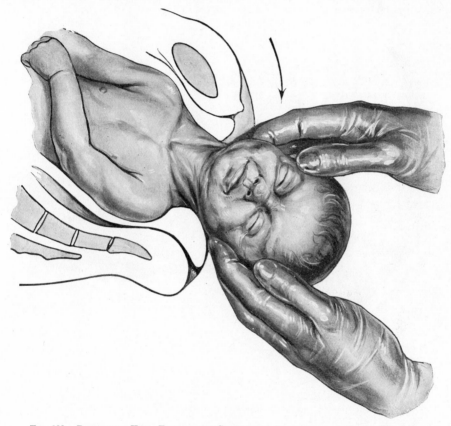

Fig. 320.—Depressing Head Toward the Sacrum for Delivery of Anterior Shoulder.
Be careful not to overstretch the neck and cause Erb's palsy. Aid this motion by outside pressure.

one may wait for the renewed action of the uterus. After a minute or two another pain comes on and the patient gently bears down until the anterior shoulder be-comes visible just behind the pubis. Now the accoucheur lifts the child up and brings the posterior shoulder over the perineum. If the child's hand is accessible, the arm is drawn out gently. Then the child is depressed as the anterior shoulder comes from behind the pubis, and now the rest of the body follows in one long pain without particular mechanism. The child must not be dragged out of the uterus. It is best if the natural powers force it out, the physician aiding the process only by directing the mechanism, as above indicated. A perineum may be torn by the shoulders or a slight tear plowed deeply by them, and the clavicles may be broken, or the nerves and muscles of the neck overstretched at this stage of the delivery unless proper care be exercised.

If the delivery of the shoulders is delayed too long, the woman is asked to bear down, failing which, the hand on the belly performs Kristeller's expression, or the child is delivered by slow traction following the mechanism here indicated. (See p. 1076 for pathologic shoulder deliveries.)

Historic.—Hippocrates recognized the importance of the prevention of perineal laceration, and sought to soften the structures by oily salves and relaxing douches, a practice which was recommended by Baudelocque and others, even by some today, in the form of hot moist applications. Van Horn (seventeenth century) dilated the perineum, pushing back the coccyx and stretching the levator ani manually, with boring or circular movements, a procedure that was used for many years by most authorities and is still recommended in a modified manner by Edgar for normal cases. The author advises such interference only in pathologic cases, and as a preparation

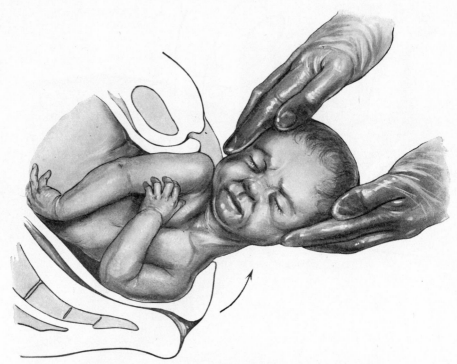

FIG. 321.—LIFTING THE HEAD FOR DELIVERY OF POSTERIOR SHOULDER.
One should use great gentleness and follow the normal mechanism to avoid damage to the baby.

for a rapid breech or forceps extraction. Various instruments were designed to lift the head away from the perineum, one of the most curious being a perineal horn, like one used for putting on shoes.

Soranus of Ephesus (about 110 A. D.) first attempted to "support" the perineum with the hand, a notion that it has been impossible to eradicate from the medical mind. Goodell tried to "relax the perineum" by pressure from the two sides toward the middle line. Various attempts have been made by some accoucheurs to lift the perineum forward with fingers introduced into the anus, or by the hand placed on the perineum from the outside. Others try to strip the vulva back over the head—all maneuvers which fail in their object, are harmful because of injury to the levator ani and rectum, and dangerous because of sepsis. Finally, may be mentioned the employment of incisions in the perineum to avoid deeper tears of the structure.

Episiotomy.—When a tear of the perineum appears inevitable, the question arises, shall it be allowed to occur spontaneously and go in whatever direction it may, or shall we seek to anticipate it, or at least direct it away from the sphincter into unimportant structures? Ould, in 1742, cut the vulvar outlet when it offered too great resistance to the escape of the head.   G. P. Michaëlis, in 1810, incised the perineum to avoid a dangerous tear.   Ritgen and Schultze made numerous small incisions in the tense vulvar ring.   Scanzoni recommended two lateral incisions, Credè, one, directed from the frenulum toward the tuberosity.   Many accoucheurs perform the operation, preferring a clean cut to the jagged tear, and claiming that the lateral structures are less important than the central portion of the perineum, and fearing that a tear beginning in the middle line only too easily goes beyond control of the attendant into the sphincter ani, even into the rectum.   Episiotomy is the name applied to the operation, which might more correctly be considered under the heading of operative obstetrics, but, because of its frequency, will be described here.   The incision is made in three ways—the lateral or bilateral (Fig. 322), where the cut is in the horizontal plane; the median, where the line lies in the raphé (a method urged by Pomeroy and Henkel) and the mediolateral, recommended by Tarnier and practised by the author.   One must be sure that he understands what is expected of episiotomy.   It simply cuts the skin, the urogenital septum, with the constrictor cunni and transversus perinei, the inter-columnar fascia, and a few of the anterior fibers of the puborectal portion of the levator ani.   Dührssen, in 1888, recommended a deeper episiotomy or perineotomy for pathologic cases, in which the incision went through the levator ani into the ischiorectal fossa. There are special indications for this extensive operation, and it is performed only when delivery must be effected before the levator has had time to stretch even a little.

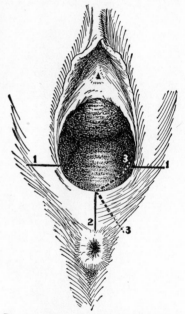

FIG. 322.—DIAGRAM OF THREE KINDS OF EPISIOTOMY.

1, 1, The bilateral; 2, the median; 3, 3, the mediolateral, recommended by author. A radial incision may be made anywhere between 1 and 2.

   The indications for the usual episiotomy are: Resistant perineum, causing delay in the exit of the head through the vulva; some pathologic con-dition of the vulva, scars, syphilis, etc.; abnormal size of the child or abnormal mechanism, causing mechanical disproportion; the necessity for rapid extraction when one may not give the perineum time to dilate, and when one sees that the perineum will surely tear, to divert the laceration away from the anus.

   One must not wait until the intercolumnar fascia is destroyed and the levator ani pillars distracted.   There is then little of the pelvic floor to save.   One blade of the scissors is laid on the vaginal mucous membrane, the other rests on the skin of the perineal body, midway between the anus and the tuberosity of the ischium, the cut-ting angle of the scissors being at the median raphé (Fig. 322).   With the finger and thumb of the other hand the sphincter is pressed out of the bite of the scissors.   The patient is given a few extra-deep inhalations of ether or local anesthesia is used (Fig. 322a) and with one or two quick motions the tissues are severed.   Hemorrhage is stopped by pressure. Usually the head issues quickly after the incision is made, and then the bleeding ceases, but if it does not, a firm tampon will check it until the sutures are applied. If a deep perineotomy is to be made, a systematic operation is performed, the structures being incised one after the other, in anatomical fashion.   The incision is repaired after delivery of the placenta, in the manner usual with perineorrhaphies (p. 786).

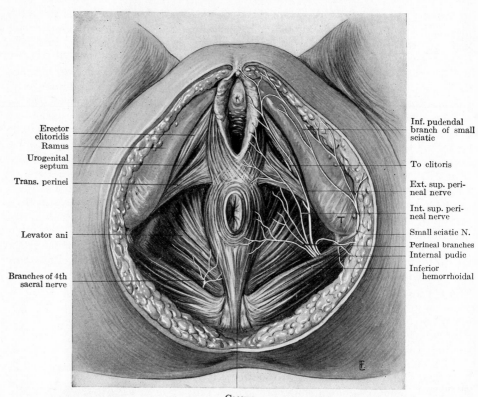

Erector
clitoridis
Ramus

Urogenital
septum

Trans. perinei

Levator ani

Branches of 4th
sacral nerve

Inf. pudendal
branch of small
sciatic

To clitoris

Ext. sup. peri-
neal nerve

Int. sup. peri-
neal nerve

Small sciatic N.

Perineal branches
Internal pudic

Inferior
hemorrhoidal

Coccyx

Fig. 322a.—The Nerves of the Female Pelvis.   (Combined from Kelly and Savage.)

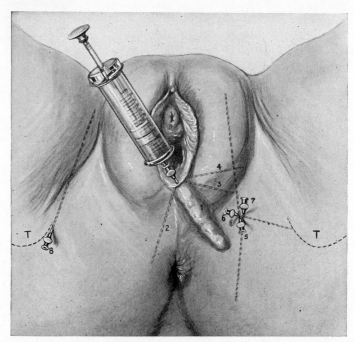

Fig. 322b.—Areas to be Infiltrated for Episiotomy.   Enter Needle in Fourchette, Infiltrate Perineum
(1 Per Cent. Novocain) in Sectors 1—2—3.   Then No. 4—Subvaginal.

For low forceps the pelvic nerves must be blocked too.   No. 5, long perineal; 6, internal pudic (the finger is
inserted into vagina or rectum to find the spine and orient the needle); 7, the branches of the fourth sacral in the
ischiorectal fossa; 8, the lesser sciatic along the ramus pubis.   Both sides must be blocked.   Use no more than 5 ounces
of 1 per cent. solution or 10 ounces of ½ per cent.

THE CARE OF THE CHILD

A warm sterile receiver is ready for the new-born individual, who, as soon as born, is placed near the vulva, so that the cord is not dragged upon, yet far enough

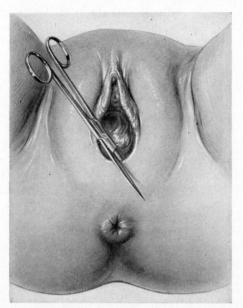

Fig. 323.—Episiotomy Incising Skin, Fourchet, and Uro-genital Septum.
This cut exposes the fascia over the left pillar of the levator ani, which may or may not be incised, depending on the size of the child and the distensibility of the tissues.

away so that he is not soiled with the blood, feces, etc., about the anus, and also safe from compression by the mother's person.

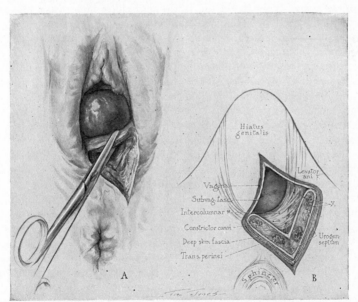

Fig. 324.—A, Second Step of Episiotomy. Cutting Vagina and Subvaginal Fascia. B, Diagram of Surgical Anatomy. Intercolumnar Fascia Not Incised. X, Deep and Superficial Layers of Fascia of Urogenital Septum. Shows How Structures Are to be Reunited.

The first attention to the child is the wiping of the face and eyelids with a sponge squeezed dry from a 1 : 1500 bichlorid solution, and removal of the mucus from the air-passages immediately after the head is born—points already mentioned.

In maternity hospitals the danger of mixing the babies is a real one, and infallible methods of identification must be practised.

Tying the Cord.—After waiting until the pulsation in the exposed umbilical cord has perceptibly weakened or disappeared, the child is severed from its mother. The fetal end of the cord is washed with bichlorid solution, then painted with tinctura iodi, and then, with a piece of linen bobbin, coarse silk, rubber band, or any sterile strong string, the cord is ligated close to the skin margin of the navel (½ inch), first being sure that there is no umbilical hernia which might allow a loop of gut to be caught in the grasp of the ligature. Another ligature is placed a few inches from the first, and, protecting the child from injury, the cord is severed with sterile, dull scissors close to the first ligature. The cut end is touched with tinctura iodi. It is important to leave as little as possible of the cord to be cast off, and, further, a short stump is easier to dress and less likely to be dragged upon. The short stump method was practised by Mauriceau and only recently revived. The first tying must be made very secure, and security is obtained by tightening the knot slowly and interruptedly, permitting the jelly of Wharton to escape from under the thread, which thus comes to constrict only the vessels.

During the four or eight minutes while waiting to tie the cord the child obtains from 40 to 60 gm. of the reserve blood of the placenta—a fact which was first shown by Budin. The blood is pressed into the child by the uterine contractions, and part is aspirated by the expanding chest. This extra blood the child needs in its first days of life, and observation has shown that such children lose less in weight and are less subject to disease. It is an error, on the other hand, to force the blood of the placenta into the child by stripping the cord toward the child. This overloads its blood-vessels, causes icterus, melena, even apoplexy. The child never had the extra blood of the placenta. The practice of waiting until the placenta is delivered before tying the cord is not recommended.

A second ligature is applied to the cord to keep the blood in the placenta and give the uterus a firm body to act on, to prevent the soiling of the bed and patient with blood which would flow from the open vessels, and to preserve a possible twin, still in the uterus, from hemorrhage, since the two circulations of twins often anastomose.

The stump and the region of the belly around it are now wiped with 1 : 1500 bichlorid or pure alcohol, a piece of dry gauze laid over the wound, and the infant, wrapped in a sterile receiver, is handed to the nurse, who puts it in a safe, warm place, delegating a relative to watch it and see that it breathes naturally.

The Care of the Eyes.—Many States have passed legislation making the antiseptic treatment of the eyes of the new-born obligatory on the part of the accoucheur. Statistics prove that about 10 per cent. of the cases of blindness admitted to the institutions supported by the State have lost the light of day through the lack of proper precaution at the time of birth. The blindness is caused by a disease known as ophthalmia neonatorum, which is a purulent inflammation of the conjunctiva and cornea, due, nine times out of ten, to the gonococcus of Neisser. The disease is highly preventable, and, even in eleemosynary lying-in hospitals, receiving large numbers of patients with gonorrheal vaginitis, it has been almost eradicated. The germs get into the eyes during the passage of the head through the vagina, or are washed into them by the attendant, or wiped into them by the mother. While the gonococcus is usually causative, the pneumococcus, the bacillus of diphtheria, and other germs may cause serious conjunctivitis. The child may be born with the disease already well advanced.

Mode of Prevention.—If the husband or wife is known to have gonorrhea, the vaginal inflammation is to be treated during pregnancy by the usual methods.

Douches of 1 : 1500 potassium permanganate, given under low pressure, and applications of 25 per cent. argyrol tampons give good results. During labor antiseptic douches and acriflavin co. instillations are used—this only in cases of gonorrhea, not for the routine delivery. The bag of waters must not be ruptured, but is to be allowed to come down and line the vagina for the passage of the head. It is best if the child of such a mother is delivered with a caul. During all vaginal examinations the eyes of the fetus (for example, in face presentation) must not be touched. When there is a purulent greenish vaginal discharge, or if there are condylomata on the vulva, the precautions are redoubled, the aim being to prevent all possibility of maternal secretions getting into the conjunctival sac. The same principle is carried out after the head is born, the vaginal mucus being removed at once from the neighborhood of the eyes with pledgets wrung dry from 1 :1500 bichlorid, and great care observed to allow no *reinfection*.

The nurse is instructed always to observe this same care while giving baths, and the first cleansing is best made by an albolene or lard rub, to remove the vernix caseosa. When gonorrhea is present, oil rubs are substituted for the baths entirely. In maternity practice the child and its mother are rigidly isolated, because the disease is highly contagious.

Active antisepsis of the eyes may not be needed if the above method is practised, but it is best to disinfect the eyes as an additional precaution. Where gonorrhea is suspected in either parent, the old Credè method is used—a drop of 2 per cent. silver nitrate solution in each eye, neutralized immediately with salt solution.

As a routine, in hospital practice, the author uses 1 per cent. nitrate of silver solution and does not neutralize it, a practice also in vogue in the New York Lying-in Hospital, the University of Pennsylvania Maternity, and the Manhattan Maternity. At the Johns Hopkins Maternity the silver is washed out with saline solution.

Other antiseptics have been recommended, as bichlorid, boric acid (useless), acetate of silver, argyrol, sophol, etc., but the author has found no reason to alter the practice outlined above.

Some practitioners use the drops immediately after the child is born, but the author prefers to wait until after the third stage is completed, so that he can do the little operation himself, under favorable conditions. Thus is assurance obtained that the medicine actually reaches the conjunctival sac.

No objections may be urged against this prophylactic antiseptic treatment of the eyes. Statistics prove conclusively that it reduces the frequency of purulent conjunctivitis to less than $\frac{1}{2}$ of 1 per cent. The frequency of "silver catarrh" under the old Credè method has been reduced by the use of a 1 per cent. instead of a 2 per cent. solution. The silver solution must be made fresh nearly every day, as it is the decomposition products which cause the conjunctival irritation. Highly to be recommended is the silver nitrate package devised and furnished free by the Illinois State Board of Health.

The writer believes that a child would be able to recover damages at law from the accoucheur if it should be blinded by infection acquired at birth and it were proved that the attendant did not use the recognized precautions.

In the author's Obstetrics for Nurses he has given in great detail the conduct of labor and the care of the child.

LITERATURE

Budin: Fasbender, Geschichte der Geb., p. 610.—*Davis:* "Painless Childbirth," Forbes & Co., 1916; also Amer. Jour. Obstet., October, 1917.—*DeLee:* Identification of Babies in Maternities, Jour. Obstet. and Gyn., March, 1923. —*Harrar and McPherson:* Amer. Jour. Obstet., October, 1914, p. 623.—*Harrar:* Am. Jour. Obstet. and Gyn., April, 1927, p. 486.—*Henkel:* Zentb. für Gyn., 1926, March, p. 769.—*Keller, M. R.:* Gyn. et Obstet., Paris, November 5, 1931, p. 650.—*Littig:* Jour. Amer. Med. Assoc., 1908, vol. l, p. 394.—*Lynch:* Jour. Amer. Med.

Assoc., March 6, 1915. Literature in same Journal, January 17, 1920, p. 195, and September 29, 1923.—*Meyer:* Zentralbl. für Gynäk., 1921, p. 1238.—*Polak:* Med. Times, December, 1914.—*Ries and Krönig:* Quoted by Holmes, Jour. Amer. Med. Assoc., December 25, 1915.—*Rongy:* Amer. Jour. Obstet., October, 1914.—*Schmidt, W. Th.:* Monatsschr. für Geb. u. Gyn., July, 1931, Lit.—*Sellheim:* Zentb. für Gyn., July 11, 1931, p. 2196.— *Ibid.:* Zentralbl. f. Gyn., 1910, No. 27; also *ibid.,* 1911, p. 1334.—*Siemerling:* Zentralbl. für Gynäk., May, 1922, p. 835, Lit.—*Sippel:* "Chloroform Death," Arch. f. Gyn., vol. lxxxviii, 1, p. 167.—*Stander:* Amer. Jour. Obstet. and Gyn., 1926, November, p. 633.—*v. Steinbüchel:* Zentralbl. f. Gyn., 1902, No. 48, p. 1304.— *Sticher:* Zeitschr. f. Geb. u. Gyn., vol. xlv, Heft 1.—*Strauss:* Jour. Amer. Med. Assoc., January 29, 1927.— *Stroganoff:* Zentralbl. f. Gyn., 1901, p. 146, No. 6.—*Strube:* Zentralbl. für Gynäk., September 8, 1923, p. 1460.

CHAPTER XXII

THE THIRD STAGE

MORE women die from accidents of the third stage of labor than during the other two combined. On a proper conduct of this part of the delivery depend the woman's freedom from postpartum hemorrhage, the expulsion of the secundines complete, the smooth convalescence during the puerperium, and even her health later in life. Postpartum hemorrhage may be directly fatal, or may leave the woman permanently invalided; retention of pieces of placenta may be the cause of puerperal infections and lay the foundation for ineradicable disease. It is important, therefore, that the accoucheur be familiar with the physiology of the third stage, and possess a good technic in its conduct. Baudelocque distinguished the *separation* from the *expulsion* of the after-birth, and this difference must always be kept in mind. The same general principle applies to the treatment of this stage as to the others, the accoucheur studies the mechanism as it unrolls under hand and eye, watches the patient, and interferes only for good reason.

Mode of Conduct.—As the child leaves the vagina the nurse or the assistant follows down the receding uterus with the hand placed lightly upon it; a procedure first recommended by John Harvey in 1767. After delivery the accoucheur himself guards the uterus through a sterile towel. *No massage of the fundus is practised; the hand simply rests on it, noting its firmness and the varying consistence, due to contraction and relaxation.* When the child has been severed from the mother, the accoucheur resumes his watch over the uterus, a warm, clean, folded sheet is laid under the patient, a sterile basin or bed-pan is pushed against the nates and perineum, taking care not to push feces upward onto the vulva, and the cord is drawn up over the thigh. The woman lies on her back, with the legs drawn up or outstretched, according to her comfort. The abdomen is covered, but the basin must be visible, for the accoucheur wishes to see if blood accumulates in it. If the woman has been delivered on the side, she is gently turned on her back for the conduct of the third stage, taking care to be certain that the legs are pressed firmly together, and that the uterus is very hard during the movement—these precautions to avoid air-embolism, which has occurred (Braun, Gough, Surg., Gyn., and Obst., 1924).

The accoucheur now sits or stands at the side of the patient, and studies the phenomena of the separation of the placenta, and, in the absence of hemorrhage from the vulva or into the uterus, has nothing else to do for fifteen to thirty minutes. The hand on the uterus notes the frequency and strength of the after-pains and the degree of advancement of the placenta; the eye notes the amount of blood accumulating in the basin. If the uterus remains firm and does not balloon out with blood; if there is no external bleeding—nothing is done; but if the uterus softens and fills up, or if there is external hemorrhage, a gentle massage is practised. The four fingers make circles on the posterior wall of the fundus, while the thumb rests in front, the motion resembling the kneading of bread. As soon as the uterus becomes firm the oozing will cease and the kneading may be discontinued. Inspection of the vulva will show whether the hemorrhage comes from some tear of the vulva or clitoris or from a point higher up in the parturient canal. In pathologic cases abnormalities of the separation of the placenta cause hemorrhage, and then the treatment of the third stage has to be altered. (See p. 840.)

22   337

The accoucheur waits for the signs that the placenta has been separated and has been expelled from the uterus into the dilated lower uterine segment and upper vagina. Strong uterine contractions themselves would indicate this to the accoucheur, but there are other signs: (1) The cord becomes limp and advances 3 or 4 inches from the vulva (diagnosed by observing the longer loop in the basin); (2) the uterus rises up in the abdomen, usually to the right side, while below, over the pubis, a soft, boggy mass appears (the placenta) (Fig. 325); (3) the globular uterus has flattened out from before backward, presents a sharp ridge at the fundus, is more movable, smaller, and harder; (4) a flat dimple is palpable on the fundus; (5) firm pressure on the fundus fails to send a wave of blood through the cord—Pinard (unreliable).

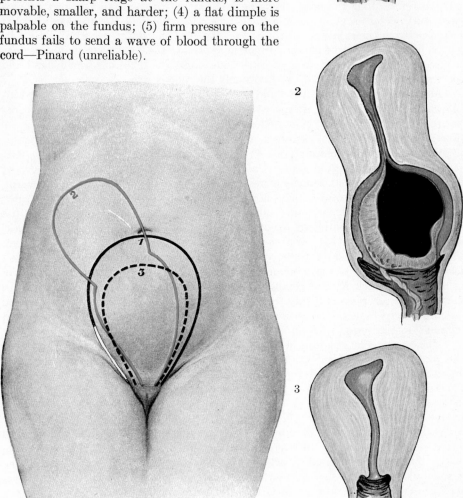

A   B

FIG. 325.—MUTATIONS OF THE UTERUS DURING THE THIRD STAGE; SCHULTZE'S MECHANISM.

1, Right after the child is born; fundus is seen and felt as a large globular mass reaching to navel; 2, placenta has left fundus which has ascended toward liver; 3, empty fundus sinks low, for a few minutes has a square shape, soon becoming globular and small. Remember, pituitary disturbs this mechanism. (See p. 137.)

In Duncan's mechanism the changes are similar, but the uterus is not so large. The numbers on the figures A and B correspond.

These phenomena are apparent in ten to forty-five minutes, depending on the strength of the uterine contractions. When the placenta is surely out of the cavity of the uterus there is no real need of waiting longer for its delivery; indeed, the author believes that it is better practice to remove it at this time, because there is less likelihood of blood-clots forming in the partially emptied parturient canal. On the average, twenty to twenty-five minutes elapse before the placenta is fully separated and comes to lie in the vagina, but of late, it being routine practice with many accoucheurs to give pituitary extract as soon as the baby is born, the uterus, under the influence of this drug, contracts powerfully and expels the placenta into the vagina within a few minutes.

Now the attendant assures himself of three things—that the bladder is empty (catheterize, if necessary); that the uterus is in firm contraction (wait for an after-

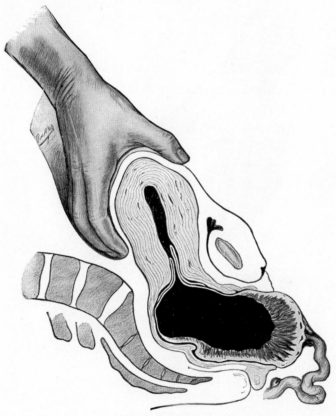

Fig. 326.—Early Expression.
Uterus is used only as a medium to exert pressure on placenta.

pain); that the uterus is in the median line (bring it there by pressure from the sides). The woman is asked to bear down, to see first if she can expel the placenta herself. If she cannot, the uterus is grasped in the whole hand with the thumb in front (Fig. 326) and gently, *without squeezing*, pushed down onto the placenta, in the axis of the inlet. The uterus is used simply as a piston, as a body through which to exert pressure on the placenta lying in the vagina, and this maneuver is called "early expression"—"early," because it anticipates nature's expulsion. As the placenta distends the vulva the woman usually bears down and expels it into the basin, into which it should be allowed to fall, dragging the membranes after it. It is best to allow the membranes to come out of their own weight, but if they should be adherent (evidenced by the placenta not falling into the basin), gentle, steady traction is made on them without twisting. One grasps the membranes near the vulva from above, to avoid contact with the possibly infected perineal and anal regions. If the membranes start to tear, greater gentleness is to be used, and if they should break off, the proximal end should be grasped with an artery forceps. Five minutes' time may be required to remove the secundines in an intact condition. Now the uterus is given a brisk massage, and the patient, an ampule of pituitary and 1 dram of ergot. This is not always necessary, but the author has never seen any harm from its use, and often felt that the uterus got harder and remained so more continuously when it was administered. Ergot is never given before the placenta is delivered, nor may traction be made on the cord before the placenta is visible in the vulva, and better not then. While in

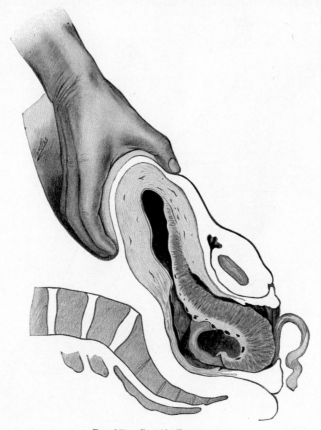

Fig. 327.—Credè's Expression.

Placenta is squeezed out of uterus, from which it has not yet been fully detached. Note the direction of the pressure.

some clinics pituitary is given to aid the expulsion of the placenta, it is inadvisable for general practice. Incarceration of the placenta sometimes results. In such a case one must wait for the uterus to relax, an hour or more if need be, unless there is bleeding.

If the first "early expression" does not bring the after-birth, a mistake has been made as to the placental separation, and the attendant waits for more definite signs to appear, when the simple expression is repeated. Unless the woman bleeds there is no danger, and one may safely wait even eight or ten hours. If, after one hour, during which time two, or at most three simple expressions have been attempted, the placenta fails to come, a Credè expression is performed, since the third stage is pathologic. Credè's expression differs from the simple form in that the uterus, at the same time that it is forced down into the pelvis, is squeezed from all sides, so that its contents are expelled "like the stone from a cherry" (Fig. 327). Being assured that the bladder is empty and the uterus contracted, the fundus is grasped in the full hand with the thumb in front, and, while the fingers are pressed together, the uterus is firmly but gently forced down in the line of the axis of the pelvis. One Credè expression properly executed will almost always force the placenta into the vagina, and now the woman expels it or it may be delivered by simple expression. The further treatment of such a pathologic third stage belongs in the chapter on Postpartum Hemorrhage, p. 845.

Other Methods of Treatment of Third Stage.—Savage tribes and the ancients pulled on the cord, pressed on the belly, gave emetics or tickled the nose, to provoke sneezing, had the woman blow into a gourd, a bottle, or into the closed fist, to evoke the abdominal pressure, or even removed the placenta by hand. Hippocrates blew irritating powders into the nose, a practice that some physicians carry out today. The French, even now, exert traction on the cord, together with pressure on the fundus, after the placenta is loosened and slipped from the uterus—a practice which is not dangerous in a skilled hand. The author would unreservedly condemn it, however, because—(1) Most of the deliveries are conducted by midwives who blindly imitate the physicians; (2) it is inefficient if the placenta is adherent or incarcerated; (3) the cord may tear off, or only part of the placenta may come with it; (4) traction on the placenta may cause inversion of the uterus; (5) there is danger of infection from the fingers inserted into the vagina; (6) it is not necessary. In 1861 Credè formulated a method which was given his name, and consisted in the rapid expression of the placenta by squeezing the uterus through the abdomen during the first after-pain, that is, from four to eight minutes after the delivery of the child. Dohrn and Ahlfeld, in 1880 and 1882, showed the dangers of this method—(a) It is unphysiologic; (b) the uterus is emptied too rapidly—it has not time to retract properly, it fills up with clots, and the tendency to late hemorrhage is increased; (c) the primary hemorrhage is great; (d) retention of the membranes, of decidua, and even of pieces of placenta are more common; (e) the uterus is bruised; painful after-pains and puerperal infection are invited.

Ahlfeld, in 1882, proposed a purely expectant plan of treatment of the third stage. The uterus is not even touched after delivery unless interference is necessary because of very profuse hemorrhage; the cord is drawn over the thigh, a bed-pan put under the vulva, or the patient is put over a hole in the mattress, the escaping blood is caught in a funnel leading to a graduated vessel under the bed, and the attendant sits at the bedside, watching her face and counting her pulse, occasionally taking note of the amount of blood lost externally. If the placenta is not born spontaneously in two hours, the woman is asked to bear down, and if she fails to expel it, the placenta is expressed as already indicated. As a rule, the placenta is spontaneously expelled in three or four hours, but without aid it might remain until putrefaction sets in. Ahlfeld claims for his method that the loss of blood is less than with Credè's; that the deciduæ are usually expelled complete; that the tearing and retention of the membranes and placenta are less frequent; that the puerperium is less likely to be morbid—with all of which the author cannot agree. In 60 consecutive cases in which this method was tried the author found the hemorrhage greater than with the method first described in this chapter, and there was no difference in the frequency of retention of pieces of membrane or decidua. Other investigators have confirmed these findings. Outside of the greater loss of blood, which may signify much to a small or anemic woman, the constant anxiety of the patient throughout the long hours of waiting, the prolongation of the possibilities of infection, and the useless expenditure of the physician's time, condemn the method. In Dublin, since 1783, and in England, since 1775 (John Harvie), a method of treatment was practised whose essentials were the guarding of the uterus with the hand and the expression of the placenta by gentle force exerted on the fundus from the abdomen fifteen to thirty minutes after the child was delivered. The plan recommended by the author is based on the Dublin method.

Mojon and Gabaston advise to overdistend the placenta with cold water to aid its separation and expulsion.

One of the important functions of the obstetrician is to save the woman's blood. Even though the obstetric patient can lose enormous quantities—as much as three liters, according to Ahlfeld—without succumbing to hemorrhage, these great losses leave the woman debilitated, anemic, neurasthenic, and, if not these, at least protract her recovery decidedly. The author aims to conduct all labors as nearly bloodlessly as possible, and is strongly convinced that the women recuperate much quicker, suffer less infections, nurse their babies better, and altogether are more healthy and vigorous than those who have suffered the losses which are given as physiologic in most text-books. Excessive hemorrhage is produced by improper conduct of the third stage. The accoucheur should hurry the process of separation of the placenta only in the presence of an indication; rough massage of the uterus is to be avoided, since it mashes the soft placenta to a pulp, and a uterus that is behaving well should not be excited to irregular action. All these conduce to retention of pieces of placenta, hemorrhage, and infection.   The same is true of improperly performed and frequent Credè expressions.

Examination of the Placenta.—This is a part of a physician's work which may never be omitted, hurried, nor delegated to another.   A minute and systematic inspection of the after-birth is made as soon as it is delivered, while the hands are still sterile and the patient ready for operation.   If postponed until the physician is about to leave the house and the patient already comfortably settled in bed, one is loath to disturb her and may neglect a small piece of placenta which may be found wanting, and trust its removal to nature, when, if everything were aseptically prepared, the uterus would be properly emptied of its contents, and late hemorrhages, polypi, subinvolution, and puerperal infection thus avoided.   It is well to repeat the inspection of the placenta before it is destroyed.   Some country women make it a practice to preserve the placenta for five days, in order that the physician may inspect it if fever develops.   Under a good light, and gently rubbing the blood-clots off the maternal surface with a piece of cotton without producing new

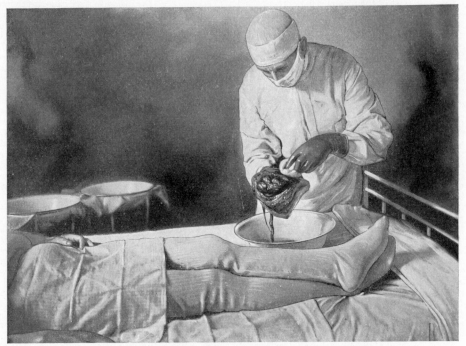

FIG. 328.—INSPECTION OF THE PLACENTA.
Before being taken from the bedside, a careful scrutiny of the placenta is made, all blood-clots being wiped away with dry gauze.   Note posture of patient and the fact that the uterus is contracting.

injuries, the accoucheur goes carefully over each cotyledon separately and successively.   Beginning at one point in the periphery, the edge is followed all around three times, and if it is smooth and even, in all likelihood nothing is missing, but the center of the placenta must also be examined carefully.   A gray, smooth, shiny surface (the decidua serotina) is a positive indication that that portion is not missing, but a rough place requires careful attention.   If the torn and roughened surfaces fit smoothly *without forcing the cotyledons together;* if the broken and jagged edges of the thin decidua serotina mortise into each other perfectly, one may decide that nothing is missing from that point.   Every roughened portion of the placenta should be washed with water, and if the villi are seen free and floating, one may be certain that a larger or smaller portion of the organ has remained attached to the uterus.

Turning the organ inside out, the fetal surface is scrutinized, the presence of cysts noted, but especially the distribution of vessels. If the vessels all disappear before they reach the edge, one may be fairly sure that a placenta succenturiata, has not been left behind. If a large vessel breaks off sharply at the edge of the after-birth, search should be made for the portion it supplied (Fig. 329).

The membranes also must be studied. If the opening through which the infant came is round and complete, usually all the membranes are delivered. The empty ovum sac may be filled with water. If the membranes are in shreds, the parts may be fitted together or spread on a sterile towel. If torn from the edge of the pla-

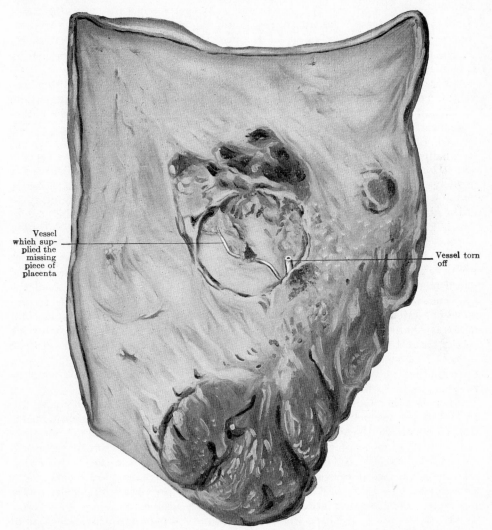

Vessel which supplied the missing piece of placenta

Vessel torn off

Fig. 329.—Edge of Placenta, Showing Aperture in Chorion Where a Placenta Succenturiata has been Torn Out.

centa, they must be readjusted and notice taken if like fits like structures. The amnion is now studied separately from the chorion. Pieces of missing chorion always carry decidua with them, and are especially important because they may also carry a placenta succenturiata or placenta spuria with them.

Discovery of the Absence of a Placenta Succenturiata.—The possibility of the retention of an extra placenta is invariably to be borne in mind, especially since even the minutest examination of the delivered portion may fail to give rise to suspicion of such an occurrence. High authorities have testified to this point in court. Still, an investigation with this particular object will rarely fail to discover the true conditions.

If the membranes are torn from the edge of the placenta, leaving the latter jagged, thick, and rough; if a blood-vessel runs to the edge of the placenta and breaks off sharply; if, with velamentous insertion of the cord, not all the vessels are accounted for; if there is an extra placenta on the one delivered; if, on holding the membranes up to light, an irregular defect in the chorion is found, with thickened and vascular margins; if the placenta is smaller than the size of the child should demand—one may feel reasonably sure that a placenta succenturiata is retained in the uterus. In cases of real doubt the uterine cavity is to be explored.

So complete an examination of the secundines requires all of ten minutes, during which time the nurse guards the uterus, stimulating it to contraction by light massage if necessary.

For experimental purposes milk could be injected into the placenta through the vein; it would flow in a large stream through the opening left by the missing portion.

When to Invade the Uterus.—Properly, this question comes up in the pathologic part, but, owing to its importance, it will bear frequent repetition. The invasion of the uterine cavity after parturition is a serious procedure, and, done as it usually is, is more dangerous than most laparotomies, done as they usually are. Done as laparotomies are usually done, the introduction of the hand is not dangerous. In his recommendations for general practice, therefore, a teacher is bound to consider the conditions there met, and the qualifications and limitations of the attendant physician.

In general practice it is safest to leave the membranes, if retained, for nature to dispose of, which she usually does—they come away with the lochia, in pieces or as a whole, by the end of one or two weeks. Severe after-pains, fetid lochia, a slight rise of temperature, a moderate bleeding, often accompany this condition, but the puerpera recovers, though a chronic endometritis may remain. Even if all the membranes are retained, the placenta being "decrowned," most authorities recommend non-interference in the absence of hemorrhage. A missing piece of placenta, unless it is larger than the thumb-nail, or unless it causes hemorrhage, is also left to the natural resources of the woman. The hand may be introduced into the uterus only under the strictest indication, vast experience having shown that, under the conditions in which most of human births occur, the woman is safer if the above rules are applied and much trusted to nature.

On the other hand, where the parturient is in an aseptic maternity hospital, and where the accoucheur has at his service all the accoutrements of aseptic operation, he may make the attempt to spare the woman the ills that follow the retention in the uterus of membrane, shreds of thick decidua, scraps of placental tissue, and firm blood-clots. Persistent oozing of blood, which sometimes causes decided general anemia before it ceases spontaneously, severe after-pains, fetid lochia, slight saprophytic infections, prolonged lochial discharge, persistence of lochia rubra, protracted convalescence, late puerperal hemorrhages, subinvolution of the uterus, which may result in chronic metritis, with sterility and permanent invalidism, mild parametritis with later shrinking of the uterine ligaments—all these may be avoided by leaving the uterine cavity empty and the walls smooth after delivery. It must be again repeated, however, that unless the conditions for aseptic operation are perfect, the primary danger of infection far outweighs the advantages to be gained.

The Asepsis and Antisepsis of the Second and Third Stages.—Antiseptic surgery has very properly given way to aseptic surgery. The principle of aseptic surgery has been carried over to obstetrics, but a few of the old antiseptic practices have been and must be retained. An example will illustrate the need for this: A parturient is ideally prepared for delivery, with sterile night-gown, sterile leggings, sterile sheets and towels, all safely (?) pinned together, with a sterile towel under the buttocks, leaving only the vulvar orifice exposed; the accoucheur is dressed as for a major laparotomy. What happens? The woman, in her throes of pain, tosses about, disarranging all the sterile covers; she grasps the hand of the attendant, or puts her hand over the sterile towels to the vulva; she coughs or expires forcibly and droplets of saliva are blown on to the sterile cloths; with the pressing efforts feces escape from the rectum, and soil the towel under her or the towel at the side of the buttock, and with her next motion these are spread all over the region about the vulva; the second stage drags on, one, two, or three hours, dust settles on the extensive area of sheets, leggings, towels, gloves, gowns, basins, etc., which are supposed to be sterile. How many of these things are really sterile when the actual time of delivery arrives and may safely be touched? In view of these experiences, and be-

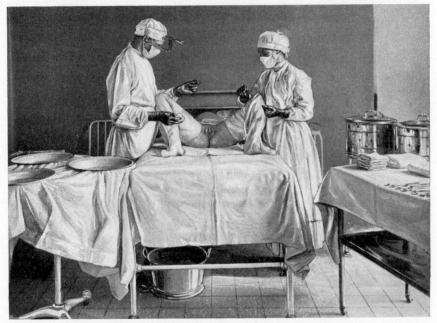

Fig. 330.—All Ready for Delivery—Maternity Practice.

Although the large area of sheets, etc., was sterile when first exposed, it soon must be regarded as not so, and may not be touched. Only the towel on the belly and the vulva may be touched by the sterile hand.

cause the immense majority of confinements must be conducted without so many conveniences, the author practises and teaches a very simple system of antisepsis. The bed is dressed with sterile sheets; the patient is in a sterile night-gown; sterile leggings are put on; a sterile towel lies under the buttocks; another covers the belly, but nothing is draped near the vulva, and the only towel which is considered aseptic, and kept so by frequent changes, is the one on the belly. If it is impossible to obtain the sterile clothes, clean ones, fresh from the laundry, are as good, for they are not touched anyway (Fig. 330). The accoucheur must put on a sterilized gown, which is not considered sterile after it is on, and use sterilized rubber gloves, but these must be considered sterile and must be kept so by very frequent dipping in actively antiseptic solutions. He wears a mouth and head cover.

The inside of basins carrying antiseptic solutions, the hands (gloved), the region immediately around the vulva, and the towel on the belly are the only objects which are considered sterile, and which the accoucheur tries to keep sterile. If feces issue from the rectum, they are caught in sponges wrung out of 1 : 1500 bichlorid, and the region of the anus washed with the same. If the woman touches the abdominal towel, a new one replaces it, and during the second stage the vulva and introitus vaginæ are frequently sponged with 1 per cent. lysol, and 1 : 1500 bichlorid solutions. Since the child is delivered "inter feces et urinam," the field can never be considered aseptic. The author has never seen ill effects from the liberal use of these antiseptic solutions on the introitus vulvæ and perineum, and, since investigations have proved that the greatest danger of infection arises from this region, the above practice is justified. Experience in his own private and consultation practice and in the large service of the Chicago Lying-in Hospital and Dispensary has also convinced him that, if the region of the vulva is kept aseptic with antiseptic solutions; if the gloves are kept sterile by frequent immersions in

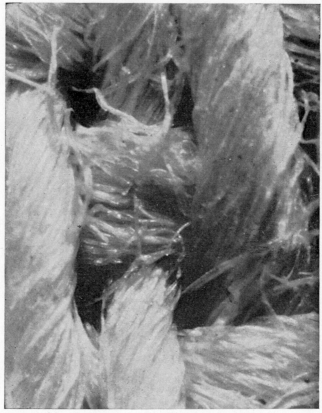

Fig. 331.—How Many Bacteria Could Pass Abreast Through the Interstices of this Sterile Gown? The Cloth is Magnified Only 90 Diameters.

the same, and if the few objects that must necessarily be introduced into the genitalia are absolutely aseptic, one can conduct the most difficult and prolonged obstetric manipulations in the dirtiest hovel with brilliant results.

Wherever possible, naturally, and in obstetric operations, the precautions and technic of the laparotomy are practised (Fig. 330*).

A popular and dangerous fallacy is that one or two layers of sheeting or towel offer a barrier to the passage of germs, and may be used to wrap up sterile supplies, to cover non-sterile tables, the patient's limbs, etc., and that one may safely touch surfaces thus protected. Figure 331 is a microphotograph of a piece of a sur-

* See article by author, "Several Every-day Obstetric Problems," Amer. Jour. Obstet., July, 1917.

geon's gown. The enlargement is only 90 diameters. If it were enlarged to a size that would permit bacteria to be seen, about 900 diameters, one hole in the mesh would cover an entire page. Billions of bacteria could pass through it.

When the child is delivered, the hand follows the uterus through the sterile abdominal towel. Before tying the cord, the gloves must be disinfected since they are soiled with vaginal bacteria which, introduced via the navel, can cause pyemia in the child. After the cord is tied the accoucheur rinses his gloves very thoroughly in both solutions (1 : 1500 bichlorid and 1 per cent. lysol), which are then made up fresh, and supplied with fresh pledgets. For the conduct of the third stage the author washes his gloves with pure lysol. New gloves are put on when one has inadvertently touched some unsterile object or perforated the first pair. After the placenta is delivered, the vulva and parts about it are sponged gently with 1 : 1500 bichlorid, taking care that nothing is washed into the perineal wound. If one is called to a case of injury to the perineum, where no preparation of the patient had been previously made, it would be an error of technic to scrub the vulva with soap and water, etc., and thus carry infection into the wound. One should treat such a case as one would a compound fracture, that is, clean well around the edges, guarding carefully against carrying anything into the freshly opened surfaces. The contiguous skin is painted with tincture of iodin.

Examination of the Parts for Injuries.—Lacerations of the outlet may be observed during the delivery of the child, but the attendant must also inspect the parts carefully after the third stage. Having sponged the blood away, the fingers, holding two dry pledgets, gently, under good light, separate the labia so that a perfect view of the vagina and perineum is obtained. In all breech, in excessively rapid, and in all operative deliveries the author insists on a careful exploration of the whole parturient canal, followed by catheterization and rectal examination, to determine the integrity of all the structures involved in the labor process. With the protection of a good aseptic technic the cervix is inspected in all cases and repaired if necessary. This is not established practice, many excellent accoucheurs believing it safer, under the conditions in which most babies are born, to repair the cervix only if there is hemorrhage from it.

SUMMARY OF THE CONDUCT OF THE THREE STAGES

During the First Stage.—(1) Asepsis and antisepsis. (2) Diagnosis of the case. (3) The prognosis of the mechanism of labor. (4) Watchful expectancy and recognition of impending danger to mother and babe. (5) Attention to bladder, bowels, and general health of patient. (6) Relief of pain.

During the Second Stage.—(1) Asepsis and antisepsis. (2) Relief of pain. (3) Protection of life of infant and watching for complications which threaten the mother. (4) The preservation of the perineum.

During the Third Stage.—(1) Prevention of postpartum hemorrhage. (2) Delivery of the placenta. (3) Asepsis and antisepsis. (4) Tying the cord. (5) Care of the eyes. (6) Examination of the placenta. (7) The search for birth injuries. (8) Examination of the child for deformities and injury.

The accoucheur stays in the house at least one hour after the placenta is delivered, time which may be profitably employed watching the mother for hemorrhage, eclampsia, etc., in cleaning instruments and packing satchel ready for the next case, the filling out of the history sheet or card and birth-certificate, weighing and measuring the baby, giving instructions as to after-care, etc. Before leaving the house the attendant must have assured himself on these seven points: (1) That the uterus is in firm tonus—that is, well retracted and not inverted; (2) that there is no hemorrhage from the vulvar orifice and no internal hemorrhage; (3) that the placenta and membranes are complete; (4) that the bladder is empty;

(5) that all perineal tears are attended to; (6) that the child is in good condition—no hemorrhage from the cord, and that it breathes freely; (7) that the mother is in good condition, with good pulse, no headache (eclampsia), no vomiting.

It is good practice to administer 1 mg. of ergotamin tartrate after delivery and if the uterus shows any tendency to relax—to repeat it after three or four hours.

RETROSPECT

Let us pause here to take a glance back at the treatment of labor as a whole. It should be regarded as a surgical operation: it really is such, and the obstetrician is really a surgeon. He considers every labor, therefore, first, as to the ability of the patient to stand the shock; second, he provides for asepsis and antisepsis; third, he carefully watches for and guards against complications.

During the labor the accoucheur observes the powers and estimates the resistances, judges whether the powers are sufficient to overcome the latter; he watches the mechanism of labor as its various phases pass under the eye and hand; he is always alert to any abnormality in the mechanism, and keenly alive to the possibility of some outside complication occurring, which may throw either or both patients into acute danger. Through all, he throws around both patients the protection from infection which, of recent years, has become almost perfect.

The conduct of labor is not a simple matter, safely intrusted to every one. Let the people know that having a child is an important affair, deserving of the deepest solicitation on the part of the friends, needing the watchful attention of a qualified practitioner, and that the care of even a normal confinement is worthy the dignity of the greatest surgeon.

CHAPTER XXIII

THE CONDUCT OF THE PUERPERIUM

AFTER the delivery of the placenta the vulvar region is cleansed of blood, etc., by the physician, and a sterilized vulvar pad applied, which is held in place by a T-binder. An abdominal bandage is generally used to hold the pad and to relieve the puerpera from the feeling of emptiness. Such a binder cannot be applied tightly enough to compress the uterus and thus prevent postpartum hemorrhage, and it should, therefore, only support the abdominal wall, and be loose enough to allow the nurse to put her hand underneath for the palpation of the fundus.

No douches are given postpartum except for some special indication, e. g., hemorrhage. When the soiled sheets are drawn from the bed and the patient's night-dress changed, the woman should be moved with great gentleness, and one must insist that the legs be kept close together and that the uterus be hard—these precautions to prevent air-embolism. If the uterovaginal tract has been tamponed, the moving of the puerpera is slowly and gently done, because of the danger of tearing the uterus over the tampon. The bed is now set to rights, the room cleared and darkened, the mother warmly covered up, a warm-water bag placed at her feet, a hot drink given, and she is allowed to get the repose and sleep she has so well earned. By this time another hour has passed, and if hemorrhage has not begun and the third stage was conducted properly, few complications need to be feared, though it is wise for the nurse to take an occasional look at the patient.

The treatment of the puerperium falls almost entirely to the nurse, but it is well for the accoucheur to have his own ideas on the subject and to be able to carry them out if necessary. For details see "Obstetrics for Nurses."

Aseptic Care During the Puerperium.—This is as important as during the labor, for many cases have been successfully delivered only to be infected in the puerperium. The vulva is treated as an open wound—indeed, it is beset by the same dangers as an open wound. This point is to be remembered when comparing obstetric with surgical practice. The pads lying on the vulva are changed as often as they become soiled with blood or lochia, and the parts are dressed after each urination or defecation, also as a routine three or four times a day. For this purpose the patient is placed on a sterile bed-pan, the nurse sterilizes her hands or wears sterile gloves, and gently pours from a narrow-lipped pitcher a solution of 1 : 2000 bichlorid over the vulva. The excess is dried off without rubbing, by touching with dry sterile cotton, and a fresh sterile vulvar pad is applied. Simple sterilized water may be used. If there is any odor to the lochia, 2 per cent. carbolic solution is more deodorant. These attentions are needed for ten days. No douches are given (see Pathology of the Puerperium, p. 947), and the patient is instructed never to touch the genitals nor her nipples. Internal examinations are not made by the physician except under strictest indication. The parts are left severely alone. If there are stitches in the perineum, extra care and greater watchfulness are required on the part of the nurse and accoucheur, since unclean bed-pans, non-sterile cloths, and filthy bed-covers may come in direct contact with the wound.

The Diet.—There is no ground for the old notion that errors of diet cause puerperal infection, but the studies of Macy et al. tend to show that a puerpera needs 60 per cent. more food than a gravida if she is to nurse adequately and retain her health.

During the first eighteen hours after the labor the patient should have liquids in amounts sufficient to quench her thirst. After a few hours a cup of broth or tea and a small slice of buttered toast may be given. Milk, plain or with seltzer, is allowable, also tea, coffee, milk-toast, oyster-stew, salt wafers, and chocolate. On the second day, after the bowels have moved freely, the amounts may be increased, and the patient may have soups, thickened with rice, barley, etc., bread and butter, cereal foods, and stewed fruits, omitting the strongly acid. In summer ice-cream and ices are allowable. On this day a small piece of meat, as a chop, the breast of chicken, or squab, may be given at noon. Fresh fish is also now allowable. The other meals are prepared from the dietary of the preceding days. On the third day a small piece of tender steak, eggs, light puddings, blanc-mange, baked apple, jellies, and other delicacies may be given. Tea and coffee are given sparingly and should not be strong. Fresh vegetables are allowed, with salt or cream dressing, not vinegar. Baked potatoes, beans, and peas are best omitted, as they may produce tympany. Stewed fruits, as prunes, dried apples, and peaches, are given for their laxative effect.

Three meals a day are served. At ten in the morning a glass of cool milk, and at three in the afternoon a cup of chocolate with a wafer, are given. Occasionally an eggnog is prepared instead of the chocolate at three. At midnight, after the nursing, a glass of hot milk or malted milk is usually administered. A nursing mother should have food rich in all four vitamins, in phosphates, and calcium in order to make them over into her milk.

Throughout the puerperium the nurse will see that the patient drinks pure water freely, to make up the loss caused by the free action of the skin and kidneys and the fluids required for making milk.

The Bladder.—The necessity for frequent emptying of the bladder during labor has been emphasized. During the third stage it may fill rapidly, incarcerate the placenta, and cause postpartum hemorrhage. The bladder must always be emptied within the first ten hours after delivery, and thereafter at least three times a day. Owing to the bruising of the neck of the bladder, the edema of the neck and the urethra, and spasm of the sphincter, plus the horizontal position, the patient may not be able to urinate. Before the catheter is resorted to these methods should be tried: (a) Have the nurse put the woman on a bed-pan containing steaming hot water, and leave her alone; (b) the same, and allow the water to run in the wash-stand; (c) let the patient, while lying on the bed-pan, smell a bottle of sal volatile; (d) lay a large pad, dripping with warm sterile water, on the pubis (the warm solution imitates the flow of urine); (e) place a hot fomentation over the bladder; (f) give the patient an enema: often the bowels and bladder act simultaneously; (g) gentle pressure on the bladder may start the flow; (h) let the patient sit up on the pan, this being less dangerous than catheterization. With all these measures a little suggestion may be used, and the patient is to be left alone. Many persons cannot urinate in the presence of another. If the bladder must be catheterized, it is wisest for the accoucheur to do this himself, unless he has a trustworthy nurse, because many cases of cystitis take origin at this time. After the bladder is once thus emptied, the patient can usually urinate herself thereafter, but if the operation must be repeated, it should not be done oftener than every eight hours, and hexamethylenamin, 5 grains thrice daily, should be administered prophylactically. Other remedies for obstinate cases are: (1) A hypodermic of pituitrin; (2) instillation of 40 minims of sterile glycerin in the bladder (after emptying it with a catheter); (3) placing a small glycerin suppository in the urethra; (4) use of a permanent catheter for thirty-six hours.

The Bowels.—Custom immemorial gives a cathartic on the third day after labor. The author prefers to give it on the morning of the second day, and usually prescribes castor oil. This evacuates the bowel, aids the discharge of the lochia, activates the pelvic circulation (indirectly preventing infection) helps to overcome a tendency to bladder retention and, it is said, favors milk secretion and detoxicates the intestine. Castor oil was cultivated and used in Egypt seventeen hundred years before Christ. The oil is administered in lemon juice and soda during effervescence, in orange juice, or in gelatin capsules. After the bowels are once thoroughly evacuated, a bi-daily enema is sufficient to unload the rectum, but these movements are often unsatisfactory, and an occasional dose of cascara at bedtime may also be given. Constipation is the rule for two or three weeks postpartum, but usually, when the patient resumes her customary duties, the condition improves. When the patient has a complete perineal laceration, the attention to the bowels becomes a very important item of treatment. (See p. 795.) If the woman has too much milk, or if the breasts are engorged and painful, salines, Rochelle salts, or effervescent citrate of magnesia may be prescribed.

The Breasts.—After the mother has slept, usually about eight hours, the nurse prepares the breasts. They are gently washed with soap and water, then with bichlorid 1 : 1500, which is allowed to dry in. A loose breast-binder is now applied, simply to prevent the glands from sagging. Tertullian tells us that the Roman women used a breast-binder made in the temples and possessing mystic powers.

A short time after this the baby is applied to the nipple. Before and after each nursing the nipple is washed with saturated boric acid solution, poured fresh from a bottle, not kept in a glass, using sterilized cotton pledgets on toothpicks, known as "applicators." The fingers do not come in contact with the nipple at all; if it is necessary to do this, the hands must be disinfected. The baby is put to the breast every eight hours until the milk comes, then every four hours during the day. The first nursing is at 6 A. M., the last at 10 P. M. When the milk "comes in," which usually occurs on the third day, the breasts need more support from the breast-binder. The treatment of cracks, engorgement, and other conditions of the breast will be taken up in the chapter on Complications. Too much care and too careful asepsis cannot be given to the breasts, as infection, with resulting abscess and impaired nipples, and resulting necessary weaning of the child, must be avoided.

The question of nursing is an important one. Every mother should nurse her child, for her own good, because it favors involution of the genitalia and develops the maternal instinct, but principally because it reduces the terrific mortality of the first months of life. Fully 25 per cent. of children die in the first year of life, and a large proportion of the deaths is due to bottle-feeding.

It has been said that a bottle-fed baby never became great, a statement which appears reasonable, but has never been proved. Without doubt the public is awakening to the importance of maternal nursing, and now it is considered by most women a real calamity if they cannot give their offspring the breast. Certain contraindications to nursing exist. General diseases, tuberculosis, pernicious anemia, cancer, contraindicate it, because the disease is likely to become very active during lactation. Severe hemorrhage in labor retards the nursing, but with full diet the patient may give her breast to the child for half or more of its feedings. Syphilis does not forbid nursing. Only its own mother may nurse a syphilitic child. A healthy child never comes from a syphilitic mother. The new serum tests for syphilis have proved this.

Malformation of the breasts, as deformed, inverted, cracked, and split nipples, may preclude nursing The latter often are healed by proper treatment. Mastitis commands the suspension of nursing for a few days, and an abscess forbids it permanently from the affected breast. A weak, puny, or hare-lipped child may not be able to nurse, and in these cases the milk is to be pumped and fed to the infant.

Remarkable as it may seem, the milk of some mothers may act like an irritant poison to the infant and may produce enteritis or even death. The milk in the next puerperium may be normal; or the milk may be poor in quality, not agreeing well with the child, but agreeing with another; or there may be a scarcity of milk. Attempts specifically to alter the quality of the milk have been unsatisfactory. The patient's general health must be improved. If there is a scarcity of mother's milk, one may try to stimulate the glands—first, by daily massage, Abt's mechanical pump, cold bathing of the whole body, giving much fluid to drink, especially milk, water, cocoa, gruels, and oyster-stews, but no tea, coffee, beer, or malt liquors. The last two fatten the patient and reduce the milk-supply. A strong baby is the best stimulant to the breasts, and if this fails to bring milk, usually there is no gland tissue there and all efforts will be futile.   Occasionally the milk-supply is not abundant until the patient is up and about and takes outdoor exercise.

Artificial feeding is not resorted to unless the mother is obviously unable to meet the demands made on her, and when it is demonstrated, by the condition of the baby, that the breasts are inefficient.   Before attempting substitute feeding it is best for the baby that a wet-nurse be obtained.

Pulse and Temperature.—The nurse should take the pulse, temperature, and respiration at least morning and evening, better, every six hours,—at 6, 12, 6, and 12,—and record the same on a carefully kept history sheet.   The pulse may be counted frequently during the first five days, and the temperature taken if it shows any increase in rate.   The pulse is a more sensitive indicator of abnormalities than the temperature, but the latter is more certain, since the pulse is very mobile.   Any temperature above 99.5° F. should be considered abnormal and its cause sought. Chills normally are absent from the puerperium.   The author is very suspicious of "nervous chills"—they usually are not nervous, but due to infection.   The pulse normally ranges from 66 to 80; a decrease below 66 is not pathologic, but an increase over 90 should direct our attention to the patient.   If the patient has no nurse, the temperature is taken by the physician during his visit, and he leaves a thermometer with the patient, instructing her to hold it in her mouth at a certain time, then to lay it aside for him to read at his next visit.

The Doctor's Visit.—A daily visit to the puerpera is desirable, but not necessary if she has a good nurse.   It is important that the patient be seen on the third, fourth, and fifth days, because these are the critical ones.   The nurse will keep a record of all the happenings to both mother and child.   The nurse is supplied by the author with special blanks for this purpose, and she also fills a card showing temperature and pulse graphs.   It is well for the physician himself to inspect the vulva, the pads, the breasts, and the nipples for evidences of disease, and to palpate the uterus to determine its state of involution.   He must watch the retrogressive changes of the puerperium, and be alert to the first beginning deviation from the normal, as infection, subinvolution.   He must study the progress of the repair of the puerperal wounds to discover early any abnormality here, like necrosis of tissue, inflammatory infiltration, exudate, and he must be acquainted with the general state of health of the puerpera, so as to be able to recognize, before they occur, impending accidents, as eclampsia, yellow atrophy of the liver, septicemia, puerperal insanity.   Of particular significance is the passage of clots, since this indicates something wrong in the uterus.   Very few medicines are prescribed in a normal puerperium—really none save cathartics and an occasional remedy for after-pains.

After-pains.—Multiparæ suffer more with painful uterine contractions than do primiparæ.   Occurring in the latter, they give rise to the suspicion of infection or the retention of clots or placental fragments in the uterus.   They are due to lack of tonus of the uterine muscle.   Unless very severe, keeping the patient awake, morphin is not given, a trial first being made with a barbituric acid preparation, or sodium bromid, or aspirin, or a little codein and aspirin, or local applications, hot fomentations, camphorated oil, or a hot saline enema.

Sleep and Mental Care.—It is highly important that the puerpera obtain sufficient real sleep as well as rest.   One of the symptoms, and perhaps a contributory cause, of puerperal insanity is lack of sleep.

After the patient has been cared for on the completion of labor, she is allowed to sleep as long as possible, and the room is darkened and quieted to favor this. Subsequently the nurse must arrange the duties of the day so that the puerpera has a little nap in the afternoon, and at least eight hours' good sleep at night.   If the puerpera is persistently sleepless, the physician should be notified.   The cause of the sleeplessness must be investigated, and if there is a family history of mental disease, the condition must be cured at once.   The author has tried suggestion with good effect, also sodium bromid in 20-grain doses, veronal in 5-grain doses, and chloralamid, 5 to 15 grains, but where the woman is tired out, nervous, excited, and evidently under a strain, a hypodermic of $\frac{1}{6}$ grain morphin with $\frac{1}{150}$ grain atropin should be given.   The danger of inaugurating the morphin habit is always to be borne in mind, and the patient properly guarded against it.   Much can be done by the nurse to procure sleep, as giving a warm alcohol sponge-bath, a glass of hot malted milk, cultivation of a regular habit of sleep, removal of the infant from the room, and a constant cheerful, hopeful demeanor, withholding worries of all kinds from the patient.

The physician should study the mind of his patient to learn if she is making the proper adjustments to her new conditions of life.

After having been the center of interest throughout the many months of pregnancy, and perhaps a little spoiled by the petting of her family and friends,

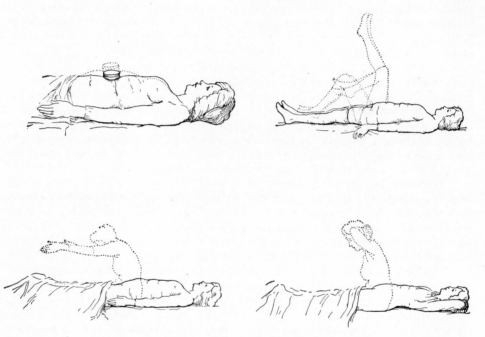

FIG. 332.—A FEW OF THE EXERCISES FOR RESTORING MUSCLE TONE.

the new mother may, unconsciously, resent the sudden transference of attention to the baby.   Indeed, she may be a little jealous of it, as was frankly confessed to me recently by one of my patients.   Then, too, the realization comes that life will never be as it was before, that now she has restrictions on her freedom and her social activities, and new responsibilities which she may fear are beyond her powers.

In normal cases—i. e., in the vast majority—the woman's mental adaptability remains with her and she quickly adjusts herself to her new outlook on life, she assumes her responsibilities gladly, and bravely begins her work as mother of the child and her household.

In abnormal cases, on the other hand, in women with a weak nervous heredity, or in those pulled down by protracted labor, hemorrhage, toxemia, or infection, these mental conflicts are not won by the patient.   Introspection develops into

23

moodiness, even melancholia; the illusion that the husband has transferred his affection to the child develops into jealousy which may result in her refusal to nurse it, or compulsive acts, even attempts at infanticide; or the illusion that her husband loves her no longer may develop into a delusion of unworthiness or persecution, which may lead to attempts of suicide. Observation of the workings of the mind may lead to the early discovery of a psychosis.

General Treatment.—This is the same as for any bed patient as regards bathing, changing bed, and so forth. Unless the weather makes it agreeable, a full bath is not needed every day, but may be given twice or thrice a week. Daily, however, the whole body may be sponged with alcohol and water, one part to three, paying especial attention to the axillæ. There should be plenty of light and fresh air in the lying-in chamber. Sun and air are not harmful by any means. In the olden time both were feared, and the puerpera was kept in semidarkness all the time, and all air excluded to prevent her from catching cold. It was thought that "catching cold" caused puerperal infection and mastitis, but now we know these complications are due to infection, and are in high degree preventable by proper asepsis. Free ventilation and light are strong opponents to infection. The nurse, while providing both, must see that at no time either mother or child is exposed to a direct draft, and that the bright light does not fall directly on the eyes of either

After the first week the nurse may give the patient a general light massage. She should avoid the inside of the legs, where there are veins, and the uterus and breasts. Passive motions of the arms, legs, and trunk are also recommended. Systematic motions of the arms and legs, such as extending and flexing them against a slight resistance, may be practised. These exercises while away the tedium of the bed, improve the circulation, strengthen the abdominal muscles, and hasten the return of the patient's strength. She is less likely to be faint and weak when first gotten out of bed. (See Obstetrics for Nurses, 1933.)

Visitors.—The lying-in room should be quiet and restful. The puerpera must be given opportunity to recover from the strain of labor and recuperate her strength from the exhaustion of pregnancy and delivery. Therefore only the nearest relatives are to be allowed in the lying-in chamber during the first week. Even these visits should be very short. Aside from the nervous disturbance caused by too many visitors, there is the danger of the introduction of contagion.

The Time of Getting Up.—The author allows a normal puerpera, after normal labor, to sit up in bed on the sixth or seventh day, get out of bed into a large chair for an hour on the ninth or tenth day, for three hours on the eleventh, and before the end of the second week she has the freedom of the floor, going downstairs on the fifteenth to eighteenth day. Operative cases, perineorrhaphies, and women who have had fever during the puerperium require special regulations—usually a prolongation of the stay in bed and slower resumption of active movements. But the women are not condemned to such absolute quiet in the bed as formerly. For the first two or three hours the puerpera should lie quietly on her back, but after this she may be turned gently on the side, the nurse supporting the heavy uterus. Next day the position may be changed oftener, and by the third day only ordinary care is necessary, and the changes may be made as frequently as comfort demands. These changes facilitate drainage and better the pelvic circulation. The puerpera after the fourth day may be propped up with pillows or back-rest for her meals, bowel movements, and urinations, may sit up straight on the sixth day, but her perfect condition and her frequent requests to be let out of bed should not lead the physician to permit it until the ninth or tenth day. It is wise, too, to forbid too early resumption of household duties, responsibilities, and social functions.

This time-honored custom of keeping the woman in bed nine days or more has been assailed by late writers. Küstner, in 1899, and White, as far back as 1775, advocated the practice of allowing the women to leave the bed as soon as they felt able to do so, and claimed that no evil results followed, but, on the contrary, the woman recovered strength quicker, had less fever, less frequent thrombophlebitis, less coprostasis, less necessity for catheterization, better lactation, and no greater frequency of prolapse of the uterus and vagina.

It is probable that those physicians who keep their puerperæ in bed two, three, or even four weeks err in the opposite direction, and it is certain that one can let the women get up too soon. The best plan will, as usual, be a compromise between the two, and the limits be applied to special cases. One must hesitate long before allowing a principle, grounded in thousands of years of empiricism, to be overthrown by a new theory, and, indeed, the early getting up does not possess all the advantages claimed, nor is it free from the dangers it is said to be. In the first place, theoretic consideration of the condition of the pelvis postpartum will indicate the necessity for rest in the horizontal position. The bruised, suggillated condition of the pelvic floor has already been referred to. It stands to reason that such an impaired pelvic floor should not be given the task of supporting the large heavy puerperal uterus and the whole intra-abdominal pressure before it has regained, in a measure, its strength and elasticity. The ancient idea that too early getting up leads to prolapse of the vagina and uterus has anatomic foundation, and, further, clinical experience proves it. Prolapse is more common in the poor women who have to get up early after delivery and do heavy work. It is common among Indians.

It is claimed that fever is less frequent. The author believes that fever is more frequent. In the service of the Chicago Lying-in Hospital Dispensary, in nearly every case where the puerpera is reported to have fever the history reads that the patient had gotten out of bed and soon after sickened. We know that the streptococcus—and a virulent strain too—normally inhabits the puerperal vagina. When the puerpera gets up, the heavy uterus falls to and fro and tears open the granulating surfaces, giving the germs access to the lymph-spaces. Statistics have not proved all the claims for the new treatment. More about this interesting subject must be sought in the literature, of which much has accumulated in the last few years. (See Mosher and Küstner.[*])

The Binder.—Ancient custom prescribes the application of an abdominal binder directly postpartum. Van Swieten (1754) recommended it for the prevention of syncope, the raising up of the uterus, and postpartum hemorrhage. It does replace the feeling of emptiness of which the women complain after delivery, but it will not prevent the uterus from rising in the belly or from bleeding, no matter how tightly applied. The women insist on the application of the binder throughout the puerperium, with a view to preserving the figure and preventing "high stomach." In the author's opinion, the binder will do neither. Enteroptosis, nephroptosis, relaxed abdominal wall, are the results of congenital deformity, pathogenic conditions acquired before or during pregnancy,—for example, overstretching of the abdominal walls,—and very little may be done during the puerperium to correct these evil effects. The author applies the binder postpartum to relieve the feeling of emptiness of the abdomen, to help steady the uterus when the patient is moved, and to satisfy her whims. Hardly any objection can be offered to its use. It is almost impossible to apply it tightly enough to force the uterus backward, but it may, if tympany develops, interfere with the passage of flatus and feces, which is especially true after cesarean section. During the second week of the puerperium a very gentle superficial abdominal massage and mild gymnastics are used to strengthen the muscles. By preventing the accumulation of gas in the bowels and providing a daily alvine evacuation, the above treatment is aided. After the patient assumes the erect posture, the abdominal binder may assist greatly, by supporting the weight of the viscera for a short time until the recti and obliqui have regained sufficient tonus and power. The abdominal binder used after laparotomy may be applied, or a jockeystrap may be worn. The latter furnishes also some slight perineal support. Corsets may be resumed after five weeks, and the variety which holds up the lower abdomen should be preferred.

Final Examination.—The patient is instructed to appear for examination at the office of the accoucheur with her baby eight weeks after delivery. By this time involution is complete, the woman has had the first menstruation, if it was to occur, and one can better judge of the condition of the parts. Special attention is directed to the size and position of the uterus, the presence of exudates in the broad ligaments, the condition of the adnexa, the firmness of the levator ani and perineum, and the state of the bladder and vaginal walls as regards prolapse. If the uterus is retroverted, it is to be replaced and a pessary inserted, which the patient should wear

* Küstner: Verh. der Deutsch. Gesell. f. Gyn., vol. viii, p. 530. White: The Treatment of Pregnant and Puerperal Women, 1775. Mosher: Amer. Jour. Obstet., 1911, vol. xliv.

three months. Cervical tears that were not repaired at the time of labor are inspected. If small and with but little eversion they may be treated by the electric cautery. If extensive and, as usual, combined with pelvic floor relaxation or tears, operation is to be recommended as soon as weaning is done. If the perineal floor is relaxed, the patient is instructed how to exercise the levator ani, to take the knee-chest position for ten minutes three times a day, and is given a prescription for hot vaginal douches. Other gynecologic treatment or operation is advised if necessary, and the opportunity is used to discover the very beginnings of post-puerperal disease and to correct them. If the woman has had a severe labor, she is advised as to a subsequent pregnancy.

The child is examined for umbilical hernia, and its nutritional state determined. These points are all to be noted on the puerperium card, which entry closes the obstetric history of the particular case and the patient is requested to report again the day after the baby is a year old, for "follow up."

SUMMARY OF THE PRINCIPLES OF TREATMENT OF THE PUERPERIUM

1. Antisepsis and asepsis of the open genital wounds.
2. Asepsis of the breasts.
3. Attention to the emunctories, bowels, urinary tract, and skin.
4. Provisions for comfort, sleep, and relief of pain.
5. Watchfulness for complications.
6. General treatment to facilitate recovery.
7. The time of getting up.
8. Final examination to prevent future invalidism.

THE DIAGNOSIS OF THE PUERPERIUM

Chiefly in legal cases is the accoucheur required to give an opinion as to the existence of the puerperal state. At postmortems on women dead after an illegal operation, as criminal abortion, it is usually easy to determine the exact condition, from the macroscopic and microscopic appearance of the parts. If a woman pleads the puerperal state for the purposes of blackmail or for the substitution of an infant, it is usually a simple matter to discover the fraud, but if a labor has actually taken place and the patient wishes to hide her condition, as, for example, in cases of child murder, it is not so easy to prove incontestably that gestation has preceded the examination. Naturally, the difficulties increase with the length of time since delivery. A full-term labor also leaves greater and more permanent traces than an abortion. No reliance may be placed on the statements of the patient or her friends.

The examination includes a search for the changes of the puerperium, especially for the presence of a functionating breast (not traces of milk or colostrum) and for the evidences of fresh wounds in the genital tract. The vulva has a quite characteristic, reddish purple, velvety, succulent appearance for the first four weeks postpartum, and the presence of the typical birth injuries undergoing the usual changes of wound healing lends great weight to the diagnosis. Absence of such injuries does not eliminate the possibility of previous delivery, because the fetus may have been small or macerated, or the parts especially elastic. The presence of vestiges of the hymen—carunculæ myrtiformes—is indicative, not conclusive. Cervical tears are usually due to child-birth, but sometimes come from instrumentation, as dilatation for dysmenorrhea or sterility. The enlargement of the uterus, directly or shortly after labor, its consistence, its contractions, and its rapid decrease in size, determined by repeated bimanuals and measurements with the sound, give valuable information, both as to the fact and to the time of a previous confinement. If the cervix is patulous, a finger may be inserted and feel the placental site. Less reliance than one would expect may be placed on a study of the lochia and scrapings. One must find ovular remnants to clinch the diagnosis. Vernix caseosa, meconium, but especially pieces of placenta or chorionic villi are positive. Decidual cells, when in very large numbers, are presumptive evidence, but one must find villi to arrive at positiveness. Opitz believed he could diagnose a preëxisting pregnancy from the construction of the uterine glands thus removed. Later investigations have disproved this, but a study of the scrapings will give very strong evidences of puerperal changes if done early enough. The presence of hyaline remnants of blood-vessels in the scrapings even six months postpartum is said to be good evidence. (See changes in the uterine mucous membrane during involution, p. 224.) Since the patient may refuse to permit a curetage on the ground that it is dangerous to her, and justifiably, we are usually without this kind of information. Abortion in progress or a fibroid may simulate the puerperium. After an early abortion it may be impossible to distinguish the puerperal uterus from one that is menstruating. The Aschheim-Zondek test of pregnancy continues eight days after delivery. Even though strongly suggestive one ought to have confirmatory evidence. It behooves the obstetric expert to be very thorough and systematic in his examination, very deliberate in his consideration of the findings, and very circumspect in his statements on the witness-stand in such cases as the above. A full record is to be made of every examination. These should be gotten up in legal form, the help of an attorney being asked if necessary.

LITERATURE

Macy: Editorial, Jour. Am. Med. Assoc., July 2, 1932, p. 36.—*Opitz:* Zeitschr. f. Geb. u. Gyn., vol. xlii.

SECTION V

THE NEW-BORN CHILD

CHAPTER XXIV

PHYSIOLOGY OF THE NEW-BORN CHILD

At no period during the life of the individual does he undergo such violent and fundamental changes as at birth and during the two weeks after it. Not a few children fail to survive the shock of delivery, and a great many succumb in the first few weeks because of their inability to meet and overcome the adverse conditions surrounding their lives. The new-born must now do its own digesting, must oxygenate its own blood from the air, which is of varying temperature, must keep up its body warmth in spite of violent external variations, and, besides other functions, must take care of hosts of bacteria which assail it from every port of entrance. True, it brings into the world certain acquired immunities against infection, but it must develop a great many itself.

Respiration.—At first the breathing is very irregular and abdominal in type; later it becomes more even and more thoracic, becoming abdominothoracic during crying efforts. The respirations are both superficial and deep, occasionally intermittent, and vary from 35 to 60, even in health. Murphy and Thorpe found that the mean tidal air of sleeping infants varied from 10 to 27 c.c. The exchange of gases in the lungs is more than twice as active as in the adult. Oxidation in the body is also more active, assimilative processes and growth being so vigorous and marked. At first only a small portion of the lung is expanded, and it requires a month or more to expand it all (Fig. 535). The chest wall is so poorly developed that when the pleural cavities are opened, the lungs do not collapse, as in the adult.

Crying is good for the child, because it expands the lungs. A whining, grunting expiration is a sign that the alveoli are not developed, as occurs in premature, asphyxiated, or injured children. Mucus in the trachea causes rattling; it may come from congestion of the throat, the result of labor, or from aspiration of vaginal or other discharges during the delivery. This is dangerous on the score of mechanical obstruction of the air-passages (atelectasis) and infection, bronchopneumonia, and enteritis.

The **blood** is more concentrated than that of adults (specific gravity, 1060 to 1080), and contains more hemoglobin and salts. The amount varies from 250 to 350 gm., depending on the size of the child and the time of ligation of the cord, being, with late ligation, about one-eleventh of the body weight. Lucas and Dearing found it varies from 10.7 to 19.5 per cent. Leukocytosis is the rule for the first few days—up to 23,000; later, an average of about 10,000 to 12,000 is attained. The polynuclears are in the majority early, but after the twelfth day the lymphocytes preponderate and there are usually 7 per cent. eosinophils. Owing to the thickening of the blood in the first days the reds are increased in number—from 5,000,000 to 6,500,000—but soon the normal is reëstablished, because of the destruction of about 10 per cent. of them. The size of the red corpuscles varies very much, there being many microcytes. Poikilocytosis also may be found, and, for four to nine days, nucleated reds, erythroblasts.

358

Halban and Landsteiner studied the serum of the child, and found that it possessed less antitoxic, bactericidal, and hemolytic properties than the adult's, and that, therefore, the blood is not complete. Its clotting time varies and, if delayed too much, may explain the frequency of hemorrhage in the new-born (Rodda). Sharpe found that it had no significance in cerebral hemorrhage.

The *circulation*, studied by Seitz, of Munich, showed marked changes. During fetal life the pulse-beats number 120 to 150; after delivery, 150 to 190; sinking to 110, then rising to 120 to 130 a minute on the fourth to sixth day, with many variations of frequency, and rhythm, and strength, caused by sleep, waking, crying, colic, etc. The blood-pressure varies from 38 to 48 mm. on the first day and 66 to 76 on the twelfth day (Seitz), and since the arteries and capillaries of the child

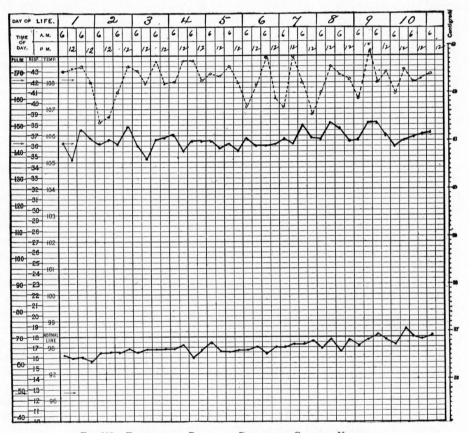

Fig. 333.—Temperature, Pulse, and Respiration Chart of New-born.

The average readings of ten apparently healthy children were taken. The pulse and respiration in every instance were counted with the stethoscope. Records were made at 6 A. M., 12 noon, 6 P. M., and 12 midnight. Dotted line is the respiration, the lowest line, the temperature.

are large, the peripheral resistance is less, allowing a more active and rapid circulation of the blood. This is needful for the rapid development of all the organs, the active digestion, and tissue growth of the child.

The Temperature.—Owing to the fetus' own metabolism, the intra-uterine temperature is one-half degree higher at birth than that of the mother (Fig. 333). As the result of the exposure following delivery, the temperature sinks 1 to $3\frac{1}{2}$ degrees—greater in premature and asphyxiated children. After twelve to twenty hours the normal, 98° F., is reached. After a week or so the temperature remains around 98.6° F. Bathing, nursing, exposure, lack of food, etc., easily alter the temperature of the child. Diurnal variations are not usual.

The Urine.—Reusing presents this table of the daily average amounts of urine:

	1	2	3	4	5	6	7	8	day
Breast-fed..................	18.9	38.6	64.9	84.0	121.5	147.0	175.5	217.2	c.c.
Bottle-fed.................	28.8	59.7	111.4	153.8	198.9	237.7	278.7	371.0	c.c

From 7½ to 9 c.c. of urine may be found in the bladder at birth. Later, daily amounts vary very much with the size of the child, prematurity, the room temperature and moisture (incubator children pass less urine), the food (mother's milk, less urine), icterus, and illness. If the baby is a water-tippler, the bed may be wet all the time. The specific gravity is from 1006 to 1008; color, clear, watery, later a light straw; reaction acid. Urea shows highest on the seventh day—0.8 per cent., from 0.1 per cent. on the first day. The percentage of uric acid is large, as is shown by the frequency of uric-acid infarct of the kidney, due largely to the destruction of red blood-corpuscles. It is nearly thrice as much as in the adult, a condition which also exists in the blood (Sedgwick). Uric-acid infarct of the kidney occurs in 50 per cent. of children, and may be assumed from a microscopic examination of the urine showing the crystals. Often the crystals (ammonium urate principally) are found on the diaper as a reddish brick-dust. When a kidney containing the infarct is cut, it grits under the knife, and yellowish or brownish streaks are seen radiating from the papillæ. The deposit occurs oftener in premature children, after prolonged or instrumental deliveries, after asphyxia, in cases of delayed lactation, with icterus and febrile complications. The granules may cause pain in their passage. Nephritis is not uncommon in early infancy (Jacobi) pyelitis, too. Albuminuria is very common—almost constant for four to seven days. Acidosis with convulsions may occur within the first few days. Both boys and girls show the Aschheim-Zondek reaction for three or four days.

The Intestinal Tract.—Shortly after birth the meconium which has accumulated in the large intestine is discharged. Occasionally a plug of mucus which filled the rectum precedes the green, thick, pasty meconium. There are 70 to 90 gm. of meconium (Camerer), and it is usually all passed by the third or fourth day. Burrage found Bacterium coli and a staphylococcus in 38 per cent. of meconium of babies just born. Meconium contains epithelium from the intestine, bilirubin, cholesterin crystals, stearic acid, fat, bile, lanugo, skin epithelium, and sebaceous matter from swallowed liquor amnii. The colostrum has a laxative action, and air and gas in the bowel aid the active peristalsis of the first days. The green discharge is followed by brown, then yellow movements, if the child is fed at the breast, but the discharges are whitish and curdy if the child is fed by the bottle.

Within twenty-four hours the whole intestinal canal is infected by the enterococcus and the Bacterium coli commune and other bacteria present in the air, the bath-water, the vagina of the mother, and on the fingers and lips of the mother and nurse. Without doubt many infections of serious nature originate at this time, and, too, the germs introduced may be beneficial, since they aid the process of digestion. Ordinarily the child's intestine is inhabited mainly by two forms—the Bacterium coli and the Bacillus lactis aërogenes.

Breast-fed children may have more stools than fully bottle-fed. In the latter the odor is not that of sour milk, as it is with breast-fed infants, and one is more likely to find clumps of casein, formerly thought to be fat, in the movement.

The stomach contains pepsin; the pancreas trypsin, and a fat-splitting ferment, but no diastatic ferment. x-Ray study shows active peristalsis (Vogt).

The Weight.—During the first four days the infant loses in weight—on the average 6 to 8 ounces. The loss is greater in bottle-fed babies, and those getting scanty food. Forty per cent. of children regain their birth weight by the tenth day, and from then on the normal, breast-fed infant should gain about an ounce a day. The initial loss is due to excretion of meconium, urine, evaporation, and to the fact that the new-born gets very little nourishment in the first few days. Such losses do not occur in animals, and they have important bearing on the diseases of early infancy. (See Bailey and Murlin.) The table from Beuthner gives the average amounts of food taken by children from the breast for the first fourteen days:

	1	2	3	4	5	6	7	8	9	10	11	12	13	14
Average birth-weight, 3126 gm..........	17	91	190	302	348	381	450	476	476	476	476	476	476	476

If more food is given the child in the first days, the initial loss in weight is not so great or may be avoided. Premature infants lose relatively more and regain their birth-weight very slowly, often requiring a month. The same is true of

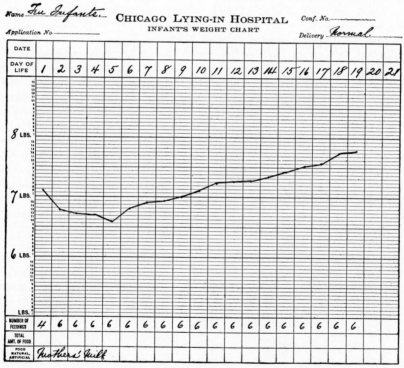

FIG. 334.—CHART SHOWING AVERAGE WEIGHT OF 10 APPARENTLY NORMAL BREAST-FED INFANTS.

excessively large children. Children fed on cow's milk lose more weight and regain flesh less rapidly than breast-fed infants. Since nearly as large a percentage of cow's milk as of human milk is absorbed (93 and 96 per cent.), there must be other reasons for the inferiority of cow's milk as an infant food. It is well known that breast-fed children grow faster, are more vigorous, resist infections better, throw off disease quicker, suffer less from rickets, etc., than the bottle-fed. Human milk is easier to digest. Fewer calories of it are required. Its albumin is partly in solution as a homologous albumin, ready for absorption into the blood without the preparatory stages of propeptone, peptone, and albumose; it contains phosphorus in very assimilable form, as nuclein, lecithin, and opalisin. It is not a dead secretion, but a live tissue, and carries ferments which render the milk easily absorbed, and which, added to cow's milk, will even render the latter much more assimilable. This fact, known clinically for many years, has been emphasized by Marfan and Escherich, who call these ferments or enzymes, trophozymases. Human milk also contains diastatic, proteolytic, fibrin- and fat-splitting ferments, also alexogenic ferments (Moro). Ehrlich proved that immune bodies pass from the mother to the fetus and from mother to child through the milk (Seitz).

General Condition.—Observing the child after birth, it is seen to be in a half-sleeping state. The eyes are opened once in a while, but immediately closed, the arms move, also the legs, sometimes quite vigorously. The difference between sleep and waking is not very well marked until the end of the first week or even later. Of the special senses, touch and taste are already well developed. Sight is probably, the light reflex is certainly, present. Hearing is sometimes determinable as early as the first day, but usually is positively present only toward the end of the first week. The sense of smell develops later.

The spinal nervous system is in a state of hyperexcitability, the infant jumping on even slight jarring, and the will is certainly developed early, as one may judge from the rapid acquisition of bad habits. Reaction to electric stimulation is slower.

The Skin.—At first the child is cyanotic, especially about the face and extremities, and the eyelids may be swollen. After thirty or forty minutes the normal rosy pink of the new-born appears, unless the infant is premature, when the color is a dusky red. Over the back and in the creases of the body a thick white paste is often found—the vernix caseosa. This consists of fatty skin secretions, epidermis, and lanugo, and is usually removed by oiling with the first bath. In many children the epidermis exfoliates in branny scales, or there may be pronounced desquamation. In the latter cases, which may be toxemic, the skin looks a little raw at first and may crack, but later a healthy pink or white appears. During the first weeks the skin is subject to various eruptions, especially vesicular and pustular. They are called strophulus—red, if the border of the vesicles is red, and white, if simply vesicular. These are usually affections of the sweat-glands. There may also be a generalized erythema. A pustular eruption is generally due to infection with the Staphylococcus albus. In summer the tendency to skin affections is marked, vesicular intertrigo being an annoying complication, and in general the skin is more sensitive to the action of soap and water, irritating clothing, insufficiently rinsed diapers, etc.

Icterus Neonatorum.—About 20 per cent. of children show slight icterus during the first week. Two varieties must be distinguished—icterus simplex and icterus gravis. The latter is a symptom of sepsis, syphilis, Buhl's disease, the hemorrhagic diathesis, congenital obstruction in the bile-passages, etc. A peculiar and fatal form of icterus affecting the ganglia of the brain is described. Here only the benign form will be considered—the simple jaundice or icterus neonatorum.

Most authors place the percentage of jaundiced infants at about 80, but the experience of the writer is that even 20 per cent. is too high. With the aseptic care of the new-born and more physiologic treatment the minority of infants develop even a trace of icterus. On the second or third day one notices a slight yellowish tinge of the skin of the body and face, which may be better seen if the usual redness be pressed away by the finger. In marked cases even the sclera may be yellow, the nasal discharges and the urine also showing the discoloration, bile-pigment having been found in them. Autopsy shows that the intima of the arteries, the cartilages, and the interstitial tissues are stained, but the brain and cord, the liver and the kidneys, very slightly, if any. The kidneys often contain the uric-acid infarct. Icteric children usually are thin, grow less vigorously, show signs of gastro-intestinal inflammation, are colicky, subject to febrile disturbances, intertrigo of the buttocks, and generally are poorer than the others, for which reasons the author cannot call the affection a physiologic manifestation. The excretion of urea and uric acid is greater, more albumin is used up, oxidation is more rapid (Hofmeier).

After the first week the jaundice has usually disappeared, but if it was severe, three to five weeks may be necessary. Much depends on the cause.

Etiology.—The cases occur with equal frequency in hospital and private practice, in town and city. Jaundice is more common in the children of primiparæ, after long and hard instrumental deliveries, breech cases, in premature or atelectatic infants; it is more common in boys than in girls, and in the children of young mothers; it may be a familial characteristic.

The jaundice is probably due to the action of several causes. Bilirubin, according to Schultz, is formed by action of the cells of the reticulo-endothelial system on the red cells destroyed by the forces of labor. Jaundice, therefore, both extra hepatic and hepatogenic, is aided by the increased destruction of red blood-corpuscles, which occurs in the first weeks.

There are many theories, for example—(1) Obstruction of the ductus choledochus by mucus or epithelium; (2) edema of Glisson's capsule; (3) changes in the circulation of the blood in the liver; (4) absorption of the bile from the intestines, which may take place directly into the blood or the general circulation, as a result of the persistence of the ductus Arantii; deficient excretion of bile (Hess); (5) imperfect action of liver cells, disturbed perhaps by injury, toxemia, or infection.

Infection has been given as a cause, and for severe cases is usually active. Gessner believes that infection of the umbilicus will explain many cases, and in this the author fully agrees. Intestinal infection will explain more of them.

The prognosis is good in the simple icterus, but one should reserve expression of opinion until the severe forms of disease are excluded. It is wise to regard all cases of jaundice as significant, and examine the infant carefully to exclude syphilis, sepsis, etc.

The treatment is symptomatic. It has seemed to the author that the cases get better quicker on treatment directed to intestinal disinfection—castor oil, followed by calomel, with gastric and colonic lavage.

LOCAL CHANGES

Separation of the Cord.—At the insertion of the cord into the belly the amnion covering the cord passes into the skin. If the skin runs up onto the cord, it is called "skin navel"; if the amnion runs down onto the abdomen, "amnion navel," the latter being rare. Vessels from the arteries of the abdomen make a circle around the navel and send up tiny branches which end $\frac{1}{12}$ to $\frac{1}{8}$ inch on the cord itself. The piece of cord not in connection with this circulation must necrose and fall off.

After a few hours one can see evidences of a reactive inflammation at the point of union of dead and living tissue, the skin around the insertion of the cord becoming red and swollen. White blood-corpuscles wander out and soften the cord at its junction with the body until a layer of granulations is fully formed separating the cord at its base. The dried stump finally drops off, the arteries giving way first, and then the vein. The surface of the navel is covered with very fine granulations; the center is retracted, the sides falling in; epithelium forms over the surface very quickly, and the navel is thus cicatrized. The cord drops off from the fourth to the twelfth day. The majority of authors give the average as the fifth day. Our experience has been much different. With the older methods of treatment of the stump it was exceptional for the cord to drop off before the end of the week. Now the cord is tied close to the insertion in the skin (but not involving it), and under aseptic treatment it falls off in three to six days—seldom later than the eighth.

There are two ways in which the cord behaves—mummification and moist gangrene.   The first occurs when the cord is kept warm and dry, the second when it is wrapped in oily dressings and evaporation is prevented.   The drying-up of the cord is more common, less dangerous, and is to be favored.   A large, thick cord dries up late, and some authors advise to strip all the jelly of Wharton from the cord, so as to favor the rapid mummification.

The umbilical vein collapses, the walls adhere, and normally there is no thrombosis.   The hypogastric arteries collapse, and, owing to the thick muscular layer, are quite obliterated, but a small clot almost always is found in them.   This should not present the appearance of pus.

The staphylococcus, streptococcus, and various non-pathogenic bacteria have been found in a large proportion of cords of healthy children.   They were much more in number and much earlier found in the days when moist gangrene of the cord commonly occurred.   The method of dressing the navel had a great deal to do with it.   Separation of the cord takes place earlier in large, strong children, later in premature children; earlier in healthy children, later in sick children; later if wet, earlier if dry, gangrene of the cord occurs.   The sinking in of the center of the wound is due to the retraction of the intra-abdominal part of the arteries.   The healing of the navel is complete on the third or fourth day after the dropping of the cord.

The **breasts** of some new-born children show an interesting phenomenon.   On the third or fourth day they enlarge, become hard, and occasionally secrete a little watery milk, with yellowish streaks.   Microscopically, it resembles the colostrum, and colostrum corpuscles may be found.   On the fifth or sixth day a fluid resembling milk in color and taste may be pressed out.   This continues for two to four weeks if the gland be irritated, but if let alone, the secretion dries up and disappears.   In rare cases a little fluid can be expressed after a year.   This condition must be distinguished from true mastitis of the infant, a disease which does occur.   The secretion is called by the Germans "Hexen-Milch," witch's milk, and occurs in boys as well as in girls—really it seems to occur oftener in boys than in girls; in weak as well as in strong children.   The cause of the action of the breasts is unknown.   Bayer believes it is due to the presence of the same ferment which causes the maternal milk secretion.   He has found also an enlargement of the uterus of the new-born girl, which he likewise ascribes to maternal influence.   The breasts should be let alone.   Wash them with soap and water, pad them lightly with cotton, and tie a bandage over them.   *Do not squeeze them.*

In about 1 case out of 100 the female infant will present a phenomenon resembling menstruation.   The flow may last from one to six days, and be very slight or profuse.   It usually is not attended with symptoms, but if very free, may produce evident malaise in the child.   This pseudo-menstruation is more common in the children of primiparæ, after prolonged and operative and breech deliveries, and may be associated as a symptom with hemorrhage into the brain. Its causes are various.   Perhaps it may be the result of stimulation of the ovaries by parturition, and have analogy with the enlargement of the breasts and uterus above referred to.   Perhaps the child has absorbed some of the internal ovarian secretion of the mother.   For a masterly consideration of the physiology and pathology of the new-born, see *von Reuss*, Die Erkrankungen des Neugeborenen, Berlin, 1914, Springer.

Literature

Burrage, S.: Jour. Bacteriology, 1927, vol. 13, p. 47.—*Lucas and Dearing:* Amer. Jour. Dis. of Children, January, 1921, vol. xxi, p. 97.—*Murphy and Thorpe:* Jour. Clinical Investigation, August, 1931.—*Rodda:* Jour. Amer. Med. Assoc., August 14, 1920.—*Schultz, W. G.:* See Edit., Jour. Am. Med. Assoc., December 6, 1930, p. 1748. Lit.—*Sedgwick:* Jour. Biol. Chem., 1917, xxxi, p. 261.—*Seitz:* Zentralbl. f. Gynäk., November 20, 1920, p. 1339.—*Sharpe:* Surg., Gyn., and Obstet., February, 1924, p. 200.—*Vogt:* Radiology of Newborn, Zentralbl. f. Gynäk., July 23, 1921, p. 1032.

CHAPTER XXV

THE CARE OF THE CHILD

WHILE the third stage of labor is being conducted, and the accoucheur and nurse are devoting their attention to the mother, the infant lies in its crib, securely and warmly wrapped up, or is given in the care of a relative or neighbor, who is instructed to look at the navel occasionally for possible bleeding and see that the infant does not choke with mucus. After the confinement room is set to rights, the nurse takes the baby and dresses it, preferably in an adjoining apartment, to avoid disturbing the sleeping mother. First the whole body is rubbed with warm, sterile, solid albolene or benzoinated lard, paying particular attention to the places where the vernix accumulates. The fat dissolves the vernix, and the little body is now smoothly rubbed clean with a soft towel. No bath is given. Next the stump of the cord and the navel region are washed with 1 : 2000 bichlorid or 95 per cent. alcohol, and the wound dressed with sterilized gauze, a sterile belly-band being put over this primary surgical dressing. Then the eyes are treated after Credè's or some prophylactic method, if this has not been done before, and the child quickly and warmly dressed, after which it is placed in its crib, with a warm-water bag at its feet. All this must be done near a fire, away from chilling drafts, and the navel must be dressed with sterile hands if the wound is touched with the fingers.

The Bath.—Long custom prescribed a daily bath for the child. This is not to be recommended, because the infant is likely to be chilled and the wash-water may get to the eyes, navel, vulva, and mouth, causing infections; further, the poor soaps often used may cause eczema and various skin eruptions.

Until the umbilicus is healed, the child should not be given a tub-bath. The head and face are sponged daily with lukewarm water, using a little Castile soap, if necessary. The buttocks. when soiled, are sponged with cool water. The body is gently rubbed with benzoinated lard; this is removed by means of a soft towel, and this is usually all that is needed to keep the infant sweet and clean. After the cord is off and the navel cicatrized, the child is given a full bath. In summer the child may be given a sponge-bath instead of the oiling, because the perspiration and fat macerate the skin.

Dusting-powders are usually not needed, as with good care the infant will not chafe. In hospitals the nurses must be made aware of the dangers of carrying skin diseases and infections, especially syphilis, gonorrhea, and pemphigus, from one child to another, and they should be instructed to report at once any evidences of disease in the child. If stearate of zinc is used, the nurse must be told that the baby can get pneumonia from inhaling it.

Attention to the Cord.—The navel is treated like any surgical open wound. While the binder is changed as often as it becomes soiled, the dressing of the cord is not disturbed unless it has been dislodged or gotten wet. After soaking off the gauze with 1: 2000 bichlorid, the stump is washed with 95 per cent. alcohol, and a new dry gauze dressing applied. Dusting-powders are not used unless the stump shows signs of moist gangrene, when a mixture of 1 part salicylic acid to 20 parts of starch (sterilized) is applied. A wet dressing of 50 per cent. alcohol applied for six hours will usually cure it, and is recommended especially for signs of infection around the stump. During all these manipulations the nurse does not touch the wound unless she sterilizes her hands. Sterile applicators are used.

The Eyes.—Only the outside of the eyelids is washed with a little sterile

365

salt solution. Unless there is some irritation or infection of the eyes, they do not need any treatment. The nurse is to be instructed to report at once by telephone or messenger the first sign of inflammation of the conjunctiva.

The Bowels.—The author recommends the routine administration of 10 drops of castor oil to the infant on the day after the day of birth. This evacuates the meconium and any matters swallowed during delivery, and does much to prevent colic. Later an occasional repetition of the dose, and salt solution colonic flushings, given with a funnel attached to a soft-rubber catheter, will keep the intestinal tract in order. The mouth and tongue are not cleansed unless required, and then with gentleness, to avoid rubbing off the delicate epithelium. Wounds thus produced may form the atrium of infection, especially at the pillars of the fauces (Bednar's aphthæ). Excoriation of the anal region seldom occurs with breast-feeding, but is usual with bottle-feeding. Absolute cleanliness of the parts, frequent change of the diaper, the invariable use of washed, well-rinsed, and ironed diapers, cool ablutions, avoidance of friction, moderate use of dusting-powders, as stearate of zinc, will do much to prevent and cure the intertrigo, but, best of all will be the procuring of a proper food for the infant.

Urination.—If the infant does not urinate within twelve hours, the parts are to be examined for congenital deformity. A tight prepuce is almost never the cause. Either the infant has not had enough water or food, or it passes water unobserved in its bath, or has an attack of renal congestion, perhaps even nephritis. In such cases uric-acid infarct is usually found. Sepsis may also cause anuria, also absorption of toxins from the bowel and all febrile affections. The treatment is on general lines—free catharsis, administration of much water, moderate use of mother's milk, warm fomentations over the bladder and kidneys, a sitz-bath, a prolonged colonic flushing, and, finally, the catheter. The author had one case where a female child, apparently healthy, passed no urine for three days. Catheterization brought a few drams of thick, highly colored urine, after which the function became normal. The brick-dust sediment in the urine and on the diaper consists of uric-acid crystals or ammonium urate. They may cause pain during voiding and they indicate the need of more water.

The Feeding.—Eight to twelve hours after birth the child is put to the breast, as usually by this time the mother has rested. Thereafter, until the milk comes in, the infant nurses every eight hours, and then every four hours, unless it is puny, when it is fed more often, alternate breasts being used. No attempt is made to sterilize the child's mouth by washing, because it is impossible and harmful, and invites the infection it seeks to avoid. The nursing lasts ten to fifteen minutes, and the nurse must be sure that the infant really swallows the milk. It is occasionally necessary to give water between the feedings, but the nurse is to be advised of the uselessness and dangers of the habit of water-tippling. The child really needs little extra liquid. If the child does not take the breast willingly, an investigation may reveal a poorly shaped nipple, a too full breast, difficult flow of milk, milk that does not agree with the child, and which it instinctively refuses, salty or bitter milk, or, finally, there may be none in the breast. Much patience is required to teach the infant how to suck, and wide differences exist in the capabilities of nurses to do this. If there is any doubt of the child getting enough nourishment, it should be weighed before and after each feeding.

For the first few days water, an ounce every two hours, and the colostrum from the breasts usually suffice for the wants of the infant, but if it should cry from hunger, a mixture of one-third milk and water may be given. In hospitals the infant may obtain an occasional feeding from one of the other mothers until its own mother has milk. The possibility of the contagion of syphilis in maternities must never be forgotten. The author is very skeptical regarding the "starvation fever" so often mentioned as occurring at this period. Probably most of such temperatures are due to infection—intestinal, bronchial, faucial, or from the navel. (See Jaschke.)

AHLFELD'S TABLE

NUMBER OF NURSINGS	AVERAGE AMOUNT DRUNK AT EACH NURSING	TOTAL GRAMS	TOTAL OUNCES
1st day.....2	2.5 grams	5.0 grams	1¼ dram
2d " 5	29.0 "	149.0 "	4½ oz.
3d " 6	41.0 "	246.0 "	8¼ "
4th " 7	58.8 "	401.6 "	13⅓ "
5th " 6	67.5 "	405.0 "	13½ "
6th " 7	73.0 "	511.0 "	17 "
7th " 6	92.2 "	553.2 "	18½ "
8th " 7	97.0 "	589.0 "	23 "
9th " 6	93.0 "	558.0 "	18⅗ "
10th " 7	86.0 "	602.0 "	20 "
11th " 6	96.0 "	576.0 "	19⅕ "
12th " 6	93.0 "	558.0 "	18⅗ "
13th " 7	86.0 "	602.0 "	20 "
14th " 7	91.0 "	637.0 "	21¼ "
15th " 6	93.0 "	558.0 "	18⅗ "
16th " 7	90.0 "	630.0 "	21 "
17th " 7	92.0 "	644.0 "	21½ "
18th " 6	96.0 "	576.0 "	19⅕ "
19th " 7	105.0 "	735.0 "	24½ "
20th " 6	112.0 "	672.0 "	22⅓ "
21st " 7	102.0 "	714.0 "	23⅝ "

Without doubt the best food for the infant comes from its mother's breasts, and if she be absolutely unable to nurse, before employing artificial food a wet-nurse should be obtained.

Weighing the Infant.—The child should be weighed directly after birth, and

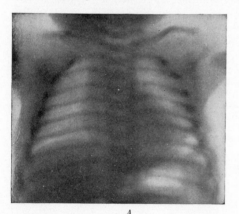 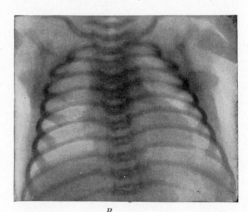

A   B

FIG. 335.—*A*, SKIAGRAGH OF A BABY TAKEN WITHIN THIRTY MINUTES AFTER BIRTH; *B*, ONE TAKEN ON THE THIRD DAY OF LIFE.
Note the increased but not yet full air content of the lungs in the second picture.

daily for several weeks. The beautiful "baby scales" on the market are quite impractical, and should be replaced by the ordinary grocers' scale with a scoop, iron weights, and a scale-bar for the ounces.

Temperature, Pulse, and Respiration.—The first of these must be taken twice daily, and the others occasionally, all of which is to be recorded on the history sheet, the same as for the mother.

General.—A quiet, undisturbed, ordered life is to be provided the new individual, as habits formed now are permanent. Plenty of fresh air is as necessary for the infant as for the adult, and without doubt most babies are cuddled too much. It should sleep in a room with a temperature of from 66°–68° F., and for the first few weeks its eyes should be protected from bright, glary light. It is not to be disturbed except for attentions to itself, and when being lifted, should be guarded against injury. The nurse must be instructed not to let the nursling get into bad habits—water-tippling, peppermint-water tippling, whisky and water and crême-de-menthe tippling, sucking on the finger, nursing-bottle, or nipple, sleeping with mother, being taken up when it cries, or rocked, held, and carried except when sick. By proper training the child can be taught regular habits, to sleep all night and between nursings, and to cry only when hungry, uncomfortable, or ill.

During his professional visit the physician pays some attention to the infant also. He must especially discover the first signs of malnutrition, because, unless this is early remedied, structural changes occur in the intestinal mucosa and the general system which may leave an impress for bad on the child's whole life. This is the reason the author insists so strongly on the wet-nurse when the mother cannot nourish her offspring. The physician watches the physiologic changes which adapt the child to extra-uterine existence, and decides each day if they are proceeding normally. The condition of the navel and eyes claims his special attention.

Pratt, Kraushaar, and Sun made some interesting studies of the behavior of newborn infants.

Summary of the Care of the Infant

1. Asepsis and antisepsis of the navel, eyes, and orifices of the body.
2. Watching for evidences of sickness.
3. Attention to emunctories—bowels, kidneys, and skin.
4. Feeding and nutrition.
5. The healing of the navel.

For details of the care and treatment of the infant the reader is referred to the author's Obstetrics for Nurses, 1930, and to works on pediatrics.

Literature

Bailey and Murlin: Proceedings Society Experimental Biology and Medicine, 1914, xi, 109.—*Chury and Langrock:* Jour. Amer. Med. Assoc., 1916, lxvi, p. 627.—*Halban and Landsteiner:* Münch. med. Woch., 1902, No. 12, p. 473.—*Hess:* Amer. Jour. Children's Diseases, May, 1912.—*Jaschke:* Zeitschr. f. Gyn. u. Geb., 1915, Bd. 78, H. 1, p. 136.—*Pratt et al.:* Ohio State Univ. Press, Columbus, 1930.—*Sedgwick and Kingsbury:* Jour. Amer. Med. Assoc., November 17, 1917, p. 1699.—*Seitz:* Die fetalen Herztöne, Tübingen, 1903; Handbuch der Geb., vol. ii, I, 306.—*Warfield:* American Medicine, September 20, 1902.

PART II

THE PATHOLOGY OF PREGNANCY, LABOR, AND THE PUERPERIUM

CHAPTER XXVI

THE PATHOLOGY OF PREGNANCY

It would be surprising if a function which causes such marked general and local changes as gestation does should be completed without the production of conditions that might be considered pathologic. Pregnancy does not confer immunity against any disease; on the contrary, it makes the woman susceptible to certain general diseases, and almost always aggravates existing general, and especially local, affections. Only seldom do we hear that patients feel better during pregnancy: the majority suffer more or less discomfort. Many conditions formerly classed as normal are now called pathologic.

In Chapters IV and V we studied the changes which occur in the woman as she adapts herself to the new condition of pregnancy. These changes, which are both general and local, must be looked upon as the response of the organism to the demands of the growing fetus. If the reader will recall these adjustments of metabolism, of the blood, of the heart, of the digestive tract, etc., and the alterations in the uterus and vagina, i. e., the provision of a nest for the ovum, and the development of a mechanism for the extrusion of the product of conception, he will be able to perceive that they border closely on the pathologic—indeed, that some, if found under other circumstances, would be called disease.

At all events gestation means a drain on the woman's system. If she can supply all the wants of the fetus she will remain well. If she herself is not endowed with a reserve of all the elements required she will suffer from "inanition" as Opitz says, or incompetence of one or the other function of the body. Animals and primitive women do not show these disturbances. Civilization, therefore, is producing a race of women in whom the response to the necessities of child-bearing is becoming weaker as time goes on, and breakdowns occur. Sellheim calls them "culture-diseases." There is much food for thought in these hints, especially if one holds in view the perpetuation of the race, but they also throw light on many every-day problems and give important leads for prevention and treatment.

The affections of pregnancy are broadly divided into those of the mother and those of the ovum. Of diseases of the mother, two grand divisions are made— the *general* and the *local*, the latter taking in all the affections of the uterus, decidua, vagina, etc. Both general and local diseases may be classified, first, as to whether they are only morbid exaggerations of conditions natural to normal pregnancy— that is, they are incidental to pregnancy, are disorders of pregnancy; and, second, as to whether the diseases are accidental complications, either preëxistent or developed during pregnancy. The general diseases *incident* to pregnancy are most likely to be disorders of those functions most concerned by gestation, for example, the general metabolism, the liver and kidneys, the blood. Examples of *accidental* diseases are smallpox, tuberculosis, and syphilis.

Local diseases *incident* to pregnancy manifest themselves in pathologic increase of the congestion of the parts, abnormal tissue growth, deformation of the uterus, displacements, unusual location of the ovum, etc.   Of diseases of the ovum, we must consider those of the child and those of the fetal envelops, the chorion, the amnion, the placenta.

Most of the diseases of the mother and child have close relations—one can hardly be ill without affecting the other.   A great many general diseases have local manifestations in the genitalia, and many diseases accidental to pregnancy aggravate the affections incidental to pregnancy.   Then, too, the mother may be apparently well, while the fetus alone is ill or dying, and furthermore, the mother may show signs of illness which are produced by the disease-products of a sick fetus.   The reader may thus appreciate the difficulties of making a classification of the morbid states of pregnancy and adhering to it in the subsequent discussion of the subjects.

CLASSIFICATION—PATHOLOGY OF PREGNANCY

Diseases of the Mother Incidental to Pregnancy.—*General.*—Toxemia; hyperemesis gravidarum; ptyalism; gingivitis; eclampsia; the kidney of pregnancy; acute yellow atrophy of the liver; chorea, blood affections; skin diseases, such as pruritus, fibroma molluscum, herpes gestationis, impetigo herpetiformis, toxic efflorescences.   A new term, gestosis (pl., gestoses), has been introduced to designate these toxemic manifestations in pregnancy.

Local.—Varicosities; relaxation and softening of the pelvic joints; extra-uterine pregnancy; angular pregnancy; retroflexion of the gravid uterus; ante-fixation of the uterus; abortion; abruptio placentæ; placenta prævia.

Diseases of the Mother Accidental to Pregnancy.—*General.*—The exanthemata—measles, scarlatina, typhoid, etc.; sepsis; syphilis; diseases of the lungs—tuberculosis, pneumonia, etc.; of the heart; of the kidneys; of the liver; traumatism.

Local.—Deformities of the uterus; the local inflammations—vulvitis, vaginitis, cervicitis, endometritis, peritonitis, gonorrhea; tumors, as fibroids, carcinoma, ovarian cysts.

Diseases of the Ovum.—The Child.—Monsters (teratology); disorders of the mother which affect the child; the injuries of the fetus.

The Membranes.—Polyhydramnion; oligohydramnion.

Placenta.—Abnormal shape, size, and number; the white infarct; syphilis; edema; calcification, hydatidiform mole.

Naturally, in a work of this size it will be impossible to treat fully all the above affections, nor will the scheme here given be strictly followed.   Diseases duplicated under different headings will be considered together—for example, syphilis of the mother, of the child, of the placenta, and of the decidua will be treated as one subject.   The author also considers it best to treat consecutively in a single chapter a disease which affects all three states—pregnancy, labor, and the puerperium—rather than to discuss it, as it influences each stage separately, in three different parts of the volume.

CHAPTER XXVII

THE TOXEMIAS OF PREGNANCY

Toxemia is a term which has obtained very general usage, though little is positively known about the conditions it represents. It means that the blood contains toxins or poisons, but their nature we do not understand. These toxins are supposed to be the result of deficient or abnormal general metabolism, or morbid processes occurring in special organs, as the liver, the kidneys, the thyroid; again, the poisons are supposed to come from the fetus or the placenta, from abnormal chemism occurring here. As a result of the deficient action of some organs of the body, for example, the liver, the kidneys, the thyroid, and perhaps others of the ductless glands, these poisons are retained in the body, or they are not sufficiently oxidized or changed so as to be rendered harmless and eliminable by the emunctories. They seem to have great affinity for the nerves of the organs of special senses, for the brain and its nuclei, for the liver, the kidneys, and the capillary walls, affecting them in variable proportions.

Such is the theory, and to explain why and how these changes originate we have other theories. Many authors believe that every pregnancy is attended by an auto-intoxication, due to the mighty changes in the general metabolism incident to its adjustments to the new condition, the active chemism required for the transfer of materials for the growth of the fetus, the presence in the maternal blood of the waste of the child, the by-products of the exaggerated eliminative action of the special organs, liver, kidneys, spleen, etc.

The constitution of a perfectly healthy woman might meet all these demands without any external symptoms or signs of disease, but such individuals are very rare, and, therefore, evidences of impaired function, of toxemia, are quite common. In other words, the woman suffers in her struggle with the parasite—the ovum. Predisposing elements for toxemia are neurasthenia, anemia, vicious heredity, especially one of psycho-neuroses, antecedent liver, kidney, intestinal, or other organic disease and allergic states. Insufficient internal secretion by the ovary has been cited as a cause, as also has abnormal functioning of the hypophysis and thyroid. Faulty diet undoubtedly has some bearing.

Veit says the transportation and dissolution of syncytial elements of the placenta produce syncytio-toxins, which, if not properly met by antibodies in the patient's blood, act injuriously. Zangemeister believes there is excessive water retention, accounting for the toxemias of late pregnancy.

Focal infection may be the underlying cause of a gestosis. Albert mentions infective endometritis. The removal of other foci, the appendix, the gall-bladder, the tonsils, abscessed teeth, etc., has sometimes worked a cure.

We have as yet very few scientific facts on which to base all these hypotheses, but, while desirable for practice, it is not unconditionally necessary to have every theory proved. The general applicability is sometimes proof itself. We recognize many groups of symptoms which can be most satisfactorily explained by this theory of toxemia, and treatment directed in appropriate lines is successful in relieving the conditions. The term "toxemia" should be supplemented by toxicosis, which means a disease caused by toxins in the blood and by gestosis.

Symptomatology.—Two groups of symptoms may be distinguished, the mild and the severe, but transition forms are common.

As mild toxemias many of the minor complaints of pregnancy may be classed. *The Nervous System.*—Headache, dizziness, hyperexcitability, lassitude, tendency to melancholia, exaggeration of reflexes, muscular twitchings, cramps in muscles, neuralgias, neuritis, aberrations of the special senses, as of taste (pica), of sight (restricted vision, hemeralopia), and of smell.

The Skin.—Edema, pruritus, pigmentation, various eruptions, for example, herpes, pruriginoid lesions, eczema, erythema, urticaria, acne, red nose. Graver symptoms will be considered later.

Digestive Canal.—Nausea, vomiting, constipation, colic.

Circulatory System.—Palpitations, syncope, varices, enlarged thyroid, symptoms resembling "formes frustes" of Basedow's disease, anemias.

Respiratory System.—Cough, asthmatic attacks.

Bones.—The puerperal osteophytes, softening of the bones, similar to osteomalacia, pains in the bones, perhaps due to alteration in the hematopoietic system (?) or endocrinopathy (?).

The Urinary System.—The kidney of pregnancy (Leyden), albuminuria, oliguria, decreased urea output.

General examination of the patients will usually show the evidences of deficient excretion, pasty or muddy skin, even subicterus, with perhaps an odor; dry, coated tongue, reddened gums, *pulse of low tension*, tympany, tender liver, and urinary findings. The pathologic anatomy of these toxemias has never been studied because they are not fatal. The severer toxicoses have been much investigated, and we may deduce from such findings the probable conditions in the milder forms.

The **treatment** of mild toxemias is symptomatic and general, directed toward the increase of elimination, restriction of nitrogenous food, and hygienic living. Prevention of the graver toxicoses, the hint of which is contained in the milder manifestations, is important. If the history, family or personal, points to such tendency, closer supervision of the gravida is needed. The consistent examination of the urine throughout pregnancy and the watchfulness over the patient, fully described under the Hygiene of Pregnancy, will disclose threatening dangers if the rules laid down for the guidance of pregnant women have not prevented such disease altogether.

The graver toxicoses of pregnancy are hyperemesis gravidarum, eclampsia, hepatic autolysis (fulminant toxemia), impetigo herpetiformis, etc.

HYPEREMESIS GRAVIDARUM

Nausea and vomiting occur, in greater or less degree, in half of all pregnant women, and are considered normal. They may be so marked as to become serious and deserve the appellation "pernicious," leading not seldom to abortion or death, or both. It is difficult, in a given case, to tell when the vomiting passes from the normal to the pathologic. The disease has been called the obstinate, the uncontrollable, the incoercible, vomiting of pregnancy, but the term "hyperemesis gravidarum," though a hybrid, is the one generally used.

Soranus, of Ephesus (20 A. D.), observed the disease, but Delorme, in the nineteenth century, called attention to the danger of the affection. Simmond, in 1813, was the first to interrupt pregnancy as a therapeutic measure, and with success. Paul Dubois, in 1852, before the French Academy of Medicine, presented a thesis on the subject which is still classic. It is said that Charlotte Brontë died of this affection. It occurs in animals, cats and dogs.

Symptoms.—The disease usually begins in the second, more rarely in the fourth, month, but may appear in the sixth month, though seldom after this, and if it does, one suspects nephritis. It lasts from six weeks to three months, but may take so violent a course as to be fatal in two weeks. It may also intermit for a few weeks, then recur, growing better, then worse.

Dubois distinguished three periods in the sickness, and while clinically the lines of separation are never sharp, such a division of symptoms is useful for purpose of description. At first attention is not called to the gravida because nausea and vomiting are such frequent occurrences in the early months, but when the intolerance of the stomach for all liquids and foods becomes apparent and the patient loses her appetite, one is forced to recognize that the state of the gravida is serious. The anorexia may become an actual loathing of food, and nausea, with retching, may occur at the mere mention or sight or smell of it. Emesis is caused by a mere change of position of the person, the entry of another one into the room, even by the sight of the husband. It continues during the night, robbing the distressed woman of sleep, and contributing to the exhaustion caused by the constant retching. Hiccup may be a troublesome symptom, as may pyrosis. Thirst is harassing. The patient complains of a constant boring pain in the stomach and of soreness of the ribs and adjoining muscles. Salivation is occasionally a concomitant, even double parotitis; constipation is the rule, but sometimes there is diarrhea. Standler reports 2 cases of hemorrhagic retinitis.

The vomit at first is composed of undigested food, mucus, and a little bile, later of mucus and bile; finally, it becomes bloody, bright, or of coffee-ground consistence. In one of the writer's cases the odor was almost fecal. The reverse peristalsis may be so active that medicines and food given per enema may be detected in the vomit. The blood may come from the mouth, pharynx, or stomach, and carries significance only if from the last. The urine, at first normal, becomes scanty, high colored as the disease progresses and later contains albumin, casts, sometimes blood, bile, acetone, diacetic acid, indican, and even sugar. It may also show the diazo-reaction. The urea may be even 4 per cent., and the ammonia excretion is high. According to Losee and van Slyke there is but slight acidosis in this form of toxemia, but the anhydremia will soon lower the alkali reserve.

During the *second stage* the symptoms become aggravated, and everything is rejected by the stomach; the patient complains of intolerable thirst, is extremely irritable and weak, has frequent fainting spells, and loses weight rapidly—in severe cases as much as a pound a day.

Examination shows the skin pale, waxy, sometimes icteric, non-resilient, shrunken, the patient emaciated (only in the chronic cases; the toxemic cases may die before emaciation is pronounced). The lungs usually are normal, the heart shows hemic murmurs, the pulse-beat is rapid—100 to 140, weak, "the pulse of empty arteries," the blood-pressure is variable—the abdomen is scaphoid; one can trace the aorta from the epigastrium to beyond its bifurcation; great tenderness is elicited over the cardia and sometimes over the liver.

The irritating vomit has eroded the lips and lower face; the gums are reddened and covered with sordes; the tongue is red, dry, brown in the middle, and cracked, sometimes to bleeding; the pharynx is dry, red, sometimes infiltrated with minute hemorrhages; the breath is fetid, and may have a penetrating or a soft, fruity odor. Fever of a low grade, but continuous, is now determinable, and symptoms referable to the nervous system usher in the third stage—delirium, polyneuritis, insanity. Korsakoff's psychosis has been observed. In some cases the temperature remains subnormal until just before death, when there is an agonal rise. Dehydration of the blood—thickening—is shown by the scarlet lips, dry skin, acidosis, hyperglobulism, both reds and whites, and, when intense, these may indicate the time for terminating the pregnancy (Devraigne).

Third Stage.—Mental aberration, delirium, headache, somnolence, stupor, and coma occur invariably. The vomiting usually ceases, leading the attendants to raise false hopes, but the pulse increases in frequency, the myocardium gives out, the general prostration rapidly augments, icterus and cyanosis appear, and the patient dies under the clinical picture of uncontrollable vomiting and acute poisoning.

The length of the three stages varies very much—the first is long; the second, longer; the third is usually short, the patient rapidly going down, and herein lies a warning—not to let the disease progress to the third stage, because then even therapeutic abortion cannot stay it; on the contrary, the interference may hasten the end.

During all this disturbance, local and general, the fetus is usually alive, and if delivered at term, may be large and fat. If the vomiting is toxemic, the fetus is more likely to suffer, and abortion is more apt to occur. The vomiting often ceases on the death of the fetus.

Causation.—Curiously, more cases of this affection are reported from the United States and France than from Germany and England. Carl Braun, in an experience of over 150,000 obstetric cases, never observed one of hyperemesis that was fatal, but McClintock was able, with a very moderate amount of search, to collect 50 fatal cases. It is more frequent and fatal in multiparæ than in primiparæ. In discussing the cause of hyperemesis, one must not lose sight of the generally increased nervous excitability of pregnancy, which would tend to exaggerate the action of any irritant located at any part of the body. Uncontrollable vomiting is more common in neurotic, neurasthenic, and hysteric women. A study of my cases of hyperemesis and of milder gastric disturbances shows four more or less distinct classes: (1) Those in which the vomiting is the main symptom of a toxicosis; (2) those in which a functional neurosis or a psychosis exists; (3) those where the vomiting is a reflex from the genitalia; (4) where it is due to some disease of the stomach or some abdominal disorder.

1. Toxemia best explains the majority of cases of hyperemesis, and the clinical picture as well as the pathology seems to show that there is here a distinct disease entity. The changes in the liver, kidneys, stomach and blood, and the findings in the urine cannot be satisfactorily explained by assuming a starvation and dehydration. We have every indication that a noxa is in the system. Accepting the belief that a toxemia exists—where do the toxins come from, what is their chemical nature, and how do they cause vomiting? No one knows, but we have many theories.

Veit and others believed that syncytium was dissolved in the maternal blood, making syncytiotoxin, causing disease. Seitz shows that the placenta is a new gland of internal secretion and may act as a disturber of all the other endocrines. Is syncytiotoxin placenta hormone? Urine from toxemic gravidæ used for making the Aschheim-Zondek test is very toxic to mice.

Abnormalities of function of the thyroid, the hypophysis, the adrenals, the corpus luteum, the mammæ, the parathyroids, have been proposed as causes of disturbed metabolism, resulting in the formation of toxins (Fieux).

Dirmoser believes they come from the intestinal canal, and many case reports indicate they may come from a focus of infection. Charpentier relates a case where the vomiting ceased when a peri-urethral abscess was drained—Talbot several where the removal of abscessed teeth effected a cure, and the author had 4 cases where treatment of pyelo-ureteritis stopped the excessive nausea and vomiting. Abscessed tonsils, diseased cervix, uterus, adnexa, appendix, gall-bladder, all seem, clinically at least, to be able to cause hyperemesis, and removal of the focus of infection may stop the vomiting. Some of these cases perhaps should be classified as "reflex," but a toxemic element is not missing in them.

Of the nature of the toxins we know nothing. If the kidney has become incompetent because its secreting cells have been damaged by the toxins it has sought to eliminate, urinary bodies, urea, uric acid, etc., accumulate in the blood. If the liver is damaged the whole body metabolism is thrown into dysfunction, with the accumulation of abnormal by-products, and to these two kinds of toxins are added those of starvation and dehydration.

How the vomiting is caused is also unknown. Do the toxins directly irritate the problematic vomiting center in the medulla? Does the stomach excrete the toxins and does the reflex start from here, or from the liver?

2. A functional disturbance of the nervous system is at the bottom of many cases of hyperemesis. In rare instances an organic nervous disease has been found—brain softening, tubercle or other tumors, meningitis, polyneuritis, which, however, may be the effect of a toxemia. Hyperemesis is not rare in hysterics, and it may be a pure neurosis, as Kaltenbach insists. It may also be a psychologic manifestation. If the pregnancy is abhorrent or fearful to the woman, she may, consciously or subconsciously, as a protest go on a "hunger-strike," and vomit. Schwab says that psycho-analysis will discover the hidden conflict in such cases, and proper suggestion will work a cure. We seldom need the intricate methods of Freud to prove that psychopathologic states are responsible for some of the abnormalities in pregnancy. A kind-hearted physician in a confidential talk with the patient will usually be able to discover any hidden fears or antipathies.

Hyperemesis is very amenable to suggestion and most of the cures we accomplish are due to it, e. g., the multitude of drugs, hypodermic medication, the dark room, isolation, electricity, quackery, gastric lavage, local treatments, dilatation of the cervix, the false assertion that the uterus has been emptied, painful treatment, etc. We might stretch a point and say that treatment of a local condition relieves the patient of a local irritant and the vomiting ceases because the whole nervous system has regained its equilibrium.

A neurotic constitution may aggravate the ordinary morning sickness to a threatening degree. By curing the neurosis and supplying water and food, we enable the woman to stabilize her metabolism and conquer the underlying toxemia, or "emesism" (see Eclampsism).

If a woman dies from neurotic vomiting, the course of the disease is very chronic and the clinical picture and pathologic findings are those of starvation. In toxemic vomiting the course is rapid, with little emaciation, and death results not from starvation, but from the profound change in the general metabolism.

3. The reflex-neurosis theory explains very few cases of hyperemesis. Many of those formerly believed to be of reflex origin are now in the toxemic class, e. g., metritis, endometritis, polyhydramnion, twins, hydatid mole, cervicitis, cervical erosions (Bennett), pelvic inflammations, and focal infections. Bretonneau believed excessive distention of the uterus, Grailly Hewitt, displacements and flexions, by pinching the nerves, could cause vomiting. Owing to the close connections between the genitalia and the stomach, via the sympathetic and vagus, a reflex through this arc is easy, but we must assume a special predisposition on the part of the gravida, because all the diseases proposed as causes of hyperemesis often exist in marked degree without disturbing the stomach. It may be that a general toxemia sensitizes the vomiting center. Vagotonic vomiting is a clinical fact. Spasmophilia in the form of pylorospasm is in this class.

4. Finally may be mentioned those conditions which are usually attended by vomiting, but in which, when pregnancy is added, the vomiting becomes pernicious. Such diseases are gastric ulcer, carcinoma, tuberculous peritonitis, gall-stones, appendicitis, chronic gastritis, helminthiasis, large fecal concretions, uremia, etc. True, these are rare, but they should be borne in mind.

In practice it is difficult to determine the exact cause in each patient, but we usually find either a toxemic or a neurotic basic quality, often the two combined. Grave situations may develop in both cases, but they are more common when the toxemia is predominant.

Pathologic Anatomy.—At autopsy on women dead of hyperemesis gravidarum the most marked changes are found in the liver and kidneys. The liver may be slightly enlarged in the acute stages, but after the degeneration has progressed somewhat it is smaller. There may be a diffuse hemorrhagic hepatitis, with all the findings of acute yellow atrophy. There may be fatty degeneration of only the cells around the central lobular veins, or extensive areas of necrosis (Fig. 336). Thromboses may occur in branches of the portal vein. Bile stasis is the rule. Hofbauer says the glycogen is limited to the periphery of the lobule. Pinard claims that slight changes of this kind are constant in pregnancy, and we should speak of the liver of pregnancy as well as of the kidney of pregnancy.

The kidney suffers all the changes from those of the so-called kidney of pregnancy to an acute parenchymatous nephritis. Figure 338 shows a marked fatty degeneration of the epithelium of the secreting tubules. The glomeruli are, if at

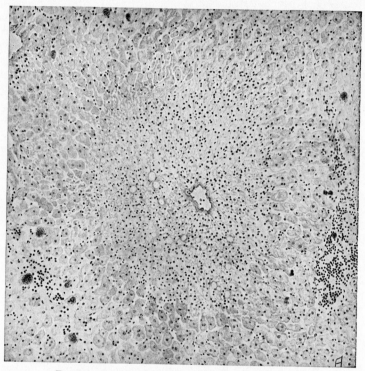

FIG. 336.—LOBULE OF LIVER IN HYPEREMESIS (low power).
Shows central necrosis. In some cases no pathologic changes are found.

all, but little affected. Hemorrhages are often found, and possibly the degeneration may never be fully corrected.

The heart undergoes fatty degeneration in the bad cases, as in sepsis. The nerves also are quickly attacked by the circulating toxins and death may be due to polyneuritis.

Diagnosis.—First one must decide when the vomiting becomes serious enough to be called pernicious. When the stomach rejects everything; when the anorexia is complete and the general health is palpably affected, one must conclude that the so-called physiologic vomiting has passed over into the pathologic. As Guéniot has shown, the diagnosis is not so simple as appears at first glance. It consists— (a) Of the diagnosis of pregnancy, which is not so easy in the first trimester, when the cases usually present themselves; (b) in determining the causes of the vomiting, basal and adjuvant; (c) the differentiation of vomiting due to, or rendered pernicious by, pregnancy, from vomiting having no connection with an existing pregnancy, such as would occur in the absence of pregnancy, *e. g.*, intestinal obstruction, acute appendicitis. The diagnosis of pregnancy is made by the usual methods, and, owing to the emaciation, bimanual examination is rendered easier. A study of the genital findings may disclose a malposition of the uterus or other pelvic anomaly which may be the adjuvant cause of the excessive vomiting—that is, the peripheral irritant. Stomach, intestinal, hepatic, renal, hemic, nervous diseases, and focal infection will require the careful general medical investigation which should be a part of the treatment of all cases. An underlying neurosis should not always be lightly assumed.

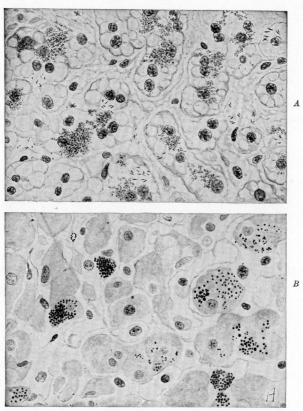

FIG. 337.—LIVER CELLS IN HYPEREMESIS (high power).
A, Cells in center of lobule, showing fat, yellow pigment, and crystals—tyrosin (? Hektoen). *B*, Cells in periphery of lobule, showing granular protoplasm, pale nuclei, and blood-pigment.

Of vital importance is the separation of the neurotic from the toxemic form of vomiting. Whereas many kinds of treatment, especially suggestive, will cure the former, toxemic vomiting is very rebellious and often requires the termination of pregnancy to save the woman's life. Rapidity of the onset of threatening symptoms, evidences of profound alteration of metabolism, such as jaundice, fever, rapid prostration, with cerebral symptoms, marked acidosis, early albuminuria, with casts, or blood, indican, much acetone and diacetic acid, tenderness over the liver, bloody vomit, indicate a toxemia, while the more gradual development of starvation symptoms leads one to suspect a reflex or neurotic cause for the vomiting.

Urinary findings are uncertain. Blood chemistry cannot be fully relied upon to distinguish the various forms of hyperemesis. If the blood shows an increase in the amounts of non-protein nitrogen, of uric acid and creatinin, one may conclude that the parenchyma of the kidney has begun to suffer and that at least a retention toxemia probably exists (Caldwell and Lyle). Tests of liver function

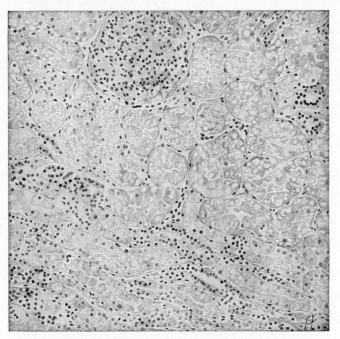

FIG. 338.—KIDNEY IN HYPEREMESIS (low power).

are not yet satisfactory. Bilirubinemia, normal in pregnancy, is increased in toxic conditions. Lennox, 1924, finds uricemia in starvation. Plass questions all this

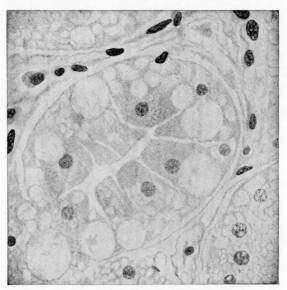

FIG. 339.—KIDNEY CELLS IN HYPEREMESIS (high power).

blood chemistry. There seems to be a perverted carbohydrate metabolism, hypoglycemia and also hypochloremia—giving hints for treatment.

That the diagnosis is not simple is proved by the mistake made by Trousseau, where, after induction of abortion for hyperemesis, the autopsy showed cancer of the stomach, and one by Caseaux, where a woman dead from supposed vomiting of pregnancy had tuberculous peritonitis, and the one of Beau, where a tuberculous meningitis caused the death. W. E. Morgan, of Chicago, relates the case of a girl who, almost in extremis from vomiting, threw up a ball of cotton which she had swallowed for the purpose of inducing abortion. Prompt recovery ensued.

Prognosis.—Guéniot collected 118 cases, with 46 deaths. Statistics are uncertain because the ideas of observers as to what constitutes hyperemesis differ. Carl Braun, in an immense experience, never saw a death from the vomiting, which is a remarkable statement, because they do occur. The disease lasts ten days to three months, depending on the variety. Not seldom, either because of some attempt at treatment or spontaneously, the patient suddenly ceases to vomit, demands food and retains it, going on to rapid recovery—this, too, when the previous condition was such as to excite real alarm. More often the disease subsides slowly, or may not be fully cured until after delivery. If the fetus dies or abortion occurs, recovery usually begins, but not invariably, and, too, such an occurrence is rare, the course of the gestation being seldom affected by the general disturbance. If therapeutic abortion is delayed too long, it cannot prevent death, rather may precipitate the impending fatal exhaustion. The toxemic hyperemesis is less amenable to treatment than the reflex or neurotic varieties, but those cases where some pathologic condition of the stomach, brain, kidneys, or liver is aggravated by the pregnancy are most fatal. Death comes from acute starvation, acute toxemia, with delirium and coma, exhaustion, myodegeneratio cordis which may come on suddenly during apparent improvement, from rupture of stomach or bowel because of the constant retching, from hematemesis, polyneuritis, and from intercurrent disease. Hyperemesis may recur in subsequent pregnancies. The toxemic varieties are usually more severe when they recur, the others less.

Treatment.—Careful search having revealed the cause, treatment is to be pursued along the lines indicated. The most important point to determine is whether or not the vomiting is toxemic. Since the exact cause is not invariably determinable, one may have to follow empiricism at first.

General.—Every mild case of vomiting during pregnancy should be cured as soon as possible with a view to preventing an aggravation of the disease. Attention to the bowels, a plain, easily digestible dietary, a gastric sedative, *e. g.*, cerium oxalate combined with scale pepsin, of each 5 grains thrice daily after eating, and suggestive therapeutics usually suffice to make the gravida comfortable. If water disagrees, Vichy may be tried. Dewees roused the patient early, gave hot coffee and crackers, and then had her lie in bed an hour or so, a plan that is often successful. She should eat small meals frequently, every three hours, during the night also, and the food should be mainly carbohydrates—cereals, sugar, bread, crackers, fresh and leafy vegetables, fruits (vitamins); fats and proteins are restricted. Coitus is to be forbidden, the wife being best given a separate room. Dyspepsia or symptoms of gastric disease are to be treated on general medical lines, and it is wise to search for and correct all abdominal conditions found to be causative of vomiting.

Some women need iodin, and Lugol's solution (℥iij t. i. d.) has cured. I have not yet used thyroid extract, though recommended. Dilute hydrochloric acid (℥x, t. i. d. a. c.) has helped a few cases. Corpus luteum has proved useless in my hands.

As soon as a given case shows itself to be obstinate and threatening, the woman should be put to bed, isolated as far as possible, and a thoroughly competent nurse put in attendance. It is best to remove the patient to a hospital. The room should be darkened (ocular disturbance sometimes causes vomiting), and the horizontal position insisted upon, even while taking food. In one chronic case, much relief was obtained by the patient living on an open porch. The bowels must be emptied thoroughly, and kept free by gentle means.

The patient then is brought quickly under the influence of bromids, ℥j being given per rectum in ℥iv of milk every four hours for 8 to 10 doses. Lately luminal sodium is being used, gr. ii hypodermically every four hours. Food is withheld for a whole day. Underhill emphasizes the need of carbohydrates. A liter of 5 per cent. glucose and one of Ringer's solution are administered under the breasts or 500 c.c. of a 20 per cent. solution intravenously. When food is given it should be dry—buttered toast, a dry chop or sliver of chicken, crackers with jelly or marmalade. Water may not be drunk before one and a half hours after eating, nor one hour before the next feeding. If dry diet is rejected, liquids or semisolids are tried, and if they fail, duodenal feeding is instituted. Water and salt in large amounts must be got into the system to replace that lost in vomiting, and sugar, too, in the form of glucose, either subcutaneously or intravenously or by duodenal tube, or nasal tube, or per rectum. The glucose is supposed to replace the depleted glycogen in the liver. At the same time measures are undertaken to reduce any existing acidosis. At least 4000 c.c. of fluid must be taken in each day. The above treatment has seldom failed the author, and the failures were in the severe toxemic cases. Insulin has hardly any place in hyperemesis—and is never given without chemical study of the blood.

Suggestion forms a large part of the treatment of cases of pernicious vomiting, many of the measures here advocated depending on it for their success. The physician should determine if the woman is suffering from a neurosis. By kindly counsels he should allay a hidden tokophobia, and he should try to discover and remove domestic and family frictions or antipathies, which may be at the bottom of the disease. On the other hand, the element of fear may be invoked, and the treatment rendered so harsh and painful that the patient stops vomiting to effect its discontinuance. Freund in 3 cases pretended, with much ado, to perform abortion, and the patients promptly stopped vomiting.

Medical.—There is no specific for this disease, as the host of remedies used with apparent success and disheartening failure testifies.

All the usual remedies for vomiting may be tried: Cracked ice swallowed whole, sips of ice-cold champagne, Vichy and water, may settle the stomach temporarily. An occasional hypodermic of morphin will produce sleep or help retain food—a temporary expedient. In spasmophilia, belladonna, calcium, and parathyroid are needed.

Kaltenbach cured many cases by frequent hot gastric lavage—neurohysterics. If toxins are irritating the stomach, perhaps lavage is real causal therapy. Mayer recommended the serum of a healthy gravida.

M. M. Portis introduced duodenal feeding in hyperemesis. It is a very valuable addition to our resources. If not well borne nasal feeding is substituted.

It is usually possible with these various measures to carry the patient along until she has overcome her toxemia or her neurosis. One must, however, not lose sight of this possibility—that while we have relieved the main symptom, the vomiting, the toxic elements in the blood may be increasing, and the patient may suddenly change for the worse, when even a hurried emptying of the uterus will not avert death—from acute yellow atrophy of the liver, acute polyneuritis, acute toxemic insanity, or, later, eclampsia.

Gynecologic Treatment.—The patient should be examined carefully with the aid of a speculum, and anything abnormal remedied if possible.

An anteverted or a retroverted uterus is replaced—in the knee-chest position, if necessary—and a pessary inserted. In one of the writer's cases, the wife of a colleague, an acutely anteverted uterus was raised with a balloon pessary, with immediate cessation of pronounced nausea and vomiting. Owing to a pin-hole defect in the bag, the air slowly escaped and the symptoms gradually returned, to disappear permanently when a perfect instrument was substituted, thus proving that the effect was not due to suggestion.

An erosion of the cervix is treated with 10 per cent. solution of silver nitrate—indeed, the method should be employed on empiric grounds even if the cervix exhibits no alteration. After irrigation of the vagina with sterile water a small Ferguson speculum is introduced and the cervix engaged in its end. The silver solution is poured in and allowed to remain five to ten minutes until the tissues are whitened, then washed out with 1 per cent. salt solution. After two days the treatment may be repeated. Its rationale is not understood, but it is often efficacious, and Carl Braun used it as a routine practice. Bennett, the inventor, used carbolic acid and iodin. M. O. Jones, of Chicago, recommended the silver, but J. Marion Sims drew general attention to the remedy. In one case where the silver applications failed the author employed Bier's suction treatment applied to the cervix. The woman was in desperate condition, and abortion was to be the next procedure, but recovery ensued and the pregnancy went to term. How much the local treatment contributed to the result is uncertain. Copeman, of Norwich, in 1875, in a case of hyperemesis, tried to induce abortion by dilating the cervix with his finger, but failed; his patient, however, ceased to vomit. Subsequently, dilatation of the cervix became a recognized method of treatment, to be employed before abortion was induced, as a *next to the last* resort. The author used it once—failure.

Obstetric.—Therapeutic abortion will cure all cases of hyperemesis if done early enough. It will cure all cases of neurotic or reflex vomiting unless the patient is too near death from starvation and exhaustion to withstand the operation. Winter's advice to empty the uterus as soon as the vomiting is pronounced toxemic, deserves serious consideration, though one may not always follow it. In the first place, a positive diagnosis of toxemia cannot always be made, and, too, many cases of toxemic vomiting recover under the usual treatment.

The delicate point to determine is *when to empty the uterus*, and the general appearance of the patient must decide it. Examination of the blood, showing intense concentration (hypererythrocytosis and leukocytosis), may indicate the degree of starvation. Dieckmann calls those cases severe where the urine is concentrated, the chlorids below 0.1 per cent., the ketone bodies $\pm$, with albumen and formed elements in abundance. Pinard says that when the pulse remains above 100 one should not delay the operation, especially if the blood-pressure sinks at the same time, and many accoucheurs interfere on the appearance of fever, hematemesis, jaundice, albuminuria, mellituria, acetonuria, indicanuria, hemorrhagic retinitis, delirium, or marked emaciation. Fieux holds that polyneuritis with icterus and the appearance of bile-pigment in the urine indicate abortion, but I believe that these findings show we are too late. Not one but all these facts must be considered, together with one's clinical experience. The progress of the case, the condition of the patient, and the effect of treatment—these will indicate the time to interrupt pregnancy. The disease is so treacherous that it is better to interfere earlier rather than too late, because often many remedies are tried in succession, using up much time, and then, when the uterus finally has to be emptied, the patient is in no condition to stand the shock of operation. Consultation must always be had, first, to verify the diagnosis and the necessity of performing abortion; second, to protect the attendant from the imputation of criminal operation, and, third, to share responsibility. All appearance of secrecy is to be avoided, the operation being performed in a hospital, if possible. In early cases the best way is to dilate and curet the uterus in one sitting. Later in pregnancy it may be better to dilate the uterus, insert gauze, and complete the operation the next day. When great haste is demanded, anterior vaginal hysterotomy may be performed, or the placenta curetted out and as much of the fetus as may be quickly removed and the uterus packed to stimulate the pains which will expel the remnants in a few days. Anesthetic: morphin, scopolamin, and local, with ethylene if necessary; preliminary blood transfusion in desperate cases.

Hyperemesis is sometimes feigned so as to mislead the accoucheur into performing an abortion. The patient will exaggerate her symptoms and falsify statements. In all cases the objective signs only should be relied upon.

PTYALISM (SIALORRHEA, SALIVATION)

Salivation is a rare complication of pregnancy. It is related to hyperemesis in that it probably has similar causation. Hippocrates noted it in pregnancy. It is to be distinguished from the "cotton spitting" described by Dewees as one of the signs of pregnancy. Stander found in one case that the fluid had the qualities of the gastric secretion. This is exceptional.

Sialorrhea combined with nausea and vomiting frequently occurs, but may occur alone. It usually begins in the second month, and ceases about the fifth or at quickening, presenting the same variations as the vomiting. It almost always ceases with parturition, but has continued for a few weeks thereafter. It usually occurs but once, but may appear in successive pregnancies, and may be absent in one and recur in the next. The flow varies in amount, excessive quantities being reported—over two quarts a day. It usually lessens during the night, but may continue unabated. The saliva is very watery, tasteless, odorless, limpid, not acid; it has little ptyalin. The patient cannot swallow it: it nauseates.

The drain of this large amount of fluid, the absence of digestive power, and the loss of appetite not seldom compromise the nutrition of the patient, and a condition of exhaustion resembling that produced by incoercible vomiting has proved an indication for terminating the pregnancy in these cases (rare). There are few changes in the mouth or gums. The salivary glands may be a little swollen and tender; the tongue is coated, with red edges; and sometimes a gastric catarrh exists. The patients feel miserable, are always thirsty, have difficulty in talking, and the chin may be excoriated.

Ptyalism has the same causation as hyperemesis, and occurs most often in neurotic women. It may be a familial characteristic.

The diagnosis is easy, since mercurial salivation is attended by fetor and stomatitis. Montgomery says that ptyalism may be a symptom of hysteria and of cancer of the uterus.

The treatment is pursued along the same lines as in hyperemesis. Of the many drugs used, sodium bromid is the best—30 grains thrice daily. Pilocarpin is less efficient, and atropin is useless and dangerous. Adrenalin and pituitrin should be given a trial. In two cases a pint of Locke's solution injected under the breast on alternate days worked a cure, in two others nitrate of silver applications to the cervix succeeded. Suggestion?

GINGIVITIS

The slight tumefaction and hyperemia of the gums so often observed in pregnancy (50 to 60 per cent.) may be aggravated to a severe affection. Sponginess of the gums, hemorrhage into them and from them, even loosening and dropping of the teeth, occur. There is no fetor, no salivation, and there is usually little pain in the parts, though mastication is difficult. There is no periodontitis in typical cases.

Redness of the gingival margins and hypertrophy are visible, and sometimes polypoid excrescences of varying size, which are subject to ulceration, appear between the teeth. The region of the molars is less affected.

Gingivitis affects primiparæ and multiparæ alike, but is more common in those who neglect the teeth and person and in women of poor health. It begins about the fourth month, disappears after delivery, but may even appear in and be aggravated by lactation. It may recur in each pregnancy. Its causation is obscure. Perhaps the altered buccal secretions play a rôle, or the altered metabolism of pregnancy (toxemia?). Such alterations in the secretions may favor the growth of bacteria which, in turn, cause caries. The treatment is hygienic; antiseptic mouthwashes, as tincture of myrrh in water, potassium chlorate, 1 ounce in 1 pint of water, weak peroxid solution, milk of magnesia, cleansing the gums with a soft cloth, rubbing precipitated chalk into the crevices, and iron and calcium tonics, combined with outdoor living. Hemorrhage from the gums is treated by a compress of gelatin or of adrenalin, or cauterization. Polypoid excrescences may be removed a few weeks postpartum if they do not shrink up.

Toothache is a not infrequent occurrence in pregnancy, and it is especially troublesome in women subject to neuralgia. Carious teeth, also common, should be cared for during gestation; even extraction under gas should, if indicated, be made, but exhausting gold fillings had better be postponed. The gravida should be given a tonic containing lime and should eat freely phosphate, lime- and iron-carrying fresh vegetables. Perhaps codliver oil and viosterol may help.

ECLAMPSISM AND ECLAMPSIA

History.—Hippocrates mentions convulsions of pregnant women and knew that they most often occurred in women who had headache and a tendency to sleep (coma). The word eclampsia means to flash, or shine out, and was introduced by Boissier de Sauvages in 1760, and Gehler, in 1776. More properly it should be eclactisma (Kossman).

In the latter half of pregnancy, women often have manifestations of some obscure disease whose surface signs not infrequently are the precursors of convulsions or coma, usually both. Naturally a gravida may suffer from the convulsive seizures to which any woman is liable, such as those due to epilepsy, hysteria, meningitis, tubercle, uremia, poisonings, etc., but there is a fairly definite symptom-complex, presented by pregnant women of which convulsions are the most prominent manifestation, to which the term "eclampsia parturientium" has been applied.

Unfortunately this symptom-complex may be produced by several well-known diseases, and also by other conditions, of whose nature we are almost absolutely ignorant. These diseases in a man or non-pregnant woman would not usually nor so easily cause convulsions and coma, but pregnancy, for some as yet only dimly known reason, confers these qualities upon them. For example, an acute nephritis in a normal adult usually runs its course without convulsions, but occurring during pregnancy it nearly always eventuates in convulsions and coma. The same is true of tumors of the brain.

We assume a toxic element in the causation of these violent motor and cerebral phenomena, and, in some cases, we think we can discern a pure and complete toxicosis. The last are the patients with true eclampsia, but at present we group all cases of convulsions and coma occurring in pregnant women, not due to extraneous medical causes, as epilepsy, hysteria, meningitis, tubercle, syphilis, poisonings, etc., under the term eclampsia. This must suffice as a definitition for the present. At the bedside we cannot always tell what is the underlying disease, even though it is desirable for treatment. Sometimes the subsequent course, sometimes the autopsy will enable us to properly classify the case.

Eclampsia, therefore, is not a disease by itself, but only the symptom, the most outstanding one, of several underlying diseases, and, before the convulsions (eclampsia) break out, we have a stage, more or less long, full of symptoms and signs of most varied nature, which serve to call our attention to what is pending.

This stage is called the pre-eclamptic state, or pre-eclampsia, and the woman is said to be threatened with convulsions.

Bar suggested the word *eclampsism* for this condition of preparedness for convulsions and limited the term to true primary toxemias. I would recommend its general adoption, but to spread its application to cover all those cases of so called toxemia in late pregnancy which may lead, if untreated, to convulsions or coma, or both. Eclampsism might be defined as that unknown state of the constitution in late pregnancy, produced by physicochemical changes in the blood (or causing them), in which state the pregnant woman is liable to convulsions or coma. A woman may die of eclampsism or get well without convulsions or coma (Lit. Dieckmann).

From a careful study of my cases I found the following diseases may underlie the symptoms of eclampsism or pre-eclampsia. They do not always reach the convulsive stage, or "accès eclamptique," of Pinard, but may subside without fits, or pass directly into coma. (See Table.)

I. *The True Toxemia.*—We believe that here the circulating poison damages the liver primarily and chiefly, and secondarily the kidneys and vascular system, or the reticulo-endothelial system.

II. *Acute Nephritis.*—This may be brought about by bacteria or toxins from focal infection, such as pyelitis, tonsillitis, abscessed teeth, cervicitis, etc., or by any one of the usual causes of nephritis, *e. g.*, exposure, acute infectious diseases, poisoning, etc., but most frequently by the toxins of pregnancy (eclampsism).

III. *Chronic Nephritis.*—When a patient with damaged kidneys becomes pregnant, the added strain may become too great, and the organs break down, or, eclampsism being superimposed, the convulsions break out.

IV. *Malignant Hypertension.*—Whatever be the cause of the increased arterial tension—cardiac, renal, arterial, capillary, hyperthyroidism, focal toxicosis—pregnancy, added to the burden already carried by the vital organs, always aggravates the woman's condition, and, if the disturbance of metabolism (eclampsism) is superadded, convulsions or coma will result.

In the last three conditions it is the unknown quantity of pregnancy—we call it a toxemia—that lends the underlying disease its convulsive qualities. We might say the eclampsia is grafted onto them, and in certain cases this is true, both clinically and pathologically. At times other than pregnancy the toxemic element does not come into play, or only slightly.

Clinical Course of Eclampsism.—This naturally will vary with the nature of the underlying disease, and the degree of the toxemia. In general the women complain of debility, a tendency to sleep or to nervous excitation, giddiness, occasionally slight mental confusion, twitchings in the muscles with cramps in the legs, anorexia or distaste for certain foods, especially meat and eggs. As the case progresses, the symptoms become more marked. Headache appears, dullness of intellect with disturbances of the special senses—spots before the eyes (muscæ volitantes)—bright lights, sometimes colored, sometimes described as spangles, dimness of vision, hemianopsia, even complete blindness due to edema or retinitis and sometimes with hemorrhages, photophobia, ringing in the ears, even deafness, and occasionally anomalies of taste and smell. These may be manifestations of peripheral or of central lesions. Prodromata are present from a few hours to several weeks before the actual explosion, and serve to draw attention to the peril of the patient. Nausea, vomiting, and *pain in the epigastrium* are most ominous symptoms, and precede the outbreak of convulsions usually by only hours, seldom a day or more.

These warnings should be heeded, and an exhaustive examination of the patient made. This will usually reveal edema of the feet and eyelids, or more or less marked general anasarca, with pasty skin, a coated tongue, fetid breath, tenderness over the pit of the stomach (the site of the pain) and over the liver,

Types.	Pathology.	Clinical characters.	Late course.
I *"Hepatic"* *eclampsia* Pure eclampsia, *i. e.*, the particular toxic state which underlies the convulsions and coma of late pregnancy.	*General:* Tissue changes. Angiospasm. Edema, etc. *Liver:* Focal necroses. Thrombi. Lobular degeneration, peripheral. Acute yellow atrophy. *Kidney:* Kidney of pregnancy. Nephrosis. Nephropathia gravidarum. Acute glomerulonephritis.	*Edema,* moderate. *High blood-pressure,* At first moderate, but mounts fast. *Symptoms:* (Late in pregnancy and stormy.) Headache. Epigastralgia. Special senses, amaurosis, etc. *Urine:* (Findings late and quickly ominous.) Oliguria. Albumin. Casts. Red and white blood-cells. Bile. Indican. *Icterus* and bilirubinemia. *Convulsions,* after brief warnings. *Coma,* after brief warnings. *Blood,* hyperglycemia; CO_2 reduced. *Eyes:* Edema retinæ, spasm of vessels. *Baby,* usually lives; if dies, instant improvement.	Recovery usually complete. Death in coma. Child usually lives. Rarely recurs. Amaurosis cured.
II *"Nephritic"* *eclampsia* Acute nephritis with eclampsism.	*General:* Tissue changes. Angiospasm. Edema. *Kidneys:* Toxic. Kidney of pregnancy. Nephrosis. *Focal in-* Acute glomerulo- *fection:* nephritis. Nephritis. Pyelitis. Tonsillitis. Tooth abscesses. Acute infectious diseases. Exposure. Poisonings. *Liver:* Late, when eclampsism is added.	*Edema,* marked. *High blood-pressure,* mounts slowly to high figure. *Symptoms:* (Earlier in pregnancy, progressive, then suddenly ominous.) Headache. Special senses, amaurosis. Epigastralgia. *Urine:* (Findings early and progressive.) Albumin. Casts. Red and white blood-cells. Oliguria, late. *Convusions and coma:* (Both slow to follow first symptoms.) Eclampsism. Uremia. *Blood:* Chemistry equivocal, late it shows N retention. *Eyes:* Neuroretinitis, abruptio retinæ, etc. *Baby,* if dies, subsidence.	Recovery usual. Not seldom a chronic nephritis remains. Will recur if the cause of nephritis is not removed. Some kidneys are supersensitive to pregnancy toxins. Baby often dies. Nephritis may recur without eclampsism.

III
Chronic nephritis
with or without eclampsism.
	Latent nephritis.
	Chronic nephritis
	  with
	Eclampsism =
	Acute nephritis
	(above)
	  without
	Eclampsism =
	Dead fetus.
	Placenta albumenurique.
	Cardiac $\big\}$
	Renal $\big\}$ Decompensation.
	Vascular $\big\}$
	Retinitis albumenurica.
		Evidences early in pregnancy.
		Edema, anasarca late.
		High blood-pressure, early.
		Symptoms:
		Mild unless eclampsism added, then
		Headache.
		Amaurosis.
		Convulsions.
		Coma.
		Urine: Usual findings and early.
		(If acute nephritis supervenes, they are identical with II.)
		Blood, N retention. Heart findings.
		Eclampsism =
		Abruptio placentæ.
		Abruptio retinæ.
		Retinitis albumenurica.
		Apoplexy.
		
		Baby, often dies; improvement slow.
			General disease aggravated permanently:
			Vessels.
			Kidneys.
			Retina.
			Almost always recurs in subsequent pregnancy, earlier **and** worse.
			("Low reserve kidney.")
			It is the underlying cause **of** obstetric complications:
			Abortion.
			Premature labor.
			Dead fetus (macerated).
			Abruptio placentæ.
			Obstetric shock.

IV *Essential hypertension* with or without eclampsism.	*Cardiorenal vascular disease,* carried into pregnancy. *Focal infection:* *With* eclampsism: Kidney lesions. Liver lesions. *Without* eclampsism: Hemorrhagia cerebri. Death of fetus. Cardiorenal $\big\}$ failure. Vascular $\big\}$	*High blood-pressure,* early in pregnancy. (180 to 240). History. *Symptoms:* Mild. Late and suddenly stormy when eclampsism is added. *Urine:* Findings unimportant until: Eclampsism. Kidney defaults. *Blood:* Negative until kidney defaults. *Baby,* if dies, only slight improvement. After delivery, slow improvement. Without eclampsism same as III.	Continues between pregnancies. Late, symptoms of cardiorenal-vascular disease appear. Is aggravated by each pregnancy. See No. III. N. B.: The reader should hold in mind that this table is only sketchy and that many permutations exist in practice.

high arterial tension with accentuated second heart-sound (the blood-pressure may reach 240), intensely exaggerated reflexes, diminished urine, high specific gravity, albumin with hyaline and granular casts, and low urea output. Occasionally the urinary findings are negative, but there is marked edema, high blood-pressure, with or without symptoms, and sometimes even edema fails, but marked subjective manifestations are present. Rarely one observes a slight jaundice, the van den Bergh bilirubin test showing a raised icteric index.

Differentiation of the four forms of pre-eclampsia is possible often enough to encourage us to try to make it, especially as we may receive guidance as to treatment. Unfortunately the laboratory does not help very much. The history may, but sometimes we must treat the patient on general principles, and let the subsequent course of the disease show us how to classify the case.

In the *true eclamptic toxemia* the symptoms usually develop late in pregnancy, and rapidly reach an acme. Lassitude, malaise, headache, stomach symptoms, especially epigastralgia, disturbance of the special senses as above mentioned, come on sometimes so rapidly that convulsions seem imminent before the physician has been given warning. The blood-pressure mounts quickly, and edema appears, albumin, casts, red and white corpuscles, and bile are found in the urine which is diminished in quantity, increased in specific gravity and darkened in color. The blood changes are equivocal, but Zangemeister thinks there is chlorid and water retention, and Stander has shown that there is hyperglycemia and decreased CO_2 combining-power. At autopsy the characteristic liver changes are found. If the patient recovers the general symptoms and edema subside quickly, the blood-pressure, urine, etc., soon returning to normal. Recurrence of the disease in future pregnancies is rare.

Many women evince only the milder symptoms of eclampsism, and these are due to the kidney of pregnancy (von Leyden). In the more advanced stages we say a nephrosis exists (nephropathia gravidarum, Aschoff) and if infection or severe toxemia is added a glomerulonephritis develops. By nephrosis we mean that the kidney changes are degenerative, not inflammatory.

Barnes said that pregnancy is the test of bodily soundness, and it is generally admitted that the kidneys are the point of weakest resistance during this period. Von Leyden described certain changes in the kidney to which he gave the above name, believing that they occurred in a large percentage of kidneys in normal pregnancy. This condition is supposed to exist when the gravida shows edema and albuminuria in the latter half of pregnancy. The kidney is large, pale, soft, cloudy, with markings obliterated, anemic or grayish-yellow in color, and shows, microscopically, fatty changes in the glomeruli and tubules, but no infiltration of leukocytes nor vascular changes.

The capillary circulation throughout the body is slowed, the vessels showing great permeability for water which is retained in the tissues (hydrops). Edema develops, first in the legs, then the eyelids and trunk, which accounts for the increase in weight, then in the brain which explains the headache and other cerebral symptoms (Zangemeister, Hinselmann). By means of the capillary microscope, the constriction of the arterial half of the capillary loop can be easily seen, and when this phenomenon is very marked one can predict the imminence of convulsions (Neverman, Heyneman).

With our present views the "kidney of pregnancy" is the result of the intoxication of pregnancy, and the causation of eclampsia would be its causation. The kidneys suffer in their effort to eliminate toxins from an abnormal ovum, or the accumulated excreta of the fetus, or undermetabolized products and proteins insufficiently oxidized by the liver. The disease may remain stationary at the hydrops and mild albuminuria and moderate hypertension stage, and disappear quickly after delivery, accompanied by profuse diuresis. It may grow worse, with high blood-pressure, much albumin, casts and blood, with pre-eclamptic symptoms, ending in eclampsia. In such cases a glomerulonephrosis occurs and it must be differentiated from chronic nephritis with acute exacerbation, which may rarely be done.

Acute nephritis during pregnancy can seldom be distinguished from the glomerulo-nephrosis, or nephropathia of true eclampsism, but it may develop from the same causes which operate outside of gestation—exposure to cold, a flagrant error of diet (a Christmas dinner, for example), chemical poisons, scarlatina, acute angina, and infections of various kinds. It is often a "focal infection nephritis," and if we can remove the source of the bacterial toxins recovery ensues. Particular mention must be made of pyelitis, which seems to prepare toxins peculiarly caustic to the kidney. Acute or chronic pyelitis is often found associated with eclampsism and eclampsia. The similarity of acute, glomerular nephritis in pregnancy to trench nephritis is mentioned by Rockwood, Mussey, and Keith. This complication may occur at any time during gestation, but, if it appears in the later months when the toxemia is developing, it may lead to eclampsism and eclampsia. The symptoms depend on the severity of the nephritis and the general damage done to the reticulo-endothelial system (Benda). Eclampsia may follow an acute angina within three days. In chronic cases it takes weeks or months. Marriott says that in children the streptococcus causes glomerulonephritis, the staphylococcus a tubulonephritis. Perhaps this is true also of gravidæ whose constitution at this time resembles that of children in many ways.

Focal infection may lead not alone to nephritis, but also to the death of the fetus—the blood-borne bacteria kill it. After pregnancy is terminated the toxemic symptoms rapidly disappear, but the primary lesion persists until nature or art removes it. This form of eclampsism obviously may or may not recur in subsequent pregnancies.

Chronic Nephritis.—(See page 545 for description.) When a woman enters pregnancy with damaged kidneys, the results are bad in four ways: First, the kidneys may break down and the symptoms are those of acute cardiac, renal, or vascular decompensation; second, there may be an acute exacerbation of the disease; third, the combination of the poisons uneliminated by a defective kidney with those of pregnancy is too much for the placenta and fetus. The placenta is infarcted and the fetus frequently dies. Fourth, the toxemic element of pregnancy may enter with force, and the gravida will have an eclampsia superimposed on her nephritis.

When eclampsism develops on a chronic nephritic basis, the symptoms of the nephritis usually appear earlier in pregnancy than in the true toxicoses. If not treated successfully, and if the fetus does not die, symptoms of pre-eclamptic toxemia may very suddenly come up and the patient have violent convulsions. Hemorrhage into the brain, abruptio placentæ, edema of the lungs, amaurosis, retinitis albumenurica, abruptio retinæ, are most common in this form of eclampsism. The blood shows marked retention of uric acid and non-protein nitrogen, and the phthalein test, the urea clearance, the guanidine, the creatinine excretion indicate renal damage (Stander).

After delivery the toxemic symptoms rapidly subside, but the chronic nephritis can be demonstrated for years. In subsequent pregnancies the process is usually repeated, but often with variations of its salient features. In very mild cases of chronic nephritis, symptoms may be absent in the interval, but when a new gestation begins to make demands on the kidney its low reserve of power becomes evident (proved experimentally by F. J. Browne). This form of latent nephritis corresponds to what Stander calls the low reserve kidney. One should search for and eliminate the cause of the chronic nephritis, if possible, so that the kidney may be able to bear the strain of pregnancy.

Essential (?) Hypertension.—There is no essential hypertension of pregnancy. The pregnant woman's blood-pressure is a little lower than that of a healthy woman of the same age, therefore, any increase above 120 is to be looked upon with question. Since the internists are not agreed on the causation and mechanism of high blood-pressure, we may as well retain the term essential or idiopathic until they do unravel the tangle. In the meantime we can say that hypertension occurs in renal, heart, thyroid and vascular disease, that it may be a manifestation of focal infection, acute or chronic, and that it may be governed by the vasomotor center at the base of the brain. It seems that the toxin in pregnancy toxemias is a vascular poison, at least it affects the walls of the capillaries, increasing their permeability to the blood-plasma. If the edema occurs in the brain, high blood-pressure results, and perhaps this is the mechanism operative in eclampsism.

A woman entering pregnancy with hypertension is immensely handicapped and even if eclampsism does not develop (rare) she is exposed to the dangers of renal, cardiac, and vascular breakdown because of the extra strain which pregnancy puts upon these organs. If, in addition to this strain, there be superimposed a toxemia of pregnancy, a vicious circle is made and eclampsism develops, which leads to convulsions, unless the fetus dies, removing the eclamptic element. The blood-pressure does not go down much in these cases after fetal death.

The course of essential hypertension in pregnancy depends on the cause of the rise in blood-pressure. If the teeth or the tonsils or a pyelitis, or gallbladder or other intoxication continues to operate, the hypertension becomes malignant. The kidneys may function quite well unless a secondary nephritis develops from progression of the vascular lesion.

It is the eclampsism which stamps all these conditions with the same clinical features and multiplies the findings at postmortem. Until we discover the exact nature of this form of toxemia, we will not be able, at the bedside, to unmask the underlying diseases, but whatever it is and whatever they are, unless they are cured, either by nature or art, convulsions will break out, and this is eclampsia. Those cases of toxemia in which the patient goes directly into coma without convulsions might be called eclampsism without eclampsia.

Causation.—In spite of the enormous amount of study that has been put upon it the real cause of this affection is unknown. The theory that has the most plausibility is that eclampsism and eclampsia are one form of toxemia, causing perversion of metabolism of a physico-chemical nature, and that some noxa circulates in the blood which upsets the water-balance, effects liver changes, and, directly or secondarily, degenerative changes in the kidneys and also convulsions by direct toxic action on the anterior cerebral cortex.

Where do these toxins originate? Many theories have been advanced.

Uremia.—Since Rayer and Lever (1843) proved the presence of albumin in the urine of eclamptics, and later students found the indications of a nephritis almost invariably in the urine, the idea gained ground that eclampsia was allied to uremia. Carl Braun said the convulsions were due to acute renal insufficiency. While at autopsy, or in the urine, one will rarely miss evidences of nephritis (Ingerslev and Charpentier have found 250 cases in the literature without them), still the weight of clinical and postmortem evidence is against the view that kidney disease is the cause of eclampsia. It is more likely a result of the action of another cause, and is secondary, not primary.

Halbertsma believed that the uterus, by compressing the ureters, produced thus a urinemia. This is disproved by the fact that dilatation of the ureters is not the rule in eclampsia and often occurs in healthy gravidæ.

Bacteriology.—Delore suggested that bacteria might be the cause of the toxemia. Various bacteria were found in the blood and the placenta by Dolèris, Blanc, and Favre. Gerdes found a bacillus which Hofmeister proved to be the common proteus, and Gley found the Staphylococcus aureus and albus. The frequency of sepsis after eclampsia, the febrile nature of the disease, the fact that it may follow an attack of tonsillitis, that it occurs oftener in cold and damp weather, would argue for an extraneous microbic origin. Acute sepsis sometimes terminates under the clinical picture of acute yellow atrophy of the liver, which brings it a step nearer to eclampsia. Stroganov states that eclampsia is an acute infectious disease introduced through the lungs. Many cases of previously healthy women, who, after a few days of prodromal symptoms, develop eclampsia, tend to make such a hypothesis very probable. However, up to the present no one has been able to isolate a germ that could be considered causative. Perhaps it is a filtrable virus. Albert and Müller believe that the infection is in the genitals, and the toxins produced there, as from an endometritis, are absorbed and cause the convulsions.

Dietetics.—That diet has something to do with the causation of eclampsia seems to be proved by the war. Fats and animal protein were almost eliminated from the diet of German women, and the incidence of eclampsia declined more than 50 per cent. (Warnekros). Stoeckel questions the connection between the diminution of eclampsia and the lack of fats and proteins. Clinical observation leads us to believe that the nitrogen metabolism is disturbed in eclampsia.

Metabolism.—Bouchard, in 1887, broke new ground when, in his "Leçons sur les Auto-intoxications," he advanced the theory that eclampsia results from the accumulation of retained waste, which the emunctories failed to get rid of. Rivière advanced the notion of pregnancy toxins irritating both liver and kidneys. Volhard, Schumacher, and Stewart disproved these theories.

Then the liver was accused. Pinard and Bouffe de Saint-Blaise argued that eclampsia was a hepatotoxemia due to liver insufficiency. Ahlfeld and Schmorl have found, in cases of typical eclampsia, pathologic conditions which strongly resemble those of acute yellow atrophy of the liver.

Studies of the maternal metabolism show that there is an alteration in nitrogenous catabolism. It has long been known that there is a decrease of the total urea output, but recent studies by Whitney and Williams show that the amount of ammonia nitrogen equals or even exceeds the urea nitrogen in the urine. Dieckmann proved that the blood in eclampsia is concentrated and recommends glucose and gum acacia as diluents—as we treat shock. The bearing of the reticuloendothelial system has not yet been determined (Benda).

Endocrinology.—Lange believed that the thyroid gland has much to do with eclampsia, and by administering iodothyrin he cured the albuminuria of the kidney of pregnancy. Nicholson and others have obtained favorable results with thyroid extract, but the theory has not awakened general interest. Eufinger found the blood of eclamptics hastened tadpole development faster than that of normal, menstruating or pregnant women—probably because of increased thyroid content. That eclampsia may be due to the disturbance of balance between the organs with internal secretions which should neutralize each other, is an attractive but unproved hypothesis. The parathyroids (Vassale) have been suggested, the ovaries (Pinard), the corpus luteum, and the mammæ—Sellheim (on the theory that eclampsia is similar to parturient paresis in cattle, which is cured by treatment directed to the mammæ), and also the hypophysis cerebri. Anselmino and Hoffman found a marked increase of the hormone of its posterior lobe in the blood and Fauvet showed that it produced changes similar to eclamptics. The urine of eclamptics used for the Aschheim-Zondek test kills the rats. Why?

Symbiologic Relations of Mother and Ovum.—The theory of Veit, the deportation and solution of syncytium, without the production of sufficient antisyncytiotoxin, remains still a theory. The Abderhalden pregnancy test is weak or negative in eclampsia. The significance of this fact is unknown.

Numerous investigators have tried to find a toxin in the placenta, but Frankl, in summing up their efforts and his own, decides that there are no toxins in the placenta, but that there may be ferments, and says that this line of study will more likely lead to useful results. (See also Holland.) Eclampsia has been held a form of anaphylaxis due to the introduction of a foreign protein, and several facts render such a theory plausible.

The idea that the child and placenta may be the origin of the toxins is not new. Ahlfeld mentioned it in 1894, and Fehling and Collman support this view. The author has delivered diseased children from eclamptic mothers, and entertains no doubt but that the fetus can sicken independently of the mother and secondarily infect her, or, after delivery, continue ill and die. It is more than probable that certain cases of eclampsia without albuminuria and other evidences of renal disease, and cases of nephritis or toxemia developing without warning in previously healthy women, may be found to be due to a diseased ovum. Frey reported seven hydatid moles with eclampsia. Hitschman saw another in a girl pregnant four and one-half months with a hydatid mole. These may be confirmatory of the above, or they may mean that a live fetus is not necessary for the production of the convulsions. Eclampsia may occur with a macerated fetus, though usually the child dies as the result of the toxemia, and then the condition of the mother improves. Poisons excreted by the fetus reach the general circulation without passing through the liver, and perhaps these unoxidized excreta irritate the kidneys, which are not able to throw them off in this state. Changes identical with those found in the eclamptic mother have been found in the fetus also dead of convulsions (Bar, Knapp, Dienst, and De Lee).

Hematology.—Much work has been done, with little practical results. We know that salt is retained, that the calcium is not diminished, that when the kidneys become involved, urinary retention begins. Zweifel has found sarcolactic acid in the urine of 17 eclamptics, in the blood, and in the fetal blood. It was absent from the urine of a case of pure uremia, but present in the blood of all children born dead and in all the placentæ examined. Zweifel has not proved that the lactacidemia is the cause of eclampsia—only that the lactic acid is present in the urine of eclamptics. This finding occurs also in cases of asphyxia, dyspnea, exhaustion from severe physical effort, some febrile conditions, and poisoning by morphin, curare, strychnin, veratrin, cocain, phosphorus, etc. Titus proved a sudden drop of blood-sugar precedes convulsions.

It has long been observed that the blood of eclamptics contains an excess of fibrin (Dienst). This is probably not the cause of the disease, but is one of the effects of the common cause. The same may be said of the high arterial tension usually found early in the disease. Fahraeus has shown the red blood-corpuscles rapidly precipitate from drawn eclamptic blood, and Hinselmann has demonstrated capillary angiospasm. Zangemeister ascribes the disease to water retention.

A most significant clinical experiment was performed by Bumm in 1922. He used eclamptics' blood for transfusions in women that had suffered hemorrhages, and noted no evil effects.

The Cause of the Convulsion.—Here again there is much room for speculation. Without doubt the nervous system of the pregnant woman is in a state of hyper-excitability. This may easily be determined by testing the exaggerated reflexes. Perhaps this is another result of the toxemia of pregnancy. Older writers classed eclampsia as a neurosis (Dubois), and, in fact, it is more common in neurotic women. Dührssen explains the convulsions as being due to a spasm of the blood-vessels of the brain, the liver, or the kidneys, from an irritation proceeding from the uterus. Spasm of the vessels of the brain causing acute anemia and edema may evoke the fits, and analogy is drawn from cases of epilepsy. The angiospasm during the convulsion may be demonstrated by the capillary microscope. One need not go

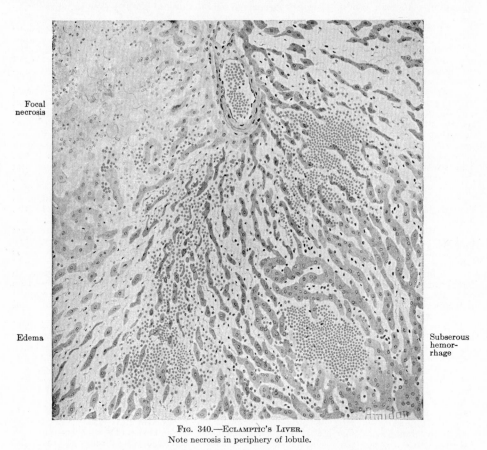

Focal necrosis

Edema

Subserous hemorrhage

FIG. 340.—ECLAMPTIC'S LIVER.
Note necrosis in periphery of lobule.

far for an explanation of the convulsions if the toxemic theory is proved—the toxins irritate the nerve-centers, as do other specific poisons, strychnin, tetanus, etc.— but the toxin of eclampsia has a special affinity for the cortex of the forepart of the brain, as is shown by the constancy of convulsions and coma and the mental symptoms. Individual convulsions in a case of eclampsia may be elicited by any external irritant, for example, jarring of the bed, slamming of doors, bright lights, external or internal examination, the induction of labor, a hypodermic injection, an enema, catheterization, delivery of fetus, etc. Zangemeister defends the theory that increased intracranial pressure causes the convulsions and all the symptoms, there being an edema of the brain similar to that occurring in other portions of the body—the legs, the eyelids, etc.—a very plausible theory and one that, if proved, would give us rational methods for treatment.

Frequency.—Eclampsia is getting rarer each year owing to the blessings of prenatal care, but even yet its incidence varies in different series of cases and

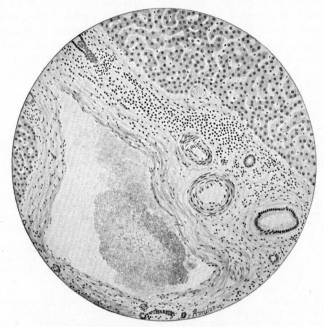

Fig. 341.—Fibrinous Thrombus in Eclamptic Liver.

localities. The cause of this variation is unknown. Stratz says that eclampsia occurs in the tropics, but seems more common in cold climates, and also in the

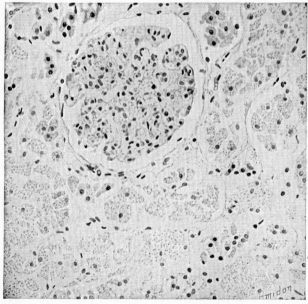

Fig. 342.—Kidney in Eclampsia.

cold raw spring months. Primiparæ are more affected than multiparæ (3 to 1). It generally appears in the last three months of pregnancy, but may occur as early as the tenth week (author's case). Fatal cases are reported in the third, fourth, and fifth months. Thaler collected 12 such cases. In Davis's 766 cases at the New York Lying-in Hospital, 54 per cent. occurred during pregnancy, 16 per cent. during labor, and 30 per cent. postpartum; at the Chicago Lying-in Hospital the percentages were 50–30–20 (Greenhill), but Essen Moeller believes most often the convulsions begin with labor, and Schroeder's figures were 62–190–64. It is not always easy to determine the time of onset of the fits, because they sometimes bring on labor, or, what seems more likely, the pains, unperceived by the patient and physician, evoke the attack.

Predisposing causes are primiparity, especially in advanced years, neurotic constitution, certain types of endocrinopathy, *e. g.*, the masculine or intersexual (Mathes), infantilism, multiple pregnancy, heredity (Elliott reports a case where a mother and four daughters died of eclampsia), and previous disease of the liver or kidneys (scarlatina, icterus and other infectious antecedents), etc.

Pathologic Anatomy.—*Brain.*—Flattening and moderate edema of the convolutions, sometimes with anemia, sometimes with congestion. Small or large hemorrhages or areas of cerebral softening with thrombosis occurred in 58 of 65 autopsies (Schmorl). Apoplexy is not uncommon, especially into the ventricles. In unusual cases other causes for the convulsions are found, as tubercle, tumors, meningitis, phosphorus-poisoning, etc.

Liver.—Here the most typical changes are found; indeed, one can almost make the diagnosis from the liver at autopsy (Fig. 340). There is albuminoid degeneration with hemorrhagic and anemic necroses. These focal necroses occur near the small portal vessels, which are often thrombotic (Fig. 341), and may be seen by the naked eye. In addition there is fatty degeneration of the periphery of the lobules, which may be so marked as to make the slide resemble one from a case of acute yellow atrophy of the liver, a fact pointed out by Jürgens, Stumpf, Ahlfeld, and others. There may be a general autolysis of the liver or only cloudy swelling. Hepatitis and perihepatitis hæmorrhagica are nearly always found. Fibrinous thrombi occur in the veins (Fig. 341). These changes show how profoundly the liver is affected by the circulating poisons if the liver disease is the primary trouble, and the general eclamptic syndrome the result of acute hepatic insufficiency. (See Ewing.) Yet, sometimes there are no liver changes.

Kidneys.—Almost always some signs of disturbance are present. In 289 cases observed from 1892 to 1900 in the Berlin Charité there were symptoms referable to the kidneys in every one, and changes were found in all that went to autopsy. Schmorl, in 73 autopsies, found only 1 with normal kidneys. Cloudy swelling and fatty degeneration of the epithelium are the rule. Thrombosis of the glomeruli and smaller veins and arteries are common. While degenerative changes in both the glomeruli and tubules are the rule, *i. e.*, a nephrosis exists, evidences of acute inflammation may sometimes be found, also, rarely, forms of subacute and chronic Bright's disease. Swelling of the kidney so that it stretches its capsule is rare, as is shown at operations of decapsulation (Edebohls). Dilatation of the ureters is found occasionally, particularly the right, but has no significance. While renal changes are almost invariably found, most authors are convinced that they are secondary either to the general toxemia, or to the disease of the liver, or a primary renal disease onto which an eclampsism has been grafted. Changes in the reticulo-endothelium system are now being studied (Benda). We believe that nephritis is only a part of a general disease affecting all the capillaries and body tissues.

Circulatory System.—The ventricles are usually contracted, the auricles full of dark blood which does not clot readily, contrary to the condition of hyperinosis which existed during life. The heart muscle is fatty, with tiny hemorrhages, necroses, and thrombi; it tears easily, and these changes may be a cause of death. Fatty heart is found especially in those cases which had been given large doses of chloroform and chloral, a fact which warns to care in the administration of these drugs. There may be subpericardial hemorrhages.

Thromboses and emboli in fine vessels are very common in the lungs, liver, kidneys, brain, and skin; they consist of liver-cells, endothelium, and syncytium. The last has no significance, being found in normal puerperæ. During life the blood contains an excess of fibrin and coagulates very quickly, so that often it is impossible to perform venesection properly. Microscopic findings of the blood in eclampsia are not constant. The reds are sometimes increased (in one instance to 9,000,000), which is due to the concentration of the blood, and there is marked leukocytosis (40,000), especially noted in the multinuclears.

The Lungs.—Almost always congestion and edema are found, and very often hemorrhages, which are usually under the pleuræ. Bronchopneumonia is not rarely found, due to admission of food-particles, blood, slime, etc., into the air-passages—aspiration pneumonia. Septic pneumonia, and, oftener in general hospitals, croupous pneumonia, may be the cause of death. Gangrene of the lung is sometimes the cause of death. Small arterial and venous thromboses and emboli of fat, liver-cells, decidual cells, and cells that look like hypertrophied nuclei of lymphoid cells of the bone-marrow, that is, syncytium, are constant findings. These are not characteristic, occurring in other conditions.

The Fetus.—Bar and others have found changes in the child which correspond very closely with those in the mother, especially when the child died of convulsions.

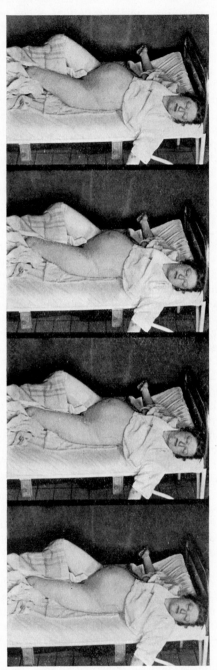 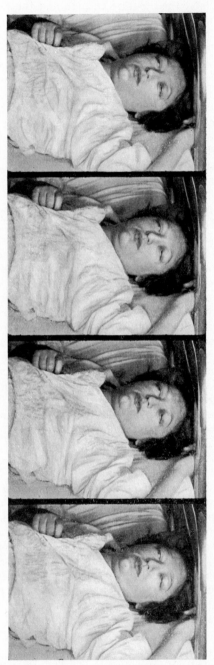

Fig. 342a.—A Strip from a Motion Picture of a Case of Eclampsia Showing the Extreme Jactitation Between Convulsions.

Fig. 342b.—Close-up of Same Patient Taken Right After a Convulsion. Note Foam on Lips.

The Attack.—Wherever the patient may be, she falls to the ground unconscious, a few seconds of quiet, a few twitchings of the facial muscles occur. The pupils dilate, the eyes are turned, and the head also, to one side; the patient opens her mouth, then the jaw is pulled laterally, and there may be a cry or a sigh. The whole body becomes rigid; the features are distorted; the arms flexed; hands clinched; the feet inverted; the toes flexed, and the whole person drawn to one side in a tonic spasm. This condition lasts for a few seconds, then the jaws open and close violently, the eyelids also, the twitchings beginning in the face, then usually one arm, then the leg, and now the whole body. This is a violent clonic convulsion, which may throw the patient out of the bed against any object. Severe injuries can result—even fractures of the skull or long bones; the tongue is protruded; the teeth may chop it up. Foam, often tinged with blood, comes from the mouth. The respiration is completely stopped, the chest being rigid. The pulse is high and strong; later it grows weaker, but may be hard to feel because of the convulsion. In rare cases the pulse is weak and the arterial tension low from the start, a fact which is explained by degenerative changes in the heart. The blood-shot eyes protrude, the face is swollen, the cyanosis is extreme, the lips are purple—altogether the picture is a horrible one. Gradually the convulsive movements remit, a few twitches or jerks take place, the patient lies quiet, the heart thumping violently against the chest-wall. For a few seconds the woman appears to be dying, but there is a long sigh, and stertorous breathing becomes established, coma supervening. Soon the respirations quiet down. In the favorable cases the patient wakes up after a short time bewildered, severely sore in all the muscles. After from a few minutes to an hour another fit occurs, or she may have no more. With recurring convulsions the intervals become shorter and the patient lies in deep coma all the time. Fever now begins; the pulse-rate rises. The fits may occur every five minutes, but usually the time is twenty minutes to one hour, and they may show some regularity of recurrence. Cases are on record of 81 (recovery) and even 593 convulsions (Spalding). These cases almost invariably die. The average number is from 5 to 15 attacks. The convulsion lasts from thirty seconds to two minutes, very rarely any longer, and these are bad cases. Between the attacks the patient may be quiet or restless, and sometimes there is great jactitation, with wild and exhausting delirium. These patients usually show signs of severe liver involvement.

Marked albuminuria with casts—hyaline, epithelial, granular—and blood are the rule in true eclampsia; reduction of the amount of urine is constant and occasionally there is anuria. Cases of convulsions without albuminuria are due to apoplexy, epilepsy, meningeal disease, or reflex irritation. Examination of eclamptic women often shows tenderness over the liver, kidneys, and stomach, with greatly exaggerated reflexes, marked leukocytosis, and often complete amaurosis.

Pains usually begin if the convulsions are at all severe, and labor is often rapid when once begun. After labor the progress of the case is generally more favorable, but the convulsions may recommence as late as the eighth day. Of great interest is postpartum eclampsia. When the convulsions begin after the delivery of the child, or a long time after the death of the fetus, it is probable that the poison was retained some place, and finally was freed so that it could unite with the brain-cells (Liepmann).

If the woman is to get well, the convulsions grow less frequent and less severe, the secretion of urine increases, the coma lightens, the temperature goes down, the pulse slows, the cyanosis disappears, the mind begins to clear, and after from six hours to three days, rarely as long as a week, consciousness returns. A recrudescence of the fever usually means that sepsis is starting. Recollection of what happened from the beginning is completely lost, and the puerpera may deny her child when it is presented to her. This amnesia may extend as far back as a week before the actual attacks began, and occasionally there is weakness of mentality for several months after delivery. Puerperal psychoses are not uncommon as a sequel to those cases having had many convulsions, especially postpartum (Thaler), but they usually offer a good prognosis. The blindness usually lasts only a few days, unless a retinitis albuminurica existed, and this betokens chronic nephritis. In pure eclampsia edema of the retina and nerve, partial spasms of retinal vessels are found.

In rare instances the convulsions cease without interrupting pregnancy, and the patient may deliver a living child at term. The author had a case where the patient had two attacks during pregnancy, with an interval of three weeks, in one of which attacks the convulsions were so severe that the jaw was dislocated, and yet a living child was born at term. More usually the attack kills the fetus, the symptoms abate, and the product of conception is expelled in due course of time.

If the woman is going to die, the attacks usually increase in frequency and force, the temperature goes up to 103° F., sometimes to 107° F., or it sinks; the pulse increases, becomes weak and running. Signs of edema of the lungs appear, with rattling and *pale cyanosis*, even between the convulsions, or death may take place at the height of a convulsion from apoplexy or heart paralysis. There is anuria or hemoglobinuria, or one obtains a few drams of thick, brownish urine from the bladder, which solidifies when heated.

Sometimes the woman is successfully delivered, but the pulse does not improve, the coma deepens, and edema pulmonum closes the scene. Some cases are bad from the start, the patient dying after one or two convulsions in a few hours. As a rule, the case ends one way or the other within three days.

Rarely the course of the disease is that of acute yellow atrophy of the liver, with jaundice, petechiæ, diminished liver dulness, the well-known urinary findings, delirium, jactitation, coma, exitus.

Occasionally, after a severe labor or during the last part of the second stage, the parturient will have a single convulsion or a second milder one, without or with very slight albuminuria. This is called *eclampsia reflectorica*, and might be likened to the discharge of an electric accumulator, the toxins being massed during labor in an especially predisposed person. Spasmophilia, tetany, anesthesia?

An acute collapse after labor, simulating internal hemorrhage, embolism, or edema of the brain, and attended by albuminuria, is of the same nature as eclampsia, and requires careful differentiation from the other conditions.

Acute toxemia, presenting all the manifestations of eclampsia *without convulsions*, has been mentioned. The patient sinks at once into coma, which is almost always fatal. Premonitory symptoms have been present, as a rule, such as headache, visual disturbances, nausea, vomiting, epigastric pain, and low blood-pressure. Fever is usually present and a slight jaundice is seldom absent, the blood-pressure sinks very low, and such cases are characterized by great asthenia. Marked liver autolysis is usually found at autopsy, but death may have been too quick for much change in the kidneys (Schmid).

Diagnosis.—Convulsions and coma during pregnancy may come from epilepsy, hysteria, brain syphilis, tumors, tubercle, cerebral thrombosis, apoplexy, meningitis, salvarsan encephalitis, pneumonia, phosphorus, strychnin and other poisonings, as by drugs taken to induce abortion, uremia, diabetes, and true eclampsia. Pregnancy exaggerates the tendency to convulsions in these diseases. Characteristic for true eclampsia are repeated convulsions with coma, or at least lethargy between them, early fever, and marked albuminuria, with other findings of renal involvement. The history of the case will almost always exclude poisoning, but medicolegally a differential diagnosis may occasionally be necessary, and this may not always be possible, even at autopsy, because, for example, the liver in cases of phosphorus death resembles acute yellow atrophy. Epilepsy is eliminated by the history of previous convulsions, but the first attack of a permanent neurosis may occur during labor, or, as happened in a case of the author's, epilepsy may be inaugurated by an attack of eclampsia, a fact which was also noted by Ferè. The contracted pupils and diminished or absent reflexes and low blood-pressure are good points in favor of epilepsy. Epileptic attacks seldom occur during pregnancy and labor, and are usually single, but the status epilepticus may cause trouble in making the differential diagnosis. Here the slight or absent urinary findings, the late presence of fever, diminished reflexes, and the history must help.

Hysteria will cause no trouble to an observer who has seen both conditions. An atypical convulsive seizure, lasting a long time, with grotesque motions and spastic contractions of muscle groups, retained consciouness, and mobile pupil, without cyanosis, or stertorous respiration, or fever, or urinary findings serve to make the differentiation easy.

Diabetic coma—history: acetone breath, glycosuria and hyperglycemia, Kussmaul's air hunger, paucity of renal symptoms.

Organic disease of the brain must be diagnosed by the usual medical methods, but mistakes are very liable to occur in cases of meningitis, tubercle, and apoplexy. Spinal puncture may be required. The Wassermann test may not be used in differentiation because it has been found positive in 8 cases of true eclampsia by Semon. The treatment must be carried out on obstetric lines.

From uremia it is impossible to separate true eclampsia unless the preëxistence of nephritis is known, but often the general picture of the case impresses the observer as one of renal insufficiency, and, again, another case gives almost indubitable signs that the liver is at fault. Delirium, jactitation, jaundice, and petechiæ point to hepatic involvement, ammoniacal breath, retinitis albumenurica, increase of urea, residual N, and indican in the blood indicate renal involvement. Treatment in all cases is the same. (See Table, p. 385.)

Prognosis.—Over 20 per cent. of women afflicted with eclampsia die, and this has been hardly affected by changes of treatment in the last one hundred years. Wyder collected large statistics, and showed a general mortality of 20 per cent. and a mortality of 10 per cent. of cases which developed in the maternities. The prognosis varies in different countries, in different years, and to a certain extent with different operators. Statistics vary from 5.31 per cent. (Stroganov) to 45.7 per cent. (Büttner) for the mother, and from 3.62 to 42 per cent. for the child. (See Peterson.) When attacked by true eclampsia multiparæ probably are no more endangered than primiparæ, but since renal disease is more common in them, the prognosis is usually worse when convulsions occur. Eclampsia occurring during pregnancy has the highest mortality, during labor less, and during the puerperium the least, but the experience of the individual observers may be otherwise, as in the author's cases the worst have been those where the attacks began postpartum. The mortality of eclampsia depends on the type. The hepatic have the highest death rate, the nephritic lower, and the hypertensive forms the lowest. In comparing statistics these facts must be considered.

For the child the chances are not good, nearly one-half of the children dying, a result that is due to—(1) Prematurity; (2) toxemia; (3) asphyxiation by the repeated convulsions of the mother, with prolonged cyanosis; (4) drugs (morphin, chloral) administered to the mother; (5) injuries sustained during birth, especially forced delivery. The child may die of eclampsia after delivery. Of viable children about 20 per cent. die, and the mortality increases with the number of convulsions the mother had before delivery.

One must, therefore, in individual cases give a very guarded prognosis, even in the apparently favorable ones, because death may occur in coma after one or two convulsions. Death comes from exhaustion, heart-failure, toxemia (the system being overwhelmed by the poison, such cases being evidenced by deep coma, with few or no convulsions), embolism, thrombosis of the pulmonary artery, fat embolism of the lungs, hemorrhage into the brain, pulmonary edema, œdema laryngis, and asphyxiation. Further, the patient is endangered by the results and accidents of severe operations undertaken to deliver her, as ruptura uteri, postpartum hemorrhage from cervix tear, from drugs administered, such as chloroform and veratrum, and from sepsis. Infection is a common cause of death, and eclamptics show a decided susceptibility to it. A large proportion of the deaths is due to aspiration pneumonia and the accidents of anesthesia mostly preventable.

In individual cases the pulse is the best index. If it remains full and hard, below 120, there is no immediate danger, but if faster, weak, compressible, or even running, with low blood-pressure, the prognosis is bad. A falling blood-pressure in the absence of hemorrhage or shock is of good omen. High fever is not necessarily a bad prognostic sign unless it runs above 104° F. and is going higher. Symptoms of edema of the lungs, rattling in the chest, bloody froth from the mouth and nose, with cyanosis, are usually precursors of death, but may respond to treatment. Prolonged and violent fits or frequently repeated attacks with short intervals, or both, give a bad outlook, but recovery has occurred after 81 attacks, though this is unusual. When the number exceeds 20, the prognosis gradually becomes worse. If the severity of the symptoms abates after delivery, the woman usually gets well. Rarely is there a recurrence of the fits after hours or days, and, if there is, recovery is the rule. Such cases are likely to show a large number of attacks, for example: Jardine, 207; Engelman, 200; Spalding, 593. It is doubtful if these were true eclampsia. Deep cyanosis between attacks is an unfavorable symptom, as also is extreme jactitation. Anuria, hemoglobinuria and intense albuminuria are of bad omen, and much hope is justified as soon as the kidneys show signs of recovery (free secretion of pale urine). Apoplexy is almost always fatal, but sometimes part of the body will be paretic or paralyzed from a local edema which disappears during convalescence. "Wet" (edematous) eclampsia is less fatal than the "dry"—perhaps the storage of fluid in the tissues is defensive and removes some of the toxins from the circulation. On this theory sweat packs would be harmful. Jaundice clouds the prognosis.

After delivery the puerpera is not out of danger. Aspiration pneumonia is not rare, the result of mucus, blood, food, etc., being drawn into the lungs by the deep stertorous respiration. It causes most of the deaths. The tongue may be so severely bitten during the fits that it may become so swollen as to demand intubation or tracheotomy to prevent suffocation. Pneumonia, too, may result from the infected bitten tongue. Sepsis is common, and usually runs a severe course, since the kidneys and liver are already diseased and their defensive powers in abeyance. The proneness of toxemics to sepsis is marked. Perhaps study of this relation may discover the causes of toxemia. Late effects may be aphasia, amaurosis, hemiplegia, and puerperal insanity (1 out of 20, Loehlein).

After delivery the albumin quickly diminishes in amount, and may have been reduced to a trace by the time the puerpera leaves her bed, disappearing entirely in from three to twelve weeks. A longer persistence of the urinary findings indicates permanent damage to the kidney parenchyma, and one should be guarded in prognosis. In subsequent pregnancies albuminuria and casts may recur, even convulsions (Dührssen, 1.5 per cent.), but we must decide that a chronic though latent nephritis has existed in the meantime. Many authors believe that one attack of eclampsia confers immunity, but such is not always the case. Even the kidney of pregnancy may recur. It has been held that the kidney of pregnancy never left permanent changes in the organs. This statement cannot be proved, because it is never possible to demonstrate absolutely that the woman did not carry into her pregnancy a latent nephritis, dating, perhaps, from a scarlatina or other infection in infancy.

Treatment.—*Prevention.*—One can speak of rational prophylaxis only when the cause of disease is known. Since we do not know the cause of eclampsia, our treatment is all empiric. Even so, more can be accomplished by prevention than by treatment, because after the convulsions have set in the nervous balance is overthrown. We cannot prevent the action of the primary cause of eclampsia, but by carefully watching the pregnant woman we may discover the first manifestations of the action of such noxious influences, and by appropriate measures either ward them off entirely or interrupt the pregnancy before the disease reaches a climax. It is the pregnancy that favors the development of eclampsia. If we cannot prevent and cure eclampsia, we can remove the pregnancy. If the earliest signs of the impending catastrophe, the *pre-eclamptic toxemia,* can be detected, emptying the uterus will almost invariably avert a fatal issue.

The prevention, in a general way, is equivalent to the conduct of the hygiene of pregnancy. Every pregnant woman should be considered a possible candidate for eclampsia, and all our efforts should be directed to save her. Greater watchfulness is imperative if the family history presages trouble, for example, if the mother had eclampsia, if the parents were neurasthenic, insane, or alcoholic, these indicating a hereditary instability of the nervous system which may lead to disorders of metabolism, especially during the crucial test of pregnancy. The personal history is important; for example, if the patient had eclampsia or declared renal disease before; if she has had diseases which may have damaged kidneys or liver, especially the acute infections; if she is of a "bilious type," one is on the lookout for the first symptoms of eclampsism which precede the convulsion.

If, in spite of the hygienic rules laid down for the patient, the symptoms of toxemia appear, if the blood-pressure begins to rise, or if the urine—which should be examined as a routine duty every two weeks in the latter months of pregnancy—shows evidences of deficient renal activity, the patient is put on a strict prophylactic regimen. High blood-pressure is the most important finding, and, in the author's experience, is never marked without toxemic symptoms. Albuminuria, small output and decrease of total solids are next in importance. Casts, unless granular and cellular, are not unusual in the urine, but they may not be numerous without exciting suspicion; white and red blood-corpuscles with renal epithelium show the acuteness of the process. The percentage of urea is not a reliable index of the nearness of the attack, but it is a valuable adjunct to the diagnosis, since when a woman passes less than half the amount of urea considered normal and has albuminuria, we can suspect derangement of the liver and kidneys. If the urea steadily diminishes while the albumin increases, the danger signs are unequivocal. Blood chemistry, while helpful, is not available for the majority of practitioners. Increase in the non-protein nitrogen, in uric acid, and creatinin may thus be discovered. Their amounts indicate the degree of kidney involvement and may give the signal for interference (Kilian and Sherwin). In suspected cases daily or bi-daily examinations of the urine and blood-pressure are made.

We have in the sphygmomanometer a valuable aid in early detecting eclampsism. A rising blood-pressure is a warning of danger, and the limit of safety may be placed at 140 mm., but a pressure above 130 should warn to greater vigilance. Although blood-pressure readings increase the work of the accoucheur, they must be taken as a routine in the latter months of pregnancy. As stated in the chapter on the Hygiene of Pregnancy, all gravidæ are requested to notify the physician if any untoward symptoms arise, and the accoucheur should give these women a large amount of personal attention, because the symptoms will show that trouble is brewing long before the urine discloses the fact. A more rapid increase in the patient's weight, indicative of water retention, will give valuable evidence of impending toxemia.

When the first signs or symptoms of eclampsism occur, treatment must be at once instituted. It is not always possible, but one should try to fit the case into some classification, *i. e.,* to place it in one or two of the columns in the Table on page 385. In practice, however, we must proceed over general lines, of which there are three: (1) The diet should be so ordered that enough nitrogenous matter is given to sustain life, in the form easiest assimilated, and that will leave the least amount of waste and by-products, which throw extra work on the liver and kidneys. (2) The kidneys should be aided to throw off the surcharge of poisons already in the blood. (3) The termination of pregnancy is to be considered.

(1) The patient is put at complete rest in bed. This favors the circulation through the kidney, which is also aided by the even warmth of the bed. For twenty-four hours only water is allowed, then a low protein and low fat diet is ordered. The salt intake is omitted for a few days, then a small amount allowed, but alkaline carbonates are increased. Fresh and cooked vegetables, fruits, cereals, breadstuffs and sugars, with a small amount of fresh cream or butter comprise the dietary. When the condition improves animal protein is added. Spices, tea, coffee, milk, and alcohol are forbidden. The French claim that the absolute milk diet will prevent eclampsia in nearly all cases. The author has had better success with the above.

(2) One may increase excretion by the bowels, the kidneys, the skin, and the lungs. A saline purge is given at the start, and the bowels are kept open by salines, alternating with vegetable cathartics. Except in very anasarcous patients liquids are freely administered, water, vichy, hot and cool orangeade, lemonade, fruit syrups with seltzer, etc. Of medicinal diuretics only liquor potassii acetatis is recommended, and glucose intravenously. A 20 per cent. glucose solution—1000 c.c. slowly given—forty to sixty minutes, will often cause the kidneys to secrete freely.

The author has discontinued the sweating treatment of toxemia and eclampsia, it being dangerous and inefficient. Werner and Kolisck having proved that the serum from edematous parts is more toxic than that of the general system, it would be illogic to sweat the patient and cause the absorption of these toxins. Jaborandi is heartily condemned, even when the patient is conscious, as it is dangerous and unnecessary. Urinary antiseptics may be used in the presence of pyelitis and bacteriuria.

Fresh air in abundance aids excretion by the lungs, and the patient is instructed to fill and empty the lungs by very deep breaths in fresh air ten times each morning and evening.

Venesection yields only temporary improvement. If there is hyperthyroidism (B. M. R.), iodin is indicated.

Glucose and insulin are not to be given without efficient laboratory control.

Fischer, in 1916, recommended magnesium sulphate intravenously for eclampsia, and through his, Lazard's and McNeile's reports, this drug has obtained wide usage in both pre-eclamptic toxemia and eclampsia. It is slightly anesthetic and dehydrating, reduces the edema of the brain which causes the headaches and the convulsions. In cases where the eclampsism is not marked 4 c.c. of a 50 per cent. solution are injected into the buttock 2 to 4 times a day. I have found that this drug helps, with bed rest and diet, to reduce blood-pressure, increase diuresis and subdue the symptoms for a variable period, and we may use it to tide over an emergency and to prolong the pregnancy for a short time, thus to aid the viability of the fetus. When the symptoms are controlled somewhat we may more safely induce labor.

If a diagnosis of acute hepatic toxemia can be made the uterus is to be emptied as soon as possible whether or not the child is viable. In acute nephritic toxemia one may try to temporize for a short time to secure better viability for the child, remembering, however, that the element of eclampsism may develop suddenly and throw the patient into acute jeopardy, and that the renal damage may be rendered permanent by delay. If a pyelitis is discovered it is treated on general principles and one may see the symptoms moderate as this disease is cured; the same may be said of abscessed teeth and other focal infections.

Chronic nephritis with eclampsism is to be treated just like acute nephritic toxemia, but here, while the danger of eclampsia is slightly less, the complications of abruptio placentæ, apoplexy, infarction of the placenta and death of the fetus are so much more frequent that interference is indicated early. Occasionally if the patient is willing to take the risk for the sake of the child, one may temporize a few days or weeks, under the closest observation, of course. I believe that the "low reserve kidney" of Williams and Stander is a larval form of chronic nephritis and should be treated as such. Seitz mentions it as a recurrent nephrosis.

Hypertension with eclampsism is treated like chronic nephritis with the toxemia element added. Even greater watchfulness, if it were possible, is necessary in these cases, because, edema, albuminuria and symptoms being absent, one is lulled into a false sense of security, when suddenly an apoplexy or acute eclampsism occurs.

Eclampsism, therefore, is what must be looked for in all these cases of late pregnancy toxemia.

The symptoms that, in my opinion, most surely indicate the near approach of convulsions are: Headache, occipital or frontal; seeing colored lights or "spangles"; amaurosis or changes in the retina seen with the ophthalmoscope; twitching of the muscles; somnolence or insomnia; nausea and vomiting; *pain in the epigastrium;* subicterus; general edema of the body; high blood-pressure (175 to 200, with 100 or more diastolic), and marked albuminuria with the appearance of casts and red cells. Rarely one symptom or the other will stand out very prominently, or several may be absent. Marked leukocytosis is also significant, and blood chemistry may reveal progressive damage to the kidney—retention of non-protein nitrogen and uric acid.

How long one should wait to see the effects of treatment depends on the individual case and on the attendant's experience, but the final proof of our deep ignorance of the nature of these affections is brought by the fact that sometimes, when these patients go untreated, eclampsia does not occur, and when treatment has produced apparent cure, the convulsions occasionally manifest themselves, as in one case, where the patient had been in bed under medical treatment for six weeks and was successfully delivered, but three days postpartum convulsions developed and death ensued. Eclampsia is not always a preventable disease, as Davis and Edgar claim, a view which is supported by Williams. Even if the symptoms subside under treatment watchfulness may not be relaxed, as recurrence is not rare.

Methods.—That method of inducing premature labor should be selected which will empty the uterus quickest and with least traumatism. The symptoms rarely are so threatening as to demand excessive haste. In multiparæ the simple rupture of the membranes is usually sufficient, pains coming on, as a rule, within twenty-four hours. In primiparæ it is better to prepare the cervix by packing it and the lower uterine segment with gauze for from twelve to twenty hours. Pains are elicited, the tissues softened, and the chances of injury to the cervix and danger to the fetus diminished. After removal of the gauze the membranes are punctured, the liquor amnii is allowed to drain off, and then a colpeurynter is inserted, which evokes strong pains and completes the dilatation, so that when the bag is expelled the child soon follows. (See Induction of Labor.) After labor has been inaugurated it should be terminated as soon as the conditions will permit, as experience has shown that eclampsia is less likely to occur postpartum after a quick delivery. Since the pains disturb metabolism and diminish excretion, increase angiospasm, and raise the blood-pressure, they seem to elicit convulsions in some cases, and if eclampsia is very imminent, it may be best to select an operation which empties the uterus in one sitting, *i. e.*, laparo-trachelotomy. Since all general anesthetics produce lesions in the kidneys and liver, local anesthesia is used.

TREATMENT OF ECLAMPSIA

Historical.—In the early part of the last century the accepted treatment of eclampsia was antiphlogistic—massive venesections, leeches to the neck and spine, hot baths with cold affusions, mustard packs to the extremities, ice-bags on the head, drastic catharsis, etc. The mortality was high—30 to 35 per cent. Ramsbotham advised induction of labor to ward off eclampsia (1832).

Chloroform was introduced by Simpson and Bouchacourt in 1850–60, and opium, recommended by Bland of London in 1794, also came into use, displacing to a certain extent both bleeding and antiphlogosis.

In 1888 Veit employed morphin in large doses, as much as 3 grains in four to seven hours, and in 1889 von Winckel proposed chloral.

In 1886 Schroeder threw his strong influence against venesection, and bleeding soon lost much of its popularity, but was not completely discarded.

The ancients usually left the labor to nature, although Mauriceau (†1709) recommended rapid delivery, and Baudelocque (1781), puncture of the membranes, even incisions in rigid cervices. Lauverjat proposed cesarean section in 1790, Halbertsma introduced it in 1889. Accouchement forcé was the usual method of rapid delivery when such was considered necessary.

In 1892 Dührssen proposed immediate emptying of the uterus, as soon as possible after the first convulsion, claiming that in 93.75 per cent. of the cases the convulsions ceased or became less severe after the early delivery. Dührssen devised the operation of vaginal cesarean section for the purpose, but the rapid delivery idea spread through the profession and the old brutal accouchement forcé methods were revived, and with disastrous results.

In 1909 Stroganoff pleaded for a more conservative treatment of eclampsia, and described his method of absolute rest, protection from outside irritations, moderate doses of morphin and chloral, elimination, etc., by which he had obtained a mortality of 6.6 per cent. in 360 cases. Since this time bleeding has again come into favor to aid all treatments.

When the pregnant, parturient, or puerperal woman has had the first convulsion, the case at once assumes a most serious aspect. The nervous balance has been upset, the damage to the vital organs by the noxa has grown too great, and one convulsion is likely to lead to another. The mortality of eclampsia is still from 6 to 45 per cent. for the mother, and 20 to 60 per cent. for the child. Such high mortalities rarely accompany surgical complications, hence the patient deserves as much, if not more, consideration than does the surgical patient. She should have at least two physicians and one or more good obstetric nurses. If a good maternity hospital is near by, she should be quickly transported thither; if not, the facilities of the maternity should be closely imitated at home.

Two divergently different methods are at present in vogue, the conservative and the radical, the one meaning that the eclampsia is treated as a medical complication and the pregnancy not disturbed, the other, the radical, being the emptying of the uterus as soon as the diagnosis of eclampsia is made. Stroganoff is the most active proponent of medical treatment, believing that eclampsia is a self-limited disease (an infection) and that if the convulsions can be mitigated for a time, immunities will develop and the patient continue safely in her pregnancy or labor will come on and she will deliver herself. Most men, however, feel that while conservative measures should be used up to a certain point, medical treatment should not be relied on exclusively, but the uterus should be emptied as soon as it can safely be done. Stoeckel of Berlin is the most outstanding radical—he does low, cervical cesarean section on all eclamptics as soon as possible after the first fit, but his results are no better than those of the more conservative. Indeed they would be worse if his material and hospital were not so good, because if there is one thing that is settled in the treatment of eclampsia it is that cesarean section, routinely performed, gives the highest maternal mortality—this being true in America as well as Germany (Küstner) and Britain (Jellett).

TREATMENT DURING PREGNANCY

Conservative treatment varies much in different clinics and with individual practitioners but the statistical results are about the same, which means that we do not yet possess the ideal, and that most eclamptics will get well if not maltreated. The best known of conservative methods is Stroganoff's.

Zweifel, after practising and praising the rapid delivery method, has gone over to the Stroganoff treatment, to which he has added venesection. He had 5.3 per cent. mortality in his last 93 cases; Lichtenstein, in collected statistics, found 12 per cent. of deaths of mothers, and 32.3 per cent. of the children. Stroganoff, up to 1923, had 9.8 per cent. mortality and since has reported a series of 230 cases with 1.7 per cent. No one else, even using his method exactly, has done as well, Edler, Lindquist, and others having had 8.5 to 20.2 per cent. of deaths.

Only the following may be called his method:

> Begin with morphin, $\frac{1}{4}$ grain hypodermically.
> One hour later, 20 to 40 grains of chloral per rectum.
> Two hours later, $\frac{1}{4}$ grain morphin, hypodermically.
> Four hours later, 30 grains of chloral per rectum.
> Six hours later, 15 to 30 grains chloral per rectum.
> Seven hours later, 20 grains chloral per rectum.

The chloral is dissolved in 4 or 5 ounces of warm water and slowly injected into the rectum. A light chloroform anesthesia is given to prevent a convulsion which might result from the local irritation. The opportunity is used to make a rectal examination to determine the progress of labor. Stroganoff stresses the importance of a dark, quiet room, careful watching, chloroform for each threatening convulsion, and non-operative treatment of the labor. If labor has begun, the membranes are to be ruptured.

As a rule the patient calms down and the convulsions cease or become very far apart. Labor may not occur, and in a few cases the patient recovers from the eclampsia and goes to term. The convulsions, however, may recur, and usually at the time of labor. The fetus may live or die. The relative frequency of these terminations cannot be given. Usually, however, labor pains come on. They may aggravate the convulsive state and require a little more of the narcotics. We do not practice "Stroganoff," objecting to chloroform and chloral.

A method having some vogue is the magnesium sulphate treatment, recommended by Fischer in 1916.

26

As soon as possible after the first convulsion 20 c.c. of a 10 per cent. solution of magnesium sulphate are injected slowly intravenously, and repeated bi-hourly until the fits are under control, the intervals being lengthened of course as the patient improves. No more than six doses are necessary, as a rule. Blood-pressure readings taken each hour will tell when to give more of the drug. Small doses of morphin or chloral and bromid per rectum may be given to meet special indications, restlessness, insomnia, etc. (See McNeile and Vruwink.) We occasionally use magnesium sulphate, but intramuscularly not intravenously, the latter being dangerous.

Measures to mitigate the convulsions until pregnancy can be terminated are numerous. Morphin is our sheet anchor, and may be given in doses of $\frac{1}{4}$ grain repeated every three to six hours. Larger doses may increase the coma, and endanger the child. One should always be sparing with drugs. Recently pernocton (sodium-butyl-β bromallyl barbituric acid in 10 per cent. solution) given intravenously has been praised by the Germans. Sodium luminal, 4 grains given intramuscularly every four hours for not more than four doses, or amytal may, occasionally, replace the morphin. In order to restore the proper water balance of the blood and thus produce diuresis, 500 c.c. of a 20 per cent. glucose solution is injected intravenously and if well borne another 500 c.c. every two hours, but no more than 2500 c.c. in one day. Dieckmann also recommends for this purpose 600 c.c. of 6 per cent. gum acacia solution. Normal saline, Ringer's, bicarbonate solutions are contraindicated.

Nowadays we do not believe it possible to get rid of the toxins by active eliminating measures—sweating, cathartics, gastric and colonic lavage, venesection, diuretics (excepting glucose)—yet the Dublin method is based on starvation, gastric and colonic lavage (frequent) and catharsis. Morphin, in very large doses (as recommended by Veit), is also given to suppress the fits. FitzGibbon's mortality at the Rotunda in Dublin was 14.6 per cent.

Be whatever the treatment, the conservative awaits the natural termination of pregnancy. Sometimes the convulsions cease, the eclampsia becoming "intercurrent" (Lichtenstein), yet the patient is not out of danger, as after a few hours to a few days increased albuminuria, higher blood-pressure and threatening symptoms warn us the attack will recur or that the woman may go into coma and slip away. It is wise therefore to induce labor after the active convulsive stage has passed, and we have to do it also if the patient does not respond to medical treatment.

TREATMENT DURING LABOR

Usually the toxemic state or the convulsions bring on labor, and the pains are likely to be strong, progress rapid. It seems as if the pains inaugurate the fits and also that the convulsions stimulate uterine action. The treatment is the same as above described but as soon as we are sure that labor has begun we may use very conservative measures to hasten its termination as there is no doubt that the woman is safer if delivered. One should puncture the membranes at once, experience proving this reduces the number and violence of the convulsions. Only if labor drags on, with evident aggravation of the disease, do we hasten dilatation by metreurysis. On theoretic grounds pituitary preparations are prohibited and may not be given to hasten labor but I have used a single dose after delivery, where needed, without any bad results.

The patient should be allowed to deliver herself if possible. A long second stage is not permitted but the process is facilitated by episiotomy done under local (procain) anesthesia. If she is in ideal surroundings and a man capable of his task is at hand, prophylactic forceps may be employed, also under local anesthesia, with ethylene as second choice.

The accoucheur must stay beside his patient throughout labor and exhibit whatever symptomatic treatment may be needful.

Radical Treatment.—The proponents of rapid delivery base their arguments on statistical, theoretical, and practical grounds. They hold that eclampsia is the result of abnormal processes going on in the ovum, and by removal of the fetus and placenta the source of the toxemia is eliminated—thus the treatment is causal. The general state of angiospasm, usually present in eclampsia, is heightened by the labor pains, and by eliminating these the convulsions (which are the direct result of cerebral angiospasm) are mitigated if not eliminated. It is a generally accepted fact that the convulsions cease or become less severe after the uterus is emptied. Dührssen claims 93.75 per cent., Olshausen 85 per cent. of such improvement, and Seitz and R. Peterson prove it in very large statistics. R. Freund collected 551 cases of eclampsia from the Berlin Charité which were delivered within an hour after the first convulsion with no mortality.

That the child has better chances for life by early delivery nearly all the statistics prove, but these come from clinics managed by competent obstetric operators. If cesarean section is the method of rapid delivery chosen, naturally the children will be spared but the maternal deaths increase. If accouchement forcé is practised, the fetal rises with the maternal mortality to great heights, and these two procedures have brought the rapid emptying of the uterus into disrepute, since the good obtained by shortening or eliminating labor has been usually cancelled by indiscriminate operating.

Methods of Delivery.—The method of effecting the delivery depends on, first, the period of pregnancy; second, the environment of the patient; third, the state of the cervix; fourth, the skill of the operator; fifth, extraneous complications, for example, contracted pelvis, placenta prævia, etc. Before the seventh month all children die, and it is, therefore, necessary to procure only enough dilatation of the cervix to perform craniotomy and extraction. After viability one must try to save the baby also.

If the cervix is fully dilated, delivery is accomplished at once by forceps if the head is engaged; by version and immediate extraction if the head is above the brim. The pains in eclampsia are usually strong, and rapidly efface and dilate the cervix. Indeed, one is sometimes surprised to find the child delivered under the coverlet.

If the cervix is effaced, shortened, taken up, so that only the thin edge remains, this may be dilated with the fingers, or by means of hydrostatic bags, or the thin portion may be incised (Dührssen's incisions). Manual dilatation in these instances is usually selected, but the expert operator chooses the incisions. After this, forceps or version and extraction of the child, depending on engagement, will follow. Version after Dührssen's incisions is somewhat hazardous.

If the cervix is tightly closed, not effaced, and the cervical canal long, two methods of delivery are available—vaginal and abdominal cesarean section. In a primipara before the thirty-second week and in a multipara with softened, usually lacerated cervix, roomy vagina, and relaxed pelvic floor, vaginal anterior hysterotomy is indicated. In a primipara, at or near term, with a long hard cervix and rigid soft parts, this operation is very difficult, and the question of abdominal cesarean section arises. It saves most babies, and the reason the maternal mortality is so high is because it is performed as a last resort in desperate cases, and because the old classic method is used, and with general anesthesia. The low, cervical cesarean, done under local anesthesia, will show a mortality more nearly like that of the conservative treatment. If the patient has, besides eclampsia, a contracted pelvis, either at the inlet or at the outlet, even of minor degree, a large fetus or one presenting unfavorably, placenta prævia, heart disease, etc., one will select the abdominal operation. (See Conditions for Cesarean Section, page 1081.)

Choice of Method of Treatment.—In a given case, which plan shall the obstetric attendant adopt, the radical or the conservative? A careful study of the following conditions will enable one to decide, and, naturally, this presupposes a thorough examination of the patient: (1) The period of pregnancy; (2) the presence of complications, such as contracted pelvis of either inlet or outlet, a large baby, placenta prævia, heart disease, etc.; (3) the degree of advancement of labor; (4) the apparent severity of the disease; i. e., frequency and violence of the spasms, the degree of coma and cyanosis, the blood-pressure, the pulse-rate, the state of the lungs, etc.; (5) the operative skill and experience of the obstetric attendant; (6) the environment—whether the patient is in a clean home, or a hovel, or in a clean maternity with plenty of help.

If pregnancy is not advanced to viability of the child, the conservative plan is chosen in the hope that the convulsions can be kept in abeyance and thus the pregnancy will continue. Later in pregnancy or close to term, the plan will depend more on the skill of the obstetrician and his environment. The conservative treatment gives such good results that it can be cordially recommended to the general practitioner. The experience of all obstetric consultants is unanimous—that if an inexpert operator attempts forceful methods of delivery through unprepared soft parts, the dangers to the mother from infection, rupture of the uterus, and hemorrhage are greater than those of the eclampsia itself, and a large proportion of the children are lost also. With morphin or sodium luminal, the convulsions are held in check and 500 c.c. of a 20 per cent. glucose solution is given intravenously. We wait as long as the patient improves but induce labor if she does not, or if she is near term. The method depends on the conditions.

If the patient is in active labor, making rapid progress, and her general condition not alarming, even the expert obstetrician should incline toward conservative treatment; at most, he will perhaps incise the cervix if it is fully effaced, and deliver a few hours earlier than nature would.

In the presence of mechanical disproportion between the pelvis and the child, laparo-trachelotomy would be the method of choice. (See page 1079.) The same may be said of placenta prævia, abruptio placentæ, and perhaps of cardiac disease or essential high blood-pressure (danger of apoplexy).

For the occasional case of a primipara late in pregnancy, or at the beginning of labor, with rigid soft parts, a long closed cervix, the head high, possibly in posterior position, the convulsions coming at rapidly lessening intervals, low cesarean section under local anesthesia may be recommended, if the patient is in a good hospital and a man capable of his task is at hand.

When the eclampsia sets in with extreme violence, the convulsions being very hard and frequent, the coma and cyanosis deep, etc., the uterus had best be emptied at once if it can be done with safety to the mother. If a gravida falls at once into toxemic coma without convulsions, even cesarean section seldom saves her, but it should be done for the baby.

Adjuvant Treatment.—Whether one employs one or the other plan of treatment, the following measures are occasionally helpful:

Venesection.—Venesection forms part of the treatment of eclampsia of all men of experience, although it is not used as much as formerly. It was basic treatment until 1890, then it was held useless and dangerous, but was revived by Lichtenstein and Bumm about 1905. We bleed only when the convulsions recur frequently and with violence, in which case the pulse is full and hard, the face flushed and cyanotic—in short, when the picture might be called sthenic or apoplectic. When the evidences of cardiac engorgement are present and pulmonary edema threatens, even if the pulse is weak, bleeding will do good, especially if combined with stimulation. Zweifel and Bumm also recommend it in such cases. Before delivery one should be a little sparing with blood because it is not possible to predict the loss during labor.

Colonic Flushing.—Many accoucheurs place great stress on irrigation of the large bowel with quantities of bicarbonate of soda and glucose solutions, on the theory that the bowel contents are toxic and the absorption of these two substances combats the toxicity of the blood. The author has little faith either in the theory or in the practice, and would permit the procedure only after delivery, as there is danger of the field of operation being flooded with liquid feces and infection resulting.

Puncture or incision of the swollen limbs or swollen vulva may be indicated, under strict antiseptic precautions, of course.

Elimination via the bowels is an old practice, but is much overdone, to the patient's harm. Cathartics should be withheld until the uterus is emptied, because of the danger of infecting the operative field with liquid feces. After delivery they should be used with moderation—mild salines being preferred.

Diaphoretics, especially pilocarpin, are to be condemned. The latter drug is a dangerous cardiac depressant and it causes edema of the lungs. Hot baths involve too much manipulation, but hot-wet packs and sweats are recommended by many accoucheurs. The author, in common with many others of experience, has given them up entirely. They are dangerous because depressing, and they seem to favor apoplexy by raising the cerebral blood-pressure, aside from which the amount of poison eliminated through the skin is negligible.

Blood Dilution.—Authorities are divided as to the amount of fluid to administer in eclampsia. Volhard and Fahr urge a thirst cure in acute nephritis, but most accoucheurs believe fluids do good if given cautiously in anasarcous patients. After delivery when the kidneys resume action, large amounts of water are needed to make up for the usually profuse diuresis.

Glucose is a favorite adjuvant in many clinics. It is given in 10 to 25 per cent. solution intravenously, in amounts not exceeding 1000 c.c. at one dose—never if there are signs of edema of the lungs or of diabetes. Dieckmann also recommends 500 to 800 c.c. of 6 per cent. gum acacia

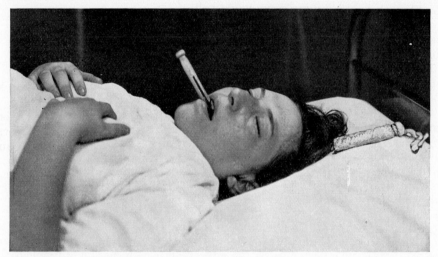

Fig. 343.—Use of Large Clothespin to Prevent Injury to Tongue in Eclampsia. Stage of stertorous respiration. Note swollen hands.

solution. One may replace the blood of venesection by an equivalent of glucose solution. One frequently observes an increase in the urinary output after the perfusion, which ought to be helpful. Sugar, besides being our only safe diuretic, also stimulates the pains.

General Advice.—Protection against injury. Since the convulsions sometimes show frightful vehemence, the patient must be quickly undressed, and put to bed, surrounded with pillows, and watched by a trained attendant, preferably a physician. False teeth should be removed. To prevent the biting of the tongue a simple device illustrated in Fig. 343 may be used. A large wooden clothespin is wrapped in a thin handkerchief and hung near the head of the bed. As the attendant sees the attack approach it is placed between the teeth, so that the elasticity of the prongs takes up the champing of the jaws. If the tongue is swollen from injury, it may be necessary, to prevent asphyxiation, to intubate, using soft-rubber tubing, or to do tracheotomy. Restraint of the movements should not be made—all that may be done is to keep the woman from injuring herself. Heart-failure may be induced by forcibly holding the patient still. For extreme and exhausting jactitation morphin may be given, or, but rarely, an anesthetic may be used. Mucus in the throat and mouth is to be removed frequently, but with gentleness, using, if available, the tonsil operation suction pump, and it is best for the patient to lie on the side, to allow the oral secretions free escape—an especially important injunction during vomiting; these precautions are taken to prevent aspiration pneumonia and lung abscess. In the side position, too, the swollen tongue falls forward and frees the respiration.

All irritants should be withheld, which means that examinations are to be omitted, if possible, and the patient disturbed only for absolutely necessary treatment. Visitors are excluded from the room, which should be well darkened, and the attendants should move about quietly, and permit no loud talking, jarring the bed, etc. As in tetanus, these external irritants may excite a convulsion.

Nothing may be given an unconscious patient to swallow since the fluid usually enters the lungs and causes pneumonia.

Oxygen in the form of fresh air is very beneficial, a point frequently neglected while the oxygen tank stands in a stuffy room. Artificial respiration may be needed to tide the patient over a syncope following a spasm, or to improve the oxygenation of the blood between attacks. Part of the coma is due to the hypercarbonization of the blood. It is a question if the ordinary oxygen inhalations do good (Stadie), but an oxygen room might help.

During the delivery of eclamptics extraordinary precautions against sepsis must be observed, because they are particularly liable to infection, the liver and kidneys being thrown out of immunizing action. The author has seen fatal infection arise in spite of the most rigid precautions. One source of trouble is feces streaming from the anus, the result of the administration of cathartics and enemata before delivery.

Without doubt, in the author's mind, some eclampsias are of infectious origin and in all cases the liver's antibacterial and detoxicating functions are in abeyance. On such conditions infection will be likely to follow any injury and thus the frequency of peritonitis after cesarean section and of septicemia after accouchement forcé is perhaps explained.

The operator should not forget that eclamptics readily go into shock, as Bailey has pointed out. Frequent blood-pressure readings will apprise one of this danger.

Choice of Anesthetic for Operation.—This requires careful thought. All the usual drugs exert a destructive action on the liver, kidneys, blood, and heart, especially when their structure is already compromised by the toxemic state. Chloroform is the worst of offenders and should never be used. In the days when it was much in vogue, fatty heart and acute yellow atrophy of the liver were the usual postmortem findings. Ether is the anesthetic most generally available, but, if procain locally cannot be used, ethylene is the next choice.

The author does not approve of spinal anesthesia. Theoretically, the paravertebral method is promising. For venesection, local anesthesia with procain is used.

Treatment of Postpartum Eclampsia.—Venesection, magnesium sulphate, narcotics, mild catharsis, moderately free administration of fluids, especially glucose solution, with general hygiene measures, constitute the treatment here.

Sundry Remedies Mentioned for the Sake of Completion.—Veratrum viride, first used by Dr. Baker, of Eufaula, Alabama, in 1859, once attained considerable repute in America and Italy as a specific, but large experience did not sustain it; thyroid extract (Lange and Nicholson); parathyroid extract (Vassale); amyl nitrite (Jenks); trephining the skull and spinal puncture, on the theory that increased intracranial pressure is causative. The latter has shown a few remarkable results and deserves trial in desperate cases (Slemons); amputation of the mammæ (Sellheim); injection of air and oxygen into the mammæ, as is done for a similar disease in cattle (Healy and Castle, Kininmonth); and renal decapsulation (Edebohls). Both theory and practice speak against the last operation. Chiriè collected 30 cases with a mortality of 46 per cent., and the clinical histories do not show that the decapsulation improved the conditions present with any regularity. Littauer reports 62 cases with 20 deaths, which is better, especially since only the serious ones were operated on. The question of permanent damage to the kidney from the shrinking of the new connective-tissue capsule requires sober consideration. Dienst recommends hirudin, an extract of leeches, given intravenously to reduce the fibrin content of the blood. Plasmaphæresis (Irving and Taylor), removal of a portion of the blood, extraction of the corpuscles, adding saline solution as a substitute for the plasma and restoring the mixture (Abel's idea) is based on purely theoretic and wholly unproved principles. The same may be said of heparmone. (See Miller and Martinez.)

The After-treatment.—Nothing may be given by mouth until the patient is fully conscious, but about 2500 c.c. of 20 per cent. glucose solution may be administered intravenously during the first twenty-four hours. When the puerpera can swallow knowingly, water, lemonade, orangeade are allowed for the first forty-eight hours. For ten days the diet should be carbohydrate—gruels, cereals, vegetables, and fruits. After this—general diet, omitting spices.

Since the kidneys now begin to act freely, often 140 to 180 ounces of urine a day being passed, it is well to watch the bladder for overfilling. Suppression of urine is serious. It is combated by (1) hot wet packs around the kidney region; (2) prolonged colonic irrigations; (3) venesection followed by glucose infusion; (4) intravenous administration of 20 per cent. glucose solution; (5) hot lavage of the bladder; (6) renal decapsulation.

Involuntary bowel movements are the rule, and, therefore, the lochial pad should be arranged so that the feces do not dam up into the vulva. Warm-water bags are to be closely watched, because eclamptics are especially liable to burns and necroses. Sometimes spontaneous necroses resemble burns.

Since the convulsions may recur even after a week, the puerpera requires constant supervision, and especially if she shows any signs of puerperal insanity, such patients not seldom making attempts at suicide or infanticide.

The temperature of the eclamptic quickly subsides, a rise after such a fall indicating sepsis, pneumonia, etc. Nursing should not be allowed until the puerpera has been fully conscious for several days and the urine has become nearly normal, and when her strength permits. In a few reported cases and one of my own it has seemed that the milk of the mother caused convulsions in the child. (See also Goodall.) One is always asked if the woman may have more children. The answer depends on the evidence of permanent renal damage. True hepatic eclampsia recurs in only 2 per cent. of cases. Nephritic toxemia is very likely to appear in subsequent pregnancies. Peckham found 23 per cent. developed chronic nephritis and 40 per cent. showed nephritis after toxemic pregnancies. A pre-existent chronic nephritis makes a gloomy prognosis. After a simple toxemia the kidney damage is not so bad. In all events pregnancy may not be allowed for two years, in order to give the kidneys and liver ample time to recuperate, and then only if the urine, blood-pressure, etc., show the perfect recovery.

LITERATURE

Ahlfeld: Lehrbuch d. Geburtsch., 3 Aufl., p. 235.—*Albert:* Arch. f. Gyn., vol. lxvi, p. 483.—*Anselmino, Hoffman, and Fauvel:* Archiv für Gynaek., 1931, vol. 147, H. 3, p. 652.—*Bell, W. S.:* Brit. Med. Jour., 1920, i, p. 626.—*Benda:* Das retikulo-endotheliale System in der Schwangerschaft, Urban und Schwarzenburg, Berlin, 1927.—*Blanc:* Arch. de Tocologie, 1889 and 1890.—*Bouchard:* Leçons sur les auto-intoxications, 1887.—*Bouffe de Saint-Blaise:* Annales de Gyn., 1891, vol. xxxv, p. 48, and *ibid.*, 1898, vol. i, pp. 343, 432.—*Browne, F. J., and Dodds, G. H.:* Jour. Obstet. and Gyn., Brit. Empire, 1930, 37, 476.—*Bumm:* Brundriss d. Geburtshilfe, 1922, p. 680. —*Chiriè:* L'Obstetrique, Juin, 1909.—*Collman:* Zentralbl. f. Gyn., 1897, No. 13.—*Corwin and Herrick:* Jour. Amer. Med. Assoc., February 12, 1927, p. 457.—*Cragin and Hull:* "Chloroform," Jour. Amer. Med. Assoc., June, 1910.—*Davis:* Jour. Amer. Med. Assoc., 1926.—*Delore:* Arch. de Tocologie, 1884, vol. ii, p. 921.—*Devraigne:* Obstetrique, May, 1909.—*Dieckmann, W. J.:* Amer. Jour. Obst. and Gyn., September, 1931, p. 351.— *Dieckmann and Wegner:* Amer. Jour. Obstet. and Gyn., May, 1932, p. 657.—*Dienst:* Zentralbl. f. Gyn., December, 1909, No. 50; *ibid.*, p. 133.—*Dirmoser:* Pernicious Vomiting of Pregnancy, Vienna, 1901.— *Dubois, P.:* Bull. de l'Academie de Med., 1852, 6 Mars.—*Dührssen:* Handb. der Geb., vol. ii, 3, p. 2403.—*Ehrenfest:* Surg., Gyn., and Obst., September, 1911; also Amer. Jour. Obst. and Gyn., November, 1920, p. 218, Lit.—*Engelman:* Zentralbl. f. Gyn., 1907, p. 306.—*Engelman and Frankel:* Zentralbl. f. Gyn., 1909, No. 18, pp. 618 and 634.—*Essen-Möller, Halban-Seitz:* Biologie des Weibes, vol. vii, p. 978.—*Eufinger:* Zentb. für Gyn., 1930, p. 2734.—*Ewing:* "Pathog. of the Toxemias of Pregnancy," Amer. Jour. Med. Sci., June, 1910.—*Favre:* Virchow's Arch., vol. cxxvii, p. 133.—*Fehling:* Verhandl. d. Deutsch. Ges. f. Gyn., 1901, p. 261.—*Fieux:* "Complete Report of Meeting of French Obstetricians," Annales de Gyn., Toulouse, December,

1910.—*Fitzgibbon:* Irish Medical Journal, Coombe Centenary Number, 1926.—*Frankl:* Praktische Ergebnisse der Geb. und Gyn., 1909, vol. i, Heft 1, p. 232; also 1910, vol. ii, p. 2.—*Freund, R.:* Zentralbl. f. Gyn., 1918, No. 47.—*Frey:* Schweiz. Med. Woch., January 31, 1924.—*Gerdes:* Zentralbl. f. Gyn., 1892, No. 20.—*Goodall:* "Should Eclamptics Nurse the Newborn?" Amer. Jour. Obstet., January, 1911.—*Halbertsma:* Münch. med. Woch., 1887, No. 35, etc.—*Healy and Castle:* Jour. Infect. Dis., 1912, vol. x, p. 226.—*Hermann:* Die Eklampsie und ihre Prophylaxe, Urban u. Schwarzenburg, Wien, 1929. Lit. to date.—*Heyneman:* Zentralbl. f. Gynaek., February 26, 1927, p. 518.—*Hinselman:* Die Eklampsie, 1925, Proceedings Int. Congress at Dublin; also Irish Journal Med. Sci., 1926.—*Hitschman:* Zentralbl. f. Gyn., 1904, No. 37.—*Hofbauer:* "The Toxicoses of Pregnancy," Zeitschr. f. Geb. u. Gyn., vol. lxi, Heft 2, p. 185; also Zentralbl. f. Gyn., 1924, No. 3, p. 74.—*Hofmeister:* Zentralbl. f. Gyn., 1892, No. 51.—*Holland:* Jour. Obstet. and Gyn. of Great Britain, December, 1909. Gives literature on causation to date.—*Jaggard:* American System of Obstetrics, vol. i, p. 421.—*Jardine:* Jour. Obst. and Gyn., British Empire, June, 1906.—*Jürgens, Stumpf, Ahlfeld:* Berlin klin. Woch., 1886, p. 875; Lehrbuch d. Geb., 1903.—*Kilian and Sherwin:* Jour. of Obst. and Gyn., July, 1921.—*Kininmonth, J. G.:* Brit. Med. Jour., March 7, 1931, p. 395.—*Kossman:* Monatsschr. f. Geb., 1901, vol. xiv, p. 288.—*Küstner, H.:* Arch. für Gyn., 1931, 145, 3, p. 577.—*Lange:* Zeitschr. f. Geb. u. Gyn., vol. xi, Heft 1.—*Lichtenstein:* Zentb. für Gyn., 1922, Nr. 5 and Nr. 34.—*Liepmann:* Zentralbl. f. Gyn., December 17, 1921, p. 1811.—*Losee and Van Slyke:* Bull. New York Lying-in Hospital, January, 1917.—*Marriott:* Ill. Med. Jour., February, 1927.—*Massen:* Zentralbl. f. Gyn., 1895, p. 1106.—*Mathes:* Halban-Seitz, Biclogie, 1924, vol. iii, p. 1.—*Mayer:* Zentralbl. f. Gyn., September, 1911, p. 1299.—*McClintock:* Dublin Jour. Med. Sci., 1873.—*McNeile and Vruwink:* Jour. Amer. Med. Assoc., 1926.—*McPherson:* Bull. New York Lying-in Hospital, January, 1917. —*Miller and Martinez:* Jour. Amer. Med. Assoc., 1929, 92, p. 627.—*Montgomery:* Signs and Symptoms of Pregnancy, 1857, p. 93.—*Murling and Baily:* Arch. of Internal Med., September, 1913.—*Opitz:* Zentralbl. f. Gyn., 1924, No. 1, p. 2.—*Peckham:* Johns Hopkins Hosp. Bull., 1929, 45, 176, 188; also Johns Hopkins Hosp. Bull., 1931, October, No. 49.—*Peterson, R.:* Amer. Jour. Obstet., July, 1911; also July, 1914.—*Pinard:* Annales de Gyn. et l'Obst., 1909, Juillet, p. 391.—*Pinard et Bouffe de Saint-Blaise:* Annales de Gyn., 1891, vol. xxxv, p. 48 et seq.—*Rebaudi:* Gaz. degli Ospedali, Milan, September 21, 1909.—*Rivière:* Auto-intoxication eclamptique, Paris, 1888.—*Rockwood:* Surg., Gyn., and Obstet., March, 1926, p. 342.—*Rosenthal, Krebs, Dieckmann:* Am. Jour. Obst. and Gyn., January, 1924, p. 89.—*Schmidt:* Zeitschr. f. Geb. u. Gyn., 1911, vol. lxix, H. 1, p. 148. Gives literature.—*Schmorl:* Zentralbl. f. Gyn., 1901; *ibid.,* Verhandl. d. Deutsch. Ges. f. Gyn., 1901, p. 303 et seq.—*Schumacher:* Hegar's Beiträge, vol. v, p. 257.—*Schwab:* Psycho-analysis of Hyperemesis, Zentralbl. f. Gyn., July, 1921, p. 957.—*Seitz:* Arch. f. Gyn., 1909, vol. lxxxvii, p. 117.—*Seitz, L.:* Monatsschr. für Geb. u. Gyn., July, 1931, p. 335.—*Sellheim:* Med. Klinik., August, 1923.—*Semon:* Zeitschr. f. Geb. u. Gyn., 1910, vol. lxvii, iii, p. 773.—*Slemons:* Jour. Amer. Med. Assoc., September 8, 1917.—*Spalding:* Calif. State Med. Jour., September, 1920, xviii, p. 325.—*Stadie:* Jour. Amer. Med. Assoc., April 22, 1922, p. 1204.—*Stander, H. J.:* Surg., Gyn., and Obstet., February, 1932, p. 129.—*Stander and Williams:* Jour. Amer. Med. Assoc., February 12, 1927.—*Stewart:* Amer. Jour. Obstet., 1901, p. 506.—*Stoeckel:* Jahreskurse f. Aertzl. Fortbildung, July, 1917, p. 9; also Zentralbl. für Gyn., January 15, 1927.—*Stratz:* Halban-Seitz, Biologie, 1924, vol. i, p. 511.—*Stroganov:* Monatsschr. f. Geb. u. Gyn., 1909, Bd. 29, p. 568; also Jour. Obst. and Gyn. of the British Empire, 1923, Spring No., p. 1.—*Thaler:* Zentralbl. f. Gyn., June 24, 1922, p. 1019.—*Titus:* Jour. Med. Med. Assoc., August 15, 1925, p. 491.—*Titus, P.:* Amer. Jour. Obst. and Gyn., 1930, 19, 16.—*Underhill:* Arch. of Internal Medicine, 1910, vol. v, p. 61.—*Volhard:* Monatsschr. f. Geb. u. Gyn., vol. v, p. 411.—*Ward:* "Thyroidism and Toxemia," Surg., Gyn., and Obst., December, 1910, p. 632.—*Werner and Kolisch:* Arch. für Gyn., v. 103, 230, 1914.—*Whitney:* Amer. Gyn., 1903, p. 180.—*Williams:* Johns Hopkins Hospital Bulletin, 1906, vol. xvii, p. 81; also Jour. Obst. and Gyn., British Empire, January, 1912.—*Winter:* Monatsschr. f. Geb. u. Gyn., July, 1922, p. 222.—*Wyder:* Verhandl. d. Deutsch. Ges. f. Gyn., 1901, vol. ix, p. 268.—*Zangemeister:* Zeitschr. f. Geb. u. Gyn., lxxix, H. 1, 1916; also Die Lehre von der Eklampsie, Hirtel, Leipzig, 1926.—*Zweifel:* Doederlein's Handbuch, 1916, vol. ii, p. 708.

CHAPTER XXVIII

TOXEMIAS OF PREGNANCY, CONTINUED, AND SUNDRY DISEASES

ACUTE YELLOW ATROPHY OF THE LIVER

Closely allied to hyperemesis and to eclampsia is acute yellow atrophy of the liver—the *icterus gravis* of older writers. Pregnancy seems to predispose to this disease, since over half the cases reported occur in pregnant women. It appears at any period of gestation, during labor, or in the puerperium. Without doubt several diseases may terminate under the clinical picture of acute yellow atrophy, and the author has seen hyperemesis gravidarum, eclampsia, sepsis acuta, and chloroform poisoning do so, also one case of secondary syphilis in a prostitute. Other authors report typhoid, osteomyelitis, diphtheria, erysipelas, anaphylaxis, phosphorus, alcohol, and ptomain-poisoning as precedent illnesses. It is sometimes epidemic. The causation is unknown, and whether the degeneration of the liver is due to infection or to a toxicosis is still *sub judice*. Bacteria, among others the streptococcus (Prochaska), and Bacterium coli (the author) have been cultivated from the liver, but since degeneration and not inflammatory changes are predominant, the theory of an intoxication is more plausible.

Pathology.—At autopsy the liver is found wasted, perhaps to one-half its volume, soft, friable, sometimes almost diffluent, yellowish streaked, and mottled with red. Rarely one finds an acute diffuse hepatitis or the evidences of other hepatic disease, in which case the liver may even be enlarged. The liver-cells have undergone albuminoid degeneration, the nuclei are indistinct or absent, and in the red portions the cells have disappeared entirely, or are found only at the periphery of the lobules. Tiny hemorrhages are sometimes found, especially under the capsule. The interlobular connective tissue appears increased because the liver-cells have dropped away from it and there is a slight wandering in of leukocytes. These probably have to do with the conversion and the carrying away of the fatty degenerated parenchyma, though it is probable that a proteolytic enzyme is also active. The heart, the muscles, and the glands of the bronchi and of the digestive tract are fatty degenerated, and all the tissues are bile stained. The kidneys are intensely involved, in one of the author's cases the convoluted tubules being completely degenerated, but the tubuli recti and the glomeruli being unaffected. This case showed no inflammatory changes, but such are reported by some authors. The spleen is large and soft, similar to that seen in the acute infectious diseases.

Symptoms.—Much variation exists in the descriptions given of this affection. If the hepatic atrophy is a termination of hyperemesis or of eclampsia, the symptoms of these disorders precede. If it follows the use of chloroform, the symptoms are very acute—may be fatal in from six hours to as many days. In the "idiopathic" cases a prodromal stage with anorexia, vomiting, constipation, headache, perhaps slight mental disturbances, extreme weakness, a tinge of icterus, and pain in the epigastrium exists, but its significance is not recognized. After a few days to a few weeks symptoms of serious illness appear, rarely with a chill and high fever (Vinay), but usually suddenly. Frequent vomiting, first glairy, then bilious and bloody, anorexia, thirst, pain in the epigastrium, acholic stools, with occasional hemorrhage, intense headache, restlessness, later extreme and incessant jactitation, with rolling the head to and fro on the pillow, insomnia, delirium, sometimes convulsions, and coma before death. In secondary chloroform poisoning I have seen the disease end fatally in six hours with all the characteristic symptoms appearing in rapid succession. Abortion usually takes place just before death, but may not occur. Otherwise uterine hemorrhage is infrequent.

Examination of the patient shows extreme exaggeration of reflexes, general icterus, sometimes of a lemon, sometimes of an orange-yellow, tint; minute petechiæ on the trunk and extremities, or an erythematous eruption; a slight cyanosis of the face, with puffiness of the features; a dry brown tongue, with sordes; a characteristic but indescribable fœtor ex ore—it resembles the fruity odor of sepsis, but has a slight pungency; the pulse is fast, weak, and numbers 120 to 140 beats; the respirations are dyspneic, stertorous, and later weak and superficial; the temperature is almost always elevated,—102° to 104° F.,—but is rarely subnormal; at first contracted, later dilated, pupils are seen, together with slight exophthalmos; toward the end, however, the eyes are sunken; there are extreme tenderness over the liver and diminution of liver dulness, which is determinable by daily measurement; enlargement of the spleen occurs (66 per cent.); the urine is diminished, containing bile, albumin, casts of all kinds, fatty renal epithelium, blood, methemoglobin (Stumpf), often leucin balls and tyrosin crystals, very little urea (which, divided, shows a large percentage of ammonia nitrogen, indicating that the liver function is in abeyance), acetone, diacetic acid, indican, albumose, and peptone, but sugar rarely.

One or more of these symptoms or findings may be absent, but always, after the prodromal stage, there are enough present to make a positive diagnosis. The disease lasts a few hours or days after the real symptoms appear, the most rapidly fatal cases being those in which the cerebral symptoms, delirium, and agitation are worst. Death is due to exhaustion and intoxication, the heart giving out first, and it occurs in deep coma.

Diagnosis.—If a pregnant woman, after a week or two of lassitude, headache, and symptoms of gastric catarrh, suddenly develops delirium, jactitation, jaundice, with epigastric tenderness and diminution of liver dulness, the diagnosis of acute yellow atrophy is almost certain. If such symptoms appear after hyperemesis, eclampsia, and sepsis, the diagnosis may still be asserted, and differentiation is not necessary, since both may be due to the same cause, which may be unknown, or at least its action not understood. The administration of chloroform should be considered in the history taking. In those cases which begin with a chill and high fever the disease may be an acute septicemia with this unusual clinical picture. Confusion will arise only with "bilious" typhoid, yellow fever, and phosphorus-poisoning, but a careful medical examination will usually procure clearness.

The **prognosis** is bad. Recoveries are reported, and while most authors claim these are mistaken diagnoses, the writer believes that he has had a case which survived the disease. The fetus is practically always lost, through either prematurity or toxemia. It is usually icteric, but in cases of simple maternal icterus the child is not jaundiced.

The **treatment** is symptomatic. In hyperemesis one should terminate pregnancy as soon as suspicions are aroused that the liver is beginning to suffer. Indeed, in all cases the pregnancy should be interrupted as soon as the diagnosis is made, unless the patient is so sick that the interference itself would precipitate the end. Vaginal or abdominal cesarean section under novocain would be the best method.

CHOREA GRAVIDARUM

Another disease which in all probability is toxemic or infectious in origin is chorea gravidarum. Pregnancy aggravates a preëxistent chorea but rarely to a serious degree. Chorea may bring on abortion. The causal connection between pregnancy and chorea is very certain, but predisposition is provided by heredity (neurasthenia, insanity, alcoholism, hysteria); previous chorea in infancy; nervous shock, as fear or anger; anemia; chlorosis; acute polyarticular rheumatism; endo-carditis; infections of various kinds. In 5 of 6 cases observed by the author the picture was one of toxemia, and in four of them treatment on this hypothesis resulted happily. In milder cases a hysteric element may be discerned; indeed, some authors distinguish a hysteric and an idiopathic form. Sometimes the movements are unilateral or involve only a few muscles.

Chorea during pregnancy often becomes threatening, the movements at first localized, rapidly becoming general, incessant, violent, and preventing sleep. One observes anemia, exhaustion, delirium, perhaps maniacal, and later torpor, then fever, coma, and death. Emaciation, bed-sores, furunculosis, erythematous or morbilliform eruptions, cardiac murmurs, and albuminuria are sometimes found on examination. All degrees of severity are noted. Incontinence of urine and feces is of bad omen, and jaundice may also occur in such cases. The disease usually appears before the middle of pregnancy, rarely in labor, and still more seldom after; it lasts from eight days to months, disappearing, as a rule, with the expulsion of the ovum, whether spontaneous or induced. Recovery often occurs before term, delivery then being natural. The child may be choreic. The toxemic forms are acuter and seldom go to full term, abortion being common. Primiparæ are most affected, especially if younger than twenty-five years, but when chorea appears in a multipara or recurs in a subsequent pregnancy, it is usually more serious.

The **prognosis** is grave, 20 to 30 per cent. of the women and over half of the children dying, the latter from prematurity. Permanent mental disturbances may follow, as after eclampsia. Death occurs from exhaustion, inanition, injury, de-cubitus, sepsis, endocarditis, and toxemia, shown by delirium and coma. At autopsy cerebral anemia, edema of the dura, thromboses of the sinuses, and emboli and softening of the cord may be found, but, again, there may be negative findings.

Treatment.—The general rules for medical cases apply here, but in view of the danger of the disease and its probable cause (toxemia), one should not temporize too long, but as soon as the movements become marked the patient is to be put in bed and isolated in a dark quiet room. A vegetable and fruit diet is ordered and much fluid, including glucose, is introduced into the system. Sodium bromid in 60-grain doses q. i. d., chloral, even morphin, may be administered, but the author was able only with hyoscin to calm the movements, and even this failed after a few days. Salicylates, sodium luminal (gr. iij t. i. d.), and elimination of infective foci form part of the treatment. By skilful nursing the nutrition is main-tained and exhaustion prevented. Normal pregnancy serum should be tried, 20 c.c. every day, for three or four days (Albrecht). When hypocalcemia is proven, give calcium gluconate, etc.

Pregnancy must be terminated when it is seen that the general health has begun to suffer, certainly long before incontinence, jaundice, fever, or delirium begins. Curiously, Wade saw recovery after dilatation of the cervix without abortion, as Copeman did in hyperemesis. If the uterus is emptied early enough, recovery is the rule. At or near term cesarean section should be considered. Willson and Preece collected 951 cases. (See also Vignes and Williamson.)

PRESUMABLE TOXICOSES

Every physician meets conditions in pregnancy which are best explained by calling them toxicoses. Truly the expression means nothing definite, but the affec-tions present the picture of intoxications and respond to appropriate treatment. Asthma in a woman who never had the disease before may have such a basis. Sometimes the asthma is due to retention of chlorids, when proper diet is helpful. Adrenalin often relieves the dyspnea, even when placed under the tongue. In one case of the author the child had hardly any adrenal glands.

Fainting spells, acute collapse, or even sudden death may have no other apparent cause. Such accidents strongly resemble anaphylactic phenomena. Peripheral neuritis may be of septic origin, but well-authenticated cases have been found as a complication of an almost certain toxemia—hyperemesis gravidarum—as in the case of Soloview, quoted by Vinay, and three of my own. The tingling of the hands and legs, with numbness, even anesthesia and paresis, of which many pregnant women complain, are probably due to affection of the nerves by some circulating toxin. The nerve-trunks are tender and sometimes determinably enlarged, especially the ulnar. Since the symptoms disappear quickly after delivery, the injury to the nerves is slight, but grave forms of neuritis and polyneuritis do occur, either on a toxemic or an infectious basis.

Psychoses during pregnancy are usually toxemic. A bad heredity is found in nearly half of the cases, but this does not preclude the idea of a toxicosis, because we have seen that such taint predisposes to other toxemias, as eclampsia and hyperemesis. It seems that disturbed metabolism is more common in women whose nervous systems are not equal to the strain of pregnancy. The mental disease may recur after delivery. Korsakoff's psychosis has been observed in pregnancy. While usually alcoholic in origin, the syndrome, polyneuritis and delusions, may appear during the early months of gestation, and a toxemia may be involved. The frequency of insanity after puerperal fevers is strongly suggestive of an infectious origin, but very often the psychosis follows an eclampsia, a chorea, hyperemesis, or a normal puerperium, and other theories must be invoked. One might divide the cases into infectious, toxic, and idiopathic (heredity, inanition, exhaustion, anemic) psychoses. It is more than possible that some of the diseases we call toxemias are in reality infections, the causal bacterium still eluding our crude methods of investigation.

Most authors do not favor the induction of abortion or premature labor in the insanity of pregnancy, but the writer believes that the cases should be treated just as any other toxemia, unless the accoucheur, after consultation with an alienist, is convinced that the mental disease is simply contemporaneous with gestation, without direct causal relation. So far as the child is concerned, no indication for abortion will lie, because if the psychosis is toxemic, the condition is not necessarily transmitted to the offspring, and, further, we have no right to sacrifice the child on the assumption of the possibility of its being mentally unfit.

In some neurotic women I have seen the occurrence of pregnancy produce a degree of terror that certainly was close to mania. During labor acute insanity is sometimes observed in women of poor nervous balance, neuropaths, hysterics, when the pain is very severe. Without doubt the strain of labor is too much for many nervous systems, and the author believes that prolonged painful labor, without infection, will explain many cases of puerperal insanity. Transitory mental aberration during the agony of the second stage is not seldom observed, and it may be infanticidal or homicidal, a point of importance in medicolegal cases. It is an indication for immediate delivery.

During the puerperium and lactation insanity is a not infrequent disease, statistics of the asylums showing from 10 to 18 per cent. of female inmates affected at this time. Puerperal infection, mastitis, eclampsia and allied toxemias, postpartum and other hemorrhages, especially if grafted on a bad heredity, exhausting labor, the drain of lactation, are the most common causes. The attack may be developed by a violent psychic shock, such as death of husband or child.

Melancholia with suicidal intent was the most common form in the author's cases, but mania with infanticidal tendencies was also observed. Vinay says that the maniacal forms are most frequent. The prognosis is fair, the majority of the cases recovering in from six weeks to six months. The treatment is along general lines. Hypocalcemia (backache, shoulder pains, claudication, restlessness, irritability, mental excitability) resulting from lactation requires the usual remedies.

Neuritis.—Pain in the nerves, especially the trigeminal, the ulnar, and the sciatic, is frequently noted in pregnancy, and is generally treated as a neuralgia, but often prickling sensations, numbness, and slight paralysis of the member or members show that the nerve is more deeply involved—that a neuritis exists. Polyneuritis with marked paralyses, even atrophy, has been observed, and has been ascribed to toxemia. The degeneration of special nerves in hyperemesis gravidarum has been mentioned. Not rarely pregnant women complain of numbness and pricking of the fingers, with lack of power in the hands, and examination shows the members to be puffy, slightly cyanosed, with diminished tactile sensibility, and occasionally tenderness of the ulnar nerve is discovered. The nerves of the special senses may be involved—neuritis optica, auditoria, etc. (*q. v.*), and the pregnancy may have to be terminated to prevent permanent blindness or deafness. After delivery the symptoms rapidly subside, having been probably toxemic. Treatment is along these lines. (See Wilson, Lit.; Berkwitz and Lufkin, Lit.)

Puerperal neuritis is of the same nature, though Bar calls it septic. Monoplegias after delivery are probably septic. They are usually radial or cubital, Möbius believing that these nerves are points of predilection in puerperal infections. Sciatic neuritis is particularly intense when a puerpera is affected. Occasionally paralysis and atrophy result. While some of the cases are acute and heal rapidly, many pursue a course of months, and recovery may be incomplete. When the connective tissue of the pelvis is inflamed, the nerves of the sacral plexus not seldom are also involved, with peripheral muscular and sensory disturbances. Recovery occurs after the inflammatory process has subsided, but scar formation may render it incomplete.

Injury to the nerves in the pelvis by the forceps may result in peripheral neuritis or paralysis, but the prognosis is good. The differential diagnosis is on general lines—here need only be mentioned the rupture of the symphysis pubis, where the pseudoparaplegia, with abduction of the thighs, at first glance, might cause confusion. The findings over the pubis and the results of the neurologic examination will always clear the diagnosis. Treatment of neuritis is given in text-books on internal medicine. For toxemic polyneuritis it may be necessary to induce labor, especially if vital nerves—phrenic, pneumogastric, or the nerves of the special senses—begin to show the least involvement.

Tetany.—A disease, discovered by Steinheim in 1830 and studied by Trousseau, characterized by tonic spasms of the muscles of the arms and legs—occasionally general and very painful, rarely with, but usually without, loss of consciousness. Minor symptoms are formication, paresthesia, muscular weakness or stiffness, and pains in the fingers during writing or sewing. Trophic disturbances may be noted, falling out of the hair and finger-nails, cataract, anomalies of the teeth. Examination shows excessive motor excitability, Trousseau's sign—contracture of the hand when the brachial plexus is compressed; Chvostek's sign—facial spasm when the facialis is percussed, etc. The disease in milder forms is not very rare, indeed, tetanoid symptoms are quite common in pregnancy, but the severe cases are rare and they may be fatal. The second half of pregnancy is the usual time, but it may appear during lactation. Recurrence is frequent. Labor is not affected, but the fetus may be macerated or die of convulsions. One of the causes of convulsions and death of the newborn is tetany, and this may be due to hemorrhages in the parathyroids the result of labor.

Parathyroid insufficiency is the cause of tetany and pregnancy develops it. The lack of calcium due to the large amount consumed by the fetus may be contributory.

Treatment.—In mild cases, calcium gluconate by mouth or by vein, or milk and calcium lactate liberally, with viosterol ♏ 20 T. I. D., the latter favoring absorption of calcium ingested. In severer cases, calcium and glucose intravenously with parathyroid feeding, or implantation, or parathormone intramuscularly. Interruption of pregnancy if refractory to treatment and patient's state alarms. Avoid ergot, pituitary, atropin, calomel, and chloroform. (See Voegtlin, Lisser, Richardson.)

BLOOD DISEASES

Pregnancy, generally held to be a normal function, produces pathologic anemia in 50 to 65 per cent. of cases (Bland, Galloway, Moore). It is a simple secondary anemia with low hemoglobin, low specific gravity (Palowe), and red count. Destruction of the red cells in the placenta and insufficient replacement due to imperfection of the reticulo-endothelial system (Benda) may be the cause. Treatment as usual, iron, arsenic, liver, etc. In the South one thinks of hookworm. Chlorosis, due probably to ovarian dysfunction, may cause sterility, but may also be improved by pregnancy. It is a not infrequent cause of abortion, which tonic treatment may prevent. Chlorotic women stand hemorrhage very poorly, a loss which may be insignificant for another being fatal to them, and, besides, they show a tendency to bleed—a point of great importance in the treatment of the third stage. Chlorosis, which is often a sign of general infantilism, may cause atonia uteri during the second and third stages of labor, and one may find a generally contracted pelvis too. (See Hüssy.)

Pernicious anemia seems to be favored by frequent child-bearing, especially if the woman is otherwise weak or anemic. Hemorrhage favors the disease, and it may follow an infection; indeed, a careful diagnosis is necessary to shut out tuberculosis, syphilis, cancer, helminthiasis, chronic gastritis, intestinal infections, and other conditions which cause secondary anemia. A toxemia could cause the disease, but, although this theory has been advanced, no proof is shown. It seems to be a deficiency disease, and is helped by feeding the patient liver. Toxemia is said to excite **leukemia** which may occur during pregnancy, but it is doubtful if there is any special relation between the two (Kosmak). If there were, one should meet the disease oftener. Esch reports 6 cases where the clinical picture resembled pernicious anemia, but the hemolysis, etc., were probably due to a toxemia. This pseudopernicious anemia is often combined with fever, leukocytosis, and heart murmurs, which render the differential diagnosis from acute endocarditis very hard, though it is still possible. True pernicious anemia is often fatal in spite of emptying the uterus. Pseudo forms are less dangerous and may be submitted to the usual medical treatment before doing abortion, but don't wait too long (Spitzer).

Labor may occur naturally in these conditions without any particular tendency to hemorrhage, but sudden exhaustion, with coma and œdema pulmonum, has been frequently noted to follow a few hours after delivery. Leukemia does not pass over to the fetus. (See Rowland.)

Hemophilia is rare during the reproductive period. Contrary to most writers, the author believes that fatal cases of hemophilia can occur during delivery. Hemophiliacs may have profuse menses, and may bleed to death from defloration; they abort frequently, and may have postpartum hemorrhage or late bleedings in the puerperium. Hemophilia, or at least a hemorrhagic diathesis, can occur in a woman who has no family history of it, and in whom the bleeding tendency has not been in evidence in previous deliveries, abortions, or menstruations. The author is convinced that a temporary hemorrhagic diathesis can occur during pregnancy, its basis being a latent hemophilia, syphilis, malaria, intoxication by chemical or hemolytic poisons, a toxemia, or a sepsis or an endocrinopathy. It is a generally admitted fact that toxemia disposes to hemorrhage. The hemorrhagic types of eclampsia, hyperemesis, etc., are particularly fatal. The blood in the cases observed by the writer was lake colored, like port wine, the clots small, soft, and black. Suggillations, petechiæ, and bloody infiltration around the vulva, vagina, and cervix, and the hypodermic punctures betrayed the fact of a dissolution of the blood. Thrombopenia (Frank) evidenced by bleedings, especially uterine, immense reduction of blood-platelets, long bleeding time, normal clotting time, purpura—a rare complication of pregnancy often fatal, may explain some of such cases. These are sometimes called morbus maculosis werlhofii.

In one case of hæmatoma vulvæ (p. 807) the woman had a gingivitis with hemorrhages and other toxemic symptoms which gave almost the clinical picture of scurvy. It is more than possible that a toxemia or infection lies at the bottom of these diseases. This subject is an inviting field for investigation. (See Mosher.)

So far as treatment is concerned, if the condition is recognized during pregnancy, the attempt should be made, by general tonic remedies, to upbuild the patient's strength. Iron, mercury, and arsenic have given the author good results. Calcium chlorid and gelatin are supposed to increase the clotting power of the blood, and may be administered for a few days before, during, and after labor. The author could not convince himself that any effect was obtained, a view also held by Robertson. The use of a heterogeneous serum, as that of the horse, has been advocated in cases of obstinate hemorrhage, as also has been human serum, and the results with the latter certainly encourage trial. The object is to supply the missing thrombin, thrombogen, and thrombokinase. In bad cases human transfusion is indicated and Bernstein recommends the blood of a menstruating woman.

The author has had 2 cases of **polyglobulism**, a syndrome with enlarged spleen, intense cyanosis, hypererythrocytosis. The spleens in both patients reached the brim of the pelvis; one woman had 8,000,000 reds and 60,000 whites, clubbed fingers, rheumatic pains, and general asthenia. One was sterile after having had two children before the disease appeared; one had two still-born macerated children, then, under iron, arsenic, and mercury treatment, a live child without trouble, followed by sterility. The pregnancy seemed to aggravate the general conditions very much. (Lit. in Jour. Amer. Med. Assoc., November 23, 1907, p. 1776.)

SKIN DISEASES IN PREGNANCY

A close relation exists between the skin and the changes in the general metabolism due to pregnancy. Virchow and Neusser believed that there is some relation between the ovaries and the skin. Of the milder manifestations of the disturbed nutrition of the integument may be mentioned the pigmentation, hyperidrosis, edema, falling of the hair, cracking of the nails, erythema, acne, etc. While most skin diseases are aggravated or even developed, some are cured by the advent of pregnancy. Pregnant women may have all the dermatoses that other women have, and, since the reaction is usually more severe, it is probable that many of the affections hitherto designated as gestational are really merely coincident. The latest and most complete exposition of the subject is given by Scheuer.

Pruritus is an affection, perhaps neurotic, perhaps toxemic, usually localized on the vulva, sometimes general, which begins in the middle or end of pregnancy, and may rarely reach such an intensity as to demand the emptying of the uterus. Diabetes should always be looked for. Neurasthenic and hysteric women more often have the itching. Genital pruritus is often a symptom of varicose veins, edema, vulvitis, vaginitis, cervicitis, with leukorrheal discharge, and in these cases the skin of the vulva is thickened, red, and shiny. Mycosis vulvæ is not infrequent in multiparæ. Lack of cleanliness is another cause of itching. Eczema and other dermatoses must, of course, be sought. The pruritus is usually worse at night and in summer because of the warmth, and the patients lose sleep. After delivery recovery promptly ensues. Subsequent pregnancy usually shows recurrence. In several cases the author found evidences of renal inefficiency, and one woman had a pruriginoid eruption on the arms, legs, back, shoulders, and chest. Besnier called this form of pruritus "prurigo gestationis." He describes an itchy eruption of tiny papules closely grouped, especially on the backs of hands and feet, appearing usually after the third month, recurring in successive pregnancies, and disappearing after delivery. Usually the skin is normal in appearance except for scratch-marks. The treatment is general and local. If diabetic, the usual treatment; if toxemic or neurotic, appropriate remedies will be employed. Sodium bromid in 30-grain doses often produces sleep. Vagotonic cases are helped by atropin, gr. $\frac{1}{150}$, t. i. d. Adrenalin is occasionally successful, ♏xv, every four to six hours by mouth. There may be other signs of hypo-epinephrinemia—low blood-pressure, marked pigmentation, sweating, edema.

Urticarial eruptions are not rare, occurring in the last trimester. Erythema exsudativum multiforme and dermatitis symmetrica may be very extensive and threatening. Sometimes called "toxic rashes," they usually respond to treatment and disappear after delivery. Remember the underlying toxemia. A bland diet, without condiments, spices, and alcoholics, and one with little protein, is prescribed—in short, general hygienic conduct. Baths may be tried, but the author has had little success with them. Very light clothing, with linen next to the skin, is good.

In cases that are obstinate one should try calcium in the form of Locke's solution, a pint daily hypodermically, calcium gluconate by mouth and viosterol failing which, the serum of a healthy pregnant woman should be given, 20 c.c. every day for three days, or horse-serum, with due regard for anaphylaxis.

For local use on the skin the author has had success with this lotion:

℞ Carbolic acid.............................. 0.5
Zinc oxid
Finely levigated calamin $\Big\}$ ....āā 15.0
Lime-water........................to make 100.0

For pruritus vulvæ the author has used with varying success the following applications: Chloral hydrate, 5 to 20 gm. per liter; bichlorid of mercury, 1 : 1000; carbolic acid, 2 per cent. solution; essence of peppermint, 4 c.c. per liter; an ointment consisting of ichthyol, 2 per cent., menthol, 0.5 per cent., ointment of rose-water, a sufficient quantity; or, carbolic acid, 0.5 per cent., menthol, 1 per cent., zinc-oxid ointment and ointment of rose-water, of each, a sufficient quantity.

The washes and ointments are to be applied cold, after cleansing the parts thoroughly with tar-soap and water, using much soap. In cases of mycosis vulvæ the white patches are to be painted with 10 per cent. silver nitrate, and the patient given a dusting-powder of boric acid. This smarts a good deal, but is helpful.

For irritating discharges the best results have been obtained with daily potassium permanganate douches, 1 : 3000, followed by one of essence of peppermint, a teaspoonful to a quart of cool water.

Excessive pigmentation cannot be combated during gestation. It may be associated with the adrenals. If the mask of pregnancy does not disappear within six months after delivery, the parts may be rubbed with pure lemon-juice morning and evening, which, failing to remove the stains, a treatment with bichlorid of mercury may be recommended, under the care of a good dermatologist.

Excessive hirsuties, very rare in pregnancy, usually disappears of itself.

Brickner describes a disease which he calls fibroma molluscum gravidarum. The forehead, chest, shoulders, arms, and hands, in the order named, present pedunculate, pinkish, warty excrescences, in size from a pin-head to a bean, which drop off before or surely after labor. A tendency to warts was known to exist in pregnancy, but no one had described this disease. The writer has seen many cases of it, but in none was the eruption so generalized as in Brickner's. Treatment is symptomatic.

Edema.—More than half of all pregnant women show some edema of the feet, the hands, or the face. Often this is an elastic puffiness which does not pit. Hydroplasmia is natural to pregnancy and increase of water accounts for most of the gain in weight. A real anasarca, with exudation of serum in the tissues, is usually due to toxemia, renal or hepatic, and is produced by the alteration of the constitution of the blood or capillaries, or both. It is present in the morning in the feet, hands, and eyelids, sometimes disappearing by night. The stagnant circulation can be shown by the capillary microscope. (Baer and Ries, Lit.)

Edema which grows worse during the day is usually due to mechanical causes —varicose veins, tight garters, cardiac disease, and obstruction to the abdominal circulation (twin pregnancy, pendulous belly, abdominal constriction). The accoucheur is warned not to conclude lightly that an edema is mechanical or of no significance because the urinary findings are negative. A nephritis may exist without albuminuria, and eclampsia may occur with no other warning than the anasarca. Edema with high blood-pressure is ominous.

The treatment is plain when the cause is discovered. General obstetric hygiene usually suffices. (See p. 243, The Conduct of Pregnancy.) Rest in bed, reduction of the salt and water intake and a non-protein diet are prescribed. Excessive edema is always pathologic, and usually preëclamptic, and, therefore, treatment directed against the toxemia is indicated. Puncture of the swollen tissues should not be done unless the patient is in labor and soon to be delivered, because of the danger of infection from the prolonged drainage and, of course, extreme antisepsis will be observed. A cross-cut above the pubis lets out the serum better and more safely.

Special skin diseases, described by writers as due to pregnancy, are very rare. *Herpes gestationis* is a form of herpes which appears during pregnancy, especially on the arms, legs, face, and chest, in the order named, passes through the usual states of grouped vesicles, small bullæ, pustules, and crusts—is of chronic nature, and liable to recurrence in subsequent pregnancies. Very probably other affections, for example erythema multiforme and dermatitis herpetiformis, have been called herpes gestationis.

Impetigo herpetiformis (Hebra), on the other hand, is a serious disease (mortality, 80 per cent.), sufficiently characteristic to be called a gestational affection, though it is rare in America. The following is a description of the author's typical case treated in conjunction with Dr. Josef Zeisler:

A quintipara, aged thirty-seven, had the disease in her third pregnancy and miscarried, but not in the fourth, a normal pregnancy. Since four weeks she has been bedridden because of general weakness, vomiting, diarrhea, insomnia, pain in the legs, and an eruption which began on the inside of the thighs and has slowly spread all over the legs, trunk, and arms. Groups of pustules, pin-head to lentil in size, appear, coalesce, form crusts which fall off and litter the bed, leaving reddened skin. The lesion extends progressively in all directions. The center of the large areas is healed, but large patches of epidermis are elevated in places, resembling pemphigus. In the genital region the crusts and excoriated skin produced a red, fetid, oozing, bleeding surface. The mouth was early affected, showing gray plaques.

The general condition of the woman is poor, but she has no fever,—contrary to Kaposi,—a pulse of about 100, and there is slight icterus. At eight months the woman aborted, whereupon the eruption rapidly disappeared and the woman quickly recovered. The child showed no eruption. Bacteriologic examination of the pustules and of the blood was negative. Polyuria was present, with a trace of albumin, diminished urea, no sugar, no peptones or indican, and no casts.

The cause of impetigo herpetiformis is unknown—an infection or a toxemia appears probable. Wolff-Eisner believe it is of an anaphylactic nature, the foreign protein coming from the uterus. Mayer believes it is a toxemia, and that the system does not react with sufficient antitoxin. He therefore injected 20 c.c. of the blood-serum of a healthy gravida to supply the antitoxin. Result, cure in three cases. Treatment is palliative, but the author, having observed the rapid subsidence of the disease following the expulsion of the fetus, if rapid amelioration did not follow Mayer's treatment, would induce labor.

During the puerperium the author has observed the following skin diseases: the skin seems to be particularly liable to disease. Sudamina; acne; furunculosis; erythema multiforme; pityriasis versicolor; drug eruptions, e. g., quinin; urticaria from too free use of cresylic acid preparations; eczema from bichlorid, which in one case became a generalized eruption with high fever, and was erroneously called by the attending physician an erysipelas. Septic eruptions will be discussed under Puerperal Infections.

LITERATURE

Albrecht: Zeitschr. für Geb. u. Gyn., 1915, vol. 76, Heft 3, p. 677.—*Baer, J. L.:* Amer. Jour. Obst. and Gyn., August 19, 1922, p. 622, Lit.—*Baer and Ries:* Capillary Microscopy in Pregnancy, Jour. Amer. Med. Assoc., February 16, 1924, p. 526.—*Benda, R.:* Das Retikuloendotheliale System beim Weibe, 1931.—*Berkwitz and Lufkin:* Surg., Gyn., and Obstet., May, 1932, p. 743.—*Bernstein, M. A.:* Jour. Bone and Joint Surgery, July, 1932, p. 659.—*Bevan:* "Chloroform Deaths," Jour. Amer. Med. Assoc., 1909.—*Bland, P. B., et al.:* Amer. Jour. Med. Sci., 1930, 179, 48.—*Brickner:* Amer. Jour. Obstet., 1900.—*Buist:* Transactions of the Edinburgh Obst. Soc., 1894, 1895.—*Charpentier:* Traite d'Obstet.—*Debreuihl:* La pratique dermat., 1901, vol. ii, p. 918.—*De Lee:* "Fatal Hemorrhagic Diathesis," Amer. Jour. Obstet., 1901, vol. xliv, No. 6.—*Duhring:* Amer. Jour. Med. Sci., vol. lxxxviii, p. 391.—*Esch:* Zeitschr. f. Geb. u. Gyn., 1916, vol. 79, H. 1; also Archiv für Gynaek., 1927, p. 788.—*Fellner:* Die Beziehungen innerer Krankh. zu Schwangersch., etc., 1903, p. 183.—*Frankl-Hochwart and von Noorden:* Die Erkrank. des Weibl. Genitales in Beziehung zu Innere Medizin, 1912–13. Gives full literature.—*Galloway, C. E.:* Jour. Amer. Med. Assoc., 1929, November 30, Lit.—*Hebra:* Wien. med. Woch., 1872, No. 48.—*Hüssy:* Die Schwangerschaft, 1923, p. 114.—*Kosmak:* Amer. Jour. Obst. and Gyn., February, 1921.—*Linser:* Arch. f. Derm. u. Syph., 1911.—*Lisser:* Jour. Amer. Med. Assoc., February 12, 1927, p. 461.—*Lynch:* Trans. Chicago Gyn. Soc., 1913, Korsakof's Disease.—*Mayer:* Zentralbl. f. Gyn., 1911, No. 9, p. 351.—*Moore, J. H.:* Amer. Jour. Obst. and Gyn., 1930, 20, 254.—*Mosher:* Surg., Gyn., and Obstet., April, 1923, p. 502.—*Müller, P.:* Die Krankheiten des weiblichen Körpers, p. 405.—*Neverman:* Zentralblatt f. Gynaek., April 22, 1922, p. 618.—*Palowe:* Amer. Jour. Obstet. and Gyn., June, 1932.—*Richardson, G. C.:* Illinois Med. Journal, June, 1931, p. 458.—*Robertson:* Jour. Amer. Med. Assoc., vol. 1, No. 20.—*Rowland:* Jour. Amer. Med. Assoc., February 2, 1924, p. 362.—*Scheurer:* Hautkrank, sexuellen Ursprungs, Vienna, 1911.—*Spitzer, W.:* Zentb. für Gyn., June 6, 1931, 5, 1933, Lit.—*Vignes, H.:* Gazette Med. de France, 1930, 3, 65.—*Vinay:* Maladies de la Grossesse, p. 249; *ibid.*, 1894, p. 584; *ibid.*, p. 485.—*Voegtlin:* Surg., Gyn., and Obstet., September, 1917, Lit.—*Whitman:* Peroneal Paralysis, Surg., Gyn., and Obst., 1922, xxxiv, 32.—*Williamson, A. C.:* Amer. Jour. Obst. and Gyn., 1930, 20, 192.—*Willson and Preece:* Arch. of Internal Medicine, April, 1932, p. 698.—*Wilson, K.:* Amer. Jour. Obstet. and Gyn., June, 1932, p. 775, Lit.

27

CHAPTER XXIX

LOCAL DISEASES INCIDENT TO PREGNANCY

Varicosities.—Varices of the legs or of the vulva or hemorrhoids are found in a majority of pregnant women. While marked varicosities are present in only 20 per cent. of gravidæ, a few dilated veins are an almost constant accompaniment of gestation. The veins of the ankles, legs, thighs, vulva, vagina, rectum, and broad ligaments are affected, in frequency and degree, according to the order given, but one or the other form may be alone present or predominant. Fine venous networks or large paquets of tortuous veins, resembling bunches of angle-worms, are observed. The vulvar lips may be enlarged and spongy (Fig. 132). They resemble varicoceles and cause much the same distress. Edema often attends varicosities. The patient complains of pain, fatigue, burning, itching, and a feeling of tension in the affected parts. In some cases the veins are so dilated and the legs so edematous and painful that the patient can hardly walk. After the delivery of the child the varicosities collapse, and they almost always disappear in three weeks. The causes of varicose veins are not known, but pregnancy surely has much to do with developing them. Women who are much on their feet and have to work hard, multiparæ with pendulous belly, women with heart disease, are most afflicted, and a special disposition can also be observed. This may be congenital. Frequent pregnancies and tight abdominal bands and garters also favor them. Varicosities are not due to pressure of the gravid uterus on the veins of the pelvis, because this is impossible, nor to increased intra-abdominal tension, because this seldom exists to such a degree. That there is some obstruction to the return circulation from the legs is highly probable, but there must be some change in the vessel-wall or of the blood which predisposes to venectasis during pregnancy. Toxemia again has been suggested, also a vasodilating ferment from the corpus luteum. It may be the same condition which causes the pelvic vessels to enlarge and dilate with the progress of pregnancy. That some such relation exists is proved by the fact that in some women the veins enlarge as soon as conception occurs, and that they collapse if the fetus dies in utero. With other abdominal tumors varicose veins of the legs are rarely observed, and this point may be used in the differential diagnosis. A woman was sent to the author from a neighboring city for her accouchement. She was suffering from carcinoma of the ovaries with immense abdominal distention. There were no varicosities, but the patient said she had had such in all her six pregnancies.

Varicosities, beyond the pain they produce, are dangerous because they may ulcerate, become infected (phlebitis and periphlebitis), may thrombose, sometimes give rise to emboli, and may burst, allowing fatal hemorrhage. Vaginal, vulvar, and broad-ligament varices may rupture also into the connective tissue, causing hematomata, which may be fatal from internal hemorrhage, or, becoming infected, from sepsis. During labor vaginal and vulvar varicosities not seldom are torn, requiring quick diagnosis and immediate suture or firm tamponade, because the bleeding is profuse. Differential diagnosis from placenta prævia, abruptio placentæ, and atony of the uterus must be made, which is done by inspection and finding the bleeding vessel. A hematoma occurring during labor may obstruct the delivery of the fetus. Treatment consists in opening and packing the cavity until the cervix is dilated, then removal of the packing, delivery, followed by repacking the cavity of the hematoma and the uterovaginal tract. Occasionally a varix of the broad ligament will burst into the peritoneal cavity, producing the symptoms of ectopic gestation, and one may thus rupture during labor, the patient dying of intraperitoneal hemorrhage without a drop showing externally to apprise the accoucheur of the cause of the fatal anemia. (See Naujoks, Lit.)

Clotting, occurring in broad-ligament varices, may lead to emboli, which may break off during labor, and this warns to gentleness in handling the uterus during the third stage or during the puerperium.

Treatment.—A hemorrhage from a varicosity is easily controlled by pressure or suture. The patient must be instructed to avoid injuring and infecting the superficial veins by scratching them or knocking against things; to avoid coitus if the varices are vulvar or vaginal, and she should be taught how to stop hemorrhage while waiting for help if one of them should bleed. Phlebitis and periphlebitis are treated by rest in bed, moderate elevation of the leg, and 30 per cent. alcohol dressings. Rest must be enjoined for three weeks, or until it is judged that the thrombosis is complete and the thrombus firmly organized—this to avoid the danger of embolism. Suppurating thrombi of the legs are to be drained. Little can be done to cure the bad cases of varicosities during pregnancy, but much relief can be had from calcium and viosterol. A rubber stocking or flannel bandage may be worn, and the feet held elevated whenever possible. More comfort is gotten from the application of adhesive strips placed spirally around the limbs while the woman is recumbent. They divide and support the column of blood.

Hemorrhoids occasionally are very obstinate and annoying to the pregnant woman, who perhaps is not affected with them under other conditions. Hemorrhages, fissures, with exuberant granulations, or extrusion and gangrene, may occur. Operation is not to be made during gestation, but the usual treatment may be pursued. During labor the hemorrhoids come out, swell up, and may bleed. They predispose to lacerations of the perineum. An attempt should be made to replace and retain them with a pad. Some accoucheurs use this opportunity to remove the masses, but probably it is best to wait until the puerperium is over. Postpartum hemorrhoids often cause a great deal of distress. If the piles are internal, they may be replaced, under ether if necessary; if external, no such attempt may be made, but the hips should be elevated and cold applied to the parts. If there is a hemorrhage into one or the other pile, it may be incised under local anesthesia and the clot turned out, but the author prefers medical treatment where possible.

Anusol suppositories or this prescription may help.

℞	Acidi tannici	2.0
	Ext. hamamelis	12.0
	Menthol	0.5
	Ext. opii aq	0.5
	Ung. aquæ rosæ	q. s. ad 100.0

Fiat unguent.

Relaxation of the Pelvic Joints.—The ancients believed that the pelvic bones separated during delivery, and labor thus was rendered possible. Later this view was dropped, and cases where such separation occurred were called abnormal. In cows the sacro-iliac joints soften, and in guinea-pigs all the joints, especially the pubis, soften and enlarge, allowing wide latitude of motion. In the human there is no doubt but that the joints soften, thicken, and thus enlarge the cavity of the pelvis. The bones become more movable on each other and thus permit the pelvis to accommodate itself to the mechanism of labor. Matthews Duncan proved this. The mobility in the joints renders the Walcher position effective in enlarging the inlet, and, by placing the parturient in the exaggerated lithotomy position, through the same conditions, some enlargement of the bony outlet is produced. That a small pelvic cavity enlarges during pregnancy the author is convinced, and that the tilting (or "nutation") of the sacrum favors the passage of the fetus is another clinically demonstrated fact.   The x-ray shows little, if any, pubic separation.

When the softening of the pubic and other joints becomes marked, symptoms resembling arthritis are produced, as follows: Pain in and about the pelvis, referred to the site of the joints, and especially to the particular one involved; difficulty in locomotion; easy tiring, with a general sense of weakness; inability to rise from a sitting posture without raising the trunk on the hands or outside assistance; relief by walking, but soon followed by pain in the pelvis, necessitating rest; the condition is worse in the morning, better in the day, and worse again in the evening; pain reflected up and down the nerve-trunks of the pelvis, simulating neuralgia, or even pains in the hypogastrium, simulating abdominal disorders.   When the patient is bedridden, the case is decidedly pathologic.   On examination no cause for the symptoms can be found until the condition of the pelvic joints is discovered.   The tenderness of the pubic cartilage is the most prominent finding.   The sides of the joint are painless, but pressure directly over the middle evokes lively expressions of suffering.   Then the groove may be found over the pubis or with the finger in the vagina.   By rocking the pelvis one can feel the bones ride on each other, especially plainly if the woman is examined while erect and stands first on one foot and then on the other.   Deep pressure over the sacro-iliac joints elicits pain, but not over the coccyx.   The gait is peculiar, waddling—"like a duck," as one woman expressed it.   A distinct rising and falling of the crests of the ilia can be seen, which is not all due to the tilting of the pelvis.   The distress in walking may sometimes be a real pain, referred to the affected joint or joints.   The affection occurs in the latter half of pregnancy, in multiparæ more than in primiparæ, is often combined with varicose veins, the joints under these conditions seeming to partake of the general imbibition of the tissues of the pelvis; it often recurs in successive pregnancies.

During labor, if the sacro-iliac synchondrosis is loose, the ilium may be dislocated on the sacrum, a condition which was noted by Madame Lachapelle.   A case of this kind is reported by Bates, of Denver.   Putschar proved that during labor the joints are distracted by the wedge-like passage of the child, hemorrhages resulting in their capsules and clefts arising in the symphysis pubis.   *The joint may rupture during operative or even natural delivery.*   After delivery the solidity of the pelvis is rapidly restored, unless the synchondroses were injured, in which case the patient may be bedridden for weeks or months.   Milder cases of injury to the sacro-iliac joints are undoubtedly commoner than is generally believed.   Such injury explains many of the prolonged backaches and neurasthenic states following parturition.   An orthopedist should be drawn in consultation in such cases.

How closely this condition is related to osteomalacia has not yet been discovered.   It bears some resemblance.   The diagnosis is easy if the disease is borne in mind.   Neuritis and paraplegia seldom need consideration, but are easily eliminated.   The prognosis is good, but the possibility of rupture of the symphysis should be remembered.   (See Chapter on Ruptura Symphysis Pubis.)   During pregnancy cure is impossible.   External applications, rest in the horizontal position, calcium, viosterol, endocrines, and general hygiene are prescribed.   A tight girdle (Osgood's brace) or adhesive straps may be tried.

LITERATURE

DeLee: "Relaxation of Pelvic Joints," Jour. Amer. Med. Assoc., January 4, 1902.—*Duncan, Matthews:* Researches in Obstetrics, 1868, p. 146; Zentb. für Gyn., 1926, October, p. 2771.—*Naujoks:* Arch. für Gyn., 1932, vol. 148, H. 3, p. 635.—*Putschar, W.:* Entwickelung, etc. der Beckenverbindungen des Menschen, G. Fischer, Jena, 1931, Lit.

CHAPTER XXX

EXTRA-UTERINE PREGNANCY

A BETTER term is ectopic pregnancy, or eccyesis, which means a gestation which occurs outside of the cavity of the uterus. Extra-uterine gestation is the term more commonly used, but this would exclude from the study those cases where pregnancy develops in the interstitial portion of the tube.

An ovum may be fertilized and remain at any point of its passage from the ovary to the uterus (Fig. 344). The most common sites of its nesting are the tube, its median or isthmial, its ampullary, its uterine or interstitial, portions, in the order named, and, lastly, the ovary. Primary abdominal pregnancy has been reported on the posterior fold of the broad ligament and on the omentum (Hirst and Knipe, Czyzewicz, Graefe, Hammacher, and Galabin), but it is of such exceeding rarity that it need only be mentioned. Hecker considered it very common, but these were secondary abdominal pregnancies. Pregnancy has developed in a sinus, possibly within a piece of Fallopian tube, following vaginal hysterectomy, and also in the stump of

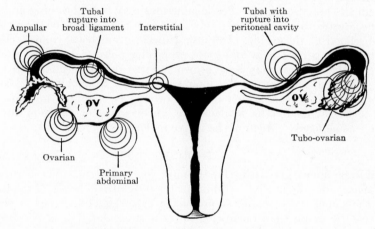

Fig. 344.—Diagram of Locations of Ectopic Ova.

a tube after partial salpingectomy. Pregnancy may occur in a closed accessory horn of the uterus and on the fimbria ovarica of the Fallopian tube. In the latter instance one speaks of a tubo-ovarian form. As the ovum distends its container other structures are encroached upon, adhesions form between them, and the primary topography of the gestation is modified. When the tubal wall bursts, the fetus escaping into the free abdominal cavity or into a mass of preformed adhesions, we speak of tubo-abdominal pregnancy; if the rupture occurs in the lower portion of the tube, between the folds of the broad ligament, an intraligamentous sac is formed; if the sac which is formed in an interstitial pregnancy bursts into the uterus (rare), we speak of tubo-uterine; if the ovarial pregnancy goes toward term, it almost always becomes ovario-abdominal—these are all secondary forms, and clinically, as well as anatomically, hard to distinguish from each other.

Causation.—The first mention of extra-uterine pregnancy is by Abulcasis in the tenth century, and Riolan, in 1626, refers to several cases. Since then the subject was frequently noted, and recently, since operative interference has become common, an enormous literature has accumulated (Werth and Shuhman).

421

Extra-uterine pregnancy is quite frequent, and occurs also in the lower animals —the ape, cow, sheep, bitch, and hare (Sutton). Many cases of rupture of the sac, or tubal abortion, and spontaneous recovery undoubtedly occur, and pass under the diagnosis of appendicitis or abdominal colic. "Prostitutes' colic" is surely often of this nature. It is more frequent in city than in country practice; oftener after the thirtieth year—frequently after a long period of relative sterility; and in women who have had an antecedent pelvic disease. Repetitions of the accident in the same tube and in the other tube have been reported, and intra-uterine and extra-uterine gestation may coexist (Novak, Lit.). Bilateral eccyesis was first noted by Noier, 1595.

The actual causes are unknown, but the following have been advanced, with more or less plausibility, in the order named: (1) Salpingitis; (2) pelvic adhesions; (3) infantile tubes with lack of cilia; (4) external wandering of the ovum; (5) diverticula and accessory tubes; (6) decidual reaction of the tubes; (7) disease of the corpus luteum, increased invasiveness of the ovum, favoring early nidation. (8) spasm of the tube, muscle insufficiency, and antiperistalsis (Lahm).

Salpingitis may act either by the loss of the cilia, which should favor the motion of the ovum to the uterus, or by gluing the folds of the mucosa tubæ together and forming blind pouches in which the ovum is caught, or by occluding the tube through the kinks or swelling or by paralyzing tubal contraction. Gonorrhea is a frequent antecedent, but puerperal infections and other inflammations like appendicitis are also found. Pelvic adhesions may bind the tubes and ovaries down and compress the lumen of the tube, or prevent the escape of the ovum from the neighborhood of the ovary. Infantile tubes are much convoluted (Freund), and have both imperfect cilia and little propelling power. In cases of external wandering of the ovum it may have grown so large that it is unable to pass the lumen of the tube, and during the long journey the trophoblast has had time to develop, so that it can attach itself anywhere, or perhaps the slow motion imparted to the ovum by the weakened or undeveloped or adherent tube gives it time to become fixed. Much of the above is purely theoretic.

PATHOLOGY

Tubal Pregnancy.—This is by far the most common form. Whether the ovum rests in the ampulla, the median, isthmic, or the interstitial portion of the tube, the course is the same, the trophoblast producing cytolysis of the cells of the tubal mucosa, and the ovum then burrowing into the muscular wall of the tube, in a way similar to that of pregnancy in the uterus. A full decidua may not be formed, but usually one finds islands of decidual reaction in and near the implantation of the ovum, and even in the other tube. As the ovum grows it bulges the wall of the tube inward, occluding its lumen, the cells of the opposing surfaces necrose, and the capsularis, if there is one, fuses with the opposite side of the tube. The villi erode their way into the blood-vessels and between the muscular fibers. Conditions in the wall of the tube are so different from those in the thick decidua of the uterus that the dangers of tubal pregnancy are easily grasped. In the uterus the ovum develops in the thick decidua and in a mucous membrane capable of strong decidual reaction, which membrane might really be considered a protective wall against the advancing army of villi. The blood-vessels are small, and the muscle of the uterus is physically adapted to stretching and hypertrophy. On the other hand, in the tube there is little or no decidua, and the advancing villi rapidly eat their way into the muscle-fibers and into the blood-vessels. These latter are large, and the muscle of the tube is not so capable of hypertrophy and stretching. Indeed, in the tube the ovum acts like a rapidly growing destructive neoplasm.

The ovum may be arrested between two folds of the redundant tubal mucous membrane, or it may attach itself to the top of a fold (Werth). Minute differences in the early development of the ovum result here, but they are of no clinical importance. In either case the growing ovum distends the tube to the point of rupture. Some hypertrophy of the tube occurs in all cases, and in rare ones the tube grows until term without rupture, these being the instances where it has been supposed that muscle-fibers could develop in an adventitious sac.

Usually the hypertrophy of the muscle of the tube is insufficient to accommodate the egg, and the fibers at the placental site being separated and destroyed by the erosive action of the villi, a weak spot here results. Any traumatism, as straining at stool, a jar, coitus, a bimanual examination, causes a slight hemorrhage at this site, with a rupture, or the tube bursts from overdistention of the thinned necrosed wall, and the villi lie free in the peritoneum. This is called extracapsular rupture. Bleeding naturally results from each of these occurrences. If the site of the rupture was on the free portion of the tube, the hemorrhage takes place into the peritoneal cavity, a hematocele forming in the pelvis. When the tube bursts into the broad ligament, a hematoma develops there. Rupture of the tube is the usual termination of isthmic and of interstitial pregnancy, and it almost always occurs in the second and third months.

When the ovum is in the ampulla, the gestation sac, in developing, may point in the direction of the fimbriated end of the tube, and a process known as *tubal abortion* is the usual termination.

The course of tubal abortion resembles that of uterine abortion very closely—a hemorrhage occurs in the placental site, loosening the ovum from its bed. The

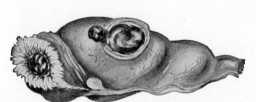

FIG. 345.—TUBAL ABORTION IN PROGRESS, WHEN A RUP-TURE OF THE TUBE FROM NECROSIS CAUSED SUCH A HEMORRHAGE THAT OPERATION BECAME IMPERATIVE. COMBINED INTRA- AND EXTRACAPSULAR RUPTURE.

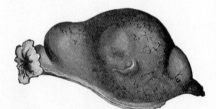

FIG. 346.—TUBAL HEMATOMA FROM TUBAL GES-TATION. INTRACAPSULAR RUPTURE.

blood and the ovum now fill the overdistended tube. The bag of waters may rupture and the fetus escape among the clots in the lumen of the tube. This is called intracapsular rupture. Blood oozes through the fimbriated end of the tube and clots around it, slowly forming a hematocele in the lower pelvis. The ovum and clots are gradually extruded through the open end of the tube into the peritoneal cavity, and they are all finally absorbed, unless the hemorrhage has been so great as to demand surgical interference (Fig. 345). If the extrusion does not take place or is not awaited, the hemorrhages into the tube destroy the ovum and it becomes converted into a mola carnosa, very like those often found in the uterus (Figs. 346 and 347). In these early moles it is rare to find the little fetus—it has been destroyed or even absorbed. Unless one finds the fetus or demonstrates villi, the diagnosis of ectopic gestation may not be made. In molar formation also a slight amount of blood may ooze into the pelvis and bind the tube to neighboring structures. The mole may be absorbed in the tube.

Hematocele.—Very soon after the blood touches the peritoneal surface it clots, and the peritoneal surface also throws out a layer of fibrin. Adhesions are thus quickly formed between the tube and the neighboring organs, and the blood is encapsulated. This is a hematocele, and the sac is composed of the fibrin mentioned, the neighboring organs, mainly intestines, bound together by adhesions. When a new bleeding occurs from the end of the tube, the newly formed sac is overdistended and may rupture, the process of adhesive reaction being continued a shorter or longer distance, in the direction of least resistance. Another hemorrhage causes a repetition of the process, and the woman may die from the repeated losses of blood. This slow hematocele formation is the rule in tubal abortion and tubal mole, but it may occur with a slow rupture of the tube as well.

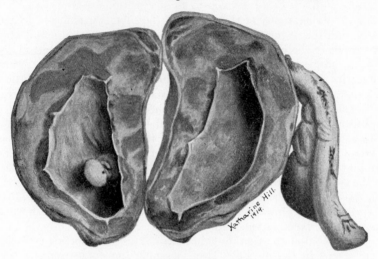

FIG. 347.—CROSS-SECTION OF EARLY TUBAL MOLE. NATURAL SIZE.
To the right is the appendix adherent to the tube.

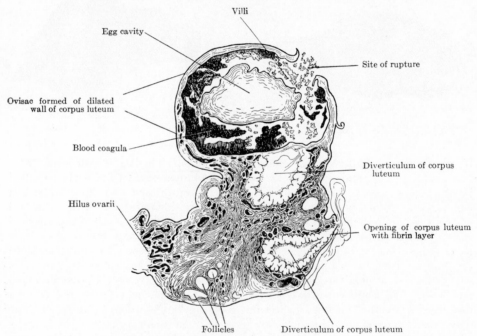

FIG. 347a.—OVARIAN PREGNANCY (C. Van Tussenbroek).
The ovum developed in the Graafian follicle, and part of this is changed into corpus luteum.

When the tube bursts, it usually does so suddenly, and a profuse intraperitoneal hemorrhage results. If the woman does not die from shock and the anemia, this mass of blood, too, is walled off and a large hematocele forms. This condition is found in isthmic and in interstitial pregnancies. Rupture of the tube may occur in any part of its periphery. Sometimes the perforation is minute, the villi seeming to have actually eaten a hole through the wall.

Hematoma.—When the rupture of the tube takes place into the broad liga-ment, the two folds are torn asunder by the blood, and one finds a mass lateral to the uterus, extending variably to the wall of the pelvis, under the round liga-ment, even up into the iliac fossa.

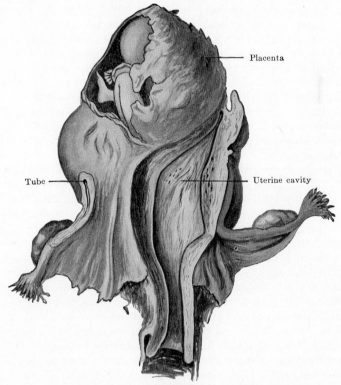

FIG. 348.—INTERSTITIAL PREGNANCY (Simon, Berlin, 1885).

The fetus does not always die. Sometimes the rupture occurs at a point in the periphery of the ovum which does not affect the placental site, and then the embryo escapes into the peritoneal cavity or between the folds of the broad ligament and continues its development. These are secondary abdominal pregnancies. Secon-dary abdominal pregnancy may also result when the tube, not rupturing, but im-mensely thinned, forms one layer of a sac, which in the main is composed of lamel-lated fibrin and adherent intestines and omentum. Such sacs may be readily pedun-culated at operation. If the fibers of the tube grow and are very slowly distracted, the pregnancy may also develop into, and between the folds of, the broad ligament, without the violent symptoms of rupture. Still, in all forms there may be late rupture of the sac.

Interstitial pregnancy (Fig. 348) has the same terminations as tubal, that is, rupture, mole, and abortion, the latter occurring into the uterus (rare). The corner of the uterus is developed, distorting the rest of the organ. Rupture is of late oc-currence, because the uterine wall is capable of more hypertrophy than the tubal, and the ovum may die, or it may develop to maturity in the broad ligament. The gestation sac may grow into the uterus and then continue as a normal pregnancy. (See Angular Pregnancy.) Such a diagnosis is exposed to much question, but cases not infrequently occur where this explanation of the phenomenon seems very probable.

Ampullary gestation pursues the same course as the others, but abortion is the usual termination, because the open end of the tube is near by. The ovum may be inserted on the fimbria ovarica, and in such an event the pregnancy is almost entirely abdominal, and the sac is made up of lamellated fibrin and adherent intestines, uterus, ovary, and omentum. The placenta spreads out over the tube, ovary, pelvic wall, and back of the uterus. It may be attached to the omentum.

Ovarian Pregnancy.—This is one of the rarest forms, but its occurrence is proved, there being over 85 cases on record (Fig. 347a). Norris, Penkert, Lockyer, and Liebe give a résumé of authentic cases, with the literature. It is not easy to decide that a given case is truly ovarian in origin, because the sac quickly makes adhesions to the tube or uterus, or a pregnancy on the fimbria ovarica may tear loose from its attachment or grow over onto the ovary, and one cannot decide if the location of placental tissue on the latter is primary or secondary. To establish the anatomic certainty of an ovarian pregnancy all that is necessary is to prove that "the tube, including the fimbria ovarica (excluding also gestation in an accessory tube), is absolutely free from any part in the formation of the fetal sac" (Werth). Werth evidently considers primary abdominal pregnancy so rare that it need not be considered.

Ovarian pregnancy pursues the same course as tubal. The impregnation of the ovum by the spermatozoid takes place before the former leaves the ovary, and if the ovum was deeply located in the ovary, the sac is evenly covered by ovarian stroma; if it was superficial, the fetal sac grows out into the peritoneal cavity. In both cases the pregnancy is pedunculated and easily removed, though it does contract adhesions with the surrounding structures. If the ovum was near the hilum, the gestation-sac may become intraligamentous, spreading the utero-ovarian ligament apart, and showing the tube stretched over its exterior, as occurs on a cystic tumor of the ovary in a similar location. Rupture of the sac, with hematocele, is the usual termination, with or without death of the fetus, but molar formation including hydatidiform is also observed. One may not say a hematoma found in the ovary is always the result of a pregnancy, unless chorionic villi or parts of a fetus be demonstrated in it. Rupture of a Graafian follicle is sometimes attended by free, even threatening, hemorrhage, and hemorrhagic ovarian cysts or twisted ovarian tumors may cause pelvic hemorrhage. A differential diagnosis of such accidents from ectopic gestation cannot be positively made before operation.

Later Course.—If a tubal pregnancy terminates by abortion, the extruded mass of clots and the embryo are rapidly absorbed. Tubal moles also disappear in the same way, but more slowly, and subsequent permeability of the tube is established. If, in rupture, the placenta became detached, torn, or disorganized by blood-clots, the fetus dies, and, unless advanced beyond the eighth week, the little body is absorbed. The blood-masses slowly shrink, harden, and are dissolved by leukocytic and ferment action, disappearing in a longer or shorter time, depending on their size.

If the child escapes alive, it may continue its development among the intestines or in the broad ligament, *i. e.*, secondary abdominal pregnancy. In either case it may have escaped inside an intact amniotic sac or naked. A new sac now forms, made up of fibrin, adherent intestines, omentum, uterus, broad ligament, etc., depending on the location in which the fetus happens to be. In the structure of the sac no traces of the original container, tube or ovary, will be found, except at one place, the site of the rupture.

If rupture of the container does not take place, but the tube or the ovary distends, accommodating the growing ovum, a large pelveo-abdominal sac is formed which becomes adherent to all the surfaces it touches—pelvic wall, uterus, bladder, rectum, intestine, omentum, liver, spleen, stomach. This sac in structure shows the tissue of the original site of implantation of the ovum, such as tube, ovary, together with lamellated fibrin, muscular fibers from neighboring organs, especially the broad ligament and the peritoneum, to which it at first adhered. The sac varies in thickness from 1 mm. to several centimeters, depending on the amount of fibrin.

The placenta is spread out over the tissues adjacent to its first point of development, is usually thin, but otherwise like a uterine placenta. The blood-vessels in the neighborhood of the placenta are enormously dilated, and many new ones are formed—this especially when the omentum is used to help nourish the placenta. In one of the writer's cases the newly formed blood-vessels in the omentum were as large as crows' quills, had very thin walls, tore easily, and were innumerably distributed over the sac.

In one or the other of these fashions the secondary abdominal pregnancy may go to term. Spurious labor now sets in, the child dies as the result of hemorrhage into, or dislocation of, the placenta, or may not die until later, and nature tries to get rid of the foreign body. The contractions of the uterus expel the decidua, and usually the attendant hemorrhage is slight. At any period of pregnancy the sac may rupture, or the child may die and the changes about to be described may be inaugurated. Spurious labor with expulsion of the uterine decidua may follow the death of the child at any time. There is always a degree of peritonitis in ectopic gestation with hemorrhage, and this, according to Dudgeon and Sargent, is due to the Staphylococcus albus, and is a conservative process. Jaundice is also frequent from absorption of more blood-pigment than the liver can take care of.

After the death of the fetus it first becomes macerated, as in intra-uterine pregnancy, then the liquor amnii is absorbed, the sac lays itself onto the body, a zone of granulations fills the interspaces, and the soft parts of the fetus are absorbed, *i. e.*, it is skeletonized. By way of the blood, or by passing through the intervening wall from contiguous structures, especially the bowel, infection may gain entry to the mass, and it suppurates, the pus finding its way out through the bladder, the rectum, or, least often, the vagina or abdominal wall. Œdema bullosum can be seen in the bladder when the perforation into this organ begins. Through the fistula are passed, first, the broken-down fluid placenta, then the soft parts of the fetus, and finally the separate bones, by a process of suppuration which may last months or years, and which the patient may not survive. Sometimes, even after months, the woman dies from hemorrhage due to rupture of the sac, sometimes from peritonitis, but rarely, since firm adhesions have walled off the danger-zone.

Another termination after death of the fetus is mummification, the child drying up, and in this state it may be found years after. Absorption of the water of the fetus takes place, and it is surprising how well its tissues are preserved. Calcium salts are deposited in the sac around the fetus, and if these are abundant, the child is incased by a shell or even partly calcified itself—*lithokelyphos*, or *lithopedion* ("stone child"). Wagner had a case where a mummified fetus was carried for twenty-nine years, and Virchow one for twenty-eight years. Smith describes a calcified fetus which was removed from a woman ninety-four years old sixty years after conception. There are many cases on record. Suppuration may occur at any time even after calcification is marked.

Changes in the Uterus.—In response to the stimulus of pregnancy, the uterus hypertrophies but not as much as if it were carrying the ovum itself, and it exhibits intermittent contractions. A decidua develops in it, and this may be as much as 1 cm. in thickness, presenting all the characters of an intra-uterine pregnancy decidua, *except that it contains no chorionic villi*. At the time of spurious labor or spurious abortion the decidua is cast off, either in one piece, as a cast of the uterine cavity, or in large shreds or plaques, sometimes accompanied by fetor. With death of the fetus the uterus shrinks.

Combined extra- and intra-uterine pregnancy is not very rare, Weibel, in 1905, having collected over 119 cases. Penkert found 17 cases in 1912 and 1913. Double tubal gestation has been observed, also two gestation-sacs in one tube. Twins, and even triplets (Baldwin), have been found in one sac. Fœtus papyraceus may also occur in combined gestations, as well as in twin ectopic gestation.

Extra- and intra-uterine pregnancy offers a very serious prognosis. Abortion of the uterine ovum precedes or follows the rupture of the ectopic sac, but death from internal hemorrhage may occur before abortion takes place. Rarely the woman goes to term, and then labor is usually spontaneous, but death frequently follows from internal hemorrhage or sepsis starting from the abdominal mass. The extra-uterine fetus rarely obstructs the passage of the intra-uterine. If the ectopic pregnancy is successfully removed, the patient may go to term with the other one normally. Both fetuses may be delivered alive at term.

Repeated extra-uterine pregnancies, after months or years, are not seldom observed, and the recurrence may be situated in the same tube originally affected or in the other.

CLINICAL COURSE

Rarely do the first months of an ectopic gestation pass without symptoms which would direct attention to the pelvis as the seat of trouble. Once in a while a woman, previously perfectly well, has sudden symptoms of internal hemorrhage and may die from the same even before a diagnosis can be made. Medicolegally, the question of foul play may have to be settled in such instances.

Usually the patient misses a period and has the ordinary concomitant symptoms of early pregnancy, but soon complains of pains in the lower abdomen, especially on the affected side—cramp-like, due to uterine and tubal contractions. There may be mild pelveoperitonitic symptoms. After a few weeks irregular bloody vaginal discharges appear, which the attending physician believes indicate a threatening abortion. External hemorrhage usually indicates that the ovum in the tube has been disturbed. On the occasion of a jar, a strain, coitus, or an examination a sudden severe pain is felt on one side, *the patient feels faint or dizzy*, and may vomit or be nauseated. Symptoms of shock may appear, and the shock may be due to the sudden distention of the tube, to irritation of the peritoneum by blood, or to the great loss of blood. The pains continuing, a piece or all of the uterine decidua is discharged. A careless attendant will now conclude that the abortion has taken place. These symptoms may indicate that a hemorrhage has occurred in the tube, or through it into the belly, or that a rupture of the tube has taken place. Rarely is the first hemorrhage so severe that the patient dies—clotting occurs at the site of rupture and the blood is absorbed, the acute symptoms subsiding in two or three days, the whole process terminating in three to six weeks. Again, because the clot is disturbed or the blood-pressure raised, the hemorrhage recommences in a few hours or days—almost never after weeks—and the patient may die from a slower anemia or from a second or third severe hemorrhage. The gradual withdrawal of blood from the general circulation may be determined by the hemoglobin estimates taken daily. Tubal mole seems to cause repeated hemorrhages, the hematocele sac breaking at different points, fresh adhesions forming, and new additions to the sac being made. If the case is not treated, nature often works a cure, the sac being bound off by firm adhesions and the clots being slowly absorbed. Nowadays, however, most cases are operated on. In rare cases the pain may be referred to the right shoulder or to another part of the abdomen—the gall-bladder, for instance—and sometimes intestinal symptoms, like an enteritis, predominate. Jaundice is occasionally observed when the absorption of blood-pigment is active (Lit., Schottmüller). Discharge of decidua means death of fetus. Pyosalpinx may complicate ectopic gestation.

The symptoms of rupture of the sac are pain on the affected side, sometimes excruciating and sudden, soon spreading all over the lower abdomen; nausea, sometimes vomiting, sometimes diarrhea plus evidences of hemorrhage and shock. That shock plays a real part in the symptoms is certain, because the author has found severe prostration without enough blood loss to explain it. The striking pallor with slight cyanosis about the lips, pearly conjunctivæ, yawning and sighing, fast, small pulse, and extreme weakness reveal the fact of blood loss. Rarely the pulse is slow—even 46—but feeble, the blood-pressure being very low.

Internal examination, if the blood is still fluid, will usually reveal only a large uterus; later, when the blood has clotted and the hematocele is forming, one can outline the mass in the culdesac. Under particularly favorable circumstances the finger may feel a soft bulging downward of the culdesac earlier. When the rupture has taken place into the broad ligament, a hematoma forming here, the pain is most intense, and shock overbalances the anemia, because of the tearing asunder of the layers of the peritoneum. Internal examination will always disclose a firm mass on one side of the uterus.

If the rupture or the tubal abortion occurs more gradually, the symptoms are proportionately less stormy, and the true condition may not be discovered.

If, after the escape of the ovum into the peritoneal cavity or into the broad ligament, it continues to develop, symptoms of peritoneal irritation arise—pain, soreness, nausea, vomiting, diarrhea and constipation (sometimes hemorrhages from the bowel), bladder disturbance, loss of strength, and invalidism. The signs and symptoms of pregnancy continue, fetal movements are more pronounced, are painful, and may distress the patient, and the signs of tumor in the belly grow with the weeks. This tumor may be asymmetric or median. If the fetus dies, the symptoms of pregnancy disappear, while those usually made by a macerating neoplasm become noticeable, evidently due to a toxemia. Subfebrile temperatures, rapid pulse, anorexia, coated tongue, loss of weight, and invalidism are almost always in evidence. Icterus with fever denotes beginning decomposition of the sac and contents. Now the patient gets really sick, since an abdominal abscess is forming, and she may die of sepsis, of peritonitis, or of exhaustion and hectic, from prolonged suppuration, the product of conception being gradually expelled through a fistula into the bladder, the rectum, vagina, or belly wall.

If the sac goes on to lithopedion formation, involution of the uterus occurs, the irritation of the peritoneum subsides, and the patient may forget that she was pregnant, and may even have children normally. Cases are on record where an extra-uterine tumor, offering an obstacle to delivery, was found to be a calcified fetus.

Rupture of the sac and suppuration may occur at any time during pregnancy, a point of practical importance in treatment. The symptoms and anatomic course of a pregnancy in a rudimentary horn of the uterus are so similar to those of ectopic gestation that these subjects should be considered together.

DIAGNOSIS

Before rupture of the tube or a hemorrhage into it the diagnosis of ectopic gestation has hardly ever been made, because the tube is as soft as an intestinal loop. Kanavel reports a case of a woman who had ectopic gestation once before, diagnosing a recurrence after going over her period one week, and operation proved she was right. Miller, of Pittsburgh, discovered a mass in a tube which he had palpated a few weeks previously, when it was empty, and proved the ectopic pregnancy by operation. Almost all the cases, however, where such a diagnosis has been reported were tubal abortions in progress or tubal moles. Tubal mole is often diagnosed. In the early part of pregnancy the diagnosis must decide if an extra-uterine tumor is an ovum or not, and during the latter half one must decide if the ovum is extra-uterine or intra-uterine. No pelvic condition gives rise to more diagnostic errors. The author has seen such mistakes made by every gynecologist and surgeon in the city, including himself. In the majority of cases the patient will give a history of previous pelvic inflammation, either gonorrheal or puerperal, and often a period of sterility elapses before the aberrant conception.

Direct Diagnosis—First Trimester.—When a woman in the reproductive period, after some irregularity of the menses, such as going over the proper time a few days or having only a small amount, or even a more profuse flow, complains of cramping pains in the lower abdomen, mostly unilateral, with irregular uterine hemorrhage, the suspicion of ectopic pregnancy is aroused. If, suddenly, an excruciating pelvic pain occurs, with dizziness, faintness, or collapse, the diagnosis is almost certain, and is confirmed by finding an extra-uterine tumor or the discharge of a uterine decidua.   The direct diagnosis of fluid blood in the peritoneal cavity is seldom easy. A sense of soft resistance is found in the posterior vaginal fornix, but the uterus is not displaced, though in one case the author found it raised up in the sea of blood. Puncture of the fornix with a long sharp needle may reveal the blood, but it usually is not necessary for the diagnosis.   Percussion of the flanks in not one of the author's cases gave dulness, even though a quart or more of blood was removed at operation. Pain in the shoulders when the blood reaches the diaphragm (Dewes); Cullen's sign (bluish-green tint of the navel), anuria, amaurosis, are not constant.   After twenty-four to forty-eight hours the blood-clots become readily palpable and now displace the uterus—that is, a hematocele forms.   When the discharge of blood is slower, a peritubal hematocele forms, which increases from day to day, and one can trace the advance of the process with the finger by successive examinations. The hematocele may be retro-uterine, before the uterus, at the side, before or behind, and the organs are displaced in typical directions.   A broad-ligament hematoma can more easily be diagnosed from the stormy beginning, the severe pain running down the leg and the firm, tender tumor at the side of the uterus, displacing it to the side and upward.   Other occasional symptoms are pressure on the rectum with frequent desire to pass stool, tenesmus and pain, irritability of the bladder, a tender pelvis.

Warning! In all cases where the history of the patient gives only a hint of the possibility of an extra-uterine gestation, the examination must be conducted with the utmost gentleness to avoid rupturing the sac.   The author witnessed an almost fatal intraperitoneal hemorrhage on the examination table.

Direct Diagnosis—After First Trimester.—When a pregnant woman complains of irregular bloody discharges from the uterus, excessively painful fetal movements very low in the pelvis, abdominal pains and distress, with intestinal symptoms and invalidism, one may strongly suspect an ectopic fetus.   The demonstration of the enlarged empty uterus alongside the fetal sac confirms the suspicion.

The direct diagnosis of the life of the ovum can usually be made, and is based on—(1) The absence or mildness of the symptoms of rupture of the tube during the second and third months; (2) the continuation of the symptoms of pregnancy— nausea, mammary signs, fetal movements, fetal heart, etc.; (3) the presence of a loud uterine souffle (in ectopic gestation, contrary to normal, this sign is of value for determining the location of the placenta); (4) the absence of symptoms of toxemia and of suppuration; (5) the continuation of the growth and of the softening of the uterus and of the vagina; (6) the gradually increasing size of the abdominal tumor.

Differential Diagnosis.—Only the most common difficulties in diagnosis can be considered, and these will be given in the order of frequency:

ABORTION	ECTOPIC PREGNANCY
1. Onset quiet, with gradually intensifying and regular pains in the lower abdomen, resembling labor.	1. Onset stormy, with irregular and colicky pains, sometimes few and excruciating, localized on one side.
2. External hemorrhage profuse or moderate, with clots.	2. External hemorrhage slight or absent and dark, fluid.
3. Symptoms of hemorrhage proportionate to visible blood-loss.	3. Symptoms of hemorrhage and shock much greater than visible blood-loss.
4. Discharge of parts of ovum.	4. Only a uterine decidua, if anything; no villi.
5. Demonstration of ovum in uterus or empty uterus and empty pelvis.	5. Finding of a mass alongside the uterus.

Before every curetage for abortion it is wise to make a careful bimanual examination to rule out extra-uterine pregnancy, and should collapse come on after such an operation, strong suspicion of rupture of an ectopic sac must be entertained. Perforation of the uterus and rupture of a pus-sac, or other abdominal hollow organ, give the same symptoms, and it may be necessary to open the belly to find out the true conditions. The blood-picture may help here and often decisive information may be gotten from exploratory puncture.

If infection of a hematocele or of a hematoma sets in, the condition cannot be differentiated from a pyosalpinx, a pelvic cellulitis, or perimetritis, unless operation or puncture shows the hemorrhagic nature of the pelvic tumor. Jaundice is an important sign, since it usually accompanies a degenerating blood-clot. Treatment is on general principles of pelvic infections.

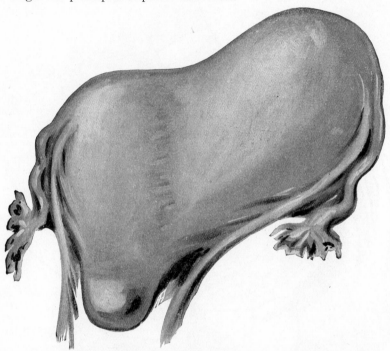

Fig. 349.—Angular Pregnancy at Four Months Simulating Ectopic Gestation (Mrs. S., twins at term).

In the early months confusion is often caused by a long cervix softened at its upper part, which allows the fundus to bend backward or *to the side*. The cervix is hard, is held to be the uterus, and the fundus is thought to be the ectopic sac. By straightening out the uterus the diagnosis may be made certain, but before attempting to do so the presence of an eccyesis must be ruled out. Or the pregnancy is situated in one horn of the uterus and distends this side, the rest remaining hard. This is an "angular pregnancy," "grossesse angulaire," and is not seldom the cause of error (Fig. 349).

Intra-uterine Angular Pregnancy	Extra-uterine Pregnancy
1. History is that of normal pregnancy, though, not seldom grossesse angulaire causes occasional slight hemorrhages and pains.	1. History of colicky pains and peritoneal irritation for several weeks; then a stormy event (rupture), with severe pain, shock, etc.
2. No expulsion of membrane, unless abortion.	2. Expulsion of decidua.
3. No anemia.	3. More or less anemia.
4. Demonstration of tube and round ligament on outside of the tumor. (See Fig. 349.)	4. Tube and round ligament not palpable, or medial to the tumor.
5. Can feel the wall of the uterus pass over onto tumor, especially during a contraction.	5. The mass is separated from the uterus by a groove. This is especially deep in pregnancy in an accessory horn.
6. The tumor is soft, feels like a pregnancy, is high up in the side of the pelvis, and movable as a part of the uterus.	6. The tumor is harder, lies at the side of the uterus or in the culdesac, and is not movable (careful!).
7. The angular portion of the uterus contracts.	7. No contractions of the sac.
8. Gradually the typical shape of the uterus returns.	8. The tumor becomes more and more asymmetric at successive examinations.

Angular pregnancy cannot be differentiated from interstitial pregnancy except by the clinical course. It is well, therefore, to place the patient in a hospital for observation.

Pregnancy in a retroverted uterus has often been thought to exist when the real condition has been an ovisac or a hematocele in the Douglas culdesac, and attempts to replace the supposed uterus have resulted disastrously.

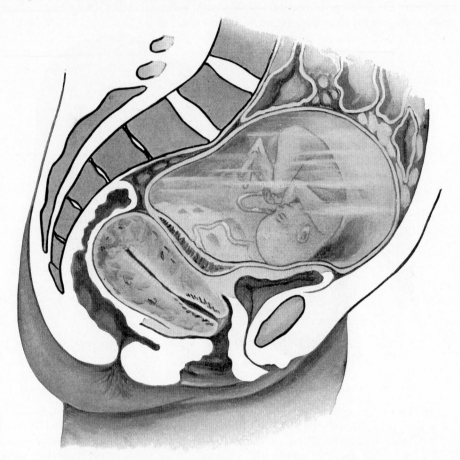

FIG. 350.—MRS. L., RETROVERSIO UTERI, WITH PREGNANCY ON TOP AND AT SIDE OF IT.
Diagnosis at first, retroversio uteri gravidi, then, when abdominal tumor did not subside on catheterization and the fetus was felt above left Poupart's ligament, correct condition discovered. Laparotomy, recovery.

RETROFLEXIO UTERI GRAVIDI	ECTOPIC GESTATION
1. History typical of pregnancy.	1. History strongly suggestive of abnormal gestation.
2. Urinary difficulties usual and marked after ten weeks.	2. Seldom bladder symptoms until after fifth month.
3. Pain and hemorrhage rare and slight.	3. The opposite is the rule.
4. The finger feels the angle at the cervix, and nothing where the fundus should be (Fig. 356).	4. The finger feels an angle, but the abdominal hand finds the fundus, and occasionally the Fallopian tubes, in front of the mass.
5. The retroflexed fundus is round, smooth, more or less movable (careful!), feels like a pregnancy, and sometimes contracts.	5. The mass in the culdesac is irregular, not movable, putty-like, does not feel like a pregnant uterus, and never contracts.
6. Late in pregnancy, condition is rare, and in cases of partial retroflexion cannot feel an adjacent, but empty, uterus.	6. Late in pregnancy may find an adjacent mass which represents the enlarged empty uterus (Figs. 350 and 351).

Pregnancy in the uterus, complicated by ovarian or other cystic pelvic tumors, may give rise to a diagnosis of ectopic gestation, especially since the accoucheur fears the danger of overlooking the latter and wishes to operate on this account. The mistake is pardonable because usually, in either case, the abdomen would have to be opened. Adnexa tumors, pyosalpinx, hydrosalpinx, and ovarian cyst may be mistaken for ectopic sacs. The main point in the diagnosis is the finding of the unchanged uterus alongside the tumor and the *absence of the symptoms and signs of pregnancy*. On the other hand, the *presence* of the early signs and symptoms of pregnancy does not speak against an extra-uterine tumor being a new-growth or inflammatory, because milk in the breasts, subjective symptoms, softening and discoloration of the cervix and vagina occur in many of the latter pathologic conditions—indeed, even under normal circumstances. The author has seen colostrum run in fine streams from the nipple of a nullipara thirty-eight years old, and has expressed milk from the breasts of a woman eight years after her last child.

Now we have an almost positive differential method, the Aschheim-Zondek pregnancy test. This will eliminate doubt of the existence of pregnancy, but it requires several days, which limits its usefulness.

Pyosalpinx cannot always be differentiated from tubal gestation, and they may coexist. The presence of fever, leukocytosis fast sedimentation time, excessive tenderness, evidences of acute or recent gonorrhea, and bilateral tumor usually settle the diagnosis, but they may *all* occur in extra-uterine pregnancy. If by

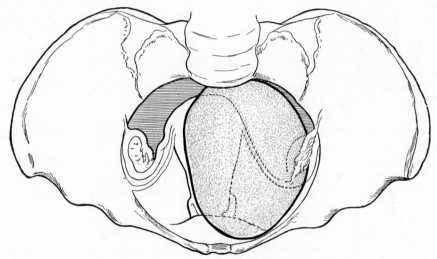

FIG. 351.—DIAGRAM ILLUSTRATING CONDITIONS FOUND IN FIG. 350.

mistake the belly is opened and an acute pyosalpinx found, it is wiser not to attempt its removal at this time, because such operations have a high primary mortality.

In rare instances the differential diagnosis of rupture of a gestation-sac with collapse must be made from rupture of a pus-tube, the twisting of an ovarian tumor, ovarial hemorrhage, bursting of an appendiceal abscess, of the gall-bladder, perforation of the stomach or duodenum, nephrolithiasis, ureteral stone, rupture of the splenic artery, but the scope of this work forbids going so far into the subject.

Acute appendicitis has not seldom been mistaken for extra-uterine pregnancy, and when real pregnancy co-exists, the differential diagnosis cannot always be made.

APPENDICITIS	ECTOPIC GESTATION
1. No signs or symptoms of pregnancy.	1. Present.
2. Pain, nausea and vomiting, fever.	2. Pain worse, vomiting less; fever absent or less.
3. Tenderness and rigidity high up.	3. Tenderness and rigidity much less and low down.
4. Leukocytosis usual.	4. Leukocytosis equivocal. The blood-count shows increase of the polymorphs and mononuclears, the basophiles with the signs of secondary anemia. Low Hb.

28

APPENDICITIS—(*Continued.*)	ECTOPIC GESTATION—(*Continued.*)
5. Patient flushed and excited. At very beginning there may have been a little dizness.	5. Pale, and faint or apathetic. (Low blood-pressure.)
6. Uterus and adnexa normal.	6. The characteristic findings.
7. Feel a tumor high up in pelvis.	7. Tumor low in pelvis.
8. No uterine symptoms.	8. Discharge of decidua.
9. Fahraeus' (blood sedimentation) test +++.	9. Fahraeus +.
10. Exploratory puncture, pus or serum with bacteria.	10. Blood or serum.

In all cases where the diagnosis is uncertain the patient should be put in a well-equipped hospital, there to rest in bed until developments occur, including AZ test, which shed enough light to allow action. Whenever an anesthetic is to be given for the examination the patient likewise must be in a hospital, to be ready for immediate laparotomy if the sac should be burst by the manipulations.

The author has never found it necessary to use a sound or to curet the uterus or create a pneumoperitoneum to make a diagnosis. Such interference is dangerous. Further, the information obtained is not always unequivocal. If the curet brings decidua and no villi, the condition may be either intra-uterine or extrauterine pregnancy, or both (v. Ott), or neither—only a dysmenorrheal membrane. A large, thick, rough decidual membrane expelled from the uterus, giving a more or less complete cast of the cavity, without chorionic villi, is almost pathognomonic of ectopic gestation. It may be expelled after the operation. Acetonuria is common in eccyesis, but not pathognomonic. Hemoglobinemia is present with rupture, and, with the spectroscope, hematin may be discovered, particularly in cases where jaundice is present.

Skiagraphy has been used to aid the diagnosis and is helpful after the skeleton is formed. A lithopedion would show well, but it could not be differentiated from a calcareous fibroid unless the outline of the fetal bones were discernible. We often use exploratory puncture of Douglas' culdesac and find it valuable and safe. Doederlein prefers posterior colpotomy.

In the later months the diagnosis is mainly concerned with differentiating whether a given fetus is intra- or extra-uterine. These points will aid the decision: History of unusual occurrences; of rupture in the early months; pelvic peritoneal symptoms; invalidism; painful fetal movements located in one place all the time; continual pain and abdominal distress; irregular hemorrhage and discharge of decidua; finding the empty uterus alongside the tumor; fetal movements active and very superficial, seeming to be almost beneath the skin; same of the fetal body, but it is not easy to make out the presentation, etc.; heart-tones exceptionally strongly audible, but sometimes not to be heard at all; sac exhibits no contractions; round ligaments are not palpable on the sac, as they are on the sides of the uterus; the tumor is not symmetric and easily definable, like a pregnant uterus; the examination is painful and unsatisfactory; skiagraphy.

PROGNOSIS

Naturally, it is impossible to give satisfactory figures in such a multicolored disease as this. Without doubt the outlook has been painted too dark, for very many ectopic ova die, are expelled from the tube as abortions or by rupture, and the patients recover without a diagnosis having been made. Many women recover under expectant treatment, but, of course, all the children die. In the cases which go to term the fetus is usually deformed or not viable. Sittner collected 179 cases and finds that, from the condition of the fetuses, one may allow the pregnancy to go on unless the symptoms of the mother are threatening. Most authorities find the opposite conditions. Fifty per cent. of the fetuses are deformed, according to von Winckel—the head in 75 per cent.; the pelvic end in 50 per cent.; the arms in 40 per cent. Pressure by neighboring organs causes compression, decubitus, impressions, infractions, etc., of the body, and disease also, as hydrocephalus, meningocele, cranioschisis. These are due to amnionitis, insufficient liquor amnii, and cramping. Amniotic bands and velamentous insertion of the cord are common, and the placenta may be thick and hard, or infiltrated with hemorrhages.

It is interesting to note that polyhydramnion can occur in extra-uterine gestation, though oligohydramnion is the rule and accounts for frequent fetal deformities. Hydatid mole and chorio-epithelioma have been observed. Hyperemesis gravidarum and eclampsia may enter as complications (Pinard, Spiegelberg, Horwitz).

Schauta found 75 recoveries and 166 deaths in 241 cases treated expectantly, and quotes Veit as saying the mortality of ectopic gestation with hematocele is 25 to 28 per cent. Death results from hemorrhage, shock, or sepsis. Nowadays operation has reduced the mortality to low figures. Prognosis as to health is also bad, because the condition leaves peritonitic adhesions, which often result in sterility; if untreated, decomposition and abscess cause hectic fever, invalidism, etc.

TREATMENT

There is no expectant treatment for a growing ectopic gestation. In the presence of threatening symptoms one does not waste time on a fine differential diagnosis. The "explosive body" (Werth) must be removed from the abdomen as soon as possible. If the diagnosis is made before rupture of the sac, or during a tubal abortion, the indication is to remove the ovum, preferably by laparotomy. Under such circumstances the operation is easy, resembling an ordinary salpingectomy.

Treatment of Rupture and Tubal Abortion.—Since the differential diagnosis may not be possible, both conditions are treated alike. There seems no doubt but that the best treatment, as soon as the diagnosis of rupture of the sac with intraperitoneal hemorrhage has been made, is to open the belly and remove the pregnant organ. Salt solution is given by hypodermoclysis, and the belly quickly opened. The author uses ether anesthesia. Blood may shoot up several inches from the incision. One grasp locates the uterus; it is pulled up into the wound, and a clamp put on the broad ligament of the affected side. Another grasp brings the sac into view, and a clamp is put on its pelvic side. Ten units of pituitary are injected into the uterine wall. Fresh bleeding is thus checked, and the removal of the sac is now undertaken deliberately. The tube is cut out of the uterine horn. If the other tube is open, it should be left. Salpingostomy may be done. A pyosalpinx should be removed—both of the latter operations only if the woman's condition warrants them. A search is made for the fetus, which is usually found very near to the site of rupture. The largest clots are scooped out, but no time is wasted in the peritoneal toilet, and the belly is rapidly closed.

We do not wait to treat shock, but in such cases give salt solution, glucose, gum glucose or blood—the one that is quickest, and operate at the same time. It requires only two minutes to get clamps onto the broad ligament. In the presence of a foudroyant internal hemorrhage one need not remove the patient from her bed. The belly can be painted with iodin, opened rapidly, and the broad ligament clamped, the rest of the operation being completed as soon as practicable.

If one is called to a case when the primary hemorrhage has ceased, the patient recovering from the shock, my own preference is for immediate operation because a second hemorrhage is often fatal.

If a hematocele forms, which is easily determined by the hardening and forming of the pelvic blood-mass, one may remove same by laparotomy, by vaginal incision and drainage, or may allow it to become absorbed. Fehling treated 91 cases conservatively with success. The patient must be kept in hospital until the mass is very hard and firm—that is, until it is certain that the fetus is dead and that there is no danger of further hemorrhage. She should stay in bed until absorption is about completed. Absorption takes four weeks to four months, depending on the size of the blood-tumor.   While most small hematoceles become absorbed, the large ones are very slow, and if they do not rupture, allowing renewed bleeding which demands operation, they not seldom suppurate, in either case causing prolonged invalidism and leaving permanent damage in the pelvis and consequent sterility.   This is especially true if the fetus had attained some size.   Such patients do better with operation, and the author prefers the abdominal to the vaginal method (Fig. 352), since it gives better control of all eventualities. It is now almost the general practice.

If a hematocele forms but the pains continue, and especially if the patient has fainting spells, one should decide that hemorrhage is recurring and operate at once. Should the temperature, chills, rapid pulse, pain, and peritonitic symptoms point to infection of the gestation-sac, it must be drained as soon as possible.   Suppurat-

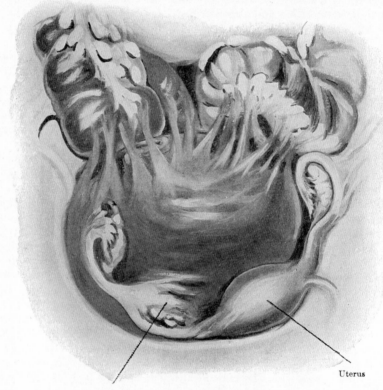

Ruptured tube forming part of hematocele

Uterus

FIG. 352.—APPEARANCE OF OPENING BELLY AFTER RUPTURE OF PREGNANT TUBE.   MRS. L.

ing hematoceles are broadly opened through the posterior culdesac as one does a pelvic abscess, and a soft-rubber tube inserted, without any attempt to remove clots and without irrigation.   If the pregnancy is further advanced, but accessible from below, the same method is employed.   If it is already an abdominal pregnancy, the belly is to be opened, the sac sewed to the edges of the incision and opened the next day with the cautery, thus avoiding infecting the general peritoneum.   Its septic contents are removed piecemeal and slowly, requiring days or weeks.

If the pregnancy is advanced beyond the fourth month, the fetus having considerable size, the adhesions of the sac to neighboring organs being extensive and firmer, and, most important, the vascular connections of the sac, especially the placental region, being much greater, the operation becomes more and more formidable.   In spite of Sittner's statistics, therefore, it is best to interfere as early as possible, and not to wait for the child to be viable.   Exceptionally, or through religious scruples, the patient may demand delay to save the child, and in this event she must be put in a hospital to await the time of operation. At the end of pregnancy it is recommended to wait for the fetus to die and operate seven to twenty days thereafter, the object being to permit thrombosis of the placental vessels and the consequent diminution of the blood-supply to the parts (Litzman). This advice is seldom followed by experienced abdominal surgeons, and the results of immediate operation compare very favorably with those of the waiting policy.

The operation should be undertaken only by one skilled in abdominal surgery, because complications, hemorrhage, injury to intestine, ureters, etc., are very common. If the pregnancy is intraligamentous or tubal, without many adhesions, it is often possible to pedunculate the tumor as one does an ovarian cyst, after tying the ovarian vessels at the brim and clamping the broad ligament at the uterus. The placenta, together with the sac, may then, little by little, be dissected off the floor of the pelvis, clamping and tying the vessels. The bleeding areas are dried by suture, cautery, packing, or sewing the peritoneum over them. When the placenta is attached to the rectum, the sigmoid, the small intestine, or the omentum, one will come upon innumerable large and small blood-vessels running from these organs onto the sac. These blood-vessels are so thin walled that they seem to have only two layers of cells, for they break under the lightest touch, and the field is instantly flooded with blood. It may be necessary in such a case to open the sac, remove the child and as much of the sac and placenta as is safe, leaving the rest, but sewing the edges of the sac to the abdominal wall after firmly packing it. While it is most desirable to remove the whole ovum, this way may lead more surely to success. The remnants or the whole of the placenta separate and are discharged by suppuration in the course of four to sixteen weeks. When the placenta is on the anterior abdominal wall, the primary hemorrhage is great, but it may be checked by pressure or compression of the aorta high above the bifurcation, as has been done by the author at cesarean sections. In one of the author's cases the hemorrhage from vascular adhesions absolutely frustrated all attempts at hemostasis by a skilful surgeon and himself. The placenta was adherent to the omentum and gut, the former being simply a mesh of brittle arteries and veins. In a similar case Sehrt's aorta compressor (Fig. 721) might possibly be tried. Many cases have been cured by simply removing the fetus and cord, sewing up the sac, and leaving the placenta for absorption, and this is usually safer than attempting its removal. (See Beck.) Pituitary reduces operative hemorrhage (Kahn, Heany).

Veit, in 1884, operated first for unruptured tubal gestation. Veit also operated first, according to Werth, for intraperitoneal hemorrhage in 1878, then Tait in 1880 and 1883, though Kiwish and Parry had suggested the idea. One of the obsolete methods of treatment of the ectopic pregnancy with living fetus was the attempt to kill the fetus by morphin injected into its body or into the liquor amnii, or by drawing off the liquor amnii, or by electricity.

Watkins recommends uterine curetage to remove the decidua, which otherwise comes away piecemeal, attended by bloody flow or fetor. In several of my cases the decidua did not come away at all. Wallace transplanted an ovum, which he unexpectedly found in the tube, to the uterine cavity from which he had removed a fibroid, and he delivered a living child at term.

The postoperative course is often marked by fever. In the absence of peritonitic symptoms this may be ascribed to absorption of blood. Some operators, Zweifel, Bröse, Werth, et al., are careful to remove all the blood from the peritoneal cavity, believing that it has a toxic action. My practice is to leave a large portion of it, on the theory that it is partly reabsorbed and used again. I have never seen any harm from this treatment, which is recommended by Veit, Martin, Watkins, Ries, et al. Halsted suggested to collect the blood in the peritoneal cavity, defibrinate it, mix it with Ringer's solution, and reinject it into the median basilic vein. Transfusion is safer, as many marked reactions follow the other.

LITERATURE

Beck: Jour. Amer. Med. Assoc., September 22, 1918, p. 963.—*Campbell:* Memoir on Extra-uterine Pregnancy, Edinburgh, 1840. Quoted by *Ramsbotham*, Obstetrics, p. 750.—*Czyzewicz:* Arch. f. Gynäk., vol. xcvii, No. 1.—*Dougal:* Jour. Obst. and Gyn., British Empire, March, 1914, p. 158.—*Galabin:* Brit. Med. Jour., March, 1903, p. 664.—*Halsted,* Garrison, American Mercury, February, 1926.—*Hammacher:* Arch. f. Gyn., 1910, vol. xcii, Bd. 2, p. 594.—*Hirst and Knipe:* Surg., Gyn., and Obst., 1908, vol. vii, p. 456; also *Richter:* Zentralbl. f. Gyn., 1912, p. 175.—*Lahm:* Zentralbl. für Gyn., 1927, No. 12, p. 752.—*Liebe:* Monatschr. für Geb. u. Gyn., 1921, Bd. 54, H. 2.—*Lockyer:* Surg., Gyn., and Obst., December, 1917, p. 563.—*Maennel:* "On the Anatomy of Hematocele," Zeitschr. f. Geb. u. Gyn., 1908, vol. lx, p. 212.—*Moller:* Acta Gyn. Scandin., 1925, Bd. 3, H. 4, p. 325.—*Noble:* Amer. Jour. Obst., 1901, vol. xliii, p. 497.—*Norris:* Surg., Gyn., and Obst., August, 1909, p. 124.—*Novak:* Surg., Gyn., and Obstet., July, 1926.—*Penkert:* Zentralbl. für die Gesammte Gyn. u. Geb., February 25, 1914. Gives complete literature to date.—*Pinard, Spiegelberg, Horwitz:* Zeitschr. f. Geb. u. Gyn., vol. ix, p. 110.—*Poorten:* Zentralbl. f. Gyn., 1922, p. 757.—*Schauta:* Lehrb. d. Gyn., 1906, p. 407.—*Schottmüller:* Münch. med. Woch., 1914, No. 5, Icterus, etc.—*Schuman:* Monograph, Appleton, 1921.—*Sittner:* Jour. Amer. Med. Assoc., 1907, p. 407 ref.—*Smith:* "Repeated Ectopic Gestation," Amer. Jour. Obst., September, 1911; *ibid.,* Jour. Amer. Med. Assoc., April 13, 1912, p. 1114.—*Sutton:* The Purvis Oration, London Lancet, 1904, ii, p. 1625. See also Waldeyer, below.—*Van Tussenbroek:* Annales de gynéc., 1899.—*Waldeyer:* Zentb. für Gyn., May 30, 1931, Nr. 22.—*Wallace:* Surg., Gyn., and Obst., December, 1917, xxiv, p. 579.—*Weibel:* Monatsschr. f. Geb. u. Gyn., vol. xxii, p. 748.—*Werth:* Handbuch d. Geb., vol. ii, p. 2.—*v. Winckel, F.:* "Über die Missbildungen ektopisch entwickelten Früchten, Wiesbaden, 1902.—Literature on Interstitial Pregnancy in L'Obstetrique, May, 1911, p. 493.

CHAPTER XXXI

DISPLACEMENTS OF THE UTERUS

ANTEFLEXION AND ANTEVERSION

NORMALLY, the uterus is anteverted, and during the first months of pregnancy this anteversion is increased, the fundus lying heavily on the bladder (Fig. 110, p. 87). Pregnancy occurring in an anteflexed uterus displaces the fundus downward, also pressing on the bladder and diminishing its capacity, but in both instances the uterus is soon directed upward into the abdomen by the obtusely placed pubis, and incarceration does not occur unless adhesion or neoplasm locks the organ in the pelvis.

Late in pregnancy the uterus always becomes anteverted, owing to the distention of the anterior abdominal wall. When this becomes pathologic, we call it *pendulous abdomen* (venter propendens, ventre en besace, Hängebauch), and in advanced cases the fundus may be inverted, pointing downward, and hanging between the knees. In primiparæ pendulous belly is very rare, and usually indicates the existence of a contracted pelvis, twins, or some condition preventing engagement of the fetal head. Occasionally, about the eighth month, the belly-wall gives way suddenly, the uterus falling forward. Striæ gravidarum are usually present in great numbers in these cases. One would naturally expect pendulous abdomen to be absent in athletic women and common in those of indolent habit, but the author's experience shows that both are equally affected. It is probable that a congenital weakness of the abdominal plates may exist and be causative of pendulous belly, as well as enteroptosis. Multiparæ suffer more commonly from this affection, and it increases with the number of children. The other factors are contracted pelvis, increased inclination of the pelvis, kyphosis, lordosis, spondylolisthesis, very large fetus, twins, polyhydramnion, frequent child-bearing, and tumors complicating pregnancy. Improper habits also cause weakening of the abdominal supports; such are constipation, wearing ill-fitting corsets or high-heeled shoes, carrying children or weights on the protuberant belly.

During pregnancy pendulous abdomen causes a sense of weight and distention, dragging pains in the loins, in the belly, and at the costal insertions of the recti, often frequency of urination, intertrigo of the lower abdomen and thighs, occasionally varices and edema of the vulva. The diastasis of the recti, which by the laity is called "rupture," may be so marked that the uterus falls forward, covered only by the peritoneum, a thin layer of fascia, and the skin, allowing the surface and the contents of the uterus to be felt with startling distinctness, and sometimes even the color of the organ showing through—*hernia uteri gravidi abdominalis*. In such cases locomotion may be hindered.

During labor pendulous abdomen may cause serious dystocia. The uterus is thrown so far forward that its axis forms an acute angle with the pelvic axis; the cervix is pulled up into the hollow of the sacrum, sometimes even above the promontory; dilatation is delayed, and the posterior uterine wall is overstretched. This, together with obstructed labor because of malposition of the fetus and disturbed mechanism, invites rupture of the uterus. Malpresentations, such as shoulder and breech, are common in these cases, because the head, in spite of strong pains, cannot get down into the pelvis. Malpositions, especially anterior parietal bone presentation, are especially prone to occur, as can be seen in Fig. 353. Prolapse of the cord and extremities may also cause dystocia, and, owing to the peculiar shape of the uterine tumor, diagnosis is difficult. In the child facial paralysis has been observed from pressure of the neck against the pubis, and the author found shortening of the sternocleidomastoid muscle, with temporary torticollis, as the result of the extreme lateriflexion of the fetal neck. Should the shortened muscle tear during spontaneous labor or operative delivery and become inflamed, a permanent wryneck may result. The child is exposed to all the dangers of the abnormal mechanism of labor, and the fetal mortality is, therefore, higher.

Treatment.—Prevention accomplishes a good deal. The corset should be removed as soon as the fact of pregnancy existing is established, and the woman's

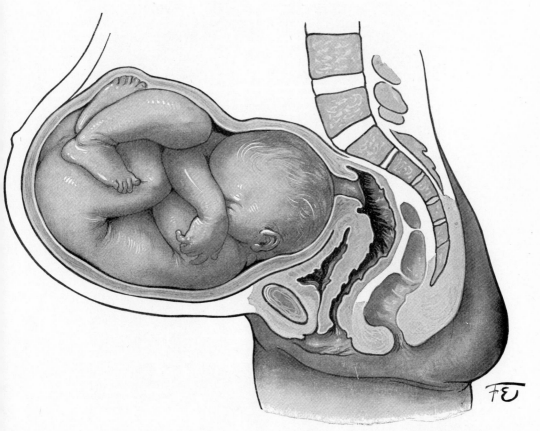

FIG. 353.—PENDULOUS BELLY.

living should be ordered as is described under the Hygiene of Pregnancy. During the latter months of pregnancy the abdomen should be supported by a properly fitting binder. Most of the "maternity corsets" on the market exert pressure on the fundus in a downward direction, when the proper action is one of support from below. The ordinary surgical binder with straps over the shoulders meets the indications best.

After delivery one should attempt to restore the tonus of the abdominal wall as fully as possible by—(a) Prevention of the accumulation of gas and feces in the bowel (these keep the muscle overdistended); (b) preventing infection, which lames the intestinal wall; (c) keeping the patient recumbent for at least a week, and letting her resume her household duties slowly; (*d*) using some sort of abdominal support after getting out of bed; (*e*) by systematic gymnastics and massage of the abdominal muscles.

In cases of fully developed pendulous belly during pregnancy an abdominal binder should be worn as soon as the uterus rises out of the pelvis; the patient should lie much on the back, and the physician should examine her in the last weeks to discover a malpresentation.

During labor the binder should be worn, or the uterus may be pulled up by a towel slung over the shoulders and held in place by another around the belly. In some cases it is best for the attendant to push the pendent fundus upward during every pain until the head enters the pelvis. The author has often accomplished

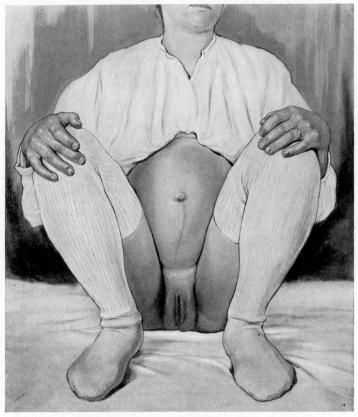

Fig. 354.—Squatting Position Used by Indians.

engagement by letting the patient squat in an aboriginal attitude (Fig. 354). This procedure is also recommended by King. The thighs force the uterus up, and the child is straightened and brought with its axis to correspond with that of the inlet. As a rule, after the head engages labor proceeds rapidly, but sometimes the widely separated recti cannot obtain a purchase on the uterus with its contents, and delay in the second stage arises or rotation stops. Unless forceps are applied, the uterus may rupture. The exaggerated lithotomy position (Fig. 495), which is the squatting position with the patient on the back, is especially useful at this stage of labor, and should always be tried before resorting to forceps. After delivery of the head the anterior shoulder may stem on the pubis and cause delay—the body of the child is to be lifted up by a hand pulling up the abdomen. In breech presentations, as soon as labor ceases to progress, the anterior foot of the child should be brought down—this adjusts the fetal axis to that of the pelvis.

Edema and prolapse of the anterior wall of the cervix as the head descends in the pelvis require treatment, which consists in gently forcing the structures up over the head by the internal fingers while the outside hand supports the fundus.

ANTEFIXATION OF THE UTERUS

Since the gynecologists and general surgeons have learned that fixation operations on the uterus during the reproductive period cause dystocia, we meet with labors, rendered difficult from this cause, very rarely nowadays.

The Alexander and allied operations, where the ligaments are shortened or transplanted, as in that of Andrews (sewn behind the uterus), usually give little real trouble during pregnancy and labor. Abortion is slightly more frequent, and abdominal pain, from the tugging of the uterus at its shortened ligaments, is usually complained of. The round ligaments grow during pregnancy, and after it undergo involution as ordinarily. Often the result of the operation is impaired by the changes wrought by gestation. Only symptomatic treatment can be employed for the disturbances during pregnancy.

Ventrofixation and ventrosuspension (often the former results when the latter is intended) and *adhesion of the uterus to the abdominal wall* following celiotomy not seldom cause serious dystocia. Lindfors, in 68 cases of labor, found the cervix was high in 27, transverse presentation in 31, and trouble in third stage in 10. There were 30 versions, 13 cesarean sections, 10 high forceps, 5 embryotomies, 5 tamponades for postpartum hemorrhage, and many other operations necessary. There were 3 deaths. It is claimed by Lindfors, if the operation is properly performed, there is almost no danger of trouble with succeeding pregnancies. In 146 cases collected by Lapthorn Smith there was trouble 36 times—10 abortions and 3 deaths. In my own experience these have occurred: Abortion, shoulder and breech presentation, obstructed labor requiring cesarean section, placenta prævia, inertia uteri and its sequences, retention of placenta, postpartum hemorrhage.

Pain in the scar is common, and occasionally hyperemesis may require interference during pregnancy. Dickinson reports 2 deaths—one from rupture of the uterus and one from late shock after cesarean section—Liesthal, 3 others.

The frequency of abortion, difficult labor, postpartum hemorrhage, and the necessity for capital operations to overcome obstruction should forbid the practice of ventral fixation in child-bearing women, an opinion also held by Cragin and Polak.

Much depends on the site of the fixation scar. If in the fundus, the worst forms of dystocia occur. Then the anterior wall can take little part in the dilatation of the uterus. It hypertrophies and forms a roof over the inlet, while the posterior wall thins and stretches to complete the cavity of the uterus. The cervix is thus pushed toward the sacrum by the growing anterior wall, and pulled up out of the pelvis by the tugging of the posterior uterine wall. One may find the external os on the promontory or above it, and the internal os up on the lumbar spine. More or less asymmetry is the rule, the fundus stretching to one side. One finds the tubes, ovaries, and round ligaments more or less parallel with Poupart's ligaments.

Vaginofixation caused such serious dystocia that its performance on child-bearing women was very soon abandoned. Now, unless the tubes are resected, insuring sterility, it is very seldom practised. Uniting the round ligaments instead of the fundus to the vagina is open to the same objections.

Since the fundus in this operation is attached to the relatively immobile vagina, the cervix points to the sacrum, and the same conditions will arise as in ventrofixation, only more exaggerated. The pelvic inlet is roofed over by the hypertrophied anterior cervical and uterine wall; the os is high up in the abdominal cavity, and can be traversed by the finger only after the whole hand has been passed into the vagina; the bladder is entirely an abdominal organ; the posterior wall of the uterus, having constituted almost solely the available uterine wall, is much thinned; the round ligaments, tubes, and ovaries converge to a common point just behind the pubis (Fig. 355). Abdominally, one finds a triangular uterine tumor with the broad base at the inlet, and can feel the round ligaments as they converge toward the pubis. Sometimes the scar is visibly retracted.

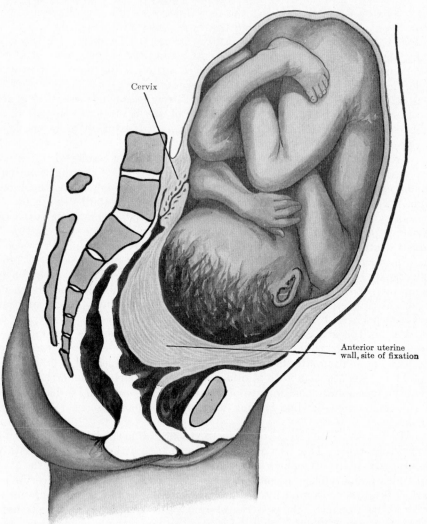

Cervix

Anterior uterine
wall, site of fixation

FIG. 355.—MRS, M, CONDITIONS AT TERM AFTER VAGINOFIXATION. CESAREAN SECTION.

During pregnancy, which is not common after the operation, the uterus tugs at its false attachments and may break them, which is more likely in abdominal fixations. This process causes much pain and symptoms of peritoneal irritation. Abortion occurs in one-fourth of the cases and annoying bladder symptoms are the rule. Labor often comes on prematurely.

Labor is complicated by premature rupture of the bag of waters and prolpase of the cord; abnormal presentation, usually shoulder; slow, weak pains, or strong but inefficient pains, because of the vault of the vagina being obstructed by the thick septum; postpartum hemorrhage. All manipulations are rendered laborious because the uterine cavity is difficult of access, since the hand has to pass a crooked canal and then operate over the border of a ledge. Even the lateral posture does not facilitate the operative procedures very much.

Treatment.—A woman who has had an operation fixing the uterus in an abnormal location requires careful watching during pregnancy. Annoying symptoms can be only partly relieved. Threatened abortion requires rest in bed and opiates; if the abortion occurs, the accoucheur must see that the uterus is absolutely empty, and that the drainage of its cavity is good. As the woman nears term frequent examinations should be made to determine the behavior of the cervix. If it is pushed backward, upward, and higher into the abdominal cavity, trouble in labor will surely arise, and appropriate measures should be instituted. Such a course of pregnancy after ventral operation may indicate reopening the belly and release of the adherent fundus, allowing gestation to go to term. After vaginofixation such an operation would be impracticable. If the woman goes into labor, a quick determination is to be made as to how much an obstruction the cervico-uterovaginal septum will make. If the hand can pull the cervix down and easily bring it into the axis of the pelvis, it is probable that nature will succeed alone or, by means of the metreurynter, version, forceps, etc., the case can be successfully terminated with ordinary methods; but if the cervix is long, high above the promontory, and hard to pull down, a cutting operation will usually be necessary.

In ventrofixations either a vaginal or an abdominal cesarean section may be selected, but the former is quite difficult of execution, because of the inaccessibility of the cervix. In cases where a typical vaginofixation has been done with the usual stripping of the bladder from the anterior cervical and uterine wall, the septum may safely be split medially from the external os almost to the pubis, without danger of injuring any organ. Since one seldom knows what operation has been done, it is wisest to open the abdomen in these bad cases. In infected cases a Porro operation is indicated, and it is usually technically difficult, because of the extensive adhesions, the immense varicosities in the broad ligaments, and the abnormal location of the bladder and blood-vessels. A word of warning is given to the operator attempting to deliver from below, to remember how thin the posterior wall of the uterus is, and that the whole organ is fixed on the pelvis, for which reason rupture is to be feared. In performing version, access to the parts which lie in the anterior pocket above the ledge separating the uterine cavity from the vagina may be obtained by turning the patient on her side and the operator inserting the hand from behind. After delivery, either vaginally or abdominally, provision for uterine drainage must be made by gauze or tube, because the fundus may be lower than the cervix, and the lochia may accumulate in the anterior pocket.

POSTERIOR DISPLACEMENTS

Retroversion and retroflexion occur in about 20 per cent. of nulliparæ, and may cause sterility, but in women who have borne children both displacements are common, and seldom are the cause of acquired sterility.

Causation.—While the pregnant uterus may become retroflexed or retroverted as the result of a sudden increase of the intra-abdominal pressure when the bladder is full, for example, through cough, fall, straining, it is usual that the pregnancy occurs in a uterus already displaced.

As a rule, the uterus slowly draws itself up out of the pelvis—that is, spontaneous restitution occurs. Sometimes, because of adhesions binding the fundus in the pelvis, or because of shrinking and inflammatory thickening of the muscle and serosa at the angle of the flexion, or because of tumors or a prominent sacrum, which interfere, spontaneous restitution is hindered and the retroflexion becomes established. It is impossible to guess at the frequency of the condition, because surely many pregnancies occur in retrodisplaced uteri and terminate unobserved, by the rising of the organ in the abdomen or by abortion.

Clinical Course.—Unless the displacement of the uterus is complicated by adhesions, no symptoms are complained of until the uterus begins to draw on the neck of the bladder. Sometimes there is a sensation of fulness in the pelvis, with bearing down, or pains radiating from the sacral and lumbar plexuses. At the end of the third month bladder symptoms appear—frequent desire to urinate, great pain, and the necessity to strain to pass water, the feeling that the viscus has not been emptied, and then, usually coming on more or less suddenly, retention of the urine. The bladder becomes enormously distended, containing, in one of the author's cases, 96 ounces of urine, and in a case reported by Blundell, nearly two gallons. Constant dribbling may occur, that is, retention with overflow—*inconti-*

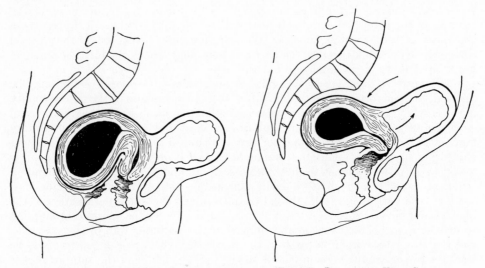

FIG. 356.—RETROFLEXIO UTERI GRAVIDI.   FIG. 357.—RETROVERSIO UTERI GRAVIDI.
Arrows show the direction of development.   Note differences in the cervix.

nentia or *ischuria paradoxa.* There may be edema of the extremities. Constipation and diarrhea are occasionally noted. Decided symptoms occur long before the room in the pelvis is entirely filled by the growing uterus, and usually bring the patient to the physician. Rarely the woman waits until the uterus is tightly wedged in the pelvis. As a rule, the symptoms begin in the third month and the case is terminated by the fifth, but sometimes the pregnancy has proceeded to the eighth month, and in partial retroflexion, to term.

Four terminations of these cases are possible: (1) Spontaneous rectification; (2) abortion; (3) partial restitution; (4) incarceration.

1. Spontaneous rectification is the rule about the third or fourth month, the fundus rising past the promontory and falling forward. Contraction of the muscular fibers of the anterior uterine wall, aided by the round ligaments, accomplishes this, and it is favored by putting the patient to bed, thus relieving the displaced uterus of the abdominal pressure. The change usually requires some days or weeks, but may occur rapidly in twenty-four hours or between two examinations. Pelvic adhesions may delay the restitution, but usually the adhesions, even when exten-

sive, are stretched, torn, and even absorbed.   If the adhesions are too strong, or
if the changes in the structure of the uterine wall are permanent, the uterus is distorted in the direction of the attachment of its wall, which portion is drawn out
sac-like, the balance of the uterus dilating to accommodate the ovum.   Fig. 361
shows such a case.   Spontaneous cure is commoner in retroflexion than in retroversion, because in the former the corpus has a firm body to pull against—the cervix.

2. Abortion is a frequent termination of retroflexed pregnant uteri; indeed,
habitual early abortion is often caused by this malposition.   The lack of room does
not cause the abortion, but the uterine action is started by disturbance in the uterine

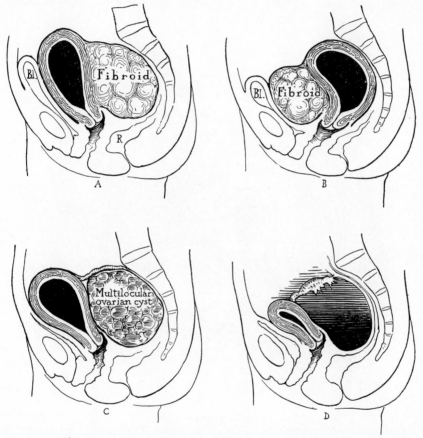

FIGS. 358, 359.—FOUR CONDITIONS SIMULATING RETROFLEXIO UTERI GRAVIDI.
A, Pregnancy with fibroid; B, fibroid with pregnancy; C, Pregnancy with any kind of ovarian cyst; D, ectopic pregnancy with hematocele.

and pelvic circulation, by chronic endometritis the result of the congestion, with
hemorrhages in the decidua, and by chronic metritis, which perhaps was the original
cause of the displacement.   Owing to the strong contractions during the course of
abortion, the uterus usually rises in the abdomen, thus hiding the cause of all the
trouble, but aiding the emptying of the ovum and the lochial discharges.   Rarely—
and in these cases there are adhesions—the drainage of the uterus is incomplete
because the fundus is lower than the cervix.

3. Incomplete restitution may result in a condition known as retroflexio uteri
partialis.   This term is applied to those cases where part of the fundus is retained

in the pelvis, the anterior wall expanding in the abdomen to form the ovum container. Many forms of the uterus are possible. (See Figs. 360–361.) They are due to inveterate adhesions, tumors, or to changes in the uterine muscle or serosa at the point of the flexion.

These cases may terminate normally at term, the deformity and dislocation of the cervix being finally overcome. Abortion or premature labor may occur, or incarceration which demands early interference, and if at term, operation.

A condition known as *sacciform dilatation of the uterus* may be confounded with partial restitution. The cervix is found behind or above the pubis; the culdesac is filled with part of the dilated cervix or the lower uterine segment (Fig. 361). It is usually a simple matter, by means of the finger or the vulsella, to pull the

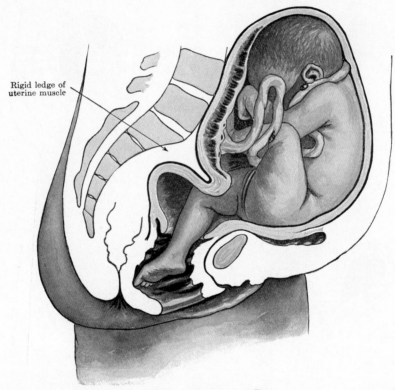

Rigid ledge of uterine muscle

FIG. 360.—RETROFLEXIO UTERI.

A retroflexed uterus had been pushed up out of the pelvis by means of a colpeurynter in the fourth month, and the pregnancy proceeded to term. Labor was normal, but because of hemorrhage the placenta had to be removed, which was difficult on account of its inaccessible location. The flexion of the uterus had persisted throughout.

cervix to the median line, and then complete delivery in the natural or ordinary operative method, but Depaul, who wrote a good paper on the subject, was unable in his case to find the os, and the patient died undelivered, though he had made an opening through the posterior uterine wall.

4. Incarceration of the growing uterus in the pelvis is the most serious outcome, and the symptoms which demand interference come from the bladder. This organ cannot be emptied properly, becomes enormously distended, reaching even to the ensiform, and becomes inflamed. The cause of the retention of the urine is compression and distraction of the urethra, and sometimes edema of the neck of the bladder from the intense congestion. Ischuria paradoxa, or constant dribbling, may excoriate the parts, especially if, in addition, the uterus becomes infected and

a septic serous discharge issues therefrom. Uremia may occur when the urine dams back into the kidneys, but, curiously enough, eclampsia has not been observed, though Halbertsma says that compression of the ureters is a cause of eclampsia. If the retention of the urine is of slow development, the bladder hypertrophies, but in all cases of any standing, with or without catheterization, cystitis and ammoniacal decomposition develop. Hemorrhages into the wall and into the bladder have been noted. The bladder may rupture into the peritoneal cavity, with acutest peritonitis and death, or into the connective tissue with septic urinary infiltration, which is almost always fatal. Or the bladder-wall becomes necrotic, in part or wholly, the intestines adhere to its outside, and if the bladder-wall is removed or broken by sloughing, the urine accumulates in a new sac formed by the adherent structures. This usually ruptures and causes general peritonitis. Gangrene and separation of all or part of the mucosa are not necessarily fatal, because, if the uterus

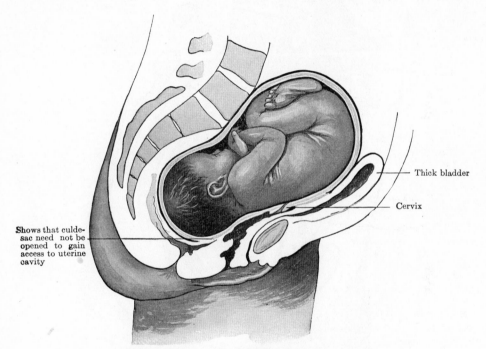

Thick bladder

Cervix

Shows that culdesac need not be opened to gain access to uterine cavity

Fig. 361.—Sacciform Dilatation of the Uterus at Term.

is emptied, the slough may be expelled through the urethra. The cause of the gangrene is infection of the necrotic mucosa, and the germs—usually Bacterium coli—gain access either through the urethra or by the catheter, or from adherent bowel. Anemia of the bladder from overdistention or rupture of one part of the mucosa, with urinary extravasation between the layers, has been given as a cause of the necrosis. Death may result from urinary sepsis (Fig. 362).

The bladder claims our chief interest, but the bowel sometimes shows symptoms, such as tympany, constipation, and vomiting. Occasionally a mucous diarrhea occurs. Ileus is exceedingly rare.

Incarceration of the uterus may lead to abortion or to septic infection of the uterine contents, the bacteria passing through from the bladder, or upward from the decomposing urine, which dribbles into the vagina continually. Perforation and rupture of the uterus, with death from peritonitis, have been noted to follow prolonged incarceration, and in rare instances the uterus was expelled through the rectum or through the posterior wall of the vagina, it and its contents being delivered outside. Even very late spontaneous restitution of the uterus may occur, but we do not wait for it in practice.

Diagnosis.—This is seldom difficult if a careful examination is made. Any pregnant woman giving a history of dysuria or dribbling urine should be examined for retroflexio uteri. Abdominally, one sees and feels the distended bladder as an elastic tumor giving a good wave of fluctuation. If the bladder-wall is hypertrophied, the tumor may be hard. After catheterization, which is invariably necessary, the changed abdomen is striking. Vaginally, one finds the cervix pressed upward

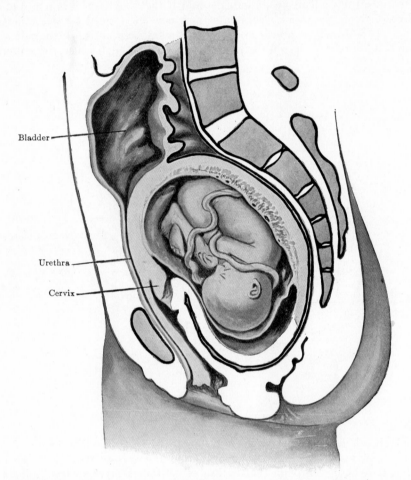

FIG. 362.—WYDER'S CASE OF INCARCERATION OF THE RETROFLEXED GRAVID UTERUS WITH GANGRENE OF BLADDER.

against the pubis or even above the pubis, while the culdesac is filled with a soft tumor which bulges into the vagina and may even (late) distend the perineum.

The differential diagnosis must be made from extra-uterine pregnancy, fibroid on the posterior wall, and incarcerated ovarian tumor. Concerning ectopic gestation, the reader is referred to the appropriate chapter, but here the warning may be repeated to be sure that one really has to deal only with a retroflexed uterus before attempting to replace it. Demonstration of the uterus alongside the tumor in the culdesac is needed to settle the existence of a neoplasm in the pelvis, but if the woman is pregnant and a neoplasm co-exists, the diagnosis is formidable.

RETROFLEXIO UTERI GRAVIDI	PREGNANCY WITH OVARIAN TUMOR
1. Symptoms of incarceration early.	1. Absent or very late.
2. Bladder symptoms pronounced.	2. Absent or inconsiderable.
3. Tumor in question symmetric and soft all over.	3. Usually asymmetric, hard, and tense all over or in places.
4. There is no other tumor above the pelvis.	4. Often can feel the pregnant uterus above inlet and to one side.
5. Moving the cervix imparts an impulse to the tumor.	5. The upper tumor (the uterus) can be moved independently of the tumor.
6. The fornices are flattened, at least not drawn up.	6. The fornices are drawn up high, sometimes even above the pubis.
7. The tumor in the culdesac may contract.	7. Never.
8. May distinguish fetal parts.	8. Never.
9. May outline the round ligaments per rectum.	9. Not positive (in one case strands simulated these).

Incarceration of a pregnant horn of a double uterus and partial retroflexion of the uterus both give diagnostic problems which may not be solved except by laparotomy, and countless mistakes have been made.

Dührssen, among others, emphasizes the differences between the clinical course and diagnostic findings in retroflexion and those of retroversion, but practically

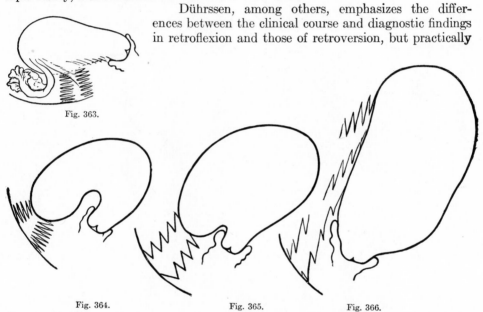

Fig. 363.

Fig. 364.   Fig. 365.   Fig. 366.

FIGS. 363–366.—MRS. F., PRIMIPARA. RETROVERSIO UTERI ADHERENTA WITH PROLAPSE OF OVARIES IN CULDESAC; PREGNANCY.

Some pain and irritation of bladder; attempted reposition in office at eight weeks failed; knee-chest position thrice daily with air into vagina; at three months could feel posterior wall drawn out and anterior wall bulging upward (very thin woman); spontaneous restitution at fourth month. The four figures indicated the process which took place.

the two conditions are the same. Retroversion may, as pregnancy goes on, become a flexion; retroversion produces symptoms of incarceration later because the cervix, pointing toward the abdominal cavity, can develop in this direction; retroversion is less likely to reduce itself and is harder to correct artificially. In retroversion one finds the cervix pointing toward the navel; in retroflexion the cervix points toward the coccyx, and one feels the angle between it and the fundus.

Prognosis.—Most cases of retrodisplacement terminate by spontaneous reduction or respond easily to art, and nowadays, when women consult the physician so readily, a neglected case is a rarity. Gottschalk, quoted by Dührssen, collected 67 cases of death in which were 16 cases of uremia and exhaustion, 7 of sepsis, 18 of peritonitis, 11 of rupture of the bladder, 3 of pyemia, 2 of rupture of the peritoneum and vagina, 5 errors of art, 1 ileus, and 4 unknown. The danger of rupture of the bladder occurs both from overdistention and from brusk attempts

29

to replace the uterus; the bladder has been punctured by the catheter and severe hemorrhage into it may result from too rapid withdrawal of the urine. The uterus may be torn by attempts to replace it, but the greatest source of danger is retention of urine, with cystitis, gangrene, or ascending infection, etc.

Treatment.—If the condition is discovered very early, one may wait a while to see what nature will accomplish. A gentle attempt to replace the uterus may be made at the first examination, and if successful, a hard-rubber pessary is introduced, to be worn until the end of the fourth month. Otherwise the patient is instructed to take the knee-chest position three times a day, and to sleep on the side, with the buttocks slightly elevated. If, after three weeks, the condition is unchanged or worse, the woman is put to bed, and a determined effort for cure is made.

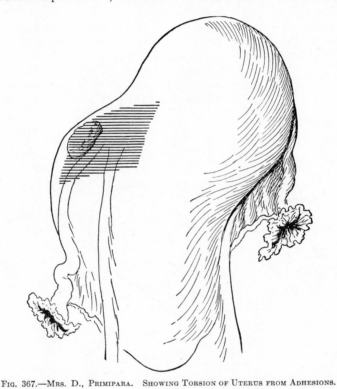

Fig. 367.—Mrs. D., Primipara. Showing Torsion of Uterus from Adhesions.
Appendicitis with peritonitis four years ago; pain at frequent intervals throughout, and painful uterine contractions at end of, this pregnancy; threatened abortion at three months, therefore rest in bed; troublesome tympany; labor at term; very severe pains and desire to urinate with each contraction; spontaneous delivery, boy, 8 pounds; incarcerated placenta; hour-glass contraction; hemorrhage; manual removal of placenta, which was partly adherent in left horn of uterus under the spleen, requiring introduction of hand nearly to elbow; uterus spirally twisted; remained open, filling with blood; tamponade; recovery. Uterus adherent to abdominal wall at point indicated by shading.

First, the bladder must be emptied and kept empty. When the uterus is incarcerated this is not so easily done, because the urethra is very long, flattened, distorted, edematous, or the bladder itself divided into two compartments, only one of which is accessible to the catheter. Care must be taken to avoid producing a false passage, and a soft catheter is the best instrument. It may be necessary for the physician, not the nurse, to use a silver male catheter. Aids to catheterization are: Sims or knee-chest position; using the right sized catheter—No. 12 to No. 15 French scale; pushing up the fundus or pushing back the cervix with two fingers in the vagina; pulling down the cervix with a vulsellum (not recommended by author); allowing warm, sterile olive oil to flow through catheter while being inserted; extreme gentleness and much patience. If the retention has been great and prolonged, all the urine should not be withdrawn in one sitting, and the rate of flow must be very slow. After an interval of three hours the bladder may be completely emptied, the reasons for this advice being that the sudden relief of so immense an abdominal distention and peritoneal stretching may cause shock, and the blood rushing into the anemic mucous membrane of the bladder may produce a hemorrhage in it.

By saline cathartics and glycerin enemata, using small amounts of liquid, the bowels are kept free and tympany prevented.

Reposition of the uterus is usually easily accomplished after the bladder is emptied, and it is aided by employing the knee-chest position, by pulling the cervix down with a vulsellum or ring forceps, and pushing the fundus upward and to the side. The fundus should be brought to slip alongside and avoid the promontory, by pressure with two fingers in the vagina or one in the rectum, aided

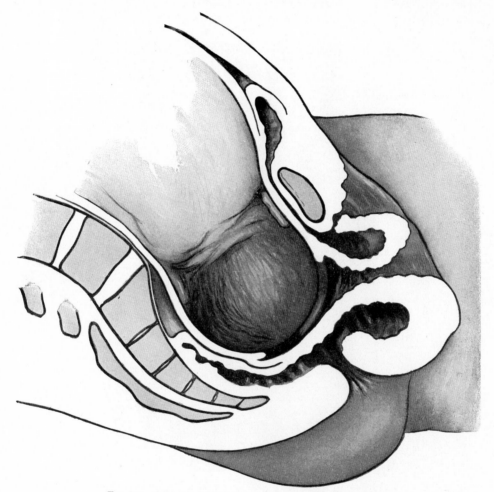

FIG. 368.—PROLAPSE OF CYSTOCELE AND RECTOCELE DURING LABOR.

by anesthesia, and using great gentleness and patience. Too great force may rupture the uterus, may tear a vascular adhesion, may cause hemorrhage into the bladder or even burst it, and may bring on abortion. Women have died because of too violent manipulations. Even after reposition bladder necrosis may occur the damage having already been done..

If manipulation will not restore the uterus, one may temporize a short time, employing the following measures: (a) Knee-chest position every four hours for fifteen minutes, with continuous rest in bed on the side, with the hips elevated, and frequent emptying of the bladder and rectum. In the absence of symptoms of cystitis, and without retention, one may wait. Urotropin, 5 grains, medicinal methylene-blue, 1 grain, in capsule, are to be given four times daily in these cases; (b) a colpeurynter with 16 ounces of water is placed in the vagina, and the foot of the bed elevated 18 inches. Some authors recommend mercury to fill the colpeurynter.

One may continue these gentle efforts for several weeks until successful, but must not delay until cystitis or aggravation of the condition indicates their futility. Laparotomy has frequently been done and the uterus easily raised, the adhesions being broken up, or—and this seems to have been overlooked—simply by allowing air to get under the retroverted fundus. The belly is opened in the interests of the child, and is permissible only when the bladder is not gangrenous, and in the absence of symptoms of acute peritonitis—this because the protective adhesions around a gangrenous bladder may be ruptured, or the softened uterus may tear.

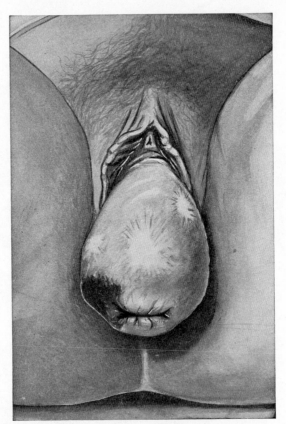

Fig. 369.—Acute Elongation of the Cervix at Eight Months (Chicago Lying-in Hospital).

The incision is to be begun high, at or above the navel, and then enlarged downward after being assured that the bladder is not in the way.

If conditions are not right for laparotomy, the uterus must be emptied, but, owing to the inaccessible cervix, this may be difficult. A sharply curved sound or male bougie may enable one to puncture the membranes, and during the resulting contractions the uterus will lift itself up and empty itself, or permit the accoucheur to do it. If one cannot reach the os, the puncture may be made through the bulging posterior uterine wall, using an aspirating needle and syringe. In one case Bumm drew off enough liquor amnii to allow the replacement of the uterus, and abortion did not follow.

Posterior hysterotomy, with removal of the whole ovum in one sitting, may also be done, and reference to Fig. 361 will show that it is not always necessary to open the peritoneal cavity. If this operation is attempted and the culdesac opened, one should try to replace the uterus by combined manipulation before incising it. If successful, the pregnancy may go to term. To prevent recurrence the vagina is tamponed for several days and then a large Smith pessary worn until the uterus is too large to fall back.

Gangrene of the bladder is diagnosed by the discharge of foul urine, with flocculi of pus and shreds of membrane, in the presence of septic fever. Cystoscopically, very little can be seen, but the severe cystitis and localized necroses with hemorrhages may be found before gangrene has set in. As soon as the diagnosis of gangrenous cystitis is made the bladder is to be widely opened from the vagina, loose pieces of tissue removed, and freest drainage provided. Urotropin, alternating with salol, is administered, 5 to 8 grains four times a day. Urinary infiltration of the perivesical spaces is to be sharply watched for, and on its discovery the whole region immediately and broadly incised, above or below the pubis, or both, and the freest possible drainage established. It is unsafe to open the uterus or induce abortion after gangrene of the bladder has begun because of sepsis; therefore it is best to drain the bladder and await developments. The uterus may be replaceable after a few weeks, or more safely attacked after the bladder has cleansed itself somewhat. When the uterus has become infected, it must be emptied, or, if this is impossible, extirpated. Nowadays these neglected cases are extremely rare, because the women consult the physician earlier.

Partial retroflexion of the gravid uterus requires treatment on similar lines if threatening symptoms arise. At term, if it is impossible to bring the cervix into the axis of the pelvis, one may have to deliver through the posterior cervical wall or do an abdominal cesarean section.

Distortion of the uterus, by its adherence to the abdominal wall, to the sides of the pelvis, the rectum, etc., may give rise to serious dystocia, as has been seen in the instance of antefixations.

PROLAPSE OF THE PREGNANT UTERUS

Procidentia may occur in the very early months, and unless replaced leads to abortion, but Wimmer reports a case of a six months' gestation outside the vulva, and this, according to Braun Fernwald, is the only authentic one on record where the pregnancy was so far advanced. Relaxation and prolapse of the vagina, with partial prolapse of the uterus outside the vulva, are not very rare. They may occur during pregnancy as the result of severe trauma, because a tendency to prolapse existed before, or a prolapsed uterus may become pregnant. (See Findley.)

Spontaneous retraction of the prolapsed portion usually occurs, and after the fourth month the tendency to fall disappears; indeed, the patient may feel better during pregnancy than at other times, since the uterus is in place. If spontaneous reduction does not take place, it is a simple matter to return the womb and hold it in position by tampons or an air pessary until it is too large to come down. Ulcerations of the cervix are to be cauterized with 10 per cent. silver nitrate and all infections cured before labor starts in. Rest in bed, with the foot elevated 12 inches, 1:3000 permanganate douches three times daily, and roborant diet will accomplish this.

An irreplaceable, completely prolapsed uterus is to be emptied.

Extrusion of cystocele and rectocele during pregnancy is a very annoying condition, the exposed parts sometimes being eroded, usually varicose, and occasionally inflamed. Pruritus may be obstinate, and the author has observed several cases of mycosis vulvæ under these conditions. Rest in the horizontal position is to be advised, also extreme cleanliness.

Eversion of the vaginal walls occurs in multiparæ in the second stage, during the strong bearing-down efforts, especially if the cervix is rigid and does not retract above the head (Fig. 368). The cervix may appear outside the vulva as far as one or even eight inches, and will not go back under pressure. Delivery is more or less difficult, depending on the degree, but usually possible, though many of the children die. If labor has to be operative, two assistants should hold back the edges of the cervix and the everted vagina with specula while the delivery is being effected. The cervix should be treated antiseptically.

Hirst collected 27 cases of *vaginal enterocele*, to which the author can add one, occurring in the service of the Chicago Lying-in Hospital Dispensary. Here the hernial opening in the posterior culdesac was 2½ inches across, but the coils of the intestine could be very easily replaced. The treatment of cystocele and rectocele during labor is symptomatic, the parts being replaced as much as possible and held back with the fingers so that the advancing head can slip through the space thus provided.

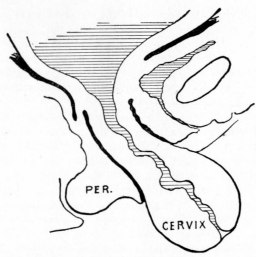

FIG. 370.—HYPERTROPHIC, EDEMATOUS, AND PROLAPSED CERVIX IN PREGNANCY.
Diagram of internal findings of Fig. 369.

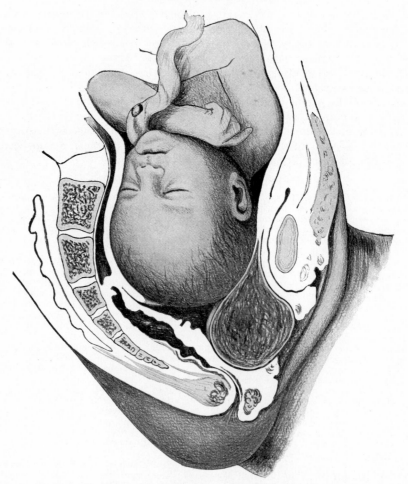

FIG. 371.—EDEMATOUS ANTERIOR LIP OF CERVIX, CAUSING DYSTOCIA.

Hypertrophic elongation of the cervix rarely complicates labor. Conception is hindered and dysmenorrhea usually calls for treatment, the cases seldom coming to the accoucheur until they have been operated on. Sometimes the scarred cervix gives trouble. In one case the author amputated three centimeters of a long cervix, which, even as late as the fourth month, the time the operation was done, was visible at the vulva. Ulceration and possible infection were the reasons for interference. Labor was uneventful. If an infected prolapsed cervix complicates labor, vaginal hysterotomy followed by hysterectomy may be indicated.

Acute enlargement of the cervix with edema, described first by Gueniot in 1872, and of which Jolly, in 1904, was able to collect 10 cases, is quite a rare occurrence during pregnancy, labor, and the puerperium. The author can add 3 cases occurring during pregnancy as the result of a sudden violent strain (Fig. 369). The fornices of the vagina were normally placed, and there were no bladder symptoms. Several days had elapsed since the accident, and the exposed portion of the cervix was dry, cracked, and partly eroded. It was disinfected, replaced, and retained by a tampon; the prolapse did not recur, and labor was normal. Williams refers the condition to an angioneurosis, but in most of the cases a history of injury has been obtained.

During labor, when the head is arrested high up, the cervix becomes swollen and may prolapse as a dark-blue, hemorrhagic, edematous mass (Fig. 371). The protuberant cervix is to be tenderly pushed up and held in position during the pains. Soon the head slips down past it. During forceps delivery it must be held back with two fingers during each traction. It may require incision. A contracted pelvis should be thought of as the cause.

Hernia of the gravid uterus in the inguinal canal, through the umbilicus or abdominal wall, and diastasis of the recti, allowing an actual hernial protrusion, have been observed.

LITERATURE

Cragin: "Ventrofixation," Surg., Gyn., and Obstet., 1908, vol. vii, p. 45; also *Muret:* Zent. f. Gyn., 1916, No. 17.—*Depaul:* Arch. de Tocologie, 1876.—*Dührssen:* Arch. f. Gyn., vol. lvii, p. 70. Gives literature. *Findley:* Jour. Amer. Med. Assoc., December 30, 1911.—*Jolly:* Zeitschr. f. Geb. u. Gyn., vol. lii, p. 396.—*Liestal:* Zentralblatt für Geb. u. Gyn., 1918, No. 24.—*Mann, Cameron, and Fry:* "Celiotomy in Retroflexio Uteri Gravidi," Amer. Jour. Obstet., July, August, 1898.—*Pinard and Varnier:* Annales de Gyn. et d'Obst., 1886, p. 339, and 1887, p. 87.—*Wimmer:* Handbuch d. Geb., v. Winckel, vol. ii, p. 355.

CHAPTER XXXII

ABORTION AND PREMATURE LABOR

It is said that almost half of the child-bearing women have had a miscarriage before the thirty-fifth year. Taussig, after proving that it is impossible to obtain exact figures of the frequency of abortion in any country, assumes that in cities there is one abortion to $2\frac{1}{2}$ and in rural districts 1 in 5 confinements.

Stumpf and Meyer collected large statistics, but they are of questionable value, as, indeed, are nearly all statistics, because one cannot get complete information. Hospital figures do not represent the conditions of private practice, because complicated cases are sent to the hospital, and statistics from both sources are, therefore, invalidated. Further, many abortions occur in the first weeks and pass under the diagnosis of delayed or profuse menstruation. Finally, very many abortions are deliberately concealed. In general, regarding abortion it may be said that it occurs more frequently in multiparæ than in primiparæ, perhaps because there are more multiparæ, but probably also for other reasons; oftener in the city than in the country, because of the prevalence of gonorrhea, the easy accessibility of the abortionist, etc.; oftener among the lower classes—but criminal abortion is probably more frequent in the educated classes; more frequent in the first three months of gestation, and, of the three, commonest during the third month; more frequent after the thirtieth year. Race, civil state, and color seem to have no influence.

The reasons for the more frequent occurrence of abortion from the eighth to the twelfth week are: The ovum is not strongly attached, and is weak and susceptible to outward influences; marked changes are going on in its circulation; since the woman is not sure of her pregnancy, she takes no care of herself; the women consider it no crime to get rid of the ovum before "quickening," and think abortion not dangerous in the early months.

Much disagreement exists regarding nomenclature. Miscarriage is a term used by the laity for every interruption of pregnancy before term, and the word "abortion" is resented as implying a criminal process. In scientific description it is best to drop the former and retain the latter. "Immature labor" has been used to designate the interruption of pregnancy from the sixteenth to the twenty-eighth week, and "premature labor" from then on, the term abortion being limited to the period before the sixteenth week. The author agrees with those writers who apply the word *abortion* to all interruptions of pregnancy before the child is viable, that is, before the twenty-sixth to the twenty-eighth week, and the expression *premature labor* to those terminations of gestation after the child is viable, but before term.

Causation.—A study of the etiology of abortion has very great importance as an aid to science, of treatment, of the prevention of subsequent accidents, and medicolegally. Therefore in all cases the accoucheur should search carefully for the underlying cause and make a note of all his findings.

A classification of the causes must be arbitrary, since they are very numerous and interact on each other. They are fetal, maternal, and paternal.

Fetal.—Death of the fetus nearly always brings on abortion, and every fatal anomaly of the fetal body or its appendages is, therefore, an etiologic factor. Mall says one-third of aborted fetuses are teratologic.

Diseases of the Chorion.—Hydatidiform degeneration almost always interrupts pregnancy, only a few cases being on record as having gone to term. Hemorrhage is usually furious when the uterus attempts to empty itself.

Placental Diseases.—Syphilis, hypertrophic endarteritis, excessive white infarct formation, apoplexies of the placenta, placenta prævia, abruptio placentæ.

Diseases of the Cord.—Torsion, knots, stenosis, which latter is usually located at the placental or navel insertion.

Diseases of the Amnion.—Acute polyhydramnion, oligohydramnion, amniotic adhesions to the fetus, causing its death.

Diseases of the Fetal Body.—Anomalies of growth; congenital weakness from ill parents,—alcoholism, anemia, saturnism, tobacco, etc.; single and double monsters (rather commonly found, and they would be oftener discovered by proper search); acute infectious diseases—typhoid, recurrent fever, malaria, measles, scarlatina, cholera, etc.; chronic infections—tuberculosis, syphilis (usually after the fifth month); asphyxia of the child from low blood-pressure (anemia, syncope, shock) or from hemorrhages into the placenta in nephritis of the mother—apoplexia placentæ; insolation, continuous high temperature being most dangerous; sudden high temperature is also dangerous, but the fetus tolerates a gradual rise better (Runge); toxemia, either autogenic or exogenic, under the former being hyperemesis gravidarum, chorea, eclampsia, etc.; under the latter, alcohol, tobacco (especially noticeable in cigar-makers), lead, carbon monoxid, etc. Infection of the fetus, acquired via the blood of the mother, the latter being apparently well, is a frequent cause of abortion. Pierrepont believes that toxins coming from septic conditions of the mother's mouth can cause abortion and premature delivery.

How does the death of the fetus cause abortion? (1) The ovum does not become a foreign body and stimulate the uterus to effect its expulsion, because the vascular connections may be kept up for months and the chorion be so well nourished that it grows. If the ovum were destroyed, this explanation would hold. (2) When the fetus dies, the stimulation of the growth of the ovum ceases and the alteration of the endometrial reflex brings on abortion—purely hypothetic. (3) The fetus and placenta may develop a hormone, which, reaching the blood, inhibits uterine action, failing which, abortion results; the corpus luteum does not grow after fetal death, and its restraining influence is lost—hypothetic.

Between the death of the fetus and its expulsion a period varying from a few hours to days, weeks, or months may elapse. The last is called *missed abortion.* Pieces of placenta may remain in the uterus as long as nine months (author) and eleven months (Playfair). Ries found villi sixteen years after an abortion.

Maternal Causes.—Next to criminal interference decidual endometritis is the most frequent cause of abortion, and especially of the habitual early interruption of pregnancy. It acts by predisposing to hemorrhages in the decidua which kill the fetus or stimulate uterine contractions; by rendering the uterus irritable and intolerant of the ovum; by raising barriers against the growth of the placenta; by not allowing the ovum to obtain a solid nidus or a well-located one (placenta prævia). The bacteria in the endometrium or in the cervix may invade the ovum and kill the fetus. Endometritis deciduæ glandularis produces a condition called *hydrorrhœa gravidarum*, attended by the sudden periodic discharge of accumulated secretions, and on one of such occasions the uterus may be urged to action. Acute gonorrhea and peri-uterine infection, for example, salpingitis or appendicitis, occasionally interrupt gestation.

Chronic metritis is the usual accompaniment of endometritis, and renders the womb still more intolerant of gestation—the "irritable uterus" of the older writers. The uterine muscle cannot hypertrophy and expand as it should.

Malformations and diseases of the uterus, infantilism, single or double-horned uteri, fibroids, polypi, lacerations of the cervix, especially with coincident cervicitis and endometritis, amputated cervix—all are sometimes causative. Retroflexion and retroversion have already been referred to as frequent causes of abortion; indeed, sometimes when abortion is threatened replacement of the uterus allows the gestation to go to term.

Acute infectious diseases of the mother often cause abortion, as was said, through the disease passing over and killing the fetus, but they act also by causing an endometritis which shows a strong tendency to become hemorrhagic. The sudden rise of temperature may stimulate the uterus to action, as also may the hypercarbonization of the blood in those diseases which are attended by cyanosis—for example, pneumonia. Hemolysis also affects the fetus through the anemia of the mother.

Sepsis should be added to the list of infectious diseases. It gains entrance to the uterus during pregnancy and kills the ovum primarily or secondarily. In cows epidemic abortion sometimes occurs, and the pathogenic organisms have been detected on the penis of the bull which had served the sick animals (Wallace). Epidemics of abortion in cows may also be caused by the Brucella abortus of Bang, which gains entrance through the mouth, lungs, vagina, or intestine (Lit., P. Morales-Otero). Abortion from such a cause occurs in the human, as cases reported by Vignes and De Forrest prove. Bacteria may reach the ovum from a neighboring focus of infection, e. g., appendix or tube, from the infected cervix or vagina, or by way of the blood-stream (Fig. 372a), analogously to other distant localizations of infection, the teeth, tonsils, so ably demonstrated by Billings and Rosenow.

Syphilis is a frequent cause of abortion after the fourth month, either by passing over to the child or by destroying it through changes in the decidua.

Trauma or violence is very frequently advanced by the patient to explain the accident, but unless it is applied to the uterus direct, we must assume that one of the predisposing causes—endometritis, etc.—is really active. A special predisposition must exist to explain those cases where a slight jar, a misstep, a nervous shock, an automobile ride, and other mild occurrences bring on abortion. On the other hand, the severest injuries, mental and physical, are sometimes inflicted on the gravida without disturbing the uterus. Thomas quotes a case where a pregnant woman jumped from an upper window, falling through a shed on to a stone flagging, but carried through to term, and reports another where a heedless boy threw a dead, bleeding black snake around his sister's neck, and in spite of the fact that she suffered from hysteric syncope and convulsions for several days, the pregnancy, then at four months, went to term. The child was not "marked."

Excessive coitus is a frequent cause of abortion in the newly married. Either the absorbed spermatoxins kill the embryo, or the corpus luteum formation is hindered by the frequent bursting of Graafian follicles superinduced by sexual intemperance, or the mechanical and vascular disturbance loosens the ovum from its bed. Operations come under the heading of trauma, but, unless some predisposition exists, usually do not affect the pregnancy. The author has removed fibroids from the pregnant uterus, in one case exposing the chorion, and has amputated the cervix, without inciting contractions. On the other hand, a slight operation on a distant organ may result in miscarriage. Ovarian tumors have repeatedly been extirpated safely (66 per cent. of cases), as have also breast and other tumors. It is usually the shock and the sepsis which bring on the abortion. Appendicitis cases are especially prone, probably because of the infection. Removal of both ovaries during pregnancy has brought out the fact that they are not needed for labor, because the pregnancy and parturition have so often proceeded naturally. It seems that double ovariotomy in the early months is more dangerous to gestation than later, and the fact is explained on the theory that the secretion of the corpus luteum is necessary for the growth of the ovum and uterus. Criminal traumatism, for example, puncture of the ovum, insertion of catheters, etc., does not come under this heading, nor does the administration of drugs— sabine, ergot, cantharides, which have to be given in poisonous doses to be effective in emptying the uterus. Overdose of x-rays, antitoxic serums, and vaccines have been known to cause abortion.

Anesthesia may cause death of the fetus if too prolonged or attended by great cyanosis, as in the continuous nitrous oxid method. Extraction of teeth under brief nitrous oxid gas anesthesia is allowable, a dentist in this city who has administered it over 12,000 times having assured the author that he has never thus caused an abortion.

Endocrinal disturbances, hypopituitarism, ovarian dysfunction, hypothyroidism, etc., are possible causes. More study of this aspect of each case is desirable.

It is necessary, especially in medicolegal cases, to decide whether, in a given instance, the accused injury really caused the abortion, and this point can seldom be determined. As criteria may be mentioned: the ovum must be macroscopically and microscopically healthy, and show no other cause for its expulsion, and the death of the ovum and its expulsion must be proved to have occurred very shortly after the traumatism.

Paternal Causes.—Without doubt some men produce a sperma which is too weak to give the ovum the necessary generative impulse. Observation of many cases of male sterility has convinced the author of the truth of this statement, and examination of the semen in these instances has shown a paucity of spermatozoids, or such as were short-lived or inactive. Syphilis, tuberculosis, general paresis, general debility, perhaps from excessive coitus or from alcoholism, will produce such conditions. It is said that abortion is frequent in cows that were covered by a sexually exhausted bull. A man with a purulent discharge in the semen may cause an infection in the uterus, with septic abortion. Men workers in lead, phosphorus, mercury, etc., are not seldom sterile. It is a well-established fact that *x*-ray operators become sterile, and it would be interesting to discover if their total sterility is preceded by a series of abortions in their wives.

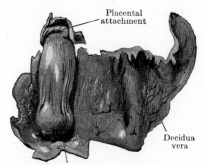

Fig. 372.—Cast of Uterus Showing Decidua Vera and Decidua Reflexa Long Drawn Out and Containing the Ovum and a Blood-clot.

Premature labor is produced by the same factors that bring on abortion, but syphilis plays an important rôle here, it being estimated that from 15 to 30 per cent. of the cases are thus caused. Next

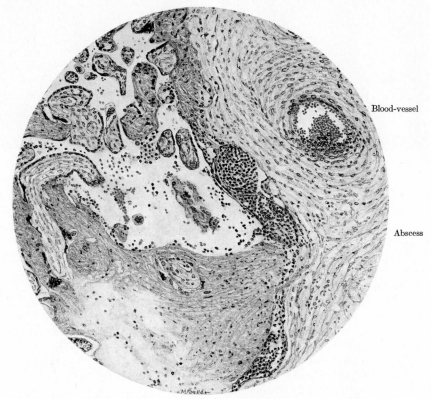

Fig. 372a.—Abortion at Five Months Caused by Suppurative Appendicitis. Note placentitis, inflammatory zones around blood-vessel and abscess.

comes nephritis, with placental hemorrhages or infarcts. Twins often come prematurely because of the lack of room in the uterus, and any tumor in the abdomen which is large enough may interfere with the development of the uterus.

Habitual abortion means that successive pregnancies are interrupted, usually at the same period of development.

Syphilis is found as the active factor in 20 to 30 per cent., and more especially in miscarriages of the later months. Each successive abortion occurs at a later period until a living child is born, but it perishes from congenital syphilis, and finally the disease has become so attenuated that a viable child is delivered. Appropriate treatment, of course, will cut the process short, and a living healthy child is delivered at term.

Chronic endometritis is more frequently a cause of repeated early abortion than in the later months, and it is not seldom combined with uterine displacement. Each abortion aggravates the endometritis, a "vicious circle" being established. Laceration and amputation of the cervix sometimes prevent carrying a fetus to term, as do fibroids and infantile uterus also.

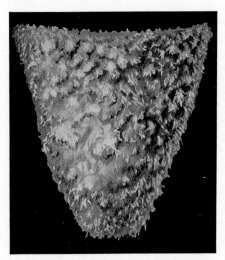

FIG. 373.—DECIDUAL CAST OF UTERUS A LITTLE FURTHER ADVANCED THAN FIG. 372, SHOWING THE SHAPE OF THE CAVITY.
Note shaggy maternal surface of decidua.

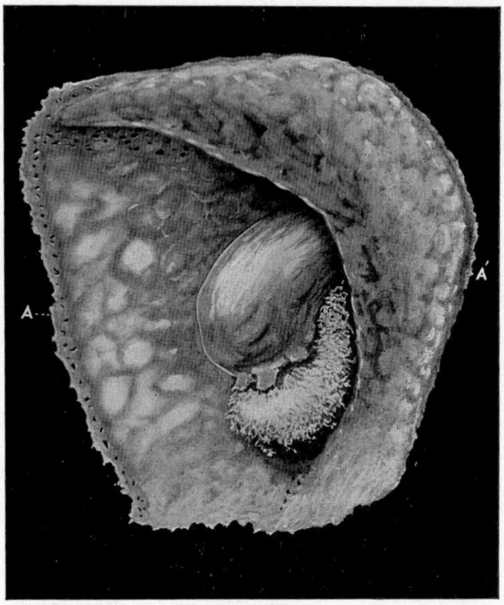

FIG. 374.—SAME AS FIG. 373, SHOWING CAST OPENED AT ONE SIDE.
The decidua is thinner at the edges, where it lay in the corners of the uterine cavity, and shows the opening of the glands. The decidua reflexa is torn, allowing the ovum partly to escape.

The author believes that infection of the ovum, as was above described, is at the root of much fetal pathology and may be active here too.

Nephritis, diabetes, or constitutional disorder, such as anemia, hypothyroidism, should always be searched for in these cases.

Deficiency diseases, lack of calcium, avitaminosis, etc. require consideration.

The influence of the father may not be forgotten. He may have gonorrhea, which keeps up a cervicitis or endometritis. He may not be capable of procreating a viable child. Chronic lead-poisoning is well known to have such an effect, and probably other poisons, especially alcohol, have similar action. Stockard has proved in guinea-pigs that the evil effects of alcohol may be transmitted to the third generation. Finally, there is a class of cases where none of the preceding conditions can be found, yet the woman cannot carry a child through to term. (See Chapter LXXIV, Induced Labor.)

Mechanism.—As in the description of the mechanism of labor, in abortion we also discuss three factors—the powers, the passages, and the passengers. Uterine action accomplishes nearly all the work of abortion except the expulsion of the loosened ovum from the vagina, which the abdominal muscles do. The bony passages practically never come into consideration, and the soft parts very seldom, but the ovum plays an important part. In the first two months the decidua is thick, vascular, and friable, the ovum small, soft, and compressible. It requires considerable effort by the uterus to separate and expel the former, while the little ovum slips out unobserved. From the eighth to the twentieth week the placenta plays the main rôle; it is relatively large, separates with difficulty, especially from the uterine cornua, and such removal is usually attended by profuse hemorrhage. After the twentieth week the fetus is the most important passenger, and the character of the labor resembles more and more that at term. Separation of the ovum ·occurs in the spongy layer of the decidua, and since the regressive changes—the

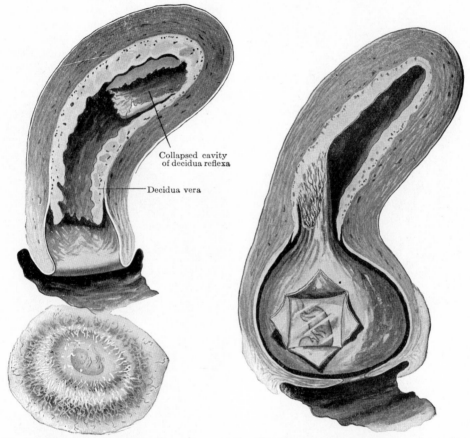

Collapsed cavity
of decidua reflexa

Decidua vera

FIG. 375.—WHEN THE NAKED OVUM, SHOWN BELOW, IS EXPELLED, ALL THE DECIDUÆ ARE LEFT IN THE UTERUS.

FIG. 376.—CERVICAL ABORTION, THE OVUM STILL IN THE REFLEXA AND THE PLACENTA DRAWN OUT, BUT ADHERENT AT ITS BASE.

necrosis—have not progressed far, this is often incomplete, and pieces of membrane or placenta are likely to be retained, especially in the tubal corners. One may, therefore, distinguish three fairly well-defined periods:

First Period.—In the first six to eight weeks the whole ovum is usually born, covered by the decidua, and it is often possible to reconstruct the conditions which existed in the uterus, as in Figs. 372, 373, 374. An ovum may be expelled naked, as in Fig. 375, or covered with portions of the decidua. Whenever the ovum alone, covered by the shaggy coat of villi, is expelled, one must conclude that the deciduæ still remain in the uterus, and will require another effort of nature, which is often attended by profuse hemorrhage. In a few cases the deciduæ dissolve and come away in pieces in the lochia. Should the external os, as in primiparæ, offer resistance and not dilate, the ovum is arrested in the distended cervix, the internal os closing. This was called cervical pregnancy by Rokitansky, but a better term is cervical abortion (Fig. 376). Simple dilatation of the constricted os is sufficient to liberate the ovum. True cervical-isthmial pregnancy occurs (Devraigne, Iolkin, 39 cases).

Second Period.—Several courses are taken by the abortive process during the third and fourth months. First the whole ovum is expelled—the fetus in an intact sac and a large part of the decidua covering it. This may be called the typical course, and offers the best prognosis for the mother, since hemorrhage is usually mild, interference is seldom necessary, and the remains of the decidua come away with the lochia.

Second, the membranes rupture, the fetus is extruded, the cervix closes, and

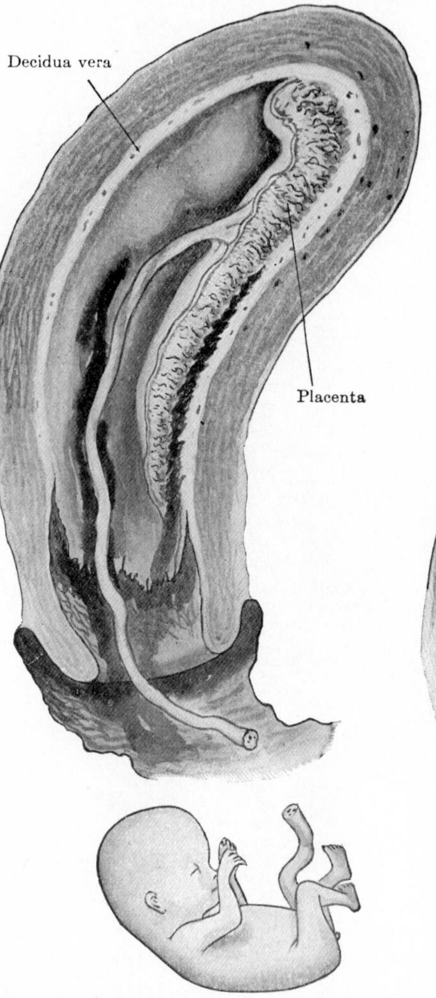

FIG. 377.—INCOMPLETE ABORTION—THREE MONTHS. When the fetus only is expelled, all the secundines remain in the uterus.

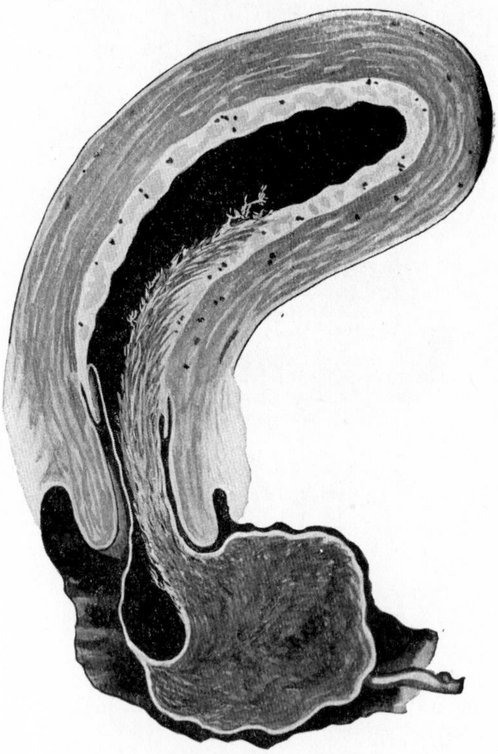

FIG. 378.—PLACENTA PROTRUDING POLYPOID INTO VAGINA AND PARTLY ATTACHED, INVITING SEPSIS. THICK DECIDUA STILL IN UTERUS.

the uterus has to make a second effort to expel the secundines (Figs. 377 and 378). During the interval, owing to partial separation of the placenta, hemorrhage is profuse, infection of the placenta may occur, and interference of some sort is usually necessary, all of which cause a worse prognosis.

Thirdly, the decidua reflexa and the chorion break, allowing the fetus in the amniotic sac to escape. A beautiful specimen is here shown (Fig. 379). The accoucheur must remember that the uterus still contains the placenta, chorion, and deciduæ.

In abortion the uterine contractions act the same as in labor, and dilatation of the cervix is produced in the same way, but, owing to the vascularity of the decidua, hemorrhage occurs as soon as the contractions begin, because the decidua loosens from the uterine wall. This separation begins at the cervix, proceeds to the fundus (Fig. 380), being latest in the tubal corners. Hemorrhages into the decidua and into the ovum occur and aid in the separation. Upon the delivery of its contents the uterus contracts down on itself and involution begins. This is slower and more likely to be incomplete after abortion than after labor at term. After-pains are sometimes observed, and milk not rarely appears in the breasts. In abortion, even before the fifth month of gestation, there may be considerable engorgement of the mammæ.

Abortion after the fifth month is really a labor in miniature, and needs no further description. Breech and abnormal presentations are commoner, and the whole ovum is not seldom extruded intact. Expulsion of an unbroken ovum is very rare in the last months of pregnancy.

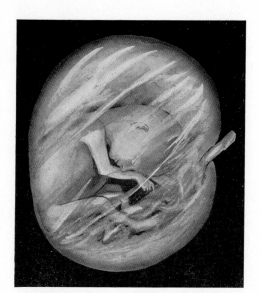

FIG. 379.—FŒTUS IN AMNIOTIC SAC INTACT.

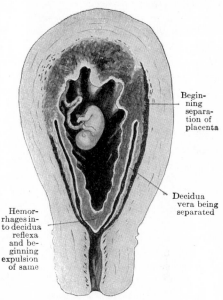

Begin-
ning
separa-
tion of
placenta

Decidua
vera being
separated

Hemor-
rhages in-
to decidua
reflexa
and be-
ginning
expulsion
of same

FIG. 380.—BEGINNING ABORTION AT SIXTH WEEK.

Symptoms.—Clinically, we speak of three forms of abortion,—*threatened, in progress* or *inevitable,* and *incomplete* abortion,—but four classic symptoms are present with all. These are: uterine pain, uterine hemorrhage, softening and dilatation of the cervix, presentation or expulsion of all or parts of the ovum.

Threatened abortion is indicated by a bloody discharge from the uterus, and sometimes by slight drawing pains in the back and pelvis, similar to menstrual sensations. The blood may come with a gush or ooze, or appear as a brownish, flaky mucus. Pain may be a slight symptom, or there may be only a sense of weight in the pelvis. On vaginal examination the uterus may feel harder than normal, which is because it is contracting. Softening and dilatation of the cervix seldom occur in threatened abortion, but the author has had several cases where the cervix opened so that the finger felt the lower pole of the ovum, and yet, after subsidence of the symptoms, the pregnancy went to term. An abortion may appear threatening for hours, days, or even months, and yet pregnancy go to full term. Again, suddenly, profuse hemorrhage occurs, pains set in, and the process becomes inevitable.

Abortion in progress presents the same symptoms, but the hemorrhage is greater, the pains stronger and more regular, resembling those of labor. Softening and dilatation of the cervix proceed from above downward, and the shortening of the neck of the womb is easily followed by the finger in the vaginal fornices, or, when the os is opened, inside the cervix, at which time also the ovum or the edges of the separated decidua may be felt. The symptoms vary, of course, with the mechanism of the abortion.

If the whole ovum is expelled complete in one effort of the uterus, the hemorrhage is usually moderate, and the pains cease as soon as the ovum escapes from the cervix. In multiparæ, because of the open cervix, the abortion is easier and quicker than in primiparæ. If the decidua remains, it is dissolved and comes away in the profuse lochial discharge, sometimes giving it an offensive odor, but seldom causing fever, though it may leave behind a chronic thickening of the endometrium.

If the membranes break, the fetus escaping naked or clothed only in its amnion, the remainder is expelled after minutes or hours, or, because of the profuse hemorrhage which usually occurs, the accoucheur has to interfere and clean out the uterus. Hemorrhage and pains may cease in the interval, during which time the case is called one of incomplete abortion.

Incomplete abortion means that the process has started, but that the uterus is not entirely rid of its contents. This does not include the retention in the uterus of a whole but dead ovum—which is "missed abortion." Incomplete abortion is a dangerous condition, because of its immediate and remote bad sequelæ: (*a*) The cervix partly closes after the escape of the fetus, and the placenta, membranes, and thick decidua gradually break down and are discharged in the lochia. In these cases the lochia are profuse and bloody, sometimes with an odor, and continue thus until the last vestige is removed. Chronic endometritis is almost always the final result of such a process (Fig. 381). (*b*) A complete interval of rest may be noted until, after hours, days, or even months, the uterus suddenly expels its contents. (*c*) Decomposition sets in, the pieces soften and are exfoliated, a layer of granulations separating the live from the dead tissue, or the bacteria break through this barrier, sepsis and sometimes death resulting. (*d*) A placental polyp is formed, the attached portion of the placenta being well nourished, layers of fibrin being deposited and organized on the outside until a pedunculated tumor is created, which may protrude from the cervix. Syncytioma malignum is not so common in these cases as in hydatid moles.

Diagnosis.—*Threatened Abortion.*—If the fact of normal pregnancy is known, uterine hemorrhage and uterine pains signify that interruption of gestation threatens. It is not easy to diagnose early pregnancy when the uterus is contracting, because then it stimulates other conditions, for example, fibroid, chronic metritis, ectopic ovum. On bimanual examination the large, contracting and relaxing uterus, the beginning softening and shortening of the cervix, and the bloody discharge show that some abnormal process is going on. The rule is to treat every case of hemorrhage, after a period of amenorrhea occurring in a woman capable of reproduction, as one of abortion.

Differential diagnosis must be made from ectopic gestation, hemorrhage from cervical erosions (not rare), varices (very rare), hydrorrhœa gravidarum, and, in addition, all the conditions not associated with pregnancy, for example, neoplasms and malpositions. When pregnancy and threatened miscarriage are associated with a neoplasm, truly complicated conditions are presented for differentiation.

Inevitable abortion is more easily determined—the cervix is shortened, its angle with the corpus straightened, the external os dilated, allowing the finger to feel the ovum, and pieces of the decidua or of the ovum are expelled; hemorrhage is more profuse, the bag of waters ruptures, and painful uterine contractions are usually present. These signs enable us to say that an abortion is inevitable, but in rare instances the cervix may close, the hemorrhage ceasing, and pregnancy goes on to term. The discharge of decidua is usually considered positive evidence of an unavoidable abortion, but the author had one case of double uterus where the decidua was discharged from one side, the other being pregnant. The rupture of the membranes may be simulated by hydrorrhœa gravidarum, or graviditas examnialis (*q. v.*, p. 524). After pregnancy is determined the differential diagnosis in abortion has to deal only with ectopic gestation, and the latter must always be taken into consideration. Rarely the extrusion of a fibroid or a polyp simulates an abortion.

Incomplete Abortion.—Is the uterus empty? Here the history of the passage of the fetus or of portions of the placenta may be useful, but unless the parts have been seen by competent eyes, the information must be questioned. We decide that something is left in the uterus when a woman who has had an abortion continues to have irregular hemorrhages, with or without pains, or discharges bloody lochia, with occasional clots or bits of tissue, for a long time. Examination will reveal a large, soft, subinvoluted uterus, which sometimes contracts, with a succulent, patulous cervix through which the finger feels shreds of decidua, placenta, or clots. Microscopic examination of discharged or cureted pieces of tissue may show chorionic villi. In some cases the diagnosis as to whether the uterus is empty or not may be impossible without a curetage. The differential diagnosis must be made from subinvolution, endometritis post-abortum, ectopic gestation, fibroids, chorio-epithelioma, polypi, and occasionally the diagnosis of a previously existing pregnancy comes up. Even the microscope may fail to settle the question. The cureted material may show large and convoluted uterine glands (Opitz), but

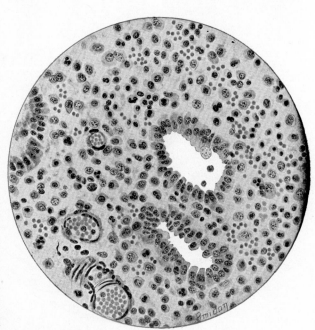

Fig. 381.—Endometritis Post-abortum.

these are not pathognomonic. Hyaline degeneration of the uterine vessels gives more information. Aschheim-Zondek persists in incomplete abortion.

Prognosis.—Few women die from hemorrhage during abortion because, if the bleeding is marked, the patient faints and clotting stops the small blood-vessels. It is much different at term. If the hemorrhage is long continued, the unavoidable small loss during the abortion may prove fatal. Death is usually due to infection introduced from without, for example, by the criminal abortionist or by the physician through a lack of asepsis. It must be remembered that coitus can cause infection of the uterus, which results in abortion, and may be followed by fatal septicemia. It is usual, however, in cases of septic abortion, to suppose that an abortionist has been at work. If the uterus has been perforated and sepsis results, death is the more common termination.

The prognosis as to health is worse than after labor at full term. Involution is slower, lasting several months, and if infection has occurred, the uterus may never be normal again, but remains the seat of chronic metritis and endometritis. Endometritis post-abortum (Fig. 381), characterized by the prolonged persistence of

30

groups of decidual cells and hypertrophy of the mucosa, is a frequent sequel of abortion, as is also pelvic peritonitis or cellulitis. In after years women who have had one or several abortions come to the gynecologist complaining of backache, sterility, and leukorrhea, and the examination shows a large, hard uterus, hypertrophied cervix, a retroversion or retroflexion, thickening of the broad ligaments, and tenderness along the sacro-uterine folds. Such women may be invalids for life or require capital operations in order to be cured.

Treatment.—*Threatened Abortion.*—It is inadvisable to examine a woman threatened by abortion because of the danger of aggravating the uterine contractions or causing hemorrhages to separate more of the ovum; therefore it is done only when a diagnosis must be made, and with the greatest gentleness. Rest in bed with foot elevated 12 inches is the best treatment, and morphin may be given to procure absolute quiet of patient and uterus. Laudanum in 20-minim doses every

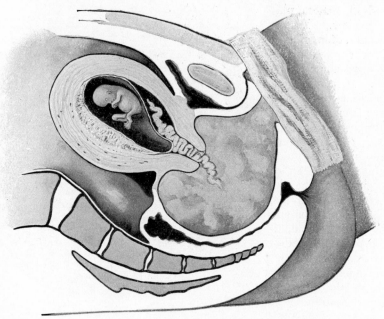

Fig. 382.—Cervix Packed with Gauze and Vagina with Cotton in the Treatment of Abortion.

four hours will usually suffice, but it may be necessary to give more, watching carefully the action of the drug. The bowels are not disturbed for the first three days, then liq. petrolatum is given, its action being helped by an olive-oil enema, the latter to avoid the patient's straining to evacuate hard feces. If the bleeding ceases, the patient may be allowed more freedom in bed, and after five days may get up, but should resume her duties very slowly, returning to bed on the slightest show of blood; if the bleeding continues, a bimanual and specular examination is made, and if the cervix is inflamed and eroded, applications of nitrate of silver (10 per cent.) and douches of permanganate of potash, 1 : 3000, are ordered. If the bleeding recommences every time the patient becomes at all active, the abortion is inevitable, a mole having probably been formed. One may not allow repeated hemorrhages to debilitate the woman. The author, in several cases of placenta prævia near term, has obtained a history of hemorrhages in early pregnancy.

How long to wait in these cases where small repeated hemorrhages occur is not easy to decide. If the local findings point to molar formation, one should not wait, but if the child is presumably alive, one will try to save it. Rest in bed, uterine sedatives, horse-serum, human serum, transfusion should be employed to stop the bleeding, and frequent blood-tests made to be sure that the gravida is not becoming dangerously anemic.

Inevitable Abortion.—Much difference exists in the treatment of abortion in progress as practised by different authors, and, indeed, no one plan will apply to all cases. A method that is ideal for the first twelve weeks must be modified toward the end of the fifth and sixth months, and again different conditions are presented for treatment, as may be seen by reverting to the pages on the Mechanism of Abortion. The ideal treatment would be "watchful expectancy," meeting the indications as they arise, similarly to our conduct during labor, but expediency may demand more active interference. The patient may live far removed from medical help, or the physician cannot remain at the bedside during the prolonged course— sometimes days—of some abortions; moreover, nothing would be gained by it, since the child is always lost and infection might invade the uterus.

If the hemorrhage is continuous, whether profuse or not, the cervix and vagina are to be tamponed. Objections to the tampon on the score of its inviting sepsis, being painful, and causing retention of urine are of little weight. The author treats, indirectly, through the Chicago Lying-in Hospital Dispensary, hundreds of abortions each year, and practises the treatment here recommended with uniform success.

Technic.—Everything needed is arranged near the bed or table, so that the operator, who usually has little assistance, may wait on himself. The patient is asked to empty the bladder, or she is catheterized before the tampon is inserted. The genital region is shaved, as for any gynecologic operation, scrubbed with soap and warm water, and then thoroughly washed with 1 : 1000 bichlorid. Painting with tr. iodi or 4 per cent. mercurochrome is recommended. The accoucheur sterilizes his hands, draws on sterile rubber gloves, and washes the vagina and cervix gently but thoroughly with 1 per cent. lysol solution. For the tamponade the dorsal, Sims' lateral, or knee-chest position may be used: the former is the usual, the last a very good one if short of help. Whenever possible the author uses a table for such work. A perineal retractor, long dressing forceps, scissors, and catheter are the only instruments needed. First the cervix is packed with a strip of narrow, plain, sterilized gauze, which extends up into the uterus (Fig. 382). Then the vault of the vagina is filled with pieces of dry, thoroughly sterile cotton, or the same, squeezed dry out of a 0.5 per cent. lysol solution. After one layer of cotton is placed around the cervix it is firmly tamped into the fornices and the second layer then put in, the packing and tamping into place being executed by two fingers. The upper two-thirds of the vagina are thus tightly and evenly plugged, but the lower third needs only a loose pack, which is good too because it relieves the urethra from pressure. A gauze pad is laid against the vulva, a T-binder applied, making moderate counterpressure, and the patient put to bed. A properly applied tampon will stop hemorrhage absolutely, and every practitioner ought to be able to insert it. Often the author has removed a "tampon" consisting of three to six lumps of cotton pulled off a roll and placed in the vagina, without any attempt at aseptic preparation of the parts.

The tampon is allowed to remain for from sixteen to twenty-four hours, and is not removed, even if the temperature rises. During the interval pains almost always supervene, which means that the uterus is trying to expel its contents. No medicine should be given to allay this pain. Quinin, gr. iij, every hour for five doses, followed by pituitary, 10 units every four hours, will sometimes hasten the expulsion of the ovum. This is especially useful when fever exists. Often the pains cease suddenly, and one surmises that the uterus has emptied itself above the tampon. A convenient hour is selected for the removal of the tampon, but preparations should have been made for curetage under anesthesia if this should be found necessary. Often the entire ovum is found lying on the tampon, its separation having been aided by the damming back of the blood, and its expulsion having been accomplished by the uterine contractions. All that is needed in such cases is to go over the uterus lightly with a half-sharp curet, to make certain that pieces are not retained—especially in the tubal corners. Some authors advise against this curetage, but the writer does it in all cases, believing that the patients make quicker and more complete recoveries when the uterus is left absolutely smooth

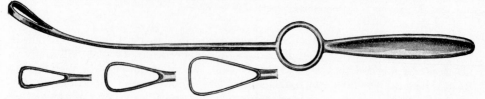

FIG. 383.—AUTHOR'S UTERINE CURET.
This is half sharp, the shank is flexible, and a ring is inserted in the handle, so that the instrument may be held securely and at the same time delicately. All curets are dangerous and should be used with the same care as a scalpel.

and clean. Without doubt much damage is caused by the curet in the hands of an unskilful practitioner, but this is no reason for condemning it—rather

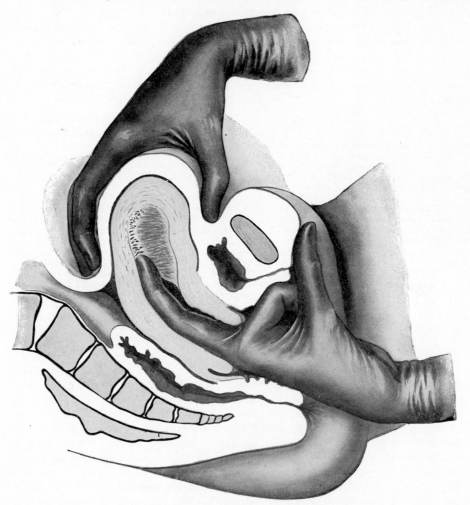

FIG. 384.—CURETAGE WITH FINGER. THE FINGER EXCELS ALL INSTRUMENTS, BUT EVEN SO, IT, AND THE OUTSIDE HAND, MUST BE USED WITH CONSUMMATE GENTLENESS!

should we seek to qualify the practitioner to use all safe means for the patient's benefit.

If, when the packing is removed, the cervix be found still closed, it is best to tampon again and empty the uterus on the following day. Forcible dilatation of the cervix is an unsafe operation, and one the author avoids whenever possible. Steel divulsors (Goodell's, Bossi's, Hegar's) even in expert hands have many times ruptured the uterus, and with fatal results. In the earliest weeks of pregnancy, after the cervix has been softened, one may procure sufficient opening with the dilator to permit curetage. Later, if the cervix is closed and rigid, vaginal anterior hysterotomy is the best method. Nowadays laminaria and other tents are rarely used because of the dangers of infection.

When the cervix is open to admit one finger, the uterus is to be emptied, preferably under ether anesthesia. If the ovum protrudes through the os, it may be

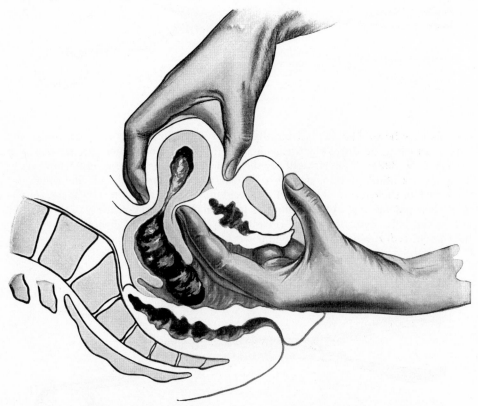

FIG. 385.—SQUEEZING OUT THE LOOSENED CONTENTS OF THE UTERUS BY BIMANUAL COMPRESSION.

grasped by the fingers or a polypus forceps and withdrawn from the uterus; then the uterine cavity is revised by the finger, and rough places smoothed over with the curet (Fig. 383). If the ovum is still in the uterus, it is completely loosened by the finger aided by the outside hand (Fig. 384). After it is freed from all its attachments, combined pressure by the two hands may squeeze it out into the vagina (Fig. 385). Should this little maneuver not succeed, *the free portion of the ovum* is grasped by an ovum forceps (Figs. 386 and 387) and gently withdrawn. Excessive care is to be observed, first, to make sure that the ovum is really floating free in the cavity of the uterus, and, second, to be absolutely certain that the forceps do not bite into the uterine wall. The latter accident has happened repeatedly and the operator been staggered to find omentum or intestine in the grasp of the instrument.

This accident may be avoided by first separating the ovum by the finger, inserting the forceps under the guidance of the finger, and then rotating the blades of the forceps during the act of closing them, a little trick which the author has attempted to illustrate in Fig. 389; on the least suspicion that more resistance is encountered than is to be expected the instrument must be released. After the main portion of the ovum is removed, the finger is inserted and the endometrium scraped clean and smooth. Since rubber gloves are used, we lose the assistance of the finger-nail. If the cervix is large enough, the finger is covered with gauze, and thus the thick

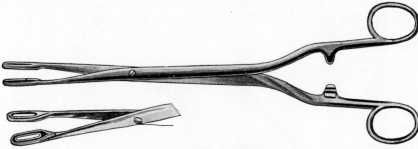

FIG. 386.—OVUM FORCEPS.

decidua may be rubbed off, but usually in early abortions it is necessary to use the curet. In using the curet the uterus is to be pulled down by means of a vulsellum forceps (Fig. 392). This straightens the canal and brings the organ within reach. Then a thick blunt sound is passed to determine the shape of the uterine canal and the length of the cavity. The curet is passed up to the fundus uteri with the gentleness of the passing of a urethral sound, being held lightly and delicately in the fingers, not in the fist. Exerting slight pressure on the scraping edge of the curet, the instrument is *drawn down and out of the cervix* with a single slow, even, gentle sweep.

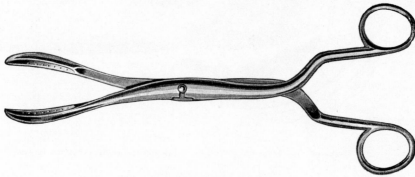

FIG. 387.—OVUM FORCEPS.

It is cleansed by moving it to and fro in a solution of lysol, then reinserted, and the process repeated, first going over the posterior wall, then the anterior, then the corners of the uterus, then the fundus from one tubal opening to the other. No to-and-fro movements are made in the uterus; each stroke of the curet must be from above downward and out. The broadest curet that will go through the cervix is to be used, but the smaller ones may be needed for cleaning out the tubal corners. By placing two fingers in the vagina one can control the movements of the curet on the anterior and posterior walls (Fig. 383), and by palpating the fundus through the abdomen one can follow it as the upper portions and tubal corners are scraped, thus avoiding the danger of perforation (Fig. 394). Now the finger revises the uterus, and any piece of tissue found adherent is loosened or removed by the curet.

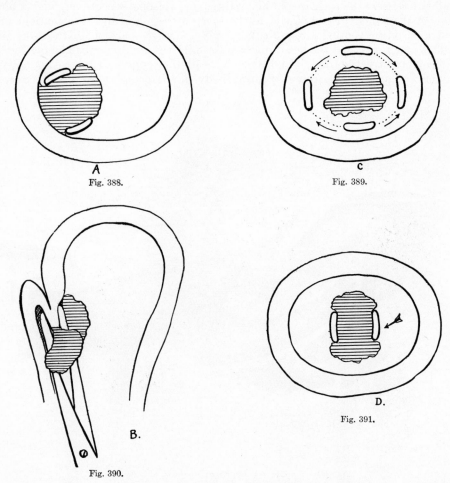

Fig. 388.

Fig. 389.

Fig. 390.

Fig. 391.

FIGS. 388, 389, 390, AND 391.—A AND B, FAULTY METHOD OF USING OVUM FORCEPS, BRINGING DANGER OF PERFORATION. C AND D, CORRECT METHOD OF USING OVUM FORCEPS.

Before the end of the twelfth week the removal of the ovum is easily accomplished, and dilatation of the cervix to admit one finger is usually sufficient. After

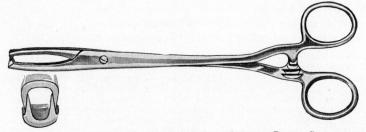

FIG. 392.—VULSELLUM FORCEPS WITH TEETH PROTECTED TO PREVENT INJURY TO RUBBER GLOVES WHILE OPERATING.

this period the fetus is larger and more dilatation is required, for which reason the tampon should be used to procure it, or a small colpeurynter is employed. Again the author warns against rapid dilatation with steel divulsors. If, at the time of operation, the cervix is not large enough to deliver the fetus entire, it may be delivered after morcellement. With the fingers in the uterus a foot is drawn down, and with scissors the body is split along the spine, grasping successively higher portions of the trunk. Heed is paid to the sharp little bones, and all attention concentrated on preventing injury to the cervix. With a sharp-pointed scissors the skull is punctured, and the head squeezed flat with the ovum forceps and delivered. If, inadvertently, the trunk is pulled off the head, the operator may have not a little trouble in engaging the round, floating body in the grasp of the ovum forceps.

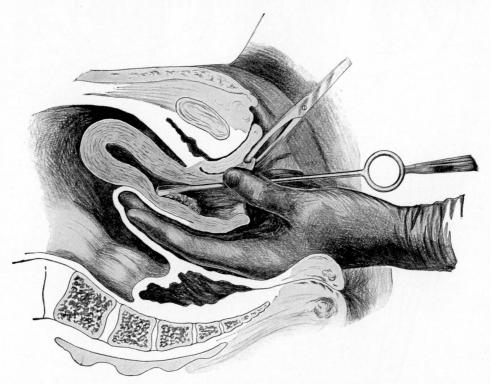

Fig. 393.—Fingers Follow Every Movement of Curet.

Fig. 387 shows a good instrument to use in this emergency—an old-fashioned stone forceps; the blades are opened in the uterus, and the head pressed into them by the abdominal hand. A better way, in difficult cases, when the cervix is very long, thick, and hard, is to make a transverse incision in the vagina at its junction with the cervix, push the bladder from the anterior wall, and incise the uterus, as in vaginal cesarean section. Any one who has attempted to remove a five months' fetus through a long, hard, closed cervix will appreciate its difficulties.

Accidents.—*Hemorrhage* is usually mild; only rarely is it necessary to pack, and the author recommends narrow gauze impregnated with a mild antiseptic (for example, weak iodin), placed with a curved dressing forceps or the tubular packer shown on p. 983. If the patient bleeds too freely during curetage, 10 units of pituitary injected into the cervix will contract the uterus, reduce the bleeding and give a firm base for the curette. If, when called to an abortion, the woman is in shock from loss of blood, the uterus and vagina are to be quickly packed, salt solution administered, and the emptying of the uterus left until the next day, by which time recovery from the effects of the hemorrhage has occurred. Transfusion.

Perforation of the uterus is a not infrequent occurrence and not seldom fatal. It is due to ignorance of the dangers of curetage and rough handling by the operator, but may also occur to the most skilful, because the uterine wall is sometimes pathologically soft and friable. This is especially true in septic cases and during the puerperium. Dührssen reports that after extirpation of a uterus inadvertently perforated, the organ was found to be so soft that the curet sank into it merely by its own weight. The placental site feels rough, and the fissures in it allow the finger or curet to enter the mucosa (Fig. 395), giving the impression that there is a piece of placenta still adherent. Thus the operator is misguided, and soon perforates into the peritoneal cavity. If the uterus is soft, the curet may be punched through its wall, especially if the operator uses force on the upstroke. Branched or bougie dilators may rupture the cervix and lower uterine segment, and the polypus or ovum forceps may grasp and tear off the inverted uterine wall, as in Fig. 390. All these accidents may be avoided by using the fingers, where possible, and by observance of the rules for their prevention. One diagnoses a perforation by the excessive freedom of movement of the end of the curet, the depth to which it disappears in the uterus, and the impingement against the bony walls of the pelvis. Not to recognize such an accident until gut or omentum is visible would be an inexcusable error of art. If a perforation occurs, the case immediately assumes a serious aspect and requires most careful consideration. Should there be the least suspicion of injury to the bowel or the omentum, the belly is to be opened immediately, the damage, if any, repaired, the uterus opened, cleansed, and sutured, after which it is drained through the vagina. Small gut is sutured or resected. The injured large intestine is drawn up into the wound and an artificial anus made. In the assurance that the viscera have not been hurt,

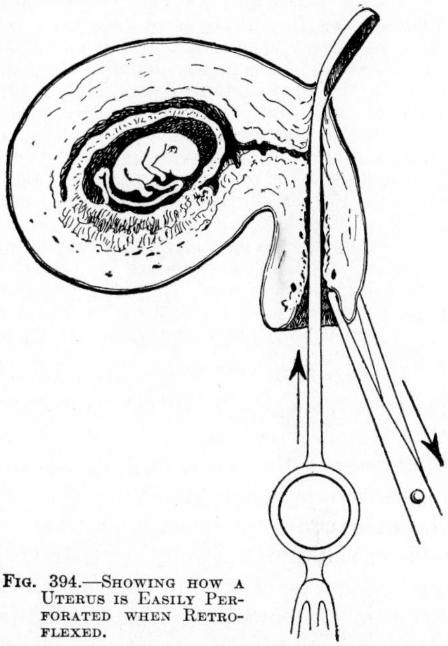

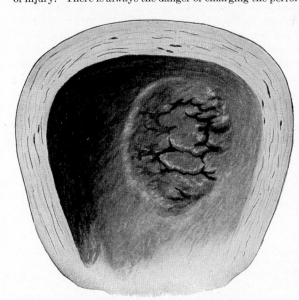

FIG. 394.—SHOWING HOW A UTERUS IS EASILY PERFORATED WHEN RETROFLEXED.

vaginal anterior hysterotomy is to be performed, the uterine cavity emptied, the rent lightly packed with gauze, leading this into the vagina, and then the uterus closed as after vaginal cesarean section. This method is safer than to attempt to curet the uterus and to try to avoid the site of injury. There is always the danger of enlarging the perforation and of injuring the bowel in thus operating blindly. A single perforation of the uterus may be treated by packing, though the accoucheur always takes a little risk here if the finger cannot confirm the diagnosis of the extent of the damage.

The above treatment is applicable only to cases where the perforation occurred in a hospital—an accident in skilful hands, but if the woman is brought in with a history of such an injury, or with omentum or gut hanging out of the cervix, the treatment must be radical—laparotomy, repair of visceral damage, extirpation of the uterus, free pelvic drainage. Only rarely, in a young woman, would one consider the risk of peritonitis, in trying to save the uterus.

Almost unbelievable reports are made of such cases. Stoeckel tells that an anesthetizer called the operator's notice to the rapid flattening of the patient's belly—he had pulled out 16 feet of gut which were found in the drainage pan: replacement through the rent, laparotomy, resection, hysterectomy, recovery, but malnutrition!

Another patient walked into the hospital her intestines trailing on the floor; resection of 17 feet, repair of uterine rent, recovery!

FIG. 395.—PLACENTAL SITE IN ABORTION.
The slightly raised cleft surface gives the impression that pieces of placenta are still adherent.

In cases of septic abortion perforation of the uterus is nearly always fatal but here hysterectomy and broad pelvic drainage must be done. An x-ray picture of the pelvis is to be taken to discover a foreign body, catheter sound, tent, etc. If such is there it must be removed, vaginally if possible, otherwise abdominally.

Acute Dilatation of the Uterus.—Occasionally, while cureting a uterus, the curet slips far beyond a normal depth and the operator fears he has perforated the organ. Examination shows no puncture, and the conclusion must be drawn that the uterus dilated suddenly, or that the instrument passed into the tube (?). The author has observed 2 cases where the uterus seemed to dilate enormously during early pregnancy. Wulff gives latest literature.

Incomplete Operation.—Rarely the accoucheur may be unable to empty the uterus completely, which occurs more commonly after the fourth month. The cervix offers unexpected resistance, or the morcellation of the fetus is impossible and preparations have not been made for a cutting operation. Whether the case is clean or not, the mode of procedure here is to pack the uterus firmly with weak iodin gauze. A leg of the fetus may be drawn down and the cervix tightly filled around it. Usually pains start up, and they may be aided by quinin and pituitrin, and after twenty-four hours, on removing the packing, the remnants of the ovum come with it. During the operation of morcellation the pieces of fetus, placenta, etc., delivered should be spread on a towel and fitted together, thus removing all doubt as to how much remains in the uterus.

Extra-uterine pregnancy must be thought of before every curetage, and a careful bimanual examination made to eliminate it. Such an operation on the uterus would almost surely cause rupture of the sac. Indeed, it is necessary to make a careful bimanual examination as a routine practice before operating, to discover the existence of adnexa tumors, for example, pregnancy, pus-tubes, appendicitis, and to determine the position and mobility of the uterus.

Incomplete Abortion.—After the diagnosis of material remaining in the uterus has been made, the best treatment is its removal, without trusting entirely to nature's efforts. Two courses are advised: one, immediate curetage, dilating the uterus if necessary; the other, packing the uterine cavity, tampon of the vagina, and waiting for the contractions of the uterus to expel its contents. The author recommends the latter course for general practice. If the patient is in a good maternity hospital, and on the first examination the cervix is found soft and open for the finger, the uterus may be cleared of its contents at once and the case thus definitively ended. After the tamponade of the uterovaginal tract the treatment is the same as that given under Abortion in Progress.

Septic Abortion.—When the cavity of an aborting uterus becomes infected, we speak of septic abortion. Most of such cases are the result of criminal interference by midwives or other abortionists, but sometimes the woman herself passes instruments into the cervix or injects fluids of some kind—usually irritating antiseptics. Thomas tells of a physician's wife who had pushed an umbrella rib up through her diaphragm. The author had a case where the belly was found full of milk, which the unfortunate woman had injected into the uterus. The diagnosis in such instances is very difficult, because the patient generally denies the facts. A thorough physical examination of the whole body will not fail to locate the trouble in the genitalia, and then the demonstration of gestation will clinch the diagnosis. The signs and symptoms of infection will be considered under Puerperal Fever.

Schottmüller, in 100 cases of septic abortion, found the following bacteria:

Streptococcus anaërobius putrificus..................... 29 times
Staphylococcus.. 26 "
Bacterium coli.. 19 "
Streptococcus vaginalis...............................   8 "
Streptococcus erysipelatis............................   6 "
Bacterium phlegmonis emphysematosæ (Fränkel).........   5 "
Bacterium coli hemolyticum........................... once
Gonococcus..   "
Streptococcus viridans................................   "
Bacillus paratyphus B.................................   "

The Streptococcus anaërobius putrificus could be frequently demonstrated in the blood, even in those cases where the process was believed, from clinical manifestations, to be purely local, *i. e.*, a sapremia, and it also caused violent salpingitis and fatal peritonitis.

Formerly, the accepted treatment of septic abortion was the immediate emptying of the uterus, by forcible means if necessary, and this practice is still quite general both here and abroad. My experience, however, taught me that this method carried certain risks with it, and I learned also that it was not a dangerous procedure to leave a uterus full of infected ovular remnants to the powers of nature. It has been found that the traumatism of curetage, digital as well as instrumental, may be fatal, a superficial and not dangerous infection being converted into one with strongly invasive qualities. Parametritis, salpingitis, peritonitis, and death oftener follow such drastic interference than the expectant treatment, and the duration of the illness is not much lengthened. The chill, and high fever which so often result from uterine manipulations in septic abortion are the expression of the flooding of the system with bacteria and toxins. After curetage in putrid infections the temperature soon becomes normal, but if the pus coccus, especially an invasive streptococcus, was present, the woman becomes very sick, and recovers, if at all, much more slowly. If we knew a virulent, invasive organism to be the cause of the infection, extirpation of the uterus would be the best treatment, but, unfortunately, science does not yet permit us to prove this in time for action. (See Puerperal Infection.)

Some operators clean out the uterus only when the streptococcus is absent from the smears and cultures, but experience has shown that it is impossible to rely upon the laboratory findings in such cases. Others rely on the local findings and abstain from cleaning out the uterus only if the pelvic organs are tender or palpably inflamed. This also is an unreliable guide.

My practice, therefore, in cases of septic abortion is as follows: First, a careful history of the cause is obtained. The physician must explain to the patient the dangers of making false statements or of hiding the truth. If there is reason to believe that she or an abortionist has passed an instrument through the uterus, or if there are symptoms of peritonitis, the belly had better be opened at once, the uterus extirpated, and the pelvis drained. If perforation is not suspected, one must decide whether there is anything in the uterus. The history, uterine contractions, continued bleeding, and the findings on vaginal examination—the large uterus, open cervix, and protruding masses—will settle this point. In cases of doubt, leave the uterus alone.

If there is no hemorrhage, place the patient in the Fowler position, clean out the bowels, push the nourishment and liquids, give plenty of fresh air, and wait and watch. Usually in a few days the temperature subsides, the pulse slows, and distinct betterment is apparent. After the temperature has been normal for ten to fourteen days the uterus is evacuated, but usually it empties itself before this time and we aid uterine activity by quinin and pituitary, gr. iij, every hour for five doses, then 5 Voegtlin units hypo every three hours for four doses. Where bleeding forces the hand, the interference must be done in the gentlest possible manner. Masses protruding from the cervix into the vagina are to be grasped by placenta forceps and withdrawn, then the uterus is lightly filled with weak iodoform or weak iodized gauze by means of a tubular packer and the vagina tamponed with sterile cotton—if possible, without anesthesia. At the end of twenty-four hours the gauze is removed, and often the ovular remnants come with it. If hemorrhage recurs on the removal of the tampon, it may be wiser to completely empty the uterus, using the finger *as a guide* and ovum forceps to remove masses, the curet only if unavoidable. *All squeezing or massage of the uterus must be omitted.* Before and after uterine interference in septic cases the author uses a douche of weak iodin solution, and when the uterus has been emptied, a light drain of weak iodized gauze is inserted to remain ten or twelve hours. This absorbs the blood, and when removed brings away shreds of membrane, leaving the endometrium perfectly smooth.

After this single cleansing of the uterine cavity no local interference with the reparative processes of nature is allowed, unless an abscess forms or other surgical indications arise.

In proposing a more expectant treatment for infected abortions the author is not alone. Ries and Watkins, of Chicago, Montgomery, of Philadelphia, Polak, of Brooklyn, Traugott, Benthin, and Winter, Bauereisen (1920), Latzko (1921), Baisch, de Bengoa, of Spain, and others published the same views. Dietrich in 1923 collected 10,000 cases of septic abortion, showing 4.8 per cent. mortality with active treatment and only 3.1 per cent. with the expectant. Veterinarians have long been aware of the dangers of forcibly cleaning out the septic uterus.

Summary of the Treatment of Abortion.—1. Threatened abortion—Rest in bed and opiates.

2. Abortion in progress—(*a*) If the hemorrhage is marked, pack the cervix with gauze and the vagina with cotton; (*b*) next day remove the tampon; if the ovum is delivered, empty the uterus with finger and curet; (*c*) if the ovum is not delivered and the cervix fully dilated, remove the ovum by traction, expression, or by the fingers, then revise the uterus with finger; (*d*) if the cervix is still closed, tampon again, aid expulsion with quinin and pituitrin; later vaginal anterior hysterotomy.

3. Incomplete abortion: (*a*) If the cervix is open, empty the uterus at once; (*b*) if closed, pack the uterine cavity with gauze and the vagina with cotton, quinin and pituitrin; (*c*) next day remove the same and treat as No. 2.

4. Septic abortion: Fowler position, roborant diet, etc.; if hemorrhage, tampon, quinin and pituitary then gynergen; when acute symptoms subside, evacuate; avoid ungentle handling of uterus.

Habitual Abortion.—This is one of the most unsatisfactory conditions the obstetrician has to treat. Women may have ten to twelve or more abortions without apparent cause and urgently demand relief, which is not always forthcoming. The author's routine in such cases is as follows: A careful examination of both husband and wife is made to discover, if possible, the cause, following closely the lines indicated on pp. 456 and 460, *q. v.* At least two Wassermann tests of both parents are demanded in doubtful cases. If the abortions occur in the early months some local cause in the wife will usually be found. If in the later months syphilis, toxemia, hypothyroidism, infantile uterus, and constitutional diseases, avitaminosis, are sought.

If a reasonable cause is determined, an attempt is made to remove it before the wife conceives again, but this is not always possible and, further, often no certain cause is discoverable. Search is made for focal infection, and if an aborted fetus is obtainable, it, the placenta, and the cord are examined bacteriologically. The husband is examined for infectious urethral discharges.

If lues is suspected salvarsan is prescribed for both parents, and in all cases, whether it is suspected or not, iron, arsenic, mercury, and iodin are administered as alterative tonics, and these are continued throughout gestation. An interval of two years is allowed before another pregnancy, and in the meantime both parents, by outdoor sports, travel, etc., get themselves into perfect physical health.

During gestation lues, toxemia, diabetes, etc., cervicitis, displacements can be treated more or less successfully. On empiric grounds give small amounts of thyroid throughout pregnancy.

The diet should be rich in calcium, milk, vegetables, cod-liver oil (vitamins A, D) and fruits.

The patient is kept in bed at the times the menses usually fall due, at the periods she has had the abortions in previous pregnancies, and she is enjoined to excessive care in exercise, and complete abstention from coitus. In aggravated cases one will prescribe bed rest for the whole nine months; no mental excitement; morphine when any threatening symptoms arise. Since Daneff proved there is an increased venous pressure in the pelvic veins (predisposing to hemorrhages in the decidua) a condition long suspected, it would seem reasonable to elevate the foot of the bed in the treatment of threatened and habitual abortion.

Changes in the Ovum After the Death of the Fetus and Missed Abortion.—If the fetus dies in the early weeks, the chorion and the decidua, which are nourished by maternal blood, may go on growing, but hemorrhages—apoplexies—are very common in the decidua, and one causes another until the whole periphery of the ovum is invaded. The cavity of the amnion is crowded

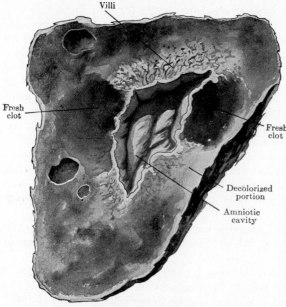

Villi

Fresh
clot

Fresh
clot

Decolorized
portion

Amniotic
cavity

Fig. 396.—Blood Mole.

together, or the blood may, in rare cases, break into the ovum itself. This is called a "blood mole" (Fig. 396). Or the membranes may undergo an eccentric hypertrophy and the amniotic cavity grows larger, fills with fluid, and may be the size of that of an ovum of two months.

Adhering to one side is found a fetus of three weeks. When the mole is older and, to a certain extent, decolorized, it is called a "fleshy mole." These moles usually cause repeated greater or smaller hemorrhages until finally the uterus expels them or the attendant interferes.

Breus describes a mole in which the amniotic cavity was invaded by smaller or larger subchorial hemorrhages, calling it a tuberous subchorial hematoma. Taussig gave it the name of hematoma mole (Fig. 397). In some unexplained cases the placenta may continue to grow after fetal death, and an enlargement of the amniotic cavity has also been found by the author.

Later in pregnancy, after the fetus has obtained some bulk, changes similar to those of a dead ectopic fetus are observed, and it may be days, months, or years before the ovum is expelled. These are cases of "missed abortion," a term first used by Duncan, and are not rare, as many authors state. (1) Maceration is most common, the fetus imbibing the dissolved blood-pigments —fœtus sanguinolentis. Its tissues are soft, the joints loose, especially the cranial, the brain is liquefied, the skin flabby, the epidermis missing in large patches, exposing the deep-red corium, and the cord thick and blood-stained; the placenta, which may go on growing even after fetal death and may attain remarkable size, is large, pale, and soft. It is impossible to decide from these changes how long the fetus has been dead, because sometimes, even after many days, little alteration of the tissues is found, and again the disintegration occurs rapidly—due to the presence of enzymes in the liquor amnii. (2) Mummification occurs more rarely. The fetus dries up, becomes leathery, and may give considerable trouble in removal by morcellation. The liquor amnii is absorbed, or represented by a thick yellow or greenish paste, the placenta being a tough white infarcted mass. This condition occurs oftenest with twins when one of the fetuses dies in the

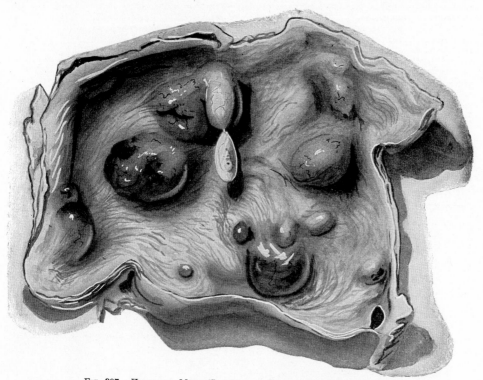

Fig. 397.—Hematoma Mole (Specimen of Chicago Lying-in Hospital).

early months and is pressed against the uterine wall by the growing twin—fœtus compressus or papyraceus (Fig. 422 on p. 513 shows the condition). (3) Lithopedion formation. This is exceptional in the uterus itself. (4) Septic infection of the uterine contents is common in ordinary but not in cases of "missed abortion," unless instrumental interference has been practised or coitus has been continued. Even after months septic infection may occur.

Missed abortion seldom gives marked symptoms. The sympathetic symptoms of pregnancy, nausea, etc., usually cease with the death of the fetus; the breast and pelvic organs retrogress; the uterus stops growing and assumes a peculiar non-resilient consistence, with frequent contractions (minus pains), and a brownish, somtimes fetid, discharge appears. General symptoms of malaise, loss of flesh, anorexia, chilliness, anemia, and afternoon |temperature are due to beginning decomposition of the ovum and demand interference. The diagnosis of missed abortion is made on two bimanual examinations with an interval of a month between them. The uterus grows smaller, not larger, harder, not softer. It is best to wait two months before deciding that the ovum is dead, because sometimes, normally, the uterus does not grow regularly, and again a hydatid mole may cause an excessive enlargement of the uterine tumor. From the history one learns that the periods have been absent for several months, that a slight bleeding, with or without pains, had occurred, since which time the signs and symptoms of pregnancy had retrogressed.

These points are very useful in the differential diagnosis which has to be made from fibroid. After one is assured that the ovum is dead, the uterus had best be emptied. The indolence of the uterus in such cases is sometimes remarkable, the author having not succeeded in days of effort in getting regular pains started, and having finally to incise the cervix to be able to clean out the uterine cavity. Hemorrhage after the curetage is the rule, and a firm uterine tampon is usually required.

Dissolution of a very early fetus and resorption, with regeneration of the decidua without exfoliation of the same, has been reported, but such an occurrence is extremely rare, and in all probability often is an error of diagnosis, the fetal and decidual structures having escaped unobserved.

Medicolegal Aspects of Abortion.—When the accoucheur has to deal with a criminal abortion, he should always have counsel, or put the patient in a hospital, avoiding all appearance of secrecy. This would excite the suspicion of connivance at the deed. While it is impossible to do so, it would be best for every one concerned if every case of criminal abortion were reported to the police authorities. Certainly if the patient dies the coroner must be notified, any other course, as signing a certificate giving a fictitious cause of death, being not alone reprehensible, but very hazardous. An antemortem statement as to whom to blame for the woman's condition is very desirable, even though the physician may not use it. The physician should obtain an accurate history, keep full records of his findings and the course of the disease, and in holding an autopsy on such a case the minutest details of the conditions found in the pelvis must be observed and noted carefully in duplicate, especial search being made for evidence of injury.

It is wise to discover, before treating an abortion case, whether any one has passed instru-. ments into the uterus, because a perforation may have been made, which later is laid at the door of the honest practitioner.

The accoucheur is often called to testify as expert in accident cases, the woman suing for damages on the ground that an injury interrupted her pregnancy. The abortion must follow very shortly on the alleged injury, or the death of the ovum must be shown to have very soon followed it, and the ovum must be otherwise normal, and the woman present none of the recognized causes of abortion, for the medical witness to be able to assert for or against the plaintiff. Indeed, in these actions the witness can usually only say that it is or is not probable that the abortion was caused by the accused injury.

Slight superficial maceration of the skin has been observed in fetuses delivered alive—due to toxemia, or the bile acids of the meconium. Must differentiate lues, impetigo, septic eruptions. The diagnosis of a previous abortion may need to be made, a subject which was discussed under the Diagnosis of the Puerperium.

Premature labor is a labor in miniature, and hardly requires separate discussion. Abnormal presentations are more frequent than at term, the breech presenting thrice as often. Shoulder presentation is also common, but usually nature terminates the case by either spontaneous rectification or evolution. (See Chapter L.) Special regard must be paid to the child, because, owing to its delicacy, it may be injured during birth. Cephalic presentation is the best for premature babies, a fact always to be borne in mind in operative deliveries before term; indeed, the indication for operation must be strict in such cases. Arrangements are to be made beforehand to receive the weak infant into a warm atmosphere—an incubator, if possible. Shock is a vital factor with them.

Anomalies in the separation and expulsion of the placenta are perhaps a little more common than at term, and the accoucheur must see that the uterus is thoroughly emptied and in firm contraction. Involution is slower than at term. Ergot is to be given for ten days postpartum.

Literature

Baisch: Zentralbl. f. Gyn., 1921, No. 11, p. 408, Lit.—*Beuttner:* Acute Dil. of Uterus.—*Daneff:* Zentb. für Gyn., April 11, 1931.—*de Snoo:* Monatsschr. f. Geb. u. Gyn., February, 1922, p. 2.—*Devraigne:* "Isthmial Pregnancy," L'Obstetrique, November, 1911, p. 961. Literature.—*Dietrich:* Zentralbl. f. Gyn., 1923, No. 27, p. 1087.— *Iolkin:* Zentralbl. für Gynaek., November 27, 1926, p. 3071.—*Latzko:* Zentralbl. f. Gyn., 1921, No. 12, p. 438.— *Meyer:* Amer. Jour. Obst. and Gyn., August, 1921, p. 140, Lit.—*Montgomery:* Jour. Amer. Med. Assoc., October 9, 1915.—*Morales-Otero, P.:* Porto Rico Jour. of Public Health, September, 1930.—*Oldham:* Rob. Barnes, Lond. Obst. Trans., vol. xxiii.—*Pierrepont:* London Lancet, June 2, 1917.—*Schottmüller:* Zentralbl. f. Gynäk., 1911, p. 83.—*Scott:* Amer. Jour. Obst., November, 1917, p. 763.—*Stockard:* Jour. Amer. Med. Assoc., October 17, 1914, p. 1400.—*Stoeckel, W.:* Lehrbuch der Geb., 1930, p. 691.—*Stumpf and Franz:* Münch. med. Woch., 1892, Nos. 43 and 44.—*Taussig:* Abortion, St. Louis, 1910.—*Taussig, F. J.:* White House Conference, Amer. Jour. Obst. and Gyn., November and December, 1931.—*Traugott and Benthin:* Zentralbl. f. Gyn., 1913, pp. 918 and 922; also *Hoehne, ibid.,* December 5, 1914.—*Vignes, Henri:* Private communication from France.— *Wallace:* Farm and Live Stock of Great Britain, p. 334.—*Watkins:* Surg., Gyn., and Obst., January, 1912.— *Williams and Kolmer:* Bacillus Abortus of Bang, Amer. Jour. Obst., February, 1917.—*Winter:* Zentralbl. f. Gyn., 1911.—*Wulff:* Acta Gynecologica Scandinavica, 1923 (German), Vol. II, Facs. 3, p. 449.

CHAPTER XXXIII

ABRUPTIO PLACENTÆ

Up to 1664 all hemorrhages occurring during pregnancy were considered as due to premature detachment of the placenta from its supposed invariable site, the fundus uteri. At this time Paul Portal proved that the placenta could be attached to the cervix at the internal os. Rigby, in 1775, differentiated between cases of detachment of the placenta situated above the zone of the dilatation of the uterus and those below that zone. He said that in the latter class of patients, owing to the fact that the placenta must necessarily separate to allow the passage of the child, hemorrhage was "unavoidable," while in the former the "separation of the placenta must be owing to some *accidental* circumstance, to violence done to the uterus by blows or falls, to some peculiar laxity of the uterine vessels from badness of habit, or fever, or to some influence of the passions of the mind suddenly excited, such as fear, anger, etc." "Accidental hemorrhage," is still used especially by British authors to designate the premature separation of the normally implanted placenta. "Unavoidable hemorrhage" is a term seldom used, but it means placenta prævia, the development of the placenta in the zone of dilatation. The author suggests the term *abruptio placentæ* to take the place of the cumbersome, generally used term, and to go with the short and expressive "placenta prævia." R. W. Holmes in 1901 suggested the term "ablatio placentæ." Abruption of the placenta means a forcible breaking off of the organ from its normal site, and, in reality, is an abortion at or near term. Clinically, it is usually easy to differentiate between placenta prævia and abruptio placentæ, but the author is convinced that many times accidental hemorrhage is due to the *detachment of the placenta situated low in the uterus*, but just above the upper boundary of the zone of dilatation. The case partakes then of the characteristics of both conditions.

Abruptio placentæ, if one includes the milder instances, occurs oftener than is generally believed. Complete separation of the highly situated placenta is rare, and probably occurs much less often than once in 500 cases. Davis and McGee found that in 40,000 confinements at the Chicago Lying-in Hospital there were 52 cases of complete placental detachment with threatening internal hemorrhage, but there were, in addition, 112 partial detachments, the placenta showing a firm antepartum clot, and the clinical course of labor having been distinctly pathologic. In practice we easily distinguish grades of severity, the grave and the mild. The grave cases occur during the last third of pregnancy, and are usually toxemic in nature; the milder ones, which are of greater frequency, occur during labor, especially near the end of the second stage, and are likely to be of mechanical origin.

Causation.—The causes, of which there are many, are divided into three general groups: (1) Pregnancy toxemia and chronic nephritis; (2) diseases of the endometrium and ovum; (3) traumatism.

1. Winter pointed out the frequency of nephritis in abruptio placentæ. Fehling had already shown the coincidence of placental infarcts and hemorrhages in chronic nephritis (the placenta albumenurique, or truffé of the French); in 58 cases collected by Hofmeier nephritis was shown in 33.

The association of pre-eclamptic toxemia and eclampsia with placental, retroplacental, and myometrial hemorrhages has been frequently noted. Faure, in 1899, Muus, in 1906, Bar and de Kervilly in 1906, reported cases which indicated that there is more than coincidence in this association. Brindeau, Essen-Moeller, the author, and many others (see Ahlström) have come to believe that a pregnancy toxemia often lies at the bottom of the pathologic local changes and symptoms found in abruptio placentæ. Portes found toxemia in 91.3 per cent. of cases in Couvelaire's clinic; in ours it was 56.6 per cent.

A discussion of the origin and nature of this toxemia would take us back to the chapter on Eclampsia, q. v., p. 383. The majority of opinions favor the belief that the ovum is the source of the toxins. Their nature is unknown, but in the disease under consideration they affect the blood and blood-vessels like a hemorrhagin. In 1901 I drew attention to the hemophilic nature of some of these cases, and Williams recently compared the pathologic changes in the uterus to the local manifestations of certain venomous snake-bites. We have known for many years that in eclampsia and other toxicoses purpuric manifestations are common.

Hofbauer believed histamin could cause abruptio but Davis could find none in the uterus of a typical case. F. J. Browne proved that bacteria could cause toxemia in animals with injured kidneys and thus abruptio.

2. Studies of the endometrium, of the uterus, and the placenta have not given much of value. Endometritis (Weiss) is rare; degeneration of the decidua (Gottschalk, Schickele) is not constant; syphilis, arteriosclerosis, myometritis have been mentioned, but the only constant local finding has been a more or less marked bloody infiltration of the decidua and myometrium, and this is probably due to some noxa which causes an abnormal permeability of the spongiosa blood-vessels. Whether a diseased ovum furnishes the noxa, or the latter reaches the uterus from elsewhere, we do not know, but the evidence points to a placenta-toxin. As in eclampsia, the rôle infection plays needs study.

3. In the presence of one of the above conditions even a slight *trauma* may cause a separation of the placenta, and a hemorrhage having been once started, the blood works its way between the soft layers of decidua and completes the abruption. A jar, turning suddenly in bed, coitus, a blow or kick on the abdomen, the action of a purge, severe coughing, have all been assigned. In Holmes' collection of 200 cases from the literature accident was given in 67, in Davis' only in 3.

Basedow's disease, high blood-pressure, even a severe mental shock causing disturbance of the local circulation may start a hemorrhage in the spongiosa. Morse sought to show experimentally that torsion of the uterus could cause abruption of the placenta, and Polak had a case suggesting such a mechanism, but I have never observed one.

During labor several accidents may cause detachment of the placenta, as sudden emptying of a large polyhydramnion, the loosening of the placenta which sometimes follows the delivery of the first twin, the retraction of the uterus above the child, stopped in its progress by an obstruction in the pelvis, the operation of version, when the uterine wall is stretched and distorted by the rotation of the child, during delivery of the trunk in breech presentation, delayed rupture of the membranes, which are pushed down, dragging the placenta along, use of bags, bougies, gauze, and, finally, traction exerted on the placenta by a cord actually or relatively too short.

Pathology.—Separation of the placenta is always accompanied by marked hemorrhage unless the fetus has been dead long enough to allow thrombosis to occur in the uterine sinuses. Since the full uterus cannot retract over its contents, the sinuses remain open and the cavity of the uterus is exposed to the full force of the arterial circulation. The blood escaping under the decidua basalis may pursue four directions: First (Fig. 398), and most rarely, it may bulge out the uterine wall toward the abdominal cavity and bulge into the cavity of the ovum, the edges of the placenta remaining attached to the uterus; second, it may dissect up the membranes all the way round, severing almost all the connections of the ovum; third, it may break into the liquor amnii, and finally it may seek a direct passage outward from the edge of the placenta under the membranes through the cervix into the vagina (Fig. 399). The first three varieties are called "concealed hemorrhage," and usually are the most serious, but in all cases the exit of the blood may be blocked by the head or membranes or a firm clot plugging the cervix. The uterus may be immensely distended by the blood, the author in one case removing almost three pints of clots postpartum. A fatal intra-uterine hemorrhage may occur without a drop of blood showing externally. A few reports are on record where the placenta, fallen from its site, has come to lie over the internal os—prolapsus placentæ (Fig. 401). Most of these cases were probably placenta prævia, but a real prolapse of the placenta occurs, and it makes a great deal of difference in the treatment. In 306 cases of abruptio placentæ collected by Holmes and Goodell, 193 showed external hemorrhage. In all the author's cases external hemorrhage followed the internal, so that the rule is that the bleeding in abruptio placentæ is first internal

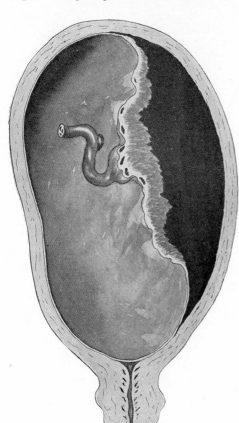

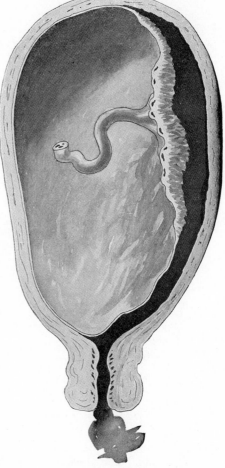

FIG. 398.—ABRUPTIO PLACENTÆ. INTERNAL OR "CONCEALED" HEMORRHAGE.

FIG. 399.—ABRUPTIO PLACENTÆ; COMBINED INTERNAL AND EXTERNAL HEMORRHAGE.

or concealed, then combined, external and internal. The mildest case and, fortunately, the most common, is the purely external hemorrhage (Fig. 400). Blood may escape into the peritoneal cavity through the tubes. Without doubt small hemorrhages under the placenta occur frequently during the latter weeks of pregnancy, and organize without producing alarming symptoms, but are discovered by the watchful accoucheur in the evidences on the delivered placenta; for example, infarcts and hard old, almost completely fibrinous clots, adherent to or incorporated in the membranes or decidua. By reverting to the history of a slight

31

trauma, a sudden pain in the belly, perhaps a slight bloody show, the connection is made clear. The placenta in cases of abruption may show the evidences of several hemorrhages or red infarcts of varying dates; it may be torn or compressed by the clots (Fig. 402), or it may show no signs save a large retroplacental hematoma similar to that which occurs in the third stage of labor.

Uteroplacental Apoplexy.—Couvelaire made an important contribution to our knowledge of the pathology of the serious cases of abruptio placentæ. He called the condition "apoplexie utero-placentaire," and likened the appearance of the uterus to that of an ovarian cyst with twisted pedicle. The surface was

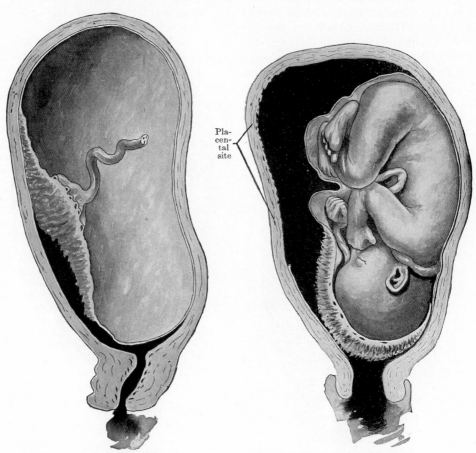

Pla-
cen-
tal
site

Fig. 400.—Abruptio Placentæ. External
Hemorrhage.

Fig. 401.—Prolapsus Placentæ.

congested, brownish, with sugillations, which extended out on to the ovaries and broad ligaments. The uterine muscle was degenerated and infiltrated with blood, there were various sized petechiæ under the peritoneum, some of which had ruptured, and the serosa was split in places, allowing blood to escape into the free cavity. In the blood-vessels endarteritic and degenerative changes with thromboses were found.

These findings would indicate a toxemic (or infectious?) causation of the primary rhexis of the blood-vessels, with consecutive abruption of the placenta, and the bloody extravasations between the muscle-fibers would explain the atony of such uteri postpartum. Louros in similar cases found active dilatation of the veins and liver necroses, which, quoting Schwarz and Franz, be ascribes to excessive vagotonia.

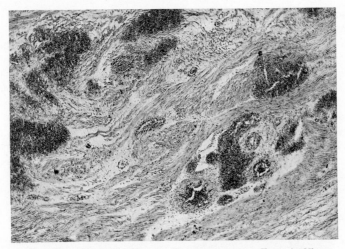

FIG. 401a.—SECTION OF UTERINE WALL OF APOPLEXIA UTERI (× 35).
Shows hemorrhage, edema, distraction of muscle fibers (Davis and McGee).

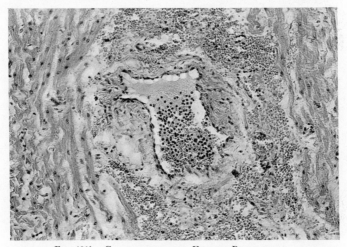

FIG. 401b.—CROSS-SECTION OF A UTERINE BLOOD-VESSEL.
Hemorrhage and edema of uterine musculature.   Many leukocytes in lumen.

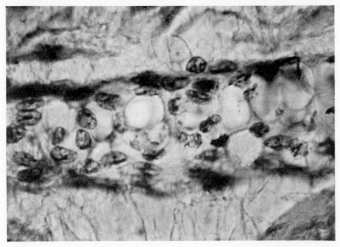

FIG. 401c.—LENGTH SECTION OF SMALL BLOOD-VESSEL (× 600).
Cytoplasm rounded and vacuolated, nuclei swollen, hydropic.   Increase in endothelial cells, size and number.

Symptoms.—*During pregnancy* a slight, perhaps repeated, hemorrhage from the uterus may indicate some disturbance of placentation which may be without apparent cause. It may follow a physical or mental traumatism, such as a blow, an automobile ride, a nervous shock. When injury is the cause a history of the same is given, but the symptoms may not come on for hours or even days afterward. Upon delivery an organized blood-clot may be found on the placenta. If a gravida presents evidences of toxemia one is on the lookout for this complication and such foresight is also indicated if she has recently suffered from a mild or severe infection, *e. g.,* tonsillitis or la grippe.

There are mild and grave cases. Sometimes the first, slight hemorrhage under the placenta sets the uterus into vigorous action, which prevents any considerable intra-uterine bleeding and quickly delivers the child—often alive. Again the accident declares itself at once as serious. The severity of the symptoms depends on the blood loss and shock. These vary with the different causes and the degree

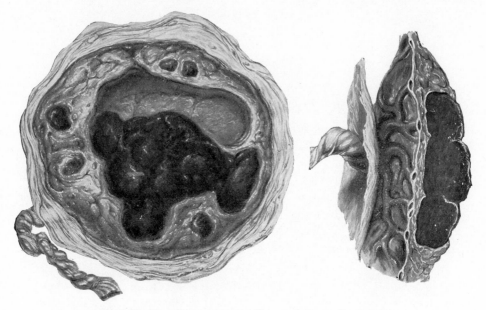

Figs. 402, 402a.—Placenta from a Case of Abruptio Placentæ.
Note the deep crater, from which part of the clot has been removed. This is pathognomonic. In 402a note the compression of the placenta by the clot.

of separation, and whether or not uterine action is inaugurated. Sudden, severe pain in the belly, often at the site of the placenta, of a tearing character at first, later a dull tense ache, interrupted by colics—these are the usual symptoms. In the concealed hemorrhages which are the severe cases and usually occur during pregnancy, the pain is often more marked, but it may be slight or absent. Occasionally nausea or vomiting occurs. Now the symptoms of acute anemia supervene, together with those of shock, from sudden distention of the uterus and absorption of toxins from wounded tissue. Dizziness, faintness, shortness of breath, precordial anxiety, and oppression appear in order; the woman yawns or sighs frequently, and complains of ringing in the ears, spots before the eyes, that she sees everything black, and is harassed by great thirst. Later she lies apathetic on the bed or may faint. This loss of consciousness may last a few moments to a half hour, and is replaced by restlessness, jactitation, or even delirium. Cramps in the legs, excessive thirst, vomiting, unconsciousness, delirium, convulsive twitchings, involuntary evacuations, coma, death—this is the usual order of the symptoms if the bleeding is not stopped. The observer will note the increasing prostration, *the growing pallor of the skin, the white cheeks and gums,* the sunken eyes, the pearly conjunctivæ, the cold extremities and face, often with an icy sweat, and in cases of shock an additional tinge of cyanosis about the lips. The pulse at the very beginning may be bounding and not accelerated, thus deceiving the accoucheur as to the gravity of the situation. In shock more than in pure hemorrhage the pulse at first is likely to be rapid, small, and compressible. Later, the bleeding keeping up, the hold of the arterial walls on the rapidly diminishing blood-stream becomes insufficient, and the heart has to pump faster to keep the small amount of blood in circulation. In some instances the pulse weakens and grows more rapid *pari passu* with the loss of blood. The pulse, therefore, is not always a sure index as to what is going on in the circulatory system. Hourly tests for hemoglobin would indicate the course of the anemia. The blood-pressure varies with the degree of shock and a complicating toxemia.

Very soon blood or serum expressed from the intra-uterine clots appears externally, but the amount of blood is entirely disproportionate to the gravity of the symptoms. Examination of the belly will show that the uterus is larger than corresponds to the given period of pregnancy and grows larger every hour, and that it has a board-like consistence, making it impossible to outline the fetus. The ligneous consistency of the uterus was noted in 63.5 per cent. of our cases. An accessory tumor, that is, the subplacental hematoma, is seldom found. Sometimes the uterus is only slightly tense, in the case of partial abruption of a low placenta. Exceptionally the uterus is flabby and dilated. One would expect the board-like uterus in the concealed cases and the relaxed uterus where the blood finds ready exit, but this is not constant. Tenseness of the belly wall because of the distended uterus and the pain is another finding. Of great diagnostic importance is a tender uterus. The patient can tolerate only the lightest pressure. Davis and McGee found this sign in only 55.8 per cent. of the several cases but probably it had not been noted—as I have rarely missed it. They believe that pain on pressure over the broad ligaments may indicate hemorrhagic extravasation into these structures. The woman says that the child is not felt, but that it was subject to violent movements at the onset. Very seldom can the fetal heart be heard, and under such conditions a partial separation of the placenta must be assumed.

Labor usually comes on at once, and, if the contractions of the uterus are strong and the os dilates quickly, the case terminates spontaneously—safely for the mother, but almost invariably fatally for the infant. Not seldom the pains are weak and the woman dies undelivered—of shock and hemorrhage—unless medical aid is rendered. Sometimes the uterus seems to be in a state of quiet tetanus, labor making no progress. These are serious cases.

During labor we also may have mild and serious cases of abruption. In the former labor is usually uneventful until near the end of the second stage, when the accoucheur, attentively observing the fetal heart beat, discovers the agitation of the child. There may or may not be external bleeding, but the signs of internal hemorrhage are wanting. The pains are usually strong and almost continuous, wherefore labor is rapidly completed. The child may be asphyxiated or dead, unless rescued by bold interference, such as a quick forceps, or version and extraction, the conditions being right. A gush of blood and clots follows the child, confirming the diagnosis.

Atony postpartum is an occasional complication, due to overdistention and myometrial disease. Exceptionally the bleeding presents a hemophilic character, the vulva, the vagina, and even the uterus, tubes, ovaries, and broad ligaments being sanguineously infiltrated. Continuous oozing of lake-colored blood defies all efforts of hemostasis. In such cases a toxic element must be assumed. Cortical renal necrosis is one of the rare complications.

Diagnosis.—Acute abdominal pain, referred usually to one side of the uterus, sudden increase of the size and hardness of the uterus, with tension of the abdominal wall, external hemorrhage, absence of the fetal heart-tones, with the general symptoms of increasing anemia and deepening shock, constitute the foundation for the direct diagnosis. In the differential diagnosis placenta prævia, rupture of the uterus, and extra-uterine pregnancy most frequently come up, but on rare occasions torsion of the uterus (Robinson) and a burst uterine varix must be eliminated and one may have to consider non-obstetric accidents, as gall-stone colic, rupture of an appendiceal abscess or gall-bladder or spleen, and intra-abdominal injuries.

ABRUPTIO PLACENTÆ	PLACENTA PRÆVIA
Symptoms	
1. Sudden stormy onset.	1. Rather quiet onset.
2. Pain, generally referred to the placental site.	2. No pain, unless uterine contractions.
3. Hemorrhage, internally or externally after a while.	3. Hemorrhage always external at start.
4. Hemorrhage, usually severe—internal or external.	4. First hemorrhage generally mild, and always external.
5. Usually only one hemorrhage.	5. Several, or history of several.
6. May find a cause—injury, jar, etc.	6. Usually no cause.
7. Symptoms of a severer hemorrhage than the amount of blood externally shows.	7. Symptoms proportionate to the amount of blood lost externally.
8. Cessation of fetal movements.	8. No change usually.
9. Hemorrhage continues after the rupture of the membranes.	9. Hemorrhage usually ceases in all but the central variety.
10. Hemorrhage continuous, sometimes ceasing during uterine contractions.	10. The hemorrhage is increased by the uterine contractions (not constant).
11. Symptoms and signs of toxemia, usual.	11. Seldom.
Signs	
1. Abdomen distended, tense, and painful to touch.	1. Abdomen as usual at time of pregnancy.
2. Uterus tense, board-like, cannot feel fetus. (Rare exception, soft.)	2. Uterus soft, unless there is a uterine contraction.
3. Fetal heart-tones absent.	3. Almost always present.
4. Vaginally, no placenta in reach of the fingers.	4. Placenta palpable in isthmus uteri.
5. Bag of waters tense—feel head easily.	5. Bag of waters loose; usually head not engaged.

Rupture of the uterus is often complicated with detachment of the placenta, and, too, it is possible that an abruption may tear the uterine wall or the peritoneal covering of the uterus. The symptoms of the two conditions, therefore, mingle:

ABRUPTIO PLACENTÆ	RUPTURA UTERI
1. Usually during pregnancy.	1. Usually during labor, unless from external violence.
2. Uterus enlarged, tense, symmetric.	2. Uterus small, at one side, with neighboring tumor—the fetus.
3. Uterus contracting.	3. No uterine pains.
4. Vaginally feel fetus through the os.	4. No presenting part, uterus contracted and empty.
5. No tear palpable.	5. May feel the rent and sometimes the gut.

With a history of violent injury it may be necessary to open the abdomen for both diagnosis and treatment.

Ectopic gestation is indicated by the history, the finding of the empty uterus alongside the eccentric and asymmetric tumor, and the absence of contractions in the tumor. In peritonitis from rupture of a hollow viscus the tenderness is more in the flanks, in abruptio it is over the uterus (Bourne).

Prognosis.—Goodell, in his 106 cases, found 54 maternal and 100 fetal deaths, but he collected only the critical ones, mostly of concealed hemorrhage. Later writers include the mild and more common abruptions, and the mortality is correspondingly less. Still, the accident is one of the gravest with which the obstetrician has to deal, and it is safe to say that one-half of the women and 95 per cent. of the babies in complete detachments with concealed hemorrhage will die, while a larger proportion will be saved with partial detachment and under skilful treatment. Abruption may recur in subsequent labors.

Treatment.—Divides itself into detachment occurring during labor, and that before dilatation of the cervix is begun. One also must separate the *mild* cases from the *serious* ones.

The *mild* abruptions usually occur toward the end of labor, and, in contrast to the grave ones, are attended by strong pains—a happy circumstance.

If a woman having apparently a normal labor suddenly begins to bleed, one thinks at once of premature detachment of the placenta, low insertion of the placenta, laceration of the cervix, and rupture of the uterus. An internal examination will tell whether the bleeding comes from the last fibers of the cervix giving way to the passage of the head, or from placenta prævia. Sometimes the placenta may be low in the uterus, but out of reach of the fingers, and here the membranes should be ruptured, which is good treatment also for detachment of the placenta—at this stage of labor—because, in the first instance, the hemorrhage will cease at once, and, in the second, labor will be so much facilitated that the danger quickly passes. If the hemorrhage continues, and especially if the fetal heart-tones become irregular or slow, a diagnosis of abruption is now made, and the child should be delivered without delay, enlarging the aperture of the cervix by manual dilatation, lateral incisions or vaginal cesarean section. If the placenta separates after the first twin is born or after the emptying of polyhydramnion, or during the operation of version or extraction, rapid delivery is indicated.

Severe cases of abruption require prompt diagnosis and treatment. In placing the indication we must consider—the apparent gravity of the situation; the presence of toxemia; the viability of the child; the state of the cervix; the size of the pelvis; the strength of the pains, and, not least, the environment, whether the patient is at home or in a hospital. Three objects must be accomplished: the uterus must be emptied, the hemorrhage stopped, and the anemia relieved. The best treatment is that which empties the uterus quickest and with the least danger to the mother.

The indication being for immediate delivery, the condition of the cervix will decide which method shall be chosen. One cannot count on good pains from a distended and blood-infiltrated uterus. If the cervix is soft and partly open, the dilatation may be completed manually and forceps or version done, depending on the engagement of the head. When the child is dead, craniotomy takes the place of forceps, certainly if the cervix is small, and in a primipara with rigid vagina.

Rapid dilatation by means of a Bossi dilator is dangerous and unsatisfactory. Accouchement forcé, the rapid, ruthless dilatation of the cervix and immediate delivery, is to be condemned as dangerous and unsuccessful. The women often bleed to death from the lacerations inflicted.

If the cervix admits two fingers but is only partly effaced we have, as in placenta prævia, five methods of treatment: Rupture of the membranes, metreurysis, Braxton Hicks' version, vaginal tamponade, and the two kinds of cesarean section. Which course is to be selected will depend on the urgency of the woman's condition, the circumstances of the case, and the personal choice of the operator.

Should the membranes be punctured? Smellie, Denman, Baudelocque, Merriman, Blundell, Ramsbotham, and Kerr (for mild cases) recommend it; Atthill, Hicks, Hamilton, Burns, and Veit (unless after complete dilatation) deny its value. Letting the liquor amnii escape may give room in the uterus for more blood to fill, or increase the shock by emptying the uterus, or interfere with the mechanism of cervical dilatation. These are theoretic objections which do not hold in practice, since experience has shown that the pains grow stronger and more efficient; that the hemorrhage is not increased, and that subsequent operative procedures are not rendered difficult by letting the liquor amnii drain away.

For metreurysis an anesthetic is not needful, which is in its favor. Under morphin and scopolamin (or if toxemia is present, magnesium sulphate), the membranes are punctured, as much as possible of the liquor amnii let off, an 8 cm. bag inserted (a smaller one if earlier in pregnancy), and very slowly inflated (to avoid rupture of the uterus), 1 pound traction being applied. As a rule the pains begin at once and quickly end labor. If pains are absent but abdominal pain and tenderness present, one suspects a Couvelaire uterus and thinks of cesarean section.

For version a general anesthetic is usually required beside the morphin and scopolamin. One should use ether. To grasp the foot one may use a long volsella, since the baby is dead. A weight of 1 pound is tied to the foot. Labor is usually quickly completed. If not, suspect a blood-infiltrated uterus.

For tamponade the morphin and scopolamin generally suffice. The membranes are not opened. The vagina is filled tight with small balls of dry cotton tamped firmly and evenly all around. Very few use this method.

In all 3 cases counterpressure from the abdomen is applied, either by the Spanish windlass (Fig. 403) or Beck's obstetric belt. A few words of caution in the

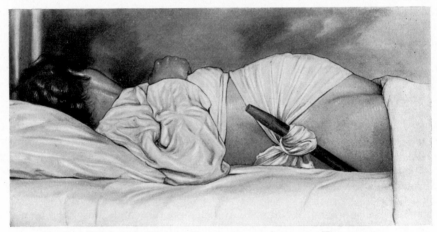

Fig. 403.—Spanish Windlass Compression for Accidental Hemorrhage.
Beck's belt is better.

use of either: If applied too tight and if the pains are strong, the cervix or even the uterus may be torn. Any spark of life in the baby is extinguished by this treatment, but this must be taken in the bargain. If pains are slow in coming on, or if the uterus seems to be enlarging from blood accumulating in its cavity one may administer a little pituitary, 1, 2 or 3 units, repeated every fifteen, thirty, or forty minutes depending on the uterine response. Ether is to be kept nearby available at once to restrain too tempestuous uterine action.

Since the causation of the bleeding in abruptio placentæ is different from that of placenta prævia, and since there are particular anatomic changes in the cervix and lower uterine segment in the latter, a vital difference exists in the treatment of the two conditions when delivery is attempted per vias naturales. In abruptio blood accumulates in and distends the uterus, it is also extravasated into the musculature, sometimes even into the peritoneal cavity. The best treatment is to empty the uterus, and enable it to close down on itself and stop the bleeding with the usual physiologic mechanism.

In placenta prævia, on the other hand, blood does not accumulate in the uterus, but runs out from the open sinuses. The most important difference is the soft, fragile, vascular, placental bed in the lower uterine segment. Simple distention of this isthmus, and certainly trauma, will open the enormous sinuses here and invite a flooding. Light pressure against the placenta and its bed suffices to stop the flow until adequate dilatation is procured to effect safe delivery. Our main endeavor is to avoid cervical and isthmial tears. Slow delivery, therefore, in placenta prævia; more rapid, but not forced, in abruptio.

The accoucheur must sit by his patient watching every change in her condition closely, while in the meantime all preparations are made for eventual operation, for the treatment of postpartum hemorrhage and the anemia. The appearance of the patient, *the degree of pallor*, the amount of pain, give more certain evidences of danger than the pulse, blood-pressure, Hb. estimations, etc. If the pains are strong the outlook is usually good and one may wait. If the uterus remains in a quiet tetanic state the muscle is probably being infiltrated and one is more likely to need section. As soon as it is possible to complete the delivery safely this is to be done.

After delivery the dangers are not past. Postpartum hemorrhage is fairly frequent, both from uterine atony, and because of the hemophilic nature of the disease. One must save blood. Immediately after the fetal head is born the woman is given an ampule of strong pituitary. If fresh blood follows the child, the placenta is removed and ergot given hypodermically. Unless the uterus contracts securely it is tightly packed with gauze, and another ampule of pituitary injected into its substance through the abdominal wall. It may be necessary even with this treatment to remove the uterus to save the woman's life. In 2 cases, both before the days of pituitrin, I stanched the inveterate oozing by packing the uterus with gauze soaked in sterile gelatin, and recently I checked the hemorrhage by means of Sehrt's aorta compressor while I repaired a bleeding lacerated cervix—the result of accouchement forcé. Here Henkel's method deserves trial. (See p. 851.)

Vaginal and Abdominal Hysterotomy.—If when first seen the cervix is closed and internal hemorrhage is going on, the case is truly formidable, the mortality very high, and brave action is needed. A skilful operator might do a vaginal cesarean section and this would offer a better outlook, but usually the abdominal route is chosen. Without question the low or cervical section, laparotrachelotomy under local anesthesia, is the quickest and safest way out of this serious situation, if the surroundings are right, and a man capable of his task is at hand. Otherwise one of the three methods previously described is to be used.

One should do the section in those cases where the baby still lives, when the pelvis might offer an obstacle to delivery, when the case is complicated by a toxemia (eclampsism or eclampsia), when an "apoplexie-utero-placentaire" (Couvelaire) is suspected and the probability or even the possibility exists that a Porro cesarean may be finally required. Supravaginal amputation of the uterus (Porro) is to be done either as an intended operation or upon indication complementing the cesarean delivery. In a multipara, in cases of fibroids, where the abdominal method is chosen after attempts at delivery from below have failed, or the patient already is infected or presumably so and where time and the amount of further blood loss are to be reckoned with, a primary Porro is recommended to the family. As a rule the laparotrachelotomy is sufficient to meet the exigencies of the case. Even with a "Couvelaire" uterus (one infiltrated with blood) contraction and retraction of the muscle may be good and bleeding not marked, but if the event shows that this is not the case after removal of the placenta, the corpus remaining flabby and bleeding keeping up, one should not hesitate to amputate the uterus. Stoeckel recommends to remove the uterus unopened, to save blood. This may be less sanguinary but it entails more shock. Operation in cases of abruptio must be rapid and definitive. Ergot and pituitrin are given intramuscularly at the start. Pituitrin is injected into the uterus as the fetus is delivered and, if the organ responds too sluggishly, again, this time directly into a vein (5 units). The large, boggy organ infiltrated with blood and toxins causes shock, and invites infection; indeed its removal is preferable in all but young primiparæ and the condition usually occurs in women advanced in years and child-bearing.

What to Do in Shock.—If the patient is in deep collapse the question of any operative interference must be carefully debated, but before doing so, a donor of blood should be sent for, while saline and glucose solutions are administered hypodermically. It may be best to give the woman a massive transfusion (800 to 1000 c.c.) and immediately perform laparotrachelotomy, under local anesthesia, if possible, with morphin and scopolamin. In most cases, however, it will be wiser to treat the shock first, and after reaction is fairly well established go to operation. If this course is decided upon the vagina is to be tightly plugged, a compression binder put on, and restoratives administered. Warmth to the body is the best, next to blood transfusion. Two liters of saline solution and one of 4 per cent. glucose may be given hypodermically. The physician seats himself beside the patient, watches her color, and, with an accurate chronometer, counts the pulse every three or five minutes. He must know whether the hemorrhage continues under his more or less blind observation. This is not always easy. Blood-pressure readings and blood-counts are not very reliable. He must be guided by the general symptoms and his clinical findings. If the hemorrhage keeps up he must operate.

Rupture of the circular sinus of the placenta, allowing maternal blood to escape externally, is a rare accident, and one which can hardly be diagnosed. Even after delivery of the placenta, and the demonstration of the opening in the sinus, one may not assert such a diagnosis because these openings are found on normal placentæ. Treatment is the same as for premature detachment of the placenta. (See Budin.)

LITERATURE

Ahlström, Erik: Monograph, Stockholm, Sweden, 1919, Lit.—*Bourne:* Recent Advances in Obst. and Gyn., 1926, Blakiston.—*Browne, F. J.:* Jour. Obst. and Gyn., Brit. Empire, Winter, 1928.—*Budin:* Femmes en Couches, etc., Paris, 1897, p. 135.—*Couvelaire:* Annales de Gyn., October, 1911; and Annales de Gyn. et d'Obst., 1912, ix, 418.—*Davis, M. E., and McGee, W. B.:* Abruptio Placentæ, Surg., Gyn., and Obst., December, 1931, p. 768, Lit.—*DeLee:* Amer. Jour. Obstetrics, 1901, vol. xliv, No. 6.—*Hofbauer:* Amer. Jour. Obst. and Gyn., August, 1926.—*Hofmeier:* Handb. der Geb., vol. ii, Heft ii, p. 1188.—*Holmes:* Amer. Jour. Obstet., 1901, vol. ii, p. 762. Gives complete literature to date.—*Kerr:* Operative Midwifery, p. 601.—*Louros:* Archiv für Gyn., 1927, 129, iii, p. 1049.—*Macan:* Dublin Jour. Med. Sci., January, 1905, p. 16.—*Morse:* Surg., Gyn., and Obst., February, 1918, p. 133.—*Portes:* Gynecologie et Obstetrique, Paris, 1923, vol. vii, No. 1, p. 56.—*Ramsbotham:* System of Obstetrics, 1865, p. 391.—*Robinson and Duvall:* Jour. Obst. and Gyn., Brit. Empire, 38, 1–226, Spring, 1931.—*Seitz:* Arch. f. Gyn., vol. lxix, p. 76.—*Williams:* Surg., Gyn., and Obst., November, 1915, p. 543.

CHAPTER XXXIV

PLACENTA PRÆVIA

PLACENTA prævia is the development of the placenta in part or wholly within the zone of dilatation of the uterus. That the placenta may be found over the os was known since Hippocrates' time, and is mentioned by Mauriceau, Deventer, Pugh, and many others, but they believed that it had prolapsed from its normal fundal insertion. Paul Portal, in 1664, stated positively that the placenta may be implanted over the os, and Giffard, Roederer, Levret, and especially Smellie, emphasized this fact. Rigby, in 1775, however, most clearly distinguished between

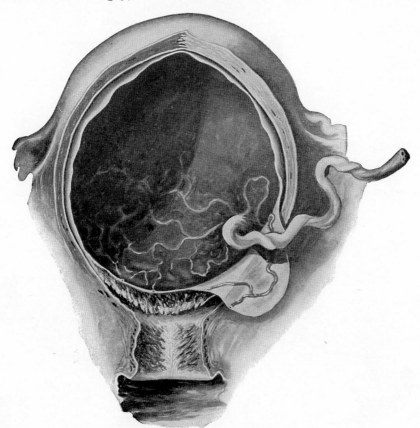

FIG. 404.—PLACENTA PRÆVIA CENTRALIS. VELAMENTOUS INSERTION OF CORD.
Specimen of Northwestern University Medical School.

placenta prævia and abruptio placentæ, although it must be conceded that some of his cases were incorrectly diagnosed. Rigby gave the name unavoidable hemorrhage to the former, and that of accidental hemorrhage to the latter, condition. Hemorrhage in placenta prævia is unavoidable because the placenta must be separated by the advancing child, and this separation causes bleeding, while in abruptio placentæ the hemorrhage is due to accidental separation of the organ. Schaller,

491

in 1709, was the first to demonstrate postmortem the attachment of the placenta over the internal os.

The placenta may attach itself to any portion of the uterus, the fundal insertion being the rarest of all, the posterior wall being the most common site, next the anterior wall, then the sides, and next to the last in frequency the lower uterine

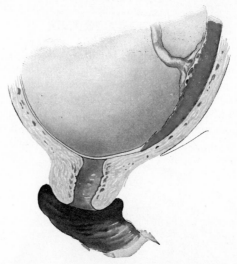

FIG. 405.—LOW INSERTION OF PLACENTA.

segment—the isthmus uteri. The lower edge of the placenta must be at least 10 cm. from the internal os, and well above the upper border of the isthmus uteri, to be normal. When the inferior border lies just at the isthmus uteri, we speak of low insertion of the placenta; when this edge just reaches the internal os, it is

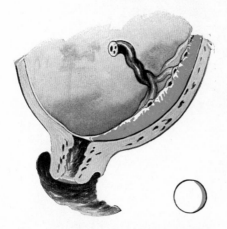

FIG. 406.—PLACENTA PRÆVIA MARGINALIS.

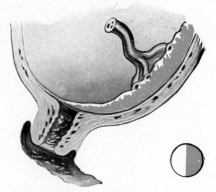

FIG. 407.—PLACENTA PRÆVIA LATERALIS.

called placenta prævia marginalis (Fig. 406); when only part of the opening of the cervix is covered, we speak of placenta prævia lateralis or partialis (Fig. 407), and when the os is completely roofed over, placenta prævia centralis or totalis (Fig. 408). Since in the last class of cases the placenta lies almost entirely in the isthmus uteri, this might be called placenta isthmialis. All these terms are relative because of changes in the digital findings produced by the dilatation of the uterus—for example, a marginalis, after the cervix is open, may become a lateralis, and a placenta that seemed to cover all the cervix with two fingers' dilatation subsequently may cover only half of the opening.

In placenta prævia cervicalis the anatomic-histologic conditions resemble placenta accreta or increta, *i. e.*, the placental villi are not separated from the muscular substratum by a reactive decidua, but have grown down into and be-

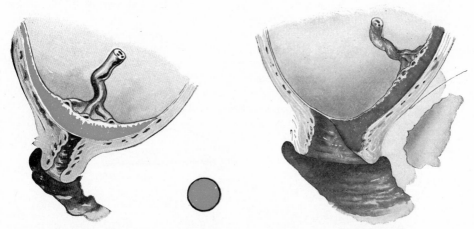

FIG. 408.—PLACENTA PRÆVIA TOTALIS OR CENTRALIS.   FIG. 409.—PLACENTA PRÆVIA CERVICALIS INCRETA.

tween the fibromuscular lamellæ of the cervix (Fig. 409). The placenta, therefore, has to be dug out of the cervix, an operation attended by much hemorrhage, indeed, often having to be terminated by hysterectomy (Zangemeister, Lit.).

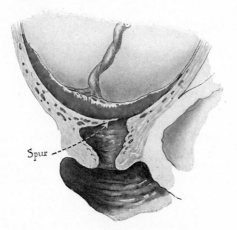

FIG. 409a.—SHOWING CRESCENTIC SPUR ON POSTERIOR WALL.

Causation.—Placenta prævia is said to occur ten times as frequently in multiparæ as in primiparæ, and in general once in 1000 cases, but no weight is to be placed on the statistics, since the figures given by various authors vary from 1 to 1500 to 1 to 200. Central placenta prævia occurs in less than one-fifth of the cases, and multiparæ are especially prone to the deeper varieties, and the tendency to the low insertion increases with multiparity and age.

Predisposing causes are chronic endometritis, multiparity, especially when the children come in rapid succession, subinvolution, and twin pregnancies.

These conditions are likely to be associated.   The author in nearly all his cases of placenta prævia has obtained a history of abortion, of slow recovery from previous confinement, of manual removal of the placenta in previous labor, of recurrent placenta prævia and other evidences of a diseased endometrium, and the findings on the placenta often confirm the endometritis as the predisposing factor—for example, white infarcts, very thick serotina, adherent placenta.

The acting causes are—(a) Primary low insertion of the ovum near the internal os or on its edge; (b) the development of placenta in the reflexa and its coming to lie over the os (Hofmeier and Kaltenbach).

(a) Owing, perhaps, to an endometritis, to lack of the cilia, or to some unknown anomaly of the ovum itself, e. g., low nidation power, the egg slips down the uterine cavity and does not succeed in attaching itself until it reaches the neighborhood of the internal os, which may be narrowed by endometrial swelling.

How the placenta grows over the internal os has given rise to much discussion. All investigators agree that the ovum must be inserted low in the uterus.   Since

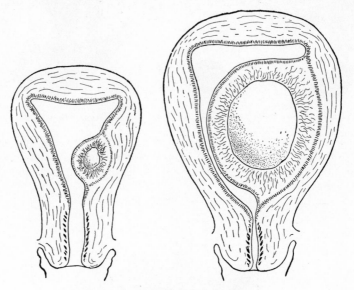

FIG. 410.—OVUM SPLITTING DECIDUA (Hofmeier).

the ovum burrows into the mucosa and then, in its growth, splits the decidua in all directions, it is easy to see how part of the placenta could come to cover the internal os (Fig. 410).   The decidua vera and reflexa are carried across the narrow cervical slit and come to lie in apposition with the vera of the opposite side, where fusion may or may not occur.   If the ovum splits the decidual membrane circularly around the os, the remaining minute hole is easily bridged over, and a horseshoe-shaped or a *placenta fenestrata* results.   The downward splitting of the decidua may not be arrested at the internal os.   Rarely the cervical mucous membrane is capable of forming decidua, and in this the development of the placenta goes on, the villi in their growth reaching even to the external os, as in the author's two cases.   In another the burrowing villi had split off a layer of mucosa and muscle (Fig. 409).   When I dug out the placenta a bleeding cavity remained in the cervix.   Krause collected 22 cases, in one of which the villi had grown through the cervix into the parametrium.   These cases resemble cervical pregnancy, a very rare condition.

(b) Hofmeier believed many placentæ præviæ are due to the development of the villi in the reflexa (Fig. 411).   Owing to peculiar nutritional conditions, the chorion læve does not atrophy, but the villi develop in the reflexa and this surface later becomes applied to the vera on the opposite wall of the uterus. In general, the nutritional power of the isthmus is not great, and the placenta of an ovum situated here, must spread out in order to obtain sufficient nourishment, thus forming a placenta membranacea.

Placentæ that have been placentæ præviæ exhibit great variety of form, two having already been mentioned. Sometimes there is a tongue of tough, fibrous placental tissue which has overlaid the os; sometimes the edge of the os is encircled by this placental tissue, more or less infarcted. Occasionally—and this in the isthmial variety—the placenta hangs across the lower uterine segment like a festoon. These are the most serious.

Symptoms.—Hemorrhage is the first and most constant symptom, occurring in the last three months of pregnancy—most frequently in the eighth. Usually no cause is assignable, the patient waking from sleep to find herself in a lake of blood, or, on arising from the toilet, sees fluid and clotted blood in the vessel. *A painless, causeless, uterine hemorrhage in the third trimester of pregnancy is almost pathognomonic of placenta prævia.* The first hemorrhage may vary from a few drops, hardly a stain on the linen, to a profuse "flooding," which may be fatal at once, but usually a few ounces are lost as the initial symptom. Each succeeding hemorrhage is greater, and unless treated, a high grade of anemia is developed. The accoucheur must not be misled by apparent recovery: this is never complete during pregnancy— the blood is only "patched up"; the system is not in a condition to withstand a new drain, one that is inevitable at labor. Some of the worst cases of secondary anemia are produced by a condition

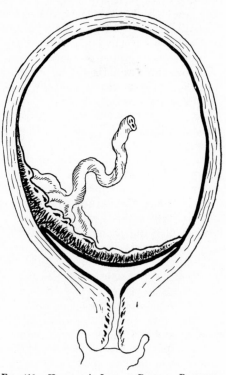

Fig. 411.—Hofmeier's Idea of Reflexa Placenta.

called *stillicidium sanguinis, i. e.,* a continuous but very slight dribbling of blood, hardly commanding the notice of the accoucheur, but slowly undermining the woman's constitution, robbing her of her ability to stand bleeding at labor and increasing her susceptibility to infection. Another important sign is a constant seepage of blood-stained serum. This indicates that a large clot is forming in the lower uterine segment and vagina. Labor usually comes on after the second or third hemorrhage.

In central insertion of the placenta the bleeding usually occurs earlier than in the other varieties, but exceptions are noted, the cervix remaining closed and there being no hemorrhage until full-term labor begins. Such cases have weak pains and are, therefore, unfavorable. In partial placenta prævia the pains of pregnancy are usually present; hemorrhage is, therefore, more constant; the cervix softens and dilates, and treatment during labor is facilitated. Marginal placenta prævia may not cause hemorrhage until the very beginning of labor, or even toward the end of the first stage, and then it is slight. One may suspect the type of placenta prævia from the above symptoms, but exceptions to the rules are very common, the author having met a severe and almost fatal hemorrhage from a marginal insertion and another case of mild bleeding in a complete placenta prævia. Ahlfeld and Edgar lost patients from one profuse hemorrhage, and only an edge of the placenta presented.   Perhaps the manner of development of the placenta prævia may explain these variations in the amount of hemorrhage.

The origin of the hemorrhage is fourfold: From the sinuses of the placental site; from the intervillous spaces of the placenta; from the circular sinus of the placenta; rarely, and then only as the result of interference, from the villi—that is, the fetal blood-vessels.   Owing to the development of the isthmus uteri and the lower uterine segment, and the constant upward retraction of the fibers of the lower portion of the uterus, the area occupied by the placenta is enlarged, but the placental growth is not in proportion.   During the painless uterine contractions of pregnancy the lower edge of the placenta, therefore, is likely to be disunited from the wall of the uterus, opening the sinuses and allowing maternal blood to escape. It is easy to see why such hemorrhage is called unavoidable.

Other symptoms of placenta prævia are both inconstant and equivocal, as pain, pressure, and throbbing in the lower abdomen, frequent urination, leukorrhea, and "carrying the child differently."

Placenta prævia affects the course of pregnancy, labor, and the puerperium. Abortion is not seldom the result of it, though Hofmeier, in sixteen years' experience, could not find one.   In several abortions the author found indubitable evidences of low implantation of the ovum.   Many cases of placenta prævia give a history of threatened abortion in the early months.   Premature rupture of the bag of waters is another sign of low insertion, usually the marginal, and is due to the adherence of the membranes around the os, from catarrhal endometritis or abnormal placentation.   Premature labor is, therefore, common.   Doranth found full-term labor in only 32 per cent.   Some authors mention that pregnancy may go beyond term in placenta prævia centralis, but I have had contrary experience.

During labor the low implantation of the bulky placenta causes malpositions and malpresentations, for example, breech and shoulder; delayed engagement of the head; abnormalities of rotation; prolapsus funis; weak pains—all these plus the inevitable hemorrhage and the injuries so commonly inflicted by operative delivery.   Air-embolism because the uterine sinuses are so near the external air, and rupture of the uterus because the musculature is weakened by the ingrowth of decidua and the placenta, are commoner than usual.

Postpartum hemorrhage is very frequent, because the lower uterine wall is thin and weak in muscle, which contracts tardily, and closes imperfectly the large venous sinuses, also often being unable to separate the placenta.   Further, the placenta is likely to be adherent because of endometritis, infarction, ingrowth of villi (placenta increta, Fig. 701), or from infection during pregnancy, the placenta being so near the septic vagina.   Did not the uterine arteries enter the uterus higher up and, therefore, in the zone of contraction, many women would bleed to death, because the clotting in the vessels is not sufficient to procure hemostasis.   No doubt many cases of postpartum hemorrhage are due to low implantation.

In the puerperium placenta prævia also makes trouble: (a) Bits of placenta may remain adherent and become infected; (b) from the close proximity of the placental site to the septic vagina and cervix infection—and that of the most dangerous kind, metrophlebitis—is invited; (c) subinvolution, and (d) finally the woman has the profound anemia to contend with which also reduces her resistance to infection.

These dangers beset the child: prematurity and atelectasis pulmonum; a much infarcted or ill-developed placenta causes the infant to be puny; prolapse of the cord; compression of the insertion of same, and dislocation of the placenta during delivery, may cause asphyxia; injury of the placenta causes fetal hemorrhage; and the infant may suffer from the forceps or version, but especially from the use of its body as a tampon to stop hemorrhage—the Braxton Hicks method.

Diagnosis.—A painless, causeless, uterine hemorrhage in the last three months of pregnancy usually enables a direct diagnosis of placenta prævia to be made, but the conclusion must be certified by vaginal examination and the finding of placental tissue over the internal os. One must bear in mind that a cervical erosion, a polyp, a varix, may bleed during pregnancy and trauma must be thought of.

The peculiar spongy, fibrous feel of the placental tissue may be simulated by a firm coagulum, by thick vernix caseosa in matted hair, by a monstrosity with exposed viscera—for example, anencephalus—by hemorrhage into the fetal membranes (which may indicate a placenta located near by), and by thickened membranes. Bogginess in the fornices, the sensation of a flat sponge between the head and the fingers, pulsating arteries, excessive vascularity, and a low and pronounced uterine souffle are all equivocal signs of placenta prævia.

In the differential diagnosis bleeding from varicose veins of the vagina and of the endocervix, hemorrhoids, carcinoma cervicis, hematuria, etc., are easily excluded, but ruptura uteri, ectopic gestation, and abruptio placentæ need more care. (See p. 486 for a table which gives the differential points concerning the last mentioned.) It must be remembered that a placenta situated low in the uterus without being actually a previa may become partly detached at its lower pole, and the point of bleeding being near the os, the blood escapes readily, not increasing intra-uterine tension and not separating the placenta entirely. In such instances the signs of abruptio may be wanting. Then, too, in the severest cases of abruptio placentæ the organ may prolapse and come to lie over the os, and, further, sometimes in abruptio the uterus is boggy.

Rupture of the uterus is easily shut out, but one must remember the tendency of the uterus to rupture when the placenta is low.

Bleeding from a vessel passing over the os from a velamentous insertion of the cord must also be thought of, and also laceration of the circular sinus.

Another point to be determined by the internal examination is whether the previal portion of the placenta is central, lateral, or only marginal—which is not always easy. Sweeping the finger delicately around the internal os, the accoucheur notes where the thin membranes become thicker, then passing into the thick placental margin. If the student will lay a placenta over a ring made by his fingers, he can practise the diagnosis of placenta prævia as on the living.

When making a vaginal examination in a case of suspected placenta prævia the patient must be in the operating room with everything in readiness for any operation—version, bag, tamponade, cesarean section.

Prognosis.—Placenta prævia is a formidable complication, and annually sacrifices more mothers and children than appear in statistics. In 1911 McDonald collected 8625 cases and found that 7.22 per cent. of the mothers and 55.5 per cent. of the babies died. In 1921 Hitschman reported 6438 cases, with 6.5 and 40 per cent. mortalities respectively. In the reports gathered from twenty different parts of the world I find mortalities that range from 1 to 19 per cent. for the mothers and 10 to 80 per cent. for the babies. The best results are gotten by individual accoucheurs, which proves that much depends on personal skill.

While these figures show the gravity of this complication they are particularly unreliable as guides to treatment, because success and failure depend on many factors, over some of which we have no control. A woman who has lost much blood or has been infected before admission to treatment is a bad risk; the stage of pregnancy is of influence, the danger being greater as term approaches because then efforts are doubled to save the child; central placenta prævia is usually more dangerous than the lateral and marginal varieties; the state of the blood (hemophilia), toxemia, and extraneous complications, e. g., heart disease, etc., may also cloud the prognosis.

Most of the deaths in placenta prævia come from hemorrhage, sepsis, rupture of the uterus, and air embolism, named in the order of frequency. The woman bleeds to death in labor usually because her store of blood has been wasted during pregnancy, or from an injury inflicted by delivery. Sepsis is invited by the proxim-

32

ity of the susceptible placental site to the field of operation, and the fact that hasty and many manipulations are necessary in the treatment. The previous bleedings reduce her resistance to infection as well as to the shock of even a small additional blood loss. Possibly the vaginal bacteria develop invasive properties, being supplied with pabulum—the decomposing blood or, perhaps, as de Snoo contends, cervical erosions form the atrium of infection. Rupture of the uterus is usually the result of violence exerted by the accoucheur, but may occur from tumultuous uterine action. Air-embolism is rare, but does occur, experiments on animals to the contrary notwithstanding. The children die from asphyxia through dislocation or compression of the placenta, tearing of the placenta and fetal hemorrhage, from being used as a plug in the Braxton-Hicks treatment, further, from prematurity. Later methods of treatment have improved the child's chances.

The prognosis as to health is also bad. Puerperal infection is of very frequent occurrence, resulting in life-long invalidism; the anemia may cause permanent changes in the blood-forming organs and in the nervous system, and the woman may be damaged by the operations performed for delivery.

Treatment.—Fortunately, we possess rational and certain methods of treatment for this formidable accident, which cannot be said of most other obstetric complications. In deciding on the course of procedure in the individual case many factors must be considered: the surroundings of the patient; the condition of the mother and that of the child; the necessity for preserving the infant (Catholic family); the skill of the accoucheur; the degree of the previa—whether partial or total; whether the patient is in labor or not; and the amount of dilatation of the cervix. From his own experience, and from thoughtful consideration of the published experience of others, the author would lay down these axioms:

1. A woman with placenta prævia should not die, except in the very rare instances of air-embolism, hemorrhagic diathesis, or spontaneous rupture of the uterus.

2. Every woman with placenta prævia should be sent to a well-equipped maternity hospital unless she is able and willing to provide the several physicians and nurses necessary in her own home. It is otherwise impossible to give the patient all the benefits of our art.

3. With two exceptions every pregnancy complicated with placenta prævia should be terminated as soon as the diagnosis is made. When the bleeding is indeed slight, and when the child is very near the border of viability, one may temporize a few weeks, *providing the patient will remain in bed in a good maternity hospital.* Should the woman refuse to go to the hospital, and also to allow the accoucheur to induce labor at her home, the attendant had better drop the case and let the patient employ a physician in whom the gambling instinct is better developed. A "flooding" may occur during the night, and the woman lose a fatal amount of blood before aid can reach her. Dr. W. W. Jaggard said, "there is no expectant plan of treatment for placenta prævia."

4. One must distinguish sharply between maternity and private practice, measures which are safe in the former being impossible in the latter. In the maternity hospital one should make a consistent effort to save the life of the child, but at the home one must use that method which will put an immediate stop to the hemorrhage, with, if necessary, less regard to the child. Also the accoucheur will select the procedure which he is best able to carry out, and must know all methods of delivery, as well as be able to suture the cervix and perform vaginal and abdominal hysterectomy, etc.

5. When labor has begun in a case of placenta prævia, the accoucheur must remain by the patient until she is delivered and out of danger.

6. At all times in the treatment of these cases the accoucheur should heed this warning— *save blood!* One can never foretell how much of the vital fluid the woman will lose in the successive stages of treatment, nor does one know what is the particular woman's ability to withstand bleeding. A loss of a pint will kill one woman, while another will recover from the loss of three quarts. Be not extravagant with her supply during the first and second stages of labor, because the normal flow in the third stage may be a fatal drain. Therefore, if, on arrival at the bedside, the accoucheur finds the woman already anemic, it is unsafe to use uncertain methods, but, regardless of all else, the hemorrhage must be arrested at once and every possible drop of blood spared. It may be wise to give the woman a prophylactic blood transfusion—at least, one should have a tested blood donor always readily accessible.

7. In deciding on the mode of delivery consider the possibility of fetal monstrosities, which seem to be a little more frequent than in normal pregnancies (Greenhill).

8. Before making an internal examination everything must be prepared as for operation, and great gentleness is to be practised to avoid separating and tearing the placenta, the dangers being maternal and fetal bleeding. It happened that the mere insertion of the finger into the cervix and even rectal examination has provoked such alarming hemorrhage that treatment had to be instituted there and then. This warning should never be disregarded.

During pregnancy, before labor-pains have begun, if one has decided to assume the risk and to temporize, the woman should be put to bed at the first indication of hemorrhage, and she should be in a perfectly appointed maternity hospital. Rarely is the first bleeding alarming, and rest, with the foot of the bed elevated, will usually stop it. If the child is not viable one may wait until it is, but on the appearance of another hemorrhage action is demanded—there is no wisdom in waiting longer. It is a wanton exposure of the mother to immediate and future danger for the sake of an infant which will probably succumb during delivery or shortly after. Hemorrhage is not the only danger—see Latent Infection, p. 941. The presence of blood in the vagina is not safe. We try to reinforce the local protective mechanism by douches of 5 per cent. lactic acid twice daily, and occasional instillation of 1 per cent. acriflavin in glycerin. One should avoid vaginal tamponade (recommended by Leroux in 1776). It is inefficient, converting external to internal hemorrhage, and dangerous—infective. If there is no other way of stopping a violent flooding (Braxton Hicks' version metreurysis), if one has started the flow at an examination and must have time to prepare for section, or, still more rarely, if a bleeding patient must be transported, one may tampon. The packing should be antiseptic, tight and removed within three hours. Counterpressure is to be applied with a firm abdominal binder, as in Fig. 403.

If the patient is near the ninth month, the child is viable and well developed, and there is no reason for waiting on its account.

During labor we have four objects to accomplish: First and most urgent, to stop the hemorrhage; second, to empty the uterus; third, to insure hemostasis; fourth, to combat the anemia.

We must stop the hemorrhage, then, first of all, and it matters a great deal whether the patient has already lost much or little blood when it comes to the selection of the method of stanching the flow.

In cases of marginal placenta prævia the hemorrhage usually begins toward the end of the second stage of labor and is very slight. The proper treatment is to puncture the bag of waters. This method is named after Puzos, who mentioned it (1759), but Justine Sigmundine had done it one hundred years before and Puzos knew nothing of the nature of placenta prævia, and, further, Mauriceau ruptured the membranes to stop hemorrhage in 1688. Both considered detachment of the placenta the cause of all the hemorrhages during pregnancy.

The puncture of the membranes allows the placenta to retract with the receding lower uterine segment, to become, as it were, part of the uterine wall, thus arresting the process of separation, and the head may now enter the lower uterine segment and apply itself against the placenta, thus aiding in stopping the hemorrhage. But rarely a case will occur in which, even in a marginal previa, puncture of the bag of waters will fail to arrest the flow. Such cases are treated like central and lateral implantation. Use a sharp needle to pierce the membranes or tear them with a bullet forceps.

If one finds the cervix fully dilated one should terminate the labor at once by forceps or version and extraction. **Be sure the cervix is fully dilated.**

The usual condition met is a more or less severe hemorrhage, with the os admitting two or more fingers. Pains may or may not be present, but some uterine action must have taken place, or the dilatation and hemorrhage could not have occurred.

There are now three methods of treatment—Braxton Hicks' version, metreurysis, and cesarean section. Which one should be selected depends on several conditions. If the woman has lost much blood; if the babe is dead or dying, or if it is very premature, so that its chances are very slim; if one has had little experience with placenta prævia—Braxton Hicks' version is preferable. Bring down one foot, make slight traction on it, so that the infant's thigh compresses the placenta

against the cervix, thus stopping the hemorrhage.   **Then leave the case to nature.**
Do not extract the child; do not give pituitary; do not put traction on the leg unless
bleeding recurs. If oozing commences, pull lightly on the leg. The object of this
method is to use the child's body as a cervical tampon to stop hemorrhage, and to

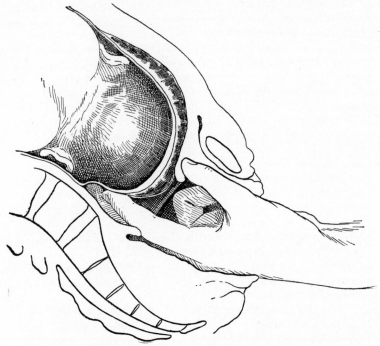

Fig. 412.—Finding a Site at Edge of Placenta for Puncture.
It is usually necessary to use a long scissors to get through tough membranes.

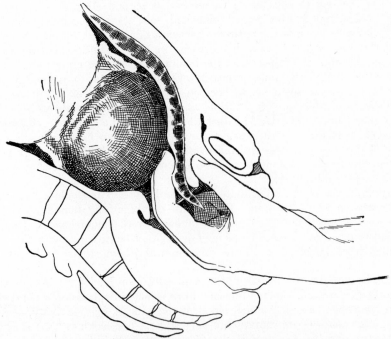

Fig. 413.—Compression of Placenta for Temporary Hemostasis.
Rubber gloves, omitted for artistic reasons in the illustrations, are used throughout.

stimulate pains *until the cervix is ready for safe delivery.* Neglect of the above advice and rapid extraction have cost many mothers their lives, and the object sought, the saving of the child, has usually been frustrated by the attempt itself.

In performing Braxton-Hick's version these points are to be noted: Puncture the membranes at the side of the cervix as far from the edge of the placenta as possible (Fig. 412). Then, disregarding the bleeding, which now commences and is sometimes furious, pass the hand into the vagina, the two fingers through the rent in the membranes alongside the head. The head is gently pushed to one side, while the outside hand presses first the breech, then the foot, down in the direction of the inside fingers. The fingers seek the foot, and as soon as this is grasped, it is led down

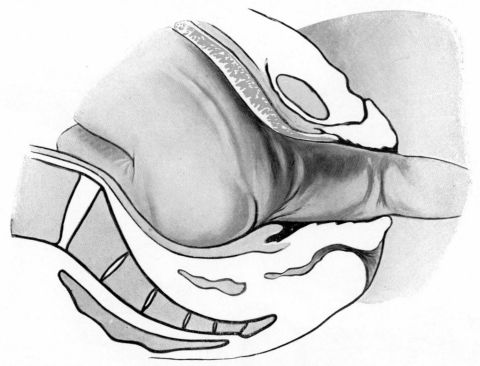

FIG. 414.—BRAXTON HICKS' VERSION COMPLETED.
Breech acts as tampon and squeezes placenta against bleeding vessels. It is essential for success to be certain that the placenta lies flat against the uterine wall, and is not bent back on itself, exposing uterine vessels.

into the vagina. It is then very gently drawn out, the other hand outside pressing the head upward toward the fundus. The secret in the performance of Braxton Hicks' version is complete relaxation of the abdomen and uterus, and dextrous aid by the outside hand in pressing the foot into the grasp of the inside fingers. The foot may be seized with a long placenta forceps. An anesthetic may be necessary for a few moments, but as soon as the foot is secured the mask should be removed, because anemic patients do not do well with anesthetics.

If the placenta covers the entire os, it is not advisable to waste valuable seconds in seeking its edge. It is better to bore through the most accessible portion.

It happens occasionally that delay is caused in performing the version after the membranes have been punctured. Perhaps the patient is unruly or rigid, or the bleeding may become so great that one fears for the mother's life. In such cases the bleeding may be temporarily checked by grasping the placenta and uterine wall, as in Fig. 413. This will give the operator time to collect himself. Another way is to grasp the whole cervix with the inside hand, press it against the head, while the outside hand forces the whole uterus down into the pelvis. We must strive to save blood every inch of the way.

After the version the case is absolutely under control (Fig. 414). If the placenta is pressed flat against the uterine wall, the woman can bleed no more, and measures may be instituted to replace the blood she has lost. Salt solution is administered intravenously or hypodermically, not per rectum, using judgment as to the proper amount. Transfusion is life saving both in critical cases, and as a prophylactic.

Unfortunately, this method sacrifices a large number of children, and to remove this opprobrium Mäurer introduced, and Dührssen urged, the second method, metreurysis.   This, in brief, is the use of a rubber balloon to take the place of the breech in tamponing the cervix and lower uterine segment.   Mäurer, in 1887, described this maneuver, but it is due to the labors of Dührssen that it has been generalized, though even now few accoucheurs are aware of its immense advantages. It is applicable at all stages of cervical dilatation, before the os is sufficiently open

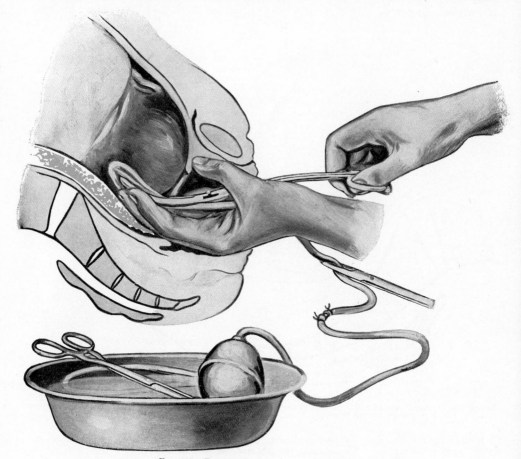

FIG. 415.—PASSING COLPEURYNTER INTO UTERUS.
Lubrication with sterile vaselin or liquid soap facilitates introduction.

to permit delivery.   It may be used to induce labor, or it may be used when version has been tried and has failed.   One may dilate the cervix sufficiently to proceed with immediate delivery, or one may dilate sufficiently for the performance of version, after which the case may be treated according to conditions as they arise.   The colpeurynter (or metreurynter) marks nearly as great an advance in the treatment of placenta prævia as did the introduction of Braxton-Hicks' version.   Metreurysis is used in cases where the condition of the mother and child is good.   When the mother has lost little blood and the child is viable, we may take a reasonable chance on a little greater hemorrhage for the sake of the infant.

Several bags are on the market.   Voorhees, of New York, made a modification of the Champetier de Ribes' inelastic conic balloon, which is very serviceable, and sizes may be gotten large enough to secure complete dilatation.   The size of the bag should be the estimated size of the fetal head.

All preparations are made beforehand.   The bag and the bulb syringe for filling are sterilized by boiling twenty minutes in plain water.   The colpeurynter is emptied of air first.   This is accomplished by filling it with 0.5 per cent. lysol solution, then inverting it so that all this fluid runs out. A clamp is now affixed 4 inches from the end of the tube. The air is all pumped out of the bulb syringe and the nozzle fitted into the end of the tube of the colpeurynter. For greater security this tube may be tied on with tape. The bag is now folded lengthwise into as narrow a compass as possible, and then grasped by the long uterine packing forceps. The whole apparatus lies in a basin of 0.5 per cent. lysol solution, from which it is to be filled.

The membranes are now punctured as for the performance of version, and, operating quickly, guided by the two fingers in the cervix, the bag (Fig. 415) is placed inside the uterus *on top of the placenta*. Be careful not to push up the edge of the placenta so that it doubles up under the colpeurynter. This would allow intra-uterine hemorrhage. The clamp is now removed from the tube, and steadying the colpeurynter on the placenta, the other hand, by slow pressures on the bulb of the syringe, injects the required amount of lysol solution (Fig. 416). The author does not recommend the extra-ovular application of the bag, putting it inside the cervix but beneath the placenta. If one could place the bag on top of the placenta, but leaving the amnion intact, as

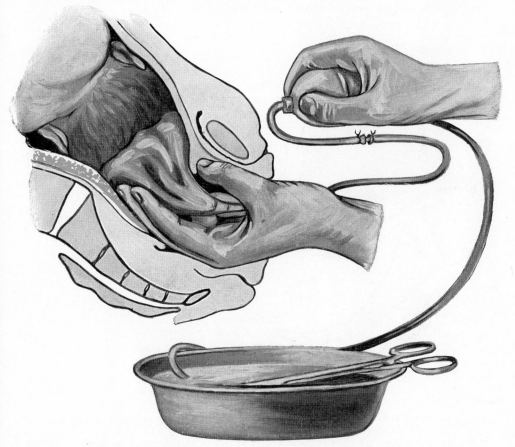

FIG. 416.—FILLING COLPEURYNTER. (Some operators prefer a piston syringe.)

happens now and then inadvertently, advantages might accrue. One must inject slowly in order not to overdistend, and too rapidly stretch, the lower uterine segment. The balloon should be full, but not overfull, which makes it hard, so that it illy adapts itself to the placenta and uterus, and it may evoke such strong pains that it is expelled precipitately, rupturing the cervix. The head, of course, is displaced by the colpeurynter, but this cannot be avoided. Since, when the bag is expelled, delivery is consummated, little harm results from displacing the head. After the bag is in position one reassures himself that the placenta is underneath it, and not doubled upon itself, and withdraws the hand from the vagina. Now the tube is clamped with an artery forceps and slight traction exerted on it (Fig. 417). Only sufficient pressure is brought to bear on the placenta and cervix as will stop the hemorrhage. This accomplished, the accoucheur seats himself at the bedside and maintains slight traction on the tube of the colpeurynter. One or at most two pounds will be required, and to determine this one may insert a scale in the line of traction, or fasten, by means of a tape, a bottle containing the proper amount of water, and hang it over the foot-board of the bed. The tube near the vulva is frequently painted with mercurochrome, to prevent bacteria from wandering upwards on it.

I prefer to hook the ordinary baby scale into the artery forceps, or pull on it myself, and thus personally watch the traction. Every three 'or four minutes one should relax the pull to allow blood to get into the cervix. An anemic cervix will tear more readily than one properly nourished.

Pains usually come on within an hour, and, while they are irregular, they accomplish the effacement and dilatation of the cervix. After an hour or so the pains become more regular. One relaxes the pull on the bag during the pain, resuming it when the contraction is over. *Avoid too powerful traction on the bag.* This may rupture the cervix and lower uterine segment directly, or it may excite such powerful uterine action that this ruptures the uterus. I have had one such accident. Indeed, the pains must not be allowed to become too strong in placenta prævia. If such a danger threatens, stop pulling on the bag, and if this does not produce the desired effect, allow several ounces of fluid to escape from the bag. Do not use pituitrin in placenta prævia before delivery of the child. The obstetrician must possess a large fund of patience, as he may be required to hold on to the colpeurynter for from three to twelve hours.

The next point of importance in the treatment is to determine the exact moment when the colpeurynter passes through the cervix. If one neglects to note this, pulling on the tube brings the bag down onto the perineum and a large quantity of blood accumulates between it and the

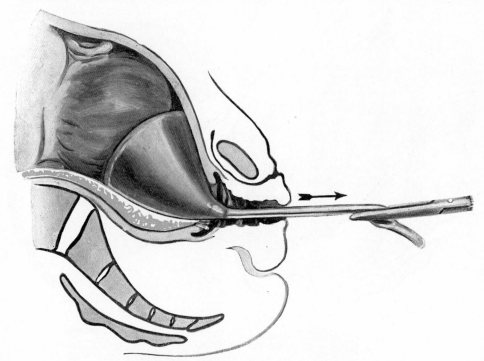

Fig. 417.—Colpeurynter in Place.
It acts like the breech in compressing the placental site.

child (Fig. 418). It is a very serious loss, because one cannot control the hemorrhage so well after dilatation of the cervix as before, unless it is possible to deliver at once. Sometimes the head follows down and takes the place of the colpeurynter, tamponing the cervix securely. These are fortunate cases, and one has nothing to do but watch and let nature take the lead. It is advisable, as soon as the head has passed the cervix, to deliver, because the child's life is in a rather precarious position, and, second, the placenta may separate and blood may accumulate in the uterine cavity.

The accoucheur determines that the colpeurynter is passing the cervix, first, by noting the steady advancement of the tube; by occasional direct rectal examination one feels the cervix slipping over the greatest circumference of the bag; third, the patient begins to bear down, and the pain has a sharp, cutting character; fourth, after the bag has passed through, the pains cease or are milder; fifth, the bag is expelled—but the two latter signs show delinquency on the part of the accoucheur. By the time the bag comes to pass through the cervix, the attendant must be ready to deliver or to do a version, as indicated. The time consumed in getting ready, after the bag has slipped through the os, may mean a fatal loss of blood.

If the head does not follow the metreurynter into the pelvis, the operator withdraws the bag quickly from the vagina, emptying it, if necessary, as quickly inserts his whole hand, and grasps the cervix and placenta until he can determine on the course of procedure. If the head is still high, he tries to force it down into the pelvis. This will stop the hemorrhage and allow the forceps to be applied. If the head does not go into the pelvis, podalic version is to be performed. If the cervix is not sufficiently dilated by the first attempt with the colpeurynter, one may insert a larger one, which will dilate the os to the size of the fetal head or perform version.

When the cervix is rigid or tightly closed, conditions more likely to be found in primigravidæ, the case assumes a formidable aspect. If the patient is in a safe hospital, in competent hands, and the child viable, cesarean section should be chosen, otherwise vaginal delivery. By gentle manipulation it is almost always possible to insinuate a small bag into the uterus, failing which, one must resort to vaginal tamponade. This, combined with firm counterpressure (Spanish windlass, Fig. 403), will usually check the bleeding and inaugurate labor. When the cervix admits two fingers the case falls into the class just described.

Regarding Delivery.—The heart-tones of the child must be carefully noted during the time the colpeurynter is in place and after a version is done. If the cord

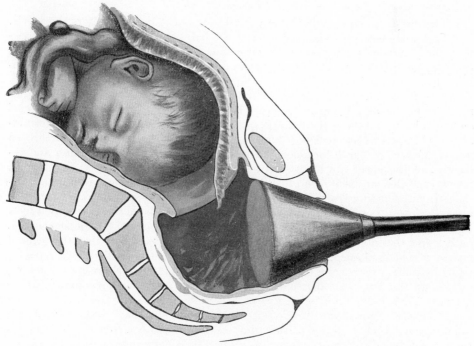

Fig. 418.—Bag has Passed the Cervix and Blood has Accumulated Behind It.

is in the area of the placenta compressed by the breech or colpeurynter, some asphyxia of the infant is unavoidable. This may not be fatal, but is very unwelcome, the more so because we are practically powerless to extract the child until the cervix is dilated. The most we can do is to try, if safe, to hasten the dilatation of the cervix somewhat. This is done by exerting a little more traction on the breech or bag, say $2\frac{1}{2}$ pounds, with, of course, the precautions already emphasized. **If an urgent indication on the part of the child for delivery should arise before the cervix is sufficiently dilated, it will have to be disregarded.** The danger of haste is too great for the mother. An indication for delivery will not arise on the part of the mother, because we can control the hemorrhage by the colpeurynter or the breech. Great hemorrhage and collapse do not indicate rapid delivery; on the contrary, the sudden emptying of the uterus may add to the shock and turn the delicate balance against the woman. In such cases of severe hemorrhage and shock the quickest and most definitive means of stopping the hemorrhage is by version and tamponing the lower uterine segment by the breech. One then has the case almost absolutely under control.

Since there is no hemorrhage, there is not the shadow of a reason for hurry. These hours should be employed in supplying the woman with fluids, as saline solution hypodermically, transfusion, food, etc. The woman recovers from the shock of her first hemorrhage. The hours are also useful for the preparations for delivery. No detail should be omitted, and everything must be gotten ready and rehearsed beforehand, so that when the delivery is to be made, not an instant's delay need be tolerated. A complete set of obstetric instruments should be sterilized, especial provision being made for the treatment of postpartum hemorrhage. Needles, long needle-holder, vulsella, specula, etc., for sewing lacerations of the cervix may be needed, as well as gauze and long uterine packing forceps for tamponing the uterus, also Henkel's museux or a Sehrt aorta compressor (Fig. 721). Good light and a table on which to place the patient for delivery should be gotten ready, and provision made for the resuscitation of the child—tracheal catheter, hot bath, hot towels, etc.

The case is much simplified if the head follows the bag and enters the pelvis. One may wait—studying the condition of the baby and the mother incessantly— until the head comes down on to the perineum. Then there is no reason for longer delaying the use of forceps. After version one also proceeds, but even more carefully, to the extraction.

As a rule, the cervix may be sufficiently prepared to permit delivery, but let me again sound the warming—*Beware of too hasty extraction through a poorly dilated cervix!* The laceration of the highly vascularized cervix is one of the most formidable accidents the accoucheur could meet. The uteroplacental sinuses are so superficial that a tear $\frac{1}{8}$ inch deep may lay one open. The contraction and retraction of the lower uterine segment are poor at best, and poorest in placenta prævia, and this means of hemostasis is not strong, so that the cases of fatal hemorrhage from even tiny tears of the placental site are easily explained. Avoid pituitary. Slowest possible delivery is to be practised. If the head is restrained by a tight cervix, the accoucheur must not use force to extract it, but must courageously allow the infant to die. The child is so often already lost that this painful advice is seldom needed. An attempt to let air into the child's lungs must be made by pulling the vagina back with a speculum, and, after cleansing the fauces, depressing the jaw with the fingers, an expedient which was recommended by Pugh, in 1754, though not in such cases.

Treatment During the Third Stage.—Many patients have been lost at this point, having been skilfully carried through the two other stages. It is necessary to save blood with every move. As soon as the child is delivered, as in cesarean section, it is handed to a competent assistant, the operator devoting all his attention to the mother. One c.c. of strong pituitary extract is given. Even a moderate hemorrhage now demands the immediate removal of the placenta. Since contraction and retraction of the bed of the placenta are imperfect, and especially since its structure may be pathologically altered, the delivery of the placenta is slow and adherences may be met with, some of which are so tough that the finger cannot break them. As soon as the placenta is removed the uterus usually contracts strongly and bleeding ceases. Sometimes the lower uterine segment remains atonic—dilated—and the contracted fundus descends into it, a sort of intussusception occurring. Watch closely, *pulling open the vagina with a speculum to see if blood continues to escape from the cervix*, and if it does, tampon the whole uterovaginal tract firmly. *Waste no precious seconds on uncertain methods of hemostasis*, but in the presence of such urgent symptoms use the most radical and definitive means we have. During the ten to twenty seconds while waiting for the gauze hold the uterus securely in forced anteflexion (Fig. 714), or apply compression to the aorta. (See Treatment of Postpartum Hemorrhage, p. 839.)

In placenta prævia a tiny laceration may give rise to a fatal bleeding. The soft, vascularized cervix is difficult to hold for suturing, and it may be impossible to sew up a laceration or to sew it up quickly enough to save an already exsanguinated woman. In suturing a laceration of the cervix it is necessary to expose the field thoroughly by broad retractors (Fig. 689). The lips are grasped with the vulsellum forceps, and the tear brought within reach of the needle. Usually the field is so flooded with blood that it is impossible to see where to sew. A heavy vulsellum forceps may be laid temporarily on each side of the uterus, seeking to secure the uterine arteries in the bases of the broad ligaments (Henkel) or Sehrt's aorta compressor applied. In one such case I packed the uterus and the rent in the broad ligament firmly with gauze, thus stopping the furious flow, after which the lips of the cervix were united over the tampon, thus closing up the uterus entirely (Fig. 722). The vagina was snugly packed with dry cotton to exert counterpressure. The sutures were removed the next day and the gauze two days later. The patient recovered.

In sewing up a bleeding cervix tear the first suture is put on an accessible part of the lips, then using this as a tractor one "climbs up" with sutures till the fornix is reached. Here a very deep bite must be taken with the needle, trying to secure the uterine artery. Failing this, a fatal dissecting hematoma may result. Hysterectomy is to be considered.

Before, during, and after delivery in cases of placenta prævia it is often necessary to treat the anemia. If the mother has lost much blood, give her saline solution under the skin, not per rectum, as this interferes with the asepsis of the local treatment. When the bowels are moving over the field of operation, it may be impossible to avoid carrying the discharges into the uterus. Saline solution is to be given even if the hemorrhage is going on, as then the patient does not lose pure blood, but blood mixed with salt solution. We do not wait for fainting to stop the hemorrhage in placenta prævia. The author has administered a gallon of saline solution under the skin and it was absorbed as fast as it could be injected, and, after the local treatment of the case was completed, 2 quarts more per rectum, with success. Such large amounts are seldom required. Nowadays transfusion has become our best friend in hemorrhage cases.

Other Methods of Treatment.—Accouchement forcé, the rapid dilatation of the cervix, tearing and cutting it, if necessary, followed by the immediate delivery of the child, has no place in the treatment of placenta prævia. The author believes it is almost criminal, and it is opposed to all recognized principles of treatment. The results condemn it, and Kerr says, judging from mortalities, it is the worst of all methods. Müller showed 44 per cent. maternal mortality and 62.7 per cent. for the children. Gentle dilatation is wanted, for even the soft-rubber bag may rupture the cervix unless properly handled.

Cesarean section, first performed by Tait, is gradually gaining reluctant recognition. Especially favored by American surgeons and gynecologists, it was condemned by American and European obstetricians—Ehrenfest, Hirst, Williams, Holmes, Schauta, Hofmeier—but very recently the operation has begun to enjoy more, and I think just, popularity. Sellheim, Stoeckel, Pankov, P. Dudley, Brouha (Liege), Zinke, Kerr, Smith, Bill, Bar, Recasens (Madrid) recommend it —of course, in well-chosen cases. Cesarean section has a general mortality of 4 per cent. in favorable cases; it should be no more than this in favorable cases of placenta prævia, and there is, in addition, the reduction of the infant mortality from 50 to 5 per cent. Placenta prævia, under the usual methods, shows at best 4 per cent. mortality, and its treatment entails great anxiety, much loss of time, and requires exceptional obstetric skill to save both mother and child. In the isthmial variety, where the placenta is implanted squarely over the internal os and hangs like a festoon above it, the maternal mortality is so high that the abdominal delivery is strongly the method of choice. I believe an indication for cesarean section will arise in cases of central and of partial placenta prævia, when the pregnancy is at or near term, with a living child and the mother in good condition. A primipara with placenta prævia and a really viable child requires laparotrachelotomy. A necessary requirement also is that the aseptic facilities of a good maternity can be had, or improvised at home, and a man capable of his task is obtainable.

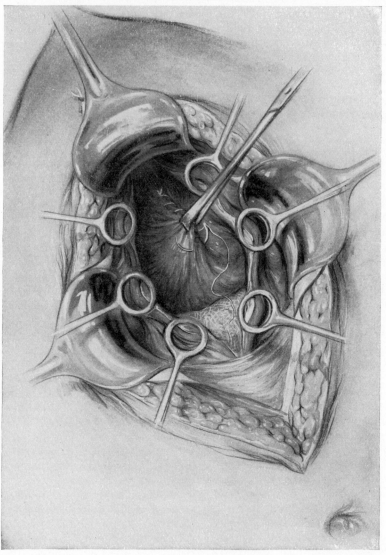

Fig. 418a.—Whipping Over Raised Bed of Bleeding Placental Site at Laparotrachelotomy.
The bleeding sinuses in the cut edges of the lower uterine segment are clamped with tongue forceps, and the wound made to gape. Any bleeding points or areas in the placental bed are thus exposed to view and are easily sutured.

While most operators choose the classic cesarean for placenta prævia, a few, including the author, prefer the low, cervical—laparotrachelotomy. If the placenta lies on the anterior wall the technic is not so easy as usual, but the difficulties are readily overcome. One has the great advantage that the bleeding field lies plainly open to view, and one may tampon or suture the sinuses of the placental site. In one case the placenta was adherent to a crescentic spur of cervical mucosa on the posterior wall and its removal was followed by a severe hemorrhage from this spot. The flow was stopped by suturing the spur. In cases of placenta prævia cervicalis (similar to the one just cited) the villi burrow deeply into the muscle. Here the low incision gives us direct access to the source of the bleeding (Fig. 418a).

If the woman has a number of children, and the bleeding approaches the danger limit, or if the intention was to sterilize her, a Porro operation meets the indications best.

Vaginal cesarean section was performed by Dührssen and is recommended by Essen-Moeller. It is condemned by most writers, among whom are Kerr, Spencer, Peterson, Newell, Hofmeier, Hannes, and the author.

In the exigencies of general practice, and in the usual bad surroundings in which these cases come to the accoucheur, it is found that the best method of treatment is Braxton-Hicks' version and very slow spontaneous delivery. Next comes the metreurynter.

LITERATURE

Bar: L'Obstetrique, September, 1909.—*Bill:* Amer. Jour. Obst. and Gyn., 1927, 14, p. 523.—*Brouha:* Gynecologie et Obstetrique, 1922, No. 3, p. 199.—*Doranth:* Chrobak's Berichte und Arbeiten, Vienna, 1897.—*Essen-Moeller:* Acta Gynecol. Scandinavica, vol. i, No. 1, 1921.—*Goodman:* "Cervical Placenta Prævia," Jour. Amer. Med. Assoc., October 14, 1911.—*Greenhill:* Surg., Gyn., and Obst., February, 1922.—*Henkel:* Arch. f. Gyn., 1908, vol. lxxxvi, Heft 3, p. 705.—*Hitschmann:* Monograph, Placenta Prævia, Vienna, 1920.—*Hofmeier:* Handb. d. Geb. v. Winckel, vol. ii, H. 2, p. 1285.—*Kerr:* Operative Midwifery, p. 591.—*Krause:* Zeitschr. für Geb. u. Gyn., 1921, Band 83, H. 2.—*Krönig:* Zentralbl. f. Gyn., 1909, No. 34.—*Leroux:* See Read, Wm.; Placenta Prævia, 1861, p. 35. Lit. Its History and Treatment.—*McDonald:* Surg., Gyn., and Obst., June, 1911, also July. Literature.—*Müller:* Handbuch d. Geb., vol. ii, 2, p. 1251.—*Pugh:* Treatise on Midwifery, 1754, p. 49.—*Sellheim:* Zentralbl. f. Gyn., 1908, No. 40.—*Smellie:* Treatise of Midwifery, 1779, pp. 120 and 143, note.—*de Snoo:* Ref. Jour. Amer. Med. Assoc., 1920, p. 777.—*Stoeckel:* Lehrbuch der Geburtshilfe, 1930, p. 495.—*v. Weiss:* Zentralbl. f. Gyn., 1897, No. 22, p. 641.—*Zangemeister:* Monatsschr. für Geb. u. Gyn., October, 1922.

CHAPTER XXXV

MULTIPLE PREGNANCY

PLACING this subject in the pathology of pregnancy might elicit comment, but the succeeding pages, showing the frequency of maternal disease and of fetal death, will prove that, in the human female, having more than one offspring at a time is distinctly abnormal. It is an atavistic reversion, and, in general, such reversions are abnormal. Twins occur, according to Greulich, who studied over 120,000,000 births, once in 85.2 cases, triplets once in 7628.7; quadruplets once in 670,734. Quintuplets occur once in 41,600,000 births (Gussoni). Over 30 cases of quintuplets have been reported. Vassali reports an authentic case of sextuplets, at Lake Lugano, there being delivered at the fourth month two female and four male children with a total weight of 1730 gm.

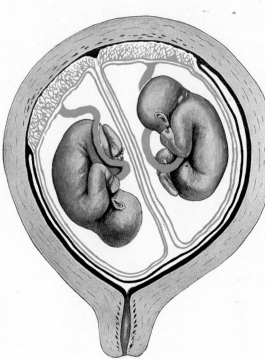

FIG. 419.—DOUBLE OVUM TWINS.
Black lines are decidua; red, the chorion; blue, the amnion.

The frequency of multiple pregnancy varies with the fertility of the people (Peuch, 1873), and the fertility varies in different countries and at different periods; thus in Ireland and Russia twin births are commoner than in France, where the birth-rate is low.

Multiparæ, especially those giving birth frequently, are more likely to have twins, and the probability increases after the age of thirty-three years in both parents. A hereditary disposition is certain, and the tendency, while usually transmitted by the mother, may also be given through the father (Bonnevie). It is also noted in the lower uniparous animals, for example, the cow (Duncan). Marriage of twins increases the potency of the hereditary impulse. Twins and triplets are likely to be repeated in the same family. Cases of unusual fertility are not rare. Geisler tells of a woman physician (Mary Austin) who, in thirty-three years' wedlock, had 13 twins and 6 triplet births, a total of 44 children, her sisters having 41 and 26 children respectively (Strassman). Sue tells of a Parisian whose wife bore him 21 children in seven years, and who seduced a servant, who then delivered triplets. (See Neugebauer et al.)

Causation.—Generally, two kinds of twins are distinguished, those coming from separate and distinct ova and those from one ovum. Two eggs escaping from an ovary at the same time may be fertilized and develop synchronously in the uterus. These eggs may even come out of the same Graafian follicle, since such follicles, and even some containing three eggs, have frequently been seen. Each ovary may furnish one of the ova. When two or more separate ova locate in the uterus, we

510

have distinct ovular formations developing side by side (Fig. 419). If the ova locate far from each other, two distinct placentas develop; if near each other, the two placentas fuse, but their circulations do not (Schatz). Since in such cases each child has its own amnion and chorion, where the membranes lie apposed, a septum will be found made up of four layers—an amnion and a chorion for each fetus. Occasionally decidual remants will be found in the septum, the relics of the deciduæ capsulares or reflexæ of the early stages of the development of the ova. Curtius showed that one egg may show two chorions. Theoretically, one might insist on finding six layers in the septum of double ovum or dizygotic twins— two deciduæ, two chorions, and two amnions (Lit., Newman).

The etiology of twins from one ovum, called homologous, or monozygotic, is still a mystery. Aristotle knew that two embryos could come from an egg with two yolks, and three embryos have been found in one egg. Two nuclei have been found in one yolk, and Kölliker, Stöckel, and von Franque found double germinal vesicles in the human egg. If such an ovum is to be fertilized, two polar bodies must first be extruded, and two spermatozoids are needed for fertilization, which theoretically is not impossible, but then we would have two chorions developed and the findings would be the same as if two different eggs had been impregnated. Perhaps we shall learn hereafter that such an occurrence has been proved. Another theory is that on one germinal vesicle two primitive streaks develop, that is, double gastrulation occurs. Two spermatozoids entering the ovum probably cannot produce this condition, because ova fertilized in this way usually die.

If the two embryonal spots develop close to each other, it is possible that one amnion will

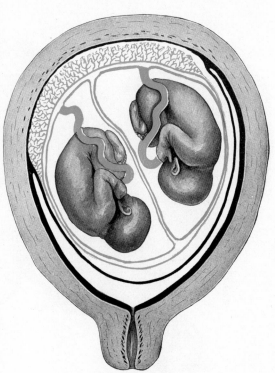

FIG. 420.—HOMOLOGOUS OR SINGLE OVUM TWINS.
Black lines are decidua; red, the chorion; blue, the amnion.

inclose the two fetuses; if far from each other, each fetus will have a separate amnion (Fig. 420). The older writers held that always two amnions developed, but that the septum atrophied and disappeared. Only about 40 cases are on record of twins without a septum between the two sacs, that is, lying in one amniotic cavity. Should the separation of the two embryonal areas be incomplete, a double monster will result (Sobotta); therefore, according to the theory that homologous twins are the result of the fission of the embryonal area into two parts, and their separate development into fully formed fetuses, we must conclude that double monsters, like the Siamese twins, are the result of incomplete fission and not of fusion. A monster with four legs would mean fission at the lower pole, and one with two heads fission at the cephalic pole of the embryonal area. It is regretable that we have little scientific foundation for these plausible theories.

Only single ovum twins should really be called twins, the others are a double pregnancy.

Characteristics.—The placenta in unioval twins is almost invariably single; there are usually two cords, but rarely only one, which bifurcates near the fetuses, and these are monoamniotic ova; the blood-vessels anastomose on the surface of the placenta, and also in the villi themselves, producing a third or intermediate circulation between the twins so that the whole placenta can be injected from either cord.   The septum of the placenta never shows traces of decidua, and only two layers, the two amnions, can be found in it.   In the rarest of cases, 2 chorions or separate placentas have been found.   The children are said to be very much alike in size and in mental and physical characteristics, including finger and sole prints (Montgomery), but the author has not found this to be constant.   (See Gesell, Newman.)   Unioval twins occur, according to Ahlfeld in 15.55 per cent., Wagner, 33 per cent.; and Orel 23.8 per cent. of cases.

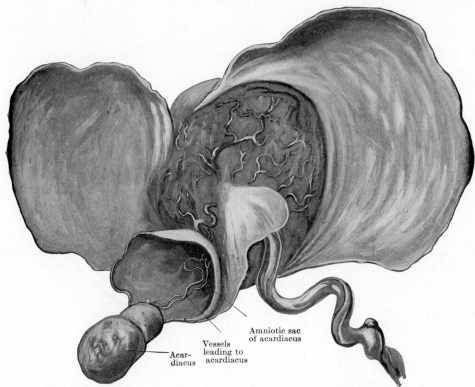

Fig. 421.—Acardiacus Amorphus.   (Northwestern University Medical School specimen.)

Triplets and even quadruplets may all come from one ovum, but usually two ova are concerned, one of which may bring forth two fetuses.   (Sasse.)

In length and weight twins usually differ more or less, 4 cm. and 2200 gm. being the limits respectively.   Twins are usually smaller than single children, but the combined weight is greater.   The same proportion of boys and girls obtains with twins as in general.   Twins from one ovum are smaller than those from two, and the difference in weight is not so great; also they have a higher mortality and are more often deformed.   The same deformity often exists in both twins, as in one of the author's cases, double harelip, and one of C. E. Black, rudimentary colon. It is said the tendency to this form of twins is not hereditary (Strassman).   Eclampsia is more common with unioval twins.   Homologous twins are always of the same sex.   The two circulations anastomose in the common placenta, artery to artery, vein to vein, and artery to vein through the third circulation, the intercommunicating villus tree.   The anastomosis of the two blood systems was known to Portal, who, therefore, advised the tying of the cord of the first child delivered to prevent the other from bleeding through the open vessels. As a result of this arrangement many anomalies arise out of the unequal distribution and size of the placental vessels and unequal nutritional conditions. The heart of one child, because of its better nourishment, may overpower that of the other through the anastomotic vessels. If this occurs at an early period, the weaker heart dilates into a tortuous vessel, the fetus remains undeveloped and becomes a parasite on its stronger brother (Fig. 421). It is called an acardiacus. If one fetus dies after being fully developed and is long retained in the uterus, it is changed into a fœtus compressus (Fig. 422). Sometimes the stronger fetus causes a polyhydramnion, according to Strassman, because its hypertrophied heart and kidneys produce more urine, while the weaker suffers from oligohydramnion. Polyhydramnion is so common with twins that when it is discovered, the existence of the latter is to be suspected. If the twins lie in one amniotic cavity, the two umbilical cords may be twisted, causing the death of one or both fetuses.

Dichorionic or double-ovum twins are also subject to abnormalities. One fetus may die and be expelled, the other going normally to term. The author delivered a woman at term of twins, and she stated that five months previously she had had, in New York city, an abortion of four months. Again the dead fetus may be retained, and the liquor amnii being absorbed, it is flattened against the wall of the uterus, a dry, shrunken mass (Fig. 422). It may present before the normal fetus, giving rise to diagnostic errors, and it may be lost in the uterus after delivery of the placenta and cause puerperal infection and late hemorrhages. The placenta of the compressed fetus is white, hard, fibrous, infarcted, and demarked sharply from that of the normal fetus, and this finding on the placenta will arouse the suspicion of the accoucheur that another fetus has been retained in utero.

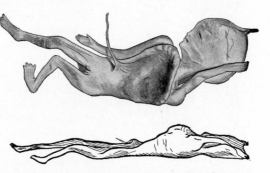

Fig. 422.—Two Views of a Fœtus Papyraceus or Compressus. The head of the second, well-developed child lay in the hollowed-out chest of the first one, the fœtus compressus.

Superfetation is the nesting of a second fetus in the uterus already occupied by one in the process of development. Its occurrence has been held possible by American and French authors, while the English and German writers usually deny it. A double uterus may carry a child in each compartment, as in the cases quoted by Ramsbotham—one, where a woman, five months and sixteen days after the delivery of a living seven months' child, delivered another of full development, and another where two well-formed, fully developed boys were born three months apart. These cases should not be called superfetation. Since the decidua reflexa does not unite with the vera until the middle of the fourth month, and since ovulation occurs during pregnancy (Rovano), theoretically superfetation is possible, but in most instances cannot be proved. Differences in the size of the fetuses may be explained by unequal development, but F. T. Andrews, Barry, and the author have seen specimens which prove the occurrence of superfetation in the human female. Dr. Zimmerman, of Cameron, Illinois found a healthy ovum of four weeks, together with a healthy fetus of ten weeks, in an aborted mass. A specimen was shown to the Gynecologic Society of Chicago of two extra-uterine pregnancies of different dates which had been removed at operation. Dr. T. J. Watkins relates the case of the delivery of twins at three months and triplets at term of the same pregnancy (Lit., Radasch, Meyer). Laboratory proof is now brought by Wislocki and Snyder, also Foederl.

Superfecundation is the impregnation of two different ova, about the same time, by sperma from different fathers. Its occurrence in animals is proved, but though doubted for the human, is possible. A negro woman gave birth to a black and mulatto child, after intercourse with a black and a white man. A white woman gave birth to a white and a negro child, but both these combinations may occur with only one father. To prove superfecundation we must ask, with Schultze, that a woman after intercourse with two men of different races and other than her own bears twins showing the characteristics of both sires. Merkel suggested blood grouping.

Clinical Course.—Plural pregnancy always gives rise to disturbances on the part of both mother and child. The sympathetic symptoms, nausea and vomiting,

33

are usually exaggerated; toxemia, varices, and edema are more marked; the **great** distention of the abdomen interferes with the bowels, urination, and respiration, especially if hydramnion complicates the condition. Softening and relaxation of the pelvic joints are sometimes extreme, which, added to the great abdominal distention and the weight of the large uterus, make locomotion difficult or impossible. Either because the several fetuses produce too much toxin or because the kidneys are laboring under mechanical difficulties the kidney of pregnancy, nephritis, and eclampsia are much more common than in single pregnancy. Edema and even ascites may occur; indeed, a pregnancy without edema is almost positively a single one. The heart has a double burden, and, if already diseased, may fail.

About 80 per cent. of duplex pregnancies terminate before term, and practically all triplet and quadruplet gestations do so. Premature labor is caused by the overdistention of the uterus, the lower uterine segment and cervix being developed earlier than usual, and the presenting part engaging in the pelvis. According to the latest theory, labor comes on sooner because of the larger amount of ferment produced by the two fetuses, stimulating the uterus to action.

Labor with twins is often abnormal. Owing to the overstretching of the uterine muscle, the pains are weak and intermittent, labor drags on, sometimes for days, effacement and dilatation of the cervix are slow, and the parturient loses sleep and becomes early exhausted. Many peculiarities are noted in the mechanism of labor. Since the children are small and there is usually much liquor amnii, we observe frequent changes of presentation and position during pregnancy, and also during labor, sometimes produced by the delivery of one of the twins. For example, while one child comes through head first, the second changes from shoulder to breech presentation. Werth gives the following table of 1688 twin births:

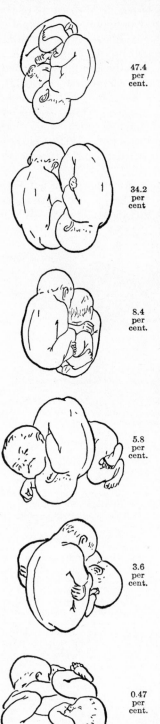

Both children in cephalic presentation. .	47.4 per cent.
Head and breech presentation.	34.2 "
Both breech presentation	8.4 "
Head and transverse presentation	5.8 "
Breech and transverse presentation	3.6 "
Both transverse presentation	0.47 "

The sacs occupied by the twins usually lie side by side (Fig. 425), but one may lie in front of the other (Fig. 424) or even on top of the other. In the last instance the second child during delivery has to pass through the empty amniotic cavity of the first, and the second opening in the membranes will be found in the septum. The children usually lie parallel, one on each side of the spinal column, but one may lie anteriorly and the other be entirely beyond the reach of the palpating hand. Occasionally, when the amount of liquor amnii is small, the children are dovetailed into each other, and, under like conditions, if the two

47.4 per cent.

34.2 per cent

8.4 per cent.

5.8 per cent.

3.6 per cent.

0.47 per cent.

FIG. 423.—PERCENTAGE TABLE OF TWINS.

heads are apposed, they may be faceted. In one of the author's cases the flattening of the foreheads of the children was noticeable after several years.

If one placenta lies above the other, it is not rare to find the lower edge of the common placenta near or over the internal os. Placenta prævia with twins endangers three lives. Transverse and breech presentations are favored by the low implantation of the common placenta.

Owing to the shape of the uterus, the child lying in its left half usually is lower and presents and is delivered first. The uterine muscle now has a chance to shorten and get a better grip on its contents. Another bag of waters forms, ruptures, and the second fetus is extruded, usually more quickly than the first, because the muscle is stronger and there is no resistance from the soft parts. The interval between the deliveries varies from a few minutes to forty-four days (Carson). Reference has already been made to the abortion of one twin while the other was carried to term.

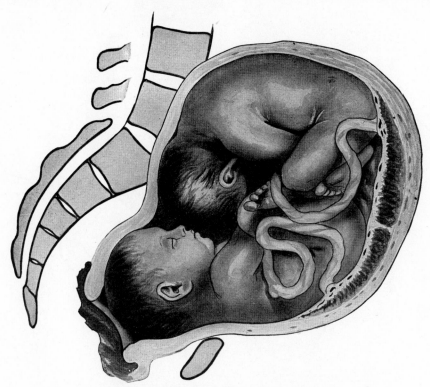

Fig. 424.—Twins, One in Front of the Other.

It is impossible to show by figures the natural interval between the two births, because, as a rule, the accoucheur hastens the second delivery. Usually the second child follows the first after thirty to forty minutes. In one of the author's cases the head of the second followed the feet of the first.

Now, the uterus contracts firmly down on the placenta, and in a small majority of cases the third stage is natural. Hemorrhage, however, is more profuse and the after-pains are harder.

Diagnosis of Twins.—Very rarely has the diagnosis of triplets been made before delivery. Pinard, of Paris, and Fletcher Bell, among others, did it. Twins may almost always be diagnosed during pregnancy if the examiner is sufficiently attentive. Extremely large and globular belly, rapid growth of the uterus, marked edema, albuminuria, motion felt all over the abdomen, excite the interest of the accoucheur and warn to greater care. The diagnostic points are:

1. A sulcus felt in the fundus or down the front of the uterus. This may occur in uterus arcuatus or distorted uteri, or even in ordinary labor, and may be absent in twins.

2. Unusually large and globular uterus. Must eliminate hydramnion and large child. Twins or large child? Treatment depends on the diagnosis.

3. Palpation of three large parts—two heads and one breech or two breeches and one head. Make no diagnosis on the multiplicity of small parts,—the extremities,—because the child can place these in many locations.

4. When one head is in the pelvis and the distance from this to the other large part in the fundus is too great to be the length of one fetus, for example, over 30 cm.

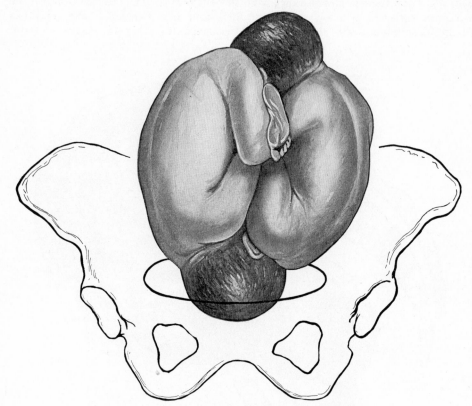

Fig. 425.—Twins Side by Side.

5. Auscultation of two sets of fetal heart-tones, with these characteristics: (1) Both asynchronous with the maternal pulse; (2) they must be asynchronous with each other, the difference being more than eight beats; (3) there must be a free zone between the two areas of greatest intensity. It is best for two qualified observers to listen at the same time; in doubtful cases it is well to use a stop-watch and take the average of many counts, and during the examination the patient may not change her position (Fig. 426).

If one child is dead, this method leaves us in doubt; again the two hearts may beat synchronously for a time. The author in such cases irritates the infant until it moves, which accelerates the heart-beat. A child with straightened spine, as in the military attitude, may have heart-tones audible on both sides of the uterus, or the placenta may divide the area of audibility. Hearing two loud uterine souffles is not conclusive, nor is hearing one fetal souffle and one fetal heart-sound. During labor one may hear normal heart-tones and feel a pulseless cord in the vagina, but even this is not positive, because the cord may be compressed temporarily while the heart goes on beating. Of course, such a condition soon kills the infant.

6. The x-ray may now be used, and its demonstration of two fetuses is positive. Edling, of Malmö, showed three in one case, the author likewise. When the differentiation must be made between one large and two small fetuses radiography is most valuable. It is important not to rely on the radiograph, but to control it by the usual methods of obstetric diagnosis. In studying an x-ray plate of twins it is not always easy to rule out a double monster.

During labor all the above signs are used, and, in addition,

7. Palpation of a fetal part in an intact sac after one sac has burst.

8. Palpation of two large parts by the vaginal examination.

After the delivery of one child the diagnosis that another remains in the uterus is easily made by one grasp of the fundus, but remember that fibroids, favorably disposed, may mimic a fetus. It may be necessary to explore the uterus.

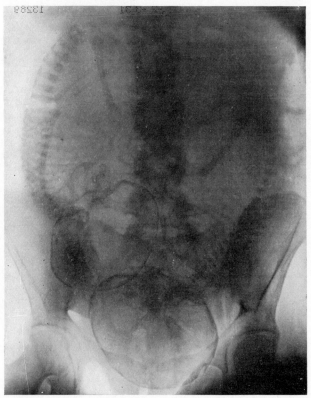

FIG. 426.—TWINS, S. L. T. AND O. D. T.

Differential Diagnosis.—In the early months the presence of twins may, by distorting the uterus, give rise to the suspicion of ectopic gestation. The differential diagnosis of simultaneous extra- and intra-uterine pregnancy from ordinary twins is possible only to a keen and experienced obstetric hand, and, even under most favorable circumstances, is rarely made before operation.

Polyhydramnion often complicates twins, and one needs to shut out ovarian tumor in these instances. (See p. 579.) Polyhydramnion may affect one ovum, the other having oligohydramnion.

Fibroid tumors complicating pregnancy may simulate plural gestation to perfection. The absence of two heart-beats upon repeated examinations; the immobility of the supposed large and small parts; their constancy of location; the history of fibroid, the x-ray allow prompt differentiation.

Prognosis.—As was said at the beginning of this chapter, plural gestation is not normal. The disturbances of pregnancy are more common, and their fatality increased, this being especially true of the toxemias resulting in eclampsia. Heart disease complicating twin pregnancy is very serious, and usually indicates the induction of premature labor. In one of the author's cases the anasarca was tremendous, hydropleura and hydropericardium developing, the patient having hemoptysis and dying of acute edema of the lungs. Owing to the longer labors and the more frequent necessity for operative deliveries, sepsis is more likely to occur, and the operative traumatisms must also be reckoned in. Postpartum hemorrhage occurs oftener,

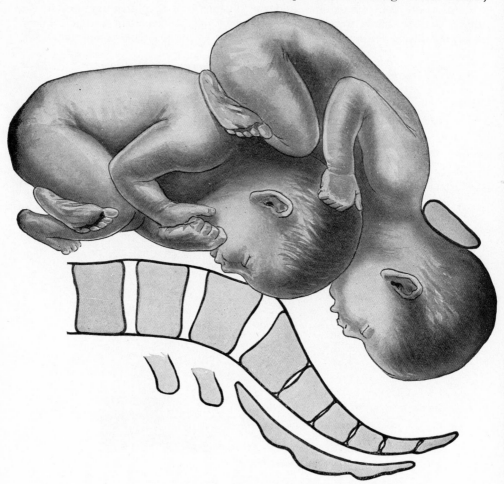

Fig. 427.—Interlocked Twins.

and it, with the danger of infection from the usual methods of combating it, must also be included.

For the child the prognosis is serious. Since the majority of twin births are premature, many infants die of atelectasis and general debility. Often one twin is larger and stronger than the other, seeming to have enjoyed better nutritional conditions in utero. One fetus may be syphilitic, the other healthy. A certain number of the second children are lost during the interval after the first is born, from abruption of the common placenta, and not a few die during operative deliveries. After birth the mother may be too ill or too weak properly to care for them, or she may have insufficient milk, and these, coupled with congenital debility, explain the high mortality in the first year of life. Ahlfeld places it at 75 per cent., but the author thinks this is too high. Triplets and quadruplets, of course, offer much higher mortalities.

Many mothers ask if twin children are mentally and physically as strong as those of single birth. The author has carefully studied his cases and other twins, and finds that all depends on the degree of prematurity. Where the children were fully developed, no difference could be noted.

Treatment.—During pregnancy, a pluriparient woman requires greater watchfulness, especially regarding her kidneys and circulation. Should she abort, the accoucheur must see that the uterus is empty. Although cases are on record of the successful carrying of the second fetus to term, the frequency of infection of the partially emptied uterine cavity is so great that the danger should not be assumed

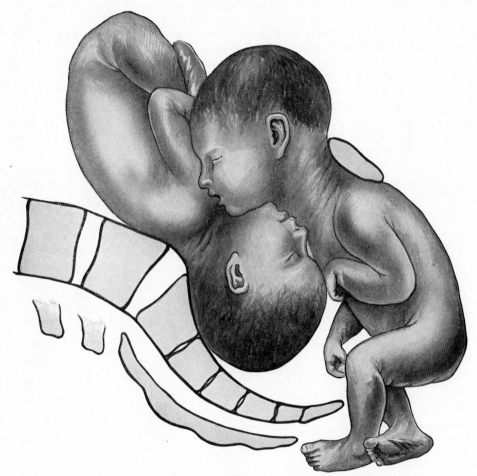

FIG. 428.—INTERLOCKED TWINS.

on so slim a chance of saving the child. During labor "watchful expectancy" is practised. One must not be deceived by the false pains of the latter weeks into assuming that labor has actually begun. Wait, if possible, for complete dilatation before rupturing the bag of waters. With frequent auscultation the accoucheur watches the welfare of the two children. It is wise not to let the first stage drag on too long, because inroads on the parturient's strength may be regretted in the third stage, when hemorrhage may set in. Preparations for operative delivery and for the treatment of a pathologic third stage must be complete.

After the first infant is delivered a careful external and internal examination will enable the accoucheur to decide on the proper treatment. The cord should be clamped or tied on its placental end. Should the cord of the second child prolapse—should the shoulder present, immediate action is required—in short, any abnormality is to be rectified. The delivery of the second twin by version and extraction or forceps or even simple Kristeller expression, is usually easy, because the soft parts have been prepared by the transit of the first infant. For the same reason the head of the second infant is not molded. If the heart-tones are normal—*and one should listen constantly*—if there is neither external nor internal hemorrhage, one may safely wait for twenty minutes before rupturing the second bag of waters. This interval allows the uterus to gather strength for the expulsion of the second child, and is also a safeguard against postpartum hemorrhage.

Owing to the overdistention of the uterus, contraction and retraction of its muscle are poor and the tendency to postpartum hemorrhage is augmented. Accurate control of the fundus and gentle massage are indicated, and expression of the placenta is usually needed earlier than in single labors. As soon as the second baby is born (the third, if triplets) a full dose of pituitary extract is given; immediately after the placenta has left the uterus, 1 ampule of gynergen. Ergot and ext. hydrastis canad. fl., āā ℥ xv are given t. i. d. for a week or more because involution of the uterus is slower. The accoucheur should remain in the house several hours to be certain that no relaxation of the uterus may occur, and to discover any tendency to postpartum eclampsia.

Anomalies of Plural Births.—(1) Pathologic presentations—shoulder, breech, brow, face, anterior parietal bone, etc.—occur in a goodly percentage of cases, and are treated on general principles.

(2) The part presenting may change several times before one finally engages and is delivered. Watch for pathogenic delay, then interfere.

(3) The bag of waters of the second child may rupture before that of the first, or the two may rupture at one time. No treatment is necessary in the first instance unless the cord of the second child prolapses before the presenting part of the second is delivered. If conditions for extraction are filled, deliver both children, otherwise replace the cord.

(4) Rarely the placenta of the first twin is delivered before the second is born. If the placenta is independent of the other, no harm results from this, but if the two are united, the necessary abruption of the placenta of the second child will be fatal to it unless it is delivered at once. The signs of asphyxia and external hemorrhage apprise the accoucheur as to what is going on. Rapid delivery of the second child will save it, and also preserve the mother.

(5) The transit of the first child may alter the position of the second, for example, from longitudinal to transverse, from vertex to face. Treatment is on general lines.

(6) Interlocking or collision may occur. The two heads may try to enter the pelvis at the same time, or one head enters, while the second head, caught in the neck of the first twin, attempts to enter with it (Fig. 427). If the children are small, such a mechanism is possible. Or the head of the second fetus enters the pelvis after the first one, presenting by the breech, has been delivered as far as the neck (Fig. 428). The second child, coming as a breech, may straddle the first in shoulder presentation, or four extremities may present, the two breeches entering the inlet at once.

(7) Rarely, after the first child is born, uterine action ceases and hours, days, or weeks may elapse before the second twin is delivered. The author does not wait more than twenty minutes for the birth of the second twin, but empties the uterus. There is little if any good in waiting, but many dangers—death of the second child, hemorrhage, and infection.

Delay in the delivery of twins should always excite the suspicion of locking, and an examination with the whole hand, in narcosis, if needed, is to be made. Much can be accomplished by manipulation aided by the steep Trendelenburg position, especially if the uterus is paralyzed by deep anesthesia, and the children may be disentangled, one of them being led into the pelvis. Should interlocking, as in Fig. 428, occur, a deep episiotomy is done, to avoid complete laceration of the perineum, the whole hand inserted, and the second head pushed up and out of the pelvis. If the heads are small, such a procedure is possible; if not, one should decapitate the first child quickly and push its head up into the uterus, then deliver the second with forceps. In such a case Lobenstine did a cesarean section and saved both twins and mother. Forceps or the cranioclast may be applied to the second child, delivering it first, but one should attempt to save at least one of the children by disentangling them under deep anesthesia. If the first one is dead, there is no occasion for hurry.

A double monster causing trouble during delivery is not so easily disposed of. First in importance, as always, is the diagnosis. The abdominal and x-ray findings almost never give reliable information, but may suggest greater watchfulness and the necessity for early exploration of the uterine cavity with the whole hand under general anesthesia.

LITERATURE

Barry: N. Y. Med. Jour., 1896.—*Bonnevie:* Ref. Jour. Amer. Med. Assoc., Heredity of Twins, 1919, p. 874; also June 26, 1920, p. 1781.—*Carson:* Zentralbl. f. Gyn., 1880.—*Curtius:* Arch. für Gynaek., 1930, vol. 140, p. 361. —*Foederl, V.:* Arch. für Gynaek., 1932, vol. 148, H. 3, p. 653.—*Geisler:* Allg. statistische Archiv von G. v. Mayr, 1900, p. 544.—*Gesell:* The Scientific Monthly, May, 1922, Mental and Physical Correspondence of Twins.— *Greulich:* The American Naturalist, March, 1930, lxiv.—*Gustetter:* "Superfetation," Jour. Amer. Med. Assoc., January 5, 1918, p. 21.—*Guzzoni:* Rassegna de scienze med., 1889, p. 19.—*Helliu:* Multiparität, Munich, 1895.—*Merkel:* Münch. med. Woch., March 27, 1931.—*Montgomery:* Biological Bulletin, vol. 50, No. 4, April, 1926.—*Neugebauer:* Zentralbl. f. Gyn., 1913, No. 29; also Jour. Amer. Med. Assoc., Queries and Answers, 1927, April 2, p. 1101, case of 69 children.—*Newman, H. H.:* The Physiology of Twinning, 1923, Univ. of Chicago Press.—*Orel:* Monatsschr. für Geb. u. Gyn., 1927, Bd. 129, 3, p. 719.—*Pinard* (of Paris): "Des Grossesse Triples," Annales de Gyn., 1889.—*Rovano:* Archiv. für Gynaek., Bd. 83, Heft 3.—*Sasse:* Acta Obstet. et Gynec. Scandinav., 1925, vol. iv.—*Schatz:* Arch. f. Gyn., vols. xix, xxiv, xxvii, xxix, xxx, liii, lv, lviii, lx.—*Strassman:* Handbuch f. Geb., vol. i, p. 742.—*Sue: Ibid.*—*Wagner:* Zentb. für Gynaek., December 22, 1926, p. 3388.— *Wislocki and Snyder:* Bull. Johns Hopkins Hosp., August, 1931.

CHAPTER XXXVI

PROLONGED PREGNANCY AND MISSED LABOR

REFERENCE has been made to prolonged pregnancy (p. 120), and here will be considered the pathologic side. Labor occasionally begins at the proper period, some degree of dilatation is attained, but for some reason the pains cease and gestation continues for from two to four weeks, when the uterus again is set in action and delivery is accomplished. This occurrence must not be confounded with the pains and changes in the cervix which sometimes occur at "lightening." When the child is thus carried over term, it undergoes certain alterations; the length increases disproportionately to the weight, the head enlarges, and the bones harden, the parietal bosses becoming prominent and pointed. The body is less fat and is firmer in consistence; the spinal column is harder and less flexible. In some cases the fetus is overgrown in every way. Oligohydramnion, with its consequences, may occur. The child may die without other cause apparently than being overripe, and this fact is known and appreciated even by the laity. Adair has found senile changes or involution in overterm placentæ. (See Adler, Lit.)

During labor I have observed these anomalies:

1. Lack of cephalic molding, from the extreme ossification; high arrest of head; prolonged and fruitless labor; forceps—hard extraction; extensive injuries; stillbirths.

2. Occipitoposterior positions, absent rotation, etc.

3. Deflexion attitudes—military attitude, forehead, brow, and even face presentations and their sequelæ.

4. More or less disproportion between the size of the passage and the passenger, prolonged labor, and operative interference.

Many irregularities in the labor apart from the above have been observed. Some of these are indirectly caused by, or indirectly influence, the mechanical factors in labor. The pains are apt to be irregular, intermittent, and ineffectual. Occasionally, on the other hand, they are tumultuous and quickly deliver the child, perhaps precipitately, injuring it or the mother. The writer had one case of complete spontaneous rupture of the uterus where the pregnancy was prolonged and labor rapid. This is the exception. Weak pains are the rule. It is possible that a fatty degeneration of the uterine muscle occurs in these weeks of prolonged pregnancy (Bossi). This invites traumatic rupture or produces inertia, necessitating the use of forceps. The lack of strong uterine contractions leaves the cervix and vagina without the softening and succulence necessary for the safe dilatation, and, therefore, lacerations of the parts are frequent and all operative intervention is rendered laborious. The same inertia is carried over into the third stage, and postpartum hemorrhage caps the climax to the succession of complications.

While these accidents are by no means the rule in women going over term, they occur so often that the question of methodically inducing labor at the normal end of gestation deserves grave consideration.

Prolonged labor is a peculiar condition. Pains begin, the cervix becomes effaced and opens, the show appears, even the bag of waters may rupture, but delivery does not occur. I have seen the os open to the size of the palm, but retract and pregnancy continue. However, intermittent pains declare that the woman is in labor. In a case sent to the author from South Dakota the woman had been in actual labor for eight weeks and came to the maternity in a typhoidal condition.

Dilatation with the colpeurynter, cervical incisions, and forceps procured a 4½ pound emaciated infant which survived. The process was repeated in a subsequent pregnancy. Occasionally labor may be completely interrupted and resumed at a later period—perhaps at the end of a menstrual cycle.

The causes for these conditions are unknown—perhaps some disease of the uterine muscle or of the nerves of the uterus or lack of endocrine gland action should be invoked. I have noticed that my cases go over term in groups, and that other practitioners are having the same trouble about the same time. This fact Bossi also mentions, and he found that the condition recurred and was hereditary. Old primiparæ, women who have had dysmenorrhea, and in whom the pelvis is of masculine type, seem oftenest affected. Fibroids have been noted in several cases. A peculiar circumstance in these patients is that, when fever begins, which is not unusual, especially if the bag of waters is ruptured and the vaginal bacteria have gained access to the uterus, the pains begin or become stronger, and delivery is completed rapidly. After delivery the temperature rapidly subsides. (See p. 865.)

Treatment.—The author does not consider it good practice to allow gestation to continue long after its natural term has passed, and, likewise, it is not safe to permit a protracted labor to wear out the woman's strength, as it is bound to do in time, through loss of sleep, much suffering, and anxiety. If labor does not set in on the day which, after careful computation, has been set for it, the accoucheur makes a careful abdominal and rectal examination of the gravida. If the fingers are to be passed into the vagina, the preparations of the patient and for the patient should be identical with those of actual labor, that is, shaving, disinfection, rubber gloves, etc. The accoucheur determines the size of the infant, using cephalometry, and of the pelvis, the degree of engagement of the presenting part, and the state of the cervix. When convinced that the end of normal pregnancy is reached, he informs the woman that unless pains begin within a week it will be deemed wise to inaugurate labor. For the details of the methods of inducing labor, see p. 1121.

Missed Labor.—This is a term applied by Oldham to the retention of a fetus, dead, near term, in the uterus. Missed labor often occurs in cows and sheep. An attempt may or may not have been made by the uterus to expel its contents. The condition is similar to the one just considered, except in the death of the child, which is often inexplicable, and is the same as "missed abortion" (p. 476), only occurring later in pregnancy. The reason for the failure of the uterus to expel the dead product of conception has been placed in a rigid cervix, for example, cancer, scars, hypertrophy, a diseased uterus, myomata, muscular degeneration, cornual pregnancy, low insertion of placenta, adherent membranes, peritonitis with adhesions, and nervous disease. More probably the cause for the uterine inertia will be found in some endocrinal deficiency. After the fetus dies it mummifies and shrinks up, its liquor is absorbed, and the uterus applies itself closely to the body. A lithopedion may form, as in extra-uterine gestation, or infection with purulent disintegration and extrusion of the bones of the skeleton through the cervix, or by ulceration through neighboring cavities—a termination which is excessively rare. Usually art interferes and empties the uterus. In Menzies' case the dead ovum was carried to the seventeenth month, and, in Hening's case, eight months after term.

Symptoms.—One finds the same symptoms here as in missed abortion (*q. v.*), but exaggerated. The woman complains of the feeling of a dead and heavy mass in the belly, and notes the absence of fetal movements. Pains of a parturient character occasionally occur, commonly at the time of the customary menstrual periods, and it is at such times that labor often sets in.

Examination shows a closed cervix, and a thin-walled, torpid uterus, of hard consistence, entirely lacking the spongy softness characteristic of normal pregnancy. The diagnosis is easy. Since the question of pregnancy is seldom uncertain, all that is needed is to prove that the symmetric tumor is the uterus and that it does not grow.   On p. 286 are the points for the determination of the life or death of the fetus.

Treatment.—If the child is dead, the bag of waters intact, and the patient not ill, it is advised to wait for the time of a monthly period or two to see if nature will not start the pains and empty the uterus.   In the interval the woman must be enjoined not to have intercourse nor to take douches.   Some authors advise the emptying of the uterus when the diagnosis of missed labor is positive, and with these I agree, because the uterine contents may become infected while waiting and this renders an otherwise safe operation extremely hazardous.   The torpidity of the uterine muscle in these cases is sometimes astonishing—one may use all sorts of local irritants—gauze, colpeurynters, etc.—for days without evoking pains.   It is, therefore, the author's practice to incise the cervix or do vaginal cesarean section if the uterus proves refractory after twenty-four hours' trial.   Since the fetus is dead, craniotomy and morcellation are indicated to save the maternal soft parts from injury.   If the mass is already infected, the case is treated as a septic abortion, with quinin, pituitrin, tampon and morcellation.   If the fetus is of considerable bulk, laparotomy and complete extirpation of the uterus might be simpler than the attempt to remove the mass from below.   If delivery from below seems better, vaginal cesarean section is performed and morcellation of the fetus if necessary. The field is exposed by broad retractors and the wound left open for drainage, to be repaired at a future time.   Prepare for postpartum hemorrhage.   v. Winckel advised a more expectant treatment of these infected cases, i. e., drainage of the uterus, lightly disinfectant douches, removal piecemeal at different sittings of parts of the fetus and secundines, the process taking weeks and sometimes months.

Graviditas Exochorialis.—Among the rare conditions met with is the development of the fetus in the uterus, but outside of the chorionic cavity.   In such cases the amnion is also torn, the membranes shrink up, the liquor amnii continually escapes, sometimes in large amounts, and the fetus may show the results of oligohydramnion—contractures, club-feet and arms, decubitus, etc.   The differential diagnosis must be made from hydrorrhœa gravidarum (*q. v.*).   Abortion is frequent.

In *graviditas examnialis* the amnion is burst, but the fetus is still surrounded by the chorion.   The amnion is found retracted around the fetus.

LITERATURE

Adair: Trans. Amer. Gyn. Society, 1923.—*Adler:* Zentbl. f. Gyn., 1927, No. 17, p. 1050, Lit.—*Bar, P.:* Bull. de la Soc. d'Obstetrique, Paris, 1898.—*Bossi:* Gynäk. Rundschau, Wien, vol. i, No. 1, p. 30.—*DeLee:* "The Induction of Labor at Term," Surg., Gyn., and Obstet., July, 1907.—*Kleinertz:* Zentralbl. f. Gyn., 1901, No. 28, p. 809.—*Krevet:* Arch. f. Gyn., vol. lxi, p. 438.—*Luther:* "Missed Labor," Amer. Gyn. and Obstet. Jour., February, 1899.—*Menzies:* Glasgow Med. Jour., July, 1843, p. 229.—*Oldham:* Guy's Hospital Reports, 1847, vol. v, pp. 105–112.—*Schneck:* "Missed Labour" and "Übertragung," Inaug. Diss., Marburg, 1903.

CHAPTER XXXVII

DISEASES ACCIDENTAL TO PREGNANCY

A PREGNANT woman is not immune to any disease which may affect her in the non-pregnant state, and, contrary to the old notion, she is more susceptible to some. Pregnancy in general aggravates the diseases which occur, and in turn the gestation is endangered by them. Abortion or premature labor occurs with varying frequency in all the infectious diseases, and also often complicates the course of constitutional, circulatory, respiratory, alimentary, and kidney affections. It is obviously impossible, in a book of this size, thoroughly to consider all the maladies from which a pregnant woman might suffer. Only the salient points of large groups, and especially important features of individual diseases, will receive mention. The reciprocal influences of pregnancy upon the disease and of the disease upon pregnancy will be studied in turn.

THE ACUTE INFECTIOUS DISEASES

Typhoid, typhus, measles, scarlatina, variola, erysipelas, diphtheria, cholera, malaria, influenza, pneumonia—all occur in pregnancy, and most of them have a very deleterious effect on both mother and fetus. The action of these diseases is twofold: first, they endanger the woman through hyperpyrexia, increased toxemia, the accompanying nephritis, and through the tendency to become hemorrhagic. Profuse metrorrhagias are often noted, some of which may be early abortions, and a differential diagnosis may have to be made from several conditions. For example, a young woman was sent to the author with a diagnosis of septic abortion with profuse hemorrhage. She was in the first week of typhoid, with epistaxis uterina, and was a "virgo intacta."

Women who have had an exhaustive siege of disease are in poor condition to withstand the pain, shock, and hemorrhage of abortion or labor, and collapse may come on in the third stage. This is especially true when the lungs or heart are much involved. Finally, some of the above-mentioned diseases lead directly to puerperal sepsis, either by blood or regional transmission of the bacteria, or by so reducing the immunities of the patient that infection easily gains foothold. Examples of these are variola (infection from the pustules), typhoid (the streptococci from Peyer's patches, and even the typhoid bacilli themselves), influenza (direct), erysipelas (direct), scarlatina (from the throat), pneumonia (direct), diphtheria (direct), etc.

Second, these diseases interrupt pregnancy, which is due to a not infrequently accompanying hemorrhagic endometritis and to the death of the fetus. Fetal death is brought about in various ways:

(a) The fetus may die from insolation. Normally, the temperature of the fetus is one-half a degree higher than that of the mother, and since it has its own heat-regulating system, it can take care of the ordinary changes, but when the mother is hyperpyretic, the child cannot do so because it has not the means to discharge heat, as by evaporation, for example. High temperature, especially a sudden rise, is, therefore, less well borne. Runge and Doré showed that a gradual rise to 104° F. is fairly well borne, and unless continued thus for a long period, is usually survived by the infant. The movements and the heart-tones are at first increased, later slowed, and death occurs. Rabbits will stand a very gradual rise to 109° F., but if it is sudden, it is always fatal. Krummaker reported a case of hysteric fever with sudden rises of 109.4° F. at intervals for seven days without effect on the child.

(b) Pregnancy is interrupted by the hot blood circulating through the uterus. This is not improbable, because heat applied to the abdomen and by hot douches causes the uterus to contract, and clinical experience in delayed labors shows that when the temperature rises, as from sepsis, the pains grow stronger.

(c) The fetus dies from *asphyxia*, brought about—(1) By low blood-pressure of the mother and consequent stagnation of the circulation in the uterine sinuses; (2) the same, because of profuse hemorrhages; (3) from hypercarbonization and deoxidation of the mother's blood, the direct result of the disease, for example, pneumonia; (4) from a hemorrhage in the placenta with separation of the organ; and (5) because of fatty degeneration of the fetal villi, which renders the respiratory exchange of gases in them impossible.

(d) The child may acquire the disease from which the mother is suffering or it may die from the toxins which it receives from the maternal circulation. The villus-wall offers no hindrance to the passage of the toxins, which, like other poisons, strychnin and potassium iodid, are known to go through, as also do antitoxins, for example, diphtheria. The villus is no barrier to the passage of the bacteria—they either pass through directly or after destroying the wall, and lesions of the latter are not hard to find. These infections have been demonstrated in the fetus: variola, measles, scarlatina, typhoid (the author in 1891), cholera, pneumonia, bubonic plague, erysipelas, pus infections, anthrax, tuberculosis, syphilis, febris recurrens, malaria, rabies. It is noted that in some of the diseases the child is not at all affected, and the author has had cases where the child alone was ill, the mother remaining free. Others have noted such an occurrence in smallpox.

Typhoid.—It is said that typhoid is rare in pregnancy. Freund found 42 cases in 3272 typhoids, which is not excessively rare when all the facts are considered. The Eberth bacillus and the Widal reaction have been found in the fetal blood, especially in the latter months of gestation. Pregnancy is interrupted in two-thirds of the cases, especially in the early months. Children of the later months almost always die after birth. Hemorrhage is usually not profuse, but the accoucheur is warned to prevent all bleeding because of the exhaustion of the patient. The soft parts are very easily torn, but bleed little. Union was good in the author's three cases. The mortality is higher than in uncomplicated typhoid. In the puerperium the differential diagnosis is most important, since the fever is usually ascribed to puerperal sepsis. The gradual rise of fever, the absence of chills, the slow pulse, the tendency to apathy, not excitement, the early splenic tumor, the stool, the roseola, and the negative findings on the genitalia usually enable the proper course to be taken, but one should always try the Widal reaction, and, if necessary, make a culture from the blood. A typhoid puerperal infection is not impossible, and typhoid may be combined with putrefactive and purulent infections. Typhoid vaccination may be done during pregnancy, but only if an epidemic exists (Kohn, Lit.).

Variola.—In the majority of cases of smallpox, abortion or premature labor occurs, and the child almost always dies. It may be born pock-marked, as was the accoucheur Mauriceau, or in the eruptive stage. Confluent and hemorrhagic variola are more common in gravidæ, and the mortality is, therefore, much higher (Vinay, 36 per cent.). Sepsis may arise from the pustules, and after recovery from the smallpox a recrudescence of the fever may occur from the resorption of toxic material from the fetus, which disappears when the uterus is emptied. Hemorrhage during labor is greater. Vaginal examination and intra-uterine manipulations are to be avoided, as far as possible, because of the danger of introducing infection.

Pregnant women, unless toxemic, may be vaccinated, but it does not always protect the child. Neonati, unless weaklings, may be vaccinated if exposed to contagion. The healthy child of a variolous mother is to be isolated (Urner). Vaccination of the child should be done immediately on delivery, but it usually does not protect. Women who have been vaccinated or who have had variola during pregnancy give birth to children, which later are immune to vaccination and smallpox (Kollock and Sawyer). Franklin reports a case where the father had smallpox; the mother, vaccinated, remained well, but the child was born dead of smallpox, which shows that the child received the contagion through its healthy mother. Pridham observed the same mode of transmission of varicella (Morawetz).

Scarlatina.—Pregnant women seldom get real scarlatina (Ballantyne), but erythemata, due to sepsis, which resemble it are not uncommon, especially in the puerperium. The relations of scarlet fever to sepsis are not yet decided upon, and will not be until the exciting cause of scarlatina is known, but probably the streptococcus has something to do with both diseases when a connection between the two is suspected. The child may have scarlatina, the mother remaining well (Liddell). The author knows of many instances of labor occurring in the same room with children suffering from scarlet fever and has seen no trouble arise therefrom. Of course, precautions were taken, but these could not always be complete, and often were largely neglected. The mortality of scarlatina in the puerperium is given as from 5 to 52 per cent., and the frequency of puerperal ulcers, parametritis, and puerperal infection in general as complications is emphasized (Tornery).

In the puerperium, unless an epidemic of scarlet fever is raging, it is best to consider the scarlatiniform eruption as due to infection, unless the other characteristics of the case stamp it distinctly as scarlet fever. (See Poesch, 1927, Lit.)

Measles.—Fellner collected 30 cases from the literature. Measles is a serious complication of pregnancy, as it generally is in adults. Gestation was interrupted in 55 per cent.; the general mortality was 15 per cent.; during the puerperium two of three women died. Sepsis explains the high mortality. The children are usually affected by the disease and show the eruption, as the one of Clarus did when removed by cesarean section from the dead body of its mother. In the service of the Chicago Lying-in Hospital Dispensary many of the puerperæ are exposed to this contagion from their sick children, but in no case has measles developed, which shows that even the imperfect isolation possible in the homes of the poor will suffice to protect. In one of my cases the child developed typical measles on the tenth day, the mother being free.

Cholera.—In the Hamburg epidemic of 1892, 57 per cent. of pregnant women affected by cholera asiatica died (Schütz). Abortion was very frequent because of hemorrhagic endometritis. The disease usually is not, but may be, transmitted to the child.

Erysipelas.—When this disease attacks any other portion of the body than the genitalia, it seems to be less dangerous, but many records are at hand to show that puerperal infection may result in such cases. The author delivered a woman suffering from facial erysipelas; shortly after birth the vulva became red, and she died under the picture of acute sepsis. At the autopsy, from the very little clear peritoneal fluid, a pure culture of Streptococcus pyogenes was recovered. A facial erysipelas is not invariably transmitted to the genitalia. Pregnancy is not often interrupted by erysipelas, and frequently the children are delivered alive, but they may have the disease. The mortality is increased. Late literature on the subject is scarce (Lebedeff). Ten per cent. chinosol ointment is said to be curative (Lusk).

Sepsis.—Under puerperal infections the usual forms of sepsis will be considered at length. Here might briefly be mentioned infections of distant portions of the body, for example, mastoiditis, frontal and other sinusitis, tonsillitis, abscesses, cellulitis, anthrax, and tetanus. These diseases are usually aggravated by pregnancy, and their bacteria may be transmitted by way of the blood-stream to the uterus and the fetus. It is possible, too, that direct transference of the virus may be effected by the woman herself with her fingers. A local infection of the uterus and fetus may occur at any period of gestation and cause abortion. Coitus in the latter weeks often causes labor to set in, and may be followed by serious puerperal infection such as gonococcal peritonitis, or general sepsis.

Pregnant cows may suffer from infection by the Bacillus abortus, which gains entrance through the mouth and lungs. Contagious abortion in cows has already been mentioned. The abortion is attended by fever, and sterility may result. The bacillus may be demonstrated in the milk for years afterward and has infected man.

Malaria.—Mild cases of malaria exert little influence on gestation. Severe cases may interrupt pregnancy through fever or cachexia. Labor may change the type from tertian to quotidian. Williams could not find the plasmodium in 15 infants, demonstrated in their mothers, yet Ter-Ossipian and Bodenhäuser report cases of such transmission, and fetuses have been delivered with enlarged spleen and pigmentation. During labor an attack may occur. Uterine action is torpid. Hemorrhages have been noted postpartum. The author had a case of hemophilia which seemed to be malarial in origin. Lardier speaks of hemorrhage in labor, and Legeois and Barker of bleeding later in the puerperium. Postpartum malaria seems to be a little more serious than usual, but its chief interest is in the diagnosis. Practitioners in malarious regions find many times that an outbreak of malaria occurs in the puerperium in a manner similar to that of a fresh attack after an operation. In such cases puerperal infection is to be excluded and the plasmodium demonstrated. Quinin is to be administered whenever indicated (Fry, Deale).

Influenza.—The recent epidemics of influenza afforded many opportunities to study this dreadful plague. Of the four waves of infection that passed over the world, the first, in 1918, showed the highest general mortality and the highest special mortality for pregnant women. The predilection for young people and the unusual malignancy shown by the influenza virus in pregnant women are not explained. They were noted in a few previous epidemics. The peculiar serologic changes in the blood may explain the virulence of influenza in pregnancy, and perhaps by studying the disease from this point of attack we may discover its nature and the pathogenesis of infections in general.

The pulmonary changes in pregnancy probably favored the development of streptococcus pneumonia which was so fatal to gravidæ. Our failure to discover the cause and learn its treatment is due largely to the natural variations of the disease itself, the multiplicity of secondary infections (strepto-staphylo-pneumococcus), and to confusion with coexistent catarrhal affections and grippe.

Even mild cases were distinguishable from common colds or bronchitis—the headaches, the red throat, the high fever, and the rapid pulse with leukopenia aiding in differentiation. Severe infection, occurring near the end of pregnancy, soon declared its malignancy. All types were observed, but the pulmonary preponderated in frequency and fatality. After a few days of fever, chilliness, sore throat, and cough the symptoms suddenly became severe and prostration threatening. Thus the advent of the secondary infection was heralded. Bronchopneumonia developed, the patient presenting a pathognomonic grayish-purple cyanosis, resembling heliotrope, and dying quickly from acute toxemia and asphyxia. After death the mucous membranes were almost black, the blood like port wine. Empyema, sinusitis, otitis were not frequent complications of the first wave (1918), but were of the later two in 1919. I observed three cases of influenzal salpingitis with symptoms of ectopic gestation—one of which was erroneously operated, and one pneumococcus salpingitis-peritonitis. The gastro-intestinal form, which is said to resemble hyperemesis, was very rare, as also were the cerebral. Some cases of encephalitis lethargica (Schulze) and a few of encephalitis choreiformis (Wein) were reported.

Upon pregnancy, labor, and the puerperium the disease had a malign influence. Abortion occurred in 25 to 40 per cent. of the cases, and premature labor in 50 to 60 per cent., and these events always increased the gravity of the patient's situation. The uterus emptied itself rapidly and without much pain and bleeding, but the prostration of the patient increased and also the tendency to acute pulmonary edema. In the puerperium profuse, fetid lochia, subinvolution, agalactia were observed. It is generally believed that influenza may cause real puerperal infection but during the 1918 epidemic the mortality in the United States from genital sepsis was relatively low (J. W. Harris, Litwak).

Prognosis.—In some localities the mortality was fearful—80 per cent. (Farrar, Seitz). Taken the world over, it was about 10 per cent. for cases of simple influenza and about 50 per cent. when bronchopneumonia or general sepsis followed. For the child the mortality was very high, since labor came on prematurely and the mothers were for days so toxemic and asphyxiated. The fetus also acquired influenza. I saw an ovum from a ten-weeks' abortion full of pus, and a child delivered at term with bronchitis (Abt). Newborn children showed a high incidence and mortality (Linzenmeier).

Treatment.—Prevention, first of the original infection and then of secondary complications, is of supreme importance. Contagion is direct by droplets of spit or indirect by carrier or through the air, the latter mode of transmission being most evident in hospitals and barracks, and especially for secondary complications. Hamburger noted a marked drop in pulmonary infections when the wards at Camp Taylor were treated by moist antisepsis.

Strict isolation of pregnant women and isolation of infected cases are demanded. We found that absolute rest in bed, in a warm, but well-ventilated room was the greatest single factor in preventing the dreaded bronchopneumonia, from which the majority of women died. The rest in bed was kept up ten days after the temperature became normal. We gave morphin sparingly, even though the cough was harassing, but alkalies and fruit acids freely. Abortion and premature labor were not induced, experience in 1892 (Vinay) and in the early weeks of the present epidemic having conclusively shown that when they occurred the mortality was doubled (Harris). Therefore, one should try to delay labor and prevent it if possible. During labor anesthetics were avoided because they favored edema of the lungs. Where possible novocain was used.

Pneumonia.—Pneumonia must be considered one of the specific infections, with localization in the lungs, and it acts in many ways like most of the diseases described in this chapter. Pregnancy is interrupted in more than half of the cases, especially if it already is in the latter months. Cyanosis and dyspnea are more marked, especially in the last few weeks, when the excursions of the diaphragm are restricted by the large uterus, and particularly if the abdomen is tympanitic. Cardiac collapse is earlier and more frequent; indeed, pregnancy and pneumonia are a dangerous combination. Vinay collected cases which showed a maternal mortality of 68 per cent. when pregnancy was interrupted, and of 15 per cent. when it went on undisturbed. Pneumonia may affect the fetus, and its chances generally are not good, though Fellner quotes 19 cases of Schauta's clinic, with only 1 death.

Pneumonia in the puerperium may be due to the pneumococcus, may result from the anesthetic (bronchopneumonia), or be hypostatic or embolic. The last two forms appear in septic cases—the one from cachexia and the other from embolism from infected pelvic veins (*q. v.*). Other manifestations of pneumococcus invasion are: Pleurisy, pericarditis, endocarditis, meningitis, otitis media, sinus infections, endometritis, and ophthalmia neonatorum, besides other fetal infections.

For further information on all these subjects see P. Müller, Fränkl-Hochwart and v. Noorden, and P. Hüssy.

LITERATURE

Abt: Jour. Amer. Med. Assoc., April 5, 1919, p. 980.—*Ballantyne:* Trans. Edinburg Obst. Soc., vol. xviii, p. 177.—*Barker:* Amer. Jour. Obstet., 1880, p. 210.—*Bodenhäuser:* N. Y. Med. Jour., 1893.—*Deale:* Amer. Jour. Obstet., 1897, vol. xxxvi.—*Farrar:* Amer. Jour. Obstet., February, 1919, Lit.—*Fellner:* Innere Krankheiten, Vienna, 1903.—*Fränkl-Hochwart and C. von Noorden:* Erkrank. des weibl. Genitales und inn. Med., 2 volumes, 1912.—*Freund:* Ergeb. der allg. Path., III. Jahrgang, 1896, vol. ii.—*Fry:* "Malaria," Amer. Jour. Obstet., 1897, vol. xxxv.—*Harris:* Jour. Amer. Med. Assoc., April 5, 1919, p. 978.—*Harris, J. W.:* Jour. Amer. Med. Assoc., 1919, 72, 978.—*Hüssy, P.:* Die Schwangerschaft, 1923.—*Kohn:* Zentralbl. für Gyn., 1927, No. 12, Lit.—*Kollock:* Amer. Jour. Obstet., 1889, p. 1079.—*Krummaker:* Münch. med. Woch., 1907, p. 1035.—*Lardier:* Lyon Méd., July, 1888.—*Lebedeff:* Zentralbl. f. Gyn., 1886, p. 423.—*Legeois:* Arch. de Tocologie, January, 1891.—*Liddell and Tangye:* Brit. Med. Jour., September 16, 1916.—*Linzenmeier:* Collective Review of Influenza, Jahreskurse für Aertzliche Fortbildung, July, 1920.—*Litwak:* Arch. für Gynaek., 1932, vol. 148, H. 2, p. 453.—*Lusk:* Annals of Surgery, February, 1922, vol. lxxv, 2, p. 143.—*Morawetz:* Wien. med. Woch., 1921, No. 34, p. 130.—*Müller, P.:* Die Krankheiten des weiblichen Körpers. Immense fund of information.—*Olshausen:* Arch. f. Gyn., vol. ix, p. 169.—*Poesch:* Zeitschr. für Gynaek., 1927, Bd. xc, H. 3, p. 609.—*Pridham:* Brit. Med. Jour., May 17, 1913.—*Schulze:* Jour. Amer. Med. Assoc., March 13, 1920, p. 732; also Zentralbl. f. Gyn., 1921, October 22, p. 1543.—*Ter-Ossipian and Markarian:* Zentb. für Gyn., 1931, September 26.—*Tornery:* La Rougeole et la Scarlatine dans la Grossesse, 1891. Book of 362 pages.—*Urner:* Amer. Jour. Obst. and Gyn., January, 1927, p. 70, Lit.—*Vinay:* Pathologie de la Grossesse.—*Wallich:* "Pneumonia," Arch. de Gyn., 1889, vol. xxxi, p. 439.—*Wien:* Zentralbl. f. Gyn., 1920, No. 43.

CHAPTER XXXVIII

THE CHRONIC INFECTIOUS DISEASES

Pulmonary tuberculosis has a marked influence on the woman during the performance of the reproductive function. In the advanced case ovulation and menstruation are usually suppressed, which may be looked upon as the conservative effort of nature, as the result of extreme cachexia with atrophy of the ovaries, or of local tuberculous disease of the genitalia. In beginning tuberculosis, amenorrhea or scanty menses may be noted, and, since the girl may be chlorotic, a difficult diagnostic problem may present itself—chlorosis or tuberculosis, or both. Every chlorotic girl's lungs should be carefully examined. A leukorrhea may substitute the menses in such cases. Sterility, fortunately, is not rare in tuberculous men and women, but only in advanced cachectic individuals.

Pregnancy is rarely interrupted, and then the infection is usually very florid, and resembles a pneumonia more than a typical tuberculosis.

During labor the degree of involvement of the lungs will determine how much trouble will be met. Mild cases go through it without causing anxiety. Advanced cases are harassed by dyspnea, cough, occasionally hemoptysis, and threatened by cardiac collapse, œdema pulmonum, pneumothorax, and, rarely, a spread of the infection into general miliary tuberculosis. Labor is slower, and the second stage is prolonged and critical. During the puerperium fever is common; a bronchitis is often added to the other troubles, but, in the author's experience, sepsis has not been more frequent. Miliary tuberculosis, not uncommon, resembles sepsis. It may result from a general anesthetic.

Tuberculosis has decided immediate and remote influence on the child. Birch-Hirschfeld (1891) first demonstrated tuberculosis in the fetus, and Schmorl showed it in the placenta in 50 per cent. of the cases, though Hardy, in 1834, mentions it (Lanz, Lit.). Bar and Renon found tubercle bacilli in blood of the umbilical cord in 2 of 5 cases. Placental tubercular foci usually precede fetal disease, but without doubt the bacilli may pass directly to the fetus through the walls of the villi. Congenital tuberculosis was held impossible for years and by many, but it occurs, and probably more frequently than is generally known. Friedman injected weak suspensions of tubercle bacilli into the vaginas of recently impregnated guinea-pigs and produced fetal tuberculosis. By men, through dirty habits, or from genital tubercular foci, the bacilli could be introduced with the semen. Baumgarten held that the disease was inherited, the germs developing at a later period, but probably a weakness of the constitution, a tendency to the malady, is inherited, and the environment of the child and the numerous opportunities for infection are the exciting causes, although Calmette has shown that tuberculosis can be caused by a filtrable virus (prebacillary), and Granzow proved that this virus can be transmitted to fetuses and children of tuberculous mothers.

The children of tuberculous women may be large and robust, especially if the disease is of the chronic type. Puny children also are born, and many die in the first weeks or months. The child may become tuberculous through the mother's milk. Counting all miscarriages and deaths in infancy Seitz found 60 per cent. mortality before one year and only 15 per cent. lived twenty years.

Much difference of opinion exists as to the influence of pregnancy on tuberculous women. Most obstetricians think it aggravates the disease and internists disagree among themselves. Robinson from a questionnaire answered by 200 specialists (tuberculosis) and health officers in Britain and abroad, learned that all deny that pregnancy benefits tuberculous gravidæ; 75 per cent. state that pulmonary tuberculosis is aggravated by pregnancy, latent infections activated, quiescent lesions lit up, active foci made more active. Förssner dissents, while various opinions were expressed by those taking part in a discussion in London, in 1931 (Marshall et al., Ingraham). A great deal depends on the stage of the infection when the gestation begins. A woman with healed tuberculosis may safely become pregnant. If a dormant tuberculosis awakens in pregnancy or a new infection occurs, the course of the disease is apt to be more rapid, being usually of the more florid type, the tendency to fever greater, and emaciation more marked. Hemoptysis occurs in 50 per cent. of the cases. Tuberculosis of the larynx, heart disease, hyperemesis, and nephritis aggravate the pulmonary condition decidedly. The chronic ulcerative varieties of tuberculosis do not usually produce such marked symptoms during pregnancy, the author having seen such women bear children repeatedly, without greater aggravation of the disease than one would expect.

Sometimes the patient does not show any untoward signs until after delivery. Owing to the changes in the lungs and heart and the drain on the system caused by pregnancy and labor, especially if there has been much hemorrhage, the caseous deposits soften and rapidly break down, hectic develops, and the course of the affection goes downward fast, which veterinarians also observed. If the patient has tuberculous laryngitis she rarely survives the puerperium (Küttner, 90 per cent. mortality).

Treatment.—Women with tuberculosis should not marry—first, because this aggravates their own disease; second, they may infect the husband; and, third, they propagate tuberculous children. The same is to be said of the husband.

If the tuberculosis is latent, or if the candidates possess only the hereditary taint, the question is more difficult, but it is only exceptionally that the doctor's advice is asked. Knowing the tendency for a latent tuberculosis to break out in pregnancy, permission is to be conditional upon the certainty and permanence of cure. If a suspect marries, she should avoid conception. Finally, if she has a baby she should not nurse it. The tuberculin tests may be made on gravidæ, but they show less susceptibility. It would be good practice to x-ray all gravidæ for diagnosis if it were certainly a safe procedure.

During pregnancy the recognized medical treatment is carried out. Should the pregnancy be interrupted because the mother has pulmonary tuberculosis? Opinions differ, three positions being held: One, that pregnancy be always interrupted as a curative measure; another, that it be never interrupted, and the third, that the cases be individually treated and the gestation brought to an end only when certain symptoms indicate it. One will need to interfere oftener in patients who cannot afford sanitarium treatment, etc. If tuberculosis of the lungs is manifest early in pregnancy; if there are fever, wasting, many bacilli in the sputum, hemoptysis, and advancing consolidation—that is, the process seems to be florid—abortion should be induced without delay. Trembley, of Saranac Lake, induces abortion in the early months in all cases, and says that the mortality and percentage of relapses are practically nil when abortion is induced before the end of the third month. Morris, from a study of 1000 cases, came to similar conclusions. If the process seems very chronic, especially if the patient comes in the second half of pregnancy, it is justifiable to wait and watch closely. If the pregnancy is near the period of viability, one may tide the woman over a few weeks for the sake of the child, or even allow her to go to term, depending on her condition. Urgent symptoms of cardiac nature, persistent hemoptysis, and dyspnea may require the emptying of the uterus. Complicating nephritis, heart disease, and contracted pelvis, which is said to be more frequent in the tuberculous, will give earlier indication for interference. Tuberculosis with hyperemesis makes the indication for immediate abortion. Laryngeal tuberculosis in the early months is a positive indication for abortion; in the later months one may temporize, unless obstructed breathing forces the hand. Be ready to do tracheotomy.

Abortion may be done in two sittings under morphin and scopolamin: the first, for insertion of a tent or packing the uterine cavity with gauze, after opening the ovum, and the second on the day following, for removing the contents of the uterus, unless these have come away spontaneously. Premature labor is performed by rupturing the membranes and metreurysis, unless great urgency necessitates more rapid operating, when vaginal cesarean section may be done. Local anesthesia with novocain is used wherever possible. General anesthetics are dangerous because they aid in spreading the disease in the lungs. During labor the patient must be spared every effort. The lungs, compressed by the risen uterus, are suddenly relieved, with occasional disastrous results. The heart has been poisoned so long, a subcyanotic condition of the blood has existed so long that the cardiac muscle is likely to be diseased; therefore, we give both heart and lungs close watch, with the aid of an internist in counsel. As soon as dilatation is complete and the head on the perineum, forceps are to be applied, no straining being permitted. The hemorrhage of the third stage is to be limited. Ethylene is best for general anesthesia, but most cases can be handled with morphin and local. In the puerperium one should keep up the heart with caffein, strychnin, and digitalis, but especially good are fresh air and full diet. Lactation is forbidden, and the child should be removed from the environment in which it was born, unless the parents are intelligent enough to carry out the necessary precautions for its safety. The woman should be instructed how to avoid pregnancy in the future. Something must be done until the woman is cured of her tuberculosis, so that she may safely go through a confinement, because every accoucheur recoils with horror from the task of repeatedly doing abortions on these tuberculous women. (See Pottenger, Lit., Bacon, Matthews, Winter on Abortion, Gross, 1927 Lit., Adair and Whitacre.)

Tuberculosis in other parts of the body is usually aggravated by pregnancy, though abortion is rarely indicated. If one kidney is tuberculous it may be removed; if both, abortion may be induced. (See Granzow.)

Syphilis.—Obstetricians should constantly be on the alert for this protean disease. Its baneful action is often discovered when least expected, and it spreads its blight on all three individuals concerned in the propagation of the species, even being transmitted to the third generation (Tumpeer). Ricord says that in Paris one in eight is syphilitic, and while in America the conditions are better, the disease is not rare, and in its lesser manifestations quite common, though often not diagnosed. R. Peterson found that 5.6 per cent. of routine gynecologic and obstetric patients showed a positive Wassermann reaction. At the Chicago Lying-in Hospital 3.6 per cent. of the ward cases gave positive results, but we do not consider the patient luetic unless the blood is repeatedly positive and with several standard tests. Negative reactions do not rule out the disease, in fact, they are more apt to occur in the pregnant syphilitic than in others and late in pregnancy and in labor a positive reaction may be obtained in the blood of a healthy woman. Control by Wassermann and Kahn tests after the puerperium. First maternal syphilis, then paternal, will be considered.

Effects of Pregnancy on Syphilis.—In olden times it was an accepted fact that pregnancy had an unfavorable influence on lues in all its manifestations, acute and chronic. In recent years syphilographers have observed a general amelioration of the severity of this disease, and this is true also when it occurs in a gravid woman—indeed, a few authors express the view that pregnancy confers a degree of immunity against lues, reducing its virulence. While this may be true of its general effects, I find that the local, especially the secondaries, are prone to be extensive,

SYPHILITIC LESIONS IN PREGNANT WOMEN

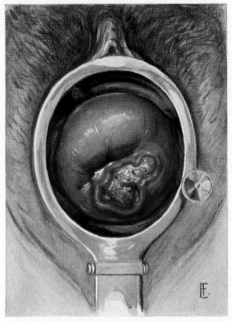

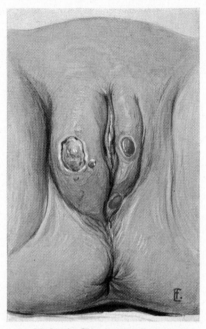

1. Confluent Chancres of Cervix in Pregnancy.

2. Multiple Chancres in Pregnancy (rarely multiple).

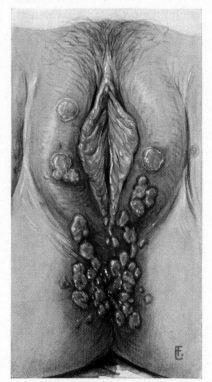

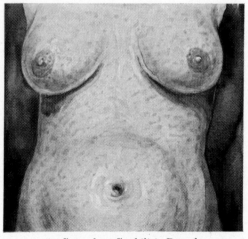

4. Secondary Syphilitic Roseola—
Circinate Type (rare).

3. Condylomata Lata (syphilitic) in Pregnancy; Above Typical Lesions: Around Anus, Exuberant, Resembling Condylomata Acuminata.

These pictures were made by Felix Eisengräber, through the courtesy of Prof. Leo von Zumbusch of the Dermatological Clinic of Munich.

ulcerative, and exuberant, forming large condylomata, due to the extreme succulence of the parts. (Plate IV.)

Effects of Maternal Syphilis on the Pregnancy.—Luetic women are often sterile, perhaps because the ovarian function is suspended in a manner similar to that of the testicle in syphilitic men. There is a syphilitic endometritis which may explain some cases. The actual effects on the pregnancy may vary with the age of the syphilis and the success of the treatment, because if the patient has been successfully treated, she may bear healthy children.

If the syphilis is more recent, the fetus dies, and abortion occurs. The subsequent pregnancies terminate the same way, but each one later, until a living but syphilitic fetus is born, and finally a living, apparently well child at term. This may develop syphilis within a few months or after years (lues congenita tarda). This course of events may be interrupted by vigorous treatment of both parents.

Apparently healthy children are born of serum-positive mothers in 61.3 per cent. of cases (Belding). One, only, of twins may be syphilitic. Why the placenta does not allow the virus access to the fetus is not known, nor is the manner of infection of the fetus settled—whether it is primarily ovular or later by placental transmission or through admixture of spirochete-laden maternal blood with the fetal, during placental separation (Esch). Spirochetæ have been found in the ova in the ovary of the fetus. Late abortion—fifth to seventh months—and early, premature labor—seventh to eighth months—are characteristic of syphilis and the fetus is usually macerated. Williams found 80 per cent. of macerated fetuses were luetic, but our experience at the Chicago Lying-in Hospital shows less than 40 per cent. Probably the difference in clientèle explains the disparity. Hydrocephalus, anencephalus, spina bifida, deformities in the nervous system, endocrinides (Henrotay), polydactylia, etc., are often due to syphilis (Rudaux, Rosinski).

If the syphilis is contracted during the early months of pregnancy, that is, post-conceptional infection, premature labor is the rule, but if the disease was acquired in the later months, the child may escape, the placenta offering a barrier to the virus. Profeta's law held the child was immune, but later studies show that these infants have a positive Wassermann reaction (Trinchese).

It is said that eclampsia is not more common, but the author had six women showing marked albuminuria while carrying syphilitic fetuses. Labor may be influenced by syphilis. The pains may be weak and progress slow. Abnormal presentations are frequent because the children are usually macerated. A chancre on the cervix may impede delivery, as also may an induration in the secondary stage of lues (Blandin), which may necessitate incisions, craniotomy, even cesarean section (Lantuejoul). Friability of the perineum was very pronounced in three of my cases, the head bursting through the vulva, tearing it in all directions like wet paper. Condylomata lata vulvæ conduce to such lacerations. Postpartum hemorrhage is usually not greater, but the author had one case of hemophilic diathesis in a syphilitic prostitute which made some such relation seem plausible. Ordinarily, if the fetus has been dead long, thrombosis of the placental site occurs.

In the puerperium the morbidity is greater than usual; the puerperal wounds, unless primarily infected, heal nicely, especially if specific treatment is given. Syphilitic fever may be mistaken for sepsis (Taussig).

Paternal syphilis is almost always transmitted to the mother, though the point of entry may be unknown. In rare cases a luetic child is delivered from an apparently healthy mother. Engman suggests that such a mother is a spirochete carrier. The history usually given is that the husband has been treated more or less successfully for syphilis before marriage. The limit of safety, that is, the time required before he can procreate healthy offspring, is variously estimated as from two to twelve years, but much depends on the success of the treatment. Even if at the time of coitus he has no infective lesions, the child is usually syphilitic, or it may show signs of the disease later in life. If the father was cured, it will remain well. If the lues is more recent or uncured, the child dies, macerates, and premature labor takes place, with a repetition of such an occurrence in subsequent pregnancies until the virus is removed by time or medicines.

How do the spirochetæ reach the ovum? They are three times larger than the head of the spermatozoid (6 to 15 microns), and surely this tiny organism could hardly carry such a load; therefore they are carried by the semen, probably as a filtrable virus or other transitional form of development (Lépine). Experience and experiment have shown that syphilis can thus be conveyed (Bab), but it is more likely that the mother becomes syphilitic and the spirochetæ settle in the ovum and decidua from the blood, i. e., placental transmission (Hochsinger, Nürnberger, et al.).

A mother carrying an ex patre syphilitic fetus sometimes develops actual lesions which may be secondary and tertiary, or even only tertiary—the "syphilis by conception." The virus has passed from the fetus through the placental wall to the mother. It is certain that the spirillum of relapsing fever may pass the placenta and infect the child, and, therefore, it is fair to argue that the Spirochæta pallida may infect the mother by a reverse process (Golay).

Abraham Colles (1837) said a woman may carry a luetic child and become immune. She probably has latent syphilis with positive Wassermann reaction.

Some syphilologists claim that all children from syphilitic parents and all parents of syphilitic children are infected, and the disease will become manifest sooner or later. Every obstetrician and pediatrist has had cases which seem to prove and disprove all these dogmatisms. The Wassermann reaction has only made confusion worse confounded. The discovery of the spirochete alone seems to allow positive conclusions, but this organism is very hard to find. All the "laws" should be discarded and the subject studied anew by a commission of obstetricians, pediatrists, syphilologists, and pathologists.

For the present, however, authorities are nearly agreed (1) that serologic tests (Wassermann, Meinicke, Kahn, Sachs-Georgi) if repeatedly positive in pregnancy are good proof of the presence of syphilis; (2) that if such women receive proper treatment the disease can be well started toward cure before delivery; (3) that the mortality rate of fetal syphilis can be decidedly lowered by intensive treatment; (4) that even if, owing to the short length of the antisyphilitic course, the child is not fully cured, the frequency of premature labor is reduced.

Syphilitic Changes in the Newborn.—The skin, the mucous membranes, the viscera, and the bones are most often affected.

1. *The Skin.*—Bullous eruptions; desquamation of large areas of epidermis, leaving deep red, macerated corium underneath; papules and vesicles, especially of the palms, soles, and face; coppery erythema of the buttocks; paronychia; pemphigus; lymphadenitis; icterus.

2. *Mucous Membranes.*—Mucous patches in mouth and pharynx, coryza, weeping papules around anus, fissures, and ulcerations of the body orifices.

3. *Viscera.*—The liver is large, feels elastic, is granular, and almost always is particularly full of spirochetæ (Levaditi). It shows the antigen reaction. Liver changes explain the frequency of icterus and infection of the child, and also, because its aid in assimilation is reduced, the athrepsia of the infant (Bar). The spleen is enlarged, sometimes to five times its normal size. The belly is distended; there is some fluid in the peritoneum. The lungs may show gummata or a peculiar interstitial infiltration which is characteristic of lues; this is called white pneumonia, and is incompatible with respiration. The kidneys nearly always show an interstitial nephritis and endarteritis and peri-arteritis, with cellular infiltration of the vessel wall, which may be generalized throughout the body, and is also found in the cord. These blood-vessel changes are pathognonomic. The placenta is large, heavy (sometimes being over one-fourth the weight of the fetus), pale, soft, fatty, edematous, but these changes are also found in other conditions. The syphilitic changes may be limited to the villi, which are thickened, club shaped (Fig. 429), obliterated by overgrowth of white cells, fatty degenerated, or calcareous and sometimes speckled with fine hemorrhages. Sometimes the changes are restricted to the endometrium and the purely maternal portion of the placenta—gummatous growths which stretch up between the cotyledons, infiltration of the deciduæ, and epithelial degeneration of the placenta materna, but usually the whole placenta is affected. The arteries, and to a less extent the umbilical vein, are much thickened, even obliterated, a fact which may be used for diagnosis. The spirochetæ

are rare in the placenta, but have been found in the cord, adrenals, liver, spleen, testicle, ovary, skin, eye, etc. The fetal blood shows a mononuclear lymphocytosis. The Wassermann reaction is likely to be negative in the fetal blood, even though the mother was luetic (Bar and Daunay), and doubtful reactions may be obtained in the absence of syphilis. From the cerebrospinal fluid the best results are obtained.

4. *The Bones.*—Osteochondritis syphilitica, described by Wegner, is the most constant and pathognomonic autopsy finding. The line of ossification is broader, with irregular edges and points running into the cartilage. There are small islands of bony matter off to the side in the cartilage, and the whole epiphysis is yellower. In advanced cases the part is swollen and the periosteum thickened. The *x*-ray shows a line of bony thickening at this point and aids the diagnosis (Pick).

The diaphysis breaks off easily. Similar changes occur in congenital rachitis.

Syphilis has been invoked to explain many diseases of the newborn, for example, icterus gravis, hemorrhagic diathesis, hydrocephalus, congenital deformities, cystic kidneys, athrepsia, overgrowth of the fetus, uniovular twins (Pinard). Perhaps the discovery of the spirocheta and the various serum reactions may bring light in these and other conditions.

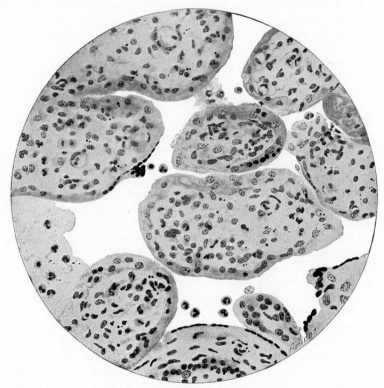

FIG. 429.—SYPHILITIC PLACENTA.
Compare with Fig. 60, p 45, normal placenta.

Treatment.—Syphilis is to be thoroughly treated as soon as discovered, and in the usual manner, regardless of pregnancy. Instituted early, abortion may be prevented. Salvarsan and inunctions seem to give the best results, but since the kidneys are vulnerable during pregnancy their action is to be watched. More than fifteen deaths of gravidæ from salvarsan are recorded. Therefore arsenic is given only in one-half of the usual dosage during pregnancy and, in the last five weeks, replaced by bismuth injections. Habitual abortion after the fifth month, or premature labor, when due to syphilis, indicate antisyphilitic treatment of both parents. In doubtful cases, too, this advice may be given. It is the author's practice to give women with such a history, during pregnancy, mercury, arsenic, and iron as alterative tonics. As soon as it is born the child also is to be treated, and it must be watched minutely for the appearance of rashes, coryza, etc. Salvarsan passes over to the child through the milk, but in small amounts. More important are the specific antibodies developed by the drug, which pass over and are curative. Baginsky warns to care with salvarsan, and prefers inunctions (0.5 to 2 daily), also baths of 1:20,000 HgCl₂ when there are profuse eruptions. Isolate the child and use rubber gloves in handling it, since the disease is very infectious. (See Wile and Shaw.)

Nursing.—Only its mother may nurse the infant, because the child is almost invariably diseased, even if it shows no evidences of lues. Latterly cases are being published in which a luetic mother infected her previously healthy child; but these cases are rare. The milk of a luetic woman is infectious. If the child is syphilitic, but the mother apparently well, only the mother may nurse the infant because she is latently luetic. *Never put a child of a syphilitic mother or father to a healthy wet-nurse.* It is criminal, though the law allows only damages from a civil suit. In hospitals and in maternities the authorities must be on guard constantly for this danger. Only after most careful investigation, including the serum reaction, has shown that the baby and the wet-nurse are healthy may nursing be allowed. In general, in maternities the physicians and nurses should constantly look for the first evidences of syphilis.

DISEASES OF THE CIRCULATORY SYSTEM

The Heart.—In the routine examination of the hearts of pregnant women the author, in a majority of the cases, has found systolic murmurs at the base and accentuation of the second aortic sound, occasionally a presystolic murmur, and displacement of the apex-beat to the left. It was not always easy to eliminate actual vitium cordis. Several real heart diseases were discovered, which, without such a routine examination would surely have passed through labor without being noticed, because they produced no trouble whatever. Heart disease in labor is certainly often overlooked. Mild cardiac abnormalities are not rare in pregnancy, such as increased rapidity, premature contractions, and sino-auricular block (irregular heart's action after exertion).

The Effect of Pregnancy on Heart Disease.—A normal healthy heart easily satisfies all the extra demands made on it by gestation and labor. Even a diseased heart, if compensation is good, often successfully carries the more than 50 per cent. additional strain. Stander and Schmidt proved that the heart must work harder beginning at the third month. (See page 110, heart changes during pregnancy.)

Pregnancy, therefore, in mild heart cases, in young, otherwise healthy women, does not seem to exert a very harmful influence on the disease, but it has seemed to the author that these women develop decompensation and die sooner than other women and men with similar cardiac disease. Naturally, it is hard to collect statistics on this point. If the disease is advanced; if the heart is in unstable equilibrium, and especially if myocarditic or fatty degeneration has occurred, the danger of broken compensation with its pernicious sequelæ is present. Pregnancy predisposes to an acute exacerbation of chronic endocarditis, especially if the latter be not too old, and with this sometimes a fatty degeneration of the papillary muscles occurs, which has a bad effect on the compensation. The anemia may weaken an already diseased myometrium, as also may pregnancy toxemia. The burden on the heart is more than mechanical. The congestion of the venous system leads to kidney and hepatic disturbances; the pulmonary congestion leads to dyspnea and carbonic acid narcosis, and the high position of the diaphragm, with the slight decrease of vital capacity, augments the respiratory difficulty and cyanosis. Near term the blood-pressure may rise. Transudations in the pleuræ may cause compression of the lungs, hypostatic pneumonia, and œdema pulmonum, and hemoptysis may also be a complication. Edema of the extremities, ascites, dyspnea, attacks of suffocation, dry cough, palpitation, insomnia, albuminuria—all these

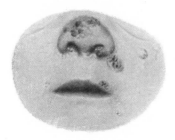

Fig. 430.—Syphilitic Child—Part of Face.

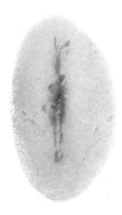

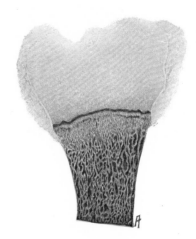

Fig. 431.—Syphilitic Child—Anal Region.

Fig. 432.—Osteochondritis Syphilitica (gross specimen from Dr. Zeit).

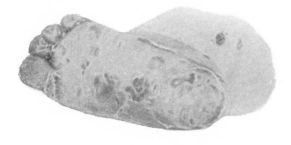

Fig. 433.—Syphilitic Child—Foot.

show that the compensation is broken and warn the accoucheur of impending danger. Occasionally symptoms of Basedow's appear—struma, tachycardia, sweating, exophthalmos, etc., and other endocrinal gland disturbances (Mackenzie).

During Labor.—There is danger from not fully compensated hearts, and, too, an apparently competent heart may suddenly prove default. Without doubt some of the cases of sudden death during labor are due to an unrecognized vitium cordis. I have seen 2 cases of acute dilatation of an apparently normal heart, but probably unsuspected myocardial disease was present. Even a strong heart may not be able to stand the strain of an unduly prolonged second stage.

Uterine action increases the arterial tension, and straining—bearing down—increases both arterial and venous pressure. The electrocardiograph shows that the heart does more work during labor. In themselves these changes are not very dangerous; it is the fluctuation of the blood-pressure incident to labor which is hard on the heart. Symptoms of a laboring organ appear, or the heart may suddenly give way to the strain, and cyanosis, collapse, œdema pulmonum, and death ensue. If the heart holds out until the baby is born, the balance of the circulation may be established rapidly, or, in not a few cases, sudden death in collapse may occur a few hours or several days after delivery.

In the puerperium some of the patients that recover from the strain of labor grow worse, and die from embolism of the brain or lungs, cardiac thrombosis, recurring endocarditis, degeneration of the heart muscle, and aggravation of the existing disease. Sepsis in the puerperium favors acute endocarditis, or may cause exacerbations of an old affection, or may start or increase myocardial degeneration.

Valvular lesions are less affected by gestation than the myocardial diseases, a point which Angus MacDonald, Berry Hart, and others have emphasized. The incidence of various forms of heart disease is given differently by observers. In 268 cases collected (Fellner, Porak, Vinay, Pardee, and my own) there were 74 of mitral regurgitation; 50 mitral stenosis; 76 double mitral; 20 aortic regurgitation; 2 aortic stenosis; 41 combined mitral and aortic; 5 myocarditis. Evidently the rheumatic forms predominate (Reid says 90 per cent.).

Myocarditis frequently accompanies valvular lesions, especially mitral stenosis, and always clouds the prognosis. Auricular fibrillation and bundle-branch block, both mentioned sparingly in the literature, are of bad prognosis. Tachycardia is frequently met. It subsides after delivery, and we often have to be satisfied with a diagnosis "nervous heart." The fetus may show the same phenomenon. Thyroid? Paroxysmal tachycardia, a cardiac arrhythmia which needs better definition, occurring in parturition will have to be differentiated from abruptio placentæ, obstetric shock, decompensation of a rheumatic heart, etc. (Meyer *et al.*).

A second class of cases is composed of those that develop during pregnancy and the puerperium. Acute endocarditis may occur during pregnancy. Acute myocarditis and fatty degeneration may occur during gestation, but they are more likely in the puerperium, as evidences of a septic process, though they may occur alone. Brown atrophy has been found in many cases of sepsis. Fatty degeneration of the heart may follow severe hemorrhages, especially if repeated, also prolonged and hard labor, protracted chloroform narcosis, and there has been observed an acute general fatty degeneration similar to Buhl's disease of the newborn. Heart cases are aggravated by the complications of pregnancy, for example, twins, polyhydramnion, contracted pelvis, tuberculosis, toxemia, nephritis, etc.

Effects of the Heart Disease on Pregnancy.—Sterility is not common in women with cardiac lesions unless in advanced stages. Profuse menstruation has been noted. Abortion and premature labor, especially the latter, occur in cases of decompensation, in from 20 to 40 per cent., and still-births in 29 to 70 per cent., giving the figures collected from various sources by Fellner. It is said that postpartum hemorrhage is frequent, but I have not found it so. Its gravity in heart cases is variously gaged, some authors even considering it beneficial. Placenta marginata is frequent. Heart disease has no particular influence on the puerperal processes. The lochia are somewhat profuse and prolonged, and lactation is imperfect.

Prognosis.—Since many women with cardiac disease pass through pregnancy and labor with the condition unknown, it is necessary to receive the published accounts with caution. Published statistics of mortality are 34, 61, 60, 55, 48, 49, 12, 6, 31, and 85 per cent., and these surely present a dark picture of the gravity of cardiopathy in pregnancy, but Fellner, who collected the above, calls attention to the fact that these are only the bad cases, and that the many mild ones are not reported. He supports the statement with the figures of Schauta's clinic, which showed a mortality of 6.3 per cent., and, if he reckoned in those cases where the vitium was accidentally discovered, it would be only 0.9 per cent. Nevertheless, my own experience has taught me to fear the complication of heart disease with pregnancy, for even though one finally brings the patient through alive, the dangers that threaten at every step are very disquieting, and when accidents occur, they require the promptest and most skilful treatment. Stoeckel, in a 1917 review of German literature, comes to the same conclusions. Mitral stenosis is generally considered the worst of the valvular diseases, so far as pregnancy is concerned, especially when complicated by myodegeneration, which makes all cases very serious. Of disturbances of cardiac mechanism bundle-branch block is most serious. Everything depends on the compensation which means the amount of reserve the myocardium has, and the various tests of cardiac muscle efficiency must tell us if the particular patient will be able to stand the mechanical and toxic effects of pregnancy. Nephritis with high blood-pressure adds much to the gravity of the situation. Death is usually from an acute exacerbation of the endocarditis with myodegeneration and it occurs after the delivery. In uncompensated heart disease many children die from prematurity, abruptio placentæ, disease of the placenta, and asphyxia, because of the imperfectly aërated maternal blood and carbonic acid narcosis.

Treatment.—A woman with uncompensated heart disease should not marry, and if married, should not conceive, and if she has a baby, should nurse it only in part. If the woman is otherwise healthy and her heart is carrying its burden well, she may marry, and if she much desires it, have children, but the dangers are to be explained to both husband and wife.

During Pregnancy.—After medical treatment has been instituted the question arises, Can this patient be carried through to viability of the child, or must abortion be done? In deciding this we must consider (1) the nature of the cardiac lesion, (2) the degree of decompensation, (3) the reserve force of the heart, (4) the condition of other organs in the body, the blood-vessels, the kidneys, the liver, the lungs; (5) whether obtaining a weak though live child is worth the permanent damage to the heart or the danger of sudden death entailed by waiting; (6) the age of the patient; (7) her parity; (8) her desire for children and her religion; (9) the advent of acute endocarditis.

The nature of the lesion itself is not the deciding factor, as many women with apparent gross pathology go through pregnancy without trouble, and others with little apparent disease may die. Combined aortic and mitral disease and great enlargement of the heart are ominous. Our decision will rest on the estimation of the cardiac reserve. Endurance tests, the spirometer, the electrocardiograph, the "pulse deficit" will help us a little, but we rely mostly upon careful clinical observation, and the aid of a cardiologist should be enlisted.

In a woman with chronic decompensation, with myodegeneration, tuberculosis, kyphoscoliosis, pernicious anemia, struma, with arterial disease, or liver or kidney insufficiency, it may be necessary to empty the uterus early because we know she will not be able to go through the process safely. Here one considers the life expectancy of the patient, weighing it against the life of the fetus, a mournful duty. One attack of decompensation does not always indicate abortion, but a second does. The earlier the break occurs, the more dubious the outlook. An attack of acute endocarditis is always ominous—tachycardia, anemia, fever. In an old woman with many children one will interfere sooner, also because such patients do not recuperate as well as young ones. Primiparæ one always tries to carry through, and the Catholic Church may forbid any interference which endangers the child.

If the attempt to preserve the pregnancy is to be made, the usual medical treatment is instituted, the details of which do not belong here. Constant watchfulness for the very first signs of decompensation is required. If rest in bed, medicines, removal of all foci of infection, etc., fail to relieve the situation, the uterus must be emptied, or the mother as well as the child will die. The method will depend on the period of the pregnancy and the urgency of the symptoms. In the first four months the usual procedures are used, a tent, or gauze packing in the cervix, and curetage on the day following, under morphin, scopolamin, and a little ethylene if necessary. If the symptoms are urgent, vaginal cesarean section under the same anesthetic, or with novocain is preferable. To be also considered is abdominal abortion with sterilization, using local anesthesia. In the fifth and sixth months puncture of the membranes and metreurysis are made or, in emergency, colpotrachelotomy. After viability the bag method of induction is usually employed if the pelvis is not contracted. The cervix is usually soft, the pains strong, and dilatation quickly effected. Lately, cesarean section is gaining adherents and has the advantages of simplicity, speed, guarantee of the life of the child, and the opportunity to effect sterilization. The author uses laparotrachelotomy. Ethylene is chosen unless the patient will allow the local anesthetic.

During labor all heart cases require close scrutiny, even if there is good compensation. Labor must be so conducted that collapse in the third stage, and sudden death later in the puerperium are rendered impossible—a task of no small difficulty. Preparations for all eventualities must be made beforehand—plenty of assistants, oxygen, salt solution, venesection instruments, hypodermic syringe with stimulants—in short, the facilities of a well-equipped maternity. All the instruments for operative delivery are to be held, sterilized, ready for instant use. If there is time the patient should be digitalized as part of the preparation for her labor. Watch the effect of the pains on the heart, such as dyspnea, cough, precordial oppression, respirations over 26, cyanosis, flagging or irregular pulse. Dyspnea between pains is especially suggestive. When dilatation is complete, puncture the membranes, but let the water escape slowly. When the head comes down on the perineum, perform episiotomy and deliver at once. Before complete dilatation, even if the dyspnea is not very marked nor the cyanosis very deep, if cough sets in, if the pulse begins to drop beats; if it gets very rapid (100 or more) or the patient gets tired and restless, one should dilate or incise the cervix and extract at once. Do not wait for actual edema of the lungs or actual cardiac failure to spur you to action, because in such cases, even if you do save the patient, the time that the circulation has been in abeyance has perhaps allowed a clot to form in the heart, or the overstrain of the muscle has caused a hemorrhage in the myocardium, and, later in the puerperium, death may occur from embolism or cardiac rupture. Extraction is done by forceps or by the breech, depending on conditions, but the actual delivery is to be executed slowly, and two strong hands must follow down the uterus, so that the intra-abdominal pressure is not reduced too quickly, since the rush of blood into the dilated veins of the abdomen would tend to leave the enlarged heart empty. Hemorrhage is dangerous in heart cases and should be prevented. Later if venesection is necessary, open a vein in the arm. Delivery of the placenta should not be hastened. Ergot and pituitrin may, if necessary, be given after the third stage. Ethylene is the anesthetic of choice, a professional anesthetizer being employed, if possible, since this will enable the accoucheur to give all his attention to the delivery of the child. In myodegeneratio cordis it is best to give no anesthetic, and I have been surprised to see how much could be accomplished by encouragement and suggestion aided by morphin and scopolamin. In many cases local anesthesia with novocain is usable.

Should collapse occur at any time during the first stage, it must be combated instantly for reasons above given, and labor should be completed by bimanual dilatation, cervical incisions, or even cesarean section. When the fetus is dead, craniotomy is to be done. While doing these, or after delivery, give hypodermically morphin with atropin, then 1 c.c. of digafoline intravenously, oxygen by inhalation, and 6 ounces of strong black coffee per rectum. For œdema pulmonum the same treatment is given. Venesection may be useful when the heart is overengorged, 8 to 12 ounces being withdrawn. Though used in other heart cases, I have never found it necessary under these circumstances. Salt solution is not to be given in these cases unless complicated by severe hemorrhage. Since the most critical period is just after delivery, a physician should remain near the patient for at least twelve hours. In the puerperium absolute rest, with the body horizontal, the head a little raised, and the exhibition of the usual remedies are advised. Nursing is to be prohibited only in bad cases, and always one should prevent too great a drain on the woman's resources.

Dysthyroidism.—In 41 per cent. of 520 patients Davis found enlargement of the thyroid. Seitz gives 80 per cent, my own cases show 60 per cent. It seems that pregnancy necessitates more thyroid activity. Cretins, strumiprivata and the myxedematous fail, therefore to respond to the demands on the thyroid and their disease usually grows worse, but sometimes it improves and here one might suspect that the fetal thyroid supplies the deficiency.

Milder evidences of *hypothyroidism* in pregnancy are dulness of intellect, sleepiness, pains in the skin and joints, constipation, pastiness of the skin, coarsening of the features, dryness of the hair, low basal metabolism, tendency to obesity. Eclampsia is said to be more frequent. Some cases of habitual abortion are due to hypothyroidism, and overgrowth of the child also (Osler).

Symptoms of mild *hyperthyroidism* are not infrequent, *e. g.*, irritability, nervousness, emotionalism, insomnia, quick exhaustion, cardiac palpitation and shortness of breath on exertion and vasomotor disturbances; occasionally nausea and vomiting. Slight enlargement of the thyroid is often found, as well as tremor, occasional high blood-pressure, increase of the basal metabolism rate and some of the eye signs. It seems that the iodin metabolism in the thyroid is insufficient and small doses of this drug often bring quick and permanent relief. (See Strouse and Daly.)

True Basedow's disease is rare during pregnancy, as also is toxic goiter, adenoma with hyperthyroidism. Sometimes pregnancy ameliorates the symptoms, the fetus taking up the excess of thyroid secretion, but oftener the effect of pregnancy is bad. In a few cases the disease makes such inroads on the heart that the pregnancy must be removed or part of the gland extirpated. Repeated pregnancies usually have a bad effect. Hirst had a patient in whom the disease recurred in three successive pregnancies. Labor does not produce serious trouble except in the advanced cases, and then the conditions are the same, and one treats them the same as heart lesions. The puerperium exerts no special influence, though sometimes the course of the disease continues downward during this time (Frühinsholz, Vignes, Lit.).

Amenorrhea and sterility are common in women suffering from exophthalmic goiter because of the atrophy of the uterus and ovaries. Pregnancy, however, has occurred during the amenorrhea. Abortion is not usual unless the cardiac decompensation is marked. In bad cases death of fetus and premature labor may occur. Labor is uninfluenced by the disease, but it is said that abruptio placentæ and postpartum hemorrhage are more frequent (White). Hyperinvolution is common. Lactation is likely to be imperfect, and only a few cases show oversupply of milk. The fetus is usually healthy. Thyroid secretion passes over to the child in the milk. Graves' disease is exceedingly rare in infants, only one case at four weeks being on record.

The *treatment* of the disease is the same as if the woman were not pregnant. Abortion may be required if the heart proves default early, and especially if toxemic symptoms predominate, though perhaps ligation of the upper poles of the gland, or partial removal, might hold the disease in check until pregnancy has been completed. Thaler reports a successful case. The administration of iodin (Lugol's solution) will enable us to carry nearly all cases successfully through pregnancy, but its action may lapse and one should not permit the best time for thyroidectomy (early months) to pass, which is especially true of adenomatous goiter with hyperthyroidism. Late in pregnancy the symptoms may demand interference, but emptying the uterus does not produce the same relief as in pure heart cases, because the toxemia and hyperthyroidism persist. The slower methods of delivery are to be preferred unless labor drags on, when cervical incisions or vaginal cesarean section may be needed. Pregnancy should never be allowed to go beyond term. Morphin, rest in bed, and an ice-bag over the heart are used to calm the cardiac action. Ethylene is the best anesthetic unless local anesthesia is applicable. (See Mussey and Plummer, Lit., Küstner.)

A simple struma usually requires no treatment, as compression of the trachea is rare. Strumectomy has been done in pregnancy, also tracheotomy. Abortion is seldom needed. Induction of premature labor relieves the symptoms of obstruction as a rule.

Phlebitis, periphlebitis, thrombosis of the heart and of the veins of the legs, all of which may occur during pregnancy, will be considered under the Puerperal Diseases.

DISEASES OF THE ALIMENTARY TRACT

Mild disturbances of the intestinal tract are very common during gestation. Nausea and vomiting have already been discussed, and, under the Hygiene of Pregnancy, the treatment of constipation has been considered.

Gastric and intestinal indigestion are of frequent occurrence, and yield very slowly to the usual remedies. For the acidity of the stomach soda-mint tablets, milk of magnesia, or effervescent phosphate of soda may be used. In a few cases slowly sucking pure rock-candy, or chewing salted nuts until fine has been helpful. The fats in the diet should be reduced and food taken (especially carbohydrates) in small amounts frequently. Sodium bicarbonate and magnesia usta are also useful for the "heartburn," also 10 ₥ of dilute HCl in water before meals. For the colicky pains a dose of Rochelle salts combined with proper dieting does the most good, but it may be necessary to give a sedative. It may not always be easy to differentiate between ureteral, intestinal, and uterine or tubal colic (ectopic gestation). Bimanual examination will clear the diagnosis. Colics due to intestinal adhesions, resulting from the so common abdominal operations of today, are very rebellious to treatment.

Flatulence causes colic, and may itself be very annoying. Proper diet and movement of the bowels will usually give relief. Diarrhea as a special symptom is rare. I have frequently observed it as a prodrome of labor. Treat according to cause.

Toothache and dental caries are common, perhaps as the result of a mild form of osteomalacia, to which reference has already been made. So common is dental caries that there is an old saying—"for every child a tooth." Neuralgia of the teeth is also noted in gestation, and is usually due to an infected cavity, or sinus disease. Before teeth are extracted the patient is to be examined by a surgeon capable of detecting these obscure causes. Dental neuralgia may indicate the toxemia of pregnancy. Teeth that are hopelessly diseased and infected are to be removed, and experience proves that nitrous oxid gas may safely be used. It is more than possible that some obscure puerperal infections have their ultimate origin in abscessed teeth.

Jaundice.—Hepatic insufficiency is now fully recognized as a cause of many of the disorders incident to pregnancy, under which heading they are considered. Icterus gravis gravidarum, or acute yellow atrophy of the liver, has been described. Epidemics of infectious jaundice have been observed, and when pregnant women are affected, they show a high mortality. Catarrhal jaundice is rare in gestation. In the service of the Chicago Lying-in Hospital, now over 40,000 cases, it occurred but seven times. No special significance attaches to catarrhal jaundice, except to call our attention to the liver and to the necessity of making sure that it is only a simple affair with which we have to deal. In ectopic pregnancy jaundice sometimes appears. Jaundice occurring just before or during labor is very significant. (See Acute Yellow Atrophy.) Jaundice may be observed after delivery when general anesthesia has been used, especially after chloroform. One should think of late chloroform-poisoning, that is, liver autolysis. The child delivered from a jaundiced mother is not icteric.

Gall-stones.—Ninety-eight per cent. of women operated on for gall-stones have borne children. It seems that pregnancy is a factor in the development of gall-stones, and it is not rare that the gravida has attacks of biliary colic. This is due to interference with the free circulation of the bile, thickening of the same, from passive hyperemia of the liver, increased destruction of the red blood-corpuscles, and the products of fetal metabolism, but infection and trauma are the exciting causes of the formation of stones. The colics seldom occur before the fifth month, and jaundice, with chills and fever, is more common than in the non-pregnant state. Labor may cause pain in the full gall-bladder, and the latter may be easily palpated during the third stage. In the puerperium attacks of gall-stones are infrequent. I have observed 13 cases, in 2 of which the symptoms were very stormy, with intense pain, collapse, and vomiting, so that suspicion of the rupture of an abdominal viscus could well be entertained. Operation should be postponed, if possible, until after delivery, at least as late in pregnancy as possible, because premature labor may occur and the child be lost. However, the later operation is made technically difficult by the large uterine tumor. Only that operation should be done which will quickest remove dangerous conditions (Peterson). Prochownick says that attacks of pancreatitis may simulate gall-stone colic. A meal of sweetbreads may incite gall-stone colic.

Bar has called attention to a syndrome of pain in the region of the gall-bladder, the ureters, and the appendix, with occasional fever, the pathologic basis being a cholecystitis, ureteritis, and appendicitis. He calls it "coli bacillose gravidique." This is a not rare condition in pregnancy. Bacteriuria accompanies it.

Acute cholecystitis may complicate pregnancy, labor (rupture), and the puerperium. The symptoms are quite stormy and jaundice common. It is better to wait until after delivery for the operation, if possible, but in the presence of a strict indication, for example, a large empyema, one may have to drain the sac before labor. In one case the author had to make a differential diagnosis between puerperal infection and pus in the gall-bladder (cf. Vineberg). Absence of local evidences of puerperal disease, signs of local peritonitis in the upper abdomen, with appropriate history, usually indicate the exact source of the trouble.

Appendicitis.—Many pregnant women complain of pain in the region of the appendix, and it is possible that the rising uterus draws on complicating peritoneal adhesions. Women who have had appendix operations almost always complain of dragging pains, especially from the fifth to the eighth months. Primary appendicitis is very rare, but recurrent disease is not rare during gestation, the latter being usually the catarrhal variety, and seldom causing real trouble. Pels Leusden found decidual reaction in the pregnant woman's appendix. This may explain the frequency of appendiceal attacks in pregnancy.

Perforation and suppurative peritonitis are very much more serious than outside of pregnancy, because—(1) Protective adhesions are less likely to be formed, the omentum and gut being pushed away by the enlarging uterus; (2) the inflammation is more stormy, owing to the intense vascularity of the parts; (3) thrombosis and phlebitis are commoner; (4) suppuration takes place higher in the abdomen (true of late pregnancy), which portion is recognized to be less resistant; (5) drainage is less free, owing to the large uterus near by, and the abscesses burrow deeply in all directions; (6) tympany compromises the respiration sooner, also pneumonia and pleurisy; (7) obstructive symptoms arise earlier; and (8) the bacteria floating in the blood may accumulate in the placenta, and even the fetus, causing abortion and sepsis. The mortality, according to Schmid, who collected 486 cases, is very high. Appendicitis offers a better outlook the earlier in pregnancy it occurs and the sooner it is recognized. During labor the contracting uterus may rupture the pus-sac or tear an adherent or perforating appendix, with resulting general peritonitis, which may be mistaken for sepsis sub partu. This danger is greatest during the third stage and during the first few days of the puerperium, at which times the uterine fundus makes its greatest excursions. In the puerperium acute appendicitis is easily mistaken for an infection of the tubes or broad ligament, and, indeed, they may coexist. The puerperal processes aggravate the appendiceal disease.

The effects of perforative appendicitis on the pregnancy are also marked, abortion, premature labor, infection of the uterine contents, and death of the new-born child being noted in the majority of cases. This might all be forestalled by early operative removal of the infective focus. Labor is very painful; the shock of it is greater, and because of the diseased uterine muscle (contiguous to an abscess) weak pains in all three stages are observed. Manual removal of the placenta is more often needed, and such brusk manipulations spread the pus. On the puerperium the worst influence is shown when the diseased appendix forms adhesions to the tube or the uterus, direct transmission of the infection being thus effected, either through the walls of the applied organs or along the surface—also through the blood. A parametritis may also be caused by the infection creeping through Clado's ligament. The relics of appendicitis may anchor the uterus in an unfavorable position, may occlude the tube, producing sterility or favoring ectopic gestation. On the other hand, I am convinced that tubal infections cause appendicitis. The frequency of appendicitis in newly married women is striking, and the gonococcus was found by J. H. Hess in the pus from an appendix.

The diagnosis of appendicitis should present no special difficulties if only the possibility of its occurrence be kept in mind. Ectopic gestation (*q. v.*) and twisted ovarian tumor come up for consideration, but most mistakes are made with ureteritis and ureteral stone (*q. v.*). All possible causes of acute peritonitis must be discussed—gastric ulcer, cholecystitis, etc. During labor, abruptio placentæ, ruptura uteri, torsion of the uterus, of an ovarian cyst, pyelitis, acute uterine infection, etc., must be differentiated from appendicitis. In the puerperium sepsis must always be thought of, and only a laparotomy may explain the equivocal symptoms. A worse prognosis than usual is to be made, because nearly 40 per cent. of perforated appendix peritonitis cases die.

Treatment.—Recurrent appendicitis should be cured before pregnancy occurs. A woman with only a history of appendicitis should not be operated on during pregnancy unless a recurrence takes place. Appendicitis in pregnancy should always indicate immediate operation—even in cases of doubt, operation is the safer course. After spontaneous recovery from an acute attack during pregnancy the appendix had better be removed as soon as possible. The incision is made higher than ordinarily, the appendix preferably removed, and in pus cases drainage should be liberal. The uterus is manipulated as little as possible, and the rule "get in and get out quickly" is observed. Every effort should be made to prevent premature labor. Should abortion occur, it should be allowed to run as natural a course as possible, the tampon and even prolonged expectancy being employed. Manual curetage is to be replaced by instrumental, should the uterus not empty itself. The reason for this is evident—the outside hand may break the protective adhesions around the abscess. During labor the same rule applies, and if manual removal of the placenta is necessary, the dangers of spreading the abdominal infection should be borne in mind. No doubt, too, genital infection is favored by all intra-uterine manipulations. If abortion is impending at the time of operation, the uterus should first be emptied, and then drainage of the abdomen carried out. The question of emptying the uterus artificially before operating on the appendix has been raised; even cesarean section has been proposed if the woman is near term. Early in pregnancy one will usually not induce abortion, but trust to drainage and nature. When one considers the high mortality of suppurative peritonitis at or near term, perhaps it would be best, in the interests of the two individuals, to remove the appendix and do a Porro cesarean section at the same time. Not enough cases are on record to definitely settle this point, but the usual cesarean section is contraindicated. Extraperitoneal section has been suggested. I believe, in cases where the uterus is opened in the presence of pelvic infection, as from ruptured appendix, pus-tube, or infected tumors, it is best to amputate the bulky organ and drain the whole pelvis freely from below. If the operation removed an acutely inflamed appendix without adhesions or abscess, it is not advisable to empty the uterus from below at once, because pregnancy may go on without further trouble, and if a walled-off abscess has formed, it is dangerous to do so, because during labor the adhesions always break. With free drainage and the use of opium one may tide the woman along for several days and thus allow the sac to get firm and the amount of pus in it to be reduced. Obstetric interference may thus be delayed until the abscess cavity is granulating safely. (See also Hilton, Rudaux, Abrahams, Murphy, Baer *et al.*, Portes, Bower.)

Ileus, a rare complication, may be due to the same causes which produce it outside of pregnancy, or may be due to compression or torsion of the gut by the growing uterus. Naturally, the gut must be abnormally adherent for this to take place. In one of the author's cases an old appendicitis was responsible for the adhesions, and the uterus at term dragged on the intestine, producing severe pain in the right iliac fossa and almost complete obstruction—induction of labor, recovery. In another, due to the same cause, the uterus had been emptied under the diagnosis of hyperemesis. If the ileus is due to a complicating suppurative peritonitis, premature labor is the rule and death very common (Gauchery).

Treatment.—Before viability, laparotomy and removal of the cause of the obstruction, then emptying the uterus or not, depending on the findings—usually not. After viability laparotrachelotomy, then treatment of the ileus on general surgical principles. When there is reason to believe the enlarging uterus alone causes obstruction, and the symptoms do not suggest peritonitis—induction of labor. Ileus after delivery may be due to the trauma of labor (intestinal paresis), to obstruction of the bowel by the large uterus incarcerated in the pelvis, to duo-denojejunal closure, and to peritonitis.

Hernia is not seldom met by the accoucheur. Unless the gut is adherent, the growing uterus pushes the contents of the sac out and away from the hernial open-ing, and makes a temporary cure, but the ring is enlarged by the distraction of its pillars, and the hernia is worse in the puerperium, though incarceration is rare. Adherent gut may be incarcerated, twisted, or stretched even to the production of ileus. During labor the opening is usually closed by the large uterus, and even dur-ing strong bearing-down efforts the rupture does not enlarge. I saw, however, an inguinal hernia develop during strong expulsive efforts. Treatment of hernia is the same as at any other time when threatening symptoms occur. During labor it is not wise to allow too strong effort if one sees the hernial tumor enlarging. Forceps should be applied soon after the dilatation is complete. It is not safe to hold the gut back during the strong expulsive straining. Umbilical and postoperative hernias are usually permanently enlarged by pregnancy, and traction on adherent omentum often causes pain (Manley).

LITERATURE

Abrahams: Amer. Jour. Obstet., 1897, vol. xxxv.—*Adair and Whitacre:* Jour. Mich. State Med. Soc., January, 1932. —*Bab:* Zentralbl. f. Gyn., 1909, p. 527.—*Ibid.:* "Congenital Syphilis," Zeitschr. f. Gyn., 1908, vol. lx, p. 161. —*Bacon:* Jour. Amer. Med Assoc., 1912, vol. ii.—*Baer et al.:* Jour. Amer. Med. Assoc., April 16, 1932, p. 1359.—*Baginsky:* Therapie der Gegenwart, 1915, Nos. 1 and 2.—*Baisch:* Münch. med. Woch., September 21, 1909, p. 1929.—*Bar and Daunay:* L'Obstetrique, April, 1909, No. 3.—*Bar and Rènon:* L'Obstetrique, vol. i, p. 69.—*Belding:* Amer. Jour. Obst. and Gyn., December, 1926, p. 839.—*Birch-Hirschfeld:* Arbeiten d. Pathol. Inst. zu Leipzig, Jena, 1891, p. 428.—*Blandin:* L'Obstetrique, 1902, No. 1, p. 43.—*Bower:* Jour. Amer. Med. Assoc., May 2, 1931, p. 1461.—*Calmette and Valtis:* Zeitschrift für Tuberculose, Leipzig, No-vember, 1930, vol. 58, p. 385; also Jour. Amer. Med. Assoc., October 17, 1931, p. 1162.—*Davis, C. H.:* Jour. Amer. Med. Assoc., September 25, 1926.—*Demelin:* L'Obstet., 1896, vol. i.—*Edgar, J. C.:* Jour. Amer. Med. Assoc., April 8, 1905, p. 1077.—*Engman:* Jour. Amer. Med. Assoc., May 11, 1912, pp. 1412, 1415.—*Esch:* Zent. für Gyn., May 5, 1923, p. 709; Value of the Wassermann, Arch. für Gyn., Band 117, 1922, p. 147.— *Fellner:* Innere Krankheiten, p. 70.—*Förssner:* Acta Gyn., Scand., 1925, vol. 3, p. 256.—*Fournier:* Syphilis und Ehe, Hirschwald, 1881.—*Fraenkel, E.:* Volkmann's Klin. Vort., 1901, No. 323.—*Friedman:* Zeit. f. klin. Med., 1901, vol. xliii, p. 11.—*Frühinsholz:* Gynecologie et Obstetrique, September 4, 1921, Lit.—*Gauchery:* Thèse de Paris, 1903. Literature.—*Golay:* Annales de Mal. Ven. Paris, 1926, xxi, p. 481.—*Gräfenberg:* Arch. f. Gyn., 1909, vol. lxxxvii, i.—*Granzow, J.:* Monograph. Die Wechselbeziehungen z. Tuberculose, etc., Karger, Berlin, 1930, Lit.—*Ibid.:* Arch. für Gyn., April, 1932, Bd. 149, H. 1, p. 38.—*Gross:* Zentb. für Gyn., 1927, No. 12, p. 744, Lit.—*Henrotay:* Gynecologie et Obstetrique, April, 1922, p. 288.—*Hilton:* Surg., Gyn., and Obstet., October, 1907.—*Hocksinger:* Monograph. Congenital Syphilis, Karger, Berlin, 1926.—*Hofbauer:* Amer. Jour. Obst. and Gyn., 1925, July 1, p. 1.—*Ingraham:* Am. Jour. Obst. and Gyn., January, 1932, p. 1. —*Küstner, H.:* Zentb. für Gynaek., March 7, 1931.—*Lanz:* Plac. Tuberculosis, Arch. f. Gyn., 1915, Bd. 104, H. 2. Literature.—*Lépine, P.:* Presse Medicale, Paris, August 19, 1931, p. 1233.—*MacDonald:* Obstetric Journal of Great Britain, 1877.—*Mackenzie:* Pregnancy and Heart Disease, Amer. Jour. Obst. and Gyn., De-cember, 1921.—*Manley:* "Hernia and Pregnancy," Medical News, 1900.—*Marshall et al.:* Proc. Royal Soc. Med., 1931, xxiv, 1123.—*Meyer, Lackner and Schochet:* Jour. Amer. Med. Assoc., June 14, 1930.—*Morris:* Amer. Jour. Obst., 1916, vol. 73, p. 997.—*Müller, P.:* Die Krankheiten des weiblichen Körpers, p. 85.— *Murphy:* Clinics, December, 1914.—*Mussey and Plummer:* Jour. Amer. Med. Assoc., August 29, 1931, Lit.— *Mussey, Plummer and Boothby:* Jour. Amer. Med. Assoc., September 25, 1925.—*Nürnberger:* Zentralbl. für Gynaek., March 20, 1926. See also Collection of References, Amer. Jour. Obst. and Gyn., February, 1926.— *Peterson:* Surg., Gyn., and Obstet., July, 1910. Full literature.—*Pick:* Roentgen Diagnosis of Syphilis, Deutsche med. Woch., No. 35, 1919.—*Portes and Seguy:* Obstét. et Gyn. Paris, 1927, vol. xv, No. 2, p. 122. —*Pottenger:* Excellent Review of Tuberculosis, Surg., Gyn., and Obstet., November, 1921, p. 354; also Amer. Jour. Obstet. and Gyn., September, 1923, p. 385.—*Prochownick:* Mon. f. Geb. u. Gyn., September 3, 1916. —*Reid, W. D.:* Jour. Amer. Med. Assoc., November 15, 1930, p. 1468.—*Renwall:* Zentralbl. f. Gyn., 1910, p. 955; 288 cases. "Gall-stones," Report of Discussion at Toulouse, Annales de Gyn., December, 1910, p. 805.—*Robinson, A. L.:* Jour. Obst. and Gyn., Brit. Empire, Summer, 1931, p. 338.—*Rudaux:* Ann. de Gyn., September, 1911.—*Schmid:* Jour. Amer. Med. Assoc., July 22, 1911, p. 349. Literature.—*Schmidt:* Deutsch. Ges. für Gyn., May, 1931.—*Schmorl:* Münch. med. Woch., 1904, vol. li, p. 1676.—*Seitz-Stoeckel:* Geburtshilfe, 1920, p. 587.—*Stander, H. J., and Cadden:* Amer. Jour. Obstet. and Gyn., July, 1932, p. 13.—*Stoeckel:* Jahreskurse für Ärztl. Fortbildung, July, 1917.—*Stork:* Monatsschr. f. Geb. u. Gyn., April, 1925.—*Strouse and Daly:* Jour. Amer. Med. Assoc., June 13, 1925, p. 1798.—*Stühmer:* Jour. Amer. Med. Assoc., 1922, p. 624.—*Syphilis:* Selected abstracts, Amer. Jour. Obst. and Gyn., September, 1923, p. 375.—*Taussig:* Surg., Gyn., and Obst., September, 1916. Full literature.—*Thaler:* Zentb. f. Gyn., 1915, No. 21.—*Trembley, C. C.:* "Tuberculosis in Pregnancy," Jour. Amer. Med. Assoc., 1909, vol. lii, p. 989, with discussion by Jewett, Edgar, Craigin *et al.*—*Trinchese:* Deutsch. med. Woch., 1915, No. 19.—*Tumpeer:* Amer. Jour. of Syph., Oc-tober, 1921, vol. v, No. 4.—*Vinay:* Maladies de la Grossesse, p. 309; *ibid.*, p. 78.—*Vignes:* Physiologie Obstet., Masson, Paris, 1923.—*Vineberg:* Medical Record, April 8, 1905, p. 532.—*Virchow:* Archiv., 1905, clxxxi, p. 150.—*White:* Jour. Obstet. and Gyn. of Great Britain, September, 1911. Full literature.—*Wile and Shaw:* Jour. Amer. Med. Assoc., December 13, 1930.—*Williams:* Bull. of Johns Hopkins Hosp., October, 1920, p. 336.—*v. Winckel:* Handbuch, vol. ii, i, p. 625.—*Winter:* Der Künstl. Abort. Enke, Stuttgart, 1926.—*Zinnstag:* Monatsschr. für Geb. u. Gyn., February, 1927, p. 498, Lit.

CHAPTER XXXIX

DISEASES OF THE URINARY SYSTEM

Nephritis.—Internists distinguish the following principal forms of renal disease: Acute nephritis, chronic nephritis, of which there are two grand divisions, the parenchymatous, with its three forms, large white kidney, large red kidney, and the secondary contracted kidney; and the chronic interstitial or primary contracted kidney, which is accompanied by cardiac hypertrophy and a general arteriosclerosis. The accoucheur, in addition to these, must consider the kidney of pregnancy, its aggravated form, the so-called pregnancy nephritis, and the kidney changes which are part of eclampsia. Since even the internists are not in perfect accord regarding the classification of their physical findings and admit that the various recognized varieties of disease may be associated or correlated, it is not to be expected that the accoucheur will be able absolutely to identify the many conditions presented to him for treatment. The symptoms of watery transudations in the parenchymatous forms give them the appellation "wet"; the interstitial varieties are "dry."

The kidney of pregnancy and the kidney in eclampsia have already been considered in the chapters devoted to Incidental Diseases. Here will be discussed the accidental complication of pregnancy with renal disease. Although only one-quarter to one-fifth of nephritics develop convulsions in pregnancy, the association of the two conditions, nephritis and eclampsism, is always fraught with grave dangers to mother and child.

Primary acute nephritis may develop during gestation from the same causes which operate outside of it, for example, exposure to cold, chemical poisons, ptomainemia, scarlatina, angina, and infections of various kinds. Antecedent septic processes make the kidney more vulnerable, which tendency is aggravated by pregnancy. Acute nephritis cannot be clinically differentiated from the "pregnancy nephritis" which often leads up to eclampsia, and, therefore, will not be further discussed here—see Eclampsia (Lit., Rockwood).

Chronic parenchymatous nephritis is always unfavorably affected by the advent of gestation, and an acute exacerbation is almost always observed. It begins to show in the early months, contrary to the renal disease incidental to pregnancy. Puffiness of the eyelids and of the ocular conjunctiva and general anasarca are marked and do not disappear in the recumbent position. The edema affects the legs, which may be elephantiasic, and the vulva, which may be transformed into two immense, white, translucent, watery, glistening tumors. Hydroperitoneum, hydropleura, œdema pulmonum may occur; pallor, a waxy, pasty skin, high pulse tension, even in this form, are to be noted. Headache, neuralgias, epigastric pain, disorders of the special senses, especially amaurosis, nausea, and vomiting, are found, but not so marked nor so common as in preëclamptic toxemia. Retinitis albuminurica is very serious, and may leave permanent blindness. Convulsions occur, but in less than one-third of the cases. The urinary findings are similar to those of preëclamptic toxemic nephritis—albumin, hyaline, granular, cellular casts, renal epithelium, white and, finally, red blood-corpuscles. Urea is diminished, the total solids reduced, the daily amount of urine much less than normal.

Labor has a noxious influence on the nephritis, and often produces alarming symptoms—œdema pulmonum, collapse, which may simulate pulmonary or cerebral embolism, apoplexy, and suppression of urine. Anemia is badly borne by nephritics. If anesthetics are given, and if the labor is protracted and exhausting, real damage may be done to the kidneys.

The puerperal processes do not exert a good influence either—sepsis is commoner and nephritics do not bear infection well. While the urine usually rapidly clears up after delivery, the restitution of the kidneys is never complete, permanent structural damage having been wrought, and the action of repeated pregnancies is so bad that death is hastened. Stander and Young (1932) confirmed these facts.

Chronic interstitial nephritis is more frequent than the parenchymatous, and is characterized by polyuria of low specific gravity, with little urea and small amount of albumin, few casts, and these usually of the hyaline variety. It is accompanied by high arterial tension (200 to 240 mm.), thickening of the vessels, and hypertrophy of the heart. The effects of this form usually appear later in the pregnancy, but the symptoms of urinemia already mentioned occur with almost equal frequency, and especially in the later months, the distinctions between the various forms become blurred. Retinitis, apoplexy, and heart collapse are more frequent with cirrhotic kidney, and convulsions less frequent.

All forms of nephritis have a very bad influence on the pregnancy, abortion and premature labor being common (66 per cent., Hofmeier); Seitz found that only from 20 to 30 per cent. of the children survived. One of the causes of habitual death of the fetus and abortion and premature labor is chronic nephritis. Labor in nephritics is slow: the uterus is indolent; the edema of the vulva predisposes to perineal lacerations, and in one case of the author's the edema of the pelvic structures prevented the head from engaging in the pelvis. Even after the delivery, which was very laborious, the cervix could not be drawn down to the vulva as usual, because it was anchored up high by the infiltrated broad ligaments. Abruptio placentæ is not infrequent. Postpartum hemorrhage is common because of atony of the uterus. Involution is slower. Many of the children are born dead and more or less macerated. The death of the fetus is caused by—(1) The hemorrhages, the white infarcts, and the sclerosis of the blood-vessels of the placenta, which cut off the fetal circulation and are frequently found (80 per cent.). Simpson and Fehling called attention to these facts, and the French call the condition "placenta albuminurique" (Fig. 488). (2) By the frequent abruption of the placenta in labor. (3) By the accumulation of toxins in the blood which alter the villi, making them unfit for the function of nourishing the child, or toxins lodge in the deciduæ, making their blood-vessels brittle and thrombotic, and the deciduæ liable to separation (a degenerative endometritis); in the first instance death of the fetus occurs; in the latter, hemorrhages into and separation of the decidua with abortion result. (4) The fetus is poisoned by the toxins which pass over from the mother. (5) Eclampsia may interrupt the pregnancy.

The children of nephritics are usually puny and pale; they thrive poorly at first, and may show albuminuria with casts. Infarcts and hemorrhages may so reduce the functionating area of the placenta that the fetus does not receive enough food—it starves in utero. The placenta may be edematous rarely, the fetus also.

Diagnosis.—The discovery of albumin in the urine at one of the routine examinations leads at once to a minute investigation of the cause. It is an error of art to be surprised into making a urinalysis by the symptoms of nephritis. The author is very skeptical about the so-called physiologic albuminurias—most often a slumbering disease is at the bottom. Before deciding that the kidneys are affected one must eliminate cystitis, ureteritis, and congestive conditions. It is usually impossible to differentiate the various forms of nephritis during gestation, because the urinary and clinical pictures are blurred, but it is not essential for treatment. A diagnosis of the functional capacity of the kidneys is of more importance.

Prognosis.—Both mother and child are seriously jeopardized by chronic nephritis, the mortalities being about 30 and 70 per cent. respectively. Care must be exercised in promising a cure by the induction of abortion or premature labor, because the condition may not be the simple kidney of pregnancy, but a real latent nephritis which has been awakened into activity. The main dangers of nephritis are edema of the lungs, hydropericardium, hydropleura, enormous anasarca, retinitis, which may lead to permanent blindness, apoplexy, eclampsia, and acute heart collapse. A combination with heart disease is very fatal.

Treatment.—Women with chronic nephritis should not marry, and if married, should not conceive. If a woman had eclampsia or symptoms of renal inefficiency in her first pregnancy, a second should not be allowed until the evidences of renal disease have remained absent for at least a year, and the modern tests of function, *e. g.*, phenolphthalein, indigo-carmin, the Schlager-Mosenthal meal, the concentration and the freshet tests, have proved the kidneys sound. Should pregnancy occur with diseased kidneys, redoubled watchfulness is required.

(*a*) *Nephritis is Discovered After the Twenty-eighth Week.*—While a cure cannot be effected during gestation, most authors advise that the patient be tided along to term if possible, but to induce premature labor in the presence of threatening symptoms. The details of the medical treatment have been fully given in the chapter on Eclampsia, to which the reader is referred. Here the imminence of convulsions or coma decides the question of the induction of labor, but in nephritis other dangers may indicate interference. Retinitis albuminurica is a positive indication for the immediate termination of gestation. Immense anasarca and a laboring heart, which do not respond to treatment, also are good reasons; then the dangers which threaten the child must be considered—abruptio placentæ and hemorrhages into it—though to discover these accidents in time to save the infant is not always possible. For this reason, and because our knowledge of nephritis is so uncertain (except that pregnancy shortens the woman's life) and our reliance on treatment so insecure, I usually interrupt pregnancy as a matter of principle when the child has fully passed the period of viability. The exceptions, of course, are those cases where very satisfactory improvement ensues under treatment. The usual methods of inducing labor are employed, but in critical cases vaginal, or abdominal cesarean section may be indicated.

(*b*) *Nephritis is Discovered Before the Child is Viable.*—Some authorities (Schröder, Fehling, Billings, Tyson, Edwards, Schauta, and others) recommend the induction of abortion, holding that the injury to the kidneys which is inevitable before the child becomes viable, and, too, the poor chances of the fetus in any case, make the continuance of the pregnancy precarious and useless. With these opinions mine agrees, but if the woman is near the period of viability, I try to tide her along a few weeks to give the child a better chance for its life. Of course, the gravida must stay in bed under rigid treatment, and a careful daily urinalysis must be made. In the early months the pregnancy is interrupted on the first indication of trouble, and, too, if the disease of the kidneys, while not retrogressing, remains stationary under treatment. Experience has shown that these cases always grow worse and require interference before viability of the child, and it is, therefore, injudicious to wait, because the kidneys will suffer irreparable damage in the meantime.

During labor nephritics require special care. It is wise to watch the heart action closely and be prepared for the same emergencies that occur with heart lesions. It may be necessary to puncture the swollen labia vulvæ (antiseptically, of course) to allow delivery. In the puerperium the usual treatment is kept up. Nursing is to be permitted only if the puerpera is in good condition and the renal symptoms disappearing. (See Fränkl-Hochwart and von Noorden, Fellner.)

Pyelitis and Ureteritis.—A not infrequent complication of pregnancy is inflammation of the kidney pelvis and the ureters. Smellie knew of it, Rayer, in 1841, recognized it, Kaltenbach in 1871 segregated the disease, and Reblaub, in 1893, reported several cases at the Congress of the French surgeons. Bacteriuria is found in a large per cent. of healthy pregnant women, probably from constipated or infected bowels. The ureters, particularly the right, with the x-ray have been found dilated and filled with urine in about 80 per cent. of gravidæ (Fig. 435a). This is caused by torsion, stretching, or kinking of the ureters, due to the enlargement and dislocation of the pelvic organs or swelling of the bladder mucosa, or atonic innervation (Stoeckel), but not to compression, since the specific gravity of the pregnant uterus is about equal to that of the intestinal mass (Luchs). A physiologic dilation of the ureters to the size of one or two thumbs may occur (Ehrhardt), at any part of their extent, though more often in the extrapelvic portions. The pressure in the pelvis of the kidney is only 10 mm. Hg, so that slight causes may stop the flow of the urine in the ureter. Owing to the stasis of the urine and the bacteriuria, a pyelo-ureteritis is easily set up, but infection can reach the parts also through the blood from a gastro-enteritis, an angina, teeth, sinuses, polyarthritis, or thrombophlebitis, through the lymph-stream from contiguous structures, for example, the appendix, the colon, and by ascending from the bladder either on the mucosa or in the peri-ureteral lymph-vessels (Sweet), or by re-

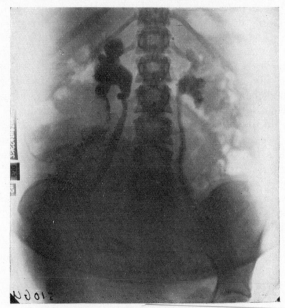

FIG. 435a.—BILATERAL HYDRONEPHROSIS OF PREGNANCY.
Multipara, seventh month. Persistence of these findings after delivery indicates chronic pyelitis. (Courtesy of Dr. Robt. A. Arens, Michael Reese Hospital.)

gurgitation of infected bladder urine into the kidney. The bacterium most often found is the colon bacillus, but the streptococcus, the staphylococcus, the Proteus vulgaris, pneumococcus, Bacillus typhosus, B. paratyphosus (Williamson), and, frequently, according to Vineberg, the gonococcus, may be associated, or even the actual cause. Pregnancy may develop the disease, or may aggravate a preëxistent inflammation which may have started in childhood or at the defloration (Wildbolz) or light up an old tuberculosis. Two varieties are found in practice—the acute and the subacute.

In the acute cases there are chill, fever of pyemic type, sometimes vomiting, pain in the back and along the ureter, and sometimes, not always, the symptoms of cystitis—dysuria, frequent urination, vesical tenesmus, and, rarely, symptoms of ileus (Stoeckel) or even of peritonitis. On palpation the kidney is sometimes enlarged and always tender; on vaginal examination the base of the bladder is sensitive, the ureter usually easily palpable, thickened, and acutely painful to touch. At first there may be suppression, but soon the urine is increased in amount, is cloudy, contains at first little, later much pus, albumin, characteristic epithelium, blood, and swarms with bacteria. If the kidney structure itself is involved—and these cases are usually mixed streptococcus and Bacterium coli infections—the general symptoms take on a septic nature, such as repeated chills, with irregular high fever, rapid pulse, sweats, and evidences of severe illness, while locally a pyonephritis may develop. One or both ureters may be involved, but the disease is thrice more frequently right sided.

Suppression of urine in the course of ureteropyelitis may be either renal or ureteral, in the former case due to inflammatory congestion, in the latter to blocking of the ureter. The diagnosis of blocking of the ureter is not easy. Renal colic, intermittent polyuria with discharges of pus and relief of pain, the results of catheterization of the ureters, access of fever at the time pus is absent from the urine—all are suggestive. The phenolsulphonephthalein test is more useful in these surgical renal affections than in nephritis. The acute symptoms last two to six weeks, but the pyuria and bacteriuria may persist until long after delivery.

When the infection is subacute the symptoms are milder; frequent urination and evidences of cystitis may exist for several weeks before the pain in the ureter and the kidney shows the ascending involvement of the latter. Rarely all symptoms are absent, the disease being accidentally discovered by urinalysis. In both cases the tendency is toward cure, requiring two to eight weeks, and recovery may be complete during pregnancy or almost certainly after delivery. In the cases where the present attack is a relighting of an old process, a cure is rare (Williams). One observes the affection most frequently about the fifth month and again near term. Renal calculi may be an additional complication. In the puerperium acute pyelitis also occurs, and may give rise to suspicion of puerperal infection, and it is possible that the infected urine flowing over the genital wounds may cause sepsis. A pyelo-ureteritis which apparently healed during pregnancy may light up in the puerperium. I have observed the association of pyelitis with hyperemesis gravidarum. Treatment directed to it cures the vomiting. I have also seen pyelitis as a cause of multiple neuritis, and, often, the preëclamptic state and

PYELO-URETERITIS AND STONE	APPENDICITIS
1. Pain goes from the kidney down ureter.	1. Pain radiates toward navel.
2. Vomiting rare—commoner with stone.	2. Vomiting the rule.
3. Tenderness in lumbar region and in the course of the ureter, and at the junction of the quadratus lumborum with the twelfth rib (Cova).	3. Tenderness over McBurney's point. Late in pregnancy the tenderness is higher up. In retrocecal appendix, pain and tenderness equivocal.
4. Abdominal rigidity not pronounced.	4. Rigidity usually marked.
5. Fever irregular and usually not high, unless sepsis present.	5. Fever more constant and continuous.
6. Pulse slow, and even if rapid, not peritonitic.	6. Pulse high, like peritonitis.
7. Rarely tympany, no tumor.	7. Both often.
8. Urination frequent and often tenesmus.	8. Rarely observed.
9. Urinalysis—pus, always bacteria, sometimes blood, tailed epithelium, and findings of desquamative catarrh.	9. Perhaps a little albumin.
10. Cystoscope shows ureteral openings, swollen and inflamed, with pus issuing, and often cystitis, or perhaps a stone may be seen. If the bladder is normal, ureteral catheterization will show the cloudy, bacteria-laden urine; pain relieved.	10. Negative. Pyelography is equivocal. Pain not relieved by catheterization of ureter.
11. May feel thickened, tender ureter (Fig. 436).	11. Negative.
12. Succussion pain in right loin.	12. Absent.
13. Leukocytosis inconstant.	13. More constant.

eclampsia. On occasion it seems epidemic in a maternity. Sometimes the pyelitis is part of the syndrome called by Bar coli bacillose gravidique—with involvement of the gall-bladder (jaundice) or appendix. The prognosis for the child is not any too good—abortion, premature labor, infection.

Diagnosis.—On the direct, the symptoms enumerated plus the urine findings will usually suffice. I have frequently noted the presence in the urine of swollen and transparent mononuclear leukocytes, the nucleus hanging on the side of the clear protoplasm. A fresh catheterized specimen is to be centrifuged for the minute microscopic examination. On direct palpation of the kidney region, tenderness may be elicited by gentle succussion with the first earlier than by pressure (Israel). In the differential diagnosis appendicitis, calculi, typhoid, puerperal infection, and all "acute abdomens" are to be considered (see p. 549).

Treatment.—Acute cases. Rest in bed, milk, buttermilk, and water diet; hexamethylenamin, 8 grains, with methylene-blue, 1 grain, four times daily. The urine must be rendered acid; acid sodium phosphate by mouth. After four days the urine is made alkaline by the free administration of sodium bicarbonate. If the urotropin should cause hematuria or disturb the stomach, salol may be substituted. Daily several colonic flushings are given and the bladder catheterized d. i. d., to remove residual urine and pus. Bladder lavage with normal saline solution at 105° F., repeated thrice daily, may start the urine flowing and help the ureters to pass the pus from the kidney. For the subacute cases the same treatment for a few days, then more freedom and food.

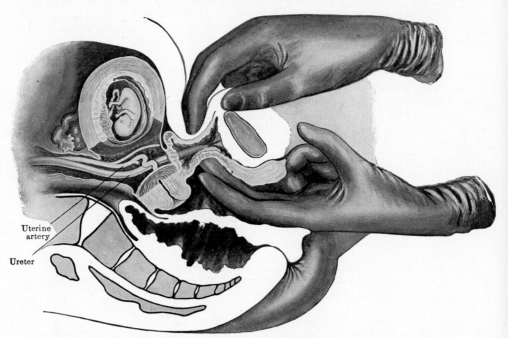

Uterine
artery

Ureter

FIG. 436.—PALPATING LEFT URETER.

Diet may have very little meat and no spices. The knee-chest position, assumed thrice daily, for ten minutes each time, and the elevated Sims' posture (Fig. 557) while in bed, are strong adjuvants, often actually curative. To aid posture in relieving the stagnation of the urine a balloon pessary may be placed in the vagina to lift the uterus out of the pelvis, and warm vaginal douches may be given. Water is to be freely administered by mouth, per rectum, and hypodermically. Ureteral catheterization, washing out the pelvis of the kidney, with or without the instillation of antiseptics, has been so successful that it should be given a trial before radical measures are instituted. Israel, Rovsing, and others do not fully approve of ureteral catheterization, but Stoeckel says it should displace therapeutic abortion. The catheter may be allowed to remain several days. Vaccine therapy has failed. Now colon bacteriophage is being tried out (Cowie). All foci of infection should be eliminated if possible; vaginal douches of 0.5 per cent. lactic acid d. i. d. if there is any leukorrhea.

It is almost never necessary to incise the kidneys (pyonephrosis), and rarely needful to induce labor. When to empty the uterus is not easy to determine. One always tries to carry the pregnancy at least until viability of the child, but interference may be imperative (1) if the fever is high and long continued with repeated and severe chills; (2) if the septic or toxemic symptoms become threatening; (3) if both kidneys are involved, or if the patient has only one kidney; (4) if repeated emptyings of the kidney pelvis do not procure permanent relief; (5) if the vomiting becomes uncontrollable; (6) if jaundice appears; (7) if nephritis or a pyonephrosis begins; in general, before the inroads on the patient's health become serious. Recovery rapidly ensues when the uterus is emptied. In operating, the infected urine should not be allowed to soil the field. The danger is not great, since the patient has developed immune bodies, and one seldom needs to do cesarean section as recommended by Deaver. A stone in the ureteral opening may sometimes be seen and extracted cystoscopically, and such an examination should always precede any operative interference. Pus in and around the kidney is to be treated on surgical principles. (See Kretschmer and Heaney, Falls, Kolischer, Opitz, Cumston.)

Pyelitis in puerperæ requires the same treatment, remembering that it may simulate a puerperal process, may accompany it or even actually cause a pelvic infection. Pituitary extract, 5 units q. i. d., may empty the ureter—given |for several days. Be a little slow with the ureteral catheter, especially with very acute cases and the streptococcus. An abrasion of the ureter may set virulent bacteria free in the peri-ureteral tissues.

Bacteriuria.—In 1895 the author found a pure culture of Streptococcus pyogenes longus in the urine of an apparently healthy gravida of the ninth month. This woman had an operative delivery, and developed double phlegmasia alba dolens on the tenth day of the puerperium. Another patient suffering from sepsis in 1896 had enormous masses of a streptodiplococcus in the urine and in the lochia. Petruschki in 1898 first showed that living typhoid bacilli could be found in the urine months after convalescence. Weichselbaum (cited by Walthard) cultivated the streptococcus from the urine in a case of sepsis (Naujocks).

Dodds found bacteriuria in 11.4 per cent. of pregnant woman, 9.6 per cent. colon. Murray found the Bacterium coli in the urine in 44.5 per cent. of gynecologic cases before, and in 93 per cent. after operation. Weibel found the urine sterile in only 25 per cent. of cases, proving present streptococci, staphylococci, and colon bacilli. It would be interesting to discover what percentage of eclamptics and nephritics show bacteria in the urine. Without doubt the healthy kidney can and does excrete bacteria, and it is more than probable that it may suffer injury in its task. I have long believed that some of the albuminurias we meet in pregnant women are due to urinary infection, and this may explain the septic mortality of operations on such patients. Cloudiness of the urine is often due to bacteria, and it is the author's practice to give such cases hexamethylenamin or soda until the condition is bettered. It is not unlikely that many instances of puerperal infection will be traceable to infected urine. During obstetric operations one should not allow the urine to drip over the field, and if it does, the parts should be washed with antiseptic solutions.

Cystitis occurs as the result of retroflexio uteri gravidi, but it may appear alone, from the usual causes, aggravated by the vascularity of gestation. Mild cystitis of the trigonum is common and induces frequent urination. Diagnosis and treatment are on general principles.

Hemorrhage into the bladder from vesical varicosities, hematuria from other causes—e. g., tuberculous kidney, acute hemorrhagic nephritis, stone, pyelitis, kinking of ureter, ulcer, papilloma vesicæ, etc.—are observed rarely. The essential hematuria of pregnancy may be toxemic, with or without a nephrosis or a glomerulo-nephritis, and may respond to hypodermic injections of Ringer's solution, normal horse-serum, or that of a healthy gravida (Becker). It may recur. A careful cystoscopic examination, perhaps with ureteral catheterization, and a bacteriologic study of the urine, are all necessary to make a diagnosis.

Pregnancy and labor after nephrectomy are usually uneventful (Matthews, Theodor).

LITERATURE

Becker: Zentb. f. Gyn., March 12, 1921.—*Cova:* Zentb. für Gyn., February 5, 1927. This number has numerous abstracts on Pyelitis.—*Cowie and Hicks:* Jour. Lab. and Clin. Med., 1932, xvii, p. 681.—*Dodds, Gladys H.:* Jour. Obst. and Gyn., Brit. Empire, 1931, vol. 38, No. 4, p. 773.—*Ehrhardt:* Zentb. für Gynaek., February 7, 1931, p. 341.—*Falls:* (Lit.) Jour. Amer. Med. Assoc., November 10, 1923, p. 1590.—*Kretschmer:* (Lit.) Jour. Amer. Med. Assoc., November 10, 1923, p. 1585.—*Kretschmer and Heaney:* Jour. Amer. Med. Assoc., August 8, 1925, p. 406.—*Luchs:* Archiv für Gynaek., 1926, vol. 127. See also Lahs, Die Theorie der Geburt, Bonn, 1877, p. 5.—*Matthews:* Jour. Amer. Med. Assoc., 1921.—*Naujocks:* Münch. med. Woch., 1925, July 11th.— *Stander and Peckham:* Jour. Obst. and Gyn., October, 1931, p. 626.—*Stoeckel:* Lehrbuch der Geburtshilfe, 1930, p. 823. Same, re Ileus, Zentb. für Gynaek., June, 1929.—*Theodor:* Ztschr. f. urol. Chir., September 24, 1921, p. 188.—*Williams, J. T.:* Amer. Jour. Obst. and Gyn., December, 1925.— *Young, Sim and Crnw:* Jour. Obst. and Gyn., Brit. Empire, Summer, 1932, p. 459.

CHAPTER XL

DISEASES OF METABOLISM—DISEASES OF THE EYE, EAR, NOSE, AND THROAT

DISEASES OF METABOLISM

Diabetes.—Sugar in minute traces is found in the urine in about 45 per cent. of gravidæ, but it is almost always milk-sugar or lactose, and when proved such, requires no further attention. True glycosuria is very rare, unless the minute traces which are discoverable with fine reagents are considered, and when it is found, is always of serious moment. Alimentary glycosuria is more easily produced in pregnancy than in the normal state, a point which must be considered in evaluating the discovery of mellituria. The carbohydrate metabolism in pregnancy is in unstable equilibrium, and if the islands of Langerhans fail to make the proper adjustments "pancreas diabetes" results. Hyperfunction of the hypophysis, the thyroid *et al.*, may cause temporary glycosuria. Transient glycosuria, sometimes to the amount of 2 or even 3 per cent., may occur in the latter weeks of gestation (Blot, 1856), accompanied by mild symptoms of diabetes. Many hold these cases as of no real significance, since recovery takes place after delivery, but the author believes that they are really the first warnings of underlying disease, and that the after-history of the women will show the same. Habitual death of the child in pregnancy and after labor is sometimes found in such women, and in two of my cases a clear hereditary tendency was proved. Kidney diabetes occurs in pregnancy. Novak reports 5 cases. The health of the patient is not affected, the amount of sugar is uninfluenced by diet, and the sugar-content of the blood is not augmented. Acetonuria is absent. Sugar, therefore, may be found in the urine as the result of (1) true diabetes mellitus, which is rare; (2) lessened sugar tolerance of pregnancy; (3) hepatic inefficiency; (4) permeability of the kidney; (5) disturbance of the endocrine system; (6) hyperfunction of the breasts (lactosuria).

Effects of Diabetes on Pregnancy.—Lecorchè found only 7 pregnancies in 114 cases of diabetes but now, with insulin, sterility is not so common, and the same may be said of amenorrhea, premature menopause, abortion, and premature labor. The mortality of the children at term is but slightly higher than normal, but after delivery quite a number die, from hypoglycemia, hydrocephalus, infection. The fetus may be born with diabetes and hypertrophied islands of Langerhans. Sugar is sometimes found in the liquor amnii, which if infected during labor (Bacterium coli) may decompose with gas formation, physometra. Polyhydramnion is frequent, but it sometimes responds to diet and insulin. Edema of the fetus, rarely, and overgrowth have been noted. Labor in diabetics is not very different from the normal unless complicated by the large edematous fetus or polyhydramnion. Hemorrhage is not a prominent symptom, nor does the puerperium show anything unusual. Sepsis is not more frequent. Lactation is not especially altered.

Effects of the Pregnancy on the Diabetes.—Without doubt pregnancy has a bad effect on the course of the disease. It may develop a latent diabetes, there being cases where severe symptoms appeared only during successive pregnancies, and others where the disease grew progressively worse each time. Since the carbohydrate control of the liver and pancreas is at fault in diabetes, and the liver is overburdened during gestation, functional overstrain is easily explained. Unless treatment is instituted the sugar in the urine increases, the malnutrition becomes marked, and the nervous system, which, as usual in pregnancy, suffers first from bad influences, begins to show signs of intoxication and acidosis appears. Coma occurs in 30 per cent. of the cases not properly treated and is almost always fatal. It may be brought on by a very slight shock in pregnancy, but more often during and just after labor. It seems that patients improve in the last trimester, perhaps, as Carlson, v. Noorden and Holzbach believe—due to the vicarious action of the fetal pancreas, and this improvement continues several months after delivery.

Diagnosis consists in determining whether the case is one of true diabetes, lactosuria, renal or alimentary glycosuria, or transient glycosuria (always to be viewed with suspicion). A true diabetes will be diagnosed when the classic symptoms are present—grape-sugar in the urine, polyuria, thirst, hyperglycemia, and malnutrition, and especially if the urine shows large amounts of sugar, acetone, diacetic, and beta-oxybutyric acids. Alimentary glycosuria will show normal blood-sugar.

Prognosis.—True diabetes if complete has a very bad prognosis, Offergeld finding over 50 per cent. mortality, of which 30 per cent. died in coma, the others of tuberculosis or coma, within two and one-half years. Such a gloomy picture may not be painted for women treated according to modern methods. In these pregnancy and labor can usually be brought up to the normal standard, and, unless the diabetes is complete, one may even permit a repetition of the pregnancy. Hansen found a mortality of 17 per cent. for the mothers and 43 per cent. for the babies, but Peckham had only 1 death in 17 cases—and this patient had neglected herself. Only 2 babies were lost. Toxemia and nephritis are serious complications.

Treatment.—Owing to the introduction of insulin, and to advances in our knowledge of dietetics, the treatment of diabetes complicating pregnancy has undergone a complete revolution. Whereas formerly we performed abortion in the early months, and induced labor after viability of the fetus, we now can almost always reduce the hyperglycemia, and combat the tendency to coma by the measures above mentioned.

It is my invariable practice to obtain the advice of an internist in the conduct of pregnancy and labor complicated by diabetes, or, indeed, simple glycosuria. Obstetric treatment is instituted when the disease proves rebellious to the medical.

A young diabetic may have a baby if she is willing to coöperate with her physician. A multipara may also be allowed to go through if she responds to treatment. Emaciated patients are bad risks and hyperemesis, late toxemias, uncontrollable hyperglycemia, marked ketosis, death of the fetus in utero, usually force the hand.

What we wish of the internist is to get the patient in the best possible condition for delivery, or if insulin and diet fail, for emptying the uterus. The points to be agreed upon are: (1) Delivery from above or below; (2) sterilization; (3) anesthetic. A long labor produces hypoglycemia; hemorrhage, vomiting, starvation, infection, anesthesia produce ketosis; for these reasons a case presenting such possibilities had best be treated by laparotrachelotomy under local anesthesia. Since diabetics should not have more than 2 children the greater certainty of obtaining a live child and the opportunity for sterilization would strengthen the argument. On the contrary a multipara with an easy labor in prospect, enjoying a good sugar balance, would be delivered from below. In either case the mind should be strongly fortified as well as the body since, in diabetes, psychic is as important as physic shock. Morphin is to be liberally used in both normal and operative delivery and to complement local anesthesia. Of general anesthetics ethylene is first choice, ether second. Ergot and pituitary may be given in small doses. Nursing might be allowed in mild cases under careful supervision. (Duncan, Schade, Joslin, Lambiè, Strouse, Peckham, Lit.)

Obesity.—Fat women are often amenorrheic and sterile. Amenorrheic and sterile women are often fat. Probably the causes of the two conditions are similar, being perhaps due to anomalies of the ductless glands. Pregnancy usually causes deposition of fat about the middle of the body, and many women put on fat during and after the puerperium. A combination of obesity with infantile pelvis is not rare. Obesity, when extreme, may cause abortion, and in some instances puny children have been noted. Edema of the feet and abdomen is often noted. Dyspnea is frequently a troublesome symptom, and in labor the heart must be considered like that of myocarditis. Rupture of the uterus is favored by fatty infiltration of the muscle-fibers. Postpartum hemorrhage is a little more frequent, and manual removal of the placenta oftener necessary, because the thick belly wall prevents a good Credé grasp for the expression. In only one case has the author noticed that the fat of the pelvis obstructed the delivery, and this was at the outlet. Perineal tears are more common, and, owing to the presence of eczema intertrigo and the locking in of the lochia, the union of the wound is not so successful. Operative procedures are very laborious, and obesity complicated with a very large fetus is a

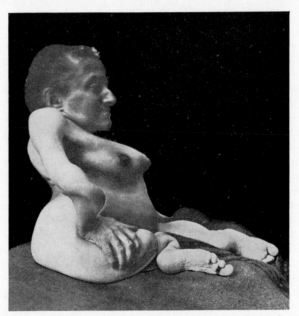

FIG. 437.—WILLARD'S CASE OF OSTEOMALACIA. PORRO CESAREAN AT FIVE MONTHS.

formidable affair. In general, it is best not to prescribe active antifat treatment during pregnancy, but where the obesity, or the condition underlying it, is the cause of frequent abortion or sterility, one should seek to establish normal conditions.

Osteomalacia, malacosteon, mollities ossium, or softening of the bones, is a disease which is very rare in this country, being found principally in Italy, the Rhine Valley, certain places along the Danube River, and in China, though no country is entirely exempt. In America but few bad cases are reported, mostly importations—Hirst, 3; Williams, 3; and the author had 1 case, an Italian woman who brought her illness from Naples. In pathology the disease consists of an osteomyelitis and osteitis progressing from the marrow along the Haversian canals outward, even to the periosteum. An absorption of the lime-salts of the bone takes place, and later the spaces are filled with an osteoid substance growing in from the marrow. As a result the bones become very much lighter in weight, softer, and sometimes so flexible that a pelvis so affected has been called a "rubber pelvis." The calcium and phosphates absorbed from the bones are excreted, probably through the urine and feces. The bones themselves are very vascular, reddish yellow or brown, and in advanced cases the periosteum remains as a sac filled with marrow and fat. If a cure results, bone salts are again deposited in the osteoid substance, and the skeleton grows very heavy, but the deformities remain. The pelvis, the vertebræ, the ribs, and lastly the long bones are affected in order.

Osteomalacia is a disease of adults, but a case occurring in a girl of eleven is on record. A similar disease occurs in men and in the lower animals. It bears some resemblance to rachitis.

Multiparæ are much oftener affected than primiparæ, and frequent child-bearing seems to be an active factor. It occurs most often in women of the lower classes of poor nutrition and unhygienic mode of life and was more frequent in Europe during the War. The actual cause of the disease is unknown. Fehling holds that the abnormal metabolism of the bones is due to dysfunction of the ovaries and the almost uniform success of castration as a cure gives a strong basis for the theory. Von Velitz found hyaline degeneration of the vessels of the ovaries, but this is not pathognomonic. Since we know more about the internal secretions of the ductless glands, and since the thyroid, hypophysis, and parathyroids have been proved to have something to do with the nutrition and growth of the bones, it seems more probable that the cause of osteomalacia may be found in some disturbance of the endocrine system. Maxwell and Miles, from a large experience in China, find that osteomalacia is due to calcium deficiency, and advise calcium and cod-liver oil in large doses with overfeeding and sunshine.

Symptoms usually first appear during pregnancy—pain in the back and legs, tenderness of the bones, muscular weakness, difficulty in locomotion, a waddling, twisting gait, intention tremor, contracture of the adductors of the thighs and of the levator ani, and, since the weight of the trunk bears heavily on the pelvis, the sacrum and innominates are distorted, the inlet narrowed, and the stature of the woman shortened. Encroachment of the bones on the thoracic cavity causes dyspnea and cyanosis. Softening and separation of the joints, especially the pelvic, have been frequently noted. After delivery, which may be spontaneous, recovery takes place, but since these women are remarkably fertile, usually a new pregnancy soon begins, and with the recurrence of worse symptoms. Finally the stature is 1 to 1½ feet shortened, the pelvis becomes impassable to the child, locomotion is impossible, and the gravida becomes bedridden. (For details of the effect of the deformed pelvis on labor see Chapter LIV, Contracted Pelvis.) Rarely spontaneous cure occurs. Fractures of the bones are common (Fig. 437).

Many women—fully one-fourth, in my experience—complain of symptoms during the latter half of pregnancy which resemble very closely those of mild degrees of osteomalacia—pain in the back and over the pelvic joints, also, but rarely, in the sternum, and the shoulder-girdle and difficulty and pain in locomotion. The softening and loosening of the pelvic articulations give the gait a waddling character, and on vaginal examination we find the pelvic bones, but especially the joints, excessively tender. It is possible, too, that the osteophytes of Rokitansky have some bearing on these two conditions.

Treatment.—Phosphorus, lime, cod-liver oil, vitamin D, and abundant nourishment are always to be administered, and if the disease is rapidly progressing, the ovaries may be removed. Bossi recommended the administration of epinephrin to limit of tolerance, and claims excellent results. Recently pituitrin has been also given (Neu). If the patient is pregnant, unless the symptoms are very urgent, wait until term and do Porro cesarean, removing the ovaries. In my case a cure was effected by simple castration at cesarean section. Great difficulty was experienced in stopping the hemorrhage at the operation, an occurrence which von Velitz also met, and which required amputation of the uterus in 2 cases. For the pseudo-osteomalacic symptoms lime and phosphates are administered (Schnell, Dieckmann).

DISEASES OF THE EYE, EAR, NOSE, AND THROAT

The Eye.—Even the ancients knew that sepsis and severe hemorrhages in the puerperium could produce blindness and strabismus, and a connection seemed to be established between the genitals and the eyes for many affections of the latter, but even yet the exact mode of interaction is obscure. Many theories were invoked, as reflex action from the genitalia, retention of poisons which should be eliminated in the menstrual blood (Charrin and Rochè), which is a disinterment of the "purification" theory of menstruation; hysteria and neuroses, demineralization of the blood, toxemia, abnormal or insufficient internal secretion of certain organs, especially the ovaries. Probably several of these hypotheses may explain the numerous ocular manifestations which seem to bear relation to gestation.

During pregnancy excessive pigmentation of the eyelids is sometimes noted in neurotic women. Tanner speaks of a chromidrosis. Ulcer of the cornea, choroiditis, and glaucoma may begin or be aggravated, and a few pregnant women complain of scotomata and dyschromatopsia. This may be due to an optic neuritis, which occurs also in the puerperium, may be associated with, and probably is similar to, the polyneuritis of pregnancy. Since atrophy of the optic nerve may result, the pregnancy should be interrupted. Weakness of accommodation and muscular asthenopia are not very rare, and may require temporary treatment. Hemeralopia has sometimes been found to precede the amaurosis of toxemia. Retinal hemorrhage and abruptio retinæ are serious complications, usually requiring interference. Teillas observed four gravidæ recover completely from retinal hemorrhages. Hypophyseal tumors may cause blindness (Winter).

Preëclamptic toxemia and renal disease sometimes produce an acute amaurosis, already referred to, which usually is transitory, disappearing more or less completely when the uterus is emptied. It may occur with postpartum eclampsia also or independently. The blindness often precedes the convulsions or coma for several days, and is of great prognostic importance. Ophthalmoscopically, nothing is to be seen on the retina. It lasts two to six days after consciousness returns, but may leave impaired vision. It is due, according to Berger and Loewy, to a poisoning of the ganglia and optic nerves, the toxins having a special selective action for them. Such selective action of poisons is well known—for example, tetanus, strychnin. This theory appeals strongly to the author. Pregnancy seems to dispose to the occurrence of neuroretinitis, with a tendency to hemorrhage and exudates. Posey and Hirst believe that the optic neuritis and retinitis, due to the toxemia of pregnancy, may indicate the basal trouble before changes show in the urine. Acute amblyopia or amaurosis occurring in the course of pregnancy demands immediate urinalysis, and if albumin or other signs of renal or hepatic insufficiency are present, the induction of labor. Another form of amblyopia and amaurosis may develop in the course of renal or hepatic disease during gestation—retinitis albuminurica. This is easily diagnosed with the ophthalmoscope by the hemorrhages and the white spots and lines which show the degeneration of the retinal vessels. These changes may long precede the complaint of loss of vision. Exophthalmos is sometimes associated (Barker). First the women complain of specks before the eyes, dimness of vision, sometimes hemeralopia, colored lights, amblyopia, and finally of complete blindness. Retinitis albuminurica may occur in all forms of kidney disease during pregnancy, but the prognosis is somewhat better than those cases which occur outside of gestation. It is more frequent in the chronic forms of disease, and it always indicates the immediate emptying of the uterus. This is to save the sight and to prevent eclampsia and uremia. Abruptio retinæ may complicate the retinitis. After delivery the sight returns, but usually incompletely, though a few cases of cure are on record. In a subsequent pregnancy the condition usually recurs, but even though it may not, one should always counsel the discontinuance of child-bearing. Edema of the lids, of the bulbar conjunctivæ, and even of the retina are found in nephritis.

During labor hemorrhages in the conjunctivæ and behind the bulb have been noted, also hysteric amaurosis and xanthopsia.

During the puerperium all the conditions mentioned may occur or be carried over from pregnancy. I have seen one case of hysteric amaurosis and several of blepharitis marginalis, of hordeolum, and one of phlyctenular conjunctivitis, which three are generally ascribed to the influence of lactation. Treatment consists of the administration of lime, phosphates, and general roborants. Muscular asthenopia has been noted, and I have seen numerous cases of headache in the puerperium from eye-strain. The women look down at the baby while it is nursing, and the eyes are unaccustomed to such prolonged action. Reading in bed and with poor light may also be causative. A true weakness of accommodation occurs also. The relation of the nasal sinuses to the eye should be remembered.

Optic neuritis may be associated with ulnar or polyneuritis, with the same etiology. In septic cases blindness may result from double retinitis septica, from panophthalmitis, or from embolism of the central artery of the retina.

Severe hemorrhage, especially if associated with other diseases which weaken the optic nerve, may cause temporary or permanent blindness. It may aggravate a myopia and favors optic atrophy. This effect may come on at once, or it may appear after several weeks. It is due to anemia of the retina and nerve or to degenerative changes in them, and lasts a few hours in the first instance, and may be more or less permanent in the latter. Choked disc with blindness has been observed after severe bleedings. It is easily seen how important is the quick restitution of the blood to a normal state, and Berger and Loewy even recommend transfusion with defibrinated blood, in addition to the other usual remedies (Runge, Silex, Shute).

The Ear.—Aurists find that pregnancy sometimes unfavorably affects diseases of the ear, especially otosclerosis (Brickner, Milligan). Middle-ear infections grow worse, chronic thickenings increase, and deafness becomes more marked, all of which is especially noticeable in repeated gestations. Ringing in the ears may be a symptom of toxemia, and even deafness may be caused by an auditory neuritis analogous to the same disease of the optic nerve. In cases of rapidly increasing deafness due to pregnancy, the induction of premature labor is to be debated with the family and attending aurist. It is possible that some of the "fainting spells" to which pregnant women are liable may be due to circulatory disturbances in the labyrinths.

The Nose.—A general hyperemia of the nose and throat has been noted by rhinologists, some even claiming that a diagnosis of pregnancy may be made from the nasal findings. Hofbauer proved clinically and microscopically that decided changes exist. The intumescent conditions of the turbinates are subject to aggravation by pregnancy. Sinus disease is not more common. Its treatment is the same as in the non-pregnant condition—indeed, all suppurations of the nose and throat must be cured before labor, because the focus of suppuration may lead to infection of the genitalia or the breasts.

Fliess claims that the anterior ends of the lower and middle turbinates, if diseased, may cause dysmenorrhea, and if cocainized during the attack, the pain ceases, and that cauterization of these areas will cure. My experience with this remedy is small but entirely negative, there having been not even an improvement which might have been ascribed to suggestive action. He also claims that the pains of labor and hyperemesis gravidarum may be favorably influenced in the same way. Epistaxis has been noted with some frequency in pregnancy. Usually an ulcerated spot is not found, the blood coming from rupture of one of the congested capillaries. An ulcer may be cauterized, even though Fliess says that abortion sometimes results from such action. Vicarious menstruation through the nose has been referred to.

Lingual varicosities are sometimes aggravated by pregnancy, and the hyperemia may lead to some hoarseness, but in general the effects of gestation are not prominent. Tuberculosis of the larynx is most unfavorably influenced, the ulcerations becoming deeper and spreading rapidly, and frequently causing edema of the glottis. Pregnancy seems even to predispose to laryngeal tuberculosis. Some singers claim that it injures the voice to sing during pregnancy, and there seems to be a scientific reason for it. It is denied by others.

As the result of violent labor efforts hemorrhages may take place in the mucous membrane of the nose and throat, as well as the ocular conjunctivæ, while after severe blood loss the parts are very anemic. Women who shriek continually during prolonged labor may show on examination redness, edema, and minute blood extravasations in the mucous membrane of the false and true vocal cords and the posterior wall of the larynx. After delivery these changes rapidly clear up.

TRAUMATISM

Pregnant women bear the effects of violence with varying resistance. Wounds heal with their usual promptness, and the old notion that bones unite poorly is incorrect. Suggillations are perhaps a little more extensive. Violence to any part of the body, but particularly to the genitals, may bring on abortion, but sometimes terrible shock may be without effect on the pregnancy, as in Waldeyer's case of fracture of the sacrum, and one of mine, where I delivered at term a woman on whom an inexperienced surgeon had performed curetage at three months. Bröse reports a case where, after laminaria dilatation of the cervix, through a uterine perforation 2 feet of intestine were pulled out. Laparotomy, resection of the gut, undisturbed pregnancy. Opposed to this may be placed the well-authenticated cases of a slight jar, as from misstep, causing abortion. Operations are to be performed on any part of the body if the indication is real and urgent, but operations of convenience, for example, simple hernia, hemorrhoids, etc., are better postponed. Ovariotomy has often been done successfully in pregnancy, also the removal of fibroids from the uterus itself. The necessity for the ovaries seems greatest in the early months, because if then removed abortion often occurs, while in the later ones both gestation and labor may be natural. Shock and sepsis are the usual causes of the abortion when such occurs, though the withdrawal of the corpus luteum hormone has been assigned. Operations on the labia and cervix have been done without disturbing the pregnancy, and even extirpation of the breast. Then, again, a slight operation on some distant organ or extremity will bring on an abortion. It is, therefore, impossible to foretell what effect a given interference will produce. It seems that operations undertaken at the time the woman would ordinarily have menstruated are more likely to bring on pains. Vesicovaginal and rectovaginal fistulas have been cured in graviditate and the local changes in the tissues seem to have improved, rather than impaired, the process of wound healing. Anesthetics may be given during gestation, but there is danger of asphyxiating the infant. Probably death of the child causes some of the premature labors recorded after operations. Ether is the safest, and the administration should be as short and as light as possible. A dentist informed me that he had given gas to pregnant women hundreds of times without injury, but in one of my cases of cesarean section, where gas-ether narcosis was used, the child was mortally asphyxiated. Previously it was in prime condition, and the actual delivery consumed less than three minutes. Operations in the presence of pus, especially if the focus of infection is near the uterus, are more than likely to be followed by sepsis.

Pregnant and puerperal women should be spared mental shocks, if at all possible. Premature labor may result, even fetal death. During labor a shock may suspend uterine action, and cases are recorded where collapse and death resulted. A shock in the puerperium has been ascribed as the cause of diabetes, acute febrile reaction, dementia, convulsions, hemorrhage, and death. (See "Sudden Death.") A shock, too, will sometimes alter the milk— either dry it up or make it unfit, even poisonous, to the child. How these changes are brought about is still a subject of conjecture.

LITERATURE

Barker and Hanes: Amer. Jour. Med. Sci., October, 1909.—*Berger and Loewy:* Augenkrankheiten sexuellen Ursprunges bei Frauen, 1906. Translated by Beatrice Rossbach.—*Bossi:* Société d'Obstetrique de Paris, June 16, 1904.—*Brickner:* Amer. Jour. Obstet., June, 1911. Literature.—*Broese:* Jahreskurse f. Aertzl. Fortbildung, July, 1916, p. 16.—*Charrin and Rochè:* Compt. Rend. des Sci., Paris, May 25, 1903.—*Cron:* Amer. Jour. Obst. and Gyn., December, 1920.—*Cumston:* Amer. Jour. Med. Sci., July, 1908.—*Dieckmann, W. J.:* Amer. Jour. Obst. and Gyn., April, 1932, p. 478, Lit.—*Duncan:* London Obstetric Trans., 1882, vol. xxiii, p. 256.—*Fehling:* Arch. f. Gyn., vol. xxxix, p. 180.—*Fränkl-Hochwart u. C. von Noorden:* Erkrank. der weibl. Gen. in Bez. zur inn. Med., 1912, 2 vols.—*Hansen, O. S.:* Minnesota Medicine, December, 1928.—*Holzbach:* Zentb. für Gyn., October 9, 1926, p. 2610.—*Joslin:* Boston, 1917.—*Kolischer:* Die Erkrankungen der weibl. Harnröhre, etc., Vienna, 1898.—*Kraul;* Zentb. für Gyn., 190, 1927, No. 12, p. 713.—*Lambie:* Jour. Obst. and Gyn., Brit. Empire, 1926, vol. 33, No. 4, p. 563. Has 256 References.—*Maxwell and Miles:* Jour. Obst. and Gyn., Brit. Empire, Autumn, 1925, p. 433.—*Milligan:* Jour. Laryngol., June, 1909.—*Mirabeau:* "Ureteritis," Arch. f. Gyn., 1908, vol. lxxxii, Band ii.—*Murray:* Jour. Obst. and Gyn., British Empire, December, 1910, p. 405.—*Neu:* Biol. u. Path. des Weibes. Halban u. Seitz, 1923, Band ii, p. 199.—*Novak:* Deutsche med. Woch., 1912, No. 40.—*Offergeld:* Arch. f. Gyn., September, 1908, vol. lxxxvi, H. 1, p. 160. Literature.—*Opitz:* Zeitschr. f. Geb. u. Gyn., 1905, vol. lv, p. 290, 1122 References.—*Peckham, C. H.:* Johns Hopkins Hospital Bulletin, September, 1931.—*Posey and Hirst:* Jour. Amer. Med. Assoc., March 14, 1908, p. 865.—*Runge:* Geburtsh. u. Gyn. u. Auge, Leipzig, Barth, 1908.—*Sant-Agnese:* Ginecologia, 1908, Fasc. 17.—*Schade:* Inaug. Diss., Marburg, 1906. Literature.—*Schnell:* Zeitschr. f. Geb. u. Gyn., 1898, vol. xxxix, p. 412.—*Shute:* Jour. Amer. Med. Assoc., June 24, 1911.—*Silex:* Monatsschr. f. Geb., 1897, vol. v, p. 373.—*Strouse:* Medical Clinics of No. America, May, 1926, p. 1491.—*Sweet and Stewart:* Surg., Gyn., and Obstet., 1914, p. 468. Analysis of 224 articles.—*Vinay, Fellner, P. Müller:* Loc. cit., p. 538.—*Vineberg:* Amer. Jour. Obstet., June, 1908.—*Walthard:* Handbuch der Geb., vol. iii, No. 2, p. 487. Bacteriology.—*Weibel:* Zentralbl. f. Gyn., 1914, 414.—*Werner:* Diabetes and Pregnancy. Full Literature. Arch. f. Gyn., 1915, Band 104, Heft 3, p. 505.—*Williamson and Barris:* Jour. Obst. and Gyn., British Empire, December, 1911.—*Wildbolz:* Zentralbl. f. Gyn., 1912, No. 1, p. 64.—*Winter, E. W.:* Hypophysen Tumor, etc., Arch. für Gyn., 1931, B'd 147, H. 1, p. 95, Lit.—*Zangemeister:* Arch. f. Gyn., 1902, vol. lxvi, No. 2, p. 413.

CHAPTER XLI

LOCAL DISEASES ACCIDENTAL TO PREGNANCY

DEFORMITIES OF THE PARTURIENT CANAL

EMBRYOLOGICALLY, the uterus and vagina are formed by the fusion of the two Müllerian ducts, the union taking place from below upward. Lack of fusion at any point or throughout the length of the two canals explains almost all of the anomalies that are observed, and rudimentary development of one duct will account for the balance. All degrees of lack of fusion are to be noted, there being one case on record where two complete, but single and distinct, parturient canals with two vulvæ were found,—*uterus didelphys*,—and it is not rare to find the fundus uteri indented in the middle,—the "uterus arcuatus,"—which is just the indication of the upper end of the line of fusion of the two ducts. In some animals the two ducts do not fuse, but two tubular uteri exist.

Not always are the two sides of the uterus and vagina equally developed, and we observe gradations from completeness of the two halves to almost entire absence of one Müllerian duct. The rudimentary side lies as an appendage to the well-developed uterus, but since its canal, four times out of five, does not communicate with the vagina, trouble infrequently ensues, such as hematosalpinx, hematometra, pregnancy in the closed horn, etc. (Ahlfeld, Munde, Santos).

General Considerations.—In all these deformities the two halves are usually not symmetric: one or the other horn is larger, or the vaginas are unequal—sometimes one of them ends blind at its lower end. Coitus is rarely interfered with, the larger vagina being used. Menstruation comes from both uteri simultaneously, but sometimes only from one at a time. Pregnancy may occur in one or both horns, twins having been found in one horn. If each horn contains an ovum, the two children may have been conceived at different impregnations and be delivered at intervals, thus raising the suspicion of superfetation. Pregnancy is ordinarily undisturbed, the side not involved growing and forming a decidua similarly to ectopic gestation. The decidua of the empty side may be cast out, while the pregnancy continues on the other side. The course of the case resembles an abortion, and unless the duplicity of the uterus is known, the accoucheur may attempt to curet, thus unwittingly destroying a living ovum. Usually the decidua comes away in the puerperium with the lochia. Müller records cases of menstruation from the empty horn during pregnancy. Abortion may occur, and it may be difficult to clean out the uterus, especially if there is only one cervix. It is doubly important to insert the finger for the curetage. In septic abortions it is necessary to empty both sides. Labor is often normal, but these complications have been observed—weak pains and atony in the third stage, with postpartum hemorrhage; the non-pregnant portion of the uterus may prolapse under the other, and act like a tumor incarcerated in the pelvis; the non-pregnant cervix may be forced down to the vulva with the head; the uterus may rupture, because of poor musculature; the septum in the vagina may be an obstruction. Septate uteri may have these complications: breech and transverse presentations; weak pains; atony postpartum; rigidity of the cervix; placenta on the septum and adherent; and, if the septum is in the cervix, obstruction to delivery. In one of my cases the child straddled the septum. (See van de Velde and Ubbens, Findley.)

Pregnancy in a rudimentary horn resembles ectopic gestation very closely.

Mauriceau and Vassal, in 1669, put the first case on record, and now over 100 have been described.   If the accessory horn is very rudimentary, it may be closed at

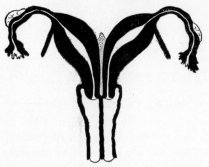

FIG. 438.—Uterus Duplex, Bicornis, cum Vagina Septa.

Uterus Duplex, Bicornis, cum Vagina Septa. —One finds two openings into two separate vaginal canals, a cervix pointing into each, and, if the os of each of the two separate uterine cavities is open, a finger passed into them will feel a septum separating the two ova. In my case, from which the diagram is drawn, the woman was eight months pregnant, with a child in each horn, O.L.P. and O.D.T., and a deep furrow could be felt between the two sides of the uterus. One horn could be rotated almost completely around the other. Fig. 439 shows the appearance of the vulva. Another practitioner conducted the labor.

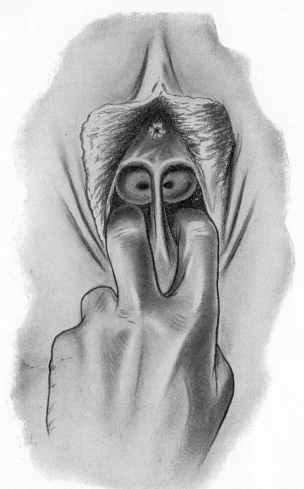

FIG. 439.—VULVA OF UTERUS AND VAGINA DUPLEX. PREGNANT IN BOTH UTERI (author's case).

both ends, making pregnancy impossible, but an accumulation of menses probable. Should the fertilized ovum be inserted in the small horn, there is no hope of its finding a way into the uterine cavity of the other, because the connecting bridge of tissue is usually imperforate, or even if the two halves are broadly apposed, the two cavities usually do not communicate, or the opening is too small. Hypertrophy of the muscle-wall of the horn may occur and permit the ovum to grow to

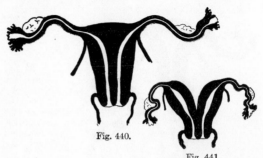

Uterus Septus Duplex, or Uterus Bilocularis.—One vagina exists, and it is capacious, with marked anterior and posterior columnæ and two cervices, with a falciform ridge between them. In the author's case the woman was pregnant in the left uterine cavity and aborted at the third month. If the fundus also shows signs of splitting, it is called uterus duplex bicornis (Figs. 440 and 441).

Fig. 440.

Fig. 441.

FIGS. 440 AND 441.—UTERUS SEPTUS DUPLEX, OR UTERUS BILOCULARIS.

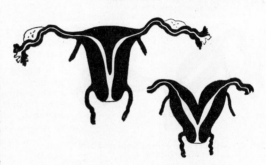

Uterus Subseptus Unicollis.—This is a simple septum in an otherwise single uterus. In one of my cases the septum came down (at term) within an inch of the internal os, which was single. The woman had had five still-births, breech deliveries, all difficult because of a flat pelvis. In the sixth, conducted by the author, the child suffered a depressed fracture of the skull, but survived. In another case the breech presented in each of two labors, and the placenta both times was adherent to the septum. This form of uterus occurs in dogs, camels, sheep, etc. If there are indications that the fundus also is split, it is called uterus subseptus uniforis, or uterus bicornis unicollis (Fig. 443).

FIG. 442.—UTERUS SUB-SEPTUS UNICOLLIS.

FIG. 443.—UTERUS BICOR-NIS UNICOLLIS.

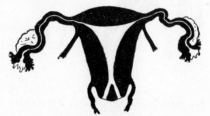

Uterus Subseptus Unicorporeus.—Consists simply of a septate cervix, the rest of the uterus being normal or presenting only an indication of double formation. In the author's case the child, presenting by the breech, straddled the septum, which had to be cut to allow delivery. Both recovered. This condition may be imitated by a cervicovaginal fistula or partial rupture of the cervix in a spontaneous abortion.

FIG. 444.—UTERUS SUBSEPTUS UNICORPOREUS. SEPTATE CERVIX.

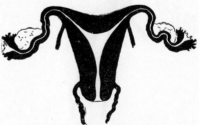

Uterus Arcuatus.—This has already been spoken of; it is the simplest and most common anomaly, often causing difficulty in differential diagnosis from ectopic gestation, pregnancy in the tubal corner, etc. It often causes transverse and breech presentations.

FIG. 445.—UTERUS ARCUATUS.

term, but more commonly rupture of the gestation-sac occurs during the middle of pregnancy, and furious internal hemorrhage ensues. Practically, what was said about ectopic gestation applies to this subject. Since there is no communication with the vagina, the spermatozoids must cross over from the open tube to the closed

36

side, to fertilize the ovum from the ovary on the side of the pregnancy, or the ovum from the open side wanders over to the closed horn before or after fertilization.

The diagnosis of pregnancy in a rudimentary horn is occasionally made, but usually the abdomen is opened for rupture of a supposed extra-uterine pregnancy.

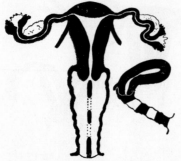

Septate Vagina.—Double hymen is frequently observed, but gives no trouble, either in diagnosis or treatment. A septum may exist at any point of the vagina, or even throughout its whole length. In these cases the lower end of the Müllerian canal failed to fuse, but the upper portions did, forming a perfect uterus. Occasionally there are two cervices. The septum is usually sagittal, but may be frontal in direction.

Fig. 446.—Septa in the Vagina, in Frontal and Sagittal Section.

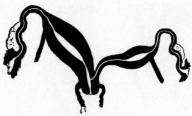

Uterus Bicornis Unolatere Rudimentarius.—Of great clinical importance, because pregnancy may occur in the rudimentary horn, and such an accident is worse than ectopic gestation, with which it is usually confounded.

Fig. 447.—Uterus Bicornis Unolatere Rudimentarius.

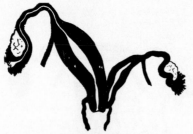

Shows the accessory horn closed at both ends, and one can see how menstrual blood will accumulate in it, causing hematometra, or, if the vagina is also partly formed, hemelytrometra.

Fig. 448.—Uterus with Closed Accessory Horn.

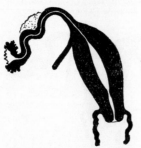

Uterus Unicornis.—Here the one Müllerian canal failed to develop. It is normal in birds. Such a uterus may bear children without trouble.

Fig. 449.—Uterus Unicornis.

On the specimen it is easy to find the connecting band between the rudimentary and the spindle-shaped larger horn, and to determine that the round ligament and the tube come off from the *outside of the gestation-sac.* The sac has much muscle at its base. Clinically, on bimanual examination the diagnosis of ectopic pregnancy is usually first made; then, when the form of the uterus (spindle shaped instead of pear-like) and the course of the round ligament—on the outside of the sac—evoke suspicion, one proceeds to palpate out the structures more minutely. Sep-

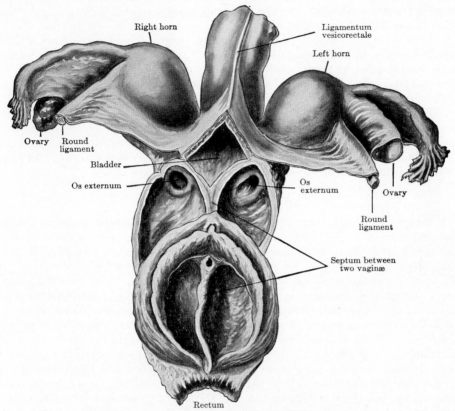

FIG. 450.—DOUBLE UTERUS AND VAGINA.
From the Lehrkanzel für path. Anat., Vienna, Handbuch der Geb., v. Winckel.

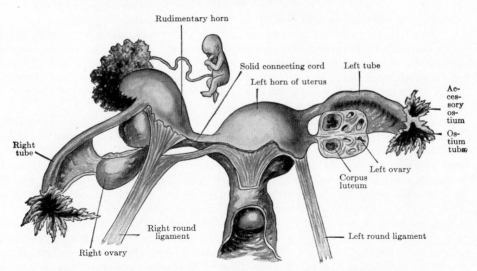

FIG. 451.—UTERUS UNICORNIS WITH RUPTURED RUDIMENTARY HORN.
The ovum wandered over from the left ovary. The horn ruptured in the tenth week. The ligaments have been dissected (Luschka, Monatsschr. f. Geb. u. Frauenk., vol. xxii, p. 32).

tate vagina or cervix may be indicative of the presence of some anomaly, and palpation of the pedicle (see Fig. 451) will clinch the diagnosis. If the fetus dies, identical changes in the ovum may follow, as in ectopic ova, and, later, owing to adhesions, shrinkage of the sac, etc., the preoperative diagnosis is usually of a fibroma or an ovarian cyst. Contractions occurring in the sac of the tumor may give the clue to a correct diagnosis.

Treatment is the same as for extra-uterine pregnancy, and even more actively interfering as soon as the diagnosis is made. Rupture of the sac is attended with more fatal results—in 82 per cent., according to Kehrer. At the laparotomy it is best to remove the whole sac, if possible; if not, or if it is septic, it is sewn into the abdominal wall and drained (Wells, Engstrom).

Diverticula of the uterus have been described, and in one case the placenta was developed in an accessory uterine cavity connected with the main portion by a passage. It is probable that these are cases of septate uterus with incomplete septum. Incarceration of the placenta in a horn of the uterus is not rare, and sometimes the placenta seems to occupy a compartment of its own.

THE LOCAL INFLAMMATIONS

Vulvitis.—Owing to the succulence and congestion of the parts and to the pronounced pelvic floor projection which exposes the organ more to injury, vulvitis is not rare in gestation. Lack of cleanliness, obesity, difficulty in keeping the parts clear of mucus and smegma, which accumulates, purulent discharges, together with the openness of the introitus, invite infection and eczema. Mycotic infection, resembling thrush of the mouth, which may cover the whole of the hyperemic and moist vulva, and pus infections, including the gonorrheal, occur. Vegetations may be seen on the labia minora or in the raphé, and they may occasionally attain enormous size. They are sometimes gonorrheal, but may as often be due to simple uncleanliness. If small, the usual treatment of vaginitis and vulvitis may be carried out. If large, they should be excised and the base touched with the thermocautery to stop hemorrhage. Even if the signs of inflammation fail, the pudendal region becomes the habitat of the Bacterium coli, the staphylococcus and the *streptococcus*, with hosts of others. For mycosis vulvæ, thrush, painting with 10 per cent. silver nitrate or tincture of iodin or 1 per cent. gentian-violet (Plass) and a dusting-powder of boric acid will be curative; the other infections are treated by antiseptic washes, after frequent ablution with tincture of green soap.

Bartholinitis is almost always due to the gonococcus, alone or in association with pus-germs. Because of the danger of puerperal infection, an abscess should be cured before labor, by exsection, if possible. Cysts of the labia, if not infected, are best left until after the puerperium is completed, because the operative hemorrhage from the dilated veins is troublesome. If they obstruct delivery, puncture and aspiration of the contents will remove the obstacle.

Vaginitis is not so common as vulvitis, but it is not rare to find a reddened, granular, thickened mucosa in the fornices—vaginitis granulosa. If great in extent and accompanied by profuse purulent discharge, gonorrhea is to be searched for. In rare cases gas (trimethylamin) accumulates in the little vesicles. Vaginitis, if marked, should be treated with antiseptic irrigations during pregnancy, but it usually disappears only after delivery. The author has had good results with douches of 0.5 per cent. lactic acid d. i. d. The reason that more women do not get puerperal infection from the septic vagina is probably because the local immunities are developed. Birth injuries, however, are poorly borne in these cases and often heal unsatisfactorily. The Trichomonas vaginalis sometimes causes a purulent vaginitis. It is easily discovered if the fresh discharge is examined in a hanging-drop under low power (Fig. 452). The vaginitis increases puerperal morbidity (see Bland *et al.*) and should be cured before labor. Gentle washing of the vagina with soap and water every fourth day, followed by painting with 1 per cent. chinasol or 1 per cent. picric acid solution. Stop two weeks before term.

Gonorrhea.—Venereal diseases are of great importance in obstetric practice. Acute gonorrhea is commoner in primiparæ, being conveyed at the time of impregnation. Unlike ordinary cases, where the inflammation is limited to or most marked in the urethra the vulvar glands and the cervix, in pregnancy, favored by the succulence of the tissues, the gonococcus attacks the vaginal and vulvar epithelium in addition to those mentioned. Profuse secretion of greenish-yellow pus results; the vulva is red, sometimes covered with grayish exudate, sometimes ulcerated, or covered with gonorrheal, pointed condylomata; the vagina is thick and granular, like a nutmeg-grater, and bleeds even on light touch; the cervix is swollen, vascular, eroded, easily vulnerable, and emits a foul mucopus in which the gonococci are most readily found. Chronic infection is the form usually met, and it has left the sur-

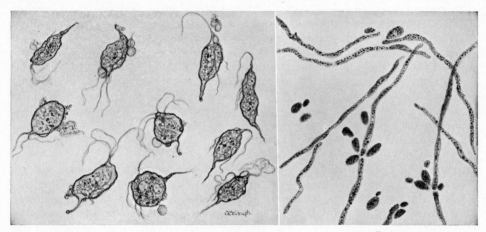

A   B

Fig. 452.—A, Trichomonas Vaginalis (from Fresh Specimen.) B, Yeast from Vaginal Cultures. Mycelia and Conidia.

faces, covered by squamous epithelium, to localize in the urethra, Skene's tubules, the crypts around the hymen, the Bartholinian ducts and glands, and the cervix, in which it is recognizable by the usual signs. Acute as well as chronic gonorrhea may affect the uterine decidua and produce abortion, but, as a rule, the gonorrheal endometritis remains latent until after delivery. Indeed, many women having a slight mucopurulent leukorrhea are delivered without the accoucheur being aware of the existence of an infection until the baby's eyes show gonorrheal ophthalmia. Through the traumatism of labor the gonococci are pressed out of the deep cervical glands, and by virtue of the open cervix and the puerperal processes, unlimited opportunities are afforded them for further virulent development. As a result, gonorrheal endometritis, salpingitis, ovaritis, and pelvic peritonitis are set up, reference to which will be made when treating of puerperal infection. Acute infections are likely to show the exacerbation in the first days of the puerperium, because of the associated streptococci and staphylococci, while chronic gonorrhea causes the "late fevers,"—on the tenth to the thirtieth day,—an ascending inflammation which results in pus-tubes or adhesive obliterating peritonitis, leaving permanent sterility and gynecologic invalidism. Acute gonorrhea in gestation can cause rheumatism, with disorganization of the joints, wrist, knee, hip, etc., or even endocarditis and general septicemia (*q. v.*).

Diagnosis.—In maternities, because of the danger of carrying infection from one patient to another, it is highly important to detect the first case of gonorrhea, but, unless it is in the florid stage, this is almost impossible. Repeated bacteriologic examination of the secretions is often required for the detection of the gonococcus—one negative result does not exclude it. The history is valuable. An obstinately inflamed single joint is strongly suggestive. Ophthalmia in the infant does not prove the existence of gonorrhea in the mother unless the gonococcus be found in the pus and other sources of infection of the child's eyes be eliminated.

Treatment must always be instituted during pregnancy, but, owing to the tendency to abortion, gentle means are adopted. Prolonged rest in bed, vaginal irrigation morning and evening with potassium permanganate, 1 : 3000; zinc permanganate, 1 : 4000; 1 per cent. ichthyol; painting the vagina with 5 per cent. silver nitrate; light packing with 20 per cent. argyrol gauze, removed after twenty-four hours—will usually quickly reduce the disease to its chronic state. Should abortion occur, curetage is not to be undertaken if it is at all avoidable.

During labor in cases of known gonorrhea we instil in the vagina, every four hours a mixture of acriflavin 1 per cent., iodin $\frac{1}{2}$ per cent., in glycerin. Vaginal explorations and operations are limited to an irreducible minimum, the bag of waters is saved, if possible, until the child's head is fully born, and every precaution is taken to prevent the entrance of vaginal mucus into the conjunctival sacs. During the puerperium no douches may be given, and the woman should be kept in bed fully eighteen days—Bumm says five to six weeks,—that is, until the involution of the uterus is complete,—this to prevent the ascension of the infection through the uterus to the tubes.

Erosions and hypertrophy of the cervix are not infrequent, and since the softened vascular structure bleeds readily, the flowing may give rise to the suspicion of abortion. The author has thrice seen a nodular hypertrophy of the cervix with ectropion and cystic degeneration of the glands, which to the touch resembled cancer, but which subsided almost entirely after delivery. Erosions during pregnancy are treated by irrigation with 1 : 3000 potassium permanganate and application of 10 per cent. silver nitrate to the patches thrice weekly. Rest in bed aids the treatment and prevents hemorrhage. Remember syphilis.

Endometritis Deciduæ.—*Acute endometritis* frequently accompanies the infectious diseases, scarlet fever, typhoid, cholera, etc. It may occur as the result of attempts at criminal or even therapeutic abortion. In one of my cases it was evidently due to external infection through a very patulous cervix, perhaps by coitus. Gonorrhea may cause it, there sometimes being tiny abscesses containing gonococci in the decidua. Abortion is probably often the result of gonorrhea, acute and chronic. Pus may accumulate in the decidua and be expelled during labor. In two of my cases a discharge of pus from the uterus followed the child, no complication resulting.

Chronic endometritis is not so common as was formerly thought. Hitschmann and Adler have conclusively shown that many of the cases of so-called glandular hypertrophic and hyperplastic endometritis are only the normal menstrual changes of the uterus. Interstitial endometritis may be accompanied by a hyperplasia of the glands, but unless the "exudate cells," especially the "plasma" cells, are found, one may not diagnose endometritis. Chronic endometritis is most often the result of gonorrhea, next of abortion, then of displacements and lacerations of the uterus.

The classifications of the various forms are not fully satisfactory, even to the gynecologists, and during pregnancy pathologic study of the uterine mucosa is doubly difficult. Most authors distinguish two main conditions—endometritis deciduæ interstitialis and glandularis. The inflammation is usually present before conception, but may arise during pregnancy, for example, from a syphilitic ovum or from gonorrhea. Figure 453 shows a piece of decidua vera expelled in an abortion at ten weeks. It is thickened, infiltrated with round-cells, degenerated in places, strewn with minute hemorrhages, and shows a lumpy, uneven, polypoid surface. Virchow first described it as endometritis deciduæ tuberosa or polyposa, or both. The glands may hypertrophy also, while sometimes atrophic areas are found. Syphilis may occasionally cause such changes.

If the glands are affected, either by hypertrophy or by inflammatory hyperemia, a profuse secretion results, which is yellowish, serous, slightly mucous or bloody. Schröder called this endometritis deciduæ catarrhalis, which may give the clinical course of hydrorrhea gravidarum. Endometritis deciduæ is of great clinical importance. It causes relative sterility, frequent abortion, and, since abortion often leaves endometritis, a vicious circle is established—abnormal insertion of the ovum (for example, placenta prævia), abnormal formation as to shape, size, and thickness of the placenta, infarcts, retarded development of the fetus, abruptio placentæ, and thickening and retention of the decidua. The earlier the disease manifests itself and the greater its extent, the more the likelihood of abortion. The ovum may be transformed into a bloody or fleshy mole.

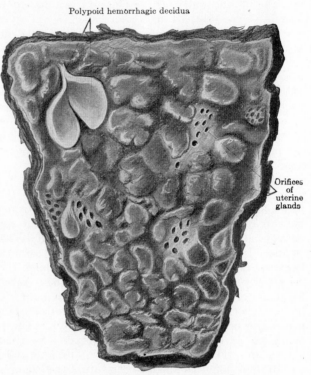

Polypoid hemorrhagic decidua

Orifices of uterine glands

FIG. 453.—ENDOMETRITIS DECIDUA TUBEROSA POLYPOSA.

Chronic endometritis affects the course of labor. Since usually the muscle of the uterus is involved, weak or painful pains are noted. Premature rupture of the membranes, hemorrhages into the decidua, sometimes at the placental site, with abruptio placentæ, abnormalities in the mechanism of the third stage, atonia uteri, from myometritis, retention of bits of placenta or membrane—all these may require obstetric interference. Pieces of thick, hard, cheesy decidua may remain in the uterus after the placental delivery and keep up a prolonged, even dangerous, oozing, requiring manual removal, the same being true of the firm blood-clots which usually surround them. If these foreign matters are allowed to come away in the puerperium they cause profuse, prolonged, bloody, sometimes fetid lochia, occasionally slight fever, and always delayed involution. (Riotte.)

Evidences of endometritis on the placenta are: Thickened serotina, which may be quite opaque and ragged in places; vascularization of the margin of the closing plate of Winkler, which may extend some distance under the membranes. One may see arteries and veins running in the thick decidua vera for 2 to 4 inches. Signs of inflammation may be missing in these thick deciduæ, which Vignes believes are evidences of absence of the normal regression, possibly due to hypothyroidism.

The maternal surface may be rough, sometimes hard, and there are numerous white infarcts. The contour of the placenta may be irregular, as if it grew easier in one direction than another; there is a tendency to the formation of placenta succenturiata and placentula succenturiata, also velamentous insertion of the cord. When the serotina, through chronic inflammation, or because of lost tissue through previous operations or disease, cannot react with sufficient decidua, the villi bore into the uterine wall and the placenta is adherent to the musculature—placenta accreta. (See Postpartum Hemorrhage.)

Diagnosis.—The diagnosis may be suspected during pregnancy, but seldom proven unless, perhaps, in glandular endometritis.

Treatment.—Prophylactically, much can be done to prevent endometritis in the early cure of gonorrhea, the proper care of abortion, the prevention of sepsis, etc. During pregnancy no treatment will reach the diseased part unless the latter be syphilitic, and here the appropriate drugs are to be exhibited. It is my custom to give all such patients, whether syphilitic or not, tonic doses of mercury—$\frac{1}{50}$ grain of corrosive sublimate in tablet three times daily. If pallor and general asthenia are present, minute doses of arsenic and iron are added. Lomer uses potassium iodid.

Hydrorrhœa Gravidarum.—A periodic, or at least intermittent, discharge of clear, yellowish, or sometimes bloody fluid from the uterus has been given this name, and the cause is almost always endometritis deciduæ catarrhalis, but similar fluids may issue from the uterus—first, from the space between the chorion and amnion, and, second, from the amniotic cavity itself, that is, liquor amnii may escape. In typical hydrorrhea the catarrhal secretion accumulates between the vera and reflexa, and periodically breaks through the mucous plug which fills the cervix, or there may be a continuous dribbling. As much as a pint may, but rarely, accumulate, and the expulsion of such an amount often provokes abortion or premature labor. The disease is most common from the third to the sixth month, but may begin or continue in the last trimester. The pathology is not fully understood, except that an endometritis deciduæ is usually back of it. It occurs in anemic and sickly women, especially multiparæ, and may, if slight, be overlooked.

In the differential diagnosis rupture of the bag of waters, rupture of the chorion, and the escape of subchorionic fluid and hydrorrhea are to be considered. The latter two cannot be distinguished from each other, but liquor amnii can often be recognized by the flocculi of vernix caseosa, if late in pregnancy, by the lanugo hairs, and sometimes by meconium. Usually it is impossible to make the diagnosis, and in all cases the patient is treated as if she were threatened with abortion.

Formerly it was held that if the ovular sac opened and the liquor amnii drained away, the uterus would inevitably empty itself within a short period. For the vast majority of cases this is true, but sometimes the membranes, after rupture, shrink up, leaving the fetus in the uterus, but outside of the chorion. Development of the child is much hindered; it is puny, shrunken, with many of its joints ankylotic, and showing decubitus over bony prominences. In addition to this form, or graviditas exochorialis, another variety exists: the amnion breaks, but the chorion does not, and the shrunken amnion is found hanging around the insertion of the cord, but the chorion is intact—graviditas examnialis.

Endometritis Syphilitica.—This was considered under Syphilis (p. 532).

Bacterial Endometritis.—Gonorrheal endometritis has already been mentioned, as also have the acute processes which complicate the infectious diseases. Tuberculous endometritis may occur in consumptives and in miliary tuberculosis. In one of my cases a tuberculous peritonitis developed acutely, after a physician, a sufferer from phthisis, had cureted the patient without sterilizing his instruments. Streptococci, staphylococci, and Bacterium coli commune (author) have been demonstrated in the uterine decidua, and, in addition, other unidentified kinds. It is generally held that while the vagina may harbor pathogenic bacteria, they live a saprophytic existence there and do not wander up into the uterus.

Under exceptional conditions (patulous cervix, husband with infected genitals) pathogenic bacteria may invade the endometrium and produce abortion and, perhaps, monstrosities. The cavity of the uterus may also become infected via the blood, or by contiguity from an organ nearby, e. g., the appendix or adherent bowel.

Le Count showed specimens demonstrating embolic bacterial endometritis. It is certain that germs can permeate the membranes both from the cervix and from the uterine wall, as in adherent appendical abscesses, thus infecting the fetus.

Under this caption should be briefly mentioned the *fever of pregnancy*. No one believes that the processes of pregnancy are ever normally attended by fever. Seitz collected numerous cases which tend to show that a bacterial endometritis can cause fever during pregnancy, subsiding when the uterus is emptied. Uterine pain, tenderness, even local peritonitic symptoms were present in a few of the cases; repeated abortion with bacteria in the decidua; eclampsia, hyperemesis, in others. Coitus carries feces and other contamination into the vagina, and it is more than probable that frequently infection of the ovum thus takes place, with consecutive abortion, which may or may not be followed by general sepsis. If Albert is correct, that a microbic endometritis can cause eclampsia, it is now easy to explain why eclamptics are so prone to puerperal infection in spite of most rigorous asepsis and antisepsis. A diagnosis of bacterial endometritis may be reached only by exclusion. The relation of such infections to puerperal fever will be taken up later.

Salpingitis causes sterility because it is almost always bilateral and occlusive. Chronic tubal inflammation may heal, but the folds of the mucosa have usually become glued together, and this is a frequent cause of ectopic gestation. Bilateral pus-tubes, of course, preclude pregnancy, but sometimes a pus-tube forms after conception has occurred, the woman having been infected and impregnated at the same time. A latent salpingitis may outlast pregnancy and break out acutely in the puerperium or on the occasion of some local manipulation. This may explain some of the cases of sepsis following criminal abortion. In rare cases a tube adherent to a gangrenous appendix may become infected. Acute salpingitis is a very serious complication of gestation, but is rare. During gestation the diagnosis is almost impossible; a peritonitis will be assumed, and if the symptoms are urgent, laparotomy will have to be performed. During pregnancy a departure should be made from the method of treatment of pyosalpinx. Labor will almost certainly rupture the abscesses, and it is, therefore, best to remove the sacs. It is a question whether it is advisable to wait for the contents to become sterile. If at operation there is reason to believe that the streptococcus is associated with the gonococcus, it may be wisest to extirpate the uterus at the same time, but the prognosis is bad in such cases. Late in pregnancy with threatening peritonitic symptoms a Porro should be considered, but if a general peritonitis already exists, free drainage alone is indicated (Kräuter). (See Brindeau and Martius.)

Peritonitis in pregnancy arises from appendicitis or salpingitis, rupture of the infected bladder in uterine incarceration, from necrosing fibroids, infected ectopic gestation-sacs, twisted ovarian tumors, and after attempts at criminal abortion. In many autopsies performed by the coroners catheters, knitting-needles, hat-pins, etc., have been found in the belly, usually embedded in pus.

Tuberculosis of the peritoneum practically always causes sterility. It is of special interest from the standpoint of differential diagnosis from pregnancy, many grievous mistakes having been made. Montgomery relates the sad case of a refined

English woman who fled to America to escape the gossip of her former friends about her growing abdomen, and at the autopsy, held in New York, the finding of a tuberculous peritonitis justified her oft-repeated assertion of innocence.

Rupture of an extra-uterine pregnancy may simulate an acute peritonitis, and there may be even fever of 102° to 103° F. to render the diagnosis difficult. In all cases of acute peritonitis in early pregnancy criminal practices are first to be thought of, and the abdomen is to be opened at once.

Chronic peritonitic adhesions have already been considered in connection with distortions and displacements of the uterus. Pregnancy, by the softening and vascularization of such bands, may be actually curative, the rising uterus stretching and breaking them. This process may be attended by more or less pain, and in several such cases the author had to prescribe rest in bed and opiates. Labor in such patients may be slow and tedious. It is believed that "missed labor" occurs more often under these conditions.

LITERATURE

Ahlfeld: Die Missbildungen des Menschen.—*Albert:* Arch. f. Gyn., 1901, vol. lxiii, H. 3, p. 487.—*Bland, Wenrich and Goldstein:* Surg., Gyn., and Obst., December, 1931, p. 759.—*Brindeau:* Arch. Mens. d'Obst. et de Gyn., January, March, 1917, p. 5.—*Cushing:* Annals of Gyn. and Ped., 1898, vol. xi, No. 7, p. 518.—*Engstrom:* Mittheilungen aus der Gyn. Klinik, Berlin, vol. iii, Heft 2.—*Findley,* Palmer, Trans. Amer. Gyn. Soc., 1926, p. 10.—*Hitschmann and Adler:* Zeitschr. f. Geb. u. Gyn., 1907, vol. lx, p. 63.—*Kehrer, E.:* Inaug. Diss., Heidelberg, 1899.—*Kräuter:* Arch. für Gyn., 1924, Bd. 122, p. 253.—*Le Count:* Trans. Chicago Gyn. Soc., February, 1918.—*Lomer:* Zeitschr. f. Geb. u. Gyn., 1901, vol. xlvi, Heft 2, p. 306.—*Martius:* Zentralblatt für Gyn., 1920, No. 49, p. 1412; also 1923, p. 393.—*Mundè:* Amer. Jour. Obstet., 1893, vol. xxviii.—*Plass:* Amer. Jour. Obst. and Gyn., March, 1931.—*Riotte:* Gyn. et Obst., 1924, Tome ix, p. 23.—*Santos:* Zeitschr. f. Geb. u. Gyn., vol. xiv. Literature.—*Seitz:* Handbuch der Geb., v. Winckel, vol. ii, 1904, 2, p. 1111.—*Ubbens:* Zentb. f. Gyn., 1916, p. 30.—*Van de Velde:* Mon. für Geb. u. Gyn., Band 42, H. 4 and 5.—*Vignes:* Comptes rendus da le Société de Biologie, Séance du 29 avril, 1922, tome lxxxvi, p. 850.—*Wells, Brooks:* Amer. Jour. Obstet., 1900, vol. xli, p. 321. Literature.

CHAPTER XLII

PREGNANCY COMPLICATED BY NEOPLASMS

TUMORS in and near the uterus may cause serious trouble before, during, and after delivery, though of late years the cases are not so frequent nor so formidable as formerly, because most of the tumors are removed when found, and, further, owing to modern asepsis, infections are almost always avoided, and operations during labor more successful.

FIBROIDS

The effects of pregnancy on myomata are well known and appreciated. It is not believed that the changes incident to gestation directly cause myomatous formations. The changes to be mentioned are usually more marked in myomata

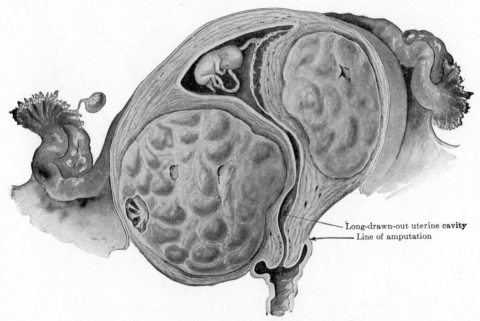

Long-drawn-out uterine cavity
Line of amputation

FIG. 454.—FIBROIDS AND EARLY PREGNANCY, MRS. G.

Tertipara. Excessive pain and irregular hemorrhages during the first months of pregnancy. Supravaginal amputation of the uterus. One ovary left. Cyst developed in it two years later.

than in fibromata. During pregnancy fibroids which were not noticeable before take part in the general succulence and hypertrophy of the uterine muscle, enlarge, and are discovered. Larger fibromata, especially if located in the pelvis, may grow so much that incarceration and dangerous compression of the pelvic organs result. Aside from hypertrophy, hyperplasia, and the increased vascularity of the tumor, cystic and other degenerations, and in rare instances suppuration and gangrene, may occur. The so-called red degeneration is one of the most serious. Peritoneal irritation, even adhesions, in the absence of gangrene, are sometimes caused. Another result of pregnancy is the dislocation and change of shape of the tumors. Myomata attached to the cervix respond to the upward traction of the fundus uteri and rise into the abdomen, which is fortunate, because otherwise they would block delivery. This retraction of the tumor above the brim may occur even during labor, and the accoucheur may be most agreeably surprised to find what promised to be a formidable case become a simple matter. The fibroid may be flattened by the growing ovum, or, if there are several tumors, they may be separated from each other. Subserous myomata may become twisted and necrose, or they may prolapse into the pelvis; interstitial tumors usually become more superficial; submucous fibroids are likely to become polypoid and may then be extruded through the cervix during the puerperium. During labor the fibroids may be crushed by the advancing head, by attempts at delivery, or by too strong "Credé" expression. In the puerperium myomata usually undergo involution with the rest of the uterus.

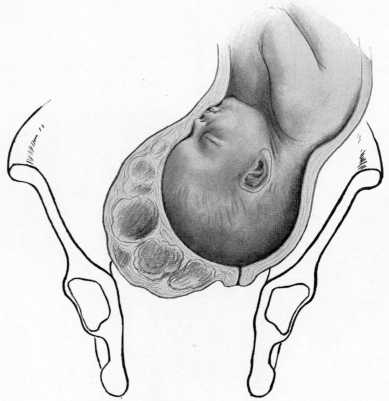

Fig. 455.—Mrs. K.   Mural Cervical Fibroids at Beginning of Labor.

Many authors report the total disappearance of the tumors as the result of involution, but I have not observed it in the few cases I have been able to follow up, the tumors all having been found as large as, or even larger, than they were before pregnancy, though smaller than they were during gestation. Landau says the same. Necrosis and infection of the tumors occur, but this accident is unusual, is favored by immense size of the growth, by bruising during delivery, but particularly by infection, which is invited by the wounding of the endometrium over the tumor. The fibroid may be converted into a necrotic, purulent mass which breaks into the bladder or discharges per vaginam, a cure thus being effected. Sometimes the uterine contractions deliver the tumor outside the cervix or vulva, the capsule breaks, and the myoma escapes through the rent, but more often gangrene sets in, requiring operation.

The influence of pregnancy on the symptoms caused by myomata is also one of aggravation. Pain was marked in all my cases, hemorrhage, simulating threatened abortion, in nine. If the tumor is large, the symptoms of abdominal overdistention result—constipation, dysuria, dyspnea—together with wasting and even cachexia.

The effects of the fibromata on the pregnancy are very variable. Women with such tumors are frequently sterile, and though Martin says this is not true, larger statistics seem to prove it. Abortion is more apt to occur, especially with the submucous varieties. The interstitial have less influence, and the subserous, unless large or near the cervix, hardly any. Placenta prævia seems to be favored by the presence of uterine tumors, probably through the concomitant endometritis or edema. Retroflexio uteri gravidi, with incarceration, has been noted; also ectopic pregnancy. In labor the fibroids usually do not give trouble unless impacted or

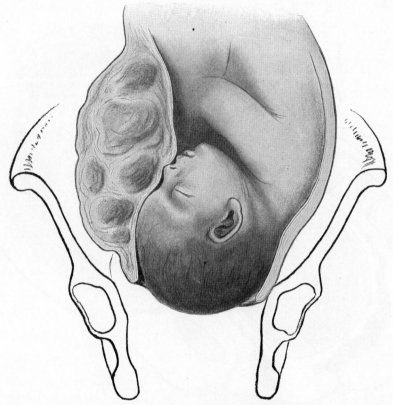

Fig. 456.—Mrs. K. Same Fibroids after Complete Dilatation of the Cervix.

adherent in the pelvis, or unless the placenta has attached itself to the tumor. A subserous impacted myoma causes the worst trouble, because it is less likely to be elevated by the contracting and retracting uterus (Figs. 456 and 457). Interstitial tumors may be flattened against the wall of the pelvis, so that they allow the child to pass; they may be retracted upward, or, if low in the cervix, they may be pushed out of the vulva, even delivered free, thus permitting the birth of the child. The last occurrence is more likely with fibroid polypi. Fibromyomata exert an influence on the mechanism of labor. The uterine contractions are usually strong and painful; indeed, when delivery is blocked by the tumor, rupture of the uterus may ensue; on the other hand, weak pains, even atony, may be present; abnormalities of position and presentation, face, forehead, breech, shoulder, are prone to occur; prolapse of the cord, interlocking of the fetus and the tumor, and inversion of the uterus have also been noted. The baby is likely to be underdeveloped.

In the third stage hemorrhage is very common because the distorted uterus has difficulty in closing the vessels of the placental site. Anomalies in the separation of the placenta are especially apt to occur when it is located on the tumor, since pathogenic adherence is the rule in such cases. If the uterine canal is kinked, the placenta may be incarcerated, and even the best operator may not be able to remove it.

During the puerperium fibroids may obstruct the lochial flow and cause lochiometra; they always delay involution; they predispose to phlebothrombosis, and when they are gangrenous or infected, the worst forms of sepsis may result.

Diagnosis.—Most complicated diagnostic problems are here presented to the

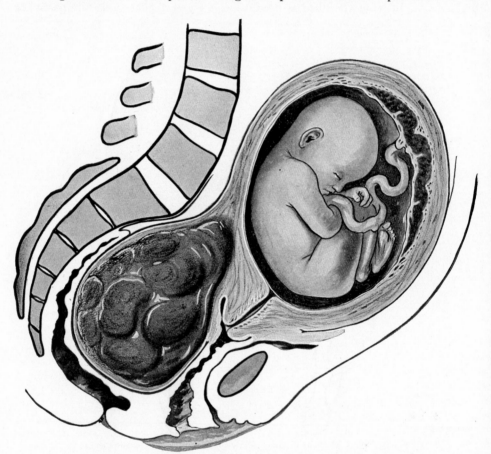

FIG. 457.—SUBSEROUS MYOMA IN PELVIS. REMOVED THROUGH POSTERIOR COLPOTOMY.

obstetrician, and mistakes without number have been made. If a woman who is known to have myomata becomes pregnant, the diagnosis is not difficult and will rest on some of these points: Cessation or irregularity of the menses or unusual hemorrhages; the sympathetic symptoms and breast signs; the rapid enlargement of the uterine tumor; the development on it of a soft area; the contractions of the uterine tumor; and the fetal heart-tones. All these may be equivocal except the last, and even the fetal heart may be inaudible because covered by an immense tumor. If the diagnosis of the existing pregnancy is made, it is usually easy to determine that there are fibroids in addition, but here, too, mistakes have occurred, a twin, an ovarian tumor, pyosalpinx, double uterus, abdominal wall fibromata, fat, hematoma, Littrè's hernia, etc., having been taken for uterine tumors. During delivery the myomatous nodules are made prominent when the uterus hardens, and unless hidden behind the uterus, are almost always discoverable. They may be mistaken for other tumors or a second child. Forceps have been applied to a myoma which imposed as a fetal head. If located in a position which causes interference with the mechanism of labor, new problems are presented for diagnosis. When the uterus is emptied, its large size and the presence of nodules will easily indicate the trouble, though on one such occasion six talented gynecologists, from external examination, diagnosed a second twin. In the puerperium the fundus remains high, involution proceeding very slowly. Infection of the tumor is announced by the usual signs of sepsis.

The differential diagnosis between a large symmetric interstitial fibroid and pregnancy is sometimes one of the most difficult to make. Times innumerable the belly has been opened and only the normal pregnant uterus found, and, indeed, it may be almost impossible to distinguish the two, even after the tumor is out of the belly, in the hands of the operator.

In such a case much weight is to be placed on careful and repeated examinations made before operation:

Myoma	Pregnancy
1. Symptoms, as nausea, etc., usually absent.	1. Present.
2. Menses present; breast signs almost always absent.	2. Menses absent; breast signs present. Rarely irregular bleedings.
3. Uterine tumor usually asymmetric or nodular.	3. Usually symmetric or characteristically deformed.
4. Tumor usually hard.	4. Soft.
5. Contractions of the tumor excessively rare.	5. Usual and involve the whole organ.
6. Round ligaments, tubes, and ovaries anomalously located.	6. Normally placed. Ligaments thickened.
7. Cervix retracted, high in pelvis, hard, and a sort of appendix to the tumor.	7. Cervix low in the pelvis, large, soft, and ' part of the uterine wall.
8. Auscultatory signs of pregnancy absent.	8. Almost always present.
9. x-Ray negative unless tumor is calcareous. (Lipiodol not to be used if pregnancy suspected.)	9. May outline skeleton of fetus.
10. Aschheim-Zondek test negative.	10. Positive.

After the belly is opened the differential diagnosis is made by the darker color of the pregnant uterus, the congested, thickened tubes and ligaments, especially the round ligaments, the presence of a large corpus luteum in one ovary, ballottement, the contractions of the tumor, which molds itself on the promontory, while a fibroid is usually lighter in color, rocks heavily on the promontory, is asymmetric, and the experienced operator usually can determine from the feel whether or not a pregnancy exists. One might listen over the tumor with a sterile stethoscope. If the doubt cannot be dispelled, it is justifiable to cut into the tumor very slowly, layer by layer and, should an ovum be discovered, unless other indications exist, the wound is to be immediately sutured and the belly closed. Pregnancy is usually not interrupted by the exploratory operation.

Prognosis.—Without doubt the dangers of myomata complicating pregnancy are misrepresented by the reports, which is due to the fact that only the bad cases are considered worthy of publication. Unless the tumor obstructs delivery, recovery is the rule, but the fetus is more endangered.

Treatment in Early Pregnancy.—Since the majority of pregnant women with fibroids go to and through labor without difficulty, it is almost never necessary to induce abortion on their account. Indeed, the interruption of pregnancy is difficult because of the distortion of the uterine canal, and dangerous because of the hemorrhage and liability of infecting the tumors. Excessive pain and repeated and profuse hemorrhages may require treatment, and if ordinary means do not suffice, an operation may be necessary. It is best, wherever at all possible, to wait until term or near it before operating. It may even be wise to try the test of labor, because nature sometimes accomplishes wonders in getting the tumors out of the way of the child's delivery. In the absence, therefore, of unbearable pain, of severe hemorrhage, of very rapid growth (the "galloping type" of Pozzi), of great distress from overdistention of the belly, and of signs of necrosis of the tumor, or torsion, or "acute abdomen," it is justifiable to wait and watch. To assist nature in elevating the tumors out of the pelvis the patient assumes the knee-chest position frequently every day. Myomectomy has been frequently done during pregnancy, but it is a very bloody operation, and is followed by abortion in 17 per cent. of cases (Winter). Hysterectomy has also been performed, sometimes when only enucleation of the tumors was intended, but made necessary because of technical difficulties, hemorrhage, etc.

Near Term or in Labor.—(a) *Clean Cases.*—Should the woman approach the end of her pregnancy, a careful examination is made to determine whether the tumors will obstruct labor, and it must be borne in mind that a degree of contraction of the parturient passage caused by a fibroid is worse than the same caused by a contracted pelvis, because of the possible sloughing of the tumor resulting from crushing during spontaneous, but especially operative, delivery. Even during pregnancy gentle attempts at reposition are allowable. Should a subserous or mural cervical myoma be so large or so firmly fixed in the pelvis that it apparently will completely block delivery, cesarean section is to be performed as soon as labor has declared itself. When the patient is anesthetized, it is justifiable to make an attempt at manual reposition of the tumor. If it succeeds, labor is allowed to continue; if not, abdominal delivery is performed. After the child and placenta are removed, an attempt is to be made to raise the tumor out of the pelvis and to extirpate it. If this is impossible because the fibroid is too densely adherent, or because it has grown out into the broad ligaments, the question of total extirpation comes up. Only a skilful obstetric surgeon may attempt such an operation. Hemorrhage is often profuse. It may be wiser to leave the tumor for future removal. If conservative cesarean section is done drainage of the uterine cavity into the vagina with gauze is to be provided.

Smaller tumors may be left for the test of labor, and, as a rule, they will be retracted or softened and flattened so as to allow the passage of the fetus. If they are very low in the cervix or pedunculated, they may be enucleated or amputated through the vagina. Labor may then be allowed to proceed naturally, or if the conditions are fulfilled, delivery is effected. Enucleation is not to be attempted unless the tumor is hard and quite superficial and its shelling-out promises to be very simple, because sometimes hemorrhage is so profuse that the belly has to be hurriedly opened to control it.

In conducting a labor with fibroids abutting on the parturient canal it is important to avoid all bruising of the tumors because necrosis and infection are so liable to set in afterward. In making a reposition of the tumor the utmost gentleness is to be practised, because its capsule may be ruptured or its pedicle injured, resulting in intra-abdominal hemorrhage or sloughing, with subsequent peritonitis. In trying to pull a fibroid out of the pelvis with the belly opened much aid is afforded by an associate pushing the tumor upward gently from below. If, now, the delivery can be accomplished through the vagina and the operation completed without establishing connection between the peritoneal cavity and the parturient canal, a distinct advantage is gained.

Operations in the uterine cavity, as version and manual removal of the placenta, may be rendered laborious by obstructing fibroid tumors, and it may be necessary to push up or even extirpate the masses before the hand can be introduced. Removal of a placenta adherent to a submucous fibroid may require the digging out of the two at once, whereby care is observed not to puncture the uterus. In such an event, or if the extraction of the placenta fails, abdominal section would be indicated. If not in position to perform major operations, and finding it impossible to remove the placenta, the accoucheur should pack the uterovaginal canal firmly with gauze. After forty-eight to sixty hours of tamponade the placenta will usually be found loose enough for easy delivery.

(b) *Suspect Cases.*—When labor has been in progress for a long time; when the woman is presumably infected; or where unsuccessful attempts at delivery or reposition of the tumor have been made—the condition becomes very formidable. Here, unless manual reposition under anesthesia succeeds, the abdomen must be opened. Now, if at all possible, the tumor is to be raised out of the pelvis, and delivery from below executed by an associate; then supravaginal amputation or total extirpation performed. If the child is dead, it is best to remove the uterus *en bloc*, without opening it to extract the child, the object being to prevent the contact of the infectious uterine contents with the peritoneum. In deciding whether or not to remove the uterus it may be necessary to consult the wishes of the patient and her husband, because if the child is dead, they may wish progeny later. In presumably infected cases the danger of peritonitis should be pointed out, and the removal of the uterus advised as a means of reducing it. (See Portes, p. 1108.)

(c) *During the puerperium*, unless symptoms are present, the myomata are not disturbed. Ergot is best omitted unless the tumor is pedunculating itself ready for extrusion and the same is to be hastened. Hemorrhage may require one or more tamponades or immediate operation. Sloughing, pedunculated tumors are removed per vaginam, but not oversoon, unless they bleed. Trust nature a little. If the tumors become infected, at first expectancy is practised, until the immunities of the puerpera are developed. Precipitate laparotomy might cause fatal peritonitis. During a laparotomy for sloughing fibroids the peritoneum is to be walled off as carefully as at all possible, and the cutting across of the pedicle, after ligation of the broad ligaments, done with the Paquelin cautery. Drainage through the vagina follows. The peritoneum must not be contaminated.

CARCINOMA CERVICIS

Of 68,000 consecutive obstetric cases at the Chicago Lying-in Hospital and Dispensary, only 5 were complicated by cancer of the cervix, and since the service here most closely resembles private practice, as opposed to an exclusive hospital service, this may be taken as a fair index of the frequency of the condition, though Sarwey, combining many statistics, gives the ratio as 1 to 2000 labors, which agrees with Kerr's figures. To the fact that cancer occurs mostly in the non-reproductive period we can ascribe its rarity as a complication of pregnancy. It occurs almost exclusively in multiparæ. It is a most unfortunate complication, since of reported cases 43 per cent. of the mothers and 60 per cent. of the children died during labor (Wertheim and Bainbridge, 1918). Cancer of the body of the uterus almost excludes the possibility of pregnancy. (See E. A. Schuman.)

The effect of pregnancy upon the cancer is generally considered unfavorable; experiments on rats and the opinion of Mayer to the contrary notwithstanding (Mundell). Rarely the growth begins after conception; usually the pregnancy supervenes after the cancer has started. Owing to the vascularization and lymphatic imbibition of the cervix caused by pregnancy the tumor grows fast and invades the lymphatics and glands very quickly. Hemorrhage and necrosis, with putrid, sanious leukorrhea, are very marked in all cases except the slow-growing epithelioid varieties. Labor may break up the tumor, the more or less deep lacerations causing hemorrhage, sepsis, and rapid extension of the neoplasm. In the puerperium the last-mentioned changes become evident, but the prostration and quick cachexia are most striking.

Upon pregnancy, labor, and the puerperium cancer of the cervix exerts a bad influence. In the first place, sterility is the rule in cancer, especially in advanced cases, for obvious reasons; second, abortion is frequent because of the endometritis

37

usually present, the infection and death of the ovum, the hemorrhages, and the restriction of the growth of the uterus by the neoplasm.   Labor is obstructed, not so much because of the size of the mass, as because of the rigidity of the cervix produced by the carcinomatous infiltration.   If the tumor is soft and takes up part of the cervix, the rest may dilate and allow the child to pass.   If the whole cervix is involved and in a hard mass, obstruction is produced, and the case is formidable. Placenta prævia is a not very uncommon complication, and because of the friability of the uterine wall near the tumor, rupture of the uterus may occur if the pains do not quickly succeed in overcoming the resistant cervix.   Should the cervix give way, the tear may extend up into the parametrium, giving rise to terrific hemorrhages, which, owing to the friable nature of the parts, cannot be stopped by suture. Missed labor has been observed, also premature rupture of the membranes, and primary and secondary uterine inertia.   Sepsis is common in the puerperium, and a cancerous puerpera is a menace to other puerperæ in the same ward.

Diagnosis.—Every woman who has irregular hemorrhages or purulent or putrid leukorrhea should be examined for cancer of the uterus, and even if the menopause has taken place, pregnancy should be suspected when the uterus is found enlarged.   The usual criteria of cancer are available, and the tumor, hard and nodular, is more easily differentiated, since the cervix is softened.   I have on four occasions found a hard, nodular, but not ulcerative condition of the cervix during the middle of pregnancy, attended by slight bleedings and fetid discharge, but which were not carcinomatous and which disappeared after delivery.   It is wise, therefore, in doubtful cases to examine a piece of the tumor microscopically.   Pregnancy will not be interrupted by exsecting a bit of the cervix.

Treatment.—If an *operable* cancer of the cervix is discovered early in pregnancy the radical operation should be done.   Since recovery is possible in 20 per cent. of the cases the life of the child is not considered.   Pinard, Pozzi, and other French authors counsel waiting, but the majority of American, English, and German advise to do everything to save the mother.   This plan is more recommendable when the woman, as usual, has children.   The Catholic Church permits extirpation of the cancerous pregnant uterus because the object of the operation is to ablate the tumor (Burke).   Spencer, Glockner, Beckman, and Küstner found 50 to 82 per cent. of the cases operable, and the abdominal route is usually selected, occasionally the vaginal, rarely the two combined.

If the carcinoma is discovered when the child is near viability, it may be justifiable to wait a few weeks in its interests.   After viability no question can be raised regarding the interference, immediate radical operation is demanded.   Up to within a few years vaginal cesarean section followed by uterine extirpation was the rule, now the abdominal route is usually chosen.   Zweifel recommended Porro cesarean followed by vaginal extirpation of the stump (vide infra).

When pregnancy supervenes upon an *inoperable* carcinoma the woman is allowed to go until viability of the child is secure.   While abortion is usually not produced by local interference, we do not perform tamponade, cauterization, or curettage unless hemorrhage or sepsis demands one or the other.   Gellhorn's acetone treatment is useful to tide over local complications.

Since labor creates a frightful (45 per cent.) immediate mortality from rupture of the uterus, hemorrhage, sepsis, exhaustion, and shock, labor pains are not to be awaited, but a Porro cesarean done beforehand, and the stump fastened to the lower angle of the abdominal incision—this to avoid peritonitis from the streptococci almost always present in the operative field.   If the cervix cannot be drawn up to the skin it is covered thickly with peritoneum *in situ* and drained per vaginam.

Now diathermy, radium, and the *x*-ray enter the field of treatment and create new problems.   Naturally one would like to treat the cancer with these new agents and await secure viability of the child, but what little experience we have had shows that in many cases abortion follows, or the child is deformed—aplastic, microcephalic, idiotic, etc.—only a few patients being free from harm. Bailey and Bagg, from their experiments on pregnant rats, warn to great care, and Mundell has collected the literature on the subject, the evidence strongly opposing radiation during pregnancy (Naujoks, Murphy). Even the use of radium and x-ray for gynecologic treatment of women in the reproductive years is forbidden by accumulated experience. They damage the ovaries, the germinal cells, the effects appearing after generations. The decision of the Deutsche Gesellschaften, Zentr. für Gyn., October 31, 1931, p. 3171, was adverse and objections were raised in the Monatsschr. für Geb. u. Gyn., March, 1932, p. 447. In inoperable cases one will await only the time of certain viability of the child, and then, a few days after the Porro, institute diathermy, radium, and x-ray treatment in accordance with modern practice. It is not quite fair to the mother to prolong the pregnancy to full term. We wish to ray the stump as soon as possible because a fair proportion of women's lives are prolonged, and in all cases much misery is avoided.

OVARIAN TUMORS

Much rarer than fibroids are ovarian tumors during pregnancy. Since cysts of the ovary are quite common, the conclusion is justified that they predispose to sterility. In 862 cases collected by McKerron, simple and multilocular cysts occurred in 68 per cent.; dermoids, in 23 per cent.; fibromata and solid adenomata, in 2 per cent., and malignant neoplasms, in 5 per cent. In 1316 cases Puech found 27 per cent. dermoids.

The influence of pregnancy on the tumor is usually not bad, most women going to term without the knowledge of its existence, and the growth of the neoplasm is not accelerated, as in the case of fibroids. While dyspnea, palpitation, etc., due to excessive size of the tumor, are exceedingly rare, torsion of the pedicle, hemorrhage into the cyst, suppuration, and necrosis have occasionally been noted. Labor exerts no influence unless the tumor lies in the pelvis, exposed to the traumatism of delivery. In this case it may be crushed or burst, or its pedicle torn, while in some instances the advancing head has forced the tumor through the rectum or the vagina outside the body—a spontaneous ovariotomy. The puerperium shows no special influence, but complications are likely to arise as the result of the bruising of the tumor. Torsion has been observed much more frequently than usual.

Pregnancy is but little affected by ovarian cysts. Abortion is commoner only with those tumors which are very large or are incarcerated in the pelvis, interfere with the growth of the uterus, or become twisted or infected. Hydatid mole has been frequently observed, sometimes with lutein cysts. Upon labor, ovarian cysts exert a bad action only when they are incarcerated in the pelvis and block the path of the child. To a certain extent, but not so much as with fibroids, nature helps herself by drawing the tumor out of the way by means of the pedicle, and a small or soft tumor may still allow the passage of the child. A soft tumor, however, when it diminishes the available pelvic cavity, is far worse than an equal amount of contraction caused by deformed pelvis. Malpresentations and uterine inertia are common. The puerperium is often stormy, since, because of the bruising of the tumor, necrosis, hemorrhages, infection, suppuration, sometimes with breaking of the pus into the neighboring organs, occur. Tumors which become adherent to the rectum are likely to be infected with colon bacilli. Dermoids, in the writer's experience, are the worst cases in all respects, and if they burst during labor fatal peritonitis may result.

Diagnosis.—In the early months it is usually very easy to differentiate the pregnant uterus from the rounded, movable, pedunculated tumor lying at its side, but sometimes great difficulties are encountered. When the tumor is intraligamentous or prolapsed in the pelvis behind the uterus, a careful differentiation from ectopic gestation and retroflexed gravid uterus must be made. Both of these have already been considered under their respective headings (*q. v.*). A large tumor may conceal the uterus and pose as a pregnancy, and since the signs and symptoms of the latter are present, the mistake is very likely to be made. Fibroids, splenic, even renal tumors must be drawn into the differential, and one should remember that torsion of an ovarian cyst produces a picture resembling ruptured ectopic pregnancy and also appendicitis.

In the later months, and during labor, the location of the tumor causes a variety of difficulties. If high in the abdomen, it may slip under the liver or spleen. If adherent to the uterus, the suspicion of twins, of fibroid, or double-horned uterus, arises. If attached to the pelvis low down, a shoulder presentation may be thought

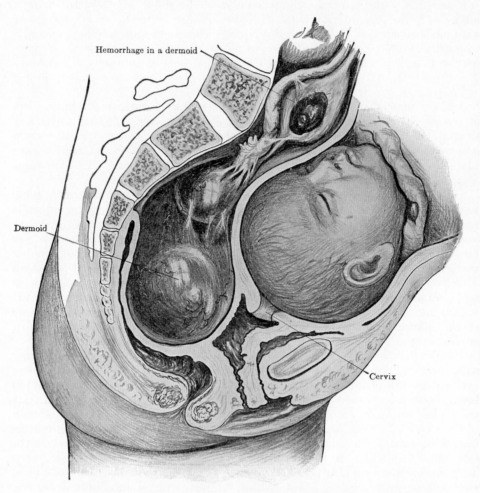

Hemorrhage in a dermoid

Dermoid

Cervix

FIG. 458.—MRS. K. THREE DERMOID TUMORS, ONE BLOCKING THE PELVIS.
Replacement. High forceps. Ovariotomy. Recovery.

of. In one of my cases a dermoid was adherent to the promontory of the sacrum and could just be reached by the examining finger. If the head had not been pushed far forward over the pubis by something behind the uterus, it is more than probable that the tumor would have been overlooked. Tumors incarcerated in the pelvis during labor are very easily discovered, but their nature and origin are not so quickly determined. A cyst under the compression of labor becomes as hard as a fibroid, and if it is adherent, may simulate a tumor of the pelvic periosteum, as occurred in one of my cases. Rectal examination will exclude this class of neoplasms. An ovarian cyst has been held to be the head of a second twin, and forceps applied; a fibroid—and enucleation attempted; a prolapsed kidney; a full rectum; a hematoma.

An important part of the diagnosis is the decision as to whether the tumor will block the delivery, and in estimating this one must never forget to measure the bony pelvis also. If possible, one should diagnose the nature of the tumor. A corpus luteum cyst enlarges rapidly to the size of a tangerine (seldom more) and then may regress. Operation not required.

Prognosis.—Nowadays few women die from this complication because the tumors are usually removed as soon as found, and because operation is substituted for the brutal obstetric deliveries of the olden time. Marshall, in the latest collection, finds a maternal mortality of only 3.3 per cent. in cases operated on during pregnancy, and 5 per cent. after laparotomy at term. Wertheim quotes two statistics—39.2 per cent. and 31.3 per cent. maternal deaths—for cases treated expectantly; Puech found 6 per cent. maternal and 23 per cent. fetal mortality. These are for cases in labor.

Treatment.—*During Pregnancy.*—Most authors are strongly in favor of immediate removal of the tumor when discovered, but the writer agrees with Fehling and Martin that here, as always, one must individualize. Operation is the rule, preferably laparotomy, though Dührssen urges the vaginal route. Abortion follows the operation in 22.5 per cent. of cases (Orgler), 16.5 per cent. (Puech), and even though it follows in 17 per cent. of cases treated expectantly, it may be wiser to postpone the removal of the tumor until the last month of pregnancy or during labor or the puerperium. Such exceptions to the rule would be: (1) Small, freely movable tumors high in the abdomen; (2) an aged primipara in whom the probability of further pregnancies is slight; (3) double ovarian tumors where the woman has no children and desires offspring. In these cases, if operation must be done, a part of the ovary and that portion carrying the corpus luteum should, where possible, be left, but only if its integrity is assurred. A damaged corpus luteum usually brings on abortion, but removal of one not always. Should the patient, after the situation in all its bearings has been explained to her, decide to wait, she must be instructed to report at once any untoward symptom, and as the time of her confinement approaches seek a good maternity hospital. If the pelvis is not obstructed, labor may be allowed to take place as usual, and the tumor extirpated with deliberation a few days afterward. Rapid growth of the tumor in pregnancy suggests malignancy.

Indications for immediate operation in pregnancy are: Suspicion of malignancy; torsion of the pedicle; signs of infection of the tumor; overdistention of the belly. If general anesthesia is employed, ethylene should be used; the pregnant uterus must be handled as little and as gently as possible, and morphin is to be given for several days afterward in an attempt to restrain uterine action.

During Labor.—A sharp distinction is to be made between cases in the hospital under the hands of the obstetric surgeon and those at home in the care of the family practitioner. The location of the neoplasm; the state of the parturient canal as regards infection, and the tumor as regards prolonged pressure, bruising from attempts at reposition, delivery, etc., are also to be thoughtfully considered. The following lines of procedure have been followed: (a) Forceful delivery alongside the tumor, mentioned first to be unqualifiedly condemned and thus disposed of; (b) reposition of the tumor, followed by spontaneous or operative delivery; (c) vaginal puncture or incision and evacuation of the cyst, succeeded by delivery from below, then removal of the sac; (d) vaginal ovariotomy; (e) abdominal ovariotomy, followed by delivery from below; (f) cesarean section, followed by extirpation of the tumor, with or without the uterus.

In all cases the first procedure is an attempt to dislodge and replace the tumor above the brim, out of the way of the advancing head.   This is to be made in deep anesthesia, the patient lying in the exaggerated Trendelenburg or the Sims position. (Fig. 557); the fetal head is to be pushed upward, and then, with the uttermost gentleness, using the whole hand, the tumor is disengaged from the pelvis.   If the manœuver is successful, the child is delivered by version and extraction or forceps, or the case left to nature, depending on the conditions present.   After the delivery of the child immediate laparotomy is performed and the tumor extirpated.   It is best not to wait to remove the cyst, because the latter may have been ruptured or injured by the manipulations or delivery, and delay might mean fatal peritonitis.

If the case is a "clean" one, that is, not infected, and without previous interference or prolonged labor, and a single attempt at reposition fails, laparotrachelotomy is to be performed, the child delivered, the uterine wound closed, and the tumor ablated or left for subsequent operation, depending upon the conditions of the particular case.   If the parturient canal is presumably infected, and the family expresses a desire to preserve the uterus, reposition failing, one must remove the obstruction from above and deliver the child from below.   (Some operators trust the laparotrachelotomy here.)   A long abdominal incision is necessary; the uterus may have to be turned out of the belly, and an assistant may have to dislodge the tumor from below before the mass becomes accessible.   After the tumor is removed, if the uterus cannot be replaced in the belly (rare), it may be covered with hot towels, delivery effected from below, and then it will be easy to replace.   Extensive adhesions, impaction of the tumor under the promontory, and solid and malignant neoplasms may render such a course impossible, as in one of my cases, and the uterus may have to be emptied in order to reach the pelvis.   In all cases a consistent attempt is to be made to remove the tumor whole because the contents, especially if dermoid, are likely to be infectious.   Should such an infected mass burst into the free peritoneal cavity, the uterus is to be also extirpated and vaginal drainage established.   In determining whether a cyst is infected or not, in addition to the appearance, pus, ichor, and the odor, the history of inflammatory attacks is important. A tumor firmly attached to the rectum or colon is frequently infected, and unusual care is to be observed in removing it.

Suspicious or infected cases are best attacked through the vagina—indeed, Dührssen, Wertheim, and most German authorities recommend this way as the rule for all cases.   Spencer, Kerr, Hofmeier, Williams, and most English and American authors advise the abdominal route.

Vaginal Ovariotomy.—A long, preferably longitudinal incision is made over the most prominent part of the tumor, the cyst grasped with vulsellum forceps, its contents evacuated through a broad incision, accessory cavities explored and emptied with the finger, and the sac then drawn down and its pedicle ligated.   Should the pedicle be inaccessible, or should the head enter the pelvis upon the cyst being emptied, the sac is fixed to the vaginal opening by a strong suture, or the opening lightly packed with gauze and delivery effected, after which the tumor becomes easily managable through the vaginal incision and should be extirpated.   It has happened that laparotomy became necessary during the vaginal operation, because the pedicle could not be ligated, or the tumor was so brittle that it could not be pulled down, or the ligature slipped, or the tumor was solid or too densely adherent.

What should the general practitioner do in the home, far from help?   In the presence of an urgent indication for delivery, the cyst is to be punctured, after opening Douglas' pouch, the sac emptied, anchored to the vaginal wall by a suture or light gauze packing, and labor completed. The sac is to be extirpated within twenty-four hours.

In the puerperium ovariotomy is to be performed in all cases, and preferably within twenty-four hours.   If operation is postponed, a minute watch is kept for the first symptoms of infection of the tumor or torsion of its pedicle.

Other Tumors Complicating Pregnancy.—Reference, only, may be made to those rare conditions which the obstetrician may meet.   They are all treated on general principles.   Enlarged and prolapsed kidneys, usually the left (Bland-Sutton) (Cragin, vaginal nephrectomy); extrauterine pregnancy combined with intra-uterine (Zinke); echinococcus cysts (Franta); parametritic abscesses and infiltrates; cancer of the rectum (Mýhoff, 26 cases, Katz and Kasper, Lit.); rectal stricture; tumors of the bladder; vesical calculi requiring lithotomy; bony tumors and enchondromata, to be considered later.

LITERATURE

Bagg: Amer. Jour. Anat., January, 1922, xxx, p. 133. Literature.—*Bailey and Bagg:* Amer. Jour. Obs. and Gyn., May, 1923, p. 461.—*Bainbridge:* Amer. Jour. Obstet., 1918, p. 36.—*Beckman:* Zeitschr. f. Gyn. u. Geb., 1910, vol. lxvii, p. 445. Much literature.—*Bland-Sutton:* The London Lancet, 1901, vol. i, p. 529.—*Burke, Rev. E. F.:* Acute Cases in Moral Medicine, 1922, p. 47.—*Cragin:* Amer. Jour. Obstet., 1898, vol. xxxviii, p. 36.—*Dührssen:* Deutsch. med. Woch., 1904, No. 42, p. 1529.—*Fields:* Amer. Röntgen-ray Journal, 1922.—*Franta:* "Echinococcus Cysts of Pelvis and Abdomen," Annales de Gyn. et d'Obst., 1902, p. 165. Full literature to date.—*Glockner:* Centralbl. f. Gyn., 1902, pp. 508 and 1446.—*Gellhorn:* Jour. Missouri State Medical Assn., February, 1922.—*Graefe:* Zeitschr. f. Geb. u. Gyn., 1906, vol. lvi, H. 3.—*Halban-Seitz:* Biol. u. Path. des Weibes, 1927, vol. iv.—*Katz and Kasper:* Arch. für Gyn., vol. cxxviii, H. 1 and 2, 1926.—*Kelly and Cullen:* Uterine Myomata, 1909.—*Kerr:* Operative Midwifery, 1908, p. 223.—*Landau:* Treatise. Fibroids and Pregnancy, 1911.—*Marshall:* Jour. Obstet. and Gyn., British Empire, February, 1910. Gives literature since 1903. —*McKerron:* Pregnancy, Labor, and Childbed with Ovarian Tumors, 1903.—*Müller:* Die Krankh. des weibl. Körpers, pp. 304–334.—*Mundell:* Amer. Jour. Obstet. and Gyn., 1927, January, p. 86, Lit.—*Murphy, D. P.:* Surg., Gyn., and Obst., December, 1929.—*Naujoks:* Zentb. für Gyn., September 26, 1931, p. 2911.—*Noble:* Amer. Jour. Obstet., 1896, vol. xxxiii, p. 874.—*Orgler:* Arch. f. Gyn., 1902, vol. lxv, i, p. 126. Literature.— *Pinard:* Annales de Gyn., September, 1901; *ibid.,* April, 1901, p. 309.—*Piquand:* "Fibroids," L'Obstetrique, Paris, July, 1909.—*Pueck:* "Ovarian Tumors and Pregnancy," Arch. Mens. d'Obst. et de Gyn., April, 1913, p. 412. Reports 1316 cases.—*Sarwey:* Veit's Handbuch der Gyn., 1899, vol. iii, Bd. ii, p. 491.—*Schuman, E. A.:* Trans. Amer. Gyn. Soc., 1928, lii, 245.—*Spencer:* Jour. Amer. Med. Assoc., 1909, vol. i, p. 1612; *ibid.,* Trans. Lond. Obst. Soc., 1905, vol. xlvi, p. 355; "Myomata," Trans. Amer. Gyn. Assoc., Washington, 1903; also Monograph on Tumors Complicating Gestation, Harrison & Sons, London, 1920.—*Werner:* Arch. für Gynaek., vol. cxxix, 1, p. 167.—*Wertheim:* Handbuch d. Geb., 1903, vol. ii, No. 1, p. 514.—*Zinke:* Amer. Jour. Obstet., 1902, vol. xlv, p. 623. Full literature to date.—*Zweifel:* Handb. d. Geb. Zweite Aufl., vol. ii, p. 84.

CHAPTER XLIII

MINOR DISTURBANCES OF PREGNANCY

THE accoucheur is often consulted about annoying, if not dangerous, symptoms during pregnancy, and it is wise to instruct the gravida to report such phenomena to him, since he may detect in them the beginning of serious illness. Most of the troubles have been considered in chapters appropriate to them; here will be mentioned only those not previously treated.

Insomnia is rare, and is usually due to digestive disturbances and neurotic tendencies. The same may be said of constant dreaming. If regulation of the diet and bowels does not suffice, simple remedies often will; for example, one or two glasses of hot malted milk just before bedtime; a hot-water bag at the feet; sleeping alone, with a superabundance of fresh air; suggestion, by means of electricity, drugs, warm or medicated baths, an electric vibrator to the back of the neck, etc. Only rarely is a dose of sodium bromid necessary, and a few drams of elixir of chloralamid or 5 grains of veronal may be used as succedanea—never morphin. If associated with high blood-pressure, look for toxemia, and if irritability, nervousness, emotionalism, rapid heart are present, search for hyperthyroidism. Three to 5 drops of Lugol's solution three times a day after meals may do more good than narcotics.

Sleepiness is a frequent symptom of early pregnancy and requires no treatment (Hypothyroidism?). Late in gestation it is always to be regarded with suspicion, as it may presage the advent of eclampsia. Mental dulness may mean the same.

Numbness and tingling of the hands and feet, usually combined with slight puffiness, not real edema, are the evidences of a mild neuritis, perhaps toxic in origin. Occasionally local anesthesia and tenderness of the corresponding nerves are discovered. While the symptom rarely has any disturbing sequels, it should be watched. Treatment is on the theory that it is due to toxemia. Neuralgias have already been considered. Milder symptoms of tetany are not very rare, e. g., cramps and spasms in the legs and arms, slight edema of legs, muscular weakness, trophic disturbances, see Tetany, p. 413.

Pain in the abdomen is frequently complained of. In the early months a careful bimanual examination is demanded to exclude ectopic gestation. Pain is a symptom of many conditions which have already been considered—appendicitis, ureteritis, pyelitis, cholelithiasis, adhesions, etc. Intercostal neuralgia is rare, the pain in the lower ribs from which so many women suffer being most often due to dragging on the thoracic cage by the recti muscles, which carry the weight of the large uterus. An abdominal supporter is indicated. Rheumatic pains also occur, and relief may be obtained from the use of a liniment of equal parts of Ol. gaultheriæ, Ol. camphoratæ, and Lin. saponis.

Most often the pain is due to constipation, with intestinal colic and flatulence. Pain associated with immense vulvar varicosities may be due to a similar condition of the broad ligaments. An abdominal binder and the occasional assumption of the knee-chest position will bring relief. Pain over the pubis and in the lower back, attended with difficulty of locomotion, is often due to softening and relaxation of the pelvic joints. This is possibly due to calcium deficiency and one may need to give calcium gluconate, viosterol, ultra-violet light treatments, etc. Relief may be given by a tight strap about the pelvis, worn over the corset. Backache and abdominal pains are often due to faulty shoes or sunken arches. An ortho-pedic study of the case will aid in treatment. Stretching of the skin and the formation of striæ gravidarum are sometimes painful. Relief may be obtained from lubricants, such as solid albolene, cocoa-butter, or rose-water ointment.

Fainting spells, dizziness, and attacks of weakness—if a thorough examination excludes organic disease of the heart, lungs, etc.—are treated symptomatically. Nervousness, hysteria, overeating, too nitrogenous diet, constipation, toxemia—all should be remembered. An iron and phosphorus tonic is often useful, but occa-sionally a small dose of digitalis does the most good. Fresh air is essential. Pal-pitation of the heart is relieved by a cold drink, but if frequently repeated and not due to organic disease, sodium bromid, 10 grains three times a day, may be given. Dyspnea is often due to unhygienic dress, indigestion, and the dragging of the uter-ine tumor on the chest. It may be toxemic, hemic, cardiac, or simply neurotic in origin.

Frequent urination is usually due, in the early months, to distraction of the base of the bladder; in the later months, to the restraint of the distention of the viscus by the large uterus, but a slight catarrh of the trigonum is not rare. The knee-chest position, a binder, and a week's treatment with urotropin and methy-lene-blue will often cure. Cloudy urine should not be present during normal preg-nancy. When it does occur, it is sometimes due to bacteriuria, and I have occasion-ally seen it precede albuminuria. Regulation of the diet, free drinking of butter-milk, and urinary antiseptics are indicated. Lack of control of the urine on making a sudden movement, as cough or a jar, is usually due to previous injury of the neck of the bladder, with cystocele or urethrocele. The knee-chest posture may help a little, but a cure cannot be effected during pregnancy. When a pregnant woman complains of urinary troubles, a careful bimanual examination and urinalysis are to be made at once.

Skin Eruptions.—Acne, mostly facial, may prove rebellious under treatment. The x-ray should not be used because the eruption disappears after labor. Wash-ing the parts with tincture of green soap, and opening the pustules with a fine lancet comprise the treatment. Urticaria is treated in the usual way. A lotion containing zinc carbonate, zinc oxide, āā 30 gm., menthol and phenol āā 1 gm. in 250 c.c. of aqua calcis is very useful for urticarial, papular, and all dry, itchy eruptions.

In addition to this a few hypodermics of Locke's solution (Oj) may be needed.

For the eczema intertrigo in the genital creases and under the breasts of fat women frequent ablution with tar-soap and water, followed by very careful drying and a dusting-powder of zinc stearate, will usually suffice. If these fail, starch and a small amount of salicylic acid may be added to the powder. Rarely, a salve con-taining boric acid, 2 per cent., carbolic acid, ½ per cent., zinc oxid and rose-water ointments, of each a sufficient quantity, will be necessary. If leukorrhea or myco-sis is present, proper treatment is needed. (See Vulvitis.)

Pityriasis versicolor, occurring principally on the chest, shoulders, and back, and due to the Microsporon furfur, is easily removed by frequent scrubbing with tar-soap and hot water, followed by washing with vinegar or 1 : 1500 bichlorid.

Edema of the extremities always commands attention, because, while many instances are due to stasis, the swelling disappearing when the woman lies down, most of them are toxemic or nephritic in origin.

CHAPTER XLIV

DISEASES OF THE OVUM

UNDER this heading will be considered, necessarily briefly, the diseases of the fetus, teratology, the pathology of the fetal adnexæ, the chorion, the amnion, and the umbilical cord.

The Fetus.—To J. W. Ballantyne is due the credit of having assembled our knowledge of the affections of the unborn child, and having really created a department of medicine—antenatal pathology.

Most of the acute infectious diseases of the mother have been demonstrated in the child, as has already been shown. Chronic infectious diseases, tuberculosis, and syphilis, the former rarely, the latter usually, pass over also. The fetus may

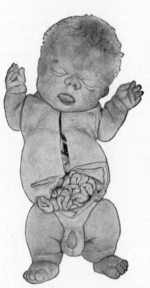

FIG. 459.—ACHONDROPLASIC **FETUS** (author's specimen).

become diabetic or toxemic from its mother, though leukemia has not yet been proved to affect it. Icterus of the mother sometimes does and sometimes does not discolor the child. Icterus from toxemic causes is very fatal to the fetus. Opium, alcohol, chloroform, ether, the iodids, methylene-blue, etc., pass over and affect the child. Methylene-blue given to the mother in the last week of pregnancy may be demonstrated in the urine and feces of the new-born for three days after birth. Most antitoxins go to the child through the placenta. Outside of these transmitted affections, the fetus has a pathology of its own. It will be impossible to do more than mention the best known maladies.

1. General fetal dropsy; fetal erythroblastosis (Schridde); cystic elephantiasis; congenital elephantiasis.

2. Congenital microcephalus, usually with idiocy; spastic spinal paralysis (Little's disease); chorea, Friedreich's ataxia, and other diseases of the nerves.

3. Ichthyosis, mild and severe; hypertrichosis; congenital absence of patches of skin, due probably to amniotic adhesions.

4. Diseases of the bones, which may be grouped under the general term "chondrodystrophia fœtalis," but are otherwise hardly to be classified. Some cases resemble rachitis; some show bone aplasia, hypoplasia, or irregular hyperplasia, usually associated with dysfunction of the hypophysis cerebri.

5. Abdominal affections: peritonitis, ascites (which may be a cause of serious dystocia), congenital stenosis of the bile-ducts, hypertrophic stenosis of the pylorus, and neoplasms of the liver.

6. Nephritis; congenital cystic kidneys (which show a familial tendency and may be so large as to cause obstruction to delivery); dilatation of the bladder, with hypertrophy.

7. Circulatory diseases: endocarditis, atheroma, goiter.

8. Congenital cataract, iritis, etc.

9. Congenital uterine prolapse and injuries to the child from without.

A minute study of these conditions would be well repaid, and probably would lead to the discovery of valuable remedies for the antenatal treatment of the diseases, or at least a recognition of some of the causes and the means of obviating their action.

The Death of the Mother.—Since the dying mother takes oxygen from the fetus, the death of the latter usually occurs first. If the mother dies suddenly, the child may live for a variable period. Brotherton reports a case where a living child was extracted twenty-three minutes after the death of the mother, and Tarnier one where the child lived twenty minutes after the death of its mother, who, while in the Maternité, was killed by a stray bullet during the Commune (Polk).

Rigor mortis may occur in utero (Fig. 460), and probably is common, though rarely observed and still more rarely published. It affects fetuses of all ages, be-

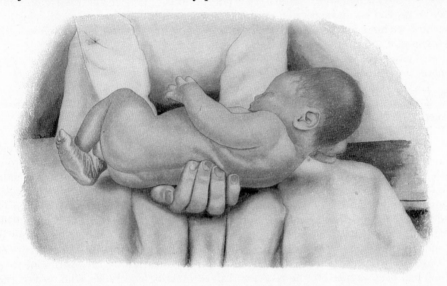

Fig. 460.—Rigor Mortis in Utero.
Child died as the result of pressure and prolonged delay during molding through a masculine pelvis. Delivery of the dead infant very laborious because of its rigidity.

gins from a few minutes to as late as five hours after fetal death, may be total or partial, and may cause difficulty in delivery. Its pathology is identical with that of rigor mortis of the adult and is due to the presence of lactic acid and colloid imbibition of the muscular fibers (Meigs). Curiously, the heart may beat a few times even after rigidity of the body has developed. Rigor mortis is found more frequently in cases of prolonged labor, eclampsia, hemorrhage, and slow asphyxia. It is not a sign that the child was delivered alive—a point of extreme importance in medicolegal cases. (See Paddock, Wolff.)

LITERATURE

Ballantyne: Antenatal Pathology and Hygiene, 1902, 2 vols.—*Brotherton:* Edinburgh Med. Jour., 1868.—*Meigs:* Amer. Jour. Physiology, 1910, p. 191.—*Paddock:* Amer. Jour. Obst., August, 1903. Literature.—*Polk:* Amer. Jour. Obst., 1885, vol. xviii, p. 1192.—*Schridde:* Ref. Jour. Amer. Assoc., May 1, 1915, p. 1506, and for Hydrops fetus see *Becker*, Zentb. für Gyn., October 24, 1925, p. 2409.—*Wolff:* Arch. f. Gyn., 1903, vol. lxviii, H. 3, pp. 549–575.

CHAPTER XLV

TERATOLOGY

For details of this subject the reader is referred to works on pathology. Only the barest outlines of classification and a few principles of treatment can here be given. (See Birnbaum, Schwalbe.)

Classification.—Congenital deformities are not rare. A child born with a deformity so marked that it interferes with the general or local development of the body is called a monster. Monsters often die in the early formative stage, which may be proved by an inspection of aborted ova, and, if delivered alive, they usually succumb within a few hours or days, being incapable of extra-uterine existence. The frequency of monsters in aborted ova is noteworthy.

Of monsters there are two classes—single and double. We distinguish three general varieties of single monsters (Gurlt):

1. Monstra per defectum—where all or part of an organ is missing.

2. Monstra per fabricam alienam—where an organ is wrongly formed or displaced.

3. Monstra per excessum—where an organ is enlarged or duplicated.

Causation.—Recent experimental work has done much to clear up the causation of monstrosities, and it is quite certain that external agencies have much to do with their formation. Heredity has indubitable influence, since we see the same peculiarity in several generations or members of the family. Sometimes a generation is skipped, and the deformity reappears in the third—atavism. We do not yet understand these internal causes, and for want of a better term they are called germinal, since they are inherent in the ovum. That the sperma has some influence in the production of monstrosities is rendered plausible by the experiments of Bardeen, who saw deformed ova result from fertilization by the sperma of toads which had been exposed to the x-ray, and those of Arlitt and Wells, who proved that repeated small doses of alcohol given to white mice produced abnormal spermatozoids and finally sterility. Levy describes monsters due to irregular distribution of the chromosomes.

Guyer and Smith produced rabbits with defective eyes by injecting the pregnant mother with the serum of fowls rendered immune by repeated injections of pulped rabbits' lenses—and the deformity was transmitted by male and female to subsequent generations!

Of external causes may be mentioned injury to the abdomen or uterus, short of the actual destruction of the fetus or ovulum; diseases of the uterus, perhaps gonorrhea; diseases of the chorion (Mall) and of the amnion; abnormal implantation of the ovum, for example, in the tube (Mall); arrest of development, and changes in the ovum during the blastula or morula stages, the result of thermic, chemical, or other physical action. It has been proved that lithium, sodium, potassium, and magnesium have a special selective action on the various cells of the morula, and produce characteristic monsters, some of the poisons affecting the nervous system and others the heart. Stockard and Lewis produced 50 per cent. of cyclopean monsters from the eggs of the common minnow by treating them with solutions of magnesium chlorid. Hertwig suggests that perhaps chemical poisons circulating in the maternal blood may affect the young embryo and cause monsters, a theory which the author has held for many years and which seems to gain some proof from the experiments of Werber. Nowadays few practitioners and none of the scientists believe the old notion that the mental state of the mother has a direct influence on the development of the child, but many careful observers are convinced that shock, worry, deprivation, etc., may produce vascular

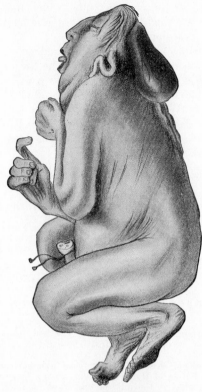

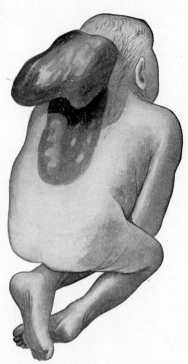

Fig. 461.—Craniorachischisis (Side).

Fig. 462.—Craniorachischisis (Rear View).

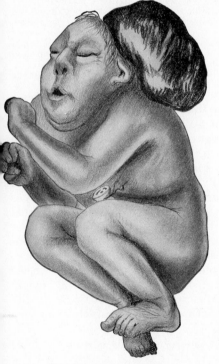

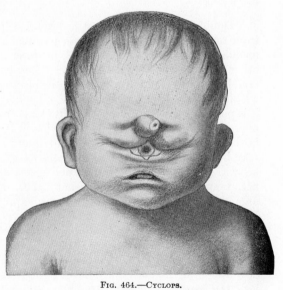

Fig. 463.—Exencephalus.

Fig. 464.—Cyclops.

These illustrations were all drawn from specimens of the Northwestern University, Medical Department.

and nutritional disturbances, general and local, in the endometrium, which may seriously affect the growth of the ovum, a position which the author has long held, and Ballantyne, one of our most authoritative teratologists, also holds.

Amniotic adhesions, formerly held responsible for many of the single monsters, Mall believes to be usually secondary, rather than primary. The author recently found a large staphylococcus in the fetal portion of the placenta from an anencephalic monster, with polyhydramnion. The rôle of syphilis in the production of monsters must again be emphasized. W. L. Williams (veterinary obstetrist) proves that monstrosities are more frequent in dairy cattle. They are unhealthy because housed, "civilized," and are also, of all domestic animals, the most subject to virulent infectious diseases. To be applied to humans?

Single Monsters.—1. *Monstra Per Defectum.*—The most common of single monsters are due to absence of closure of the medullary canal, which may be due to primary agenesis or aplasia of the medullary canal, to early hydrocephalus or hydrorachis, or to adhesion of the delicate, newly formed medullary canal to the amnion. The deformities resulting from this are grouped under the name "craniorachischisis." The splitting may be partial, either involving only the cerebral vertebræ, when we have cranioschisis, or only the spine—rachischisis. If all the structures covering the medullary canal are missing, the back presents a smooth, shining groove, with or without traces of brain or spinal cord (Figs. 461 and 462). If only the bony arch is missing, we have a meningocele, or hernia cerebri, hernia spinalis, or spina bifida.

When there is a mass of brain, more or less large, we call the condition *acrania;* when all the brain is missing, *anencephalus.* If the cranium is closed but smaller than normal, it is called *microcephalus.*

Irregularities in the closing of the branchial clefts produce deformities about the face and neck, the simplest of which are harelip, and the severest may show absence of large parts of the face.

The anomalies resulting from deficiency of closure of the lateral plates of the body walls are hernia umbilicalis, hernia abdominalis, ectopia vesicæ, ectopia cordis, etc. These are grouped under the name "thoracogastroschisis."

The splitting may go so far as to involve the intestine, showing that the two layers of the celom failed to fuse. Absence of fusion of the lateral halves of the genital and urinary organs produces deformities here of utmost variety. Hypospadias is the mildest and most common, ectopia vesicæ with split pelvis more marked, deformity.

Agenesis of the extremities, fusion of the extremities or of fingers and toes, and deformities due to amniotic bands occur, but are rare. If the anterior cerebral vesicle does not divide, we have a cyclops developed, or a *cyclocephalus.* Cyclops monsters are among the easiest to produce artificially (Fig. 464).

2. *Monstra per fabricam alienam* are mainly cases of situs inversus viscerum, abnormal position of the kidneys, testicle, colon, and sometimes of the joints, and congenital luxations and deformities. These latter are not seldom in the first class.

3. *Monstra Per Excessum.*—Increase in the number of a part or organ and increase in the size of same.

Double Monsters.—Monstra duplica come from one ovum, and are developed from one germinal vesicle. Two germinal spots, two primitive streaks, or two medullary grooves may be formed, or, later in growth, a duplication of one or the other end of the germinating zone takes place. Experiments have shown that double monsters can be produced in the blastula stage by separating the blastomeres, which is accomplished mechanically or chemically. If two embryonal areas appear, it is possible that two complete individuals (homologous twins), or, if the two areas are not entirely separated, united twins, will result. If the two areas are unequal in size, one of the individuals is stunted and attached as a parasite to the other, or may be included in the other. The etiology of such monstrous formations is unknown. Entrance of more than one spermatozoid into the ovum is not the cause, because eggs so impregnated usually die. Kohlbrügge has shown that in some animals the accessory spermatozoids supply food for the germinating ovum. Whether there is a splitting of one primitive streak or the fusion of two primarily developed is unknown—probably fission occurs. Double monsters are thus classified (Foerster).

Terata Anadidyma.—In these beings the fission or doubling is from the head downward, in the most fully developed specimens there being one pelvis and two legs, the trunks being separate (Figs. 465–469).

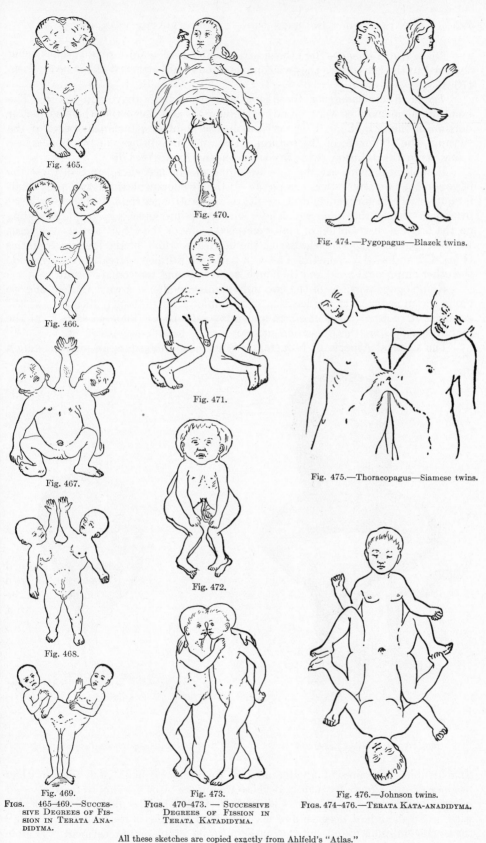

Fig. 465.

Fig. 466.

Fig. 467.

Fig. 468.

Fig. 469.

FIGS. 465–469.—SUCCESSIVE DEGREES OF FISSION IN TERATA ANADIDYMA.

Fig. 470.

Fig. 471.

Fig. 472.

Fig. 473.

FIGS. 470–473. — SUCCESSIVE DEGREES OF FISSION IN TERATA KATADIDYMA.

Fig. 474.—Pygopagus—Blazek twins.

Fig. 475.—Thoracopagus—Siamese twins.

Fig. 476.—Johnson twins.

FIGS. 474–476.—TERATA KATA-ANADIDYMA.

All these sketches are copied exactly from Ahlfeld's "Atlas."

Terata Katadidyma.—Here the splitting is from below upward, all grades being observed to the last, where the two complete bodies are attached at the head (Figs. 470–473).

Terata Kata-anadidyma, the fission being from both above and below. The bond of union may be very broad, extending up and down the whole venter or dorsum of the two children, or very small, the point of attachment being at the sternum, the abdomen, or the sacrum. Rotation may bring the two bodies into a line, as in the Johnson twins from Wisconsin (Figs. 474–476).

Homologous twins are the best examples of the last class, since in these the fission of the two streaks was complete. If the development of the two individuals is equal, two well-formed children result; if one is stronger than the other, its heart overcomes that of the other, which later shrinks up into an acardiacus. Depending on the original distribution of embryonal cells, one or the other portion of a fetus will be represented in the acardiacus, the head, the trunk, or the lower extremities (Figs. 477 and 478). Sometimes all or a part of a primitive streak develops inside the other embryonal area, and thus inclusio fœtalis and teratomata result.

Homologous portions of the two individuals are almost always united, and we name the monster after the location of the union; for example, when it is at the sternum, *sternopagus;* the ensiform appendix, *xiphopagus* (Siamese twins); at the sacrum, *pygopagus* (the Bohemian sisters); at the head, *craniopagus,* etc.

The Clinical Aspects of Monsters.—Since single monsters are more common

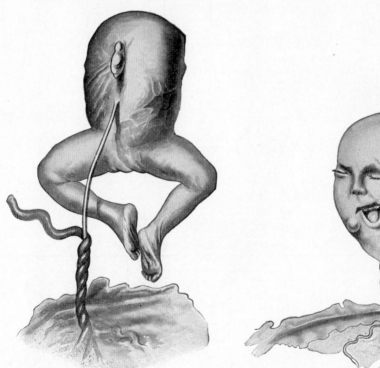

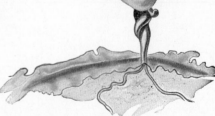

FIG. 477.—ACARDIACUS ACEPHALUS.   FIG. 478.—ACARDIACUS ACORMUS (Ahlfeld).

than double, they present greater interest to the accoucheur, and, further, they produce dystocia more frequently because they more often develop to maturity and because enlargement of the parts is so often met. Hydrocephalus, anencephalus with broad shoulders, hernias, and accumulation of fluid in the body cavities are the usual conditions found, but they present simple problems of treatment. Double monsters, curiously enough, are frequently expelled spontaneously, but when they do give rise to dystocia, dangerous and most complicated operations are often needed to effect delivery.

Diagnosis.—Even before labor one may suspect the existence of an abnormally formed child. Hydrocephalus could be diagnosed, and an acephalous monster too, if the examiner were on the alert. A woman who had delivered one of the latter was much relieved when, at the seventh month of a subsequent pregnancy, it was possible to assure her that the fetus had a large, well-formed head. Under the same circumstances the absence of a cranium would as easily have been determinable. The x-ray is now available. Since recurrence of monstrous children is not rare, the history is of service in the diagnosis.

During labor the possibility of a monstrous formation is to be considered, with other things, when the internal examination reveals atypical findings. Before attempting cesarean section it is wise to consider the shape of the child, as well as its size and viability, for it might be humiliating to deliver a monster by this serious operation. It has happened to clever accoucheurs. On the other hand, one would prefer cesarean section to delivery from below if the x-ray should prove the existence of a double monster. I make it a rule to x-ray twin pregnancies and all cases set for abdominal delivery unless the usual findings are unequivocal.

An anencephalic monster, as shown in Fig. 462, presenting by the head, might easily cause confusion with placenta prævia, prolapse of the cord, simple face presentation, or breech presentation. The frequent association of deformities will help in diagnosis; for example, when in a breech delivery a spina bifida is found, hydrocephalus may be expected, or if the delivered head shows harelip and delay in delivery of the trunk ensues, one should think of a monster, single or double. Polyhydramnion is so frequently present with fetal anomalies that one should always look for the latter when it exists.

Double monsters have never been diagnosed before labor; at most, twins have been suspected. Two bags of waters exclude a double monster. The rule has been that only after labor stopped was the obstruction recognized to be due to joined fetuses, but inspection of the part delivered may give a hint as to the cause of the delay, for example, harelip or atresia ani (Lyell). If delay in delivery, not overcome by the usual manipulations, should occur, an examination with the half hand or, if necessary, with the whole hand, is to be made. For the sake of deliberation and thoroughness an anesthetic had best be given, and in primiparæ a deep episiotomy is advisable. Such an exploration must decide the presence of enlargement of a part of the fetus, a tumor of the uterus or the fetus, a double monster, and, if the last, the location and extent of the area of fusion, the number of arms and legs, and the movability of one child on the other.

Treatment.—*Prevention.*—Can anything be done to prevent a recurrence of the delivery of a monster? Syphilis can be treated; if the uterus is diseased (*e. g.*, endometritis), one may try to cure it. In two instances where this question was put to me, the patients having had anencephalous monsters before, I prescribed a hygienic life for both parents before the impregnating coitus, quiet for the mother in the early months, and a pill, to be taken throughout pregnancy, containing carbonate of iron, gr. 3; hydrargyri iodidi rubri, gr. $\frac{1}{20}$; arsenous acid, gr. $\frac{1}{60}$; t. i. d. Both women had healthy children. One patient also received calcium lactate. On the theory that monsters are caused by dysfunction of the endocrines one may try thyroid, corpus luteum, and hypophysis, but these are wholly unscientific recommendations. Experience with breeding animals in captivity would advise a selected diet, generous in vitamins, calcium, phosphorus, etc.

Nature helps in the delivery of monsters by interrupting the pregnancy while the fetuses are still small, but cases are on record of united twins weighing 15 and 17½ pounds, causing formidable dystocia. In general, breech presentation is most favorable for all monstrosities, and if duplicate, it is best if all three or four legs are accessible. Single monsters with enlargement of parts are to be reduced in size; a hydrocephalus is punctured (never forceps); a full abdomen is emptied, etc., and if delivery is indicated, version and extraction are preferable. No consideration is to be shown either a single or a double monster when the mother's life is in danger. Since the necessary mortality in labor and afterward is enormous, all our efforts should be directed to saving the mother. Experience has shown that it is best to deliver the children whole, and not to amputate a head or trunk which has been expelled. It may be necessary to amputate the delivered portion in order to gain access to the rest or to render the balance of the mass movable, but such occasions are rare.

38

Extremities should not be removed, because they do not interfere with our manipulations; further, they provide a grasp on the locked-in fetuses, and, thirdly, their removal destroys the relations of one twin to the other and adds complications in the diagnosis and treatment. Cesarean section may be necessary if attempts at delivery from below fail, but it has very rarely been done—indeed, the patients, when they come to this point, are the poorest possible subjects for abdominal delivery. Contracted pelvis, as a complication, would, of course, indicate it, and, too, if a double monster were recognized at a time when an abdominal operation could be performed under ideal conditions—an occurrence not yet on record.

For clinical purposes the various double monsters may be divided into three forms, as follows (Veit):

1. Those which offer obstacle to delivery by the increase of the size of the body at one or the other end; for example, diprosopus, cephalothoracopagus, dipygus parasiticus—such as an epignathus. Most of these monsters belong to the classes terata anadidyma and terata katadidyma (Figs. 465 to 473).

2. Those monsters where fusion is at one or the other end, the two having a tendency to form a straight trunk—ischiopagus, pygopagus, craniopagus.

3. Where the monsters are well formed and have freedom of motion at the point of fusion, for example, thoracopagus, xiphopagus, or where there are two or three heads, well developed, on one trunk.

In the first class, if the two heads present and engage, one after the other is delivered by forceps; if not engaged, version is performed, then exenteration and craniotomy in succession, if necessary. If one head is delivered and the shoulders do not come, the delivered head may have to be amputated, by which access is gained to the double trunk. The second head is led into the pelvis, delivered, and then the double trunk reduced in size by cleidotomy and exenteration. If the duplicity is caudal, all four extremities are to be delivered at one time, and evisceration of the trunks performed, after which the extraction of the common shoulders and head is simple.

The second class of monsters, united by the head or breech, seldom causes trouble, the long, sausage-shaped trunk slipping through with no difficulty. Root and Bartlett, of Chicago, found an ischiopagus, bent like the letter U, with the two fused breeches presenting. The junction was severed and delivery quickly effected, one fetus at a time.

Of the third class of cases, the Siamese twins are a good example. One of these was delivered by the head, the other by the breech. The connecting band may be so elastic as to allow version of the second twin after the delivery of the first. It is fortunate if the two children present by the breech, and the posterior one should be delivered first, then the anterior child. If the bond of union is firmer, by unequal traction the head of the posterior fetus is to be drawn into the neck of the anterior and both delivered together. Exenteration will be done or the bond of union severed whenever necessary. If one child presenting by the head is delivered to the trunk and labor stops, the other may be turned by the breech and the two then delivered side by side. If two heads present and neither engages, version on both twins is performed.

As a rule, the operator is not required to hurry, but may proceed with calmness and deliberation. He should study carefully the kind of monster he has to deal with, its size, the shape and size of the pelvis, etc., and have the proposed procedures completely worked out before operating.

Overgrowth of the child will be considered under the Pathology of Labor.

LITERATURE

Arlitt and Wells: Ref. Jour. Amer. Med. Assoc., December 22, 1917, p. 2149.—*Ballantyne:* Antenatal Pathology, 1904, vol. ii.—*Birnbaum:* Klinik der Missbildungen, Berlin, 1909, Springer.—*Guyer and Smith:* Editorial, Jour. Amer. Med. Assoc., 1920, November 13, p. 1346.—*Hertwig:* Gegenbauer's Festschrift, 1896, vol. ii.—*Levy:* Zeitschr. f. Geb. u. Gyn., 1922, vol. lxxxiv, Heft 1, p. 276.—*Mall, Franklin P.:* Jour. Morph., February, 1908, vol. xix, pp. 3, 368. Full literature.—*Schwalbe:* Die Morphologie d. Missbildungen des Menschen, Jena, p. ii, 1907.—*Stockard and Lewis:* Jour. Amer. Med. Assoc., March 6, 1909. Gives literature of monsters.—*Werber:* Bull. Johns Hopkins Hosp., June, 1915.—*Williams, W. L.:* Cornell Veterinarian, January, 1931.

CHAPTER XLVI

DISEASES OF THE FETAL ENVELOPS

THE CHORION

CLINICALLY, myxoma diffusum and fibrosum, which pathologists describe, are of little importance, but vesicular degeneration of the chorion is not uncommon, and requires the earnest attention of the accoucheur. Hydatidiform or vesicular degeneration of the chorion, vesicular mole, or grape-mole, is due to a proliferation and degeneration, with edema, of the stroma of the chorionic villi and increase of the syncytium. (See Caturani, Turazza.)

Kossman showed that Hippocrates knew of this condition, and ascribed it to a mucoid degeneration of the villi, a theory which Virchow propounded and which was generally accepted until the minute and convincing work of Marchand and Fränkel was published. Aëtius of Amida, in the sixth century, described it, and Vega, in 1564, and Valleriola, in Turin, in 1573, reported typical cases. The latter believed the disease to be due to abnormal development of the, at that time, described "female semen." The vesicles were considered "bladder worms," "pseudohelminths," or Acephalocystis racemosa (Cloquet, 1822). Velpeau (1827) called the cysts degenerated villi, as we now know them to be; Meckel (1847) showed the hyperplasia of the connective tissue with edema, and Virchow (1853) called it a mucoid or myxomatous degeneration.

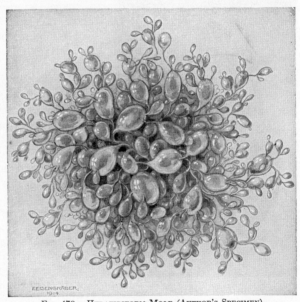

FIG. 479.—HYDATIDIFORM MOLE (AUTHOR'S SPECIMEN).

A **hydatidiform mole** cannot be mistaken (Fig. 479). It resembles a bunch of Catawba grapes of most irregular size, varying from that of a pin-head to that of a hen's egg (rare), but usually the size of a pea or bean. A loose mass of thick decidua, and cheesy cellular material with blood-clots interspersed with these bladder-like bodies, is usually delivered, but the specimen may be a compact, egg-shaped cast of the uterus, fibrous, and filled with vesicles. In these cases the growth had ceased some time prior to expulsion. The vesicles hang to parent stems and to each other (Fig. 480). Ordinarily, all traces of fetus and amnion have disappeared, but cases are on record where both have been preserved, and then the mass may be expelled entire and be covered by decidua. All the chorion may be changed, which is the usual finding, and means that the degeneration began early in gestation, but either the chorion frondosum or the chorion læve may be alone affected. Even parts of the placenta may be intact, and a living child may be born, or only one ovum of a twin pregnancy may be thus degenerated, as in the case of the famous anatomist, Béclard, whose mother, at the fifth month of gestation, expelled hydatids (Parvin). The case of Depaul was similar. Ectopic gestation may undergo this form of degeneration. It is not certain whether the degeneration precedes the death of the child or follows it—

probably both occur.   The author has frequently found, in aborted ova, one or more villi degenerated and forming vesicles.

Microscopically, the stroma of the villi is hyperplastic, and has become edematous and necrotic, so that only at the periphery of the vesicles can the fibrillary structures and cells be distinguished (Fig. 481).   Very few vessels can be found, and these are empty.   Particularly marked is the proliferation of Langhans' layer, which may invade the syncytium and grow into the intervillous spaces.   Its cells are enlarged and degenerated, staining badly.   The syncytium also hypertrophies and undergoes necrosis, it, as well as Langhans' layer, showing numerous vacuoles. This process may be so marked that the syncytium may grow through the decidua into the uterine musculature.   Even the vesicles may burrow into the veins and between the muscle-fibers, sometimes as far as into the peritoneal cavity, causing peritonitis and peritoneal hemorrhage.   If the uterine wall is honey-combed by the advancing growth of the proliferating villi, it may rupture during the process of abortion, or be punctured by the finger or instruments, or the woman may die of external hemorrhage because the diseased uterus cannot contract properly.   These forms are called destructive moles, and clinically are much feared.

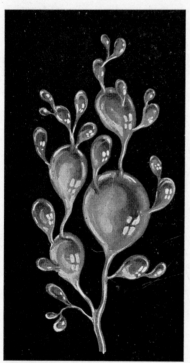

FIG. 480.—DETAIL OF HYDATIDIFORM MOLE.

Special mention is to be made of those destructive hydatidiform moles which eventuate in chorio-epithelioma or malignant syncytioma.   Meckel, before 1795, recorded an instance of grape-mole which resulted in the woman's death by metastases of a tumor formed in the uterus, and recently it has been found that a history of cystic mole is obtained in over half of the cases of syncytioma malignum which come to treatment.

The syncytioma may develop in the uterus, in the cervix, or in the vagina (local metastases), or, if the vesicles and masses of syncytium are carried by the blood-stream to distant organs, a general syncytiomatosis may ensue, but usually the lungs are first and most involved.   Local and general metastases may occur while the grape-mole is still in the uterus.   Since so many cases of chorio epithelioma malignum give a history of mole, one might think that the hydatidiform degeneration of the chorion was very frequently the cause, but it must be remembered that grape-mole is not very infrequent, and that a case of syncytioma will almost always be published, while the mole, being so much more common, is not.   For example, the author had 23 cases of vesicular mole, not published, and none, as far as known, has developed metastases.   König's 12, Giglio's 13, and Kehrer's 50, followed up, did not develop chorio-epithelioma. Unfortunately, it is impossible to determine when a given mole will become malignant.

A *polycystic degeneration of the ovaries* has, in a large proportion of cases, been found coincident with this condition, an observation made by de Gregorini in 1795. Both ovaries may be changed into tumors as large as a fist, composed of immensely proliferated and sometimes edematous ovarian stroma, full of cysts which vary in size from a few millimeters to 6 cm., and which are lined or partly filled by a variegated layer of lutein cells, that is, the ovaries are changed into lutein cysts.

While the two conditions are often associated, we cannot draw a causal connection between them nor can we explain their frequent coincidence.

Etiology.—Multiparæ are oftener affected than primiparæ. Such moles have been found in women fifty-two and fifty-three years of age, indeed, the frequency of their occurrence after thirty-five is remarkable when we consider the smaller

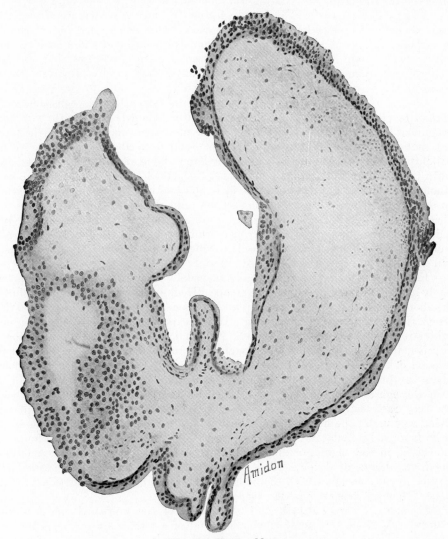

FIG. 481.—HYDATID MOLE.
Compare with normal placenta, p. 39.

number of births at this period. Molitor records the birth of a vesicular mole in a girl nine years old. Syphilis, heart disease, and general affections have no direct bearing, but the association with nephritis has often been noted. The actual exciting cause of the degeneration is unknown, and probably several exist. It is possible that the ovum is primarily diseased, because cases are on record of one twin being healthy, the other changed into a vesicular mole, and secondly, aborted ova often show a mild hydropic disease not enough to cause the death of the fetus, and probably secondary to the latter. The ovarian lutein cysts have been used as an argument for the theory of the ovular origin of the mole; a notion which may be supported by the not infrequent finding of several corpora lutea in the ovaries. Abnormal secretion from a diseased corpus luteum producing a diseased ovum is suggested by Fränkel and I might add the possibility of dyspituitarism. That the change is the result of maternal influences, and especially an endometritis, was believed by Virchow and supported by Waldeyer, Veit, and Aichel. The latter exposed the uteri of pregnant dogs, injured the placental site by pressure, and observed the formation of hydatidiform mole in 7 of 13 experiments.

Diseased decidua is usually found with moles, and the recurrence of the affection also points to the endometrium as the cause. One woman had vesicular moles in 11 pregnancies and another in 4, while the latter's husband had a healthy child by another woman. Probably endometritis will explain most cases, and we know that the nutritional conditions of the placental site are vitally important to the health of the ovum. (See Marchand, Hoerman.)

Clinical Course.—Enlargement of the uterus faster than is consistent with normal pregnancy, and atypical, irregular, uterine hemorrhages, are the two most prominent symptoms. Serous or sanguineous discharges may persist in the interval, and exceptionally hemorrhage may not occur until abortion begins. All my patients were ill, complaining of pain in the lower abdomen, general weakness, and, when the floodings were profuse, showing the effects of anemia. Two women were albuminuric and edematous up to the hips, and two had hyperemesis gravidarum. In one case, during the therapeutic abortion, undertaken for the cure of the pernicious vomiting, the vesicular mole was discovered, no bleedings having preceded. All my other cases except one terminated in abortion before the sixth month, and in the one the mole ceased growing and was expelled at term. Depaul and Madden had cases which went over term.

Expulsion of the vesicular masses is usually complete when once started; rarely does only one vesicle or cluster escape. Hemorrhage is always marked during the abortion unless growth has ceased and the mass has become shrunken and dry. Death from acute anemia is not rare. In my experience the blood has been of a lighter red than normally and showed less tendency to clot. Uterine action is sluggish, the abortion sometimes dragging on for days, and contraction and retraction of the organ unsatisfactory after it is once emptied. Destructive moles, where the proliferating syncytium and vesicles burrow into the uterine wall, or even through it into the peritoneal cavity, causing intraperitoneal hemorrhage, are very rare, but the possibility of a weakened, honey-combed musculature giving way under the finger or curet is always to be borne in mind. Sepsis seems to be favored by hydatidiform mole. Occasionally purplish tumors are found on the cervix, in the vagina, or about the vulva, which on section show syncytium, blood, and degenerated villi. These usually occur after the uterus is emptied, but may be found coincident with the mole, and are probably local syncytioma metastases. They are generally benign (*vide infra*).

Diagnosis.—Rapid growth and globularity of the uterus, atypical uterine hemorrhages, absence of fetal movements and of a fetal body on palpation and *x*-ray, with or without lipiodol in the uterus (Bortini), a soft, elastic, not doughy, feel of the uterus, irregular contractions, albuminuria, edema, and the general evidences of illness allow the accoucheur to make a strong assumption of the presence of a vesicular mole. Rarely does a piece of it escape, but here the diagnosis would be positive, and the same may be said if the mole is felt through the cervix. A vaginal metastasis will indicate a mole in the uterus. The Aschheim-Zondek test is stronger than normal, except in moles carried many months in the uterus (Bleuler). In the differential diagnosis polyhydramnion might be considered when the distention of the uterus is acute and great, and grape-like sarcoma of the cervix if part of the tumor should hang out of the uterus. In two of my cases the uterus got smaller, not larger, before the mole was expelled.

Prognosis.—In very rare instances is the child viable, which means that only part of the chorion is involved. The rule is that the fetus dies early and is absorbed.

Combining the statistics of Dorland and Gerson, Hirtzman, and Williamson we find a maternal mortality of 19 per cent. One of my 23 cases died from acute sepsis. The dangers are uncontrollable hemorrhage, perforation of the uterus (spontaneous and instrumental), infection, which is quite common, and the development of syncytioma malignum.

Treatment.—As soon as the diagnosis is made the uterus must be emptied. Dilatation of the cervix sufficient to admit two fingers is necessary, and should be obtained by cervical tamponade with gauze or a small colpeurynter. (See Chapter LXIX.) A firm vaginal pack of sterile cotton should be inserted as a safeguard against hemorrhage while the os is being dilated. At the time of operation all preparations should have been made for hemorrhage and the treatment of anemia. Curets and placenta forceps should never be used because of the danger of perforating the uterus whose walls may have been weakened by a destructive growth. Even the fingers may perforate the thinned uterus, all of which should warn to caution, yet every safe effort is to be made to remove all the masses, thus to eliminate the danger of the development of a neoplasm and of sepsis. As in placenta prævia, blood must

be spared at every move and the uterus firmly tamponed if it shows a tendency to relax and bleed. Findley advises curetment after several weeks to assure the cure, but this is seldom feasible. Certainly the woman is to be kept under close observation for two years, and the uterus removed if signs of a malignant tumor develop in it. A negative Aschheim-Zondek reaction is proof that neither hydatids are retained nor a chorio-epithelioma developing. It is claimed that chorio-epithelioma develops in $7\frac{1}{2}$ to 33 per cent. of cases of hydatid mole (Frankl), but these figures are useless in making a

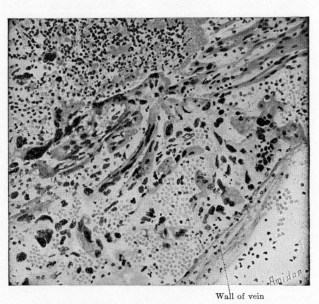

Wall of vein

FIG. 482.—CHORIO-EPITHELIOMA—MASS OF SYNCYTIUM IN A VEIN.

prognosis, as the vast majority of cases of hydatid mole are not reported, and chorio-epitheliomata usually are. Essen-Möller believes that chorio-epithelioma follows hydatid mole more frequently after the age of forty years, and, therefore, asks if the removal of the uterus, useless at this time, would not be the best treatment.

Chorio-epithelioma.—Sänger in 1889 described the case of a woman who died from metastatic tumors seven months after an abortion. The large cells found, he thought, were decidual, and he, therefore, called the tumor sarcoma deciduocellulare. Since then over 400 cases have been reported, and a mass of literature on the subject has accumulated. Only recently have our ideas regarding the nature of the affection crystallized, and the confusion which existed may be appreciated after a glance at the names which have been suggested for it—sarcoma deciduocellulare, carcinoma syncytiale, deciduoma malignum, blastomo-deciduo-chorion-cellulare, syncytioma malignum, invasive placental polyp, chorion epithelioma. Marchand's views of the nature of the tumor are now generally accepted, and the name Fränkel and Pick proposed, chorio-epithelioma, is the one most employed.   Fränkel first called attention to the chorio-epithelial nature of the growth.   (See Veit, Frank, Ewing, Sunde, Novak.)

Chorio-epithelioma is a tumor developed from the fetal ectoderm, which may begin during pregnancy (normal or abnormal) or after the uterus is emptied, and which is characterized by exuberant growth, early and extensive local and general metastases, and rapid cachexia, often combined with sepsis.

Its causation is unknown.   We know that syncytium has invasive power, that the villi erode their way into the uterine wall, into the blood-vessels, but what keeps this power in normal limits and what permits the growth of the cells to pass all bounds cannot even be conjectured.   Hydatidiform mole preceded the development of this disease in 33 to 44 per cent. of reported cases, which shows that some connection exists between the two (Fränkl).

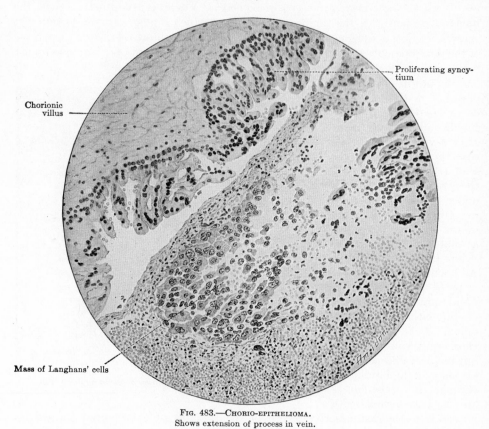

FIG. 483.—CHORIO-EPITHELIOMA.
Shows extension of process in vein.

Pathology.—The growth begins at the placental site and protrudes into the uterus as a very vascular, soft, purplish mass, usually sharply differentiated from the mucosa.   It may grow through the uterine wall and make tumors which project into the peritoneal cavity or the broad ligaments.   More often the veins are invaded, and thus general metastases brought about.   Vaginal metastases—the most frequent—are probably local, from surface implantation.   In appearance such a nodule resembles a hematoma.

Microscopically, the tumor is made up of masses of syncytium and proliferated Langhans' cells, which often form blood-spaces, and even structures which resemble villi.   Round-cells and polynuclear leukocytes abound; the whole tumor is very bloody.   Masses of syncytium may be seen advancing in the veins, and if hydatidiform mole was present, hydropsically degenerated villi may be found.   Marchand distinguished an atypical and a typical variety, both equally pathogenic, but in the latter the tumor cells resembled exactly the chorionic cells of early pregnancy. The syncytium, with its large, irregularly shaped masses of protoplasm, with sharply staining nuclei, is especially well represented, but Langhans' cells are also present. In the atypical varieties, which more resemble sarcomata, there is a more diffuse infiltration of the tissue by closely packed, deeply staining, irregularly shaped cells, with large nuclei, which may form clumps resembling syncytium, and are probably altered Langhans' cells (Fig. 483). Sometimes one kind of cells predominate and again the other. Combined forms exist. Lutein cysts of the ovaries develop in a large proportion of the cases of syncytioma, as in vesicular mole.

Curiously enough, malignant chorio-epithelioma with all its characteristics, even with structures resembling villi, has been found to arise from teratomata of the testicle. It probably originates from fetal ectoderm, included in the congenital teratoma.

Clinical Course.—After an abortion, especially of a vesicular mole, or after labor, the patient complains of irregular uterine hemorrhages. Usually a curetage is performed, but, since the masses thus obtained resemble placental tissue, a microscopic examination is often omitted. In half of the cases a vulvar or vaginal nodule first drew attention to the condition, and in my case the uterus enlarged enough to be felt by the patient. The growth may be found during pregnancy,

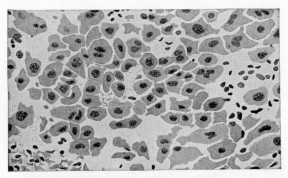

FIG. 484.—CHORIO-EPITHELIOMA.
Mass of Langhans' cells resembling decidua.

before expulsion of the mole, as early as a week after delivery (Williams' case), but usually several months later, and in three cases, two, three and one-half, and four and one-half years after delivery (Krösing), at a time when the causal gestation had been almost forgotten. Repeated hemorrhages rapidly exhaust the woman, weakness and the symptoms of anemia become pronounced, pallor, subicterus, albuminuria, edema of the feet, and puffiness of the eyes, that is, the signs of cachexia, supervene, and very often, since the tumor masses in the uterus possess such a tendency to necrosis, a vaginal discharge with gangrenous odor and general septicemia with fever occur. Metastases in the lungs may be diagnosed when cough, bloody expectoration, and pulmonary findings are present. Examination of the sputum has thus far been negative. Metastases occur in the lungs, vagina, liver, spleen, and brain. Vaginal tumors may eat into the bladder, like cancer.

Prognosis.—Later writers distinguish a less malignant type of chorio-epithelioma, one that disappears spontaneously or after the removal of the vaginal metastases and uterine curetage. As a rule, however, unless early operation is performed, these patients die within a year after the first appearance of the neoplasm. This is the most rapidly destructive growth with which we have to deal.

Death occurs from intractable hemorrhage, cachexia, infection, septicemia, and occasionally from hemorrhage into the peritoneal cavity or peritonitis, both the result of perforation of the uterus by the invading tumor.

Diagnosis.—Repeated hemorrhages after abortion are usually due to a placental polyp. Curetage is indicated, and the scrapings should be studied by a competent pathologist. Recurrence of a uterine growth after successful curetage for removal of the products of gestation is often due to chorio-epithelioma. A vaginal metastasis will usually, but not always, indicate the cause of the symptoms. Removal of part of the tumor and its microscopic study are essential for positive diagnosis, which an expert pathologist can readily make. At some point in the section the characteristic syncytial formations will be found. In the differential diagnosis fibroids, other neoplasms, and pelvic exudates must be considered. The Aschheim-Zondek test remains positive as long as relics of chorio-epithelioma persist in the body, which is true also of the male (Hady).

Treatment.—In view of the treacherous nature of the disease and its enormous mortality, radical extirpation of the uterus, adnexa, and accessible metastases is indicated. Since it is propagated along the veins, it is well to ligate the vessels as far outward as possible. Radium and the x-ray are yet on trial.

DISEASES OF THE PLACENTA

Variations in Shape.—Variations from the typical round shape of the placenta are common, and generally have no practical significance. (See p. 50.) These variations are due to irregularities in the nutritional conditions of the uterus. A placenta nested in the horn of the uterus is likely to be round and show a marginal ring. One near the os may encircle the orifice in a horseshoe form. One attached at the side of the uterus may spread on both anterior and

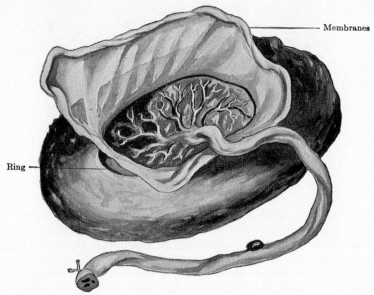

FIG. 485.—PLACENTA CIRCUMVALLATA (Northwestern University Medical School Museum).

posterior walls and be bilobate, etc. Without doubt the placenta may be bisected or trisected by white infarct formations, and I believe this is the commonest cause of irregular shapes.

Placentæ and placentulæ succenturiatæ, already mentioned, have great importance for they may be left in the uterus and give rise to hemorrhage and sepsis. They are supposed to be due to— (1) The development of some of the villi of the chorion læve; (2) to cutting off of a portion of the placenta by white infarcts; (3) to development of villi in the decidua vera with missing reflexa. Placenta membranacea, which is normal in the pachydermata, has, in excessively rare instances, been observed in the human—nearly the whole of the envelop of the egg was converted into thin, membranous placental tissue. Moderate degrees, that is, extensive thin placentæ, are occasionally observed, but are usually due to infarct formation. The thickness of the placenta is in inverse proportion to its size.

Heart disease, nephritis, anemia, diseases of the uterus, favor abnormal development of the placenta, and also make pathologic changes in the uterine musculature, such as hyaline degeneration, which in turn causes atonia uteri, even rupture, etc.

Infarcts.—Nearly every placenta will show, on careful inspection, whitish, nodular, hard areas, occupying the fetal or maternal surface, or both; and varying in size from a pin-head to several centimeters. Other names for these formations are hepatization, scirrhus, placentitis, apoplexy, cirrhosis, and phthisis. These structures are called *infarcts*, and several varieties are found, having different causation, though little is positively known on this point. Montgomery calls them necroses. The different kinds will be considered in the order of their frequency.

1. At the edge of the placenta, at the site of the subchorial decidua, a more or less complete white ring is found, which varies in width from 2 to 16 mm., and in thickness from 1 to 4 mm. This is called *placenta marginata*.

Sometimes the ring is raised from the surface and the attached membranes are doubled back over the edge of the placenta, as in Fig. 485. This is called *placenta circumvallata* or *nappiformis*. There are many views as to the manner of

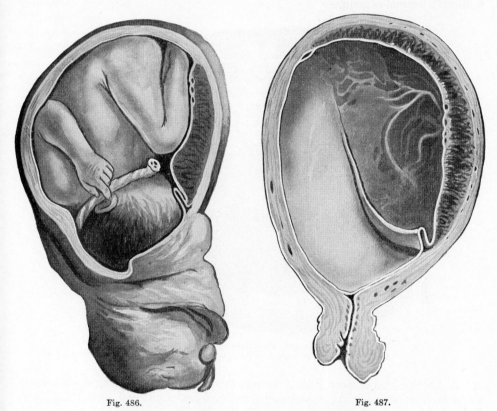

Fig. 486. Fig. 487.

FIGS. 486 AND 487.—PLACENTA CIRCUMVALLATA IN FORMATION.
Shows development of the fold in membranes (from Bumm).

production of this anomaly: (*a*) The placenta is located in a tubal corner of the uterus, or over the internal os, and the area of the placental site grows more rapidly than the rest of the uterus, the latter constricting the former at their junction (Fig. 485). (*b*) Owing to inflammatory changes in the decidua, the closing ring of Waldeyer and the decidua subchorialis, whose nutrition is precarious, become necrotic, and temporarily hinder the splitting of the decidua and the growth of the placenta in this direction. (*c*) Endometritis causes early adhesion of the reflexa to the vera, and changes at the site of the closing ring of Waldeyer prevent the growth of the placenta in the marginal reflexa, the placenta, therefore, splitting the vera. We sometimes find that the cotyledons extend 1½ inches beyond the insertion of the membranes (v. Herff). (*d*) Hitschman believes that, as the result of a sudden diminution of the liquor amnii, the coverings of the ovum must shrink, and naturally there would be an infolding at the edge of the placenta (Figs. 486 and 487) (Funck, Sfameni). (*e*) There is primary deep imbedment of the ovum (Lahm). (*f*) Williams believes there is too scanty original development of the chorion frondosum, and considers it only a developmental anomaly.

Placentæ marginatæ and circumvallatæ have some clinical importance. Tubal corner placentas might be called a distinct clinical entity, causing pain, bleeding, abortion, premature labor, puny children, postpartum hemorrhage, and difficulties in diagnosis. (See Angular Pregnancy, p. 431.) In placenta marginata adhesion of the membranes may occur, and the placenta may be delivered naked or decrowned of its membranes. As the result of this retention hemorrhage and sapremic fever sometimes ensue. Abnormal mechanism in the third stage, with retention or adhesion of the after-birth, requires the introduction of the hand in the uterus oftener than with normal placentas.

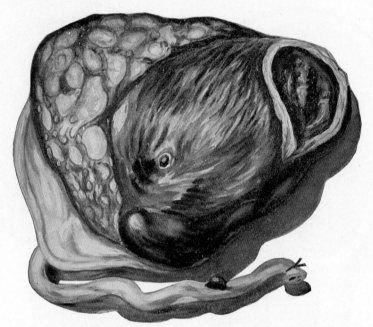

FIG. 488.—PLACENTA FROM CASE OF SEVERE NEPHRITIS.
On the left, masses of infarcts, on the right, an immense hemorrhage.

2. On the fetal surface of the placenta we find nodular infarcts, which vary in size from those scarcely visible to the eye, to 3 to 5 cm. across and up to 1 cm. thick. The smaller ones preponderate and may be bunched, or there may be a thin, nodular layer of fibrin which covers a good part of the fetal surface.

3. Some infarcts take in the whole thickness of a cotyledon and may involve one or more of them. In Fig. 488, which came from a nephritic, nearly one-half of the placenta was involved in infarct formations in various stages of development. Such a condition may compromise the nutrition of the child, which is born weak and puny, or if, as often happens in Bright's disease, more than half of the area is involved, the child will die. Such placentas are likely to be prematurely detached (abruptio), and Fig. 402 shows a hemorrhage causing a separation. This last form of infarct bears the most resemblance to the Cohnheim infarct; the other two can hardly be called thus, though Ackerman gave them the title "white infarcts." Clemenz believes they should be called "white necroses."

In general there are three views as to their causation. Ackerman believed a peri-arteritis or endarteritis existed in the villi and produced obliteration of the vessel lumen, with consecutive necrosis of the villus' stroma, then of the villus' wall, and consequent clotting of the blood in the adjoining intervillous spaces. Steffeck, von Franquè, and many investigators believe that endometritis and decidual overgrowth and consequent necrosis of the villi with fibrin deposition are the cause. Primary alteration or desquamation of the chorionic epithelium, which is not abnormal in the last weeks, causes deposition of fibrin and infarct formation, according to Hitschman. It is probable that there is truth in all these theories, and that the first explains the multiple infarcts on the fetal surface; the second, the infarcts on the maternal side and placenta marginata; the third, the microscopic infarcts made up of necrotic ectodermal cells which are constantly found in ripe placentas. Perhaps the general vascular changes of nephritis are also present in the newly formed placental blood-vessels, and, through endarteritis,

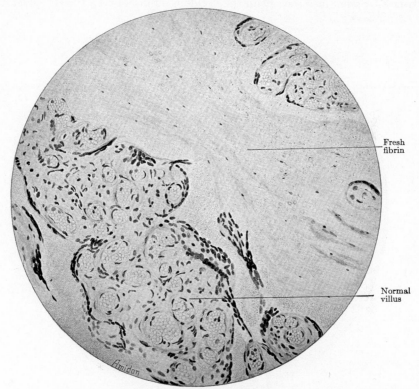

Fresh
fibrin

Normal
villus

FIG. 489.—PLACENTAL INFARCT. YOUNG.

obliterate their lumen, causing infarcts and hemorrhages, and, finally, the typical albuminuric placenta. May not these infarcts be one expression of a toxemia? The author in one case found a large staphylococcus in the infarct and Talbot tries to establish a relation between focal infections and infarction. Browne has experimentally produced placental infarcts and abruptio placentæ by intravenous injection of oxalates and coliform bacteria.

Microscopically, we find circumscribed areas of placental tissue which have undergone coagulation necrosis (Figs. 489 and 490). In the advanced stages the whole mass is changed into fibrin with only traces of the previously existing villi. Sometimes there are evidences of obliterating endarteritis and peri-arteritis, and, when endometritis existed, large numbers of decidual cells undergoing necrosis and even small-cell infiltration, which may affect the villi, will be found.

Clinically, infarcts cannot be diagnosed, but their existence can be expected in cases of nephritis, heart disease, syphilis, endometritis, and when they were present in previous pregnancies. Mention has been made of the fact that those infarcts which take in one or several cotyledons, may reduce the oxygenating area of the fetus, and also the nutritional functions of the placenta, so that the child is puny or even starved to death. Cognizance is taken of this fact in deciding on the induction of premature labor in nephritis. Extensive infarct formation is often associated with adherent membranes and the retention in the uterus of masses of thick decidua, which often give rise to annoying oozing after the third stage of labor, and even severe postpartum hemorrhage (Lit., Siddall, and Hartman).

Hemorrhages.—No structure in the body possesses blood-vessels as friable as those of the decidua, and as a result hemorrhages are not rarely found in it. These are almost always in the serotina, and produce a varying degree of separation of the placenta. Sometimes they lie in the decidual septa between the cotyledons. (It is

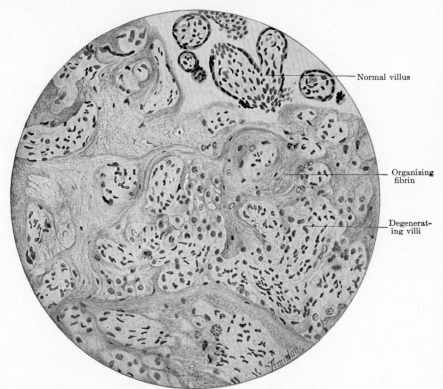

FIG. 490.—PLACENTAL INFARCT. ADVANCED.

not probable that these septa are of fetal origin.) In the latter instance they impose as intraplacental hemorrhages. It is not clear to the author how bleeding can take place into the intervillous spaces. They are blood sinuses and communicate freely with each other, so that a sudden increase of arterial pressure would be distributed evenly through the whole placenta, and would not, as Seitz believes, cause the blood to burst into the surrounding tissues. Another form of placental hemorrhage comes from rupture of the marginal sinus, already referred to.

It must not be forgotten that a hemorrhage can occur in a red or white infarct. Hemorrhages have also been observed on both surfaces of the placenta. Organization of the clot occurs, and it is possible to trace the changes through the stages of— (1) Soft, red-black clot; (2) brick-red, firmer mass; (3) fibrin formation in the periphery, with some liquid content, to (4) through-and-through hard fibrous nodule. These nodules resemble white infarcts.

The causes of these hemorrhages are acute and chronic congestion, increased blood-pressure, stagnation of the venous blood-current, disease of the villi, of the decidual blood-vessels (endometritis), and the blood changes incident to Bright's disease, toxemia, hemorrhagic diathesis, and syphilis. Physical or mental shock and local injury also may cause them. I believe there is some relation between the toxemia of pregnancy, hemorrhages in the decidua, even abruptio placentæ, and the hemophilic conditions which arise during gestation.

Clinically, placental hemorrhages are of great importance. If they occur early in pregnancy, abortion may result, and, perhaps, fetal monsters. Later, abruptio placentæ may ensue. Smaller clots may not be found until after delivery, but the history of attacks of pain, slight external bleeding, and uterine contractions which subsided may serve to show the accoucheur that some disturbance of fetation had occurred at some time during pregnancy.

Rarely coagulation of the blood in the intervillous spaces takes place. Thrombosis of the sinuses of the placental site may be looked upon, in the later weeks, as a normal process, and preparatory to involution of the uterus. It has been found

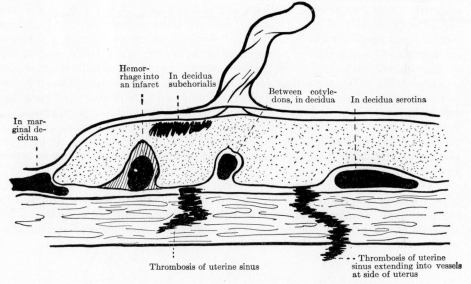

Fig. 491.—Diagram Showing Location of Hemorrhages into Placenta and Thromboses.

as early as the second, third, and fourth month, but it is then pathologic. It may overstep the bounds of the normal by going through the uterine wall into the veins of the broad ligaments, and, especially if these are varicose, may lead to the development of phlegmasia of the limbs, both before and after delivery.

Edema.—An edematous placenta may resemble a syphilitic one, and the microscope may have to decide. The villi are club-shaped and swollen, with irregular contour. Usually the syphilitic placenta feels fatty, while one can squeeze water from the edematous placenta, which is pale, thick, soft, shaggy, and mushy, with torn serotina. The causes are maternal and fetal heart disease, nephritis, diabetes, and general anasarca from any source, polyhydramnion, and fetal blood diseases. Abortion is the rule. If the child is also edematous, formidable dystocia may result.

Atelectasis.—Sometimes a placental cotyledon is completely infiltrated with fibrous material, solid, dark red in color, and hard to the touch. It occurs occasionally in placenta prævia, the piece overlapping the internal os being in this condition, and it may make the diagnosis difficult.

The fibrous change may be concrete, or may be somewhat diffuse, giving the whole placenta a fibrous character. It may, therefore, interfere with the nourishment of the fetus, and probably has a pathology analogous to that of white infarct.

Calcification.—Not infrequently the serotinal surface of the placenta is strewn with white, sandy deposits. These may be discrete or, rarely, may be fused together into little plates of hard, brittle masses. They are composed of calcium carbonate and phosphate and magnesium phosphate, lie in the upper layers of the decidua serotina, especially around the "anchoring villi," are due to the deposition of the salts in areas which had undergone fibrinous degeneration, and are, therefore, associated with white infarcts; they have no clinical significance, are not syphilitic, though they may be found in luetic placentas—usually in the vessels' wall—do not always indicate that the gestation has been prolonged (since they are found in abortions), are not tuberculous, and do not occur with especial frequency in any particular condition. It has seemed to me that they render the placenta stiff, which facilitates its separation and expulsion, and that usually no piece of a calcareous placenta is retained.

Cysts of the Placenta.—On the fetal surface, underneath the amnion and just under the chorial membrane, cysts are not seldom found. They vary in size from the microscopic to that of a goose-egg, and are oftenest found on ripe placentas, but have been noted at all times after the twenty-second week, have clear yellowish or cloudy and bloody content, contain albumin, mucin, fat, detritus, and various sodium and chlorin salts. Often a white infarct is found underneath the cyst, and, on opening the latter, the lining is seen to be of soft, whitish, shaggy, necrotic material resembling decidua. This is generally admitted to be degenerated Langhans' cells, which are large, hydropic, with a big nucleus and all fatty degenerated. It is believed that a few of these cysts may be due to degenerated decidua or the end-products of large white infarctions or hemorrhages. Clinically, they are of no importance. If a large marginal cyst ruptured, one might think the bag of waters had opened (Seitz).

Various tumors are found in the placenta—myxoma fibrosum, angiomata, hyperplasia of the chorionic villi, but especially chorio-angiomata. All are exceedingly rare. Clinically, they are of little importance; only rarely do they affect the child or the delivery (Vignes). The placenta can become infected and inflamed, obeying the laws usual to these conditions.

Literature

Aichel: Verh. der Deutsch. Ges. f. Geb. u. Gyn., 1901.—*Bleuler, M.:* Zentb. für Gyn., November 21, 1931, p. 3370.—*Bortini:* Zentb. für Gyn., March 26, 1932, p. 784.—*Browne, F. J.:* British Medical Journal, April 17, 1926.—*Caturani:* Amer. Jour. Obst., 1911, p. 617. Literature.—*Clemenz:* Zeitschr. f. Geb. u. Gyn., 1922, Bd. 84, Heft 3, p. 759.—*Essen-Moeller, E.:* Monatsschr. für Geb. u. Gyn., June, 1925.—*Ewing:* Surg., Gyn., and Obst., April, 1930. Literature.—*Findley, P.:* Amer. Jour. Med. Sci., 1903, p. 488; *ibid.*, Amer. Jour. Obst., January, 1915, p. 53; also *Pestalozza, ibid.*, p. 161.—*Frank:* Amer. Jour. Med. Assoc., 1906, vol. xlvi, p. 248.—*Frankl:* Liepman's Handbuch der Frauenheilkunde, Band ii, p. 136.—*Funck:* Annal. de Gyn. et d'Obst., September, 1910.—*Hady:* Zentb. für Gynaek., Ergäng., Heft, 1931, No. 11a, p. 912.—*Hoerman:* Monatssch. f. Geb. u. Gyn., 1908. Over 200 literature references.—*Kossman:* Arch. f. Gyn., vol. lii, p. 153.—*Kroesing:* Arch. f. Gyn. u. Geb., 1909, vol. lxxxviii, H. 3. Literature.—*Lahm:* Arch. für Gyn., 1924, vol. cxxi, Bd. ii, p. 306.—*Marchand:* Zeitschr. f. Geb. u. Gyn., vol. xxxix, p. 215; *ibid.*, H. 3, pp. 405, 472. Gives literature.—*Molitor:* Handb. d. Geb., vol. ii, 2, p. 1067.—*Montgomery, T. L.:* Amer. Jour. Obst., February, 1931.—*Novak:* Jour. Amer. Med. Assoc., June 10, 1922, p. 1771.—*Parvin:* Amer. Jour. Med. Sci., October, 1892.—*Philips:* Jour. Obst. and Gyn., British Empire, December, 1911. Chorio-epithelioma of Tube.—*Siddall and Hartman:* Amer. Jour. Ob. and Gyn., November, 1926, p. 683.—*Sfameni:* Monatsschr. f. Geb., 1909, vol. xxvii, No. 4, p. 65.—*Sunde:* Acta Gynekol. Scandinavica, 1921, vol. i, p. 16.—*Talbot:* Surg., Gyn., and Obst., July, 1922, p. 42.—*Turazza:* Centralbl. f. Gyn., 1893, p. 948. With living child.—*Veit:* Handb. d. Gyn., 1898, vol. iii, No. 2, p. 539. Literature to date.—*Vignes:* Summary of Literature. L'Année, Obstet., Paris, Masson, 1926.—*Williams, J. W.:* Amer. Jour. Ob. and Gyn., January, 1927, p. 1. Lit.

CHAPTER XLVII

ANOMALIES OF THE CORD AND OF THE AMNION

ANOMALIES OF THE CORD

Knots.—Since the umbilical vein is longer than the arteries, and the vessels longer than the cord itself, twisting of the vessels occurs, and the vein is twisted around the arteries. The veins especially, but the arteries also, form loops, and the jelly of Wharton is thicker at such places, causing nodes on the cord which are called false knots. These have no clinical significance. *True knots* occur in the cord, but they are uncommon. They are single or complicated, and may even cause the death of the fetus. While they usually form during labor as the result of the child passing through a loop and have no clinical importance, if they form early in pregnancy the active movements of the fetus may draw the turns so tight that death of the child results. (See Browne, full Lit.)

Torsion of the cord is often found in aborted fetuses, but one can seldom assert that the torsion caused the death of the child. As many as 380 turns have been counted when the whole cord is affected. Occasionally the cord is twisted—almost off—right at the navel, or at any one point of its length, and in these cases stenosis of the vessels with fetal death may follow. In a given case it may be impossible to determine whether the death of the fetus resulted from the stricture of the cord, or whether the torsion of the cord was produced by the active movements of the fetal death agony, or whether the twisting occurred after the child's death. Probably all three occur. In medicolegal cases this uncertainty is to be borne in mind. The differential diagnosis between torsion of the cord which occurred after the fetal death from that occurring before may be made certain if there are adhesions between the coils of the cord, and if, when the cord is untwisted, this is found difficult and the shape of the cord seems to be permanently altered.

Coiling of the cord around parts of the fetus affects the child only when it produces an abnormal shortness, or when the coils are so tight that the circulation in the vessels is compromised. It is said that such coiling around the neck may cause hydrocephalus, atrophy, and cerebral disease, by impeding the return circulation, and that extremities may thus be amputated. Usually the fetus will die from asphyxia, the result of the compression of the cord before such effects would be produced. Lesser degrees of compression make circular depressions in the limb and sometimes peripheral atrophy, telangiectasis, and edema. Fracture of the extremities may result during labor when the cord entangles them. Twins in one amnion usually have their cords intertwined. Coiling of the cord around the neck is found in fully one-fifth of all deliveries. As many as seven loops have been found, and this may make the cord relatively too short. In order to explain the coiling of the cord around the neck it is assumed that the loops lie over the internal os, and in delivery the child passes through them. It is more probable that, in its active movements, the child throws the cord around the body and down to the neck, and that the condition exists for weeks before delivery. One of my patients was terrified by a fire in an adjoining dwelling, noted excessive fetal movements, and then aborted. The left thigh of the five months' fetus was caught in a tight knot of the cord. It is possible that the mental shock caused hemorrhages into the placenta, and the dying child was entangled in the cord, or the maternal impressionists might say the child partook of the mother's fright and by its excited motions tied itself in the cord, which caused its death. Coils of cord around the neck may interfere with the mechanism of labor, causing deflexion attitudes, delayed rotation of the head or shoulders, and even shoulder presentation. Compression of the cord behind the pubis, between the neck and the bone, may cause asphyxia of the child, which occurs especially in primiparæ, and is another reason for carefully watching the heart-tones in the second stage of labor.

As will again be mentioned in the discussion of forceps, the coiling of the cord around the neck and the presence of a loop hanging down alongside the head have caused very many fetal deaths. Compression by the blades of the instrument asphyxiates the child; diagnosed by slowing of fetal heart.

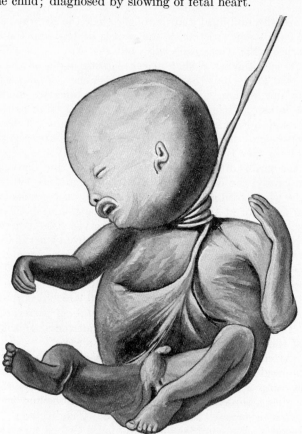

Fig. 492.—Child Strangulated by its Cord at Four Months.

Diagnosis.—During labor it is sometimes possible to feel the cord in the nape of the neck by abdominal palpation, and sometimes the funic souffle can be plainly and constantly heard in this location and digital pressure will slow the fetal heart. During the forceps operation the fingers should be passed all around the head as far as they can reach, and a maneuver, which is more successful than one would think at first, is to pass a finger behind the pubis up the nape of the neck to the back. One can feel the low lying cord. (For treatment see Forceps.)

Most authors advise, after spontaneous delivery of the head, to feel for the cord around the neck. This is not absolutely necessary unless the child seems to be held back by something. One may be required to cut the cord before it is possible to deliver the trunk, and this is always advisable when it seems that there will be traction on the placenta—this to avoid abnormalities in the third stage.

Short Cord.—Cases are reported where there was no cord at all, the fetus being applied to the placenta through an umbilical hernia. Bayer reported a cord 10.5 cm. and Naegelè one of 6.7 cm. Clinically, cords are either absolutely or relatively short, the latter being those where one or more turns around the neck or extremities make a normal cord too short for the mechanism of labor.

A cord must be long enough to reach from the placental site to the vulva, and, if the placenta is located in the fundus, a length of 32 cm. is necessary, not 35 cm., as Kaltenbach puts it. It must be remembered that the uterus follows down the child as it expels it. Too short cord may lead to—(a) Delay in the second stage of labor, the head coming down with difficulty and receding quickly as if it were drawn back by a rubber band; (b) rupture of the cord if the pains are strong, with death or asphyxia of the child; (c) tearing of the cord from the placenta; (d) tearing of the placenta from the uterus, causing abruptio placentæ or pathologic third stage; (e) inversion of the uterus; (f) painful uterine contractions and secondary inertia. A diagnosis of too short cord may not always be made. In one of my cases the patient complained of a dragging sensation about the navel during each pain, and in Brickner's case there was a desire to pass urine after each uterine contraction. In another of my cases a small amount of urine was squeezed out with each pain. Some authors have mentioned a depression,—that is, partial inversion in the uterine wall,—but most often the excessive and quick recession of the head after the pain has led to the diagnosis.

Special treatment is seldom required because of the rarity of the affection. If diagnosed, one should watch the condition of the child narrowly and deliver it on the first sign of asphyxia. As soon as the head is born the cord is to be cut between two clamps.

Long Cords.—The longest cord found in a service of over 50,000 deliveries was 156 cm., but one of 198 cm. has been recorded. The average is 55 cm.—about 22 inches. Aside from the tendency to prolapse and to coil about the fetus, they do not claim our interest. Most of these figures are from Gardiner.

Rupture of the cord is a curious accident, for it may occur with a long cord, and when we can find no reason for it. Stowe, after reporting a case of spontaneous rupture of the cord which occurred in the Chicago Lying-in Hospital Dispensary service, reports the results of his tests to discover the tensile strength of the cords. They carried weights varying from 8 to 22 pounds. In a case of mine the child was delivered, deeply asphyxiated, with the cord broken eight inches from the navel. The broken ends were not jagged, but cut as if with dull scissors, and the thickness at the point of rupture was 8 mm. In another case the brittle cord was caught between the blade of the forceps and the head, and sharply severed, as with a knife.

Neoplasms occur exceedingly rarely in the cord. Myxoma, sarcoma, and dermoid have been reported. Rupture of a varix of the cord, with hematoma, especially near the belly of the child, is occasionally observed. Immense increase of the jelly of Wharton may change the cord to a heavy, thick, glassy rope—in one of my cases it was thicker than a large thumb. Cysts, relics of the ductus omphalomesentericus or of the allantois, may rarely be found, and sometimes a cyst seems to result from liquefaction of the Wharton jelly.

Syphilis of the cord has already been mentioned. The thickening of the tunica media of the vessels and calcification, with obliteration of the lumen, found here, have also been found in other conditions, and, therefore, they are not pathognomonic of lues.

Abnormal Insertion of the Cord.—Ordinarily, the cord is inserted at or near the center of the placenta. Eccentric insertion, even attachment at the margin, is not rare. Battledore placenta has no clinical importance. When the cord is attached to the membranes and the vessels course a greater or less distance between the amnion and the chorion to the body of the placenta we speak of velamentous insertion—insertio velamentosa (Fig. 493). Embryologists are still at variance as to mechanism of the production of the aberrant insertion of the cord. Von Franquè's idea that the exceptionally good nutritional conditions of the reflexa lead to the insertion of the abdominal pedicle here seems quite plausible, but is unproved (Peiser).

Velamentous insertion is often found with other anomalies of the placenta, as infarcts, placenta succenturiata, bilobata, and prævia. It is common with twins and the rule with triplets. To the child this abnormal insertion of the cord is dangerous only when the vessels run across the lower uterine segment; then its life may be lost through hemorrhage, from tearing of one or more of the vessels when the membranes rupture, or asphyxia from compression of the vessels and the cord during the passage of the head. Both twins may bleed to death from the tearing of one vessel. Occasionally a diagnosis may be made before rupture of the mem-

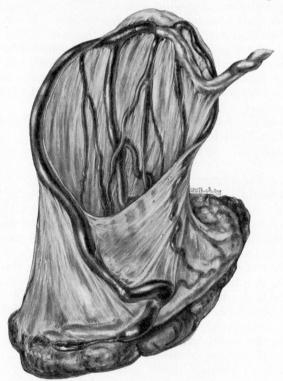

FIG. 493.—AUTHOR'S CASE OF VELAMENTOUS INSERTION OF CORD.
Note immense vein on left alongside the rent through which the child passed. It was asphyxiated, but not anemic.

branes—the pulsating vessels may be felt inside the cervix coursing over the pouting bag of waters. These vessels are not in the forelying cord, because light pressure upward would displace the latter. A slight but continuous hemorrhage after the rupture of the membranes, with weakening and rapidity of the fetal heart-tones, is diagnostic. Placenta prævia and other maternal causes of bleeding are easily eliminated and by exclusion the true condition recognized.

Treatment.—If the diagnosis is made before rupture of the membranes, the latter must be delayed until dilatation of the cervix is complete, which is accomplished by placing a soft elastic colpeurynter in the vagina and putting the woman in the elevated Sims position. When the os is fully opened, the membranes are to be punctured between the vessels and delivery effected as rapidly as is consistent with the safety of the mother.

Hernias into the cord are not so very rare. This must always be thought of while tying the cord.   Hernias, if operable, should be closed immediately, to avoid peritonitis.   Occasionally the skin of the belly runs up for a varying distance on the cord, called "skin navel," and after the stump has fallen off the retraction of the center inverts this skin, making a deep retracted navel.   Sarcomphalus is likely to result in such instances.

ANOMALIES OF THE AMNION

Beside certain minor pathologic findings on the amnion, as caruncles, epithelioid deposits containing lanugo hairs, cysts near the insertion of the cord, scratchmarks from the child's nails, and adhesions to the fetus, the amnion presents two important conditions for study—polyhydramnion and oligohydramnion, the first meaning an excessive quantity and the latter an abnormally small amount of liquor amnii.   Normally, the amount varies within wide limits, from 600 to 2000 gm. We do not know the exact source of the liquor amnii, and, therefore, it is impossible to give a scientific etiology of the anomalies of the fluid.

Polyhydramnion, hydramnion, or hydramnios, is more common than oligohydramnion, and occurs about once in 200 cases.   As many as 15 and 30 liters of fluid have been reported, but such cases are exceedingly rare.   In one of my cases we measured 8 quarts, and much more escaped into the bed and onto the floor. Ovular and maternal causes have been invoked.   Of ovular, the fetus, the cord, the amnion, and the placenta may be involved.   (1) Malformations of the child, especially those showing absence of closure of fetal cavities, harelip, anencephalus, ectopia vesicæ, spina bifida, etc.   Internal deformities are sometimes associated with the polyhydramnion, for example, occlusion of the esophagus, stenosis of the pylorus.   In the former instance the liquid is supposed to be due to transudation from the insufficiently covered blood-vessels of the deformed part.   (2) Diseases of the child involving obstruction of its venous circulation, and causing stasis, edema, and exudation, for example, stenosis of the cord, stenosis of the aorta, of the ductus Botalli, heart disease, cirrhosis of the liver, white pneumonia (syphilis), placental disease, obliteration of the placental blood-vessels, chorio-angioma.   In these cases the fetal kidneys increase their action, and there is perhaps more urine in the liquor amnii.   (3) Hydramnion in unioval twins is not uncommon, and one or both of the ova may be affected equally, or one more than the other, or there may even be oligohydramnion in one ovum.   In homologous twins, when one child is stronger than the other, its heart forces blood through the intermediate or "third" circulation into the vascular system of the other.   (4) Increase of the fetal urine may cause hydramnion, but we know no cause for the former.   Jaggard reported a fetus with deficient kidneys and oligohydramnion (Wilson).

Older writers spoke of an amnionitis, and later investigators have found inflammatory and degenerative changes in the amnial epithelium.   Ahlfeld believes that an early amnionitis produces adhesions to the fetus, with resulting deformities, such as craniorachischisis, gastroschisis, amputation of the extremities, etc.   The amnion offers promise of great results from scientific investigation.

Maternal diseases are seldom the cause of polyhydramnion: (1) All those affections which make general anasarca—cardiac, lung, liver, and kidney;   (2) syphilis, leukemia, chronic anemia—in such cases the fetus usually has hydrops universalis.   The role of infection, reaching the ovum from the vagina or via the blood, deserves recognition.

Clinical Course.—Two varieties are distinguishable—the acute—very rare—and the chronic, the commoner.   *Acute hydramnion* is graver, and usually leads to abortion.   It begins during the fourth or fifth month, and rapidly expands the uterus to colossal size, pressure symptoms being early and pronounced.   There are pain in the abdomen, back, and thighs, feeling of great distention, dyspnea, especially in primiparæ, with attacks of suffocation when the attempt to lie down is made, nausea and vomiting, and symptoms referable to the kidney of pregnancy or even of nephritis. Emaciation may be marked, fever present; edema of the legs, thighs, and even the abdomen, with enormous distention of the latter, will be found. The uterus may be larger than at term, the belly so tight and tender that palpation is rendered negative, but fluctuation is usually obtainable. Striæ gravidarum cover the skin, and often minute hemorrhages bestrew it; fetal parts are not palpable, and the heart-tones may be inaudible. Vaginally, the cervix is found high up, effaced, and the os usually opened. As a rule, acute hydramnion terminates in abortion before the sixth month, or the symptoms become so threatening that the attendant must interfere. Twins are often found in such cases, and a spontaneous cure may follow if one of them should die.

Diagnosis.—If a diagnosis of pregnancy had already been made, the rapid enlargement of the uterus with abdominal symptoms will be easily explained. Hydatidiform mole causes not such rapid growth of the uterine tumor, and, further, it is almost always complicated by hemorrhages. Generally, the first duty is to diagnose pregnancy, which is usually not difficult if all the aids are called upon. Contractions occurring in the abdominal tumor on one occasion enabled me to diagnose the condition when all other findings were equivocal. Ovarian cyst oftenest requires differentiation, but in this condition the uterus is usually found below the large fluctuating tumor, the cervix is closed and hard (open and soft, with palpable membranes in hydramnion), and the symptoms and other signs of pregnancy are absent. Ascites shows the characteristic area of tympany around the navel, which changes with position. Encysted (tubercular) ascites was once mistaken for polyhydramnion. In critical cases, where a diagnosis must be made, it is justifiable to use the uterine sound because, if the case really is acute hydramnion, the puncture of the membranes is the proper treatment.

Treatment of acute hydramnion is abortion, by letting off the waters, which must be done slowly to avoid shock, the case being then left to nature, and other interference being made only on special indication.

Chronic Hydramnion.—This differs from the acute in that the course is much less stormy—it does not lead so often to abortion, though premature labor is frequent. It is commoner and a little more amenable to treatment. It may occur in ectopic gestation, which renders diagnosis very difficult. Causation and symptoms are the same as in the acute form, but the latter are less marked and of longer duration. Enormous distention of the uterus may occur, with resulting cardiac distress and kidney insufficiency. The patient may be annoyed by false labor pains for weeks before delivery. The diagnosis lies most often between hydramnion and twins, but it must be remembered that they are often associated. In one of my cases the bag of waters, felt over the internal os, was relaxed, while the uterus, felt abdominally, was very tense, a fact which Rémy and Ahlfeld noted, and which they used for the diagnosis of hydramnion of the upper twin. Fluctuation is demonstrable only in the hydramniotic sac; it does not pass through the septum between the twins.

The *prognosis* of acute hydramnion is good for the mother, because abortion usually terminates the case early. In general the prognosis is not bad, but one should remember the dangers—kidney lesions, cardiac collapse, respiratory failure, hydroperitoneum, and hydropleura. Labor may bring added troubles—for example, a tedious first stage, sometimes lasting days, prolapse of the cord when the membranes rupture and the sudden rush of the waters takes place; abnormal presentations and positions of the child, weak labor pains, the last three requiring operative interference; atonia uteri and postpartum hemorrhage, which often is hard to stop. The sudden rush of the waters, besides causing the mentioned anomalies, may leave so small a uterine cavity that abruptio placentæ results, or the heart cannot stand the shock of the sudden diminution of intra-abdominal tension. Finally, the cause of the polyhydramnion may have a bearing on the prognosis, for example, syphilis, anemia, heart and kidney lesions.

For the child, the prognosis is bad in acute hydramnion, but in the chronic forms it is fairly good. An expression of opinion should be guarded, because of the frequency of prematurity and of fetal deformities, which may make extra-uterine existence impossible. In the higher degrees, the mother being very cyanotic, the child or children may die of asphyxia before delivery, and many succumb during operative procedures necessitated by prolapse of the cord, etc.

Treatment.—Syphilis, anemia, renal and cardiac disease, of course, are to be appropriately treated, though much success is not attained. When the symptoms become marked, the patient should stay in bed, on an antinephritic diet, and should be carefully watched. Should the heart begin to suffer or the kidneys prove default, labor is to be induced, the best method being to let off the excessive waters through a small trocar, such as is used for ovarian cysts. It is important to drain the waters slowly to avoid shock from sudden decrease of intra-abdominal tension, and to prevent the prolapse of the cord or extremities. The patient should be in the Sims position for this operation. Delivery of the child should also be slow, to enable the uterus to get a better hold on itself by retraction of its fibers. Preparations for postpartum hemorrhage are to be made beforehand, and the placenta removed on the first indication, after which the uterovaginal tract is to be firmly packed with gauze. Pituitrin is useful here. Bumm and Henkel recommend to relieve the uterus by abdominal paracentesis. I believe this would be of only temporary benefit, if not risky.

Oligohydramnion.—Decrease of the amount of liquor amnii is rare, and in such cases there may be a few spoonfuls of thick, viscid or cloudy, yellowish-green fluid, insufficient to fill the interstices between the fetal parts and the uterus. If the condition occurs early in fetation, it results in more or less adhesion of the amnion to the fetus, causing deformities, for example, hemicephalus, cranioschisis, gastroschisis, spina bifida, amputation of extremities, curvatures, ankylosis of joints, and skin defects. If the liquor amnii is lacking in the later months, the skin of the child becomes dry and leathery, the fetal body is cramped together, club-foot, drop-wrist, skin defects on the shoulders, trochanters, malleoli (decubitus), curvature of the spine, shortening of the muscles, such as wry-neck, talipes calcaneus, etc., are found —all the result of limitation of the confines of the child and of pressure of the uterine wall on its body.

These same conditions are found in extra-amniotic development of the child and in extra-uterine pregnancy.

Nothing is definitely known of the causation of oligohydramnion. Jaggard's case of absence of urethra and kidney has been referred to. Oligohydramnion can affect one twin, there being an excess of fluid with the other.

During labor, which is often premature, painful uterine contractions, weak pains, protracted first stage, a tendency to abruptio placentæ, and increase in the dangers to the child have been noted.

LITERATURE

Brickner: Amer. Jour. Obstet., 1902, vol. xlv, p. 512.—*Browne, F. J.:* Jour. Obstet. and Gyn., Brit. Empire, vol. xxxii, No. 1.—*Gardiner:* Surg., Gyn., and Obst., February, 1922, p. 251.—*Henkel, M.:* Deutsche med. Woch., July 25, 1930.—*Peiser:* Monatsschr. f. Geb. u. Gyn., 1898, vol. viii, p. 619.—*Wilson:* Amer. Jour. Obstet., 1887, vol. xx, p. 1.

SECTION VI

THE PATHOLOGY OF LABOR

AN obstetric case is a surgical case, with more than the usual surgical aspects. Older writers used to speak of eutocia and dystocia, the former meaning normal, the latter abnormal, labor. No two authorities are agreed as to where eutocia ends and dystocia begins. Most authors believe that labor in the human female borders very closely on the pathologic, but I am convinced that, today, measured by our present standards, labor cannot be called a normal function. To mention only one reason for so considering it, the almost invariable injury to the pelvic floor may be cited. No other function of the body, normally executed, is attended by permanent damage to structure. Should such damage occur, we call the process pathogenic and pathologic. "Normal" comes from *norma*, a rule, and means conforming to a law or principle. Most of us use it in a narrower sense, *i. e.*, harmless, nonpathologic. We have done the same with the word "natural." I believe that the notion that labor is normal in the usual sense is a fallacy, and that this fallacy is fundamentally responsible for the still high mortality and morbidity which attend the parturient function. Taking for granted that parturition is normal, the State allows ignorant midwives and half-instructed medical students to assume the heavy responsibilities of its conduct. Since the public is taught to believe that labor is physiologic it refuses to recognize the dignity of the science and the high degree of art, of obstetrics, and, as a result, the field of its practice is not made inviting to the best men of the profession. Such a state of affairs naturally explains why 20,000 women die every year in our country from the effects of childbirth, why nearly every mother carries the marks of injury inflicted during labor, and why a hundred thousand infants are annually lost during delivery.

It is best to regard every labor case as a severe operation. Like the surgeon, the obstetrician should consider the strength of the patient in standing the shock, the asepsis and antisepsis, the nature and technic of the operation, and, finally, all the complications which are likely to arise.

So, during labor, it is necessary and our duty to have a clear knowledge of the patient's condition, especially of the heart, lungs, kidneys, and blood; second, we must know accurately what is going on during the labor, that is, we must be thoroughly acquainted with the mechanism of the particular labor, the strength of the powers, the greatness of the resistances, and the relation between them; third, we must be aware of all possible complications and the particular ones likely to arise in this particular case, and know how to prevent and treat them; and, finally, we must know and practise the strict principles of asepsis and antisepsis, that the latest standards demand. To meet all these obligations is the duty of the obstetrician, and a conscientious man will find little time for idling at a labor case. It requires studious regard of the patient during her pregnancy, and getting her into the best possible condition for the ordeal of parturition. It requires a prompt response to the call to the labor, a careful and painstaking examination on arrival, and a proper valuation of all the conditions found. It requires attentive conduct of the case from the beginning to the end, and a preparedness for doing the usual work of a delivery, plus far-reaching provision and ability for all emergencies.

Since labor is largely a mechanical problem the attendant must be a good engineer, who particularly studies the motor (the uterus and abdominal muscles) and the load (the passages and passengers). At the same time the nervous system (to carry the simile further, the ignition), requires watching. The obstetrician should always remember Barnes' admonition: "We seek to determine not what the woman can endure, but what she can accomplish."

If, when its course is abnormal, the case is studied analytically, the accoucheur will usually find one or rarely two, pathologic conditions coursing through the picture like a scarlet thread, or as the "leit motif" of a musical composition. There is some fundamental irregularity, e. g., contracted pelvis, or weak pains, which affects the course of the labor throughout, lending its quality to every feature of the process, and one must discover it for successful treatment.

In general, the abnormalities of a labor may be classed under four heads: (1) Anomalies of the powers; (2) anomalies of the passengers (fetus and placenta); (3) anomalies of the passages (hard, soft); (4) complications on the part either of the mother or of the fetus or placenta.

It is convenient to study the pathology of the first and second stages together, leaving that of the third stage for separate consideration.

When, in the course of his study of a labor case, the accoucheur notes that one or the other of the four irregularities is present or threatens, he decides that he must do something to save the mother or the child from disaster—in other words, he finds an indication for interference. An "indication," therefore, is a reason for interference in the course of a given case. However, certain circumstances, characters, or phases of the case may demand consideration and put a certain light on the indication which may make its modification necessary. In other words, the accoucheur must consult the conditions of the case in determining the course of procedure. A "condition," therefore, is a prerequisite or requirement which governs the indication. For example, in asphyxia of the child in utero the indication is for immediate delivery. The state of the cervix is one of the conditions which will determine what mode of delivery will be selected. The study of the case, and the determination that this or that remedy or course of procedure is required, we call "placing the indication." After this the conditions are consulted. If they are all fully met, the line of procedure is carried out; if not, the plan of procedure is to be revised until it does meet and satisfy all the conditions, or, if the indication is imperative, the conditions are forced to meet it. It is here that the judgment of the accoucheur comes to the test, and, speaking generally and reflectively, I affirm that there are no situations in all medicine and surgery that require broader knowledge, finer discernment, more logical reasoning, and more courageous purpose for their control than do the problems of obstetrics.

CHAPTER XLVIII

ANOMALIES OF THE POWERS

In the first stage of labor the uterus does all the work. Regularly, with increasing frequency and strength, its muscle contracts, slowly reaching an acme and then relaxing. In this way the development of the lower uterine segment is completed, the hydrostatic bag of waters formed, the cervix effaced, and the os dilated. In the second stage the larger part of the work is done by the abdominal muscles. The uterus by this time is well drawn up over the child and can exert but little power. While in some instances the uterus expels the child unaided, its main action in this stage is forcing the presenting part against the pelvic floor, which, reflexly, elicits the action of the abdominal muscles—the bearing-down efforts. In discussing this subject, therefore, we will consider, first, anomalies of the uterine and second those of the abdominal action.

Anomalies of the Uterine Action.—The pains may be too weak or too strong, too seldom or too frequent, too short or too long, and they may be irregular in time and in character, too painful, or, rarely, painless. Even normally, much variation may be noted as regards the time, rhythm, and strength of the labor pains in different women. Knowledge of the character of the pains in preceding labors will enable us to predict the kind of uterine action in subsequent deliveries, since they are usually much alike, but exceptions are not rare.

False pains are the contractions of pregnancy, which, toward the end of gestation, become perceptible, even painful, to the gravida. They are especially marked at the time of lightening, and may force the head down into the pelvis. According to Schatz, they recur with a certain periodicity, the intervals being less by one-half as term approaches. All the usual symptoms of an actual labor pain may be present, that is, pain, hardening of the uterus, regularity, even dilatation of the cervix and rupture of the membranes. Most authors regard the last two as indicative of the beginning of actual labor. Indeed, it is often impossible to say when pregnancy ends and labor starts, but these points may help in the diagnosis: false, or pregnancy, pains are of even intensity, while true pains grow stronger apace; they cease after a day or so; they are out of the time of the expected labor, and if their type, *i. e.*, whether they appear at intervals of three, four, or six weeks, is known, they will recur on the days which would correspond to the end of one-half of the previous interval; while the cervix may open, it is not shortened nor effaced, the membranes rarely rupture, and the bloody show does not appear. False pains are not strengthened by pituitrin (Hofbauer). It is important to recognize the false pains and treat them as such, because if the woman were considered to be in labor, when actually she is not, much unnecessary and harmful examination and interference might be instituted. Treatment consists of rest in bed, narcotics, and expectancy. The author does not agree with those who would allow such a case to continue far beyond the normal term of pregnancy. (See Prolonged Pregnancy and Induction of Labor at Term.)

Weak Pains.—Inertia uteri, atonia uteri, or uterine atony may show itself in, first, infrequent contractions, feeble contractions, and too short contractions; usually the three are combined. Clinically, we must describe the condition as it affects the first stage, or the dilatation of the cervix; the second stage, the expulsion of the fetus; and the third stage, or the period of the after-birth. In the first stage labor is unduly prolonged, the pains are feeble, at long, irregular intervals, and last only a few seconds. Sometimes they intermit for a few hours or days, reminding one

618

of the false pains just considered. After a rest, uterine action is resumed, but usually with more force. Dilatation of the cervix may require several days, and the patient is exposed to the dangers of sepsis and exhaustion. Should fever arise, which is especially likely if the bag of waters is ruptured, the pains start up with vigor and terminate the labor, if this is possible. Ordinarily, the child is in no danger at this time. As long as the bag of waters is intact, serious trouble is unlikely. Should it rupture early, the uterus may retract firmly on the fetus, and for the mother there is then danger of infection of the cavity of the uterus. Either the germs wander upward or are carried up by the too frequent examinations. Further, the restrictions on the growth of the vaginal bacteria seem to be removed and they become virulent, and finally the germs resident in the vestibule, all possessing invasive powers, wander up into higher parts of the parturient canal. They may be saprophytes or gas formers, but also dangerous streptococci, and they may pass through amnion and chorion into the intervillous spaces (Warnekros). Harris has shown that even with an intact bag of waters, streptococci could be found in the lower uterine segment six hours after labor began. This change in the bacterial flora of the parturient canal is most ominous, and while it may occur spontaneously, is facilitated by vaginal examinations, even with perfectly sterile gloves. This means we cannot prevent carrying vestibular infection to higher zones. The superiority of the rectal examination is thus proved. In two cases of the author the children came to the world already infected, one with gonorrheal ophthalmia and one with gastro-intestinal sepsis and acute pneumonia is not very rare.

During the second stage weak uterine pains are responsible for weak abdominal action, because the presenting part is not forced against the perineum strongly enough to arouse the abdominal muscles. Expulsion is slow or stopped, causing danger to the mother from pressure necrosis of the pelvic viscera, which may eventuate in fistulas. The child in utero is endangered by asphyxia. In the third stage weak, infrequent, or short pains are grave, because of imperfect separation of the placenta, retention of membranes, and hemorrhage from insufficient closure of the vessels at the placental site.

Etiology.—Primarily weak pains may be due to poor general health, chronic wasting disease, tuberculosis, or anemia, though in acute affections the uterus generally acts well. The nervous mechanism may be disturbed, the muscle being poorly innervated, or the nervous balance being imperfect or the endocrinal system may be at fault. A shock may frighten the pains away, or fear of an operation hasten them. In hyperesthetic women the suffering they cause may be inhibitory, and, contrary to what would be expected, morphin will sometimes strengthen weak pains. Local causes are: infantile uterus, fibroids, and other tumors in or near the uterus; peritoneal adhesions, which interfere with the muscle action; full rectum and bladder, which act like the last; abnormal position of the uterus: retroflexion or anteversion (pendulous abdomen); disease of the uterine wall; scars from previous operations; chronic metritis, with increase of fibrous and decrease of muscular tissue; endometritis; too frequent child-bearing, with overstretching anomalies of the cervix; old primiparity; conditions of the ovum which overdistend the uterus, for example, polyhydramnion, twins; physometra; abnormal positions of the child—breech, shoulder, face, occipitoposterior, which prevent it from pressing on the great cervical ganglion; generally contracted pelvis; adhesion of the membranes around the os, a poorly shaped bag of waters being formed. Secondary weak pains are due to fatigue from overwork and to retraction of the contractile portion of the uterus above the child. Sometimes they are due to stricture of the uterus (*vide infra*).

The *diagnosis* of atony of the uterus is easy—the organ does not harden firmly with the pain, and the contraction, timed with a watch and feeling the fundus with the hand, lasts only a few seconds. With Crodel's tokometer we can now measure the pains and think more scientifically. There is no progress in labor, very little suffering, and the pains have no effect on the fetal heart-tones. An important part of the diagnosis is the determination of the point when the mother and child begin to be endangered. For the child, this is usually late in the second stage, is due to asphyxia from the reduction in size of the placental area, and is discovered by auscultation, but the child also suffers the danger of infection. For the mother, it depends largely on the cause, the worst cases being those of weak pains in the presence of disproportion between the head and the pelvis. Here the parts beneath the zone of compression become edematous, sometimes bloody, later anemic necroses begin, and in all cases the tissues lose their bactericidal power, which invites infection. Swelling, transudation, edema, fetid discharge, pain, nausea and vomiting, fever, etc., indicate the time for interference.

Prognosis.—This depends on the cause. The greatest dangers are sepsis from too long waiting, from too many internal examinations and manipulations, and the injuries inflicted by too early and unnecessary operating. The same for the child.

Treatment should be varied with the cause, and is medical or mechanical. One of the best remedies is to put the patient to sleep, and morphin, $\frac{1}{6}$ grain hypodermically, with 40 grains sodium bromid per rectum, may be used. Morphin is safe for the child only early in the first stage of labor. The effect is better if the parturient is given a full warm wet pack (no bath) beforehand. After a good sleep the patient usually has regular, vigorous pains. Ergot is never used, and quinin seldom. Several times the latter seemed to cause the premature discharge of meconium and annoying postpartum oozing. Much patience is to be exercised, and suggestion, with mental and moral support, must be given the parturient. In many instances a large dose of castor oil will prove effectual.

Pituitary extract is being used extensively for weak pains both in the first and second stages of labor. It is a powerful oxytocic and one of the most dangerous medicines we have, doing untold damage to mother and child. Rupture of the uterus, lacerations of the cervix and perineum, death of the child from asphyxia and cerebral hemorrhage occur so often that the author cannot too strongly condemn its indiscriminate use. Fortunately, of late its evil qualities are being recognized and we are being supplied with a standardized preparation of more uniform strength. Pituitary preparations vary in strength, some ampules containing 3, others up to 10 Voegtlin units. One should prescribe "units" as one does insulin. Its nasal application is safer than the hypodermic.

Pituitary extract, pitu-glandol, hypophysin, pituitrin, glanduitrin are all names for the solution of the active principles of the posterior lobe of the hypophysis cerebri. The action of this glandular secretion upon the uterus was discovered by Dale in 1906, and Fränkl-Hochwart and Fröhlich in 1909 called attention to its strong oxytocic action. W. B. Bell in 1909 first used it in labor, but it became better known as an oxytocic when Hofbauer recommended it. The drug seems to affect all unstriped muscular fiber, the blood-vessels, intestine, and bladder, as well as the uterus, but it contracts the latter most markedly. From two to eight minutes after the hypodermic injection of 1 c.c. of hypophysin the uterus contracts strongly. The pains are both strengthened and made more frequent, the effects lasting from thirty to sixty minutes, depending on the quality of the preparation used and the patient. Sometimes there is none or feeble action, sometimes an unusual effect, such as tetanus uteri. Kahn says it has another action, increasing the coagulability of the blood. It does not stimulate the lacteal secretion, and has only slight action on the bladder. Sometimes it seems to aid peristalsis and the removal of flatus. Lately the two principles have been isolated for separate use, the oxytocic and the pressor.

Indications.—(1) In a case of pure atonia uteri, uncomplicated otherwise, a few drops, 1 to 3, of pituitrin, might stimulate the flagging muscle. In two such cases the author had to give ether to quiet undesired tempestuous uterine action. (2) Some accoucheurs use pituitrin in the second stage, when the powers give out as the head must be driven over the perineum, but the author believes that episiotomy and forceps are a safer procedure for both mother and baby. (3) Watson and a few others use pituitrin, with or without quinin, to induce labor-pains at term, stopping the drugs when uterine action has been established. The author does not approve the large doses given. (See p. 1122.) (4) In abruptio placentæ an occasional indication for pituitrin may exist. (5) After the child is delivered, one may safely give pituitrin, indeed, the author does so as a routine in all labors. In several cases the placenta was incarcerated by the strongly acting oxytocic and manual removal was necessary. Therefore, one may recommend this practice only where ideal maternity conditions are available. (6) In atonic postpartum hemorrhage, pituitary extract is our sheet anchor. It sensitizes the uterus, powerfully aiding the action of ergot which is given at the same time. (7) At cesarean sections, sometimes injected into the uterine muscle if the uterus does not act promptly. (8) In cases of early abortion in progress and septic abortion, together with quinin to help empty the uterus. (9) After laparotomies (not classic cesareans) to reduce tympany and for gas-pains. (10) For late puerperal hemorrhages. (11) To prevent and combat shock. (12) For puerperal sepsis. (13) Pyelitis in puerperio.

Conditions and Contraindications.—The following accidents have been reported: (1) Tetanus and strictura uteri with incarceration of fetus and death; (2) too prolonged uterine contractions with fatal fetal asphyxia; (3) ruptura uteri (many cases, Mendelhall, 89); (4) pressure necrosis of soft parts; (5) atony of uterus postpartum and hemorrhage; (6) deep cervical and perineal lacerations (frequent); (7) eclampsia (?); (8) collapse, especially when injected intravenously, and even stenocardiac attacks; (9) necrosis of uterine wall (given at cesarean section) and fatal peritonitis (Süssman); (10) toxic convulsions in the infant (?); (11) cerebral damage in the child. In the last century ergot was widely used to hasten delivery. It was called the *pulvis ad partum* for the mother, but also blamed as the *pulvis ad mortem* for the baby. Cotret, after studying the answers to a world-wide questionnaire, gives pituitary extract the epithet, *pulvis ad mortem* for mother and infant.

Pituitrin should not be given where there is any danger of rupture of the uterus, *i. e.*, in contracted pelvis, malpresentations and malpositions, tumors blocking the passage, fibroids, diseased uteri, *e. g.*, scars from previous section, placenta prævia, old multiparæ. It may not be used early in labor or when the cervix is closed or undilatable. If the head is not engaged it may be exhibited only after the accoucheur is convinced that feebleness of the pains is the sole cause of the head remaining high. Heart disease and the dangers of a sudden increase of blood-pressure, cerebral hemorrhage in eclampsia, atheroma, contraindicate, also threatened asphyxia of the child *in utero*. Thymophysin carries identical disabilities with pituitary.

Mechanical measures are: hot-water bag to the fundus; uterine massage; letting the patient change her position or walk about; a hot milk and molasses enema (very effective); hot vaginal douches (115° F.), repeated every three hours (not recommended); insertion of a bougie into the lower uterine segment; application of a small colpeurynter above the cervix, and traction on it so as to irritate the cervical ganglion, or its use in the rectum filled with hot water; packing the cervix or vagina or both with gauze saturated with boroglycerin; separation of the membranes around the internal os and lower uterine segment, to form an effective hydrostatic bag of waters; and puncture of the membranes and allowing the liquor amnii to escape, which permits the uterine fibers to shorten and obtain a better grasp on the child.

Occasionally, in a primipara, the head will be deeply engaged, but the cervix is far back in the hollow of the sacrum and very thin. The membranes are tightly stretched over the head, and there are no forewaters. By pulling the cervix gently to the middle of the pelvis, separating the membranes around the lower uterine segment for 2 inches, and pushing up the head a little to allow some liquor amnii to run down and make a pouch, the mechanism of labor is started right and the pains improve at once. The practitioner, after carefully studying the aspects of the individual labor, will have to select the remedy which offers the best hope of stimulating the uterus. Internal manipulations should be avoided as far as possible, and expectancy carried only to the point of threatened danger.

Anomalies of the Abdominal Powers.—Weakness of the abdominal powers may be primary or secondary. Either the woman has poorly developed abdominal muscles, the result of tight lacing or insufficient exercise, or the muscles are prevented from contracting by—(1) Inflammatory conditions in the belly; for example, appendiceal abscess; (2) hernias; (3) cardiac and pulmonary disease with dyspnea; (4) tumors in the abdomen—fibroids, cysts; full bladder; tympany; fat; (5) kyphoscoliosis. Women with pendulous belly have insufficient abdominal action because the diastatic recti cannot get a purchase on the uterus, which has fallen forward between them. Comatose and narcotized women, the reflexes being abolished, do not bear down, but when the coma is not deep, the abdominal muscles act reflexly and sometimes powerfully, as may be seen in eclampsia and obstetric anesthesia. Hypersensitive women sometimes will refuse to bear down because it hurts too much, and in such cases anesthesia to the obstetric degree, by abolishing the pain, will apparently strengthen the abdominal muscles. Sometimes the parturient actually does not know how to use the abdominal muscles, and needs to be taught how to bear down effectively. Again, she bears down strongly enough, but the antagonistic muscles of the pelvic floor contract spasmodically and hold the head back. The woman must be shown how to relax the outlet while bearing down. Secondary weak abdominal action arises either from exhaustion, the woman having used up her stock of strength in fruitless bearing-down efforts in the first stage, when they could do no good and much harm, or the resistances of the delivery have proved too much for her. She may have had too little reserve power, or the weak

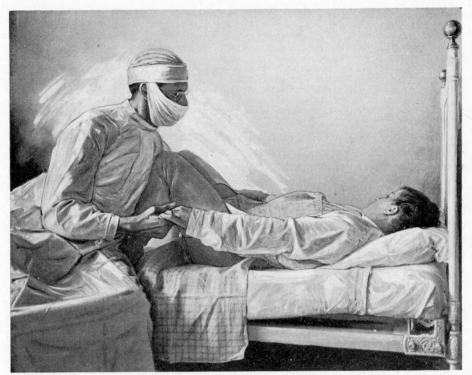

FIG. 494.—PHYSICIAN INSTRUCTING PARTURIENT HOW TO USE HER POWERS TO BEST ADVANTAGE.

uterine contractions have been unable to evoke sufficiently powerful response in the abdominal muscles. Voluntary bearing-down efforts are never so strong nor so effectual as those elicited by the uterine contractions. Curiously, sometimes a weak uterine pain will produce a strong bearing-down effort. A prolonged first stage is thus sometimes followed by a quick second stage, but in such cases atony of the uterus in the placental period is often to be anticipated.

Prolongation of the second stage is the result of insufficient abdominal action, and ordinarily neither patient runs much risk unless the delay exceeds five hours. This condition must be sharply differentiated from resistant outlet with strong pains. Owing to the pressure exerted by the head on the pelvic viscera, fistulas may possibly result, though they usually do not, the vulva becomes edematous and friable, and aid may have to be rendered simply because of the delay and the depressing effect on the woman's nervous system. For the child, such a stoppage in the labor may become dangerous from asphyxia, the placental area being diminished since the uterus has retracted; the caput succedaneum becomes very large, which, incidentally, indicates that the fetus is suffering from cerebral congestion, and the cord, if it is in the pelvis, may suffer injurious pressure.

Treatment.—First in the order of procedure is a careful diagnosis of the cause of the delay in labor, which includes the determination of the location, the station, or the degree of engagement of the head or presenting part. Weak uterine contractions in this stage require the same treatment as in the first stage (*q. v.*). In cases of inflammatory conditions in the belly, and in cardiac and respiratory diseases, the woman should not be allowed to bear down too much, but extraction is to be performed. Pendulous belly is treated with a binder. (See p. 439.) If the patient is tired out, a short respite is given her by means of light ethylene anesthesia, after which she may work to better advantage. Ethylene given to dull the pain in the stretching perineum may remove the inhibition on the abdominal muscles. A change of position from side to back, or back to side, or to the sitting posture, or even a short walk, may be useful. A multipara, however, may not go far from the

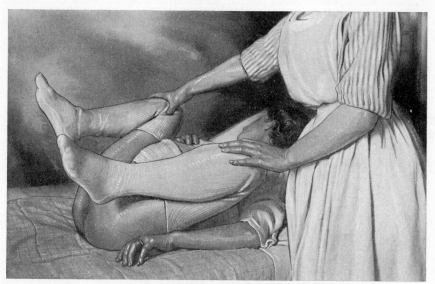

Fig. 495.—Exaggerated Lithotomy Position.

bed. Ergot is never to be given to stimulate the uterus. A valuable help is the instruction of the parturient as to the best way to bear down, and the physician, in a sterile gown, may sit on the edge of the bed, and, grasping the woman's hands, with each pain show her how to get the most out of her efforts. Another plan which has been of inestimable service in my practice is to place the woman in the exaggerated lithotomy posture (Fig. 495). The thighs support the abdominal muscles and thus strengthen them; any tendency to pendulous belly is corrected; the fetus is straightened out, the levator ani tightened (which facilitates anterior rotation of the occiput), and the outlet of the bony pelvis is enlarged.

By putting the patient in a squatting Indian attitude against either a wall or the bed, as King recommends so highly, the same results are obtainable, but it is not so easy nor so comfortable (Fig. 354). A hot enema may hasten delivery by unloading the bowel and by stimulating the forces. If the head is well down on the perineum, Kristeller's expression may be employed (Fig. 496). Both hands are evenly spread over the fundus, and during the pains gently applied, but firm pressure is exerted in the axis of the inlet. As the contraction of the uterus diminishes, the

force applied is to lessen.   It is impractical to keep up the pressure between pains.
Kristeller's expression is not without dangers—rupture of the uterus, abruptio
placentæ, injury to the abdominal viscera, and for this reason it should seldom be

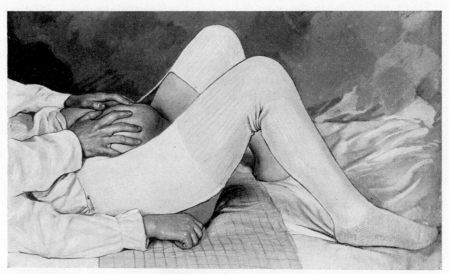

FIG. 496.—KRISTELLER EXPRESSION.

used in multiparæ, never when there is the least sign of thinning of the lower uterine
segment, and always with only moderate force.

If the head is so low that the forehead has passed the coccyx, Ritgen's manœuver may be used, that is, pressing the head out with two fingers working from

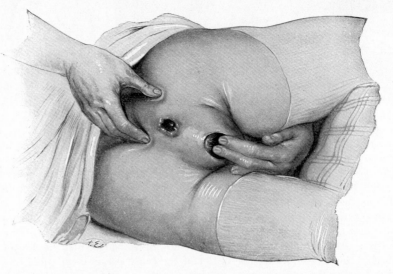

FIG. 497.—MODIFIED RITGEN'S MANŒUVER, PRESSING THE HEAD OUT WITH TWO FINGERS AT EITHER SIDE OF RECTUM.
Drawn from a photograph.   The four-ply sterile towel is not shown.   In practice patient lies on her back.

the rectum.   While the objection on the score of infection could be removed by the
use of rubber gloves, there is still danger of injury to the rectum, and cracks, fissures,
infiltrates, bruises, with subsequent stricture, are to be considered.   By placing the
two fingers outside, on the perineum, one on each side of the coccyx, with the flat-

tened rectum between them, sometimes one can obtain sufficient purchase on the forehead to aid materially in the delivery (Fig. 497). This operation may be advantageously combined with episiotomy. Incision of the perineum is a very useful operation, and, if all that is needed to complete the labor is overcoming the resistance of the vulvar outlet, episiotomy shows brilliant results. Indeed, the author often performs it to save the pelvic floor from excessive stretching.

If encouragement and instruction of the parturient and the above measures fail, forceps are to be applied, and easily 75 per cent. of the forceps operations in America are done for indications of this nature.

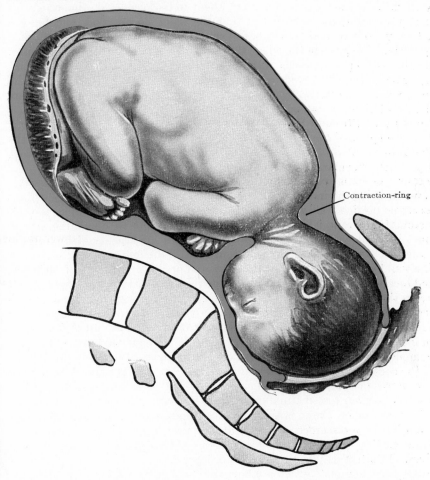

Contraction-ring

FIG. 498.—CONTRACTION-RING AROUND CHILD'S NECK. (CONTRACTION OF BANDL'S RING, STRICTURA UTERI).

The above remarks apply to the treatment of weakness of the abdominal muscles, when the second stage is well on, and the head deeply engaged in the pelvis—even visible in the vulva. If the head is not engaged, but still above the inlet, the case is much more formidable. What was said regarding the treatment of weak pains in general applies here. Unless the head can be gotten to enter the pelvis by the usual means, a high forceps operation or version and extraction will be required, both of which are dangerous under such circumstances, because of the frequency and extent of the necessarily inflicted lacerations, and the usually severe and sometimes intractable atony of the uterus postpartum. Manual removal of the placenta is often necessitated, which adds to the danger of infection. Hofmeier recommended pressing the head into the pelvis from the outside, using two

40

hands, and under favorable special conditions this may succeed. The Walcher posture has been used, but with only moderate success. (See Treatment of Contracted Pelves.) In some cases the squatting posture favors the passage of the head through the inlet, especially with pendulous abdomen. Should operative delivery be imperatively demanded, all preparations must be made to avoid the above-named dangers.

Myoclonia Uteri or Cramp Pains.—When the action of the uterus is irregular, painful, and inefficient, even though the force apparently exerted is normal or even greater than normal, we speak of cramp pains or myoclonia uteri. The condition is closely allied to tetanus or spasmus uteri, about to be considered. Labor is very painful and prolonged; the women feel that the pains do no good, and become nervous, highly excited, and sometimes even delirious. The constant suffering, with inappreciable progress in the labor, throws the parturient into a sort of frenzy. The danger of cramp pains, besides their bad effect on the morale of the parturient, lies in asphyxia of the child, and in the possible injuries and infections from the operations rendered necessary by the delay. Cases of real myoclonia uteri are rare; strictura uteri occurs oftener.

Tetanus Uteri. Strictura Uteri.—When the uterus passes into a state of tonic contraction, we speak of *tetanus uteri*. If the spasm involves only one zone of the organ, the term *strictura uteri* is applied. Older writers called it "hour-glass contraction." Such irregularities denote a dyssynergia uteri.

The causes of cramp pains, tetanus, and strictura are much alike, an unstable nervous system being the most frequent predisposing factor. Locally, any irritant to the cervix or uterine wall will evoke tempestuous action, for example, too frequent examinations, especially if combined with attempts to dilate the cervix; chronic metritis and cervicitis; the improper use and application of hydrostatic bags; premature attempts at delivery through an ill-dilated cervix; irritation of the uterine wall by the hand, bougies, douches; and premature rupture of the membranes and escape of the liquor amnii, which permit the uterine wall to apply itself too firmly on the irregular and knobby fetal body. In abruptio placentæ with concealed hemorrhage the uterus is sometimes in a tetanic state. It will be noticed that the remedies recommended for the treatment of atony of the uterus may send the organ into tempestuous action or cause stricture. Obstructed labor produces a condition analogous to tetanus uteri, but here the uterus is moderately firm all the time, and the contractions are regular and powerful—sometimes sufficiently so as to burst it. A uterus in tetanic spasm will not rupture, but operations undertaken during the contraction will tear it if too much force is used. (See Contracted Pelvis.)

Ergot, in the olden times, was frequently responsible for tetanus uteri, but now, since it has been discarded as the result of almost universal condemnation by obstetric authorities, one rarely meets such a case, except perhaps in the practice of midwives. Pituitrin may cause these conditions.

Tetanus uteri completely stops labor; the woman complains of continuous pain; the child dies as the result of asphyxia, the contracted uterus preventing the oxygenation of the fetal blood, and soon, because of the same circulatory disturbance, infection of the uterus and contents occurs. When sepsis begins, the pulse and temperature mount rapidly, the skin becomes dry, the face cyanotic or red, and great tenderness in and around the uterus is noticeable. The liquor amnii takes on a bad odor, is discolored—a cloudy green or gray—the vulva reddens and swells, while any abrasions on the labia become covered with a gray exudate. Gas may accumulate in the uterus, paralyzing it, after which the organ balloons out—that is, tympania uteri develops. In such cases the Bacterium coli is usually found. Unless relief is brought, the woman dies of sepsis or exhaustion, or both.

Strictura Uteri.—A spasm of a zone of circular fibers of the uterus may imprison the fetus. Sometimes the constriction is around the child's neck, as in Fig. 498, and sometimes around the trunk or breech, a groove around the arms and chest having been demonstrable in a case delivered at the Chicago Lying-in Hospital. Ordinarily, the contraction of the remainder of the uterus is not strong enough to rupture the lower uterine segment, nor, indeed, to overcome the resistance of the constricting ring. Therefore labor comes to a standstill, and we find the same clinical picture as in tetanus uteri (*q. v.*), though not so aggravated nor so quickly fatal. The contractions are irregular both in frequency and in strength, are very painful, and the woman is frenzied by the delay in labor in spite of constant and prolonged suffering. The lower part of the uterus is hard, the fundus soft (between pains), and the lower abdomen is very tender. Attempts at version may be rendered futile by the stricture if they do not rupture the uterus. In one of my cases the whole fetus was locked in above the stricture, which was so narrow that I could not insert more than three fingers (Fig. 499).

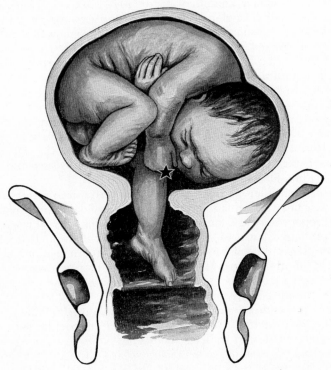

Fig. 499.—Strictura Uteri (Spasm of Bandl's Ring). Star Indicates Location of Navel.

Strictures are oftenest found in primiparæ of neurasthenic type and in women in whom the bag of waters ruptures early in labor. After a while progress ceases, the head remains high up and in the transverse diameter, the cervix becomes edematous, infiltrated with leukocytes, and infected with bacteria (Couvelaire), and the vagina hot and dry. Attempts to rotate head succeed easily, but occiput turns quickly back, as on a pivot, shoulders being locked in position by uterine spasm.

In the third stage, strictura uteri, or hour-glass contraction, is of great significance, being a frequent cause of postpartum hemorrhage with incarceration of the placenta, and even producing anomalies of uterine contraction after the placenta is delivered.

Diagnosis.—Tetanus uteri is easily determined from the board-like consistence of the organ, the continuous pain, and suspended labor. Spasm of Bandl's ring is suspected in all cases of cramp pains, irregular and painful uterine action, excessively slow dilatation of the cervix, in the absence of disease of the latter, but it can be positively diagnosed only when the ring is palpable internally or abdominally. Tetanus uteri must be differentiated from the simple emptying of the organ of the liquor amnii and the passive application of its walls to the child.   In tetanus the uterus is very hard, ovoid, and the fetal parts are not palpable, while the hand introduced from below can only with the greatest difficulty, and sometimes only with the risk of a rupture of the wall, be passed up to the fundus.   In simple retraction the uterine wall is firm but pliable, the uterus has the shape of the fetus, and varies according to the attitude of the latter; fetal parts are readily felt, and the hand is easily passed up to the fundus and version or other manipulations performed.   If the reader will recall the mechanism of the formation of the lower uterine segment, he will find that the junction of the contractile with the dilating portion of the uterus has been given four names: The contraction ring, the retraction ring, Bandl's ring, Braune's ring.   Since stricture usually occurs at this level of the uterus, the physiologic and pathologic conditions have been confused.   American teachers use the terms contraction ring and retraction ring interchangeably, but White and others give the first a pathologic, the latter a normal connotation, unless the ring, as the result of obstructed labor, rises too high (Schmid).   Practitioners also believe that a high Bandl's ring is an obstruction to labor and to intra-uterine manipulation.   It is the strictura uteri, sometimes called "contraction of Bandl's ring," that is an obstruction to labor, but the high Bandl or retraction ring only indicates the dangerous thinning of the lower uterine segment.   Differentiation is necessary and possible.   In obstructed labor, the child being delivered largely into the lower uterine segment, the contracting and retracted fundus uteri may be thought to be in tetanus.   Here the shape of the tumor, the hard fundus, the soft, dilated lower uterine segment, regularly recurring pains, and the internal exploration will clear the diagnosis (Fink, Demelin).

Treatment.—Irregular and cramp pains and stricture of the uterus require sedatives, first among which is the influence of a confident and capable physician and nurse.   Proper encouragement will help the nervous, excited woman to become quieted.   A prolonged hot pack, followed by a hot drink of malted milk, and $\frac{1}{4}$ or $\frac{1}{6}$ grain of morphin will produce sleep and a better uterine action.   Atropin has a sedative effect in dysmenorrhea, and likewise in uterine overaction and "cervical spasm" during labor.   It may be combined with the morphin, in fairly large dosage, after inquiring about idiosyncrasy.   Rucker says 0.3 c.c. of 1/1000 epinephrin will stop uterine action for ten to thirty minutes.   Sodium bromid up to 120 grains may be exhibited.   Change of position from back to side, the elevated Sims, or the knee-chest, and walking about may be tried.   Vaginal examinations are restricted, and all attempts to dilate the cervix omitted.

A tetanically contracted uterus seldom responds to the above treatment and delivery is indicated.   A prime requisite for any and all intra-uterine manipulations in tetanus uteri is profound anesthesia.   Ether is to be preferred because the patient must be brought close to the danger-line of narcosis, and the operation must not be begun—not even the hand introduced—until the uterus has relaxed.   In very rare instances a prolonged, deep chloroform narcosis failed to quiet the uterus; delivery from below proved impossible, and laparotrachelotomy had to be performed.

Spasm of the Cervix; Strictura Cervicis.—Many authors deny the existence of spasmodic rigidity of the cervix.   Fieux claims that there are practically no muscular fibers in the cervix around the external os near term.   Nevertheless, a few cases in the author's experience have shown that occasionally the cervix will contract, either in front of the presenting part or, more commonly, around the neck after the head is through it, or after the body is delivered in breech presentation, and thus create an obstacle to delivery.   Most of the cases of so-called rigidity of the cervix are not spasmodic, but anatomic, due to some alteration of structure and most cases of "rigid os" are the result of improper contractions of the uterus.

The causes, diagnosis, and treatment are on the same lines as those of strictura uteri. Stricture of the cervix around the after-coming head is often more apparent than real, though the effect is serious, just the same. The slender body slips through the unprepared cervix, but the head is arrested. Such a cervix, not dilating with gentle efforts, may have to be incised. Greenhill had a case of stricture at the external os.

Precipitate Labors—Too Strong Pains.—Too strong uterine action and too strong abdominal action are sometimes observed, and they lead to the too rapid delivery of the child. Since the abdominal action is mostly reflexly excited by the uterine pains, when the latter are strong, the former will also be strong. Then, too, even after long labor, the first stage having been very slow, characterized by either atonia or myoclonia uteri, when the head finally has reached the perineum, its presence here may evoke such powerful abdominal action that labor is finished entirely too quickly.

Precipitate labor is the forcible, violent expulsion of the child in a period of time disproportionate to that normally required for the safe overcoming of the resistances. Sometimes the woman has pains for several hours, but does not recognize them as true labor pains, and sends for the accoucheur too late. These labors should not be called precipitate. Many cases are on record where the uterus, without warning, suddenly became violently active and expressed the child in a few minutes to an hour. The woman may be thus overtaken on the street and not have time to run to shelter. In her excitement she may forget to lie down, and the child may fall to the ground, the cord breaking. In a case in the dispensary service of the Chicago Lying-in Hospital the mother was lying down and the child was hurled against the foot of the bed, the cord breaking, but the child was not injured. In another from the same service the child fell to the floor and died from a fractured skull. Very important are these cases from a medicolegal point of view, since the mother, if she was delivered alone, may be accused of having killed the child. The best authorities (Freyer) are now agreed that the excitement and pain incident to such an event can produce a state of mental aberration which may persist during the last few minutes of labor, and for a variable period after it, certainly long enough for the child to drown in the mass of blood, feces, urine, liquor amnii, and meconium, in which, under such circumstances, it is likely to be born. The actual causes of too strong pains and precipitate labor are not known. Pituitrin may act thus. Heredity, habit, neurasthenia, multiparity, large pelvis, small child, cervicitis, and old cervical and perineal lacerations have been cited as predisposing factors. Various uteri have varying contractile power—just as men have greater or less musculature and better or worse muscle, and, usually, the conduct of the uterus in a given labor may be anticipated to be like its action in previous deliveries.

Dangers of Precipitate Labor.—In the author's experience these accidents have occurred: complete and incomplete lacerations of the perineum, clitoris tears, laceration of the cervix, postpartum hemorrhage, rupture of the uterus with fatal hemorrhage, obstetric shock, puerperal sepsis, asphyxia neonatorum, fracture of the child's skull, intracranial hemorrhage, drowning of twins in the discharges, and rupture of the cord. It must be said that these are very rare, with the exception of mild and moderately severe perineal tears, and represent isolated instances from private practice and the large service of several hospitals. Other authors have noticed postpartum hemorrhage, but not fatal, emphysema of the neck, fracture of the sternum, hæmatoma vulvæ. Hirst records an instance of marvelous endurance on the part of the infant. A woman on an express train going 40 miles an hour dropped the infant through the water-closet, and it was picked out of the snow an hour later, alive and uninjured. Winckel records 20 children delivered in winter and exposed for hours without harm. These facts are exceptional—many children have died from cold and injury.

Treatment.—If the pains are coming on tempestuously, one following the other in rapid succession, the woman's face becoming turgid, and the bearing-down efforts prolonged and powerful, the accoucheur must do something to prevent the too rapid expulsion of the child and the injury to the soft parts. The patient is to be turned on the side, and ether given until the uterine action has moderated. Admonitions to the woman to not bear down are usually useless, because she cannot help it. If the head is coming through the vulva in spite of mild measures, it should be allowed to come. Under no circumstances should an attempt be made forcibly to hold the head back with a view to saving the perineum. The danger of rupture of the uterus thus arises, the conditions thus artificially produced resembling obstructed labor. Episiotomy is to be performed if there is time. Care is to be exerted to save the rapidly emerging child from injury. After precipitate labors it may be necessary to make an internal examination to find if there are deep injuries. External and internal hemorrhage and the general aspects of the case will decide this point. In cleaning up a case where the child has been delivered without the usual aseptic preparations, the open vulva is to be treated on the same principles as a compound fracture. A physician called in emergency to a partus præcipitatus should not express the placenta unless there be hemorrhage, but should institute proper arrangements for the conduct of the third stage, or provide for the transportation of the patient to a hospital or home. Pending the arrival of the woman's own accoucheur, he should do only that which is absolutely necessary for the safety of the mother and child, and should turn the case over to him upon his arrival.

Literature

Bell: British Med. Jour., December 4, 1909.—*Cotret:* Revue Int. de Med. et de Chir. Mars., 1926.—*Couvelaire, Boissel:* L'Edeme du Col. Thèse de Paris, 1922.—*Crodel:* See Lenthold, Arch. für Gynaek., 1932, vol. cxlviii, Heft 2, p. 520.—*Dale:* Jour. Phys., 24, No. 3, 1906.—*Demelin:* Monograph de la Contraction uterine et des dyskinésies Corr., Paris, 1927.—*Fink:* Zeitschr. für Geb. u. Gyn., 1926, vol. xc, S. 1–13.—*Freyer:* Die Ohnmacht bei der Geburt, Springer, Berlin, 1887.—*Greenhill:* Jour. Amer. Med. Assoc., January 14, 1922.—*Harris:* Amer. Jour. Obst. and Gyn., February, 1927, p. 135.—*Hofbauer:* "Pituitrin," Zentralbl. f. Gyn., January, 1911, No. 4.—*Jardine:* Jour. Obst. and Gyn., British Empire, July 1, 1911.—*Kahn:* Jour. Amer. Med. Assoc., January 23, 1915.—*Mendenhall:* Jour. Amer. Med. Assoc., April, 1929. See also Roques, Jour. Obstet. and Gyn., British Empire, Summer, 1932, p. 320, re Thymophysin.—*Pituitrin:* Complete literature, Jour. Amer. Med. Assoc., May 2, 1914. Also Yearbook on Obstetrics, DeLee, 1914, p. 95.—*Rossa:* "Contraction Ring and Mechanism of Labor," Monatsschr. f. Geb. u. Gyn., 1900, vol. xii, p. 457.—*Rucker:* Jour. Amer. Med. Assoc., May 21, 1921. Literature to date.—*Schmid:* Zentb. für Gynaek., October 23, 1926, p. 2760.—*Süssman:* Zentb. f. Gyn., 1917, No. 17.—*Watson:* Transactions Amer. Gyn. Soc., 1922.—*White:* Lancet, London, 1913, i, 604.

CHAPTER XLIX

ANOMALIES OF THE PASSENGERS

Classification.—Under this caption are to be considered irregularities of the mechanism of labor due to the child. While those due to the placenta might belong here, it is best to take them up with the study of postpartum hemorrhage. Anomalies of the mechanism of labor are due to errors of attitude, of presentation, and of position of the child, and also to the overgrowth of the fetal body as a whole or as a part. Before taking up this branch of the subject the student is advised to read what was said about the mechanism of normal labor, for the following pages will deal mainly with descriptions of the factors of labor gone wrong. For quick and clear orientation regarding the relations of the fetus to the mother, and the various movements executed in the mechanism of labor, a pelvis and fetal head are almost absolutely necessary, though the little models and paper manikins on the market will aid very much. It is also necessary to have clear notions regarding the terms used in describing all phases of the subject.

"Attitude" or posture means the relation of the parts of the fetus to each other; "presentation" is the part of the fetus which lies over the os, or is bounded by the girdle of resistance, and "position" means the relation of any given arbitrary point in the presenting part to the four quadrants of the mother's pelvis. The name of this arbitrary point is the "point of direction." It might also be called the "denominator." To a certain extent attitude determines presentation; for example, when the head lies over the inlet, not in its usual condition of flexion, but with the chin extended, face presentation results. If the head is less deflexed, brow presentation, and if only partly deflexed, the vertex being felt over the os, median vertex presentation is diagnosed. These might be grouped together as "deflexion attitudes." In addition to these, the result of errors of attitude, there are abnormal presentations produced by errors of polarity of the fetus, such as breech and shoulder presentation. Other anomalies of attitude are prolapse of the feet in breech presentation, of the arm in head presentation, of the cord in all presentations, etc. Just as in occipital presentations, each of the abnormal presentations may lie in different positions. Following Baudelocque and Hodge, six positions were distinguished in occipital presentations—O.L.A., O.L.T., O.L.P., O.D.A., O.D.T., O.D.P.—and six may be described for most of the abnormal presentations, though not all are observed in practice; for example, Sac.L.A., S.L.T., S.L.P., S.D.A., S.D.T., and S.D.P. In breech presentation S.L.A. and S.D.P. are the ones almost exclusively observed.

Finally, errors in rotation of the presenting part occur; either rotation ceases before its completion, or the presenting part turns backward into the sacrum, causing severe dystocia. It is thus evident that an almost infinite variety of combinations of presentations and errors of attitude and position may be presented to the accoucheur for study, and when it is considered that, in addition, a contracted pelvis, a large child, twins, or monsters may coexist, not to mention all superadded complications incidental and accidental to parturition, one must concede that truly formidable problems of deep complexity are offered for solution.

Unusual Mechanisms of Head Labors.—In order will be discussed errors of rotation in occipital presentations and the deflexion attitudes—median vertex, forehead, brow, and face presentation.

Persistent Occipitoposterior Position.—Normally, when labor starts with O.D.P. or O.L.P., anterior rotation occurs, and the delivery terminates as in

O.L.A. and O.D.A. Sutugin, of Russia, believes that in the majority of cases the head enters the pelvis in the transverse diameter, which agrees with my experience. After it has passed the inlet the occiput turns either toward the front or the back—almost always toward the pubis. Should the occiput turn toward the sacrum, or should the head enter the pelvis in an oblique with the occiput behind, an occipito-posterior position results. In rare instances the head may enter the pelvis with the occiput pointed directly behind, with the chin palpable above the pubis, or the occiput may rotate into the hollow of the sacrum after engagement. These are called occipitosacral positions. Peculiar dispositions of the soft parts and of the fetal head probably explain why the occiput commits these vagaries of engagement.

In still rarer instances the head enters and passes through the pelvis with the occiput directly anterior, and no rotation is needed in the mechanism of its delivery. Prolapse of an arm was the cause of this anomaly in the one instance the author observed. Labor may be difficult or impossible. High assimilation pelvis may cause engagement of the head in the sagittal diameter of the pelvis.

Since, in the large majority of cases of occipitoposterior position, anterior rotation finally occurs, a search into the cause of its persistence is necessary: (a) Flat pelvis in minor degrees, the occiput meeting resistance first and deflexion occurring; (b) primary brachycephalia, the two head levers being of the same length and flexion not occurring; (c) pendulous abdomen, the convex back of the fetus fitting better to the posterior arched wall of the uterus; (d) large pelvis, small child, the natural mechanism of labor of balanced resistances becoming inoperative; (e) prolapse of an arm in front of the occiput—if it lay behind the occiput, anterior rotation would be facilitated; (f) anything that would mechanically prevent anterior rotation of the head, or that would hold back the child's trunk and thus keep the back posterior, for example, the placenta, tumors in the wall of the uterus, scars in the uterus which give the lower uterine segment an irregular shape, dysharmony of the segmental actions of fundus isthmus and cervix, a full rectum or bladder, etc.; (g) exhaustion of the powers before rotation has been completed; in such cases "arrest" of rotation occurs at any point in the transit of the occiput; (h) vices of configuration of the bony pelvic cavity, for example, poorly developed spines of the ischia—funnel pelvis, transversely contracted pelvis (Thoms); (i) abnormal pelvic floor, which gives a wrong bend to the parturient canal or does not form a good gutter; (j) persistent asynclitism. (See Figs. 194, a, b, c, p. 180.) Not all the causes are known or understood. Given a cause, the child soon becomes molded to the abnormal position, the uterus adapts itself to the child, and the condition is less easily corrected as labor goes on.

Course.—Two varieties are distinguishable: first, those where the head remains high up and will not engage, and those where the head enters the pelvis with the occiput behind. In the first class, which, fortunately, are rare, labor comes to a standstill, and occasionally a brow presentation develops, a little deflexion occurring. In the second type the occiput sinks in either the transverse or one of the obliques, and comes to the second parallel plane of Hodge. Now four terminations are possible: (1) Under strong pains the occiput sweeps forward through the 135 degrees and comes to lie under the pubis (commonest); (2) it comes forward more or less, usually to the transverse diameter, and stops—"deep transverse arrest"; (3) it may come down in the transverse, and the head may even be delivered in the transverse, the occiput rolling out under one of the descending rami pubis; (4) it may rotate backward to the hollow of the sacrum, becoming an occipitosacral position. If the head rotates backward into the sacrum, nature manages the delivery in two ways: First, extreme flexion occurs, and the pains force the head downward and backward against the perineum, which is much overstretched and nearly always torn; descent is continued until the forehead stems behind the pubis and the occiput has escaped either over or through the torn perineum, the perineal region coming to lie on the nape of the neck; now the face appears from behind the pubis, extension occurring (Fig. 500). Secondly, as the head descends deflexion occurs, the forehead takes the lead and becomes the point of direction, and descent continues until the brow appears in the vulva, the glabella stems behind the pubis,

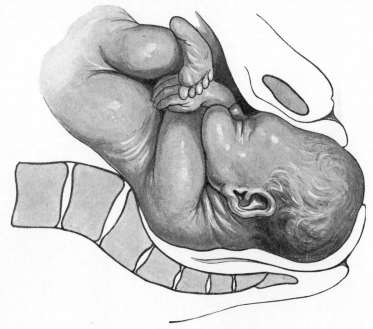

FIG. 500.—OCCIPITOSACRAL. FIRST MECHANISM, FLEXION.

and now the occiput appears over the perineum, which is more endangered than in the first instance; lastly, the face comes from behind the pubis (Fig. 501). In this

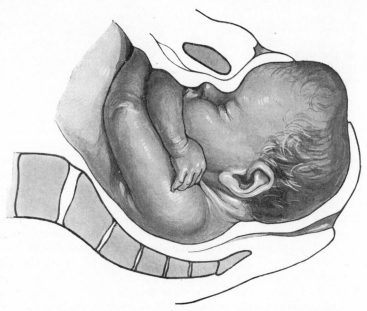

FIG. 501.—OCCIPITOSACRAL. SECOND MECHANISM, PARTIAL EXTENSION.

form it is almost impossible clinically to differentiate the mechanism from that of brow presentation. External rotation or restitution of the occiput to the rear is the rule, the face looking upward, but when the shoulders start to come, they usually descend in an oblique or even in the sagittal diameter, and then the face turns slightly toward one side.

Molding of the head with the first mechanism is that of extreme dolichocephaly (Fig. 502), the occiput being more than usually pointed, while with the second mechanism the shape of the head resembles more that of the brow presentation (Fig. 503). In multiparæ naturally the head does not suffer as much distortion as in primiparæ. The caput succedaneum in the first mechanism is found over the sagittal suture, anterior to the small fontanel; in the second mechanism it lies over the large fontanel. Lateral asymmetry of the head is usually absent.

Clinical Course and Diagnosis.—In occipitoposterior positions labor is generally slower and longer, the pains being weak and irregular both as to time and as to strength. Such pains may serve to draw the accoucheur's attention to the condition. Early rupture of the bag of waters is frequent, and in general things do not go smoothly. The head stays high up longer than in anterior positions, requires

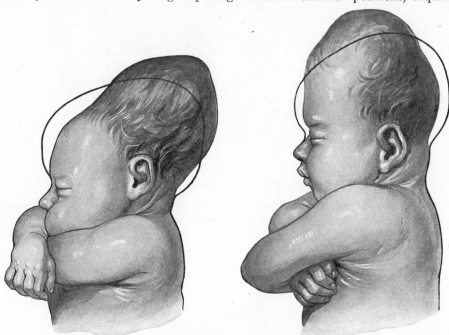

FIG. 502.—MOLDING IN OCCIPITOSACRAL. FIRST MECH-ANISM.　　　FIG. 503.—MOLDING IN OCCIPITOSACRAL. SECOND MECHANISM.

stronger pains to bring it well down in the pelvis, and, after anterior rotation has started, the uterus and abdominal pressure may prove unequal to the task of forcing the head all the way round, labor coming to a standstill with arrested rotation. Dilatation of the cervix is incomplete because the head does not fit well into the pelvis, and it does not press equally on the internal os all around. Spontaneous delivery in occipitoposterior positions requires great uterine and abdominal effort, because—(1) The head traverses the pelvic floor with its largest diameters. Instead of the small suboccipitobregmatic and suboccipitofrontal planes, the occipitofrontal and the occipitomental planes pass through the vulva. (2) When the chin is strongly flexed on the sternum, the nape of the neck is stretched and the child forms a solid, unbendable cylinder, which cannot accommodate itself to the angular birth-canal. The birth-canal, therefore, has to either stretch or tear, to allow the cylinder to pass through. (3) The back and the head have to pass through the pelvis together (Fig. 500). Perineal lacerations are the rule unless the child is small or the woman multiparous. They are due to the fact that the head passes through, presenting larger planes than usual, and also to the fact that the perineum is much and forcibly dislocated downward—torn off, in fact, from its bony and vaginal attachments.

Abdominally, in thin women, the diagnosis may sometimes be made by a glance—over the pubis there is a distinct hollow. Palpation reveals the shoulder far back from the median line, and the forehead and chin may be felt over the opposite ramus pubis. The heart-tones are deep in the flank and distant from the ear, although if, as sometimes occurs, there is a moderate deflexion of the head, the chest is pushed forward against the abdominal wall and the heart-tones are very loud and distinct. They are then on the same side as the forehead, opposite to that on which the back may be felt, and this finding may give rise to erroneous diagnoses of face presentation or of occiput presentation, the accoucheur believing the occiput is on the side other than the one truly present. Internally, early in labor the head is felt high up, usually partly deflexed, the small fontanel being higher, or on a level with the large, which is nearer the center of the pelvis. Unless the pelvis is contracted or the belly pendulous, the head is synclytic. If anterior rotation is going to occur, flexion takes place with descent. The palpating finger will discover the

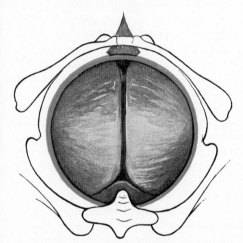

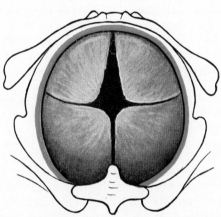

FIG. 504.—TOUCH PICTURE OF OCCIPITOSACRAL POSITION. FIRST MECHANISM: FLEXION.

FIG. 505.—TOUCH PICTURE OF OCCIPITOSACRAL POSITION. SECOND MECHANISM: EXTENSION.

tendency of the small fontanel to turn to the front during the pains, or will find it easy to push the occiput in this direction. If posterior rotation is to be the mechanism, the head descends in moderate extension, this attitude of the child having been called "military," that is, the head is set squarely on the shoulders. As the occiput turns into the hollow of the sacrum, the finger feels the small fontanel deeply on the rectum, and the large one behind the pubis, the sagittal suture running nearly anteroposteriorly and from above forward, downward, and backward. If the first mechanism of delivery, that of extreme flexion, is the one selected by nature, the large fontanel is felt just under the pubis; if the second, that of extension, the large fontanel lies in the center of the pelvis, and the glabella will be felt behind the pubis (Figs. 504 and 505). Owing to the usually large caput succedaneum, it is not always easy to outline the sutures, and under these difficulties the finger is to be passed to the side, until the ear is found, when the direction of the tragus will bring clarity. Not seldom the accoucheur is surprised by the head being delivered with the occiput over the perineum, when he was anticipating a normal mechanism. A *bimanual* examination, discovering the chin above the pubis, would have averted this humiliation.

Prognosis.—Mortality and morbidity are higher for both mother and child in occipitoposterior positions. For the mother, exhaustion and sepsis from prolonged labor, and the frequently necessary operations, with the almost inevitable lacerations, are to be feared. Postpartum hemorrhage from secondary inertia uteri is not rare. For the child, asphyxia and the operative delivery bring danger, and without doubt, in the author's opinion, more children are lost from this complication than are lost from the effects of contracted pelvis.

Treatment.—When the head is high, "floating" above the pelvis, "caput ballitabile," it is best not to interfere. A complete examination is to be made to determine the existence of a contracted pelvis or other anomaly which may require treatment for its own sake, and also, if possible, the cause of the occipitoposterior position. During the usually prolonged first stage the woman should walk around, or lie on her back in bed, until the head engages. Rupture of the bag of waters retards, rather than hastens, labor in these positions, both by interfering with the mechanism of labor and by removing the hydrostatic cervical dilator, and besides loss of the liquor amnii makes version, if the case comes to it, much more difficult or even impossible. Watchful expectancy is the treatment until an indication for interference arises. Morphin and scopolamin may be given. If the labor drags on, and danger to either mother or child, while not imminent, is to be anticipated, dilatation of the cervix may be hastened by the use of the colpeurynter or by packing the vagina tightly with gauze saturated with 10 per cent. boroglycerin (Polak). If the head remains high long after complete dilatation, it may be advisable to anesthetize the woman, change the position to one anterior, impress the head into the pelvis by combined manipulation or draw it down with forceps, and then leave the case to nature. In primiparæ this method is far more preferable than version unless the attendant is very skilful.

After the head has engaged, watchful expectancy is still practised, because the vast majority of cases terminate in anterior rotation, or at least in rotation to or beyond the transverse diameter, and thus become easy forceps operations. Change in posture, even the knee-chest, may be tried, but most of the time the woman should lie on the side to which the occiput points. By this means the breech is thrown over to the side, the spinal column is straightened, the occiput is forced down, flexion increased, and, therefore, rotation favored. Sometimes a change to the side position will strengthen uterine action. Hodge's manœuver may be helpful—upward pressure on the sinciput during pains. This, by increasing flexion, favors rotation. Tarnier advised direct rotation of the head with the fingers or half-hand, operating from behind the ear, at the same time pressing the forehead to the rear from the outside. Older writers, among whom Hodge may be mentioned, recommended the vectis for these cases. Objections to all these manœuvers may be urged on the score of danger of infection and inefficiency. In multiparæ they occasionally succeed, and may shorten the labor somewhat. At all events, they should not be persisted in, and much force may not be used, but if an indication arises for interference, it is best to make the manual correction of the malposition under anesthesia, as is described in Chapter LXX, page 1009. Failing the last, recourse is to be had to forceps.

Occipitosacral positions often require assistance. If the head is descending in flexion, the perineum is not endangered as much as when the forehead comes down. In either case a deep episiotomy is indicated unless the patient is a multipara. (See Chapter on Forceps.)

Internal Super-rotation.—In roomy pelves, or when the child is small, anterior rotation of the occiput may be exaggerated, the small fontanel passing beyond the middle line to the opposite side of the pelvis. An O.L.A. may, in the course of labor, become an O.D.A. The accoucheur will be surprised to find the back on one side and the occiput on the other, but sometimes the back rotates too and the attendant will imagine his first diagnosis was wrong. Indeed, occasionally the head will rotate through the hollow of the sacrum from an O.L.P. to an O.D.P., and the back, which at first was on the left, later lies on the right side. In internal super-rotation the head in the course of delivery may turn back again, or may escape in an oblique diameter of the outlet, the back pointing to the side opposite that of the occiput, but sometimes the trunk follows the rotation of the head, and may escape with the back looking directly upward, or even to the side to which the occiput had rotated. A turbinal movement is thus imparted to the child.

Again, though the head comes out in the normal mechanism, the shoulders may super-rotate, the back coming out on the side opposite that to which the occiput originally pointed. A knowledge of these variations of the mechanism of delivery is necessary for the proper conduct of the end of the second stage. As a general rule nature needs no help. When the delivery of the trunk is too slow, the woman should be asked to bear down; a moderate pressure may be exerted on the fundus, but traction on the child is made only when absolutely necessary. In doing this the accoucheur should aid and supplement the mechanism evidently intended by nature. For example, if, after delivery of the head, external restitution does not occur, but the shoulders show a tendency to turn in a direction opposite to that which was expected, the attendant should favor the movement, because if he sought to impress a contrary one, the child would stop in its rotation and the back would

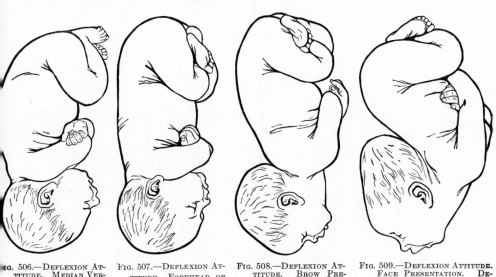

FIG. 506.—DEFLEXION ATTITUDE. MEDIAN VERTEX, "MILITARY." FIG. 507.—DEFLEXION ATTITUDE. FOREHEAD OR BREGMA PRESENTATION. FIG. 508.—DEFLEXION ATTITUDE. BROW PRESENTATION. FIG. 509.—DEFLEXION ATTITUDE. FACE PRESENTATION. DEFLEXION COMPLETED.

come out transversely, with injury to the perineum or fracture of the child's clavicle, or, indeed, the delivery of the body would be arrested, requiring strong traction in order to free it.

Deflexion Attitudes.—Often, during an examination early in labor, the head is found lying over the inlet with the large fontanel lower than the small, or even with the root of the nose and the eyes palpable. After regular uterine action is established, or if the parturient adopts a favorable posture, the small fontanel will sink and labor will assume a normal mechanism. Should the cause of the abnormal attitude of the child persist, the body of the child will remain in the wrong posture, the uterus will fix the trunk and adapt itself permanently to the abnormal conditions, a pathologic mechanism resulting. All degrees of deflexion of the head may be found, but it would be useless and confusing to describe them all. Clinically, four of these deflexion attitudes deserve mention as distinct presentations, having a clearly defined course and mechanism. Named in the order of the degree of deflexion, they are: (1) Median vertex presentation, or "military" attitude; (2) forehead presentation; (3) brow presentation; (4) face presentation. In all these the trunk of the child passes, in a varying degree, from its natural condition of flexion or C shape to one of extension or S shape, face presentation representing the greatest change (Figs. 506–509).

Causation.—All cases of deflexion attitudes cannot be explained by one cause, and often several factors combine to produce the abnormal presentation. In general, primary and secondary factors may be distinguished, *i. e.*, those active during pregnancy and those showing in labor. The primary factors are anything that will cause a straightening of the child's trunk, abnormality of the cervical spine (Kermauner, Mayer*) as tumors of the fetus, tumors of the uterus pressing in the fetal back, a congenitally long uterus which cannot adapt itself well to a curved fetal back, obliquity of the uterus, tumors of the neck of the fetus, as

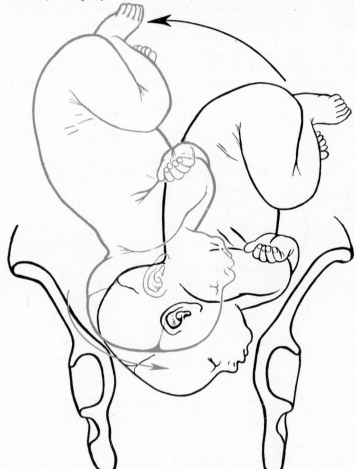

FIG. 510.—SHOWING CORRECTION OF FACE PRESENTATION BY POSTURE.

goiter, a short, deep-chested child which does not allow the chin to flex fully, and the spontaneous nutatory movements of the child. Should the pains come on when the infant happens to have his head extended, the lower uterine segment may lock the child in this position. Baudelocque called attention to the wrong direction of the uterine forces when the uterus was oblique to the inlet—if, before engagement, the back falls too far over to the side of the occiput, the chin extends, and if, now, uterine action commences, the fetal axis pressure is exerted in the direction of the chin, increasing the extension, even to the production of a face presentation. Anencephali usually present by the face—snout labors (Ahl-

* Mayer, A.: Zentr. für Gyn., November 28, 1931, p. 3438, Lit.

feld). Congenital dolichocephalus (Hecker)—elongation of the head—may favor face presentation. Polyhydramnion, by conferring a high degree of mobility on the fetus, is a predisposing factor. Secondary causes are: (1) Those conditions which prevent or delay engagement of the head, as contracted pelvis, large head (face babies are often large), pendulous belly, tumors occupying the lower uterine segment, as the placenta, or narrowing the inlet—the full rectum, full bladder; (2) rupture of the bag of waters when the head happens to be in extension; (3) occipitoposterior positions; (4) a cause of deflexion attitudes not generally appreciated is weak labor pains. With a normal pelvis the cervix exerts a certain influence on the mechanism of labor. The head presenting to it with the broad flat vertex will, under strong vis à tergo, adapt itself so as to bring the longest diameter of its ovoid into a position parallel with the axis of the passage, so that it can go through with the least friction. With weak pains the head will not apply itself to the cervix and thus come under the latter's influence.

Nearly always the cause of deflexion is maternal, and operates during labor, but the author would emphasize the rôle that the child plays. Nutatory movements are often felt during vaginal examination, and it is easy to understand that, should labor come on or the membranes rupture while the child has the chin ex-

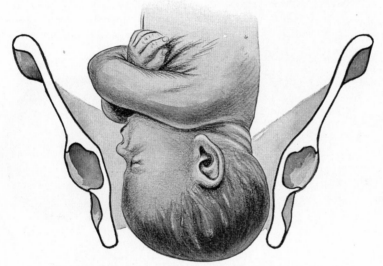

Fig. 511.—Median Vertex Presentation. Military Attitude.

tended the attitude will be fixed, and the deflexion may become exaggerated as labor progresses. For example, in occipitoposterior presentation a slight extension will throw the forehead over the inlet. Should the patient turn on the side to which the venter of the fetus points, the trunk will fall over to that side and the brow will sink lower, and if pains come on strongly, the bregma will stem on the edge of the inlet and a full-face presentation result. Often early in labor the examining finger feels the brow or the forehead high over the inlet, but by properly placing the patient—that side to which the occiput points—the breech will fall into the flank, the occiput will sink, and flexion result. If the obliquity of the uterus is marked and not corrected, a face presentation may be made. These passing deflexion attitudes should not mislead to hasty interference.

Mechanism of Labor in Median Vertex Presentation.—Most authors do not recognize this form of anomaly, but Baudelocque, Velpeau, and Hodge have described it, and Hirst, among other modern writers, mentions it. I believe it is a frequent cause of dystocia. When the deflexion is only moderate, the child presenting with its head in the "military" attitude, labor is very similar to that in occipitoposterior positions. As the point of direction, or denominator, the occiput is still employed, although sometimes in abnormal mechanisms the forehead descends and becomes the point of direction—a fact of great importance in the forceps operation.

Engagement of the head is slow, because the largest plane, the occipitofrontal, is presented to the inlet. Descent continues with the large and small fontanels on the same level,—that is, flexion remains absent,—and with the sagittal suture in the transverse, until the median vertex reaches the pelvic floor (Fig. 511). Now four terminations are possible: (1) Flexion occurs, the occiput rotates anteriorly under the pubis, and labor terminates normally; (2) delivery takes place with the sagittal suture in the transverse diameter—requires strong pains, large pelvis, small child, the perineum being much endangered; (3) the occiput rotates into the hollow of the sacrum, the forehead turns to the pubis, and the mechanism is similar to occipitoposterior positions, second mechanism, deflexion; (4) labor comes to a standstill with the head in the transverse diameter, deep in the pelvis, and, unless art is called, the mother and child may die. These last cases can hardly be distinguished from arrested rotation in occipitoposterior positions. They are both "deep transverse arrest," and require the same treatment. Molding in median vertex presentation closely resembles that of forehead presenta-

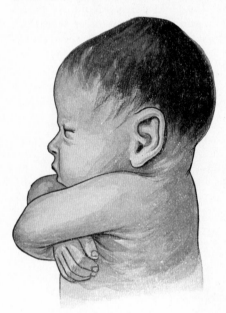
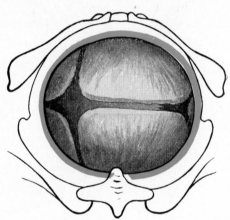

FIG. 512.—MOLDING IN MEDIAN VERTEX PRESENTATION.

FIG. 513.—TOUCH PICTURE. MEDIAN VERTEX PRESENTATION. O.L.T.

tion. The caput succedaneum is on one parietal bone, close to the posterior third of the sagittal suture (Fig. 512).

Clinical Course.—Labor is longer and tedious. The pains are weak and infrequent, because the presenting part does not press firmly against the cervix. Dilatation is slow, and the cervix must be opened wider to allow the head, presenting its biggest planes, to pass through. After the head reaches the pelvic floor the pains usually become augmented, and one of the terminations mentioned occurs, but in all cases strong pains are needed. These may fail, and the assistance of art is often required.

Diagnosis.—Abdominally, the usual points for determining presentation and position are to be sought, and the examiner will notice that the trunk of the child is very straight, the fundus applied to the ensiform, the heart-tones near the median line, and heard over a large area—distant in O.L.T., louder in O.D.T. The shoulder is in the median line, just above the pubis, and the occiput and chin are on about the same level. Internally (Fig. 513), the finger discovers the two fontanels on the same level, the sagittal suture running across the pelvis. Usually the head is synclitic, but anterior asynclitism has been observed, especially in pendulous abdomen and flat pelves. Naturally, the findings change as the various mechanisms unfold. Rectally the experienced finger can feel the sagittal suture crossing the pelvis.

Treatment.—This is the same as that of occipitoposterior positions.

Forehead Presentations.—These are primary or secondary. Primary forehead mechanisms are very rare because, if the deflexion has proceeded thus far, the forces of labor almost always complete the process, a face or at least a brow presentation resulting. The forehead is the point of direction—it takes the lead, descent occurs, usually in one of the obliques, until the presenting part reaches the pelvic floor. Now three mechanisms occur: (1) Under strong pains and late, flexion of the head, descent of the occiput, and anterior rotation of the latter under the pubis (rare); (2) anterior rotation of the forehead under the pubis while the occiput turns behind, the glabella stemming under the arch, the occiput coming over the perineum, in all respects similar to the second mechanism of occipitoposterior positions; (3) cessation of progress with the forehead on the perineum.

Secondary forehead presentations are the result of deflexion of the head and descent of the forehead in occipitoposterior positions, to which the reader is referred for a description of the mechanism and for diagnosis and treatment.

Primary forehead presentations closely resemble the brow, but an internal examination will show the large fontanel in the line of direction (Fig. 514). The configuration of the head is shown in Fig. 503, and the caput succedaneum over the bregma exaggerates the tower-like raising of the vault of the cranium In the treatment of primary forehead presentations it must be remembered that often, in the beginning of labor, the forehead is to be felt over the inlet, but when the head enters, flexion occurs and the occiput comes down, rotating anteriorly. By keeping the patient on the side on which the occiput lies, flexion and descent of the head are favored. King advises the squatting posture, claiming that the pressure of the thighs against the abdomen and uterus affects the position of the child. If it is

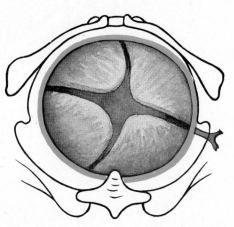

FIG. 514.—TOUCH PICTURE IN FOREHEAD PRESENTATION.

desired to exert pressure on the back of the child, the woman kneels on one knee, the other foot resting flat, and the corresponding thigh being pressed firmly against the abdomen, where the back lies (Fig. 654). Should the forehead not change its location, labor does not progress, and the case is to be treated as a brow presentation, with which, indeed, it is often confused in practice.

Brow Presentation.—Transitory presentation of the brow in the beginning of labor is occasionally observed, and as the head engages in the pelvis descent of the occiput occurs, and a more normal mechanism results. More frequently the deflexion is completed, and a face presentation is produced. Brow presentation is distinctly pathologic, and if the child is normal or above normal in size, becomes very formidable. Small or macerated fetuses may pass through the pelvis spontaneously, though labor is usually difficult and much prolonged.

The frequency of brow presentation is variously given—perhaps once in 3000 cases is as near accurate as is possible to get. In the Chicago Lying-in Hospital brow presentation occurred 24 times in 35,113 labors. Its causes come under the general etiology of deflexion attitudes, but the frequency of contracted pelvis must be emphasized and this may explain, in part, the extraordinary difficulties

41

encountered when the child is above normal in size. The posture of the child is shown in Fig. 508. It will be noticed that the S shape of the back is more marked than in forehead, but less than in face presentation, which, however, it closely approaches.

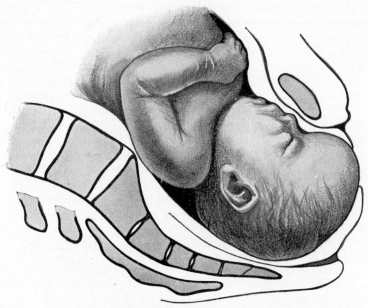

FIG. 515.—MECHANISM IN BROW PRESENTATION. BROW ROTATED.

Mechanism.—The point of direction is the brow, and although six positions are theoretically possible, two are most commonly observed in nature—frontolæva

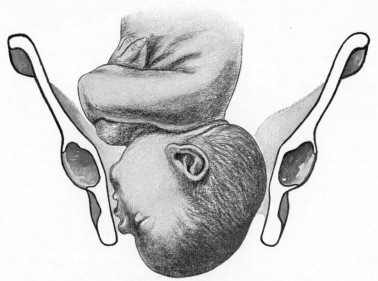

FIG. 516.—MECHANISM IN BROW PRESENTATION. BROW IN TRANSVERSE DIAMETER. NOT ROTATED.

anterior and frontodextra posterior. During the progress of labor, of course, the brow will be felt in other pelvic diameters, that is, it is found at any point of its arc of rotation. Descent of the head is slow, and starts only after complete dilatation, with the rupture of the membranes. Since the preparation of the cervix is poor, delay in the first stage is the rule. Unless the attitude is to change to either a face or an occiput presentation, the brow descends in the middle of the pelvis, the head holding itself midway between flexion and extension. During the descent the frontal suture usually takes the transverse diameter and is synclitic (Fig. 516), unless the pelvis is flat. When the pelvic floor is reached, the brow rotates to the front, and the occiput to the hollow of the sacrum. The factors producing this rotation are the same as those operative in normal cases—the pelvic floor, the guidance of the converging rami pubis, and the accommodation of the fetal cylinder, which is easily flexible only in certain directions—to the bent birth-canal (Sellheim). In the brow attitude the fetal cylinder can bend best in its sagittal diameter. The sagittal diameter, therefore, is brought to correspond with the sagittal diameter of the pelvis. The brow, therefore, comes down and turns to the front until the face rests behind the pubis. In the rima vulvæ the brow, covered by a large caput succedaneum, first appears; then, under very strong expulsive pains, by a movement

of flexion, the large fontanel, the vertex, and the occiput successively pass over the perineum, the nape of the neck coming to rest upon it, after which the eyes, nose, mouth, and chin come from behind the pubis with one movement. Sometimes the head is delivered up to the mouth before the occiput escapes,

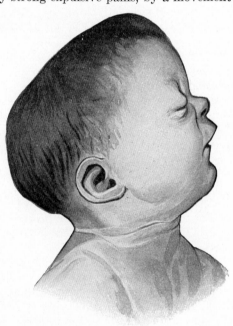

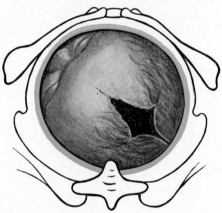

FIG. 517.—TOUCH PICTURE IN BROW PRESENTATION (FR.D.A.).

FIG. 518.—MOLDING IN BROW PRESENTATION.

and, rarely, the head may escape with the frontal suture in the transverse diameter of the outlet; that is, internal anterior rotation has not occurred. It will be seen that the accomplishment of such a mechanism must be slower, harder, and more dangerous to mother and child than any other. The perineum is almost always lacerated, and often tears high up into the rectum, because the largest diameters are offered to the outlet. Clinically, it is very difficult, at this stage, to distinguish a brow presentation from terminal occipitosacral and forehead mechanisms If the child is large, operation is almost always necessary to effect delivery.

Diagnosis.—Abdominally, the findings are the same as in face cases (*q. v.*). Internally (Fig. 517), the bregma is the lowest point, occupies the center of the pelvis, the large fontanel being palpable on one side, the root of the nose and orbital ridges on the other. The nose, mouth, and chin are high up, out of reach unless the patient is anesthetized, to allow deep insertion of the four fingers. The frontal suture runs in the transverse diameter or a little obliquely, and the amount of the facial line which is palpable determines the degree of deflexion. In true brow presentation the nose is not to be felt, the orbital ridges being on a level with the posterior border of the large fontanel, the two demarcating the girdle of resistance.

Molding is characteristic (Fig. 518), the head having acquired a three-cornered outline. The face is flattened out, the distance from chin to top of forehead very great, and this is exaggerated temporarily by the large caput succedaneum.

The *treatment* of brow presentation must be active unless it seems certain that spontaneous correction will occur. First study the conditions to determine whether a contracted pelvis may not indicate cesarean section, or other mode of delivery. To favor flexion the patient is put on the side to which the occiput points, but if this does not speedily bring about the desired result, it is best to correct the presentation under ether before the head engages and molding commences. Before the rupture of the bag of waters nothing but the use of posture need be done. When the cervix is fully dilated, the membranes may be punctured, the head flexed and led into the pelvis either by the two hands or the forceps, after which the case is left to nature. (See Operative Obstetrics.) Should it be impossible to change the brow into an occipital presentation version is to be performed. The change to full-face presentation is debatable.

After the engagement of the head in brow presentation all manœuvers are rendered more difficult and dangerous. It is astonishing, however, what may be accomplished under deep anesthesia. When the abdomen and uterus are fully relaxed, it is often easy to push the head out of the pelvis, flex or extend it, and draw it back in proper attitude and position. Version at this stage is very risky, because the lower uterine segment is usually much stretched in brow cases, and, further, version is always to be avoided in primiparæ if possible. Should version be out of the question and manual correction fail, the attendant has two alternatives —a cutting operation, suprasymphyseal cesarean section or hebosteotomy, and expectancy, in the hope that strong pains will so mold the head to the pelvis that it will finally go through or can be delivered by forceps. If the child is large or the pelvis small, the latter process is not to be expected, and if the mother and baby are in perfect condition—cesarean section is preferable as a primary operation.

What has been said acquires greater force in labors with the brow in posterior position. Here spontaneous delivery is impossible unless the infant is very small, which is also true of face presentation. Symphysiotomy has been performed by H. F. Lewis and Montgomery for the relief of dystocia due to brow presentation. Should nature's efforts suffice to bring the head well down on to the perineum, the additional power required for delivery may be applied by the forceps. (See Operative Obstetrics.) Forceps operations in brow cases are nearly always very difficult, and, should the hazard be too great, craniotomy is to be performed.

Face Presentation.—When the deflexion is carried to its highest degree, the full face comes to lie in the line of direction, or is bounded by the girdle of resistance and is felt by the examining finger. This is face presentation, and it occurs, in round numbers, about once in 200 cases. In face presentation the chin is the point of direction or denominator, and the six positions of presentation may, in individual cases, be distinguished. Mentodextra transversa is the most frequent, mentolæva anterior the next, mentodextra posterior, dextra anterior, læva transversa, and læva posterior in order. The various statistics show differing frequencies of the several positions, but, in general, face positions occur in the order of the frequency of the occipital positions from which they were developed; for example, since O.L.T. is the usual position which the head takes on entering the pelvis, the deflexion of the chin will bring the face down in M.D.T.

As a rule, face presentations are fully developed only after labor has been in active progress for some time, and most often a brow presentation can be discovered early in the first stage, but in 4 cases I distinctly felt the full face lying over the inlet in the last month of pregnancy, an observation which was also made by LaChapelle, Naegelè, Fieux, and others. I have also seen it in x-rays.

Mechanism.—Figs. 519 and 520 show the attitude or posture of the fetus in two of the common positions. The head is completely extended on the back, the forehead is flattened, and the occiput long drawn out. The neck is stretched; sometimes there are cracks in the skin from overstretching. The chest is protruded and is convex. The back is sharply incurved to receive the occiput, while the breech

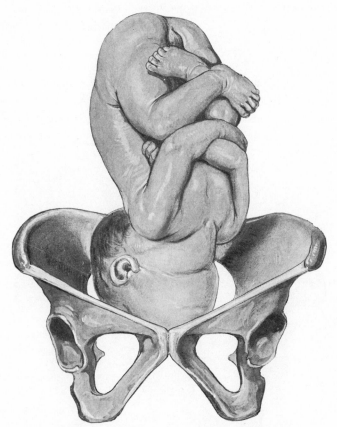

FIG. 519.—FACE PRESENTATION. M.L.A. (M.L. 45°.)

is turned to the back. The fetus is lengthened, while its axis takes the shape of the letter S.

At the beginning of labor the head lies high, with moderate anterior asynclitism, the anterior malar bone and orbit being nearer the middle line and lower. Instead of flexion, as descent begins, we observe an exaggeration of the extension, the chin becomes more accessible, and the brow recedes a little. Descent occurs, with the facial line usually in the transverse diameter of the pelvis. In M.L.A. the chin points to the obturator foramen, that is, lies in the left anterior quadrant of the pelvis; in M.D.P. the chin points to the right posterior quadrant, and the facial line runs in the right oblique diameter of the inlet. Anterior rotation of the chin, the third movement, does not begin until the face is well applied to the pelvic floor and is brought about by the same factors as operate in O.L.A. The greatest flexibility of the fetal cylinder in face attitudes lies in the sagittal plane, but in a direction opposed to that of occipital attitudes. In occipital presentations the fetal cylinder can accommodate itself best to the angular birth-canal by breaking at the fetal neck and the occiput bending backward—that is, extension occurring. In face presentations the same bending occurs, but reversed, and the chin flexes. In order, therefore, for the fetal cylinder to accommodate itself easiest to the birth-canal, it rotates so as to bring the chin forward under the pubis (Fig. 522). Anterior rotation must have begun before the face reaches the second parallel plane of Hodge, because the head, if normal in size, cannot enter the pelvis with the chin behind. This would bring the occiput and the upper chest and shoulder region into the inlet at the same time, and, under normal conditions, progress in this fashion would be

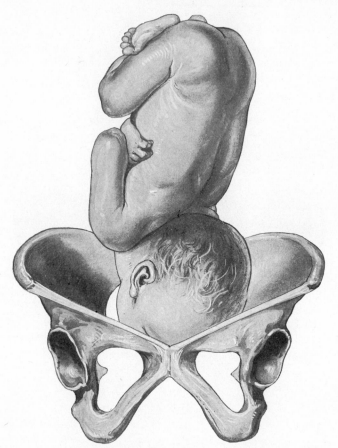

FIG. 520.—FACE PRESENTATION. M.D.P. (M.D. 135°.)

impossible. Under the exceptional combination of large pelvis, small child, and strong pains, labor may progress and terminate spontaneously with the chin posterior. Usually in those cases of spontaneous labors with the chin behind, the head entered the pelvis with the chin transverse or anterior, and, after engagement, the chin rotated to the hollow of the sacrum, the shoulders entering in one of the obliques. Further, mentosacral positions terminating happily for mother and child are so exceedingly rare that, for practical purposes, it is best to consider them as absolutely impossible and as always requiring interference from art.

Anterior rotation being completed, or nearly so, the chin comes to lie behind the pubis near to the urethra, the forehead is behind the fourchet, and the occiput occupies the hollow of the sacrum. The fourth movement is not extension as in

O.L.A., but flexion (Fig. 522), the hyoid bone of the fetus being applied to the posterior surface of the pubis, the chin, mouth, nose, eyes, forehead, and occiput

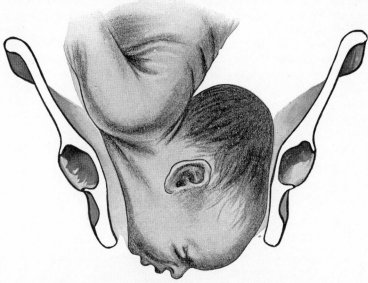

FIG. 521.—MECHANISM IN FACE PRESENTATION. FACE IN TRANSVERSE DIAMETER. NOT ROTATED. (M.D. 90°.)

appearing successively over the perineum, the chin flexing toward the sternum, but riding on top of the symphysis pubis. Internal anterior rotation may be completed

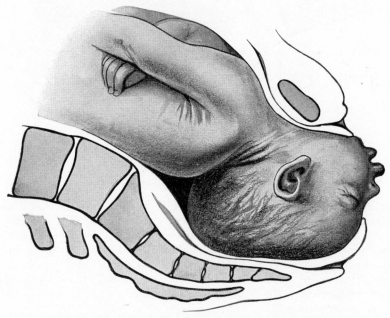

FIG. 522.—MECHANISM IN FACE PRESENTATION. FLEXION BEGINNING.

only as the head passes through the vulva. External restitution occurs as usual, the chin turning back to the position it occupied in utero, and delivery of the trunk takes place according to general principles.

Abnormal mechanisms can occur in the rotation. (1) Deep arrest of rotation, the face coming deeply into the pelvis, and even pressing firmly on the perineum, but not turning to the front, the facial line resting in the transverse diameter. Under favorable conditions—large pelvis, small child, relaxed pelvic floor (multipara), and strong pains—the head may escape in this position, the flexion of the chin taking place over one descending ramus pubis. Otherwise, unless aid is rendered, labor ceases, and both mother and child will die. (2) The second anomaly is where the chin remains at the sacro-iliac joint, or even rotates into the hollow of the sacrum. These are called persistent chin posterior positions, and are very formidable (Fig. 525). It has already been shown that the head cannot enter the pelvis with the chin behind, and it is easy to see how difficult labor will be, should, after engagement, the mentum turn back toward the sacrum. Then the broad oc-

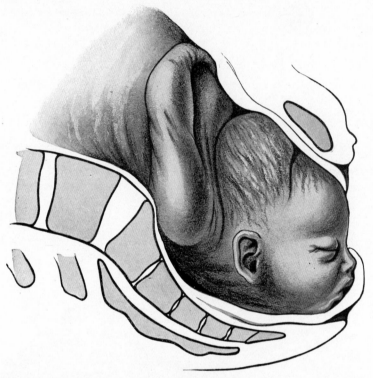

FIG. 525.—FACE PRESENTATION. CHIN ROTATED TO HOLLOW OF SACRUM. (M.D. 180°.)

ciput and the chest must pass the inlet together, which is possible only under most favorable conditions. Rarely, nature terminates these cases, first, by anterior rotation even as late as this; second, by delivering the head as a brow presentation with posterior rotation, the occiput coming down from behind the pubis, and, third, the face is forced down and out in the abnormal position, without regard to the soft parts, which are torn most extensively in all directions. Should none of these occur and art be absent, the baby dies from asphyxia and the mother from ruptured uterus or exhaustion.

Clinical Course.—Labor in face presentation is usually longer—by three or four hours in primiparæ and one or two hours in multiparæ. Since the soft face does not press so hard nor so evenly as the occiput on the cervix, the pains are weaker, especially in the first stage. Dilatation of the cervix is, therefore, delayed, and this is often enhanced by the early rupture of the bag of waters, which is favored by the maladaptation of the presenting part on the cervix, allowing the full force of the general intra-uterine pressure to act on the membranes. The cause of the face presentation, for example, contracted pelvis, tumors,

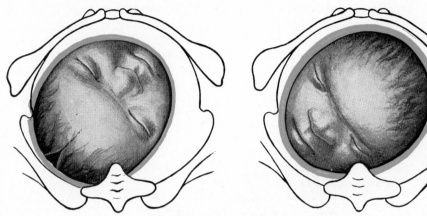

FIG. 526.—TOUCH PICTURE. FACE PRESENTATION.
M.L.A. (M.L. 40°.)
FIG. 527.—TOUCH PICTURE. M.D.P. (M.D. 130°.)

placenta prævia, may also be responsible for other anomalies. Engagement of the head is slow, but anterior rotation comes on suddenly and is usually quickly accomplished, as is also the delivery. Primiparæ less often have face presentations, and naturally in them the mechanism is slower and more arduous. Owing to the extreme

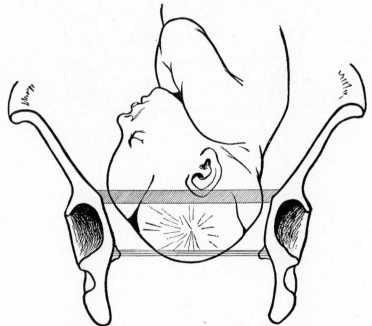

FIG. 528.—DIAGRAM. OCCIPUT ENGAGED.

lengthening of the fetal ovoid the lower uterine segment is put on the stretch, which must be remembered during the treatment.

Diagnosis.—Abdominally, the ovoid is longitudinal and very long, the flanks being quite flat. The shape of the uterus alone may sometimes suffice to make a

diagnosis. Over the inlet the head is felt, and in the fundus the breech with small
parts, the latter unusually easily outlined. It is often difficult to map out the
back, what first impresses one as being the dorsal plane not having the proper
consistence and not showing the triangular area pictured in Fig. 302. This is the
chest of the infant, and in one case I could feel the child's heart beat, which has
also been found by others. The back may occasionally be felt by deep pressure.

Above the inlet, to one side, is felt a hard, round prominence, the occiput, and
this is separated from the back by a deep furrow. On the other side the inlet is
empty, but if the patient is docile and the abdominal wall relaxed, with deep
pressure the fingers may come upon the horseshoe-shaped jaw. Great importance
is to be attached to the finding of the feet, the heart-tones, and the chest all on
the same side. If on the other side, over the inlet, a large, hard prominence is
felt with a sharp groove above it, the diagnosis of face, or at least brow, presentation
is assured. The heart-tones are unusually loud.

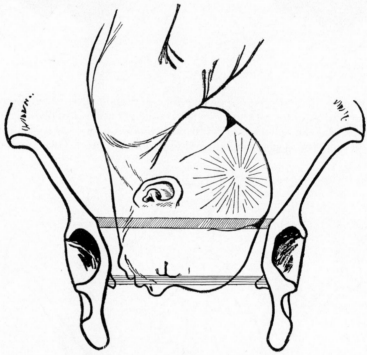

Fig. 529.—DIAGRAM. FACE NOT YET ENGAGED.

Vaginally, early in labor the pelvis is empty, the bag of waters is large, square,
at least not of the watch-crystal form observed in occipital presentations. One
can feel how it receives the full force of the uterine contraction during the pains.
High up, even in primiparæ, and generally quite movable, the brow is felt, and also
the anterior orbit, if not the root of the nose. As soon as the bag of waters ruptures there is usually no difficulty in recognizing the eyes, nose, mouth, and jaw.
Only late in labor, when the caput succedaneum has disfigured the parts, does the
face feel like the breech. An irregular surface, one with prominences and depressions,
is felt by the finger, which at once notifies the examiner that the vertex does not
present. The facial line lies in the transverse or the oblique diameter (Figs. 526
and 527), turning as rotation progresses. In differential diagnosis breech presentation, brow, and lesser degrees of deflexion, and anencephalous monsters must be
considered. Any practitioner who will hold the possibility of such confusion in
mind will easily avoid errors. If the face is so swollen that the landmarks are

obliterated, two points will always remain—the saddle of the nose and the gums. If the child is alive, it may suck the finger. An important point in the diagnosis is the determination of the degree of engagement. The head is engaged only when the biparietal diameter has passed the inlet. In occipital presentations the parietal bosses have just sunk below the plane of the inlet when the lowest part of the head, the vertex, comes to lie in a line drawn from one ischiatic spine to the other. In face presentation, however, when the brow or the root of the nose, that is, the lowest portion of the presenting part, comes to lie in this line, the parietal bosses are still several centimeters above the plane of the inlet (Figs. 528 and 529). Only when the face is deep down on the pelvic floor may we say that the head is engaged.

When making internal examinations in face cases great care is to be taken to avoid the introduction of vaginal mucus into the eyes of the child. If gonorrheal, a blinding ophthalmia may thus be caused. Similar precautions are advisable with the use of antiseptic solutions. Rectal examination often suffices for the diagnosis, but usually doubt exists and a vaginal is necessary.

Plastic Changes.—If the labor has been prolonged after rupture of the membranes, the face is horribly disfigured. Over the anterior cheek and eye the caput is always found, and the whole face is involved, the eyes bulge out, the lids are swollen, a mucoserous discharge escaping from them; the mouth is held open by the tumid lips, the tongue sometimes protrudes, and the child may not be able to nurse for several days. Minute hemorrhages under conjunctiva and skin, sometimes with bullæ, intense venous congestion, the tumefaction of the thyroid, and the cracks in the skin of the neck already mentioned, give the child a most discouraging appearance. The shape of the head is extremely dolichocephalic, the occiput being long drawn out, and there may even be a saddle-shaped depression near the large fontanel. The child lies in its crib on the side, with the head extended, the back straight, and may keep this attitude for at least two weeks. The mother may be reassured that the child's features will soon regain their proper appearance.

Prognosis of Face and Brow Presentations.—Without question both face and brow presentations must be considered pathologic. The mortality is higher in both because of the longer labor, the greater danger of infection, the frequently necessary operative interventions, and also those unnecessarily undertaken. While the majority of face cases will terminate spontaneously or with a little help from art, brow presentation is always dangerous.

For the child mortality is also higher, which is due to—(1) Prolonged labor and cerebral compression; (2) compression of the neck against the pubis, interfering with the return circulation from the head; (3) compression of the trachea and larynx against the pubis, with suffocation or even fracture; (4) injury from forceps or other operation, done to effect delivery. Fully four times as many children die from face presentation as in occipital, and fully ten times as many in brow. It would be interesting to follow up these children to see if the extreme molding which the brain suffered affects their mentality in any way in later life.

Treatment.—Not all face presentations require special treatment. The majority terminate spontaneously and happily for the mother and babe, without the assistance of art. Moschion (A. D. 100) recommended that all such presentations be changed to occipital; Mauriceau (1663) and de la Motte (1721) taught the same. Paul Portal (1685) and Deleurye (1770) took the opposite side, and left them to nature. Baudelocque (A. D. 1810) advised immediate interference, a teaching which is still felt, in spite of the efforts of modern obstetricians to dispel it. Perhaps the fact that Hodge, and more recently Schatz, recommended it, does much to explain the present frequency of operative measures in face cases. In 1789 Zeller, from 40 cases, and in 1791 Boër, in Vienna, from an experience of 80

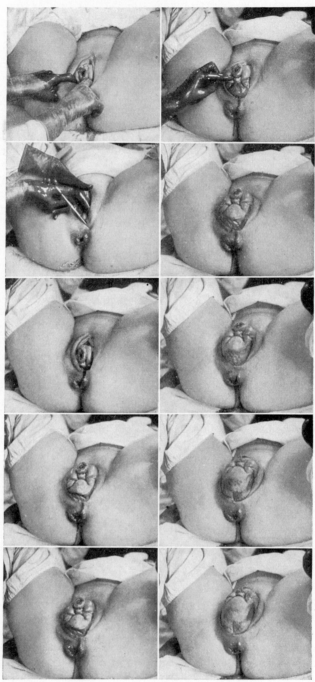

Fig. 530.—Strips from a Motion Picture of a Spontaneous Face Delivery after Episiotomy.
Note flexion.

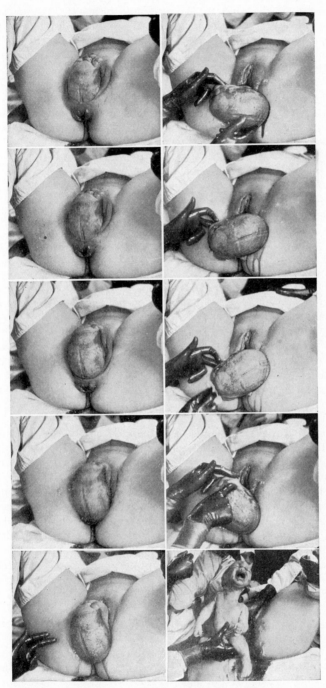

FIG. 531.—FLEXION OF HEAD, POSTERIOR ROTATION OF OCCIPUT AS SHOULDERS TRAVERSE RIGHT OBLIQUE OF
PELVIS, AND EXTERNAL RESTITUTION.
Note depression of large fontanel and sagittal suture.

cases, showed that these presentations may safely be left to nature, 79 of Boër's 80 cases having terminated spontaneously with only 4 fetal deaths. Jaggard, of Chicago (died, 1896), declared in the strongest terms that watchful expectancy should be the treatment of face presentation. No one nowadays claims that it is good practice to correct every face presentation, but when the cases are carefully differentiated, many will be found where the interests of mother and child are best served by early interference.

Before Engagement.—If discovered during pregnancy or early in labor, it may be possible to alter the attitude of the child by Schatz's method of abdominal manipulation. First determine, if possible, the cause of the face presentation. A contracted pelvis may require cesarean section, an anencephalus would preclude it. During labor all measures which preserve the bag of waters are to be employed, for example, the side position, abstention from bearing-down efforts by the patient, and care during examinations by the accoucheur. It may be very advantageous to put a colpeurynter in the vagina, filling it moderately. If the head is found in transition from vertex to face, the woman should lie on the side to which the occiput points; if the face presentation is fully formed, she should lie on that side which will favor descent and anterior rotation of the chin, that is, the side to which the chin points. As a rule, in the absence of special indications, watchful expectancy is the treatment to be pursued, and the general practitioner will do best for his patient if he gives her plenty of time to force the head well down into the pelvis and onto the perineum. Then he may wait as long as six hours for internal anterior rotation, and almost always his patience will be rewarded by either a spontaneous delivery or sufficient descent and anterior rotation that the forceps may be easily and safely applied.

If the position is one with the chin in the transverse diameter, or, better still, in the anterior quadrants of the pelvis, this is the invariable treatment, in the absence of other indication, but if the chin is posterior to the transverse diameter of the pelvis, a more active conduct may be advisable, in the interests of the child and in the hope of reducing the length of the labor and its attendant distress and dangers. If the head remains high with the chin posterior, in spite of good pains, the malpresentation may be changed manually to one of the occiput, or podalic version may be performed. There is no unanimity of opinion among the authorities regarding the selection of these procedures. Baudelocque, Schatz, Thorn, and Hodge prefer the manual correction, as do most modern writers. Bumm prefers version. The writer has had almost uniform success with the conversion of face presentation to occipital, the only cases in which his efforts failed being those in which labor had progressed too far, extreme molding of the head had taken place, and the uterus had become strictured around the child's neck. Chin posterior positions are particularly favorably altered by conversion into occiput presentations, because an anterior occiput is obtained, for example, M.D.P. becomes an O.L.A., and M.L.P. an O.D.A. (For the methods of manual correction see Chapter LXX.) Should it be impossible to correct the presentation, podalic version may be done, and, failing in this, craniotomy would be necessary.

After Engagement.—When the head is engaged in the pelvis with the chin in the transverse diameter or even anterior to it, given a strict indication for delivery, forceps is the operation of choice. Before applying the instrument an attempt is to be made to complete the rotation of the chin to the front by manipulation with the fingers or half hand. A purchase is obtained on the posterior malar and frontal bones, and, during the pains, the fingers make gentle traction upward and forward, trying to bring the chin under the pubis, aiding the manœuver by pressure on the occiput from the outside over Poupart's ligament. Occasionally a little pressure on the chin to exaggerate extension and slight traction forward will help rotation. If rotation can be thus completed, nature may terminate the case, or, at least, the forceps operation becomes at once easier, simpler, and safer.

Should the chin lie behind the transverse diameter, or have even turned toward the sacrum, the family is to be advised that, with the usual methods of delivery, a dead child is almost a certainty, and if the mother and child are in prime condition, the question of cesarean section is to be considered. When the conditions are not ideal for an abdominal delivery, the accoucheur should try to change the chin posterior to an occiput anterior, even though the head is engaged. Under deep anesthesia so much relaxation of the uterus occurs that a surprising degree of mobility is conferred on the fetus. It is then possible, and if it is done gently it is safe, to push the head up and out of the pelvis sufficiently far to enable the author's method of manual conversion to be practised. Occasionally the conversion may be effected by means of vulsellum forceps. Naturally, the operation requires the greatest circumspection, but the end will justify the risk, and the latter is very little in competent hands. If conversion fails or appears too hazardous, manual rotation of the chin through an arc of three-fourths of the half-circle is to be attempted. Unless the chin can be brought into the anterior half of the pelvis, forceps are a most dangerous and destructive instrument, being at the same time inefficient. Craniotomy is a more humane operation, and has hardly a higher fetal mortality than the forceps used in such instances. Hodge lauds the use of the vectis in these cases, but modern accoucheurs hardly know the instrument. In the treatment of face presentation the forceps are to be employed only when absolutely unavoidable. Before doing a craniotomy on a living child with the chin posterior a gentle attempt with the forceps is justifiable, but it must stop short of maternal injury. For these impacted cases pubiotomy has been recommended. In all face deliveries, spontaneous and operative, the fact must be remembered that the diameters and circumferences presented to the pelvic floor outlet are not so favorable as in occipital deliveries, and that the pelvic floor is pushed further downward and torn from its bony attachments. Deep episiotomy, sometimes going through the pillar of the levator ani, is almost always needed, and is to be strongly recommended to save both the pelvic floor and the baby's neck. After the conversion into an occipital presentation, unless there is an urgent indication for delivery, the case should be left to nature. A spontaneous delivery may now occur—at all events the head will be molded by a few hours' labor into a favorable shape, and brought low into the pelvis, sometimes even onto the perineum, making the eventual forceps delivery easy and safe.

Every face and brow case demands a comprehensive diagnosis of all adjuvant conditions which may govern the methods of treatment. As such may be mentioned contracted pelvis, placenta prævia, tumors, eclampsia, etc.

It is advisable to observe the children carefully for several days, since edema of the glottis may occur. Fracture of the larynx has resulted from too forcible pressure of the trachea against the pubis, a point worth remembering while conducting the delivery. The scratch-marks on the face require antiseptic treatment. The tumefaction of the eyelids will subside quickly under a warm salt solution dressing.

CHAPTER L

ANOMALIES OF THE PASSENGERS (Continued)

BREECH PRESENTATION

In about 3 per cent. of cases the child presents itself for delivery with the breech as the advancing portion of its body. Most authors consider breech presentations eutocia, but since the fetal mortality is three times as high as in O.L.A., and the maternal morbidity, from lacerations and sepsis, decidedly greater, the author believes, with Eden and others, that they should be considered dystocia.

Breech presentation is the first of the errors of polarity of the fetus to be discussed, the normal polarity being a parallelism of the fetal axis with the long axis

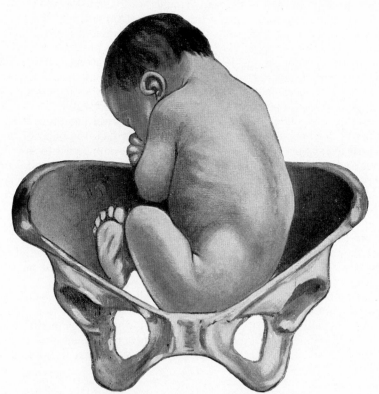

Fig. 532.—Breech Presentation. S.L.A. (S.L. 45°.)

of the mother, the cephalic pole presenting at the inlet. Reversal of the normal polarity is breech presentation; lack of parallelism between the two axes produces the varieties of transverse presentation.

Etiology.—Little is positively known of the causes, because neither the mother nor the babe may show anything unusual, but the presentation has been more frequently found in the following conditions: (1) Abnormally shaped uteri, especially uterus arcuatus and subseptus; (2) anything that will prevent engagement of the head, as contracted pelvis. tumors, low insertion of the placenta, the most

frequent cause; (3) polyhydramnion, the child being very free to move around;
(4) multiparity, which acts in the same way; (5) on the part of the fetus, hydro-

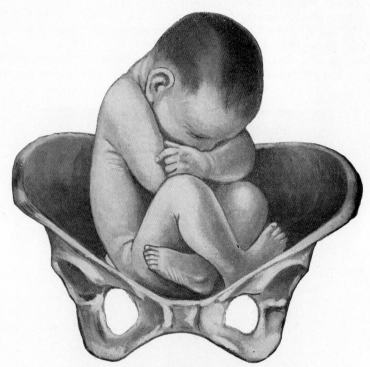

FIG. 533.—BREECH PRESENTATION. S.D.P. (S.D. 135°.)

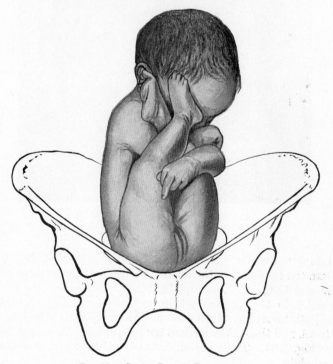

FIG. 534.—SINGLE BREECH PRESENTATION.

42

cephalus, tumor of the neck or head, making the cephalic pole larger than the caudal, and thus rendering it better adaptable to the large fundus uteri; (6) prematurity, a very common predisposing cause; (7) twin pregnancy.

Breech presentation is very frequent about the seventh month of pregnancy, but it usually changes to a head, and the process may be repeated several times, and even take place under one's eyes during labor.

Mechanism of Labor.—There are several varieties of breech presentation, depending on the attitude or posture of the child: (1) Complete or double breech,

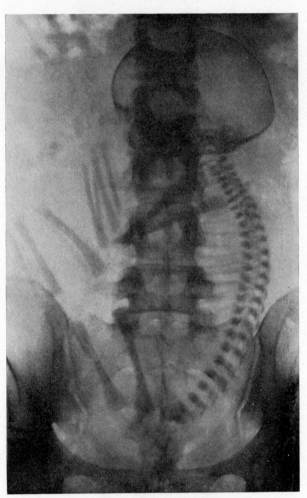

Fig. 535a.—Breech Presentation, S.L.T.
In late pregnancy. Note C-shaped spine.

where the infant maintains the same attitude as in vertex, but with reversed polarity. Here the buttocks, with the feet alongside them, present at the internal os (Figs. 532 and 533). (2) Incomplete breech, where—(a) One foot or two feet have prolapsed into the vagina—single or double "footling" presentation; (b) where one or both knees have thus prolapsed; and (c) where the legs are extended against the trunk and the feet lie against the face, sometimes called "single" breech presentation (Fig. 534). These are all errors of attitude and increase the dangers to mother and child.

In conformity with the system employed in the other presentations it is possible here, too, to distinguish six positions of the presentation, but in practice two are mostly observed—S.L.A. and S.D.P.—though in the latter usually the back tends somewhat more to the side than behind. The point of direction is the sacrum, and in following the mechanism of labor the genital crease is used for the purpose of orientation, in the same way that the sagittal suture and the facial line are used for occipital and face presentations.

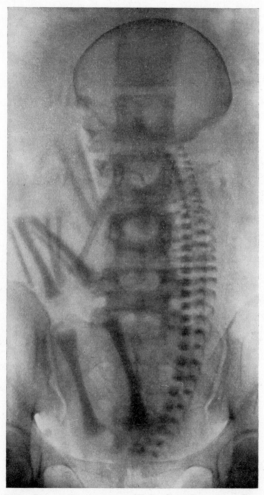

Fig. 535b.—Breech Presentation, S.L.T. Same Patient as Fig. 535a.
In advanced labor. Note lengthening and straightening of spine—part of the mechanism of fetal axis pressure.

Mechanism of Breech Presentation.—With very little variation the mechanism of labor is the same whether the complete breech presents or there is an error of attitude, as footling or single breech. For purposes of study sacrolæva anterior (S.L.A.) will be selected. The movements of the breech and lower trunk, of the shoulders and of the head, must be considered, those of the shoulders and head being more constant and important.

Even in primiparæ the breech remains high up until labor is quite well advanced, often until dilatation of the cervix is completed and the bag of waters ruptured.

The feet accompany the buttocks, but at a slight distance, being held back by the cervix or pelvic brim. *Descent* is slow in primiparæ because the soft breech cannot wedge itself into the vagina so firmly as does the head, and, further, when the head presents, the upper vagina, the cervix, and the bases of the broad ligaments, with the pelvic connective tissues, are already dilated and prepared by the descent of the broad cephalic wedge in the latter weeks of pregnancy. *Flexion*, the second movement, takes place as soon as the breech strikes the perineum; the posterior buttock is held back; the anterior one stems under the pubis (Fig. 536). This movement is always associated with the third—*internal anterior rotation*. In S.L.A. the breech descends in the left oblique, that is, the bisiliac diameter lies in the left oblique diameter of the pelvis, the genital crease lying in the right, the anterior hip pointing to the right iliopubic tubercle, and being a little lower than the posterior. This is anterior asynclitism, and is analogous to the obliquity of Naegelè. Anterior rotation occurs by the anterior hip rotating to the front from the right anterior

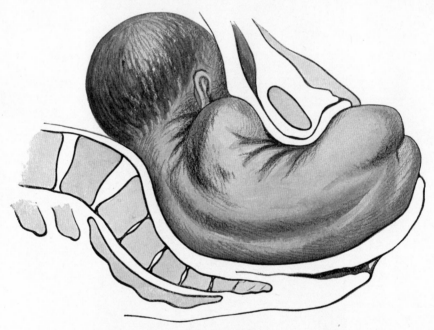

Fig. 536.—Mechanism of Breech Labor. S.D.P. Lateroflexion at Outlet.

quadrant of the pelvis, the sacrum looking directly to the left side, the other buttock turning behind, the genital fissure now lying in the transverse. The causes of this movement are the same as in the other presentations (*q. v.*). The fourth movement is continued *lateroflexion;* the anterior hip stems under the pubis, the posterior hip rolls over the perineum, the whole pelvis rising up over the pubis, a tight pelvic floor increasing this elevation. *External restitution*, the fifth movement, is not constant. Usually the anterior hip turns again to the right side, and the sacrum comes directly anterior, but sometimes the back remains in the transverse and the shoulders come out in this position. Now the legs drop down and the back again lies in the oblique (Fig. 537).

The movements of the shoulders are precisely similar to those of the breech. Descent occurs with the bisacromial diameter in the left oblique. If no attempt to aid delivery by traction from below is made, the arms lie folded closely against the chest. Stronger pains and more abdominal muscular exertion are needed for delivery of the shoulder-girdle. The anterior shoulder rotates in the right anterior quadrant of the pelvis toward the pubis and stems behind it, while by a process of lateroflexion the posterior shoulder and arm are delivered. Then comes the anterior shoulder from behind the pubis, and if no assistance is given, the body drops down with the neck against the perineum, the nape against the subpubic ligament. If the head is arrested high, the fifth movement, *external restitution*, now takes place, the back rotating again to the side. If the head follows the body closely and sinks into the pelvis, the back may rotate to the front.

When the shoulders are passing the vulva, under normal circumstances the head has entered the inlet. If the inlet is contracted, the head is held back, and the stretching of the neck permits the escape of the shoulder-girdle, but not completely, unless the soft parts are pushed back a little around the fetal neck and up into the bony pelvis. When the head is well flexed on the sternum, the same diameters are opposed to the girdle of resistance as in O.L.A., but in inverted order. A difference is also seen in the shape of the wedge—in occipital presentation the blunt occiput advances; in head-last deliveries the narrow planes from the neck to

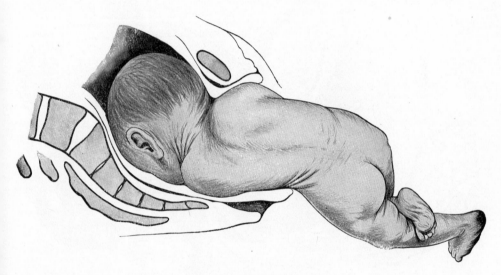

FIG. 537.—DELIVERY OF BREECH TO NAVEL. S.D.P.

the biparietal go first, a fact which explains in part why the head goes through the pelvis easier and quicker when it comes out last. Descent, flexion, anterior rotation of the occiput to the front, occur in order (Fig. 538), all explained by the usual mechanisms. The sagittal suture enters in the right oblique, just as it does in O.L.A. When the chin has rotated to the hollow of the sacrum, *flexion*, the fourth movement, occurs, the nape of the neck being the center, and the chin, face, and forehead coming successively over the perineum, after which the occiput escapes from behind the pubis.

In back posterior positions the mechanism is nearly the same. The anterior buttock needs to rotate only one-fourth of the half-circle, 45 degrees, in order to get under the pubis, whereupon the mechanism is as above described. It has happened in such cases that the back rotated in front of the sacrum to the opposite side, and before delivery is completed has traversed three-quarters of the circumference of the pelvis. I have never seen this occur except when the posterior foot and leg had prolapsed and had guided this abnormal rotation (*vide infra*).

Unusual Mechanisms.—Occasionally, after the breech is delivered, the back rotates beyond the pubis to the other side of the pelvis, an overrotation, which has likewise been observed in the mechanism of the shoulders in head cases. The remainder of the child may come out with the back on the side opposite that in which it started. Even excessive internal anterior rotation of the breech has been observed, the body of the fetus issuing with the belly to the pubis. Subsequently the shoulders enter in an oblique diameter and the proper mechanism is resumed. It is not usually possible to discover the cause of these irregular mechanisms.

Footling presentation has the normal mechanism, unless by chance the posterior foot has prolapsed. In all labors the tendency is for the lowest portion of the presenting part to slip under the pubic arch. The construction of the front part of the pelvis and the arrangement of the sacrosciatic ligaments and the levator ani, resemble the ways of a ferry-boat, and any movable body placed on these inclined

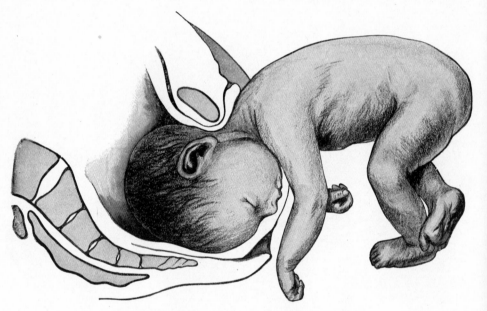

Fig. 538.—Delivery of After-coming Head in Flexion.

planes, propelled from above, would tend to go in this direction. Thus the breech, when the anterior leg has prolapsed, glides without difficulty along the ways. It is different, however, when the posterior leg has prolapsed. Here the breech is held higher, the anterior buttock impinges on the horizontal ramus of the pubis, and the posterior leg is prevented from reaching the anterior inclined plane. It finds an easier way on the other side of the pelvis, and often, not always, as some authors claim, the back rotates in front of the sacrum, the posterior limb now becoming anterior and following out the favorite mechanism, but on the other side of the pelvis. This mechanism might also be explained on the theory of Sellheim. The anterior limb fixes the lower trunk so that it cannot bend easily toward the front, but does so toward the sacrum. Rotation then takes place in the direction in which the fetal cylinder can most readily bend. After the breech is on the other side of the promontory, lateroflexion of the fetal spine is most favored in an anterior direction, and, therefore, the fetal cylinder rotates anteriorly to accommodate itself to the birth-canal. In several instances I have observed the usual mechanism, anterior rotation, even though the posterior limb had been brought down.

Abnormal rotation of the back is infrequently observed, unless the accoucheur is hasty and makes premature traction on the trunk, or ignorantly interferes with nature's methods. If the back does not rotate to the front, but to the sacrum, the child descends with the belly to the pubis of the mother. Usually the natural powers are insufficient to deliver the infant in this position, and art has to aid. (See Chapter LXXI.) Nature may accomplish the birth, the shoulders being forced out in the transverse, the elbows and arms falling from behind the pubis, and anterior rotation of the trunk is effected late. As a rule, the head gives the most trouble. If it turns with the occiput in the hollow of the sacrum, the chin to the pubis, labor may stop, and unless art aids the infant will perish. Nature sometimes terminates

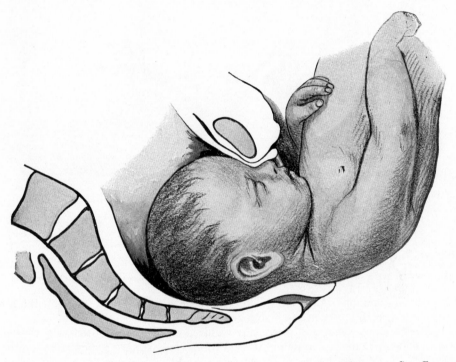

Fig. 539.—Delivery of After-coming Head with Occiput Posterior. First Mechanism, Chin Flexed.

these cases in one of three ways: (1) If the head comes down well flexed, the chin applied to the sternum, anterior rotation of the occiput may occur very late. Usually in these instances the occiput did not lie directly behind, but more to one side. (2) If the head is flexed (Fig. 539), delivery with the occiput posterior occurs, the root of the nose stems behind the pubis, the nape of the neck, occiput, and vertex coming over, or through, the perineum, the face then falling from behind the pubis. This mode of delivery is facilitated by lifting the child up. (3) If the head is extended, the chin may catch on one pubic ramus (Fig. 540). Artificial aid is almost always necessary here. By lifting the child up the occiput, vertex, and forehead in order may pass over the perineum, the neck forming the center of rotation. Nature, however, alone cannot do this; the trunk depends, and the occiput must come over the perineum, pulling the face after it, which can seldom be accomplished quickly enough to save the infant.

Single breech presentations have a more laborious delivery, because the legs, extended against the body, act like a splint and rob the fetal cylinder of its flexibility. Descent and flexion are, therefore, very slow and difficult. To be considered also are the smallness of the advancing wedge, which results in imperfect preparation of the soft parts, and delay and danger in the passage of the shoulders and head; the frequency of the early rupture of the bag of waters, and the usually weak labor pains, because no firm body presses on the cervical ganglia.

Labor may be complicated by the arms leaving the chest and being stretched up over the head, or even crossed behind the occiput in the nape of the neck. Nature cannot terminate these cases satisfactorily. Art must step in. (See Chapter LXXI.)

Clinical Course.—During pregnancy breech presentations sometimes cause symptoms which attract attention. Pain and distress in the epigastrium may be complained of, and if the fetus changes its position, these will be relieved. Pendulous

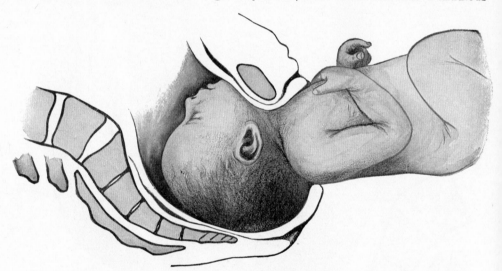

Fig. 540.—Delivery of After-coming Head with Occiput Posterior. Second Mechanism, Extension.

abdomen is common. Lightening does not occur. The fetal movements are perceived low in the belly in the iliac regions.

Since so many small and premature children come by the breech, the time of labor is shorter than with cephalic presentations, but, counting only full-sized infants, labor is actually longer in breech cases, and this is especially true of primiparæ. This increase of the length of labor is all in the first stage, the second stage progressing very rapidly, seldom taking more than eight minutes, and usually less than four. The breech remains high and relatively immobile until the cervix is completely dilated; then, with the rush of the waters, it comes quickly down to the perineum. The actual delivery is shorter and less painful than head labors. Premature rupture of the membranes is common, and this renders still slower the dilatation of the os. In primiparæ labor may be very tedious, and the second stage, owing to rigidity of the vagina and perineum, may be so prolonged that the life of the fetus is much endangered. In cases of complete breech the large foregoing part prepares the cervix and pelvic floor for the passage of the head. In footling or single breeches these parts are poorly dilated, and while the slender trunk slips through easily, the head is almost always arrested, the child's life being lost, or the tissues being torn as a result. Meconium may escape freely during breech deliveries, but it has no significance unless it shows before the breech has engaged or other signs of intra-uterine asphyxia are present. It has the same cause as the formation of the caput succedaneum; the meconium is pressed out in the direction of the least resistance, which is the anal region lying over the os.

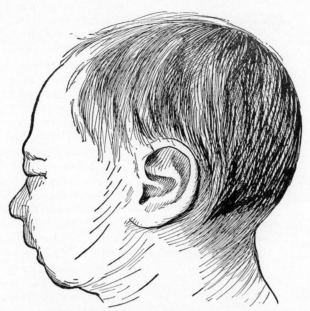

FIG. 541.—UNMOLDED HEAD; O.D.P.; CESAREAN SECTION.

In the third stage of breech labors complications due to anomalous separation of the placenta occur, also a tendency to atony of the so rapidly emptied uterus.

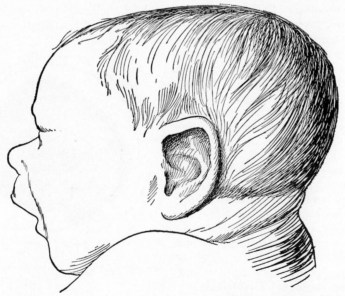

FIG. 542.—HEAD FLATTENED ON TOP. BREECH PRESENTATION IN A PRIMIPARA (Hecker).

Postpartum hemorrhage is, therefore, slightly more frequent than usual, and the rôle of lacerations must also be considered in this connection.

Plastic Changes.—The caput succedaneum is found on the anterior hip, but may spread all over the buttocks. In boys the penis and scrotum may be enormously edematous and black and blue from extravasated blood. In girls there may

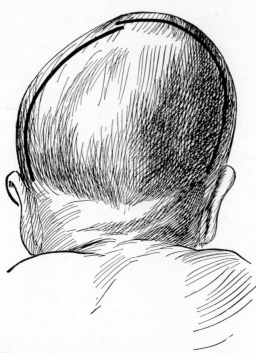

be a moderate vulvitis, with leukorrhea, for a few days. If the leg has been down for any length of time, it swells and shows minute hemorrhages besides the severe congestion. All this disappears within a week. Ordinarily, the child's head is not molded, but presents the round shape it had in utero—this in multiparæ and when the breech presentation was developed just before labor began. If the child had lain a long time in this position, especially if the mother was primiparous, or if the labor had lasted a long time after the rupture of the membranes, distinct evidences of molding will be discoverable on the head. This may take the form of a dolichocephalus, which was especially brought out by Fritsch, the head having been pressed down by the fundus uteri or one or the other side of the head may be flattened. If the mother had a pendulous abdomen, the side of the head which

Fig. 543.—Head Flattened on Side.   Breech Presentation.

lay posterior will show the flattening, as in this case the head will be inclined toward the anterior shoulder. If the abdominal wall held the head up firmly, the side of the head which lay anteriorly will be flattened, the lateral inclination then being onto the posterior shoulder. The sterno-cleidomastoid and other muscles on the side opposite that showing the flattening may be shortened and atrophied (Sippel) producing a wry-neck. In cases of oligohydramnion this is the rule. Great importance must be attached to this congenital shortening of the neck muscles, because if, during delivery, too much traction is made on them, they will tear, hematoma or myositis resulting. Permanent wry-neck, while hardly due to injury of a normal muscle, and seldom following a hematoma of the muscle, is often the result of this congenital shortening, either with or without injury. These acquired deformities are an argument for external version during pregnancy (see Kehrer).

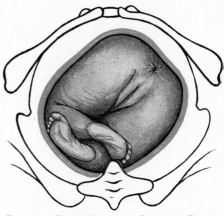

Fig. 544.—Touch Picture.   Complete Breech.
S.L.A.   (S.L. 45°.)

Diagnosis.—Unless labor is advanced and the pains are very strong and frequent, rendering the uterus rigid, the external examination will be sufficient for diagnosis. The ovoid is longitudinal, but the upper portion of the uterus is broader than the lower and runs to the side on which the head lies, a three-cornered effect being produced. Over the inlet no hard, round body is to be found, but, instead, a soft, yielding, irregular mass which glides upward from between the hands, leaving the inlet empty, and the hands to come almost together. In the fundus the head is usually easily felt, under either the liver or the spleen. If it is in the middle line, the examiner may surmise that the body of the child is straightened and that the cause of the extension may be the legs, stretched up toward the face—that is, single breech presentation. On one side the back is felt, and the shoulder is usually easily outlined above the navel and median. Between the shoulders and head a deep sulcus is found. The heart-tones are loudest on the side where the back lies, and are always above the level of the navel, an important diagnostic point. Often the head can be grasped between the two hands, or even measured with a cephalometer, but other times it can be felt only by tapping-palpation—and occasionally it is to be recognized as a body showing ballottement. *Rectally*, the diagnosis may often be made, using the points about to be mentioned. If any doubt exists, however, a vaginal examination is needed. *Vaginally*, the fingers have to be deeply inserted before the presenting part can be touched, the pelvis being empty. A convex hard tumor in the vaginal vault is not felt; instead, a roundish, soft mass of prominences and depressions, in which the examiner can distinguish the buttocks with a crease between them, and at one end a pointed bone—the sacrum. Three or four small prominences on this will identify the bone and show the direction of the pelvis, but for additional assurance the finger may follow the genital crease to the child's genitalia, when the scrotum or vulva will be distinguishable. The finger at the anus may feel the tuberosities, and, if inserted, may be covered with meconium, of course, after the membranes are broken. Higher up and to one side one or both feet may be felt, though usually only the heels are within reach of the finger. Suspicion having been aroused by the empty pelvis, the accoucheur ought to have no difficulty in recognizing the breech, but mistakes are very common, the breech being confused with the shoulder, the face, and the bag of waters. The closed axilla and the costal gridiron will identify the shoulder, and the saddle of the nose and orbital ridges, the nostrils, and the gums, will prove the face. The diagnosis of the position of the breech is made from the location of the sacrum. It is advisable not to introduce the finger into the anus or into the vulva of the fetus.

In single breech, when the feet are extended up to near the face, they may often be felt there from the outside. The uterus is longer and straighter compared with the rounded outline when the child is normally flexed. Vaginally, the feet cannot be felt; the anus is nearer the middle of the pelvis, and the straightened thighs disclose the direction of the extremities.

In footling the accoucheur should follow the prolapsed extremity up to the pelvis and make the diagnosis on general lines, the direction of the big toe and the flexure of the knee giving added information. One should not hastily diagnose breech presentation if a foot is discovered—it may have prolapsed with the head.

Prognosis.—Statistics give the maternal mortality as slightly higher than in occipital presentations, the reasons being: (1) Labor is longer and internal examinations are more frequent, both increasing the dangers of infection; (2) effacement and dilatation of the cervix are not so perfect, hence lacerations are more common; (3) since the head comes rapidly through the unprepared pelvic floor, rupture of the perineum is frequent, extending often through the rectum, and these are not always errors of art; (4) disturbances of the mechanism of labor are frequent, and since they demand the introduction of the hand or other operative measures, the prognosis for the mother is doubtful; (5) postpartum hemorrhage is increased. Most of these dangers may be eliminated by good obstetrics.

For the child, breech presentation is certainly dangerous, the mortality tables showing from 6 to 15 per cent. of deaths. With proper treatment, not over 5 per cent. of children should die in uncomplicated cases. Asphyxia causes many of the deaths. It is caused by compression of the cord between the body and the cervix after the breech is born, or by its being stretched upward from between the child's legs, by premature detachment of the placenta, by compression of the placenta by the hard head, and by delay in delivery due to rigid soft parts. In vertex presentations the soft breech lies against the placenta and exerts no compression, and if the placenta loosens before the delivery of the trunk, the head is already out, or nearly out, so that the child may breathe, whereas in breech presentation the first inspiration sucks in liquor amnii, blood, or anything which lies near the mouth. It is possible, too, that the cold air striking the body, or the manipulations of the attendant, excite premature respirations. A child will live five to twenty minutes after the breech is delivered. It is advisable, therefore, not to allow the progress to be too slow after the breech has passed the vulva; on the other hand, undue haste must be avoided because of the danger of injury to the fetal person. Fracture of the femur, of the pelvis, rupture of the filled colon, of the liver, fracture of the humerus, of the clavicle (common), overstretching of the cervical spine, even fracture of the spine, pulling the nerves out of the spinal cord (Erb's paralysis), rupture of the sternocleidomastoid, dislocation of the atlas—all these and more have been observed. The most frequent cause of fetal death is rupture of the tentorium cerebelli and tears of the falx cerebri (Fig. 734) (seventy-five per cent. Holland). In old primiparæ or such parturients as have rigid soft parts, these dangers are augmented and require special treatment for their prevention.

Treatment.—If breech presentation is discovered during the last few weeks of pregnancy, it is advisable to make gentle efforts to bring the cephalic pole over the inlet. The patient is instructed to assume the knee-chest posture several times daily, and, when reposing, to lie on that side to which the head points; for example, in S.L.A. on the right side. The accoucheur may also try, by gentle external manipulation, to bring the head down, though his efforts are not always rewarded by a permanent change of the presentation.

Watchful expectancy is the treatment during labor. Older writers usually advised version, changing the breech to cephalic presentation by internal and external manœuvers, and especially in old primiparæ. While admitting that a head presentation is highly desirable, and particularly in aged primiparæ, unfortunately the operation in them is more than usually difficult and unsuccessful. Lately cesarean section is advanced as the treatment of breech presentation in primiparæ. In the absence of other complications—very large fetus, contracted pelvis, aged primiparity, etc.—the author does not approve of this, nor does McPherson, after a study of the large material of the New York Lying-in Hospital.

Where the soft parts appear very rigid, and when the child is large, it is wise to prepare the former for the rapid stretching they are about to receive. This is done by colpeurysis, a Carl Braun colpeurynter being placed in the vagina and filled with 12 to 16 ounces of weak antiseptic solution. By the stretching it causes, and by its presence, the pains are strengthened, the tissues softened and dilated, and if it is expelled by the powers, the pelvic floor outlet is enlarged as by the passage of the first twin. Another favorable action of the colpeurynter is the preservation of the bag of waters, which is so highly desirable in breech cases.

Otherwise the treatment of the first stage is not at variance from the usual. When the second stage draws near, the accoucheur should have everything ready for all the emergencies of an operative delivery. This provision consists of a set of instruments—forceps, perineorrhaphy instruments, etc., hot bath, towels, and tracheal catheter for treating the asphyxiated child, a table on which to place the parturient for delivery, and sufficient assistants. (To avoid repetition, the reader is referred to the chapter introducing the subject of Operative Obstetrics.)

When the breech begins to distend the vulva, the woman is placed on the table, her limbs supported by assistants, and, in the absence of trained help, by courageous neighbors—not the husband, as he is likely to faint. As the breech emerges the accoucheur should restrain the desire to aid by traction, but should encourage the woman to bear down strongly. The foot, if it is down, or the breech is to be wrapped in a warm towel as it comes out. Nothing more is done, the operator sitting by with sterile hands. By means of the head stethoscope he listens to the heart-tones almost continuously, and any weakening or irregularity is the signal for rapid delivery. If the foot is out, the baby's pulse may be felt in the anterior tibial artery. Anesthesia is not used unless the patient is very unruly, because her efforts are needed safely to expel the infant. In primiparæ with rigid pelvic floor, or with a big baby, it is my own practice to perform a deep unilateral episiotomy even before the head is to be born. I prefer it to a perineal tear for reasons that have been mentioned. It saves delay in the delivery of the shoulders and the head, and surely has saved many babies' lives, as well as prevented complete laceration of the perineum.

When the navel appears, the rest of the birth must be rapidly, but not precipitately, completed. The woman is told to bear down with all her power. If she is anesthetized or cannot, the assistant, spreading his hands evenly over the fundus, exerts pressure in the axis of the inlet. This strengthens the uterine and abdominal action, and keeps the arms against the chest, preventing their ascent alongside the head, which would much complicate the delivery. If both fail, *manual aid* is rendered. Manual aid means the delivery of the shoulders and head, after nature has accomplished the expulsion to the navel. It must be very sharply distinguished from "breech extraction," which means bringing down the breech in some way and delivery of the whole child from within the birth-canal. (For the details of these maneuvers see Chapter LXXI.) Should the natural powers be successful, the accoucheur receives the child as it emerges, and when the mouth is visible in the vulva, he sponges the mucus from it and restrains the head from making a too rapid exit through the pelvic floor or if there is delay at this point Ritgen's maneuver may be used. After delivery of the child the accoucheur should be prepared to treat postpartum hemorrhage and all kinds of lacerations.

TRANSVERSE PRESENTATIONS

Another error of polarity of the fetus is transverse presentation. Here the long axis of the child crosses the long axis of the mother. It is rare that they cross at a right angle: almost always the fetal cylinder is oblique to the mother's spine. Usually the head is the lower pole, but in some cases the breech is nearer the inlet. Often early in labor the head is found deviated from the inlet and lying in one iliac fossa. The breech may be found similarly placed. These are called "oblique presentations," or "deviated head," or "deviated breech" presentations, and represent a stage of the transition from longitudinal to a transverse presentation. By external manipulation and proper posture of the woman the abnormal mechanism may be corrected.

Since the shoulder is the part that usually enters the pelvis first, most authors call the cases under consideration "shoulder presentations," but the back, the side, the belly, or the four extremities may present. True, all the last four are exceedingly rare.

Etiology.—Shoulder presentations occur about once in 200 cases, in multiparæ oftener than in primiparæ, and in premature labor oftener than at term.

In general, anything that will prevent the engagement of the head in the pelvis, also any condition conferring an extraordinary degree of mobility on the fetus, will cause transverse presentation. The causes may be primary, and lie in some malformation of the maternal parts or of the fetus, or secondary, being produced by some act or accident during labor. The most important are:

1. Contracted pelvis. Transverse presentations occur twice as often in con-

tracted pelvis as in normal pelves. So constant is this that when called to a case of transverse presentation, the first thought is of some obstruction.

2. Anything in the pelvis preventing the engagement; for example, ovarian tumor, fibroid, the placenta, full bladder, or rectum. It sometimes happens that after emptying a full bladder the fetus turns of itself into a normal position.

3. Twins displacing each other.

4. Multiparity, hydramnion, premature labor. Here the child is free to move, and the factors making for a longitudinal presentation are absent.

5. Uterus bicornis, uterus arcuatus, partly septate uterus. A cause of repeated shoulder presentations.

6. Anomalies of the fetus, for example, double monsters.

Of the secondary causes, accident plays the stronger rôle. The fetus happens to be in an unfavorable position when the bag of waters ruptures; the shoulder is forced into the pelvis, and a transverse presentation results. The dislocation

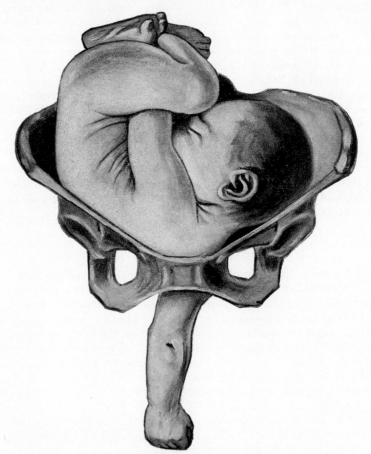

FIG. 545.—SHOULDER PRESENTATION. SC L.A.

of a second twin by the first is also to be reckoned here, and dislocation of the child by an overfilled or badly placed colpeurynter also.

Often several of these factors will combine to cause the malpresentation. In some cases the fetus seems to keep its embryonal position in utero, or the uterus is not tense enough to adapt the fetal ovoid to itself.

Mechanism and Clinical Course.—Although the back or the belly may lie across the inlet, the shoulder is the part which most often enters the pelvis first, so that usually we speak of shoulder presentation. On the shoulder these landmarks are to be distinguished, and they are useful for diagnosis—the scapula, the acromion process, the axilla, and the clavicle. The scapula is selected as the point of direction.

Four positions of the child in utero are observed (Figs. 545 and 546):

Scapulolæva anterior (Sc.L.A.): Head to left, back anterior.
Scapulodextra anterior (Sc.D.A.): Head to right, back anterior.

These are more common, are called back anterior positions, and are easier to deal with.

Scapulodextra posterior (Sc.D.P.): Head to right, back posterior.
Scapulolæva posterior (Sc.L.P.): Head to left, back posterior.

These are rarer, are called back posterior positions, and are much more difficult to deal with. The relations of the back and of the head to the inlet are most important in the study of the mechanism of labor.

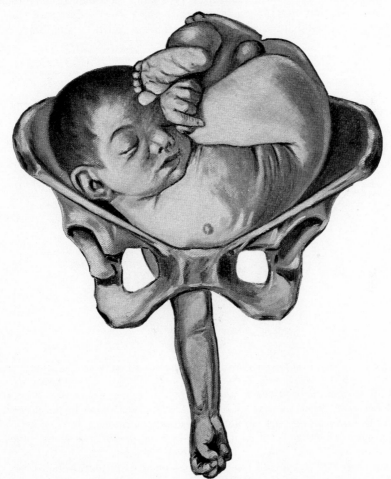

Fig. 546.—Shoulder Presentation. Sc.D.P.

Attitude.—Early in labor we find the usual posture of flexion common to O.L.A., the chin on the sternum, arms crossed over the chest, legs crossed over the belly, but later many changes are observed. Commonest is the prolapse of the lower arm, rarely the two, and still more rarely the upper one alone. Prolapse of the cord is not infrequent. When the uterus has worked on the fetal ovoid for any length of time, the latter is compressed from side to side, the head nears the breech, and the ovoid is made more globular. Occasionally the fetal body is twisted on its long axis, so that, while the shoulder lies deep in the pelvis, the belly, instead of looking to the sacrum, looks directly upward, and the legs also are turned forward. The neck may also be twisted; in one of my cases the child's head was deflected, resembling the attitude of face presentation. Ahlfeld noticed this in a case of breech presentation.

Course.—Shoulder presentations are always pathologic. True, they sometimes terminate spontaneously, but with rare exceptions the children all die, and often the mother, too, so that they are cases of dystocia and demand the aid of art. Early in pregnancy transverse presentation is the rule. Even in the last month, in multiparæ, it is occasionally found, but rectifies itself before labor begins, the process, of which the accoucheur usually has no knowledge, being called *spontaneous rectification.* This means that the contractions of pregnancy have changed the polarity of the fetal ovoid, and the process may be aided by proper position of the mother. If it does not take place during pregnancy, a longitudinal presentation may be brought about spontaneously during the first stage of labor, or even at the beginning of the second stage (very rarely). This is called *"spontaneous version,"*

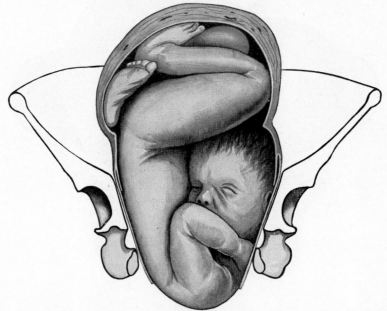

Fig. 547.—Labor in Conduplicato Corpore. Roederer's Method (Zangemeister).

is not at all a constant occurrence, and in practice is *never relied on.* Both of these processes are more likely where the fetus is freely movable, as in polyhydramnion, and where the presenting part cannot easily enter the inlet, as in contracted pelvis. As a rule, when a change of presentation is brought about, the head comes down, but sometimes the breech may come to lie over the inlet.

In order to study the mechanism of transverse presentation a case will be assumed where no aid is rendered. The pains are likely to be slow and weak, since no hard part presses on the cervix, but the bag of waters often ruptures early, because the membranes are exposed to the full force of the uterine contraction. The lower uterine segment is not cut off from the general cavity of the uterus, so after the rupture of the bag of waters all the liquor amnii escapes, since there is nothing to hinder. This is a bad accident, especially if the cervix be undilated.

When the uterus has no more liquor amnii, the walls apply themselves to the fetus very closely. Two conditions may now be observed: first, there may be no pains at all, the uterus simply lying apposed to the fetus in a condition which was called by Kilian "passive contraction." The walls are distensible; the hand can be easily introduced, and even version performed. This condition carries no danger to the fetus or the mother, may last a few hours or a few days, but generally passes over into the other state, either spontaneously or as the result of brusk manipulations. This first condition has nothing to do with the so-called tetanus uteri, to be described presently.

Sooner or later, usually the result of improper treatment, the pains begin, and very soon acquire a dangerous violence. They force the shoulder into the pelvis,

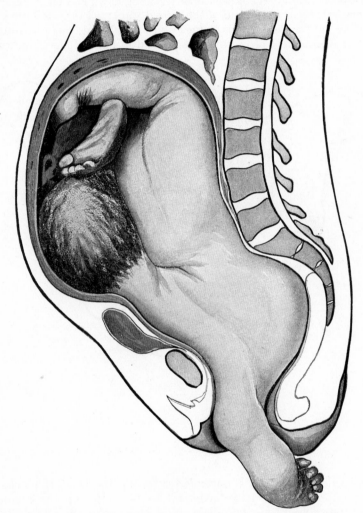

Fig. 548.—Spontaneous Evolution. Douglas' Method. Chiara's Frozen Section.

the fetus is folded together, the breech nears the head, the ovoid becoming more globular. If the fetus is small or macerated and the pelvis large enough, the uterus, aided by powerful efforts of the mother, may succeed in expelling it. This is called "spontaneous evolution," and is the last, least likely, and most dangerous method nature has of overcoming the malpresentation. Spontaneous evolution pursues three methods, named respectively, after the men who first accurately described them, Roederer's, Douglas', and Denman's. According to the first, which usually occurs without prolapse of the arm, the child is folded like the letter V, the shoulder and back advancing, the head pressed deep into the chest and abdomen (Fig. 547).

43

In Douglas' method, which oftener occurs in back anterior positions with prolapse of the arm, the fetal mass, under the influence of strong pains, becomes pointed, the head is arrested above the inlet and rotates to the pubis, the neck is applied to the brim, and very much lengthened. Now the chest, abdomen, and breech roll down alongside the shoulder, the legs drop out, then the other arm, and finally the head appears (Fig. 548). In the rarest of all three mechanisms, Denman's, which is usually taken by back posterior positions, the head rotates behind, and, as the breech descends, the shoulder ascends in the pelvis, a sort of version taking place in the pelvic cavity, the breech finally coming down and out (Fig. 549). All three mechanisms occur at the end of the second stage; all three require exceptionally favorable conditions—that is, large pelvis, small, soft, molding fetus, strong pains, and great integrity of uterine muscle, and in none of the three will a full-

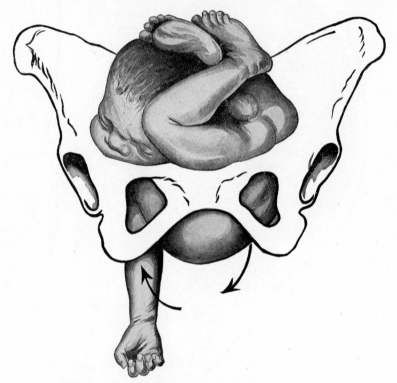

Fig. 549.—Late Spontaneous Version (Denman's Method).

term child be delivered alive. Zangemeister reports the heaviest child delivered alive—weight, 2700 gm. Usually the fetuses are macerated or very small. Death is due to compression of the vital organs in the chest and head, interruption of the placental circulation by the almost constant uterine contractions or by dislocation of the placenta in the retracted fundus uteri. Since the child is almost invariably lost and the mother exposed to risks of imminent death during these processes, they are never to be relied on in practice (Lit., Marshall).

Daily experience shows that nature is generally powerless safely to accomplish delivery in full-term cases, and labor is arrested with the child forced together in a compact mass, solidly blocking the pelvis. If the arm hangs out, it swells up, sometimes to the size of a man's wrist, shows blisters or even peeling skin, the child dies, and the vulva becomes edematous, bluish black, and even gangrenous.

The pains become irregular and tumultuous, the distinction between pain and pause is not marked, and the uterus is in a state of constant contraction. The patient becomes anxious, and complains of continual pain and great tenderness over the lower part of the uterus. Pulse and temperature begin to rise. The uterus draws up over the child; the muscle becomes thick above the contraction-ring; the lower uterine segment is thinned out until it is as thin as a blotter, and here the uterus is *likely to rupture* (Fig. 550).

This condition is called a *"neglected transverse presentation,"* and the uterus is in a state of *threatened rupture*. Where the fundus, thick and contracting,

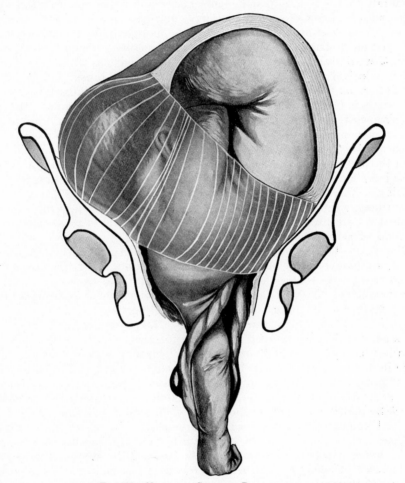

FIG. 550.—NEGLECTED SHOULDER PRESENTATION.
Uterus on point of rupturing. Above is shown the thick, retracted uterine wall. Below the thinned, lower uterine segment, the white lines indicating the direction of greatest thinning.

passes over into the lower uterine segment and the thinned and dilated cervix, a groove or depression can be seen and felt on the abdomen, running from side to side about the level of the navel. This is the ominous retraction-ring, sometimes called contraction-ring (Fig. 697). Above this groove the parts can be poorly felt; below this groove the fetus is easily felt. Unless aid is given, the uterus ruptures and the mother dies of shock, hemorrhage, or peritonitis. The uterus may rupture during an attempt at version or from the action of pituitrin. Death of the child occurs from the interruption of the placental circulation and from compression before rupture. If not, it dies after the rupture, and may be in part or in toto extruded through the rent into the abdominal cavity. Or the woman may die of shock and exhaustion before the rupture takes place.

If the uterus should not rupture soon,—and the tendency varies with different women (in primiparæ there is not so much tendency as in multiparæ),—the pains grow weaker and irregular, the cavity of the uterus becomes infected—from the vagina, from the air, from the exposed arm, or from the examining fingers; the fetus and the little liquor amnii left begin to decompose; gas is developed in the uterus and distends it. The condition is called tympania uteri or physometra. General infection is soon apparent, temperature and pulse mounting rapidly, the features change, a subicteric hue develops, and the poor woman dies in septic collapse. If successfully delivered, the sepsis may continue, but recovery is unlikely when much damage has been done to the structure of the parturient canal.

Another condition that occurs, as well with cephalic as with transverse presentation, is called *tetanus uteri*. It is due to too early, brusk, and unnecessary manipulations on the uterus or cervix, and especially to the administration of *ergot*. The uterus is in one continual spasm. Occasionally a pain will increase the spasm. One finds the uterus hard all over, very tender, and the woman in continual pain; the cervix is red, dry, and hot; the vagina also is dry and hot. Labor is at a standstill, since in this condition the cervix will not dilate, and it is generally impossible to turn the baby so as to extract it. There is no danger of spontaneous rupture, but the baby dies, due to the interruption of the placental circulation, and unless something is done the mother dies of sepsis.

Fortunately in this country, and also in Europe, cases of "neglected transverse presentation" are becoming rare. The evil results of neglect must emphasize the importance of early diagnosis and consistent treatment.

Diagnosis.—During pregnancy abdominal palpation gives the best results, while vaginally nothing but the empty pelvis is felt. During labor the conditions are reversed because the contracting uterus covers up the fetal parts.

Abdominally.—(1) No longitudinal ovoid, but one more or less transverse, and, in contradistinction to uterus arcuatus, the broad portion is just above the inlet, not above the navel, as with arcuate uterus. (2) Over the inlet, nothing—the space is empty and the finger-tips may come together over the pelvis. (3) In the fundus likewise nothing; at most, some small parts or a deep furrow. (4) The back is in neither flank, and the hand must search elsewhere. Three of the four cardinal principles of the diagnosis of presentation being negative, the diagnosis must rest on the first, plus other, special findings. In scapulolæva anterior the head will be found on the left side, low in the flank, and it is recognized by its being large, hard, rounding, sometimes with ballottement. The breech is high up to the right behind, the small parts in the fundus to the right of the median line, the heart-tones loudest a little to the left and below the navel. It is easy to outline the dorsal plane in front. In Sc.D.P. the head is deep in the right flank, the breech under the spleen, no back can be outlined, but, instead, the region of the navel seems filled with small parts, and the heart-tones are to the right of the navel, about on a level with it.

Rectally, little can be felt unless the shoulder is forced down into the pelvis or the arm has prolapsed. It is better to make a vaginal examination.

Vaginally.—An empty vaginal vault immediately awakens suspicion of something abnormal. Sometimes the bag of waters hangs down like a stocking, filling the pelvis, and the attempt to feel something through it may rupture the membranes, which would be very unfortunate. The cervix hangs down like a cuff, and collapses in the interval between pains. After labor has progressed a short while the shoulder is more accessible, and, especially if the membranes are ruptured, all the landmarks may be discovered. These are the acromion process, the scapula, the clavicle, and the axilla. The direction in which the axilla is closed, that is, its apex, points to the fetal head. By noting whether the hard edge of the scapula looks to the pubis or to the sacrum we are enabled to say that the back lies to the front or to the rear. In Sc.L.A. the apex of the axilla points to the left, the edge of the scapula lies to the front, and the costal gridiron to the rear. Prolapse of the arm or elbow will aid in diagnosis. When the hand is down, the direction of the thumb and the bend of the elbow will be toward the child's abdomen. By trying to shake hands with the child it is possible to decide which hand is prolapsed. In Sc.L.A. the right arm— the lower one—almost always falls down; therefore if you find the head on the left side and the right arm down, it is safe to diagnose this position. While much can be learned from the position of the arm in living fetuses, preserving the tonus of the muscles, it is safest to follow up the member to the thorax and try to discover the axilla, the ribs, the pipe-stem-like clavicle, and the scapula,—even the rosary-like spinal column,—which gives absolute information. In scapulodextra posterior the axilla points to the right behind (Fig. 552), the costal gridiron to the front, the clavicle also to the pubis, the edge of the scapula is behind, and the arm, if down, is the right one. Since in very rare instances the upper arm prolapses, one must be careful in making diagnoses on the direction of the hand.

After labor has been in progress for a long time the parts become so swollen that diagnosis is difficult, and if the back or belly is forced down into the pelvis, the difficulties encountered may be very great and should warn to unusual care,

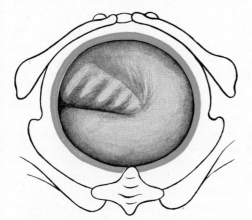

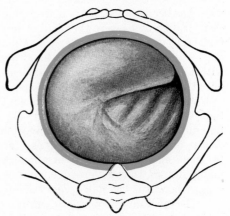

FIG. 551.—TOUCH PICTURE. Sc.L.A.
Apex of axilla points to left. Note costal gridiron.

FIG. 552.—TOUCH PICTURE. Sc.D.P.
Apex of axilla points to right.

because even very skilful accoucheurs have made costly errors. In the differential diagnosis breech, face, and vertex presentations, with prolapse of the arm, have to be considered, and confusion will be avoided by carefully searching for the landmarks peculiar to each.

Of great importance is the diagnosis of the state of the uterus as regards the imminence of rupture and the presence of tetanus, and no examination is complete without thorough study of the size of the fetus and of the cavity of the pelvis. In neglected shoulder presentations the accoucheur must discover if nature intends to terminate the case unassisted, and if so, which of the three modes will be chosen. If these points are properly evaluated, the accoucheur will be able to lay out that course of procedure which will most likely lead to a happy ending of the case.

Prognosis.—Transverse presentation being always dystocic and requiring the intervention of art, the prognosis depends on the ease and safety with which such intervention may be made. If an early diagnosis is made, the outlook for both mother and babe is excellent. In neglected cases the existence of infection, traumatism from ill-directed interference, and even of rupture of the uterus, indicate a very grave situation, and to all these must be added the dangers of the inevitable operation. In a recent article Schultze shows that in Germany alone fully 400 mothers and 4000 children annually lose their lives in consequence of transverse presentation. For the child the outlook is always bad unless its precarious position is recognized early. In neglected cases the infant almost always dies, from compression of the chest, abruption of the placenta, or asphyxia from obstructed placental circulation. Added to this is the mortality attendant on the operations of version and extraction or even decapitation performed in the interests of the mother.

Treatment.—Version, not expectancy, is the treatment of transverse presentations. The child must be brought into a longitudinal presentation—it must be turned. During pregnancy version by posture is tried, and the woman should, when abed, lie on the side to which the head points. Sometimes the breech will sag over to this side, forcing the head over the inlet. Examination at the end of three weeks may show a longitudinal presentation, when a binder, with pads on each side, may be applied, though success is not constant The French recommend a girdle, or "*ceinture eutocique,*" for this purpose, and the Japanese use daily massage and kneading to keep the fetus straight. During pregnancy cephalic version is preferred.

During early labor version by posture may be tried, but it is better to aid gravity by external manipulation. By gently leading the head over the inlet and pulling the breech up into the fundus much may be accomplished. Each manipulation is executed between pains, and when the uterus contracts, the hands hold what has been gained. An anesthetic may be advantageous and advisable. Many cases will be met where the head or breech has only slid off into the iliac fossa, and for these, external manipulation almost always suffices. Wiegand's method of version consists in placing one hand over the breech, the other over the head, and, with alternate pushing and stroking movements, striving to bring the head down over the inlet.

Version during early labor means cephalic version, but there are three conditions which govern the operation: (1) There may exist no immediate nor prospective indication for the rapid termination of labor; (2) the fetus must possess a high degree of mobility, the pains being weak and few, and the bag of waters intact; (3) there may not be too great a degree of pelvic contraction. Version by external manipulation, thus governed, should be persisted in until the second stage of labor is on, when, if it has failed, more definitive treatment is to be instituted.

The most unwelcome accident in shoulder cases is the rupture of the membranes before the cervix is completely dilated. As has been shown, conditions are particularly favorable for it. The accoucheur seeks to avoid or delay the rupture of the bag of waters by keeping the patient on the side,—that one on which the head lay,—by forbidding her to bear down with the pains, and, best of all, by placing a Braun soft-rubber colpeurynter in the vagina and filling it nearly full of solution. This exerts counterpressure on the membranes, and also prevents the shoulder from wedging into the pelvis. After complete dilatation of the cervix has been achieved a great deal has been accomplished, and the question now arises, which shall be done, cephalic or podalic version? Without doubt the child's chances are best in head-first deliveries, and the attendant will do well to consider the advisability of cephalic version, although few authors recommend it, and it is very rarely performed in practice. Generally, the foot is brought down, with a view to, with one stroke, both correcting the malpresentation and obtaining a good purchase on the child, so that its delivery can be effected at will. In the cases now cited Wright's method of cephalic version would almost certainly lead to success, and it is to be recommended for trial. Should it fail or prove too hazardous, or should the cord prolapse, as occurred once to me, the attempt is to be given up, and without withdrawing the hand a foot grasped and podalic version performed. Should the first attempt succeed, the head is to be led into the pelvis or drawn down with long forceps, held in proper position for a few uterine contractions, and *the case then left to nature,* or subject to a new indication demanding extraction. The procedure just detailed would be most desirable in primiparæ, but, unfortunately, it is this class of patients which present the greatest resistances to intra-uterine manœuvers, especially those which would change the location of the fetus.

Transverse presentation cases seldom come for treatment under the favorable conditions thus far considered. Usually the bag of waters has ruptured, the os is imperfectly dilated, the shoulder wedged more or less deeply into the pelvis, and the uterus retracted on the child. Truly neglected cases, with tetanus uteri, are nowadays, and certainly in this city, exceedingly rare. Since the rupture of the membranes has deprived the uterus of its best means of procuring sufficient dilatation of the os, nothing is more rational than to try to substitute the bag of waters. This is very successfully accomplished by the colpeurynter, and this useful instrument should be applied in all cases of shoulder presentation where the bag of waters has ruptured and the cervix has not opened sufficiently for the introduction of the hand. For such cases Braxton Hicks' method of bipolar version (combined manipulation by two fingers inserted through the os, assisted by the outside hand) has been recommended. In the author's experience the operation is very difficult and often impossible when the uterus has lost the liquor amnii, while, besides, the cord may prolapse, the placenta may be detached, or some other indication arise for immediate delivery. This indication could not be met because the cervix is not dilated. It is, therefore, better to apply a colpeurynter inside the uterus, resting against the cervix. As a rule, the pains now improve, becoming more regular and effective; what liquid remained in the uterus is prevented from escaping, the shoulder cannot wedge itself further in the pelvis, and the cervix is dilated by a fluid wedge much resembling the bag of waters. Sufficient dilatation should be procured so that extraction may be performed if necessary after the version.

It is dangerous to wait in these cases for the pains to dilate the cervix for the introduction of the hand, because the labor will become a "neglected" one under the very eyes of the accoucheur. If, on the arrival of the attendant, the cervix will admit the hand, version is immediately performed, and, usually, by the breech. Cephalic version is likely to be unsuccessful in these late cases, and, too, often an indication for delivery coexists with that for version; further, a slight degree of pelvic contraction may determine the choice of method, and finally the operator may not have had sufficient experience with Wright's operation. A point of immense practical importance is that after version has been performed the indication for the operation has been satisfied, and the accoucheur should study the case carefully to see if anything in the mother or the child creates a new indication for the extraction of the child. In other words, the operations of version and extraction must be separated, unless, at the same time, indications exist for both. Since the operation of version, by separating the placenta or causing entanglement of the cord, may create an indication for delivery, it is advisable to begin the version only after complete dilatation of the cervix has been procured by means of bags. The heart-tones must be auscultated continuously after version.

Neglected shoulder presentations, especially those where one of the modes of spontaneous expulsion is in progress, present truly intricate situations for the accoucheur to solve. The tetanically contracted uterus may foil every attempt at version, even in profound anesthesia, and to force it would inevitably cause a rupture of the organ. The stretched vagina, tightly filled with the large bulk of the presenting part, may not permit the fingers to gain access to the uterine cavity. The child may lie in the dilated lower uterine segment, which may be so thinned that the introduction of the hand may rupture it, or the uterus will tear when the woman's position is changed—and the tear may even have already begun. No consideration need be given to the child in this class of cases because it almost invariably has long succumbed. Decapitation and exenteration are the operations of choice. If the neck is within easy reach, decapitation by means of Carl Braun's hook may be done, but the author prefers the operation of exenteration. Even the most skilful accoucheur, in performing a decapitation, will twist the head against the thinned lower uterine segment and precipitate its rupture, while by exenterating the fetus it can be delivered without subjecting the uterus to any additional strain. If the chest of the child is wedged deeply into the pelvis, the accoucheur will find the neck stretched up above the inlet on one side, and the spinal column on the other, but almost parallel to the axis of the pelvis, and, of course, not placed so that a hook introduced from the vagina could operate at a right angle to them. Here exenteration is the operation of necessity. Should the accoucheur observe that nature herself is terminating the case in one of the three modes described, he may, though it is contrary to most teachings, exert tentative traction on that part of the fetus which seems to advance most, or at least seek to aid that mechanism which is occurring under his eyes.

Prolapse of the arm is not a complication of shoulder presentation. It does not interfere with any treatment. It is wise to put a sling on the wrist, and lay the end, sterile, over one groin. The arm need not be replaced in the uterus, nor should it be amputated under any circumstances. A physician amputated both arms of a presumably dead child and delivered it later alive!

What shall be done in neglected transverse presentations when version is impossible or too hazardous and the child still alive? From the nature of the case, cesarean section is contraindicated, because it jeopardizes the mother too much, and the child, though living at the time of delivery, in the majority of cases dies soon after from the effects of the compression. In the author's opinion, embryotomy should be done. While it sacrifices what little life the child has and is a painful task for the accoucheur, it offers the mother the greatest safety. (See p. 776.)

Preceding all operations in shoulder deliveries a painstaking examination is to be made to discover the existence of a complication which might affect the treatment—e. g., contracted pelvis or placenta prævia may indicate cesarean section—and, after delivery, the uterus and vagina must be explored to determine the integrity of the parturient canal—advice which cannot be too frequently reiterated.

PROLAPSE OF THE CORD

This error of attitude occurs in about 0.8 per cent. of cases (Schiller), and has been observed as early as the fourth month of pregnancy. It was first mentioned by Louise Bourgeoise in 1609. During labor it is most unwelcome, because the life of the child is so intimately concerned. Three degrees of prolapse of the cord may be distinguished: (1) An occult form, where the cord is at or near the girdle of resistance, but not within reach of the fingers during the ordinarily careful examination. Here the condition is not suspected, and the child may die from compression of the cord in natural delivery or by the blade of the forceps (Fig. 553). (2) The cord may be forelying, that is, palpable through the os, but in the intact bag of waters (Fig. 554). (3) The cord may be prolapsed into the vagina or even outside of the vulva, the bag of waters being ruptured (Fig. 555).

Etiology.—Anything which causes a maladaptation of the presenting part to the lower uterine segment or prevents engagement of the head will favor prolapse of the cord. In normal presentations the lower uterine segment is so evenly applied to the head that there is no room for the cord to slip down. Mechanical causes are: (1) Contracted pelvis, the head being arrested high and free spaces being left at the sides; indeed, the discovery of the cord must evoke the suspicion of a contracted pelvis. In Hildebrand's 126 cases of prolapsed cord one-third had contracted pelvis; (2) malpositions and malpresentations; occipitoposterior, face and brow, breech and shoulder presentations; (3) low attachment of the placenta, with marginal insertion of the cord; (4) preternaturally long cord, though a short one may also prolapse; (5) displacement of the cord as an error of art during obstetric operations; (6) prolapse of an arm. Other causes are twins, polyhydramnion, the cord being rushed out with the bursting of the membranes, and especially since the head is usually high in such cases; the accidental floating out of the cord when the waters break before the head is engaged, as occurs in multiparæ otherwise normal. It has occurred to the author that perhaps the specific gravity of the liquor amnii may have something to do with the prolapse.

Course and Prognosis.—So far as the mother is concerned, prolapse of the

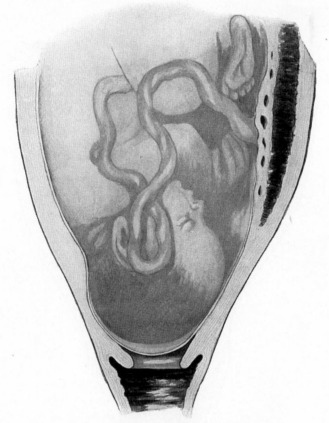

Fig. 553.—Occult Prolapse of the Cord.
In the unruptured membranes hardly any pressure is possible.

cord does not affect the course of labor, except inasmuch as the cause of the prolapse might do so, and, moreover, she is not endangered except by these causes, and by the operations which might be undertaken on account of them, and to save the life of the child.

For the child there is great danger, since the soft blood-vessels easily suffer compression and asphyxia results. The cord is most easily compressed in head presentations when it lies in front, behind the pubis. When it has slipped down at the side, near the sacro-iliac joints, it finds some little protection behind the jutting promontory, though the soft parts alone can exert fatal compression. Compression of the cord affects the vein first, reducing the amount of blood going to the fetal heart, and causing placental congestion. As the result of the anemia, lack of stimulation of the sino-auricular node in the auricle, and the asphyxia the fetal heart slows, sometimes to 50 or 60, during the contraction of the uterus, and, when the compression is relieved, the heart bounds up to 130 to 160 a minute. But this does not mean that the circulation has recovered, because in many instances minute hemorrhages in the lungs and even heart-clot have been produced, which render extra-uterine existence impossible. If the cord hangs out of the vulva, it may congeal from cold or the mother may lie on it. In breech and shoulder presentation the danger of compression is not so acute, though still serious, and if an extremity has also prolapsed, the cord may find protection by lying alongside and parallel with it. An additional danger to the child will arise in the operations undertaken for its rescue—all of which explains the 40 to 50 per cent. mortality in operated cases and the 80 per cent. in those left to nature.

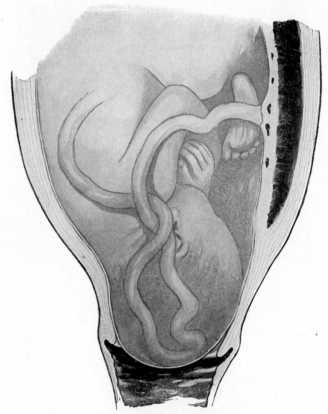

FIG. 554.—THE FORELYING CORD.
This cord may be compressed.

Diagnosis.—Occult prolapse of the cord should be thought of when, in an otherwise natural labor, the fetal heart-tones are irregular or arrhythmic, and when, as in the forceps operation, auscultation reveals cardiac tumult during the tractions. A persistent funic souffle with irregularity of the heart is very significant. Auscultation of the fetal heart is an indispensable routine in the conduct of labor. By deep insertion of the fingers behind the pubis it is often possible to discover the knuckle of cord as it lies—usually above one ear—alongside the head. (See Forceps.)

Rectally, the prolapsed cord can usually be recognized, but when suspicion of such an occurrence arises this method may not be trusted. Vaginally, a forelying cord in the intact bag of waters will escape only the careless diagnostician, and it will also be easy to differentiate it from velamentous umbilical vessels, from pulsating arteries in the fornices, and from polyps.

After rupture of the bag of waters no difficulty is experienced—it is often possible to see the cord. Palpation of the umbilical cord to determine if it pulsates must be the gentlest possible, because it is a shock to the child to have its placental circulation stopped, and, too, the vein is compressed first, shutting off the supply of oxygen. Pulsation in the cord may be absent, or so slight that it is impalpable, and yet the child be living. Auscultation of the fetal heart must always be practised before pronouncing the child dead.

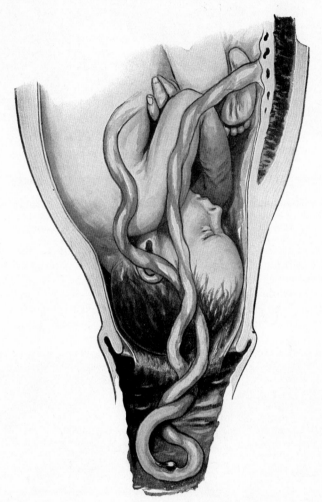

Fig. 555.—Prolapse of Cord. Greatest Danger of Compression.

In the differential diagnosis maternal intestines fallen through a rent in the parturient canal and fetal intestines in abdominal hernia are to be considered.

Treatment.—As has been stated many times on similar occasions, all treatment must be preceded by a careful obstetric examination, including pelvic mensuration, to discover the cause of the prolapse, and all adjuvant factors which may alter and direct the course of procedure demanded by the indications. For example, a contracted pelvis may indicate cesarean section, or a low-lying placenta Braxton Hicks' version.

The Forelying Cord.—When the cord is felt in the intact bag of waters, the accoucheur should attempt its replacement by posture, the elevated Sims' position (Fig. 557), the Trendelenburg (Fig. 556), even the knee-chest, being employed. **To** prevent the rupture of the membranes before complete dilatation has been secured the patient is forbidden to bear down, is kept abed in one—the most comfortable—of the attitudes mentioned, and a Carl Braun soft-rubber colpeurynter is placed in the vagina. All preparations are made for quick operative delivery, and the accoucheur stays by the bedside. When complete dilatation of the cervix has been obtained, nine-tenths of the danger has been obviated.

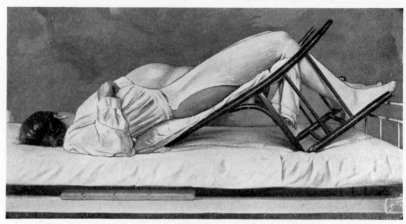

FIG. 556.—TRENDELENBURG POSITION IN TREATMENT OF PROLAPSE OF CORD.
Note concavity above pubis caused by the head leaving the inlet.

When Prolapse Has Occurred.—First, if the cord is outside the vulva, it must be sterilized (washed with warm water and soap, then painted with 4 per cent. iodin) and replaced within the vagina, the head being lifted off the cord by a finger per rectum while this is being done. Now one of two things must be accomplished: either the child must be delivered or the cord must be put in a place where it will not be compressed. Naturally, if conditions are right for immediate

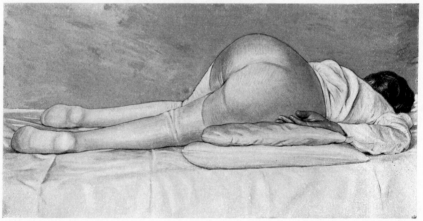

FIG. 557.—PATIENT IN ELEVATED SIMS' POSITION IN TREATMENT OF PROLAPSE OF CORD.

extraction, this is the most advisable procedure, because it instantly extricates the child from its precarious position. For rapid extraction the cervix must be effaced and completely dilated, conditions which are seldom present. Everything depends on the cervix.

(a) If the cervix is not open enough to admit the hand, the accoucheur must relieve the cord from the danger of compression. Braxton Hicks' version has been proposed, but the results are bad, because often the cord does not recede with the change of polarity of the body, and, further, during the long wait for complete dilatation the child usually dies.

It is better to replace the cord above the head and put a metreurynter in the cervix, to prevent its falling down again. H. M. Stowe advised to fill the uterus with salt solution after replacing the cord, and invented a metreurynter for this purpose. Replacement of the cord may be accomplished with a catheter and stilet, as shown in Fig. 559, *g* and *h*, the catheter being left in place until complete dilatation has been obtained, or the two fingers may be employed to push the cord up. All these manœuvers are carried out with the woman in the knee-chest posture, in order to get the benefit of gravity, and, before the hand is withdrawn, a metreurynter is inserted in the lower uterine segment and filled with 12 ounces of weak antiseptic solution, or the cervix is packed with gauze—this precaution to hinder the cord from falling out again and to keep the head away from the inlet. After the cervix is thus thoroughly plugged, the woman may be placed on her back or side. Neither of these methods is uniformly successful. The repositor may kink or injure the cord or wound the uterus, and the fingers may not be able to push the loops above the globe of the head, and in both instances the cord is likely to pro-

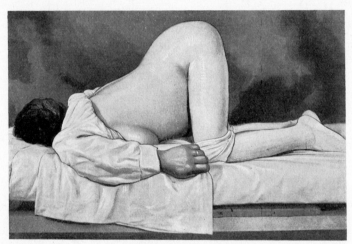

FIG. 558.—KNEE-CHEST POSITION.

lapse again as soon as the woman is laid on the back or when the colpeurynter comes out. Then, too, the cord may not be relieved of compression by the operation, and even the bag may press on it. In one case where the cord could not be replaced I pulled the arm down alongside the head and tucked the cord beside it, thus protecting it from injury. A thick rectal bougie might be used for this purpose.

(*b*) If the cervix will admit the hand, there are two methods to choose—version and reposition of the cord. Equally good results are obtained from both operations; the choice, therefore, will depend on individual skill and preference, plus the conditions presented by each case. Version will be selected when—(1) Other indications for version are present; (2) when a contracted pelvis of minor degree coexists; (3) in face, brow, or other abnormal presentation; (4) when an indication for delivery on the part of the mother or child arises or is to be anticipated; (5) when reposition has failed or the cord fallen down again.

It is always desirable to secure complete dilatation before turning, because it may be necessary to follow the version with the complementary operation of extraction. In favorable cases (soft cervix and small child) it may be possible to dilate the parts manually and complete the labor in one operation.

Reposition is practised as follows: If the woman will permit the operation without an anesthetic, the knee-chest posture is employed; if not, the exaggerated

Trendelenburg is used. Passing the whole hand into the vagina, the cord is allowed to coil in the palm, which is hollowed out for its reception, the fingers making a sort of cage for it (Fig. 560). Then, pushing the head up and to one side, going in the direction indicated by the cord itself, the loops are quickly carried to the highest point attainable in the uterus, and, if possible, the cord is hung over one leg. While doing this the other hand pushes the head away from the inlet. After the cord is replaced, the inside hand, acting with the outside hand, brings the head over the inlet, and a few pains are awaited to force it down. It may be advisable to pull the head into the pelvis with forceps and then leave the case to nature. By keeping the woman on the side the cord is prevented from coming down again.

Reposition is not likely to be successful nor advisable when the pelvis is con-

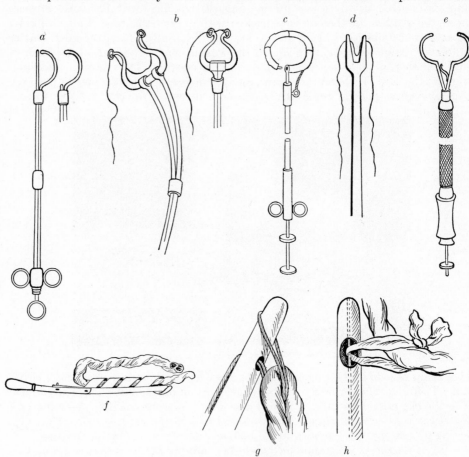

FIG. 559.—VARIOUS CORD REPOSITORS.

a, Schoeller's; b, Heyernaux's; c, Ducamp's; d, Favereau's; e, Murphy's; f, Poullet's; g, Braun's; h, Dudan's, an ordinary linen catheter with stylet and a loop of tape.

tracted, and it is usually not practised in the presence of an indication for immediate extraction. When the child is in bad condition, both reposition and version are usually powerless to save it, but in these cases the author prefers reposition for primiparæ and version for multiparæ.

In all cases, after Braxton Hicks' version, after version and after replacement, the heart-tones of the fetus must be continuously observed, in order to detect the first signs of a threatening asphyxia. Even after apparent successful replacement the cord may be compressed at a point not suspected.

When the head is engaged, reposition and version are usually impossible, and the safety of the child lies in its quick delivery. If the cervix is fully opened, no difficulties are met; if it is not, manual dilatation, Dührssen's incisions, even vaginal cesarean section, may be employed, and then forceps applied. Which method will be selected depends on the condition of the cervix as regards effacement and dilatation and the accomplishments of the accoucheur.

If, when called to the case, the cord is found pulsating feebly or not at all, the accoucheur's first duty is to determine, so far as possible, the actual condition of the child and its chances for ultimate recovery even if delivered alive. It is no feat to be proud of to deliver a child at the expense of extensive maternal injuries when it dies after a few minutes or hours from late asphyxia or cerebral hemorrhage. If a prolapse of the cord finds the accoucheur unprepared for its proper treatment,

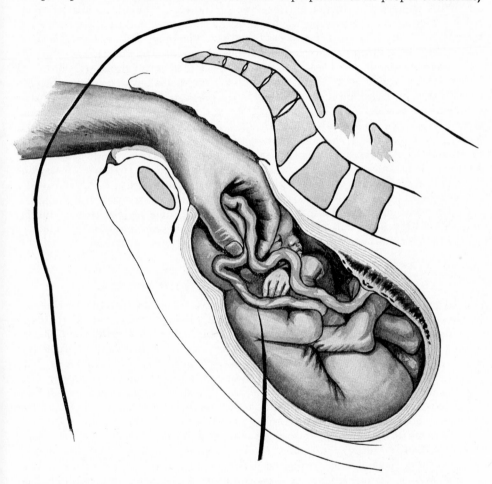

Fig. 560.—Replacement of Prolapsed Cord with Whole Hand. Patient in Knee-chest Posture.

the head may be held back and the cord protected for several hours by the hand inside until assistance can be procured.

What to do if the baby is dead. Craniotomy is recommended to the skilful accoucheur to save the pelvic structures from the injuries incident to normal labor. Lacking skill the attendant leaves the delivery to nature. Forceps and version on a dead child are contraindicated. Of course, if there is doubt of the life of the child, it should have the benefit of the doubt. What to do when the cord is pulsating only feebly and there is reason to believe the death of the child is not far distant is not easy to decide. If the child can be quickly brought to light without the danger of serious maternal injury, it ought to get this chance for its life, but if the operative delivery promises to be hard—a primipara, for example—or tedious, it is more than likely that the child will perish during the attempt to save it, or shortly afterward. The almost inevitable cervical and perineal lacerations will then make the accoucheur regret his futile and perilous operations.

Breech and Footling Presentations.—Prolapse of the cord complicating these presentations carries a degree of danger slightly less than with head presentations. Most authors say that the cord is not easily compressed by the soft breech, but this is not my experience. It is best to replace the cord, hanging it over the shoulder, and then put in a metreurynter.

With transverse presentation prolapse of the cord requires no special treatment. During the preparations for version the cord is to be kept clean and warm by putting it into the vagina and applying a vulvar plug. If the cervix is to be dilated by a metreurynter, the cord is first pushed up into the uterus.

Cesarean section has been proposed for the treatment of prolapsed cord. At first breath it would seem that such an operation would never come up for consideration, since it is done almost entirely in the interests of the child, but the author can think of several conditions in which the abdominal delivery would command serious attention. These are: (1) An aged primipara, very desirous of a child. Here, if the parturient canal is unprepared, the child is almost invariably lost; (2) mild degrees of pelvic contraction, insufficient of themselves to indicate cesarean section; (3) where the religious scruples of the family demand that in all operations the child be given equal chances with the mother. Couvelaire and Potocki report successful cases. When cesarean section is considered in the treatment of prolapsed cord, two conditions must be insisted upon: the child must be in perfect condition and the mother have not even the suspicion of infection. The cervical method should be done and the cord not drawn upward through the uterine wound.

PROLAPSE OF THE ARMS AND FEET WITH THE HEAD

In general, the same causes which produce prolapse of the cord may permit the hands or feet to come down alongside the head. Voluntary motions of the child may also be mentioned. On several occasions the author has felt the child present a hand at the os and then withdraw it. If the bag of waters should break at this moment, the extremity would be floated out. Contracted pelvis, small or dead fetus (lack of tonicity), and sudden rush of liquor amnii are the usual causes. The complication occurs once in about 350 labors. We speak of the presenting or forelying hand or foot when the extremity is felt in the intact sac at the os, and of prolapse when the membranes are broken and the part is in the vagina.

Prolapse of the arm may influence the mechanism of labor. In the first place, it may stiffen the fetal cylinder and confer a rigidity which is harmful to normal rotation, and, secondly, by occupying a portion of the pelvis which the occiput should traverse, it may prevent anterior rotation of the same. For example, if in O.L.A. the posterior arm lies alongside the forehead, it will aid anterior rotation; if the anterior one comes down behind the pubis, it will delay or prevent it. An arm lying in the anterior half of the pelvis will obstruct labor more than if in the hollow of the sacrum, where there is more room. The anterior arm is the one usually found, and prolapse occurs oftener with occipitoposterior positions. The diagnosis is simple, but the accoucheur should always remember that the hand may be that of a shoulder presentation or of a second twin, and that sometimes the foot may be mistaken for the hand.

Treatment.—Before rupture of the bag of waters, while the head is still above the inlet, posture will usually suffice. Place the woman on the side on which the hand does not lie. As labor advances the head pushes by the arm. After the membranes rupture, as a rule, the head enters the pelvis, the arms being held back, but sometimes the arm prevents the engagement of the head. Here the extremity must be replaced, using the half or the whole hand, under anesthesia, if necessary. If this fails, or if the arm falls down again, version is performed. Version is also done when, in addition to the arm, the cord is down or the placenta is low in the uterus, or any other indication for changing the polarity of the fetus exists.

After the head has engaged with the arm nothing is done because there is evidently enough room in the pelvis for the two. Since labor is longer and anomalies of rotation commoner, forceps are more often needed. In applying the forceps care to see that the blades do not grasp the arm is necessary.

Arms in the Nape of the Neck.—Figure 561 shows a rare anomaly of attitude. It was described first by Simpson, and the author has met with only two instances of it. About 25 cases have been reported, mostly English. After the engagement of the head the arms, crossed above the brim, effectually stopped the attempted forceps delivery, and the author being under the impression that a distended chest was the cause of the obstruction, it was only after the half-hand, under deep narcosis, was passed up, that the real reason was discovered. With considerable difficulty the arms were gotten into proper position and then the instrumental delivery was easily completed. Unless such replacement of the arms is possible, the case will be formidable. Version was successful in Simpson's, Gray's, and Lambert's cases. Craniotomy may have to be done; then, when sufficient room is procured alongside the crushed head, the arms may be reached and either pushed out of the way or drawn down.

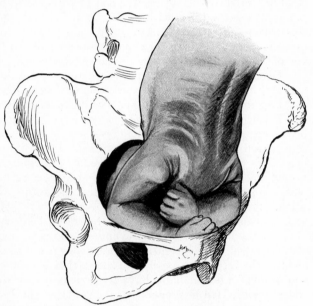

FIG. 561.—ARMS IN NAPE OF NECK.
Mrs. L. Primipara. Eclampsia. Heart disease. Readjusted arms. Forceps.

Prolapse of the foot alongside the head is very rare, and only 7 such cases occurred in the author's experience. Version in each instance was easy, though most authors say it is difficult under the circumstances. Since the fetal cylinder is made rigid, slow advance and delayed rotation are usual, and, therefore, forceps oftener needed. If the foot prevents engagement of the head, it may be pushed away and the head led into the pelvis by combined manipulation; if this does not succeed, version is the treatment. If the foot and head have engaged in the pelvis, watchful expectancy and forceps, if needed, are recommended.

LITERATURE

Couvelaire and Potocki: Annales de Gyn., February, 1910, p. 111.—*Gray:* Med. Record, New York, 1894, vol. xliii, p. 589.—*Kehrer, E.:* Zeitschr. für Geb. u. Gyn., 1932, Band 101, H. 3, p. 497. Lit.—*Marshall:* Amer. Jour. Obst. and Gyn., 1921, p. 15.—*McPherson:* Bull. New York Lying-in Hosp., 917.—*Sippel:* Zentb. für Gyn., November 12, 1921, No. 45, p. 1634.—*Schiller, W.:* Monatsschr. für Geb. u. Gyn., 1931, vol. lxxxviii, p. 52.— *Schultze:* Monatsschr. f. Geb. u. Gyn., August, 1909, vol. xxx, No. 2, p. 137.—*Simpson:* Obstetric Memoirs.

CHAPTER LI

ANOMALIES OF THE PASSENGERS (Concluded)

DYSTOCIA DUE TO EXCESSIVELY LARGE FETUS

OLDER writers report the birth of children weighing 23 and 24 pounds (Ortega, Rachel, and Neumer, quoted by Dubois in 1897). Beach reported a giantess's child weighing 10,773 gm., about $22\frac{1}{2}$ pounds, and being 76 cm. long; Belcher, one of 25 pounds; Moss, one of 24 pounds, 2 ounces, and 35 inches long. It is best to accept the stories related by patients as to the immense size of their previous children with much reserve, because they are usually exaggerated or mere guesses. The largest child delivered by the author weighed 14 pounds and necessitated cesarean section. It was diseased and died with high fever in sixteen hours. One weighing $12\frac{1}{2}$ pounds was delivered by forceps and survived. In the service of the Chicago Lying-in Hospital in 35,113 cases only 5 children weighed over 13 pounds, 5900 gm. All but one of these children gave rise to marked dystocia. Brodhead gives the literature.

Given a normal pelvis, normal powers, and a normal presentation, position, and attitude, nature is usually capable of accomplishing the delivery of children weighing up to 9 pounds without very great difficulty.

Etiology.—(1) Partus serotinus, prolonged pregnancy, carrying overterm, has been recognized as a cause of overdevelopment of the child, and, though questioned, was proved by von Winckel (see p. 120). In addition, my own studies show that the bones become harder, less malleable, the spine stiffer, the fat and muscles firmer, and the head actually larger and more square in shape, with pointed parietal bosses. The fontanels are smaller, the sutures almost closed and in apposition. Sometimes children carried overterm are lighter in weight relatively to their increased length, but the difficulties of delivery, rather than being diminished by the long narrow fetal cylinder, are really augmented, because of the lack of moldability. (2) Overeating in pregnancy is not a common cause of overdevelopment of the fetus, but experience shows that women of the better situated classes and those of indolent habit have larger babies than those that have to work hard and are poorly fed in pregnancy. Evvards, of the Iowa State College, by experiments on pigs and sheep, has proved that a diet rich in proteins and calcium makes large and strong offspring. If at the same time the mother be prevented from getting proper exercise, dystocia will result. In France and Germany special maternity provision is made for these women with a view to improving the offspring. The war diet in Germany, contrary to what was expected, has resulted in larger children than in times of peace (Momm). (3) Multiparity—children of later pregnancies are usually larger than that of the first, but an exception is to be noted in old primiparæ with male children. These are likely to be large and a frequent cause of dystocia. (4) Large parents usually have large children, which is fortunate only if the mother exceeds the normal size, because then her pelvis will accommodate the child. A large father may procreate children which the mother cannot deliver. In one of the author's consultations the third wife of a very large and powerful man died, as did the other two, from obstructed labor. (5) Finally, no particular cause being found, it is supposed that some factor producing a large ovum may be the reason for the overgrowth of the fetus, or perhaps the endocrine glands should be invoked. Osler says babies over 9 pounds suffer from hypothyroidism. The children in placenta prævia and other placental anomalies are usually small. Overgrowth does not mean overterm (Schmid).

Course.—During pregnancy, overdistention of the belly may cause the same disturbances as twins (which are usually suspected); these are: a feeling of great weight, dyspnea, edema, albuminuria, pendulous belly, etc. If labor is postponed, intermittent false pains may annoy the woman for several weeks. Labor is slow, and usually characterized by weak pains (from overdistention), with early rupture of the membranes, because the head engages late. Cephalic presentations are the rule. Occipitoposterior positions are very common. In general, the course of labor resembles that in contracted pelvis of the justominor type. If the head is not too hard, it molds into the pelvis and is delivered under strong bearing-down effort or by the aid of art. The broad shoulders then cause delay. Girls have broader shoulders than boys when compared with the size of the head. After the head is out, it snaps back against the perineum, pressing this upward into the pelvis, due to the elasticity of the fetal neck. Unless the shoulders can be brought down, the child quickly dies. Anomalous mechanisms are very common, but delay in engagement of the shoulder-girdle is the usual cause of the trouble, and this is because it is too large or incompressible. Rupture of the uterus may occur in the dystocia due to the delivery of voluminous shoulders. Even the breech may be so voluminous that its delivery is slow.

Postpartum hemorrhage and anomalies of placental separation are more frequent than usual, because the large uterus needs time to retract on itself and may not do so perfectly. Lacerations must also be expected, especially if any manipulations were required.

Diagnosis.—A very large, protuberant belly will excite the suspicion of an overgrown child, of twins, or of hydramnion. Absence of fluctuation will exclude the latter, and the recognized methods will usually suffice to discover two fetuses. Cephalometry (q. v.) is giving better results since it is being practised more. If the accoucheur will, in every case, endeavor to determine accurately the size of the child before the birth, and control his findings by later measurements, he will acquire a degree of accuracy in estimating the size of the fetus which he would not have believed possible. The size of the fetus is just as important a matter for the obstetrician to know as the size of the pelvis. Of nearly equal moment is the hardness of the fetal head. This is determinable by bimanual palpation, from the size of the fontanels, and by noting how well the bones of the head overlap as the latter enters the pelvis under the influence of the pains. After delivery of the head a stoppage of labor usually results from the big trunk, but the possibility of anomalous mechanisms of the shoulders and of tumors of the fetal body, or dorsal displacement of the arms, must be remembered. In a breech presentation the size of the part will give a good indication, and especially if the foot is down. A large leg and foot usually means a large child. The x-ray will help.

Prognosis.—For the mother, it depends on the degree of disproportion between the child and the pelvis, and if this is very great and goes unrecognized, the mother may die—of ruptured uterus, sepsis, exhaustion, or inflicted injuries. Ordinarily, however, the mother may be successfully delivered if the child weighs not over 5000 gm. (11 pounds) and other conditions are favorable. The delivery of an enormous child through a normal pelvis is harder than the delivery of a normal child through a contracted pelvis, even when the proportions are the same. For the child, the prognosis is not so good. Many more die in labor, from asphyxia, compression of the brain, and from the injuries inflicted in operative delivery. Intracranial hemorrhage, fissure-fractures of the skull, cephalhematomata, spoon-shaped depressions, Erb's paralysis—all are more frequent. It must be remembered that sometimes these large children are diseased—for example, suffering from anasarca, universal hydrops, or myxedema. After delivery the large children lose more in weight, even proportionately. Winter, upon examining 785 mentally deficient children, found that 9 per cent. were born after prolonged pregnancies.

Treatment.—As was already said, the author considers it unwise to allow women to go far overterm, and when, after careful consideration of all obtainable information, subjective and objective, he decides that the usual period of gestation has been completed, he induces labor. (See Prolonged Pregnancy.) This procedure is still more necessary, and may be done several weeks before term, when the woman gives a history of large children and difficult labors. Prochownik instituted a special dietary for such cases, hoping thus to diminish the size of the child, but in my cases it was not successful, which failure other authors also admit (Ballantyne), and the experience with war food blockade in Germany confirms.

During labor the important thing is to discover early that the infant is large, because a cesarean section may be the easiest and safest for both patients. Hebosteotomy is not advisable as a primary selection, because of the dangers to the soft parts. If the disproportion is recognized only after the favorable time for cesarean section is past, a high degree of expectancy is to be employed. Occipitoposterior positions are to be early corrected, and then labor allowed to proceed until the head is firmly engaged. High forceps operations are bad in these cases, but not so bad as version, which should be avoided, if at all possible, and especially in primiparæ. If nature fails, and the accoucheur with his forceps cannot bring the large and often stony-hard head into the pelvis, extraperitoneal cesarean section, pubiotomy, and craniotomy are the alternatives.

Difficulty in the delivery of the shoulders is overcome as follows: (1) Have the woman bear down strongly in lithotomy position forcing the thighs against the abdomen; (2) aid gently by Kristeller's expression; (3) try to tuck the shoulder down behind the pubis, aiding by the internal hand; (4) failing, try "tight ring maneuver No. 1," i. e., put two fingers on the anterior scapula or one into the anterior axilla behind the pubis and gently twist the body ventrally so as to bring the bisacromial diameter into an oblique of the pelvis, then down; failing this, try the tight ring maneuver No. 2, i. e., operating on the posterior shoulder, one or two fingers are hooked into the posterior axilla, and, giving the torso a turbinal movement, dorsally this time, the shoulder is brought around behind the pubis and out. (See Fig. 880.) (5) Bring the posterior arm down and out, going up into the uterus with the whole hand; failing this, try to bring the anterior arm down from behind the pubis. Lubricate parts well and be very gentle, but if this does not succeed, use force, well applied, of course, risking a fracture of the extremity. In one case I deliberately fractured the humerus and saved the child's life. After one arm is down the extraction is usually possible; if not, get the other arm also. Should the child have died during these prolonged manipulations, all haste should be at once abandoned; cleidotomy and evisceration are now in order. A deep episiotomy is almost always necessary in these cases, otherwise the perineal floor, including the sphincter and rectum, will be injured, often extensively.

Morcellation of a giant child is one of the most formidable tasks that can confront the accoucheur, and on several occasions the vaginal operation had to be abandoned and cesarean section resorted to finally. Amputation of the uterus should be done in such cases to forestall sepsis.

RIGOR MORTIS

Should the child die before delivery, the rigor mortis may be a cause of dystocia. Few such cases are reported because it seldom happens that the birth occurs during this temporary condition, and many times it is not recognized; finally it is not constant. The child figured on p. 587 gave rise to real difficulty in labor; the forceps operation was very laborious; it was necessary to insert the whole hand for the purpose of pulling down the shoulders, and even the trunk came hard. Fractures of the extremities have occurred in such deliveries.

ENLARGEMENT OF PARTS OF THE CHILD

Hydrocephalus may give rise to severe dystocia. Both external and internal forms are observed, and the skull may contain several quarts of fluid and have a circumference of 80 cm. (Fig. 562). Nothing is positively known of the causes, but syphilis seems to have some effect, and in general what was said in the chapter on Monsters applies here. The frequent association of hydrocephalus with spina bifida, club-foot, fetal rickets, ascites, etc., is to be emphasized.

Course.—Pregnancy may be interrupted because of a non-viable hydrocephalic fetus. Labor is usually a little premature, and is often notable because of weak pains, but, owing to overdistention and thinning of the lower uterine segment and the mechanical obstruction to labor, rupture of the uterus is a frequent complication. For example, in Schuchard's 74 cases 14 had uterine rupture. Breech presentation is much more frequent than usual, and the soft head comes through easier than when it leads the way. A small hydrocephalus may be delivered easily, or with only slight help from art; a larger one always gives trouble, but, curiously, a very large head not strongly distended and with soft bones may mold its way through the pelvis. A dead and macerated fetus may also pass easily, especially if the pains are good. Pressure necrosis and fistulas, from prolonged labor and operative errors, are sometimes observed. The head remains

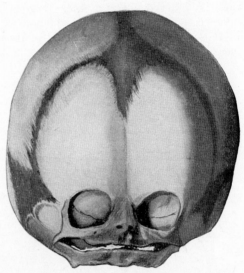

Fig. 562.—HYDROCEPHALUS (Museum of Northwestern University Medical School).

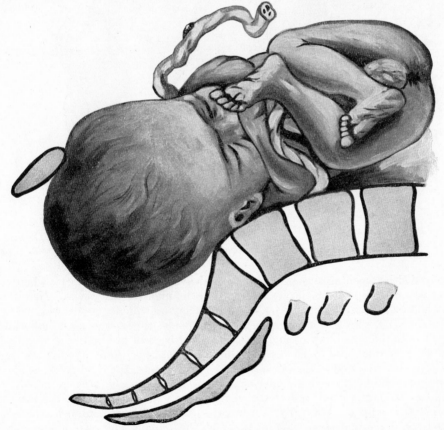

Fig. 563.—HYDROCEPHALUS, MOLDING ITS WAY INTO PELVIS.

high a long time, and the signs of thinning of the lower uterine segment are early and marked. Sometimes the head bursts under the action of strong pains or during extraction. The fluid may escape outside or under the skin, or a spina bifida bursts and lets it out.

Postpartum hemorrhage from atony of the uterus and from the frequent lacerations is observed. The mother, therefore, is much endangered by hydrocephalus unless it is recognized early, in which event the only mortality and morbidity should be those of normal labor. Since the disease is so fatal to the child, our operative measures usually do not consider it, but many cases are recorded where the child

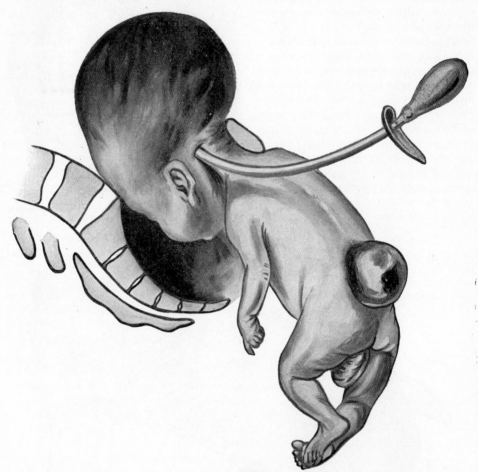

Fig. 564.—Puncture of Hydrocephalus with Trocar. Note Spina Bifida (author's case).

survived either spontaneous or instrumental delivery. Even in one case where the head was perforated to facilitate delivery the infant lived six weeks. Nearly all the children die within a few years, and hardly any are cured.

Diagnosis.—From the accoucheur's standpoint, this is the most important, and if only the possibility of such a complication be kept in mind, it is very easy. Mistakes are due more to carelessness than to ignorance. Abdominally, the large size of the uterine tumor, the tense lower uterine segment, the rigidity of the abdomen, the broad head (over the inlet or in the fundus), the lack of engagement, the tendency to inertia uteri, call attention to some anomaly. Rectally, the vault of the pelvis is empty. Vaginally, the broad sutures and large fontanels, the large flat elastic dome that seeks to enter the inlet, but remains high, will almost clinch the diagnosis. If the bones of the cranium are thin, the crackling craniotabes will be felt, and by bimanual palpation, the use of which is too much neglected in obstetric diagnosis, the immense size of the head is easily distinguishable. In the differential diagnosis a small hydrocephalus must be separated from a large but normal head and here even the x-ray may prove faulty though otherwise invaluable. A thin-walled hydrocephalus may simulate the bag of waters or the urinary bladder. Macerated and edematous fetal scalp, cystic tumors on the head, encephaloceles, and tough membranes have been wrongly diagnosed. A hydrocephalic child presenting by the breech is usually not discovered until the head is arrested at the inlet. Occasionally a spina bifida or other deformity will excite suspicion of an associated hydrocephalus.

Treatment.—Since the child almost invariably dies and is doomed to early death even if delivered alive, all effort is directed to save the mother. Perforation of the head with a trocar is the operation recommended by almost all writers. A long scissors will do if a trocar is not at hand, and the hole is made in the most accessible part of the head. In breech cases a spot beside the ear is usually the best, but the operation has been performed through the mouth and the spinal canal.

After the fluid is evacuated the collapsed cranium offers little resistance to the soft parts and is usually quickly delivered. Should an indication for rapid delivery arise in a head case, traction may be exerted on the collapsed sac, and if this tears, as is usual, the cranioclast may be applied to the base of the skull and the cervical spinal column. Version might be done but it is unwise to expose a uterus, already endangered by overstretching, to an additional strain.

DISTENTION OF THE ABDOMEN

This may result from ascites, enlarged liver, neoplasms and cysts of the liver, congenital cystic kidneys, dilated bladder or ureters, and a few other isolated conditions. Ascites accompanies most of those mentioned. Syphilis plays an important rôle in the causation of ascites, fetal peritonitis, and liver diseases. The diagnosis of excessive abdominal distention of the fetus is seldom made until delay in the exit of the child is manifest. Great abdominal distention of the mother or polyhydramnion will only direct attention to the possibility of a fetal anomaly. In head cases, after the shoulders are ready to escape from the vulva, progress is arrested, and in spite of strong traction delivery may not be effected. Examination with the whole hand will clear the diagnosis. Fig. 565 shows a case of labor arrested by congenital cystic kidneys. Since the breech did not advance, the hand was inserted and the large belly easily circumscribed with the fingers.

Treatment.—In head presentation, after the head is born and the distended trunk will not come, several ribs and the sternum are to be exsected with Siebold's scissors, the lungs and heart removed, the diaphragm punctured, and the abdominal contents thus evacuated. When the breech presents, simple puncture of the belly suffices in ascites, but if there is a solid tumor also, it is removed by morcellation. Dorland gives literature.

TOUGH MEMBRANES

The membranes are sometimes a source of obstruction to labor, and a slightly increased resistance here may be the cause of great delay. They may be either adherent over the internal os and lower uterine segment, thus preventing the dilatation of same, or they may be so tough that they do not rupture when the cervix is dilated. In either case labor is retarded: in the one at the beginning, in the other at the end, of the first stage. The second is easily recognized—delay after complete dilatation.

Lack of progress in the first stage of labor, due to adherent membranes, may be suspected when the os dilates very slowly in spite of good contractions, the head being well down in the pelvis, the completely effaced cervix fitting it closely like a cap, and the membranes stretched tightly over the scalp, with no, or hardly any, forewaters. The adherences may be felt. Labor may be delayed one or two days by such a condition.

Treatment.—In the first stage it is advisable to push up the head a little, loosen the membranes all around the margin of the internal os to the extent of one inch, and allow a little liquor amnii to come down, to make a good hydrostatic dilator. After several hours, if delay is still manifest, it is justifiable to rupture

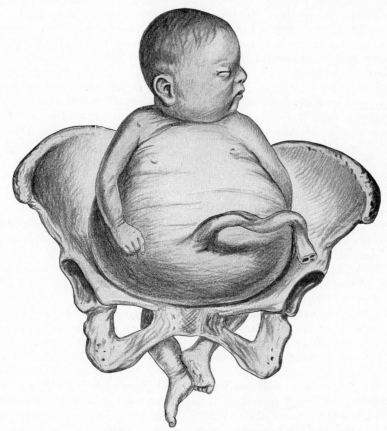

Fig. 565.—Congenital Cystic Kidneys with Ascites Obstructing Labor (author's case).
After the ascites was let off the large kidneys still gave difficulty. Patient's sister had a similar anomaly, but not so marked.

the membranes. Indispensable conditions for this little operation are: Occipital presentation and engagement of the head, effacement of the cervix, normal pelvis and soft parts.

When tough membranes do not rupture after complete dilatation of the cervix, but delay is manifest for one or two hours, it is justifiable to rupture them   Conditions are: the pelvis may not be contracted; the child not too large; the head must be well fixed on the inlet; the presentation and position must be normal. Special additional indications are required in those cases where these conditions are not fulfilled.

The parturient is placed in the elevated Sims, or knee-chest position, if the head is not deeply engaged, so as to prevent the prolapse of the cord and extremities, the membranes are pierced with a pointed instrument—scissors, for example—and the finger immediately placed against the opening. This is to permit only the slow escape of the liquor amnii, which guarantees the safety of the cord. As the liquid slowly trickles away, the assistant from the outside forces the head into the pelvis. Should the waters start to come with a rush, the operator holds the labia together, thus closing the vulva. When performed for the proper indication and under filled conditions, labor usually terminates very quickly. Always pierce membranes gently—don't plunge—danger of uterine rupture.

DRY LABOR

At any time during pregnancy the membranes may rupture. Pains almost always come on within a few hours or days, and the uterus empties itself.

If the accident occurs in the early months the membranes collapse, the fetus develops outside of them, and pregnancy may continue for as long as one hundred and twenty days (Meyer-Rügge). This condition has already been considered (see p. 524). It is called graviditas exochorialis, and the main symptom is hydrorrhea gravidarum. Breech presentation is almost the rule in such cases, the child is usually deformed, is seldom viable, and the placenta shows a "margo" in nearly all cases, the shrunken membranes hanging around the insertion of the cord. Abnormal third stage has nearly always been noted.

Rupture of the membranes in the later months of pregnancy, with few exceptions, is followed by labor within three or four days. I observed one case where labor was delayed ten days. Ahlfeld observed one of thirty-three days; Coston, of fifty days, but lacking microscopic proof. It sometimes requires other agencies to get the uterus into action after the membranes are open.

The causes are mechanical maladaptation of the presenting part to the cervix, abnormal thinness of the membranes, hyaline degeneration (Belosor), cervicitis and vaginitis, the last having a bearing on the clinical course of labor and prognosis.

The treatment of premature rupture of the bag of waters is expectancy, rest in bed, and sedatives. Coitus, douches, and examinations are forbidden in order to preserve the amniotic cavity from infection. In the later months of pregnancy, owing to the patulousness of the cervix, rupture of the membranes is often succeeded by fever, and, therefore, I usually do not wait for pains to supervene. If the child is surely viable, and the uterus does not assume action within two or three days, I usually start it by quinin and castor oil or by inserting a colpeurynter.

When the membranes burst shortly before or early in labor, it is a very unwelcome accident. The case is then called a "dry labor." Special disadvantages attach to it in cases of shoulder, breech, face presentation, occipitoposterior positions, and in contracted pelves. While the dangers and discomforts of dry labor have, no doubt, been exaggerated, indeed some observers claiming the opposite is true, most accoucheurs of experience feel that premature rupture of the membranes is an undesirable happening and would be so adjudged if not alone the immediate but also the future of the mother and baby were thoughtfully considered. The gentle cervical dilator is lost (see p. 128) and the cervix may suffer injury; the hard head pressing on the cervix causes more pain; the increased friction of the child against the dry uterus delays progress. The uterine wall applies itself to the irregularities of the fetus which irritate the muscle to irregular contractions, constriction rings being prone to form. All these factors tend to prolong the labor, and make anomalous and inefficient pains. Rotation is often arrested, the cervix remaining undilated, swollen, edematous, the patient becoming discouraged and exhausted, or getting into a highly excited state. The child suffers from injurious compression, since the brain is exposed for hours to the full power of the forces of labor. Since frequent internal examinations are required, and very often operative interference, the dangers of infection are added to those of injury. The amniotic cavity becomes infected, and Warnekros has shown that a temporary bacteremia occurs. Slemons found bacteria under the epithelium of the amnion, and also showed that the child may die during or shortly after labor from infection thus acquired—a contention the author has held for many years.

The mortality and morbidity of both mothers and babes are increased in dry labor. In primiparæ premature rupture of the membranes is more serious than in multiparæ, indeed, in an aged primipara at term, with a hard resistant cervix and perineum, with dry labor, one might well consider laparotrachelotomy.

Treatment.—In general, one tries to prevent the premature rupture of the membranes by proper conduct of labor, care during examinations, etc. To reduce the danger of infection, as few internals as possible should be made, and rectal exploration done instead. To preserve as much of the liquor amnii as possible and aid dilatation of the cervix a colpeurynter may be employed, only, however, in healthy vaginæ. Bauer in 1902, and Stowe in 1905 invented colpeurynters with a channel through which the lost liquor amnii could be replaced by salt solution (Wieloch., Lit.). While expectancy will have to be long, one must not outstay the patient's strength, psychic as well as physical. It may be wise to give the woman a few hours respite by a hypodermic of $\frac{1}{6}$ gr. morphin, $\frac{1}{150}$ gr. scopolamin, and 30 gr. bromid of soda, per rectum or luminal. Upon awakening, the pains may be better. After constriction rings have formed in the uterus, labor usually comes to a standstill. The cervix is now found edematous and undilatable—tearing under attempts to stretch it, and soon the child begins to suffer.

If rotation has been arrested, under deep anesthesia the child may be properly placed, the head drawn into the pelvis with forceps, the case being then left to nature or to respond to a new indication for delivery. The accoucheur should remember that a forced forceps delivery through unprepared soft parts always results in deep cervical and broad-ligament injury as well as vaginal and perineal damage—functionally, nearly always irreparable. If forceps delivery becomes necessary, episiotomy, indeed, perineotomy, had better be performed, both to limit the lacerations and relieve the baby's head from compression. Postpartum hemorrhage, not infrequent, requires the usual treatment. One should make sure that the uterus is empty, since a slight rise of temperature is not rare during the puerperium, and one wishes to be on this point, at least, secure.

LITERATURE

Belcher: Jour. Amer. Med. Assoc., September 23, 1916, p. 950.—*Belosor:* Zentb. für Gynaek., Nr. 12, 1925, p. 644.—*Brodhead:* Amer. Jour. Obst., June, 1917, p. 993.—*Coston:* New York Med. Jour., 1919, p. 683.—*Dorland:* Amer. Jour. Obstet., April, 1919, p. 475.—*Momm:* Zentb. f. Gyn., 1916, p. 545.—*Moss:* Jour. Amer. Med. Assoc., November 11, 1922, p. 1720.—*Ortega:* Nouvelles Arch. d'Obstet. et de Gyn., 1891, p. 481.—*Schmid, H. H.:* Monatsschr. für Geb. u. Gyn., December, 1931.—*Slemons:* Jour. Amer. Med. Assoc., October 9, 1915, also March 14, 1915.—*Wieloch:* Zentb. für Gynaek., October 30, 1926, p. 2816.—*Warnekros:* Arch. für Gyn., 1913, vol. c, p. 180. (See Editorial, Jour. Amer. Med. Assoc., January 31, 1914.)

CHAPTER LII

ANOMALIES OF THE PASSAGES

DYSTOCIA due to anomalies of the soft parts is more frequent than that due to the bony pelvis. Both give the accoucheur many intricate problems, especially since he is required to manage labors after the numerous operations performed for the relief of gynecologic complaints. In order will be considered: (1) Dystocia due to anomalies of the parturient canal; (2) that due to diseases of the bladder—(3) of the rectum.

ANOMALIES OF THE PARTURIENT CANAL

Most of these have already been studied under the Pathology of Pregnancy. Reference has been made to the relation of tumors to pregnancy and labor, to hematoma of the pelvic cellular tissue, to varicosities, hemorrhoids, etc., and the congenital deformities of the genitalia have also been described under the heading of Local Diseases Accidental to Pregnancy.

Rigidity of the Cervix.—Older writers distinguished two kinds: the spasmodic and the anatomic, in the latter there being an organic change in the cervical tissue. Spasmodic rigidity has already been described under Anomalies of the Uterine Action. Rigidity of the cervix due to disease is rather rare, which is remarkable when one thinks of the number of diseased uteri which make up the clientêle of the gynecologist. During pregnancy the extreme softening of the tissues provides for the great dilatation required in labor. Causes of such rigidity are: chronic cervicitis, scars from cautery, nitrate of silver treatments, Emmet's operations, or amputations; scars from old ulcerative processes, especially those following infections postpartum—carcinoma, etc.; syphilis, senility of the tissues (old primiparæ); adhesion of the membranes around the internal os, conglutination of the external os.

Conglutinatio Orificii Externi (Fig. 566) is a condition where the few circular fibers around the external os refuse to dilate; as a result, the cervix is not opened, but thinned by the head, and it may be delivered externally, still covering the head. The condition is not a true conglutination, and a better name should be selected for it. The os cannot always be found by the finger, but the opening can be seen in the speculum as a tiny hole with a little mucus, and surrounded by a very red ring. By pressure with the finger the resistance of the external os is overcome, and then the dilatation usually goes on rapidly.

Old primiparæ often have hard cervices. Dilatation is very slow and sometimes incomplete. The cervix contains muscular and elastic fibers, the muscular strands drawing the cervical walls actively apart. If the fibrous tissue predominates, there is no autogenous dilatation of the cervix, and the hydrostatic effect of the bag of waters is not enough. Since the membranes in old primiparæ often rupture early, the mechanism of the first stage is deprived also of this help. Further, the uterine pains in old primiparæ often leave much to be desired.

Adhesion of the membranes around the internal os is a not infrequent cause of delayed dilatation, since it prevents the action of the dilating fibers. Mild forms of rigidity or apparent rigidity are due to inefficient pains. Owing to the delayed labor and occasionally to circulatory disturbance, the cervix gets thicker, harder, inelastic, and sometimes edematous. No progress may be noted for hours, and, unless relieved, the case passes into the dangerous class of obstructed labor.

699

Syphilis causes a very serious form of cervical rigidity, and is, fortunately, rare; the whole cervix is changed into a tough, fibrous, undilatable tube. Cesarean section and craniotomy have been found necessary. Scars from ulceration may close up the cervix so that the finest probe may not discover the passage, and if, as sometimes happens, the cervix has sloughed off, the vault of the vagina may be one arched, smooth scar, in which the opening into the uterus cannot be found. One of my Porro cesareans was for this condition, complicated by a rectovaginal fistula—all the result of a previous puerperal septic process. Obstruction of the cervix is one of the causes of "missed labor."

Labor, in cases of cervical disease, shows delay in the first stage, and a great

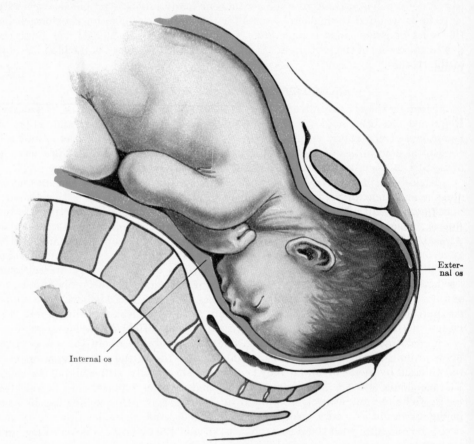

Internal os

External os

FIG. 566.—CONGLUTINATIO ORIFICII EXTERNI.

deal depends on the site and extent of the stricture. If it is in the supravaginal portion of the cervix, the worst forms of dystocia arise; if in the vaginal portion, the case is easily handled, and there are intermediate forms. Under the action of the pains the cervix dilates up to the point of obstruction. If the pains are strong, the uterus healthy, and the stricture not too rigid, nature finally succeeds in procuring a passage for the child. If not, labor stops, the child dies, the cervix may tear, the child being born through the rent, or the uterus may rupture and the child escape into the abdominal cavity, or (rarest) the cervix may tear off circularly in part or in toto. At the Chicago Lying-In Hospital a colpeurynter, put in the uterus to facilitate delivery through a scarred, indurated cervix, was expelled, bringing the cervix torn off circularly with it. Usually the posterior cervix is torn, the child escaping through the rent, the ring-like piece hanging alongside it. Severe dystocia due to pathologic cervices is rare. Slight induration, which lengthens labor but allows spontaneous termination, is fairly common. A large number of children are lost through delay caused by rigidity of the cervix (Seitz).

Diagnosis.—Not every hard cervix is caused by anatomic disease. As was said, abnormal uterine action can produce secondary cervical rigidity. The diagnosis must comprise the cause, the nature, the location, and the extent of the stricture, also the relation of surrounding organs; for example, as in one case where the cervix in toto was missing, the bladder lay close to the rectum, and a rectovaginal fistula coexisted. It is most important to distinguish between anatomic rigidity and that due to functional disordered labor, both sometimes named "rigid os" (p. 629).

Treatment.—Cesarean section as a primary operation is to be performed where a careful examination has proved that obstruction exists, unamenable to the ordinary methods. If the stenosis of the cervix is very marked, the Porro operation should be done, because the passage will be too small to permit the escape of the lochia. In cases where the stricture does not appear to offer an insuperable obstacle to labor, the action of strong pains is to be awaited. When it is evident that nature has accomplished as much as she is able, art steps in to aid in overcoming the rigidity. Five methods of dilatation of the cervix are practised: (1) By means of the hands, advocated since the time of Celsus, and perfected by Bonnaire and Harris; (2) the use of rubber balloons; (3) instrumental dilators of the glove-stretcher design, of which Bossi's is the best known; (4) the incisions of Dührssen—hysterostomatomy; (5) the vaginal cesarean section of Dührssen.

In mild cases, where the cervix is effaced and the os more or less dilated, the fingers usually are able to stretch the opening sufficiently to permit delivery. Almost invariably the cervix tears more or less. If the ring is too tough to be stretched, clean incisions radiating to the fornices may be made. When the cervix is not effaced, these methods are dangerous and inefficient. If an indication for rapid delivery on the part of the mother or child does not exist, a metreurynter is to be put into the uterus and the effect of the hydrostatic dilatation tried. Often the cervix will soften sufficiently. If it does not, or if delivery is required, the vaginal cesarean section is the operation of choice. (See Chapter LXIX.) In cases of annular rupture of the cervix nothing can be done if the amputation is complete except to whip the vaginal edge over the raw surface as much as possible. If incomplete, the detached portion may be sutured in place if the accoucheur considers its nutrition not too much compromised; otherwise it should be removed, always cutting off as little as possible, to avoid stricture of the cervix, and covering the raw surface with the vagina if it can be gotten into place.

Stenosis of the vagina is an occasional cause of dystocia.

Etiology.—Congenital deformities, duplicity (already considered), atresia (usually causes sterility), vaginal bridges or septa (the relics of congenital duplicity), tumors in and near the vagina, hematoma of the neighboring cellular tissue, cicatrices from previous ulcerative processes, puerperal sepsis or injury following labor, scarlet fever, diphtheria, measles, variola, syphilis, and gonorrhea. In one of the author's consultations the cervix and vagina sloughed out in toto after a hard, high, forceps delivery, leaving a narrow, tortuous passage, hardly sufficient for the menstrual discharges. In another, after measles, a portion of the vagina became sacculated and contained pus, and the cavity burst during delivery. (See also Brindeau.) Sometimes, in small women, the vagina is too narrow for safe delivery. In women who have been married a long time without children, and in prostitutes, the vagina may be constricted and tough, so that it will not dilate, but when forced, tears. Old primiparæ also are likely to have rigid vaginas, and in cases of frigiditas sexualis the author has often found a short, dry, indistensible passage. Finally, the vagina may be relatively too small; that is, it may be normal, but in the presence of some indication for immediate delivery it is unprepared for rapid dilatation.

Labor in cases of vaginal atresia is not delayed until the head reaches the point of obstruction. Congenital septa or bridges are usually pushed aside or torn through by the presenting part; rarely is discission required. Tumors may be flattened or even extruded before the head, as occurred in one case of large vaginal cyst in the author's practice. Vaginal rigidity is usually overcome by the powers of nature, the vagina softening or dilating, though sometimes splitting longitudinally—the last oftener during operative interference. Even a scar may sometimes soften and dilate under the influence of the pains, but scars often give rise to obstinate dystocia. A very rare condition, conglutination of the vagina, may or may not require interference.

Diagnosis.—This is easy, the finger meeting a hard ring or narrow passage beyond which the cervix is felt, but care is required to determine how much the contiguous organs are involved. Sometimes the vagina folds up before the oncoming head and a stricture is simulated (Fig. 118). Such a fold is soft and easily pushed open. Even rectally a hard rigid cervix may be recognized, but probably not vaginal anomalies.

Treatment.—Cesarean section is performed when the first examination shows an insuperable obstacle to delivery, and if the passage is apparently too small to allow the escape of the lochia, the uterus must be amputated. A cicatricial septum may be split by three or four radial incisions, care being exercised to avoid opening the rectum or bladder. Occasionally a stricture may be dilated with a colpeurynter. A rigid or small vagina may be better prepared for the dilatation it has to undergo by means of the colpeurynter. During operative delivery a narrow, tight vagina must not be allowed to burst: it is better to incise it. Since the tears almost always occur in the lower half, a deep vaginoperineal incision will usually suffice (*vide infra*). A vaginal tumor may be enucleated, or at least enough of it removed to permit extraction of the fetus. A cyst may be enucleated or, if need be, punctured. A hematoma may be punctured, the clot evacuated, and, after delivery, the cavity packed with gauze.

Rigid Pelvic Floor.—Two forms of rigidity of the pelvic floor may be distinguished, anatomic and spasmodic. Disease of the muscles or connective tissue may compromise the dilatation of the parts—for example, syphilis, scars from injury or from previous labors, the cicatrices following repair operations, hematoma, and hypertrophy of the muscle. Bicycle-riding hardens the perineum, and old primiparæ will often present such a complication in addition to rigid vagina. Spasmodic rigidity may be found in those women subject to vaginismus; it is a spasm of the levator ani muscle, and in one of Benicke's cases necessitated the use of forceps. Sometimes a nervous, apprehensive parturient will contract the outlet of the pelvis and stop labor. Here a narcotic, by relieving the pain, aids delivery.

Labor progresses until the presenting part is on the perineum, and then delay is manifest. If the parturient has a good reserve store of strength, she will be able to overcome the added resistance. If not,—if it has been wasted by premature bearing-down efforts or if the woman has an oversensitized nervous system,—arrest of the head now occurs and exhaustion begins, the life of the fetus also coming into jeopardy.

Seitz (*loc. cit.*) shows the importance of rigid pelvic floor in his statistics from the Munich Maternity, by proving that one-third of the fetal deaths in head presentation are due to delay in labor at this point. Our own experience confirms this and emphasizes the strong necessity to listen to the fetal heart-tones every few minutes toward the end of the second stage. By following this practice a very large number of children will be saved.

Diagnosis.—Delay at the end of the second stage demands careful examination.

One will diagnose a rigid pelvic diaphragm only when it is manifest that the head presses firmly on the pelvic floor but does not advance. To be eliminated as causes of delay are contracted bony outlet (funnel or masculine pelvis), overgrowth of the child, faulty rotation (deep transverse arrest—occipitoposterior), enlargement of the trunk of the fetus, a short cord, and primarily weak pains. The diagnosis of an asphyxia threatening the child forms part of the accoucheur's duties at the same time.

Treatment.—When the parturient has shown her inability to overcome the resistant pelvic floor, or when the child begins to show signs of asphyxia, delivery must be accomplished. One should not wait until the mother is exhausted or until her nervous system is tried to the limit; rather one should determine how much nature can accomplish, not how much she can endure. Resistance at the outlet may often be overcome by a deep episiotomy, and this little operation will obviate many applications of the forceps. If the birth does not now occur, forceps are applied and nothing has been lost, because in all probability episiotomy would have been done in any case to avoid deep rupture of the perineum. Tetanic spasm of the levator ani is treated by anesthesia, failing which the forceps are used.

Stenosis of the Vulva.—Congenital closure of the vulva is usually complete, and, when an opening exists, it leads to a deformed uterus and tubes, so that conception is almost unknown. As a unicum may be mentioned the case of von Meer, of pregnancy in the uterus connected with the bladder, coitus, and abortion per urethram. Acquired closure of the vulva may result from injury—burning with fire or acids (author's case), inflammation with ulceration in childhood. A pin-hole hymen may offer a distinct resistance to the exit of the head. In one of the author's cases, when cut, the hymen was one-fourth inch thick. Hymenal septa may offer a slight barrier to progress, but they usually break, or can be easily snipped in two. Edema of the vulva resulting from prolonged and obstructed labor may sometimes be very great, and the labia may even slough off. This is usually due to concomitant infection. Sometimes the edema seems to aid the dilatation of the vulva; again it seems to predispose to lacerations of the tissues. Varicosities do not delay labor, but they comport the dangers of hemorrhage and hematoma.

Treatment.—When it is plain that the vulvar outlet is holding the presenting part back, the resisting ring is either to be stretched with the fingers or incised (episiotomy). A closed hymen is incised radially. In the author's case of stenosis of the vulva due to carbolic acid burn the child was delivered outside the bony pelvis under a tough, glistening scar, which, with the skin, dissected itself off the perineum and thighs to the extent of 6 inches. After a long median incision had released the dead fetus the flaps were readjusted and sewn in place so as to form a new vulva and a shallow vagina.

Infantile Genitalia.—Infantilism of the genitalia is not very rare, and often leads to absolute or "one-child" sterility. It is one of the findings of the status hypoplasticus. Dysmenorrhea, dyspareunia, frigiditas sexualis, nervous weakness, and a syndrome which resembles Basedow's disease are the usual symptoms, and a tendency to firm obesity is noticeable. The vulva is small, with little hair; the vagina narrow, short, and hard, with little secretion; the fornices flat, the uterus being either normal in size, but infantile in shape (large cervix with small fundus), or very small and undeveloped. Not seldom it is found bent or curled on itself in sharp, retroposed anteflexion. Bossi called the cervix "tapir nosed." The pelvis is either generally contracted, of infantile type, or it is large, with masculine lines and a funnel outlet. It is very probable that the thyroid gland or the anterior lobe of the hypophysis or both are concerned in this hypoplasia (Goetsch). Marasmus of enteric origin in early life and prematurity are sometimes causative. Should pregnancy ensue, abortion in the early months is frequent, and this often ends the reproductive effort of the individual. Labor is characterized by weak pains and delay in the second stage. This comes from both the rigid vagina and perineum and the bony outlet. Instrumental delivery is often required, and it is usually attended by extensive lacerations. Postpartum hemorrhage is common, and because of the oligemia a small loss of blood may be serious or fatal. Because of the vascular hypoplasia accidents of narcosis must be watched for. It is highly important to preserve the fetus in these cases, since the first is so often the only pregnancy. Later effects, as pointed out by Pfannenstiel, are retroflexio uteri from overstretching of the isthmus, and prolapsus from injury and overdistention of the levator ani with subsequent atrophy.

Dystrophia Dystocia Syndrome.—There is a more or less clearly defined class of difficult labors to which Dr. Horner drew attention and the author has given the name "dystrophia dystocia syndrome." Its main features are: (1) Slightly justominor or masculine type pelvis, with girdle obesity and other signs of dystrophia adiposogenitalis (hypopituitarism); small cervix, narrow, rigid vagina; (2) aged primiparity; (3) overmaturity of the child (prolonged pregnancy); (4) non-engagement of the fetal head when labor begins; (5) occipitoposterior position; (6) premature rupture of the membranes; (7) weak pains with protracted first stage; (8) familial dystocia; (9) tendency to eclampsia.

Many mechanical difficulties have to be overcome in such cases during the course of labor. Owing to the hypoplastic genitalia atony of the uterus is common, cervix tears frequent, and lacerations of the soft parts extensive. Often, upon labor's completion, one feels that if these could have been foreseen, cesarean section would have been a better choice at the beginning.

Labor in Old Primiparæ.—The best years for women to bear children are from eighteen to twenty-five. After thirty the function is attended with increasing difficulties, although these are all exaggerated by both doctor and patient (Quigley). Exceptionally labor is surprisingly easy. I had a primipara aged forty-one whose precipitate delivery lasted one hour, and with little laceration. Delamotte mentions one of fifty-one years whose labor lasted only two hours.

In general it may be said that in older women the pregnancy disorders—hyperemesis, eclampsia, abortion, and premature labor—are more frequent. Contracted pelves, usually the justominor, the infantile, or the masculine types, are oftener met. Labor is longer in all three stages. Premature rupture of the membranes, cervical and perineal rigidity are more common; the pelvic fascia is less distensible (see p. 173); indeed, the soft parts may be so inelastic that they tear in all directions, like old rubber, when stretched. (See p. 699.)

Face, breech, and shoulder presentations, occiput posterior positions, and deep transverse arrest are more frequent, while the action of the uterus may leave much to be desired. Since the pelvic synchondroses are rigid, the nutation of the sacrum is absent, and thus delay in delivery occurs. All these retard labor and necessitate frequent recourse to forceps. They increase the danger to mother and child: for the one, lacerations and infection; for the other, cerebral injury and death from asphyxia. Postpartum hemorrhage from lacerations and uterine atony have also been noted. The after-effects on the nervous system are more pronounced, such puerperæ requiring a longer time for recuperation. Nursing is less likely to be adequate and breast troubles are prevented with greater difficulty. Prolapsus uteri is more prone to develop in later years. Primiparity in advanced years has lately become a factor influencing the indications for many operations, often, in borderline cases, swinging the decision toward abdominal delivery (Spain). One finds differences as regards dystocia between the cases of women marrying late in life and those who conceive after many years of marriage (Lundh).

Labor in young primiparæ shows little variation from the usual. Eclampsia, premature delivery, atonia uteri, and breech presentation are slightly more frequent. Labor is shorter, somewhat easier, and has less hemorrhage. The pelvis is larger than one would expect. General rules for treatment apply (Specht, literature).

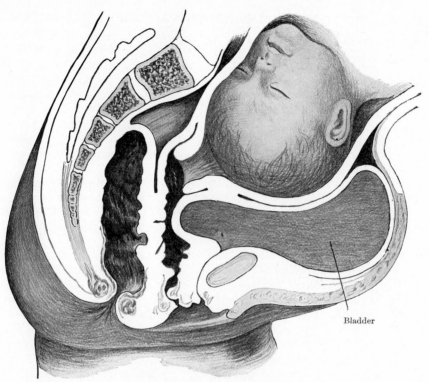

Fig. 567.—Full Bladder Causing Dystocia.

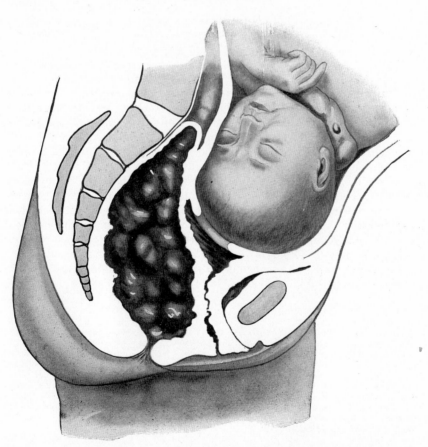

Fig. 568.—Full Rectum as Obstruction.

DYSTOCIA DUE TO OBSTRUCTION OFFERED BY OTHER PELVIC ORGANS

Bladder.—A full bladder (Fig. 567) prevents the engagement of the head, and labor may not proceed until it is emptied. It may cause deflexion attitudes and predispose to prolapse of the cord. In one case it appeared to me to favor an occipitoposterior position, because the back at once came to the front after the viscus was emptied by catheter. It causes weak pains and interferes with bearing-down efforts, and thus increases the number of forceps operations. A cystocele may delay the head, and itself run the danger of severe contusion or bursting. After the birth of the child the full bladder may obstruct the delivery of the placenta or weaken the uterine contractions, in either case causing postpartum hemorrhage or retention of the placenta.

The diagnosis is easily made, there being a soft, fluctuating, rounded tumor stretching from the pubis toward or to the navel. It resembles the thinned-out lower uterine segment, but catheterization will settle the diagnosis if the presence of distinct fluctuation has not already done so. The treatment is catheterization with a soft-rubber catheter, pushing up the head if necessary.

Tumors of the bladder have seldom been known seriously to complicate delivery—two cases of fibroma are on record. Vesical calculi may cause serious trouble; the traumatism of labor may crush them or crush the bladder-wall, resulting in fistula. It is best to remove the stone per vaginam late in pregnancy. If labor has started, it may be possible to push the stone and the bladder out of the pelvis and lead the head into it, but it may be necessary to perform lithotomy during labor. The diagnosis is easy if all the possibilities are considered. A stone may be mistaken for a pelvic exostosis, cervical fibroid, or other tumor.

The Rectum.—A full rectum may act very much like the full bladder in preventing engagement and modifying uterine action. One danger of the full rectum which is not sufficiently emphasized is infection from feces expelled during the birth of the child. In spite of extraordinary precautions on the part of the accoucheur, particles of feces may be carried into the genitals and give rise to fatal puerperal infection. When the head is held above the pelvis by the full viscus, faulty presentations, positions, and attitudes may result. Ofttimes a colonic flushing will, by emptying the pelvis, permit engagement, which is followed by rapid delivery (Fig. 568). Cesarean section has been necessitated by megacolon.

Tumors of the rectum may cause sufficient dystocia to require cesarean section. In one of my cases a large gonorrheal stricture of the rectum, with its surrounding cellular tissue infiltration, caused obstruction and prolonged delay in delivery, during which the child became asphyxiated. Forceps were employed to overcome the obstacle, but the child succumbed in eighteen hours.

Hemorrhoids are forced out and enlarged during delivery. They should be smeared with an emollient and returned within the sphincter.

Fissures of the anus are a common sequence of the great stretching of the anus during labor. They cause painful defecation and bloody and purulent discharges in the late puerperium. A few applications of 10 per cent. nitrate of silver, with perhaps a little stretching of the muscle, usually suffice to cure them.

Third degree tears and fistulæ may be repaired after labor; they seem to heal better than after operation done in the interval.

LITERATURE

Brindeau: L'Obstetrique, 1901, vol. xl, p. 95.—*Dohrn:* Cent. f. Gyn., 1908, p. 530.—*Fränkel:* "Missed Labor," Volkmann's Klin. Vort. No. 351.—*Goetsch:* Surg., Gyn., and Obstet., September, 1917. Literature.—*Lundh:* Acta Obst. et Gyn. Scand., 1925, vol. iv. Fasc. 3. Lit.—*Mayer:* "Infantilism," Beiträge f. Geb. u. Gyn., 1911, vol. xv, H. 3. Literature.—"Labor in Young and Old Primiparæ," Jour. Obstet. and Gyn., British Empire, December, 1909, p. 408.—*Meyer-Ruegge:* Zeitschr. f. Geb. u. Gyn., 1904, vol. 51, p. 424.—*Pfannenstiel:* Münch. med. Woch., May, 1909.—*Quigley, J. K.:* Amer. Jour. Obst., and Gyn., February, 1931, p. 234.—*Seitz:* Arch. f. Gyn., 1910, vol. xc, H. 1.—*Spain:* Labor in Elderly Primiparæ, Amer. Jour. Obstet., March, 1922. Literature. See also Daichman, Amer. Jour. Obstet. and Gyn., July, 1932, p. 127.—*Specht:* Zentralbl. für Gyn., 1916, p. 74.—*Theilhaber:* Monatsschr. f. Geb. u. Gyn., vol. lx, p. 496. Literature on Cystic Kidneys.—*Winter:* Amer. Jour. Obst., December, 1912.

CHAPTER LIII

ANOMALIES OF THE BONY PELVIS

As much variation is found among female pelves as in female features. A perfectly symmetric pelvis is the greatest rarity. Tramond, of Paris, who prepared many thousands of them, found hardly one in 5000 that was nearly perfect. The variations are individual, racial, pathologic. Large women usually have large pelves, women of masculine habitus have masculine pelves, small women usually have small pelves, women of delicate, effeminate constitution have slender bones, while the muscular individual develops a strong, rigid pelvis. Racial differences also exist, but have not been sufficiently studied. In general there are four forms, judging from the shape of the inlet: The transverse ellipse, the heart shape, the round, and the anteroposterior ellipse. European women have the large transverse elliptic, with a tendency to heart-shaped inlet. The Bush women of Australia, the African negress, and the Indian women have a round pelvis, but also with a tendency to lengthening of the anteroposterior diameters. English, Irish, and German women have large cordate pelves, the French a large pelvic canal with tendency to small bones. Jewish women have small pelves.

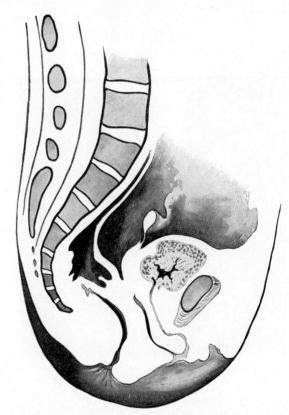

FIG. 569.—Sagittal Section of Pelvis of New-born Girl (Northwestern University Medical School).

The study of the adult pelvis is much facilitated by following its development from the fetal stage, and the study of the effects of disease in early childhood upon the configuration of the bones would throw much light on this complicated subject. Here exists a fertile field for investigation. The pelvis of the new-born child (Fig. 569) is long, narrow from side to side, and converges, funnel shaped, toward the outlet. The sacrum is long and straight; the bodies of the vertebræ do not project from between the wings, which are small. The promontory is high and not prominent; the pelvic inclination is marked. Fehling was able to distinguish differences between the male and female pelvis even in fetal life, but the greatest changes occur during the years of most active skeletal development. Since the time of Denman the factors in the development of the shape of the adult pelvis have been under discussion, and the names of Litzmann, H. von Meyer, Schröder, Fehling, Bayer, Balandin, Freund, Breus, and Kolisko might be mentioned as a few of the many who took part in it. We cannot go into the details of the discussion, but briefly may give the results, which are now quite well established. In general, there are two factors which form the adult pelvis, the first and most important being the inherent property of growth of the bones, which the latest researches tend to prove lies in a proper reciprocal functioning of the hypophysis cerebri, the thyroid, and the ovary, i. e., is constitutional; the second, the mechanical influences exerted on the growing child. That the inherent growth-tendencies of the bones are the determining factors is proved by—(a) The pelvis of the new-born girl already differs slightly from that of the boy; and (b) though subjected to the same mechanical influences, assumes, in its maturation, a much different shape; (c) even when distorted by disease, after the cause is removed, nature tries to correct the deformity for example, in rachitis; (d) when other anomalies of growth are present abnormality of the pelvis often coexists, for example, aplasia of the genitals with infantile pelvis.

Mechanical influences after birth are auxiliary in the production of the developed pelvis. Litzmann (1861) and H. von Meyer emphasized the action of the pressure of the trunk, and considered also the resistance of the pelvic bones and cartilages and the dragging force of the muscles and ligaments of the pelvis.

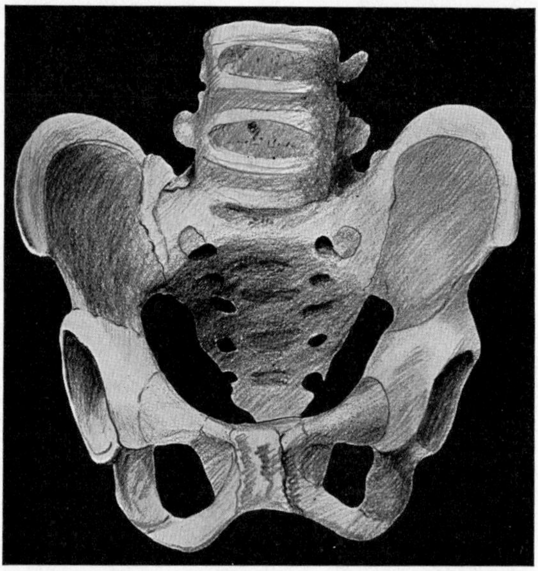

FIG. 570.—PELVIS OF NEW-BORN GIRL (Northwestern University Medical School).

The three bones of the pelvis are put together so that the sacrum does not act like a keystone or wedge. The sacrum is movable, being held in place by the ligaments, aided by the interlocking of the roughnesses of the apposed articular surfaces of the ilia.

In the growing child the line of direction falls through a point somewhat anterior to the sacrum. This causes pressure to be exerted on the first sacral vertebra when the child is erect or sitting. The lower end of the sacrum is prevented from going backward by the strong sacrosciatic ligaments. A bending of the sacrum, therefore, occurs in the sagittal diameter, which is most marked at the third sacral vertebra.

A tendency of the sacrum to become concave from side to side, which might result from the same factors, is counteracted by the weight of the body, transmitted through the spinal column to the sacrum (the "body or trunk pressure"), forcing the bodies of the sacral vertebræ downward. In pelves softened by disease this forcing down and forward of the vertebral bodies is very pronounced. Another effect of this trunk pressure is the flattening of the posterior portions of the bodies of the vertebræ.

The *body pressure* also forces the whole sacrum, and, of course, the promontory, more into the pelvis; when the sacrum goes down, it puts the iliosacral ligaments on the stretch, and this gives the posterior iliac spines the tendency to approach each other. This would be attended with a separation of the symphysis were this joint loose (Fig. 571). Let us call this tendency of the innominate bones to separate at the pubis, because of the iliosacral ligaments tugging at the posterior spines, "transverse tension." A marked tension posteriorly with soft bones, but fast symphysis, would result in the approach of the symphysis to the promontory. But this is counteracted by the pressure of the heads of the femora in the acetabula, which forces the bones upward and inward. Let us call this pressure "lateral *pressure*" (Figs. 571 and 572).

Transverse tension would be increased by the active growth of the sacrum in the breadth. Lateral pressure would be increased by the carrying of heavy

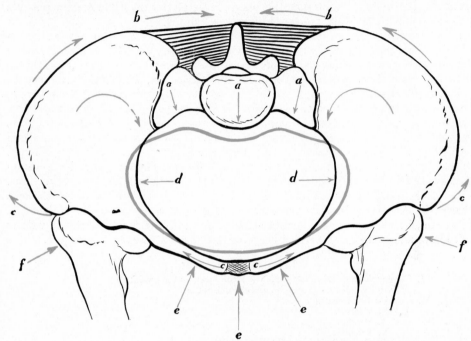

FIG. 571.—DIAGRAM TO ILLUSTRATE TRANSVERSE TENSION AND LATERAL PRESSURE.

a, a, a, Trunk pressure; *b, b*, drawing together of posterior superior spines; *c, c, c*, tendency of ilia to part; *d, d*, transverse tension or thrust, the result of *c, c, c, c; e, e, e*, resultant flattening of pelvis; *f, f*, lateral pressure exerted by the femora, which tends to counteract *d, d*.

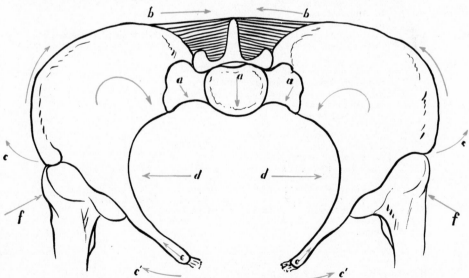

FIG. 572.—DIAGRAM TO ILLUSTRATE ACTION OF TRUNK PRESSURE IN CAUSATION OF FLAT PELVIS.   (Lettering same as Fig. 571.)

The weight of the trunk falls on the sacrum, as is indicated by the arrows *a, a, a*.   As a result, the sacrum, which has no wedge action, tends to fall downward and inward into the plane of the inlet.   This tendency is resisted by the stout sacro-iliac ligaments, *b, b*, and the posterior superior spines of the ilia, to which they are attached, tend to come together.   If the pubic joint were open, as in Fig. 572, the rami pubis would tend to separate more and more, a condition which is actually observed in the rare cases of split pelvis.   Since the symphysis prevents the divulsion of the ends of the pubes, the resultant of all the forces is to cause the symphysis to approach the promontory.   To a certain extent the lateral inward pressure exerted by the femora, *f, f*, counteracts this flattening action of the trunk pressure.

weights during the formative period. All these mechanical results would be exaggerated if the resistance of the bones and cartilages were reduced, as in rachitis and osteomalacia, or removed, as in split pelvis.

Muscular action has a decided influence on the formation of the pelvis; for example, the outward rolling of the lower edges of the descending rami pubis is probably due to traction by the adductores femoris.

A harmonious operation of all the above factors is necessary for the production of the normal pelvis, and, in the study of the pathologic, we shall see how abnormal tendencies of growth, abnormal endocrine action, abnormal application of body pressure, reduced resistances, diseases of bones and joints, etc., produce distorted pelves.

Classification.—Scientifically, the best way to classify abnormal pelves would be according to their etiology or pathology. Kolisko presents 12 different systems, proposed by various German, English, and French authors since 1840, but admits that all, including his own, are unsatisfactory. This is because the genesis and pathology of most of the pelves is either unknown or not universally agreed upon, so that they can be given a settled place in any classification, and, further, a system that would suit the anatomist would not aid the obstetrician in his daily practice. The latter would prefer a system based upon the dimensional and morphologic characters of pelves, because these are what he has to consider at the bedside. Litzmann, in 1861, proposed such a classification, and nearly all obstetric writers since have adopted it, at least as a basis for their presentment of the subject.

LITZMANN'S SYSTEM

I. *Pelves with normal shape,* but either too large or too small:
   Pelves æquabiliter justomajor and justominor.
II. *Pelves with abnormal shape:*
   (a) Flat pelvis.
       1. Simple.
       2. Rachitic.
       3. Generally contracted, flat pelvis.
   (b) The transversely contracted pelvis.
   (c) Irregularly contracted pelvis.
       1. The scoliosis.
       2. The coxalgic.
       3. Amputation.
       4. Dislocation of femur.
       5. Asymmetric sacrum, as the Naegelè pelvis, tubercular hip disease, etc.
   (d) Crushed together pelves, the osteomalacic and pseudo-osteomalacic pelves.

SCHAUTA'S SYSTEM

I. The results of developmental anomalies.
   1. Generally contracted, not rachitic, pelvis.
       (a) Infantile pelvis.
       (b) Masculine pelvis.
       (c) Dwarf pelvis.
   2. Simple flat, not rachitic, pelvis.
   3. Generally contracted flat, not rachitic, pelvis.
   4. Funnel-shaped pelvis, fetal type.
   5. Insufficient development of one wing of the sacrum (Naegelè).
   6. Insufficient development of two wings of the sacrum (Robert).
   7. The generally too large pelvis (justomajor).
   8. The split pelvis. Absence of closure of the symphysis pubis.
II. Anomalies the result of diseases of the pelvic bones.
   1. Rachitis.
   2. Osteomalacia.
   3. Neoplasms.
   4. Fracture.
   5. Atrophy, caries, and necrosis.
III. Anomalies of the pelvic joints.
   (a) Synostosis of one or more.
   (b) Softening of one or more.
IV. Anomalies caused by diseases of the trunk.
   1. Spondylolisthesis.
   2. Kyphosis.
   3. Scoliosis.
   4. Kyphoscoliosis.
   5. Assimilation.

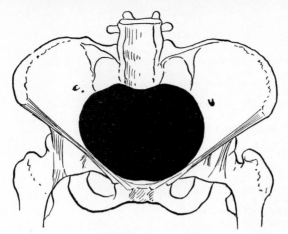

Fig. 573.—Normal pelvis.

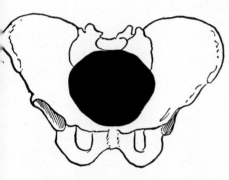

Fig. 574.—Generally contracted pelvis.

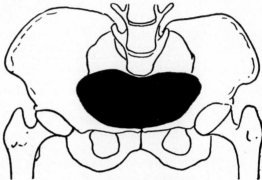

Fig. 575.—Flat pelvis.

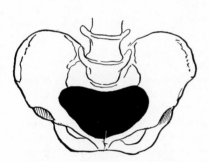

Fig. 576.—Flat and generally contracted pelvis.

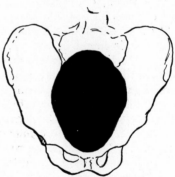

Fig. 577.—Transversely contracted pelvis.

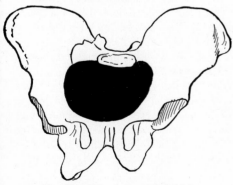

Fig. 578.—Obliquely contracted pelvis.

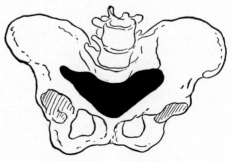

Fig. 579.—Crowded together pelvis.

FIGS. 573–579.—DIAGRAMS TO SHOW THE VARIETIES OF DEFORMED PELVES, ALL DRAWN FROM SPECIMENS OF THE NORTHWESTERN UNIVERSITY MEDICAL SCHOOL.

V. Anomalies the result of diseases of the supports of the pelvis.
1. Coxitis.
2. Dislocation of one or both femora.
3. Club-foot.
4. Absence or inefficiency of one or both legs.

Tarnier.—Budin.—Bonnaire.

I. Deformities due to excess of malleability of the bony tissue.
  (a) Rachitic pelvis.
  (b) Flat, non-rachitic pelvis.
  (c) Osteomalacic pelvis.
II. Anomalies in the application of the spinal pressure.
  (a) Lordotic pelvis.
  (b) Scoliotic pelvis.
  (c) Kyphotic pelvis.
III. Anomalies from displacement of the spinal column, spondylolisthetic and spondy-
  lolizematic pelves.
IV. Anomalies due to misapplication of femoral counterpressure.
  (a) Unilateral lameness.
  (b) Bilateral lameness.
V. Anomalies of the initial development of the bones of the pelvis.
  (a) General large and small pelves.
  (b) Local and asymmetric, oblique oval pelves.
  (c) Local and symmetric, double oblique oval, split pelvis, arrest of development of
  sacrum, etc.
VI. Atypical deformities, as tumors, fractures.

It must be remembered that several causes can combine to produce a pelvis which may be fitted into no classification—for example, a child born with a dislocation of one hip becomes rachitic, or a rachitic child develops a tubercular hip, etc. If the deforming disease appears late in life, the pelvis is altered in a way differing from that resulting from early changes; variations in degree of deformity, also of location, occur, and these, with many other factors, sometimes produce pelves of most bizarre shapes and irregular sizes.

Too Large Pelves.—Dystocia may arise from the pelvis being too large, and usually this is found in large women, but as these, as a rule, have big babies, the proper proportion is reëstablished. Often enough a large, apparently well-built woman will have a difficult delivery, even resulting in the death of the child, and on investigation the accoucheur is surprised to find a large inlet, but with a small pelvic outlet, that is, a large funnel-shaped pelvis. If the pelvis is too large, all the diameters exceeding the normal by 2 cm. or more, the mechanism of labor may be influenced. During pregnancy the head sinks low down and causes pressure symptoms in the bladder and rectum. In labor the soft parts are exposed to the full force of the powers, and often tear or stretch too much, permitting the rapid exit of the fetus. Subsequent relaxation of the pelvic floor and prolapse of the uterus may result. Flexion and rotation of the head are not so marked, and occipitoposterior positions are common—all of which may cause serious dystocia if not promptly recognized. It has seemed to the author that such women have a tendency to postpartum hemorrhage.

Anomalies of pelvic inclination may cause dystocia by influencing the direction of the uterine axis. Engagement of the head may be delayed by too great inclination, and the pelvic floor is endangered by the direct pressure of the head when the outlet lies in a way to receive the full force of the uterine action. On the living it is very difficult to measure the pelvic inclination, except with Neuman and Ehrenfest's complicated cliseometer, but the skilful accoucheur can usually discover the abnormality if it is causing dystocia, and, by raising or lowering the parturient's trunk, bring the axis of the uterus into parallelism with that of the pelvic canal.

Literature

Breus und Kolisko: Die pathologische Beckenformen. Five volumes, 1900–1912.

CHAPTER LIV

CONTRACTED PELVIS

Definition and Frequency.—Authors generally state that a pelvis which shows a diminution of $1\frac{1}{2}$ to 2 cm. in an important diameter should be called contracted, but clinically every pelvis should be so designated when it is certain that the anomaly has produced a disturbing influence on the parturient function. It is also a general practice, since contraction at this point is the most common, to use the conjugata vera as the determining diameter, and to say that a pelvis is contracted when the conjugata vera is shortened, and, too, the degree of the contraction is measured by the amount of the shortening of the conjugata vera. Thus Michaëlis, who really founded the scientific obstetric study of pelves, placed the beginning of contracted pelvis at a 10 cm. C. V. in the justominor types, and at 9.5 cm. in those of the flat variety.

Litzmann, who published Michaëlis' posthumous book, proposed four grades, according to the length of the conjugata vera, thus: If the conjugata vera was less than 5.5 cm., absolute contraction; a second degree, from 5.5 to 7.3 cm., a third degree, from 7.4 to 8.3 cm., and a fourth, 8.4 cm. to normal. Schröder proposed a simpler division. As the shortest conjugata vera which would permit the delivery of a normal-sized child through the natural passages 6.5 cm. was set, and pelves smaller than these were called *absolutely* contracted. If the conjugata vera was from 6.5 to 9 cm. long, the pelvis was called *relatively* contracted, because a living child could be gotten through in a large proportion of cases, and a mutilated fetus always. A third grade took in those with a conjugata vera from 9 cm. to the normal, and labor in these cases was complicated more often by errors of mechanism than by spacial disproportion between head and pelvis. These measurements applied to flat pelves. In generally contracted pelves, since there is diminution of all the diameters and the area of all the planes is smaller, 0.5 cm. is to be added to the upper limit of each division.

A moment's thought will show how artificial and futile such, or any, division of pelves is, but for purposes of description and discussion some standard must be used, and this one is the best of all yet proposed. The size of the child, the hardness and moldability of its head, the presentation, position, and attitude, all make the pelvis smaller or larger as far as the question of spacial relations is concerned. Add to this the difficulty of measuring the pelvis and the inaccuracies always present, and it becomes apparent why authors vary so much in their estimate of the frequency of contracted pelves and in the division into degrees or grades of obstruction.

In Germany, considering a pelvis contracted when the main diameter is $1\frac{1}{2}$ to 2 cm. shortened, it is estimated that from 14 to 20 per cent. are thus to be designated, and, considering contraction to exist only when serious dystocia results, 3 to 5 per cent. One element of irregularity is the lack of standardization of contracted pelves.

One author reports all pelves contracted with a conjugata vera less than 10 cm., another with less than $9\frac{1}{2}$ cm., another uses the conjugata diagonalis and calls all pelves contracted with a conjugata diagonalis less than $11\frac{1}{2}$ cm. Another author relies on the external measurements, and we already have shown how uncertain these are. Statistics collected by Dohrn in 1896 show a total frequency varying from 5 to 27 per cent. In Austria a variation of from 2.15 to 16 per cent. exists; in Switzerland, 7.9 to 20.07 per cent.; in Holland, 3.51 to 33 per cent.; in the United States, 11.45 to 25 per cent. (Dobbin, Williams, Flint, Davis).

These figures carry the stamp of unreliability on their faces Most of them were collected in clinics, to which a large proportion of obstructed labors is brought,

713

which, of course, increases the percentage, and the others are from out-maternities, in which only those cases exhibiting delay in labor are accurately measured, or, practising among the poor, disclose a higher proportion of deformities than the whole community would show. In America it is impossible to obtain accurate information of the frequency of pelvic contraction. In American-born women high degrees are very rare, many practitioners meeting few in a lifetime. Milder degrees, insufficient to provoke serious dystocia, are not infrequent and may be unobserved, the delay in labor being ascribed to malpositions, etc. Among our foreign-born and colored population high grades of contraction are not infrequently observed, but here again statistics furnished by the obstetric specialist and the clinic or the hospital are useless, because the difficult labors are referred to these institutions and swell the percentages.

Still greater uncertainty exists regarding the frequency of the various forms of contracted pelves. It seems to the author that the abnormal pelvis most commonly met with in general practice is a mild degree of the funnel, infantile, or masculine type, i. e., those caused by constitutional anomalies. In consultations on obstructed labor the generally contracted has been more frequently encountered than the flat type. In Germany the simple flat and rachitic flat pelves predominate, but even there the authors are not agreed. Osteomalacic deformities are exceedingly rare in America.

THE GENERALLY CONTRACTED PELVIS

Other names for this type of anomaly are: Pelvis æquabiliter justominor (Stein); pelvis nimis parva (Deventer, who first described it). Several varieties are to be considered: The simple, equally contracted pelvis, the infantile, the masculine, and the dwarf. Fig. 580 shows an equally contracted pelvis. It has beautiful lines, and is a normal pelvis in miniature. This pelvis is found in women of small stature and gracile, never in large women, and is in proportion to the rest of the skeleton. All its diameters are shortened, though rarely is the relation of the conjugata vera to the others absolutely correct—usually a slight flattening exists. This seems to indicate that perhaps rickets had something to do with the production of the general hypoplasia. Fig. 582 shows a justominor pelvis of the infantile or juvenile type. The inlet presents an anteroposterior oval; the sacrum is high and long; the pelvic inclination marked. Compare it with Fig. 570, a child's pelvis. This pelvis is deep, and the tuberosities are close together, giving the excavation a funnel shape. A woman bearing this pelvis will have narrow hips, the female escutcheon (the hairy portion of the mons veneris) will be long, narrow, and sparsely covered, the posterior superior spines of the ilia close together, the rhomboid of Michaëlis short and narrow, the labia majora small and undeveloped, the same being true of the breasts, and altogether the person will show a child's habitus. Frigiditas sexualis, sterility or pregnancy late in marriage, and other general evidences indicate that the individual was not completely developed.

If the bones are very heavy and thick, the cavity of the pelvis may be encroached upon and the pelvis may partake of the characters of the male. The sacrum is long and narrow, the arch of the pubis high, the sides of the pelvis close together, and the inlet even an anteroposterior oval. This masculine type of contracted pelvis will be again mentioned under funnel pelves.

Minor degrees of general pelvic contraction are very common—those with a conjugata vera between 9 and 10 cm. are moderately rare, while those below 9 cm. are almost always combined with rachitis, the dwarf pelves alone showing a true conjugate of 7 cm. or less.

Dwarf pelves are very rare in this country. Breus and Kolisko distinguish five varieties of dwarfs:

1. The chondrodystrophic dwarf, the result of achondroplasia fœtalis, which formerly was

called congenital rickets. The development of the long bones is hindered by pathologic changes in the epiphyseal cartilages (Kaufman), but the head and chest may be well formed. A tendency to obesity is the rule. In the author's case the ovaries were as large as hen's eggs and through and through cystic. Is it possible that the changes in this organ had something to do with the production of the bony deformities and the obesity, both of which began in the tenth year?

The pelvis of such a dwarf is usually very small and flat, but signs of rachitis are absent. The flattening is due to insufficient development of the iliac portions of the ossa innominata (Fig. 584).

2. In the "true" dwarf pelvis growth ceased at an early period of life and the pelvis shows it, the ossification of all the pelvic synostoses being absent, and the pelvis itself retaining infantile shape and characteristics. Of the two such female dwarfs known, Boeckh's is the one usually

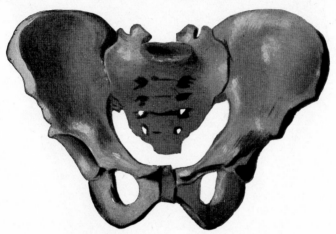

Fig. 580.—Pelvis Justominor (author's collection).

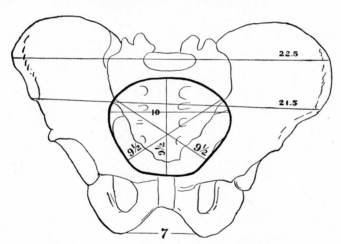

Fig. 581.—Pelvis Justominor. Measurements of Fig. 580.

described. Her age was thirty-one years, height, 108 cm., conjugata vera, 8.6; transverse diameter, 9.5.

3. Cretins often have dwarf pelves. They are characterized by general lack of development of the bones and delay or absence of ossification of many of the epiphyses, the latter point differentiating them from true dwarfs, where all the epiphyses fail to fuse, even very late in life. A cretin's pelvis is often flat, with thin bones, but thickened junctions of the ossification areas; the foramina are large, and the sacrum is short and well curved. Other evidences of insufficient thyroid secretion are always present.

4. Rachitic dwarfs are of two kinds—first, those showing general hypoplasia due to disease; second, those reducing the size of the individual by the excessive bending and shortening of the long bones. Only the first kind should really be called dwarfs, because here the bones are actually shorter and, in addition, bent in a moderate degree. The pelves of such individuals come under the classification of generally contracted flat pelvis (q. v. Fig. 585).

5. Hypoplastic dwarfs are persons whose whole skeletal system shows a quantitative restriction in growth. This may be combined with rickets. The author has observed it in the later development of very premature infants.

Causation of Justominor Pelves.—Little is positively known about the causes

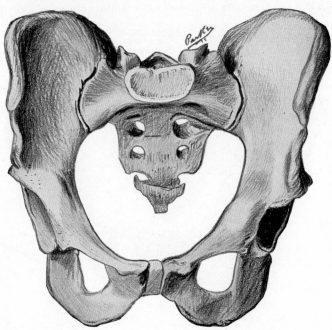

FIG. 582.—Generally Contracted Pelvis. Infantile Type (Chicago Lying-in Hospital Museum).

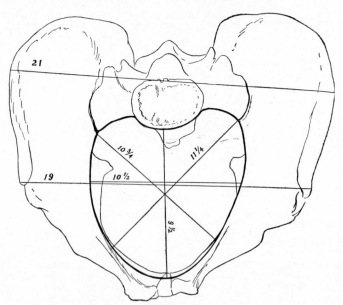

FIG. 583.—Measurements of Fig. 582.

and their manner of action, but these may be mentioned as having some influence: heredity (small parents); prematurity at birth; bottle-feeding; marasmus; improper hygiene at the time of puberty (overcrowding the growing girl with studies, social demands, etc.); improper dress. Four sisters in the author's practice have generally contracted pelves, and symphysiotomy, induced labor, craniotomy, and forceps have been rendered necessary in their labors. Since the ovary and thyroid are known to have an influence on the osteogenetic processes, we may look to their pathology for the explanation of some of the cases.

Diagnosis of Justominor Pelves.—All the external pelvic measurements, including the circumference, are smaller than normal, but it is not safe to diagnose pelvic contraction on these figures, because the canal may, nevertheless, be very roomy. The stature of the patient is usually small, but a large woman may have

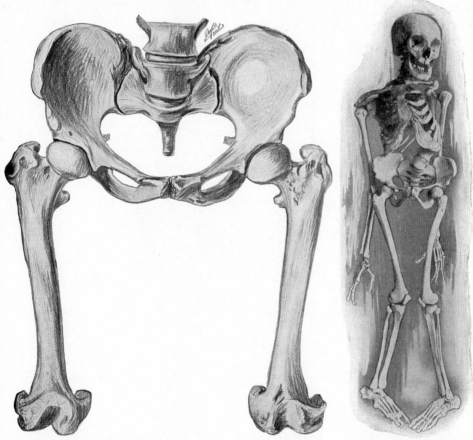

FIG. 584.—PELVIS OF CHONDRODYSTROPHIC DWARF.
The femur is nine inches long.

FIG. 585.—PSEUDO-OSTEOMAL-
ACIC (RACHITIC) DWARF
(Northwestern University
Medical School).

a heavy pelvis of the masculine type, with a much reduced lumen. The rhomboid of Michaëlis is small and short. Women with infantile pelves show other evidences of hypoplasia—small face, small breasts, long thorax, visceroptosis, straight spine, small vulva, narrow hips, and generally one gets the impression as of a grown-up child. Dysmenorrhea, sterility, and neurasthenia are frequent symptoms.

On the internal examination the general reduction of all the diameters will make the diagnosis, and only on these may reliance be placed. The sides of the pelvis are very easily reached with two fingers, and one can often palpate the linea terminalis throughout its entire length. The spines of the ischia are close together; the tuberosities usually still closer, and the arch of the pubis narrow.

THE FLAT PELVIS (PELVIS PLANA) (Fig. 586)

This is a pelvis contracted in the anteroposterior diameters, and many authors distinguish two kinds—the simple flat and the rachitic flat. The writer is inclined to the opinion expressed by Ahlfeld and Sellheim, Breus and Kolisko, that the so-called "simple flat" pelvis is really rachitic in origin. The absence of the characteristic rachitic landmarks on the pelvis induced Betschler, who first described it, and Michaëlis to separate it from those of known rickety origin. It was believed that the carrying of heavy weights in early childhood or putting the child too early on its feet caused the simple flattening of the pelvis, but in all probability the cause, if not due to rickets, will be found in the abnormal tendency of growth of

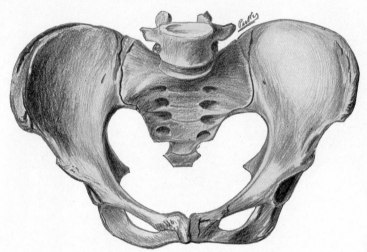

FIG. 586.—SIMPLE FLAT PELVIS (author's collection).

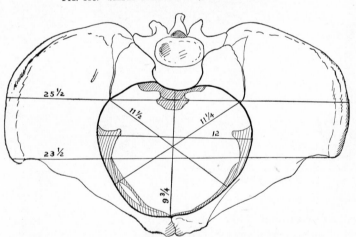

FIG. 587.—SIMPLE FLAT PELVIS.

the bones. In all respects save two the simple flat pelvis looks like a normal one—the sacrum has sunk downward and forward, giving the inlet a broad, kidney-shaped outline, and the pelvic cavity also is slightly flattened. Schröder says this pelvis never is highly contracted, and that it is very frequent in Germany. There is no widening of the outlet, and the distance between the anterosuperior spines bears the usual relation to that between the crests. Among the large number of flat pelves of the Northwestern University Medical School, not one could be found that did not at the same time show positive evidences of rachitis. Flat rachitic pelves are not rare in any obstetric museum (Fig. 588).

Pierre Dionis (1724) first called attention to the association of rachitis in childhood with the flat pelvis.

Rachitic flat pelves are usually smaller than normal ones because the bones

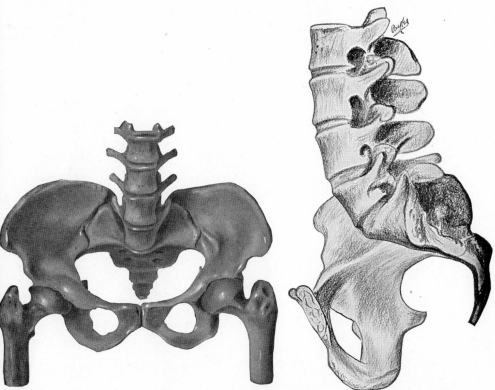

FIG. 588.—RACHITIC FLAT PELVIS (Northwestern University Medical
School Museum).

FIG. 589.—SAGITTAL SECTION OF FLAT RACH-
ITIC PELVIS.

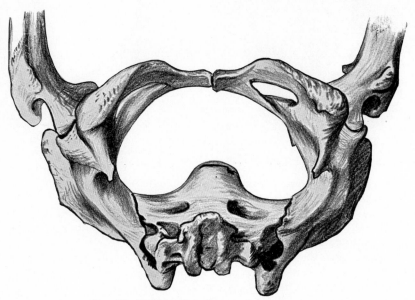

FIG. 590.—RACHITIC FLAT PELVIS, VIEWED FROM BELOW.
Shows large, flaring outlet.

are smaller and thinner.   Rarely the bones are heavier.   The ilia flare outward and are flattened so that the distance between the anterosuperior spines is equal to, or greater than, the distance between the crests.   The pelvic inclination is increased, the pubic arch broad, the angle which the pubis makes with the inlet obtuse, the tuberosities widely separated, and the acetabula look more anteriorly than is normal.   This peculiar insertion of the femora gives the patient a remarkable gait, the feet being thrown outward.   The most characteristic changes are shown by the sacrum.   This bone is forced downward into the pelvic cavity; the concavity of its anterior face is changed in both directions, so that it becomes flat,

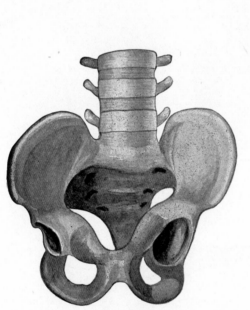

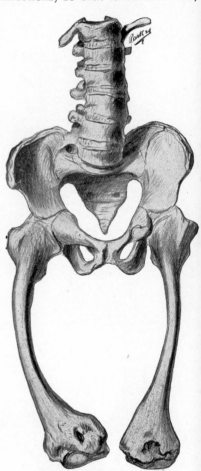

Fig. 591.—Pelvis of New-born Girl, Showing Rachitis
(Northwestern University Medical School Museum).

Fig. 592.—Pelvis of Rachitic Girl Aged Three.
Had the child lived, her pelvis would probably be
like Fig. 593.

and in advanced cases convex from side to side, and straight from above downward, the bodies of the sacrum protruding from between the wings, and the sacrum being bent on itself.   A second, or false, promontory is sometimes found below the true one (Fig. 589).   Important alterations result in the shape and size of the pelvic canal, most prominent of which is the flattening of the inlet from before backward. The inlet may have the shape of a kidney, and the highest degree of contraction may exist in the conjugata vera.   The transverse and oblique diameters may be normal or even larger.   The true pelvis is shallow, the outlet usually much enlarged (Fig. 590), and this gives labor a character different from that in generally contracted pelves.   In the latter, because the pelvis is usually uniformly contracted throughout the length of the canal, the head has to overcome resistance all the way down, while with the flat pelvis, after the inlet has once been passed, the rest of the distance is quickly and easily traversed.   Rachitic pelves often show exostoses on the posterior surface of the symphysis pubis.   One of my cases had such a bony crest 8 mm. high.

Mechanical factors have been invoked to explain the formation of the rachitic pelvis, but one must not forget that the inherent tendencies of growth, perverted by the disease of the bone, may have much to do with it.   When the rachitic child sits or stands, the trunk pressure forces the sacrum downward into the pelvis, tilting the promontory forward, increasing the transverse tension, and drawing the pubic symphysis backward, as is shown in the diagram (Fig. 571). The lower end of the sacrum may not recede backward because of the strong sacrosciatic ligaments; the sacrum, therefore, is bent in its lower portion, and the bony edge of the sciatic notch and the spine of the ischium are much developed.   The lateral pressure of the heads of the femora, acting on the softened bone, tend to force the acetabula inward, as is clearly shown in Fig. 571.   In exaggerated cases the pelvis is pressed together from all sides, as in Fig. 593, presenting the shape

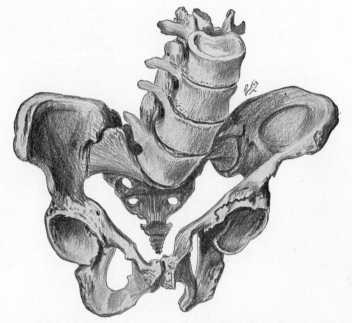

Fig. 593.—Pseudo-osteomalacic Pelvis (Northwestern University Medical School Museum).

of an osteomalacic pelvis, and is called "pseudo-osteomalacic pelvis."   That these changes in shape are not due to the trunk pressure alone is proved by the occurrence of similar pelves in new-born children (Figs. 591 and 592).   In rickets the osteoid substance near the epiphyses remains soft and unossified for a long time, and, therefore, the bone at these points bends under the influence of the trunk pressure and muscle action.   Then, too, the apposition-relations of the various ossification centers are disturbed, and, as a result, when the rachitic disease later abates, nature is unable to restore the proper balance in the various lines of ossification.   The adult rachitic pelvis, therefore, is the result of the disturbance of bony growth and of the deformation of the pelvis by misdirected or relatively too powerful mechanical forces.

Diagnosis.—In the routine history the fact of delayed walking and dentition-illness when a child, bottle-feeding, etc., may be noted.   An inspection of the whole person will not fail to reveal stigmata of rachitis—the square head, distorted clavicles, rachitic rosary, bowed tibiæ and femora, "bow-legs," short and broad hands and feet, etc.   The spine is usually scoliotic, Michaëlis' rhomboid low and broad—indeed, it may be a triangle instead, with the base upward.   The vulva is usually retroposed because of the exaggerated pelvic inclination.   There is often so much compensatory lordosis that the hand can be run under the spine

46

when the woman lies on her back. The area between the thighs is broad, the escutcheon squarer.

The characteristic of rachitis is the flattening of the pelvis, and the experienced accoucheur may feel this at once by grasping the hips in both hands. The distance between the spines of the ilia is usually equal to, or even more than, that between the crests, a fact which also can be determined by palpation; the iliac bones flare out and appear smaller than usual. Baudelocque's diameter is short, running from 19 down to $15\frac{1}{2}$ cm., and when scoliosis exists too, the external oblique diameters are very unequal, but seldom is there a difference of more than 3 cm.

On internal examination will be noted the shallowness of the pelvic cavity; the startling prominence of the sacral promontory; the projection of the ischiatic spines, with the tense sacrosciatic ligaments; the possibility of palpating the linea terminalis all the way, and, near the sacrum, its sharp bend forward; the presence

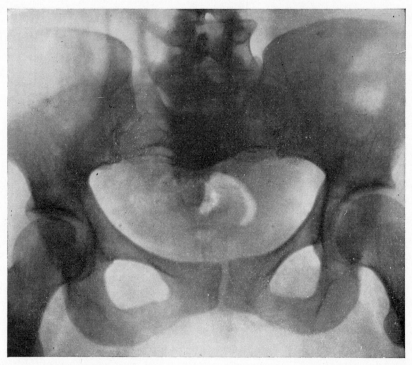

Fig. 594.—Mrs. S. X-ray of Obliquely Contracted Rachitic Pelvis.

of an exostosis on the posterior wall of the pubis; the low and broad pubic arch, with distant tuberosities of the ischia; the flat or even convex sacrum when palpated from side to side and from above downward (but here one may note that the lower third of the bone is sharply incurved); and the reduced conjugata diagonalis. It is the rule to deduct 2 cm. from the length of the diagonal conjugate to obtain the true conjugate, but this is not always reliable. If the angle which the symphysis makes with the inlet is very obtuse; if the pubis is very high; if there is a high exostosis or bony ridge on the posterior surface of the pubic joint—it may be necessary to deduct 3 cm. Fig. 594 shows an x-ray picture of a rachitic pelvis. It is of more scientific interest than practical use. The information it gives was more easily obtainable by palpation.

Finally, the course of the labor will often disclose the nature of the pelvic contraction, but this will again be discussed (see p. 745).

THE GENERALLY CONTRACTED FLAT PELVIS

When rachitis is very severe and prolonged, the bony growth is so stunted that the pelvis does not attain to normal size. Added to this insufficient development are the deformations of the pelvic bones, the sinking down of the sacrum, etc., all of which combine to produce the generally contracted and flat pelvis. We find

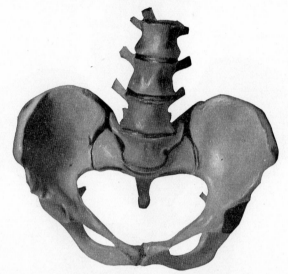

Fig. 595.—Generally Contracted and Flat Pelvis.
Conjugata vera, 5.3 cm. (Northwestern University Medical School Museum).

the smallest pelves in this class, and the inlet may be so narrowed that it will hardly let a six months' fetus pass through (Fig. 595). Rachitic dwarfs have such pelves, and in the chondrodystrophic dwarf pelvis of the author's collection much flattening exists.

OBLIQUELY CONTRACTED PELVES

A perfectly symmetric pelvis is a great rarity—as rare as a perfect face or head. One oblique diameter is always a little larger than the other. When this difference in size of the two halves of the inlet is marked, we speak of an obliquely distorted pelvis. Several varieties are to be described, but the general effects of such pelves on pregnancy and labor are about the same.

The most common of the obliquely contracted pelves is the result of scoliosis of the vertebral column, and, of the various forms of scoliosis, the rachitic causes the most marked alterations in the pelvis. Much depends on the location of the curvature, because if it is high up, compensation takes place below, and the effect on the pelvis is hardly noticeable. The rotation of the spinal column and the torsion of the vertebræ are distinguishable in the sacrum when the deformity is located low down. Another point is that the pelvic asymmetry may cause the scoliosis. Fig. 596 shows a pelvis with simple scoliosis, probably due to muscular weakness. Only the slight flattening indicates the possible rachitic origin. Mild cases of such scoliosis are not uncommon, but very rarely do they give rise to dystocia. Fig. 597 shows a pelvis with a large lumen, but distorted as the result of a scoliosis due to infantile right spinal paralysis. It is easy to see that the bones of that side are smaller than the healthy side.

Fig. 598 shows a pronouncedly rachitic pelvis, the flattening of the inlet, the sinking and frontal rotation of the sacrum, the development of the spines, the flaring of the ilia, all being well in evidence.   Common to all these pelves are these points: (1) The inlet is smaller on that side to which the convexity of the lumbar

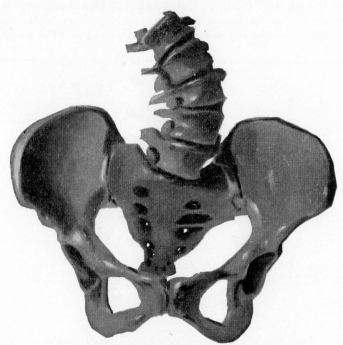

FIG. 596.—ASYMMETRIC PELVIS DUE TO SCOLIOSIS FROM MUSCULAR WEAKNESS (Northwestern University Medical School Museum).

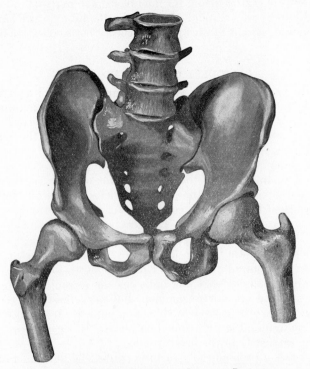

FIG. 597.—ASYMMETRIC PELVIS FROM INFANTILE PARALYSIS.
Also shows high assimilation (Northwestern University Medical School Museum).   Note difference in size of femora.

scoliosis points, this being due to the fact that the sacrum is pushed over onto that side, and, the trunk pressure being greater here, the sacrum sinks lower; (2) since the trunk pressure comes to bear on one wing of the sacrum more than on the other, the part of the bone which suffers the pressure is less well developed, the foramina are smaller and closer together, even the iliac portion of the sacro-iliac joint sometimes taking part in this atrophy; (3) the pelvis is tilted so that the more contracted side is higher than the larger side; this is due to the fact that the line of direction of the body falls, not through the middle line of the sacrum, but to the side, away from the greatest convexity of the scoliosis; this throws the weight of the trunk almost entirely on one leg, and, therefore, this femur is forced upward, inward,

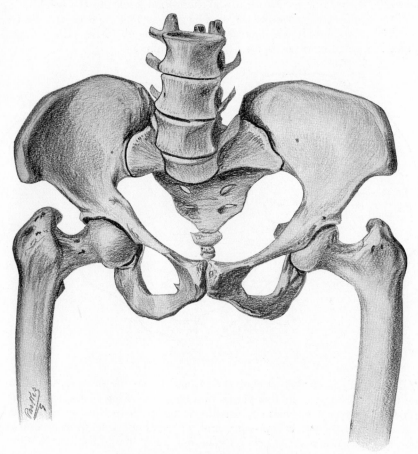

FIG. 598.—OBLIQUELY CONTRACTED FLAT RACHITIC PELVIS.

and backward; (4) the sciatic notch is narrowed; (5) the arcus pubis points to the contracted side; (6) the conjugata vera runs obliquely backward; (7) the obstetric transverse diameter is always shortened; (8) the oblique diameters are very unequal; (9) one ischial tuberosity is higher than the other.

The Coxalgic Pelvis.—Disease of the hip-joint in infancy almost always leaves marked pelvic deformity, but rarely does sufficient encroachment on the lumen result to cause serious dystocia. Fig. 600 shows a coxalgic pelvis. Since the diseased side of the pelvis is painful, the patient throws all her weight on the well side, and, as a result, the head of the femur flattens this half of the pelvis and the whole pelvic girdle is distorted. The bones of the diseased side are smaller because

of atrophy from disuse of the muscles, and, owing to irregular muscular and ligament traction, the diseased half of the pelvis is enlarged and pulled outward. Since
the patient tries to spare herself pain by keeping that leg off the ground, she pulls
up the diseased side of the pelvis, which, therefore, is higher than the well side—
an action which is aided by the crutch worn under the corresponding axilla. The
asymmetry of the pelvis obtains throughout the whole pelvic canal, the tuberosity
of the ischium of the affected side being usually drawn upward and outward.

Similar pelvic changes, but less pronounced, occur with tuberculosis of the
knee, amputation of the thigh, or other disturbance of function of one limb.

Naegele Pelves.—One of the most typical of this class of pelves—the obliquely
contracted—is that due to disease of the sacro-iliac joint and the neighboring portions of the ilium and the sacrum. F. C. Naegelè, in 1839, first described it, having
collected 37 cases, but it was mentioned by various obstetric writers long before
this, and Naegelè found one in an Egyptian mummy.

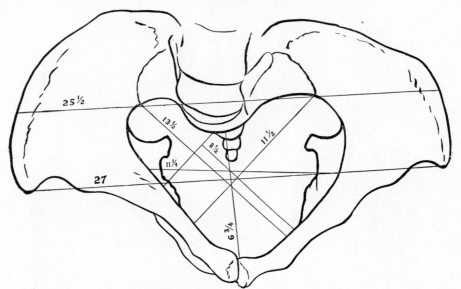

FIG. 599.—MEASUREMENTS OF FIG. 598.

All the findings of oblique contraction, and those due to exaggerated pressure
of one thigh, are present in this pelvis, and since one wing of the sacrum is often
atrophic, aplastic, or even missing, in addition to the distortion actual reduction in
the size of half of the pelvis is present, and, what is important from a clinical point
of view, the narrowing of the pelvic lumen extends down to the very outlet. The
innominate bone of the affected side is dislocated upward and backward, while the
pubic joint is pushed to the healthy side. The linea terminalis of the healthy side is
given an exaggerated curve, being straightened on the diseased side. In nearly
all cases a firm synostosis is found in the affected sacro-iliac joint, and a sharp
polemic was waged among the students of this pelvis as to whether this was primary
or secondary. Naegelè believed that, most likely, a primary congenital deformity
of the joint existed, and he did not deny that the entire change could be due to
acquired disease. Hohl proved that the wing of the sacrum could be congenitally
absent, but other specimens were exhibited which showed that characteristically
deformed pelves could be produced by acquired disease of the sacro-iliac joint.
Fig. 602 shows a pelvis from the author's collection, and it presents positive evidences of disease of the sacro-iliac joint. Disease of the right hip-joint coexists,

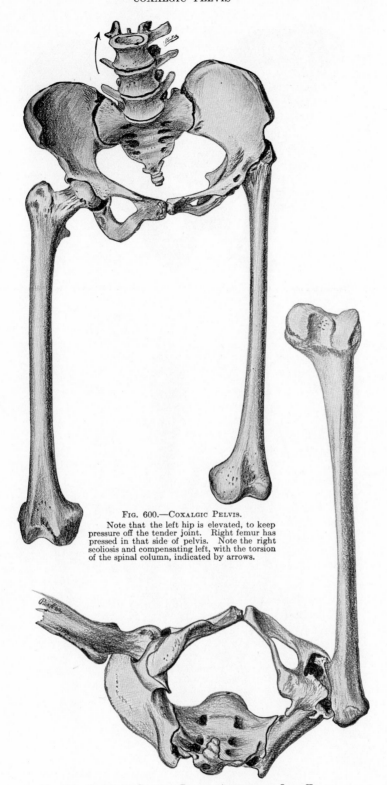

FIG. 600.—COXALGIC PELVIS.

Note that the left hip is elevated, to keep pressure off the tender joint. Right femur has pressed in that side of pelvis. Note the right scoliosis and compensating left, with the torsion of the spinal column, indicated by arrows.

FIG. 601.—OUTLET OF COXALGIC PELVIS. ANKYLOSIS OF LEFT HIP.

Delivery is best accomplished by placing woman on left side and bringing occiput up over right ramus pubis.

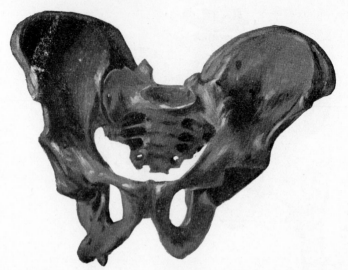

Fig. 302.—Naegelè Pelvis. Osteo-arthritic Type (Northwestern University Medical School Museum).

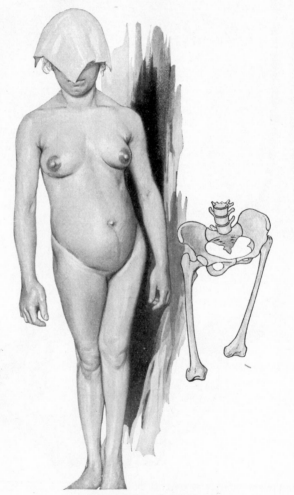

Fig. 603.—Left Coxitis.
Sketch at side is from a pelvis almost identical with that of the living patient.

a point which Litzmann emphasizes and draws into the causation of the Naegelè pelvis. Breus and Kolisko find traces of ostitis in all so-called Naegelè pelves, and insist that the deformity is always due to arthritis, caries, or trauma of the sacro-iliac synchondrosis or other portions of the pelvis. Pelves with congenital defects of the wings of the sacrum exist, but they do not produce such great deformity of the inlet nor do they show contraction of the whole length of the pelvic canal, as do these pelves with disease of the sacro-iliac joints. Here the sacral and iliac portions are wasted, absorbed, and ankylotic. If the disease occurs in

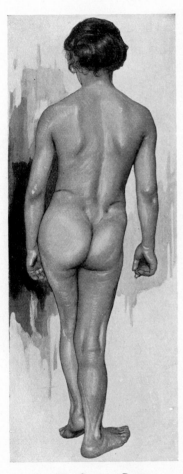

FIG. 604.—COXALGIC PELVIS.
Tilting of the pelvis is shown by the rhomboid of Michaëlis.

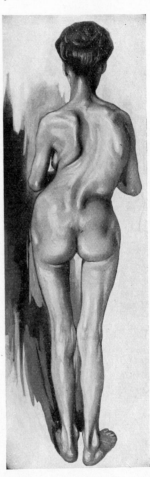

FIG. 605.—SIMPLE SCOLIOTIC PELVIS.
Compensation not complete, and pelvis, therefore, tilted as shown by rhomboid. Normal labor.

early life, the developmental portions—the ossification centers—are destroyed, and growth of the bone, of course, is rendered impossible. Now come the mechanical factors, the pressure of the trunk, the lateral pressure of the femora, and the characteristic changes are brought about.

Diagnosis.—It is usually easy to discover an obliquely distorted pelvis, but not so easy to decide on the actual pathology of it, nor on the degree of spacial contraction. Attention may be called to the deformity by an uneven, limping gait, a scoliosis, or by the unequal length of the legs. Scars from old sinuses point to disease of the hip or sacro-iliac joints, and the history will usually show some infantile disease or injury. Spinal paralysis, rachitis, habit scoliosis, coxitis, gonitis, amputation of the leg, and spina bifida, have been the causes of the asymmetry in the cases which came under my observation, and it was possible to decide in all of them how the deformity was produced. Fig. 603 is a photograph from a marked case of coxitis, and Fig. 605, one of a simple scoliotic pelvis. A rachitic kyphoscoliotic dwarf pelvis is shown in Fig. 606 by an x-ray picture. In addition to the scoliosis and the apparent shortening of the leg, one will notice the hip of one side higher and retroposed, the pubic region displaced to one side, and the hair-line

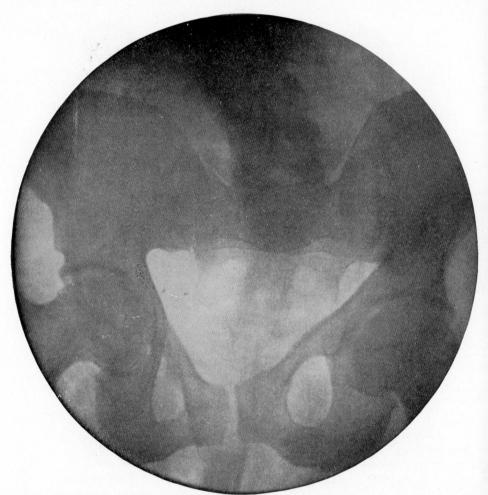

FIG. 606.—KYPHOSCOLIOTIC ASYMMETRIC RACHITIC PELVIS. CESAREAN SECTION (x-ray by O'Donnell).

oblique. The rhomboid of Michaëlis is asymmetric or tilted, and the gluteal fold lower on one side. Palpation of the bones confirms the above findings, and, in addition, discovers that the ischial tuberosity of one side is higher and the ramus of the pubis has a different direction on that side. Examining first with one hand and then with the other, it is usually possible to distinguish the flat linea terminalis of one side and the bowed arc on the other, and the fact that one-half of the pelvis is less roomy. External measurements from corresponding points may show a discrepancy between the two sides, but it is almost impossible to diagnose the kind of a pelvis from them. By excluding all the other varieties we may make a diagnosis of a Naegelè pelvis, and this may be confirmed by finding the corresponding half of the rhomboid of Michaëlis reduced in size, the spine of the last lumbar vertebra lying close to the posterosuperior spine of the ilium. On internal examination the corresponding half of the pelvis is very small and the encroachment of the ischium on the lumen persists even to the outlet. Ankylosis of the sacro-iliac joints may be palpated by the fingers per vaginam or rectum if exostoses and pericapsular thickening exist.

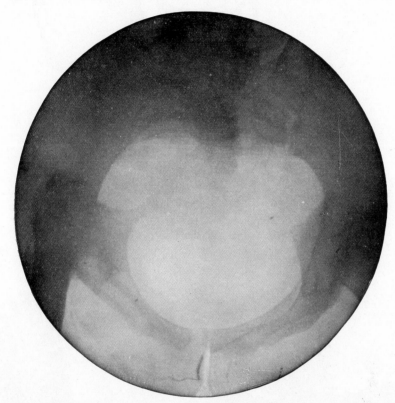

Fig. 607.—X-ray of Left Coxitis. Craniotomy, First Labor. Subsequently Two Spontaneous Deliveries. Note general smallness of outlet, also reduction of space of left side. Reproduction has reversed the x-ray picture.

After the fact of *pelvic distortion* has been discovered, the degree of *pelvic contraction* must be determined.

A few cases of dislocation of the ilium upon the sacrum are on record. It is easily diagnosed if its existence is suspected. It causes persistent backache, difficulty in locomotion, and, if it occurs in labor, occasional dystocia.

TRANSVERSELY CONTRACTED PELVES

It has been generally taught that contraction of the superior strait is the most common of the pelvic deformities, and of these, anteroposterior shortening is the most important. From the pathologist's standpoint this may be true, but clinically the justominor and transversely contracted pelves are more commonly found as the cause of dystocia. Pelves much contracted transversely at the inlet are very rare.

Mild degrees of contraction are found in the kyphotic, the infantile, and some varieties of high assimilation pelves. Contraction of the pelvic outlet is found in the funnel pelvis and those of the masculine type.

The Robert Pelvis.—Only 10 or more of these, the classic transversely contracted pelvis named after Robert, who in 1842 first described it, are in existence.

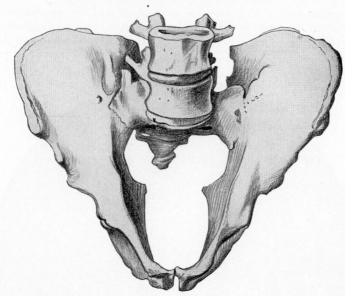

FIG. 608.—ROBERT'S PELVIS (after Robert's Dubois' pelvis in Paris).

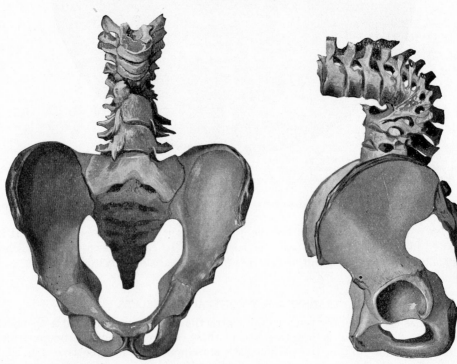

FIG. 609.—KYPHOTIC TRANSVERSELY CONTRACTED PELVIS   FIG. 610.—LEFT VIEW OF SAME.
(Northwestern University Medical School Museum).

This deformity is due to the same cause which produces the Naegelè pelvis, that is, an osteo-arthritis, but acting on both sacro-iliac joints. Both sides of the pelvic cavity are compromised, and the inlet assumes the form of a narrow wedge (Fig.

608). The narrowing of the pelvis usually extends to the very outlet, and in one case described by Breus and Kolisko the distance between the spines of the ischium was only 2 cm.

The Kyphosis Pelvis.—Fig. 609 shows a pelvis contracted in the transverse diameter, and possessing also some of the characteristics of the funnel type. It is from a young girl, ossification still being incomplete. If the kyphosis is situated in the upper part of the spinal column, a compensatory lordosis lower down restores the line of direction of gravity to its normal position in the statics of the person, and, therefore, the pelvis suffers little, if any, change. If, as in Fig. 610, the knuckle or "gibbus" is in the lumbar spine, marked alteration of the pelvis occurs. The sacrum is, as it were, drawn upward and out of the pelvis; at the same time it rotates on a transverse axis so as to throw the promontory up and back, the coccyx forward and inward. As a result of the rotation of the sacrum the innominate bones are rolled around the sacral articular surfaces, so as to bring the ischia together and exaggerate the forward dip of the crests, that is, increasing pelvic inclination. This action is produced by the patient throwing her head and shoulders back to counteract the tendency of the body to fall forward when the bodies of the vertebræ soften and break down under the tubercular caries (Fig. 612).

The extreme pelvic inclination of these pelves is easily understood. The patient throws the lower abdomen forward and holds the chest high and the shoulders backward. Pendulous belly is more marked in these women than in all others.

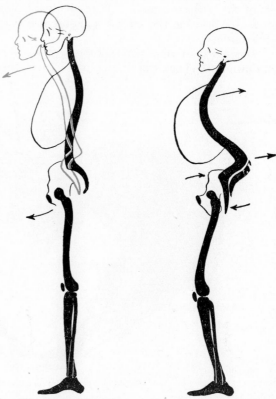

Fig. 611.—Normal Stature, Black; Kyphosis, Red. Body Falls Forward and to Prevent Toppling, Patient Throws Head and Shoulders Back.

Fig. 612.—Shows Rotation of Trunk on Hip-joints, with Backward Propulsion of Promontory and Forward Movement of Lower Sacrum.

If the caries of the vertebræ is in the lowest lumbar or in the first sacral vertebra, the upper arm of the knuckle comes to lie over the inlet, roofing it over—*spondylolizema*, as Herrgott called it, or *pelvis obtecta*, a better term, offered by Fehling. While the inlet may be large, the spinal column roofs it over so that the head cannot gain entrance to the pelvic canal.

The Funnel Pelvis.—When the lumen of the pelvis grows smaller from the inlet to the outlet, we speak of funnel pelvis. Most pelves of the generally contracted type belong in this class, as do also several of the other varieties already considered—the kyphotic, the Naegelè, the Robert's, and some of the rachitic. The causes of the convergence of the pelvic bones toward the outlet cannot always be determined. Figure 613 shows a pelvis normal in every other particular, but the sacrum and the ischial portions of the innominates converge toward the outlet.

Women of masculine habitus, who have large, leonine features, hirsuties, a tendency to firm obesity, and who are often sterile, frequently have heavy bony funnel pelves. Infantilism of the genitalia sometimes is associated with funnel pelvis. Williams emphasizes the frequency of high assimilation as a cause of funnel pelvis, and my own observation tends to confirm this view. (See Dystrophia Adiposogenitalis, p. 704.)

High degrees of funnel pelvis are exceedingly rare, but moderate contraction of the outlet is, in the author's experience, a pelvic deformity very commonly met. True this is not usually recognized, the dystocia being ascribed to some anomaly of the soft parts or of the presentation and position, the size of the fetus, or weakness of the powers of labor. Without doubt many of the forceps operations performed for delay in the second stage are necessitated by contraction of the bony pelvic outlet.

Diagnosis.—Funnel pelvis of the kyphosis type is easily recognized—the gibbus low down in the back will point to it. Not so easy is the recognition of the mascu-

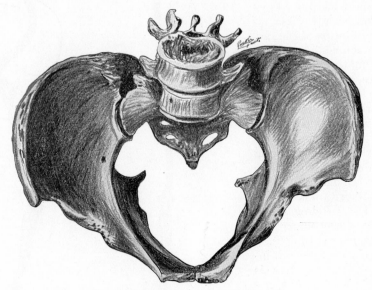

FIG. 613.—FUNNEL PELVIS (author's collection).

line pelvis, and the attendant is usually only apprised of the latter's existence when a stop in the labor occurs with the head low down in the pelvic canal. If in the routine pregnancy examination the accoucheur will take care to palpate the descending rami of the pubis as in Fig. 276, p. 262, and measure the distance between the tuberosities, as in Fig. 274, such surprises will come to him very seldom. During labor, if the palpation of the side walls of the parturient canal does not indicate narrowing, the pelvimeter used as in Fig. 269 will give positive information. A masculine pelvis may be looked for if the patient is large, with a tendency to firm adiposity, with large leonine features, and hirsuties of the face. Often such women are married late, are sterile for many years, have frigiditas sexualis, early menopause, and often develop fibroids. If they do become pregnant, it is often the only reproductive effort (single child sterility), for which reason special care should be exerted to preserve the child.

Schauta found funnel pelves in about 6 per cent., Stocker in about 26 per cent., and Klien in 24 per cent., of the cases examined.

Assimilation Pelves.—In the embryo the iliac bones develop in the region of the twenty-fifth to the twenty-ninth spinal vertebræ, which five vertebræ later are fused together to form the sacrum. The sacro-iliac joint is usually made with the twenty-sixth spinal vertebra at first, but soon the twenty-fifth and twenty-seventh are involved. If the iliac bones are united with vertebræ higher up in the spinal column, that is, the twenty-fourth, twenty-fifth, and twenty-sixth, we will find the sacrum long and narrow, and the first sacral vertebra presenting the characteristics of a transitional stage from the last lumbar. The sacrum has six segments instead of five and five foramina instead of four. The last lumbar vertebra, therefore, seems to be "assimilated" with the sacrum, i. e., has helped to make up this bone, and such a pelvis is called "upper assimilation pelvis"—upper because the union of the ilia with the spinal column is higher up than normal.

If the union of the ilia with the spinal column occurs with the twenty-sixth, twenty-seventh, and twenty-eighth vertebræ, we find six lumbar vertebræ instead of five, the last lumbar (sixth) having many of the characteristics of the first sacral.

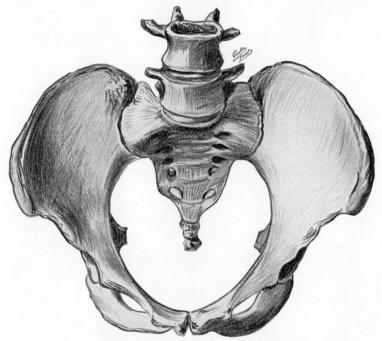

FIG. 614.—HIGH ASSIMILATION PELVIS. ROUND INLET.
Drawn from a specimen Professor Kolisko gave to the author.

Such a pelvis is called a "lower assimilation pelvis"—lower, because the union of the ilia with the spinal column is lower than normal and the sacrum is short, usually broad, and has four foramina.

In many instances the insertion of the ilium is normal on one side and higher or lower on the other, asymmetric assimilation pelvis resulting. Only half of the last lumbar vertebra then goes to help make up the sacro-iliac joint. Scoliosis is a frequent result of this deformity. Unless one has the whole spinal column for study, it may be difficult to determine where the assimilation occurred. Indeed, in many cases it is not easy to recognize the abnormality.

Sometimes the coccyx is assimilated with the last sacral vertebræ. This is of little practical importance. Perhaps fracture of the coccyx is more common, and, too, since assimilation sometimes causes funnel and transversely contracted pelvis, the delay in labor at the outlet may be prolonged by the abnormal bony formation, which latter, too, predisposes to fracture.

Breus and Kolisko, of Vienna, to whom we are indebted for the most thorough study of these pelves, distinguish five kinds: (1) The high assimilation pelvis; (2) the transversely contracted; (3) the midplane contracted; (4) the low; (5) the asymmetric.   The terms high and low have nothing to do with the site of the union

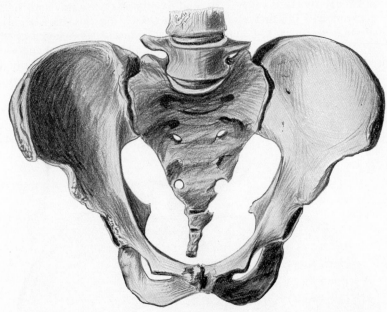

Fig. 615.—Transversely Contracted Assimilation Pelvis (Breus and Kolisko).

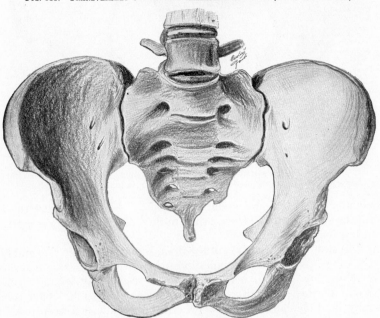

Fig. 616.—Midplane Contracted Assimilation Pelvis (Breus and Kolisko).

of the pelvic girdle with the spinal column, that is, upper or lower assimilation, but refer to the height of the pelvic canal.

Fig. 614 shows a high assimilation pelvis, which, with those of Figs. 615 and 616, Kolisko kindly presented to me. Its characteristics are: a very high promontory, long sacrum, composed almost always of six vertebræ and with five sacral foramina, the first of which may lie above the plane of the inlet; almost perpendicular wings of the sacrum, which are thin; pelvic canal deep, conjugata vera lengthened, conjugata transversa sometimes shortened.

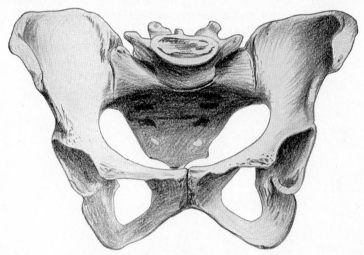

Fig. 617.—Low Assimilation Pelvis (Breus and Kolisko).

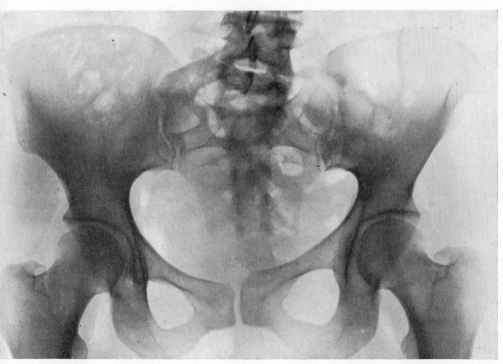

Fig. 618.—X-ray of Partial Unilateral Assimilation (University of Chicago, Prof. Hodges).

Figure 615 shows a transversely contracted assimilation pelvis from the same source. The promontory is very high, and another, or double, exists. The sacrum is long and narrow, the wings being poorly developed, and the transverse contrac-

47

tion may continue downward to the outlet, giving this pelvis a funnel shape or masculine type.

Fig. 616 is one of Breus and Kolisko's midplane contracted assimilation pelves. The forward prominence of the sacrum is evident, and this causes a shortening of all the sagittal diameters, especially that of the second parallel of Hodge. This pelvis has two promontories, and the uppermost sacral vertebra, carrying the sacral foramina with it, seems to be bent backward, to get into alinement with the lumbar spine. All these pelves have extreme inclination to the horizontal.

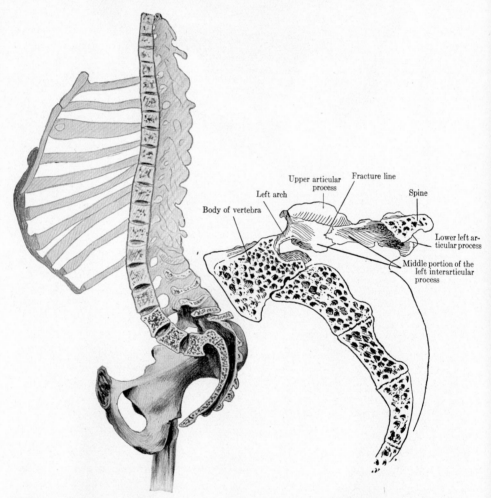

FIG. 619.—CHIARI'S SPONDYLOLISTHETIC PELVIS   FIG. 620.—DETAIL OF SPONDYLOLISTHETIC SACRUM (Breus and
        (Breus and Kolisko).   Kolisko.)   (From the "large Vienna pelvis.")

Fig. 617 shows a low or shallow assimilation pelvis; its promontory is very low and projects forward, the pelvis being shallow, but roomy.

Fig. 597 (p. 724) shows an asymmetric assimilation pelvis from the author's collection. It was combined with scoliosis. Since the pelvic lumen is not seriously encroached upon in the assimilation pelves, much practical importance is usually not attributed to this deformity by most authors. I am convinced, however, that many of the lesser irregularities of labor, such as occipitoposterior, occipitosacral positions, arrest of rotation in the midplane, deep transverse arrest, extensive pelvic floor lacerations, etc., are due to the irregular shape of the pelvic canal produced by these peculiarities. Transverse contraction can be so pronounced as to cause real dystocia, and if the child is large, it may die in delivery or even craniotomy may be required.

Diagnosis.—It may be possible to feel six sacral vertebræ in exceptionally favorable cases, but usually the diagnosis of assimilation pelvis on the living is only a surmise. When distinct narrowing of the outlet exists and signs of infantilism are absent, one may suspect that such deformity exists. A very high or double promontory with normal measurements is suggestive, and a scoliosis which has no other apparent cause may also lead one to think of assimilation. The x-ray might discover it (Fig. 618).

Spondylolisthetic Pelvis.—Kilian, in 1854, first named this pelvis, the term being derived from the Greek, which means a sliding of the vertebra. F. L. Neuge-

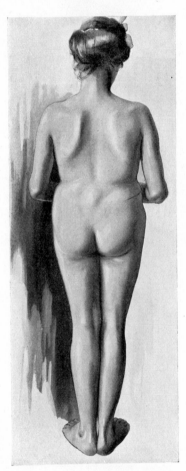

Fig. 621.—Spondylolisthetic Pelvis.
Shows the hump of last lumbar spine.

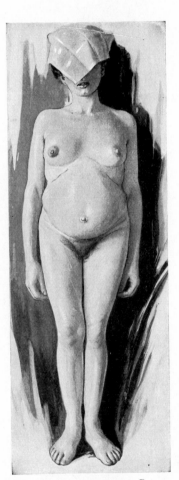

Fig. 622.—Spondylolisthetic Pelvis.
Shows pubis rotated upward.

bauer is entitled to the greatest credit for his thorough investigations, and many monographs have placed the subject in a very clear light (Williams, DeLee).

The essential feature of this pelvis is a sliding of the body of the last lumbar vertebra over the first sacral and into the pelvis, carrying, of course, the spinal column with it. The articular processes of the vertebra and sacrum are not dislocated, the slipping of the body of the former being permitted by a stretching or fracture of the interarticular processes. The last lumbar vertebra thus comes to be much elongated from before backward, and may even be bent over the sacrum like a clamp and the apposed portions of the two bones are compressed and often synostotic. Severe injury, a congenital lack of fusion of the ossification areas of the anterior and posterior ossification centers of the lateral portions of the vertebra, and carrying of heavy loads (coal heavers' spine) are given as causes.

On the pelvis spondylolisthesis has a very deforming action: (1) The inclination of the pelvis is obliterated, in marked cases the inlet being almost horizontal; (2) the lower lumbar spine projects over and into the inlet—pelvis obtecta—in a way similar to that of lumbosacral kyphosis, and the promontory becomes

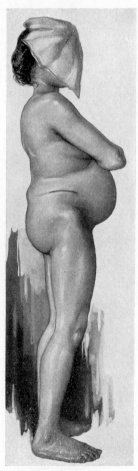

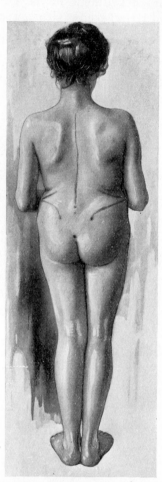

Fig. 623.—Spondylolisthetic Pelvis (Side View). Shows spine of last lumbar and horizontal crest of ilium.

Fig. 624.—Spondylolisthetic Pelvis. Ribs almost rest on crests of ilia. Upward curve of crests is shown by lines drawn on the skin.

the fourth, third, or even the second lumbar vertebra; (3) the available true conjugate of the inlet may be reduced to even 5 cm., and the rest of the pelvis tends to become funnel shaped.

Diagnosis.—The history of injury will indicate a careful study of the pelvis; note the horizontal iliac crests and close proximity of ribs (Fig. 623), the broad rhomboid of Michaëlis, the sharp hump presented by the last lumbar vertebra, the compensatory dorsal lordosis, including the thrown back head, and the tightrope walker tread (Fig. 625). Internally the lumbar spine overhanging the sacrum and encroaching on the inlet can be easily felt, but it is not always so marked as in

Fig. 619.   The sacrum, with its lateral wings, is easily distinguishable from the last lumbar vertebra, the sharp angle can readily be felt, and the bifurcation of the

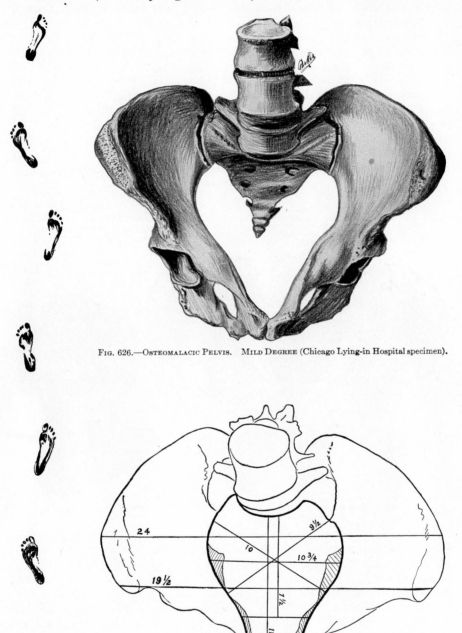

FIG. 626.—OSTEOMALACIC PELVIS.   MILD DEGREE (Chicago Lying-in Hospital specimen).

FIG. 627.—MEASUREMENTS OF FIG. 626.   OSTEOMALACIC PELVIC INLET.

FIG. 625.—TREAD OF SPON-
DYLOLISTHETIC   PA-
TIENT.   "TIGHT-ROPE
WALKER'S TREAD."

Patient's   feet   were
painted with red ink and
she walked on a strip of
wall-paper, which was then
photographed.

common iliac artery may be distinctly palpable on the left side, but not on the right. Von Winckel proved that this last finding was unreliable, being found also in kyphotic pelves. See Monograph, Meyer-Burgdorf, Meyerding, Chandler.

The Osteomalacic Pelvis.—Part of the general affection, osteomalacia, which has already been considered (p.554), is the deformity of the pelvis, and, from the obstetrician's point of view, the most important. As the result of the action of the trunk pressure, the pressure of the heads of the femora, the traction of the muscles and ligaments on the softened bones, the pelvis is crowded together in an astonishing manner. Figs. 626 to 629 show these deformations, and description is unnecessary. The sinking downward and forward of the sacrum, the beak-like distortion of the horizontal pubic rami (due to the inward pressure of the femora), the approach of the tuberosities of the ischia, the rolling inward of the iliac crests, must be emphasized. On the pelvic lumen this invasion from three sides and above produces very decided effects—indeed, the cavity may be almost obliterated.

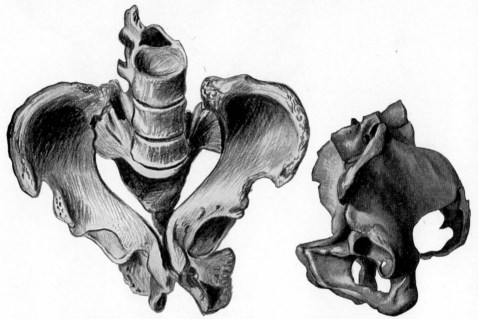

FIG. 628.—OSTEOMALACIC PELVIS. HIGHEST DEGREE.   FIG. 629.—LEFT VIEW OF FIG. 628.

Labor is rendered impossible if the process is at all advanced, but if it occurs when the osteomalacia is in the florid stage, the soft bones may give way to the head advancing under the influence of strong pains, and dilate enough to allow the child to pass through. This dilatation of the pelvic canal has been found in 17 to 30 per cent. of the cases, but in practice it is best not to depend on it.

Diagnosis.—From the history of the patient one will learn that the body has gradually grown shorter, with complaint of rheumatoid pains in the back and the pelvis, difficult and painful locomotion (duck-gait), contraction of the adductor thigh muscles, muscular trembling, paresis, asthenia, and progressive invalidism. Previous labors have grown successively more difficult. Tenderness is found over most of the bones, and the incurvations of the spine, the ribs, and the extremities are usually present in sufficient degree to be found. On the pelvis the most decided changes are discoverable, the most notable being the beaked pubis, the narrow pubic arch, which in the author's case hardly permitted two fingers to pass; the sharply curved sacrum and low promontory. All the external measurements are diminished.

In the differential diagnosis the pseudo-osteomalacic rachitic pelvis need be mentioned, but the history, the disease appearing in childhood, will at once eliminate this. Spondylolisthesis is also easily determined.

DOUBLE DISLOCATION OF THE HIPS

Congenital dislocation of the hips is not a very rare deformity, and only recently have the efforts of the orthopedists been successful in correcting it. When such

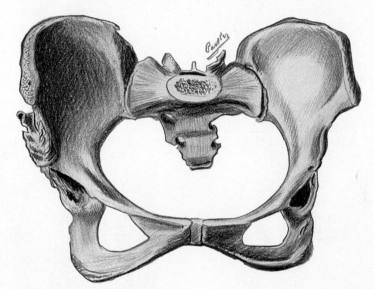

FIG. 630.—DOUBLE DISLOCATION OF HIPS.

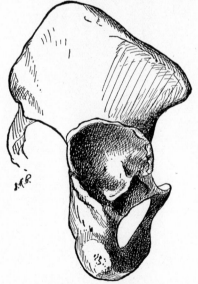

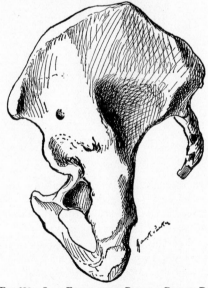

FIG. 631.—RIGHT ELEVATION OF PELVIS. DOUBLE DIS-
LOCATION OF HIPS.
Shows new acetabulum.

FIG. 632.—LEFT ELEVATION OF PELVIS. DOUBLE DIS-
LOCATION OF HIPS.
Shows contracted acetabulum and new socket.

a child begins to walk, the trunk pressure forces the whole pelvis onto the iliofemoral and capsular ligaments, the line of gravity is anteposed, the spinal column is thrown back to preserve the balance, the result of all this being a forward tilting of the pelvic girdle and increase of pelvic inclination. Since the transverse pressure exerted by the heads of the femora fails, distinct flattening of the pelvis results (Fig. 630). The outlet is very large.

Diagnosis.—In the accompanying photographs the characteristic appearance of such a woman is to be seen. The high trochanters, the broad hips, the lordosis

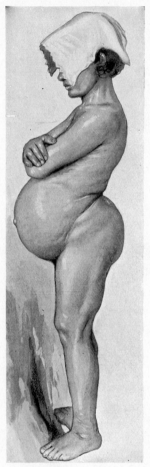

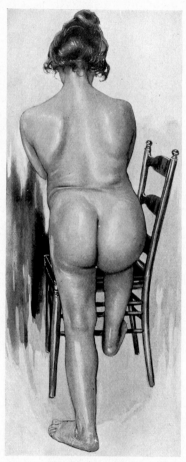

Fig. 633.—Double Dislocation of Hips.

Fig. 634.—Double Dislocation of Hips.
Shows downward and backward rotation of head of femur when leg is flexed.

with increased pelvic inclination, the folding of the skin at the hips, the loose-jointed gait—all strike the eye at once. On internal examination the shortening, if there is any, of the conjugata vera is easily determinable. Labor has the characteristics of that in flat pelves.

For the sake of completion may be mentioned the pelvis split at the pubis, an accompaniment of ectopic bladder,—gastroschisis,—and the case of absence of the sacrum, both scientific curiosities.

Literature

Breus and Kolisko: Die pathologische Beckenformen, 1902 to 1912.—*Chandler, F.:* Surg., Gyn., and Obst., September, 1931, p. 273, Lit.—*DeLee:* Obstetrics, 4th ed., p. 720.—*Klein:* Volkmann's Samml. klin. Vort., N. F., No. 169, 1896.—*Meyer-Burgdorf:* Untersuchung über das Wirbelgleiten, Georg Thieme, Leipzig, 1931.—*Meyerding:* Surg., Gyn., and Obst., February, 1932.—*Williams:* Amer. Jour. Obstet., July, 1911.—"The Rhomboid of Michaelis," L'Obstetrique, January, 1910, p. 65.—"Spondylolisthesis," Arch. f. Gyn., vol. lii, p. 101.

CHAPTER LV

CLINICAL ASPECTS OF CONTRACTED PELVES

During Pregnancy.—Certain varieties of contracted pelvis may interfere with coitus, for example, the double coxalgic, with ankylosis. Very large pelves allow the uterus to sag down onto the pelvic diaphragm, and such women show increased pelvic floor projection. It has seemed to me that they suffer larger tears in labor and are liable to develop prolapsus uteri. Retroversion of the uterus may be maintained by an overhanging promontory, and if pregnancy supervenes, an operation may be needed to restore the uterus to its place.

As a rule, it is later in pregnancy that the effects of pelvic obstruction become apparent. Since there is no room in the pelvis for the growing uterus, it forces itself upward, the abdomen is overdistended, the anterior wall stretches, or the recti part and the fundus uteri falls forward, the condition being known as pendulous abdomen (Fig. 353, p. 439).

If the muscles retain their integrity, the uterus is forced upward against the ribs and forms here a high plateau. Another effect of contracted pelvis is the conferring of a great degree of mobility on the uterus. The organ, since its pelvic attachments are overstretched and it lacks the support of the side walls of the pelvis, is free to sag from side to side with every turn of the patient. Some women complain much of this, and require the support of a firm binder. From the same causes the position and presentation of the fetus change readily and frequently. The cephalic pole does not remain so constantly over the inlet, hence when labor begins quite often the child is found in an unfavorable attitude and presentation, which, becoming confirmed by the uterine contractions, causes serious dystocia. Varicose veins of the vulva and limbs, especially if one or more severe operative deliveries have preceded, are often particularly marked. Occasionally, in primiparæ, the head enters a contracted pelvis in the later weeks of pregnancy, and labor is unexpectedly easy. The head, by its configuration, may show the shape of the pelvic cavity. Subsequent labors may be difficult.

During Labor.—*General Considerations.*—Labor is likely to be a little premature in contracted pelves of the flat variety, and to be prolonged in those of the generally contracted, funnel, and masculine types. Reasons for this I cannot advance, but such has been my experience. When labor has frankly declared itself in a woman with contracted pelvis and at term, it early becomes evident that the process is not going as it should, and the observant accoucheur soon perceives that it is not alone the spacial disproportion which causes dystocia, but many other factors—abnormal presentations, positions, attitude, the size and hardness of the fetal head, irregular uterine action, premature rupture of the bag of waters, etc.

Abnormal presentations—breech, face, brow, shoulder—are four times as frequent with contracted pelvis, Litzmann having found the cephalic pole presenting normally in only 84 per cent. of his cases (usually in 96 per cent.). The reason for this is that the head, finding the entrance into the superior strait blocked, glides off into one iliac fossa, producing an obliquity of the fetal axis to that of the inlet. It is now easy for a partial or even a complete rotation of the fetal ovoid to occur, and the pains coming on, the child is locked in its unfavorable position. Prolapse of the arm, foot, and cord are also much more common in all forms of pelvic contraction, but particularly in the flat varieties. The reason for this is that the head does not lie firmly in apposition on the lower uterine segment, but is held away by the jutting promontory of the sacrum, which leaves unfilled spaces at the sides, through which the small parts easily slip. All these accidents are commoner in multiparæ with their flaccid and flabby uteri.

A great deal depends on the size and moldability of the fetal head and of the trunk. If the bones are soft, they easily give themselves to the shape of the inlet, and apparently great disproportion may thus be overcome. If the child is small, the pelvis, relatively, may not be at all contracted, while if the infant is large, the contraction of the pelvis must be rated higher.

Of prime significance in all labors with contracted pelvis is the action of the uterus. Speaking broadly, the strength of the uterus is proportionate to the amount of work required of it. In some cases the uterus acts regularly and with increasing power as it finds that the child does not progress through the birth-canal. Within well-defined limits this augmented action of the uterus is healthy and very desirable, because by this means nature often overcomes spacial disproportion between the head and the pelvis which no one would have thought possible. The recurring pains adjust, compress, mold, and propel the head through the narrowed canal in a fashion that the finest art absolutely fails to imitate. Further, good pains dilate the cervix and prepare the soft parts for the passage of the fetus. Weak pains are a most unwelcome complication of labor in contracted pelvis. They may be primary or secondary. Primarily weak pains frequently accompany generally contracted pelvis and are another expression of the infantilism which caused it. Again, other causes of weak pains may exist. Weak pains from exhaustion, tetanus, or infection of the uterus are much more significant and correspondingly serious. To weak uterine action are often added weak abdominal muscles, so common with pendulous belly, a frequent complication of contracted pelvis. If the passage is not too markedly contracted and the child is of moderate size; if the presentation and position are good and the pains strong, the large majority of labors will terminate spontaneously and happily for both mother and child. Even experienced accoucheurs will often be surprised to see what nature can accomplish if properly supported and not interfered with. On the other hand, the contraction of the pelvis may be negligible, as far as spacial disproportion is concerned, but it has caused an abnormal presentation—for example, brow or shoulder, which results in perhaps fatal dystocia.

The First Stage.—At the beginning of labor the head is high up, not engaged, as so often happens in healthy primiparæ and in multiparæ with strong abdominal walls. It does not even project into the pelvis with a large segment, but floats high, almost out of reach of the finger. It does not fit the lower uterine segment accurately, hence the membranes over the os are exposed to the full force of the uterine contraction. If they are delicate, they burst and the liquor amnii drains away; if they are tough, they are stripped off the lower uterine segment and pouch down into the vagina or even to the vulva, stocking shaped, and are of little service as a fluid dilating wedge. The evil consequences of early rupture of the sac are: Loss of the hydrostatic cervical dilator; (2) increased danger of pressure necrosis of soft parts lying between head and pelvis; (3) increased possibilities of prolapse of cord, arm, and feet; (4) infection may gain entrance to uterine cavity and cause physometra, fetal death, and sepsis. If the membranes rupture before complete dilatation has been secured, the lower uterine segment and cervix collapse, and it requires prolonged effort on the part of the uterus to open the passage again. Von Herff's experience must have been contrary to that of most observers, for he finds that rupture of the bag of waters in contracted pelvis is not an event to be feared; that the dilatation progresses just as satisfactorily as before, or often better.

True, the pains may be stronger after the waters have drained away, but experienced accoucheurs will find it hard to admit that the head makes as efficient and as safe a cervical dilator as the bag of waters, or that the mother and child are not in more danger after the sac has been opened, and they will be loath to dispense with the natural water-bag dilator until the cervix is open enough to permit natural or operative delivery.

Many differences are observed in the way the lower uterine segment is formed and the cervix dilated in cases of obstructed labor. In a healthy primipara the usual mechanism occurs, but in a multipara, especially if she has had several difficult labors, the contraction ring ascends very early, the lower uterine segment quickly forms under the influence of the pains, and the os soon dilates. Now, unless the head quickly passes into and through the pelvis, the expanded parturient canal will give way and allow the fetus to escape into the peritoneal cavity. If the cervix is tough, it may long resist the action of the uterus and require the intervention of art. Sometimes the cervix is compressed between the head and the pelvis. The part below the area of compression then may become edematous and even slough off. Particularly the anterior lip, in flat pelves with pendulous belly, is liable to be caught between the head and the pubis, becoming enormously swollen (sometimes to the size of one's wrist), suggillated, even necrotic, leaving cervicovesical fistula. Previous deep lacerations of the cervix and of the lower uterine segment predispose to fresh rupture. Dilatation of an old, much-lacerated cervix is usually rapid unless the scars are very extensive.

The Second Stage.—Up to this point labor in nearly all forms of contracted pelvis is the same. When the head is to pass through the inlet, different mechanisms are developed, and these will be considered separately later. Certain general features are common to all obstructed labors, and they may be divided into two groups: first, the absolutely impossible labor, where the disproportion is so great that the child cannot pass, and, second, the labors where the child can pass, but it requires prolonged effort on the part of nature, without or with the help of art.

If the head is arrested, the uterus is stimulated to redoubled vigor, the pains become stronger and stronger, the intervals shorter, but no advancement is perceptible. The vagina becomes hot, swollen, blue, and dry, the vulva dark blue and edematous, often with small suggillations, and in much neglected cases gangrenous. A large caput succedaneum replaces the bag of waters, and the scalp may be visible at the vulva when the head has not yet passed the inlet. The child dies because the violently acting uterus cuts off its oxygen supply, and sometimes also from cerebral injury or hemorrhage, the result of nature's attempt to crowd the head through a passage too small for it. Gauss calls attention to the slowing of the fetal heart as the head traverses the superior strait, it being greatest just after the excavation is reached. He explains it as the result of positive and negative commotio cerebri. If aid is not rendered, the woman inevitably dies and death occurs from rupture of the uterus, with intraperitoneal hemorrhage or shock, from sepsis, or exhaustion. (For the symptoms of rupture of the uterus the reader is referred to Chapter LIX.) Infection during prolonged labor may be autogenous or exogenous. In the vast majority of cases the physician introduces the infection from the vulva, or from without entirely, or by repeated examinations inoculates the patient with the bacteria normally present in the vagina, the frequency of the various modes being, in the author's opinion, in the order given. In a small percentage of the cases the bacteria wander upward from the vagina through the opened membranes into the uterine cavity. In either event the woman develops fever, the first effect of which is to stimulate the pains, but soon the uterus is paralyzed, with or without the formation of gas in its cavity (physometra). Women in labor stand infection not at all well, and the temperature and pulse rapidly mount high, while delirium, subicterus, and prostration quickly follow. There is a foul discharge from the vagina, and the vulva is swollen, reddened, and superficially necrotic in places. Acute dilatation of the heart is a not rare termination of too prolonged labor.

Exhaustion is an infrequent cause of death, but without doubt it will explain many cases of shock and of gradual, uncontrollable asthenia terminating fatally after operative delivery. The operation may have been quick and skilful, without undue hemorrhage, and with little anesthetic, but the woman does not rally, the pulse mounts higher and higher, the vital powers slowly sink, and in from four to twenty-four hours death supervenes in quiet coma. In the differential diagnosis internal hemorrhage, uremia, and shock from injury are to be considered.

If the disproportion is not absolute, nature often accomplishes the delivery, and even the experienced obstetrician must marvel when he sees all his preconceived notions set at naught.

At first the head is high up, separated from the bony inlet by a pad of thick cervix, the bases of the broad ligaments, the bladder, and the pelvic connective tissue in general. After the uterus has been in action for a while all these structures except the base of the bladder are drawn upward with the retraction of the lower uterine segment out of the pelvis, thus allowing the head to apply itself to the inlet. If one examines the woman now during a pain, peculiar phenomena are observed. The head flexes and deflexes, and sometimes rotates on its transverse axis, or even in a horizontal plane, and one feels the large fontanel advance, recede, turn from behind forward, and the head rolls on either shoulder. It is important for the

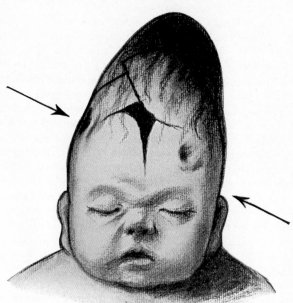

Fig. 635.—Head After Four Days' Labor in a Generally Contracted and Flat Pelvis.
Arrows show direction of compression and point to areas where the scalp subsequently sloughed out.

accoucheur to study these motions with great care, because they are the evidences of the intended mechanisms of the head, that is, that manner in which the head is to overcome the resistances of the passage. Nature seems to be fitting the head to the pelvis as a key is fitted to the wards of a lock, until a combination is secured which will best allow the head to pass.

Now the process of molding or configuration begins, and the general intrauterine pressure, together with the fetal axis pressure, gradually forces the head through the narrowed superior strait. Owing to the nature of things the head cannot be reduced in size by compression, and only a minute quantity of cerebrospinal fluid can escape through the foramen magnum into the spinal canal—not enough appreciably to affect the size of the head. Now, owing to the softness of the cranial bones and their movability on each other at the sutures, the head is capable of being changed in form so that it accommodates itself to the shape of the superior strait. That parietal bone which first meets with resistance is pressed under the other, and the plate of the occipital bone lies under the two parietals. The overlapping may be so marked that the dura mater begins to strip off, and a row of minute hemorrhages will be found on either side of the longitudinal sinus. Fig. 635 shows the head of a child spontaneously delivered after four days' labor. This length of time is very seldom required for the process; indeed, nowadays such cases are not allowed to take so long, but interference is thought necessary after giving the natural powers reasonable opportunity to show how much they can accomplish. From four to ten hours of good strong pains will almost always suffice for the test, but even here great watchfulness is indicated lest mother or babe suffer harm from the experiment.

As soon as the head has been molded so that it is ready to pass through the inlet the pains assume an expulsive character—the parturient bears down, the head drops into the excavation, and the occiput begins to rotate to the front.

Three signs indicate that the head is descending: (1) The patient begins to bear down; (2) feces are discharged, or the woman expresses a desire to go to stool; (3) cramps of the muscles of the legs occur—usually the left leg in left occiput positions and vice versâ. The first two symptoms are due to the pressure of the head upon the rectum; the last one, to irritation of the sacral plexus by contact of the advancing head. In flat pelves, in which the resistance is met only at the inlet, this part of the labor is completed with surprising quickness. In multiparæ one or two powerful expulsive pains procure anterior rotation and the birth of the head; in primiparæ the soft parts have to be overcome, and this requires the usual time. The head may be given a shape different from that acquired in the passage of the inlet by the molding caused by the pelvic floor. If the pelvis is generally contracted, the resistance continues all the way to the outlet, and labor is unduly prolonged and tedious. In addition the uterine action in this class of pelvis is often weak, the uterus partaking of the general hypoplasia. Women with funnel and masculine pelves are also prone to uterine inertia. Occipitoposterior positions, imperfect dilatation of the cervix, and strictura uteri (hour-glass contraction) are also more common in them.

After the head is delivered the main difficulty is overcome, but if the child has broad shoulders, they may cause much trouble, especially in the generally and transversely contracted pelves. Many an infant has been lost during the prolonged attempts to deliver impacted shoulders. At any point the uterus may give out and labor comes to a standstill, requiring the assistance of art. It is as often the nervous system of the woman or the condition of the baby which demands interference as the uterus proving default.

The third stage does not present any conditions which are peculiar. Postpartum hemorrhage is rare if the pains have been good, but if the delivery has been operative, lacerations and bleeding must be expected.

CHAPTER LVI

MECHANISM OF LABOR IN FLAT PELVES

An experienced accoucheur can diagnose the nature of the pelvis by observing the mechanism with which the head passes through it. Many of its motions are characteristic of flat and of generally contracted types. In flat pelves abnormalities of position and presentation are very common. Owing to the jutting forward of the promontory, the head cannot enter the pelvis and, therefore, slips off to one side, which often allows the cord to prolapse in the free space thus provided. The

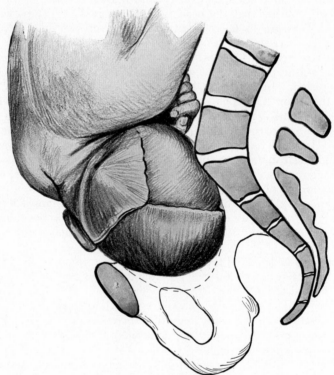

Fig. 636.—Anterior Parietal Bone Presentation. Head Molding its Way Into Flat Pelvis (adapted from Smellie).
Dotted line shows caput succedaneum.

head tries to enter the pelvis flexed, as in the usual mechanism of labor, but the biparietal diameter is too large to pass through the conjugata vera, the diameter of greatest contraction. As a result the head slides off to the side, the bitemporal, a smaller diameter, comes to lie in the conjugata vera, while the biparietal lies in the larger space opposite the sacro-iliac joint. As soon as the head sinks the forehead descends, because the resistance offered the occiput is greater—deflexion, instead of flexion, the first movement, occurs. Owing to the long transverse and short sagittal diameters of the inlet the head seeks the position which will easiest allow it to advance—that is, the sagittal diameter of the head will lie in the transverse of the pelvis. Since the jutting promontory forces the head forward the available—or obstetric—transverse diameter of the inlet lies anterior to the true or anatomic transversa. The available space, therefore, for the passage of the head is much reduced, the pelvis, though large, going into the class of justominors.

A third and most important abnormality of the mechanism is the almost constant lateroflexion of the head, that is, the parietal bone is inclined on one or the other shoulder, or, in other words, the head enters the pelvis in exaggerated asynclitism. This is called parietal bone presentation. Normally, although some authorities deny it, the head often enters the pelvis with slight anterior asynclitism, that is, obliquity of Naegelè. In flat contracted pelves this is exaggerated, and sometimes the lateroflexion is so great that the anterior ear is palpable behind the pubis—ear presentation. In the subsequent course of labor the posterior parietal bone rolls over the promontory into the pelvis, the anterior bone forming a sort

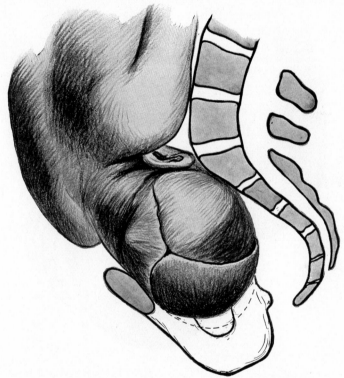

FIG. 637.—NEXT STAGE OF THE MOLDING. POSTERIOR PARIETAL ROLLS OVER THE PROMONTORY. HEAD NOW ENGAGED.
Sagittal suture comes near middle line.

of sliding fulcrum on the posterior wall of the pubis. The amount of molding of the cranial bones needed to allow the descent of the head according to this mechanism depends on the size and hardness of the head and the roominess of the inlet, and the time required depends also on these factors plus the strength of the uterine contractions. The process may be completed in a few hours, or may last over a day (Figs. 636, 637, and 638). That part of the head which rubs over the promontory often shows a pressure mark—a red streak. In right positions the red mark (in bad cases, real pressure necrosis) lies over the right parietal bone, parallel with the coronary suture; in left positions, in a corresponding location over the left parietal bone. The configuration of the head is sometimes remarkable. In one of the author's cases the head, viewed from above, had the shape of a kidney, and was almost a mold of the pelvic inlet. If the head remains long in the pelvis after having passed the superior strait, it acquires another shape from the secondary molding produced by the pelvic floor.

As soon as the greatest periphery of the head has passed the region of the inlet, or even just as it is about to pass, the occiput sinks, the large fontanel ascends, descent of the head takes place, and, as a rule, anterior rotation follows at once. The head undergoes a complicated movement, consisting of descent, flexion (the chin on the sternum), laterodeflexion, that is, the synclitic movement and anterior rotation of the occiput all simultaneously. Now the mechanism is as usual—flexion, descent, extension, external restitution. Even in primiparæ a few pains often accomplish the delivery; in multiparæ it is usually done with one or two.

Findings.—Abdominally, one may determine the deflexion of the head by noting the straightening of the fetal spine. The lateroflexion at the neck may

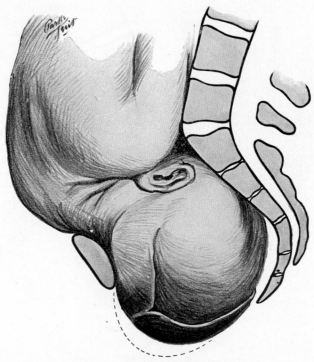

Fig. 638.—Head Has Sunk onto Pelvic Floor and Has Almost Completely Rotated to Front. Some lateroflexion of head persists even as late as this.

also be felt. On internal examination the sagittal suture lies in the transverse diameter, but *very close to the sacrum;* the small is on the same level as the large fontanel, sometimes even higher, so that the brow comes down; the sutures are at first plainly felt, because the cranial bones overlap so strongly, but later in labor the caput succedaneum obliterates the lines (Fig. 639).

Another mechanism, and an important variation, is the posterior parietal bone presentation (Fig. 640). Here the head is inclined on the anterior shoulder; the posterior parietal bone occupies the vault of the pelvis,—posterior asynclitism, —and if the lateroflexion is very decided, the posterior ear may be palpable in front of the promontory—"posterior ear presentation." The mechanism here is the reverse of that just considered. The posterior parietal stems on the promontory and the anterior rolls down from behind the pubis into the pelvis.

Findings.—In posterior parietal bone presentation one can often feel the angle which the shoulder makes with the head just above the pubis, and often the round parietal bone can be felt here—in one case the ear was indistinctly outlinable.

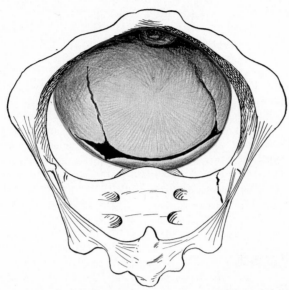

Fig. 639.—Touch Picture. Anterior Parietal Bone Presentation. Naegelè's Obliquity.
Sagittal suture near sacrum, ear near pubis. This picture also shows how the jutting promontory crowds the head forward, rendering useless a large part of the area of the inlet, the rear part of pelvis being empty.

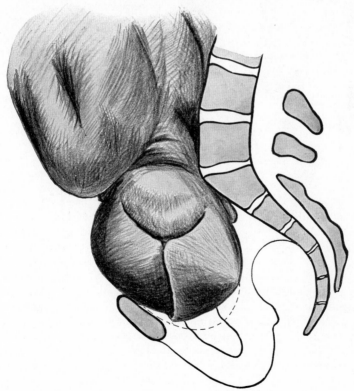

Fig. 640.—Posterior Parietal Bone Presentation. Flat Pelvis.
Dotted line is caput succedaneum.

Internally, the sagittal suture runs just behind the pubis, usually transverse, or the least bit obliquely, the small and large fontanels on a level or the small one up high, out of reach, and, by passing the fingers well up above the promontory, the ear is sometimes to be felt. As the head descends the sagittal suture leaves the pubis and comes to lie nearer the sacrum, but then descent and anterior rotation of the occiput bring the sagittal suture into an oblique. Sometimes the lateroflexion is kept up until the head escapes, and then the occiput is likely to remain in the oblique and the nape of the neck stems, not directly behind the pubis, but behind one ramus, and the head is delivered in the oblique. Use may be made of this fact in the conduct of such a labor, and the processes of nature imitated by art.

Why the head enters the pelvis in one or the other of these attitudes is not known. Probably pendulous abdomen will explain the anterior parietal variety, but I have seen the posterior parietal present, and pendulous belly was also a complication. A high sacrum might predispose to the anterior parietal, especially if there is a double promontory. Litzmann says that the anterior parietal bone presentation is three times more frequent than the posterior. In general the more contracted the pelvis, the closer the sagittal suture runs to either promontory or the pubis.

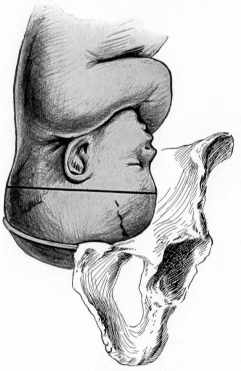

FIG. 641.—HEAD ABOUT TO ENTER A GENERALLY CONTRACTED PELVIS. PARTIAL FLEXION.

Labor is much more difficult and more often impossible in posterior parietal bone presentation, since in the latter the child is bent almost to a right angle at the neck. The uterus acts at a great disadvantage also, and is liable to excessive thinning on the posterior wall, a point of utmost practical importance, since here spontaneous rupture may occur, and the greatest danger from traumatism lies.

MECHANISM OF LABOR IN GENERALLY CONTRACTED PELVES

Labor in this class of pelves also bears marked characteristics. Since the head fits the inlet well, abnormal attitudes, presentations, and positions are not so frequent as in flat pelves. Prolapse of the cord is rare because the head fits the lower uterine segment accurately. Early in labor one notes that the head lies in flexion, and as soon as descent begins this flexion becomes extreme, the small fontanel being the first reached by the finger, and the sagittal suture lying in an oblique diameter of the pelvis and running almost perpendicularly. After labor has been in progress for some time and molding is advanced, the small fontanel lies almost in the center of the pelvis, and is covered by the caput succedaneum. The extreme flexion is due to an exaggeration of the same mechanism which produces flexion in normal labor—the sincipital end of the lever, being longer, meets with greater resistance and rises higher. Nature finds this the easiest way to force a head through a pelvis contracted in all diameters. Generally contracted pelves, unlike flat ones, have the narrowing all the way down, and, therefore, progress is not rapid after the inlet has been passed, but the head has to bore its way slowly through the canal (Figs. 641, 642, and 643).

Pressure marks are unusual because the resistances met are broad, not sharp, as in flat pelvis, and when they are present, owing to the flexion of the head, are found on the frontal bone, which lay against the promontory. Excessive length of the occipitofrontal diameter characterizes the molding in these cases, the occiput is peaked, the forehead and face are flattened, the neck is almost in a line with the back of the head, and the chin is buried in the chest. Lateral asymmetry is also marked. Extreme overlapping of the bones and minute cracks and fissures of the parietals or frontals are very common.

Labor in this form of pelvis is usually very slow and tedious. The uterus, partaking of the general hypoplasia, acts poorly, and often gives out before the head has passed all the narrow straits, instrumental interference being required. This is especially dangerous to both mother and babe

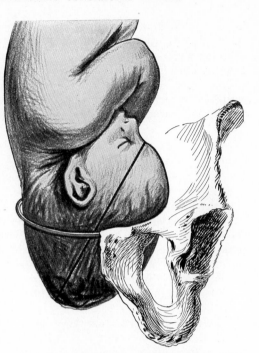

FIG. 642.—HEAD ENTERING A GENERALLY CONTRACTED PELVIS. FLEXION MARKED.

because of the inevitable injuries to the soft parts and the great compression of the child's brain. If the delivery is spontaneous, laceration of the perineum seldom occurs, because the head is so long drawn out.

The **diagnosis** of labor with generally contracted pelvis is usually easy. Abdominally, the extreme flexion is indicated by the high forehead, easily palpable over one ramus pubis, and the deep occiput, usually not palpable, even when the hand is pressed deeply into the groin. Vaginally, the small fontanel lying almost in the axis of the pelvis and the vertical position of the sagittal suture disclose the extreme flexion so characteristic of this form of labor.

Labor in pelves, both generally contracted and flat, partakes more of the nature of the mechanism of flat pelvis. Most authors say that labor partakes of the characteristics of both forms—combined in degrees varying with the preponderance of either deformity, but in my experience the head never could get into the pelvis far enough to meet the resistance all around and thus exaggerate the flexion. High transverse arrest is the condition

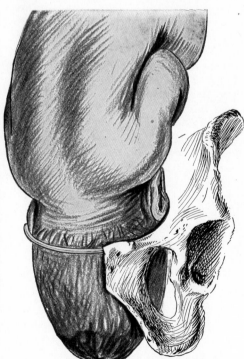

FIG. 643.—HEAD ENGAGED IN GENERALLY CONTRACTED PELVIS. ROTATION COMPLETED.

usually found, and, even in moderate degrees of contraction, cesarean section or, on the dead or dying child, craniotomy is often necessary. Not seldom the accoucheur, thinking he has to deal with a flat pelvis, meets unexpected difficulty, and investigation will show that moderate lateral contraction exists in addition. Since such contraction of the sides of the inlet leaves no place for the head, compressed in the conjugata vera, to expand in, these difficulties are easily explained, and generally contracted flat pelves present the most formidable complications unless early recognized.

MECHANISM OF LABOR IN FUNNEL PELVES

At the pelvic outlet the resistance begins, and the head comes to a stop at this point. Now extreme flexion occurs, and the labor resembles that of generally contracted pelves. If the funnel shape of the pelvis is due to kyphosis, as an additional complication the spinal column may overlie the inlet (pelvis obtecta) and prevent the entrance of the head into the superior strait. If spondylolisthesis exists, the same obstruction may present, and then labor is usually impossible without cesarean section. Klien emphasizes the frequency of occipitoposterior positions and forehead presentations. Such malpositions are probably due to the pendulous uterus, the fetal back fitting best to the posterior uterine convexity and its belly being bent over the pubis.

Pelves contracted transversely at the outlet are not so rare as was formerly thought. Klien has shown their immense clinical importance. Since the contraction lies between the descending rami of the pubis and the tuberosities of the ischia, the broad occiput cannot use this space during its passage under the symphysis, but is forced backward onto the perineum and against the sacrum and coccyx (Figs. 644, 645, and 646). As a result the perineum and levator ani are often torn, the coccyx broken, and if the sacrum curves too far forward, labor becomes impossible. The author is convinced that a large number of forceps cases with deep pelvic floor injuries and tearing of the vagina over the spines of the ischia, often to the walls of the pelvis, come in this class but are unrecognized.

The **diagnosis** of labor in funnel pelves will vary with the engagement or non-engagement of the head. When the head reaches the pelvic floor it is arrested, impacted between the ischia, but usually anterior rotation of the occiput has been completed. Strong bearing-down efforts produce no advance, *the perineum is not put on the stretch*, bulging does not occur, and the parturient, soon perceiving that her bearing-down efforts produce no real effect, gives up trying and calls for relief. Internal examination will disclose the head in exaggerated flexion, lying closely packed between the spines of the ischia and covered with a large caput succedaneum. Rotation is usually complete, but sometimes the sagittal suture lies in the transverse diameter—that is, "deep transverse arrest" has occurred. If the measurements of the pelvis have been taken in the routine pregnancy examination, such a course of labor will bring no surprise. In determining whether the head will or will not pass the outlet the accoucheur must know two distances—first, that between the tuberosities of the ischia, and, second, that from the center of this diameter to the tip of the sacrum—the "posterior sagittal" of Klien.

Klien says a normal outlet has a transverse diameter of 11 cm., an anterior sagittal of 6 cm., a posterior sagittal of 9.95 cm., but my own measurements are a little smaller.

The determination of the bi-ischiatic diameter is made as shown in Fig. 274 (p. 261), and is more easily measured in labor than at any other time. By holding a short rod in this diameter and applying one end of the pelvimeter to its center and the other over the end of the sacrum, the posterior sagittal is obtained. One centimeter must be deducted for the thickness of the bone and soft parts. Several special pelvimeters are on the market (Klien's, Thom's), but this method is satisfactory. One may also obtain the posterior sagittal diameter by geometric methods, since the hypothenuse and the base of the two outlet triangles can be measured. It is apparent that, even if the narrow pubic arch forces the head back against

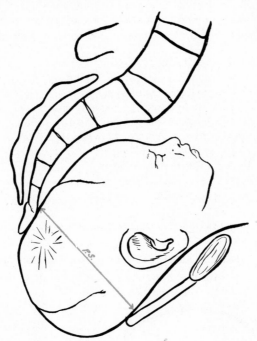

FIG. 644.—HEAD ARRESTED AT OUTLET BY CONTRACTION.
Note how head stems against descending ramus of pubis and is thrown against coccyx.

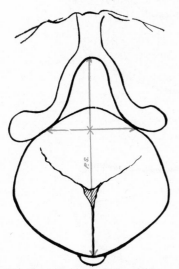

FIG. 645.—HEAD PASSING THE TRANSVERSELY CON-
TRACTED OUTLET.

Space under arch of pubis cannot be utilized. Perineum much endangered. *P.S.*, Posterior sagittal diameter

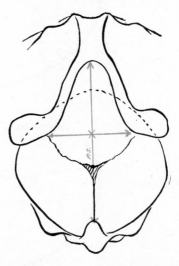

FIG. 646.—ABSOLUTELY IMPOSSIBLE LABOR. HEAD
STOPPED BY NARROWING OUTLET. SACRUM JUTS
FORWARD AND PREVENTS HEAD FROM ESCAPING
IN THE POSTERIOR SAGITTAL DIAMETER.

the perineum and sacrum, if the latter does not curve forward too much, there will still be plenty of room for the passage of the hyperflexed head—only the soft parts will be much endangered. If the bi-ischiatic diameter is less than 8 cm., it is the rule to experience trouble with the delivery and forceps are often needed. If, in addition, the posterior sagittal (Fig. 646) is less than 9 cm., labor is very difficult or even impossible, and craniotomy is usually finally resorted to. General experience shows that a pelvis with a diameter of less than 7.5 cm. between the tuberosities and a posterior sagittal less than 8 cm. with a normal child, offers insuperable obstruction to labor and demands cesarean section, pubiotomy, or craniotomy.

Breech labors are especially bad in funnel and transversely contracted pelves, because the head has no time to mold, and forceps on the after-coming head are very often required. Even then many babies are lost. If the patient is a very old primipara, and if it seems likely that the present will be the only pregnancy, the high infantile mortality and the severe pelvic injuries which are inevitable with forceps delivery should be given great weight when deciding for or against cesarean section. Forced operative delivery in such cases often results in deep lacerations of the vagina, pelvic floor, and rectum, even rupture of the pubis, and shows a painfully high infant mortality (Lit., McCormick).

Coccygosacral ankylosis with the coccyx pointing upward may cause serious delay in delivery of the head through the outlet. Usually the bone is fractured by the passing head or the operator may have to break it deliberately. Eymer sawed the bone off in 2 cases.

LABOR IN OBLIQUELY CONTRACTED PELVIS

Everything depends on the amount of contraction of the conjugata vera, and, of course, on the forward protrusion of the promontory. If the promontory pro-

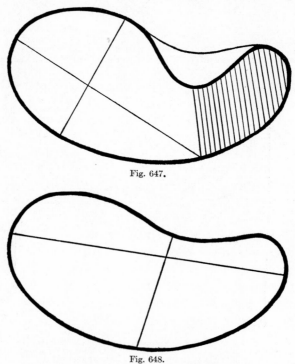

Fig. 647.

Fig. 648.

FIGS. 647 AND 648.—DIAGRAMS SHOWING HOW, WHEN THE PROMONTORY JUTS INTO THE PELVIS ON ONE SIDE, THAT SIDE IS RENDERED USELESS FOR THE ENTRY OF HEAD, AND CHANGES THE INLET TO ONE OF THE HIGHLY GENERALLY CONTRACTED TYPE. SHADED PORTION IS USELESS FOR LABOR.

jects low toward one iliopubic tubercle, it will eliminate that half of the pelvis, as far as using it for the passage of the head is concerned (Figs. 647 and 648). This is equivalent to a generally contracted pelvis of highest degree. A very sharp clinical distinction must be made between pelves which are simply distorted, but with little or no reduction in the area of the inlet, and those which are actually contracted or are so much distorted that actual contraction results. Generally it is best for the occiput to come down in the large half of the pelvis (Figs. 648 and 649), but sometimes it is best for it to enter pointing toward the contracted half. Then the biparietal diameter will lie in promonto-iliopubic diameter, and the forehead come down over the opposite sacro-iliac joint. In Naegelè pelves the labor is further complicated by the reduction in size of the passage all the way to the outlet. In rachitic pelves this does not obtain, and, once the head passes the inlet, labor is quickly ended.

In several of the author's cases the occiput did not rotate to the front, but re-

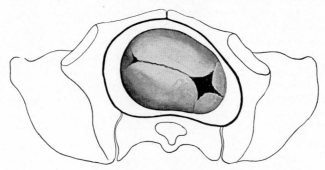

FIG. 649.—HEAD MOLDING INTO AN OBLIQUELY DISTORTED PELVIS.

mained in the oblique, and the head escaped over one or the other ramus pubis, the latter acting as the fulcrum against which the nape of the neck stemmed, while forehead and face appeared from behind the opposite ischial tuberosity. Breech labors are unwelcome in obliquely contracted pelves, and it is most desirable for the occiput to come down on the side *not* contracted. Such a mechanism should be brought about, if possible, during operative delivery.

CHAPTER LVII

PROGNOSIS OF LABOR IN CONTRACTED PELVES

The Mother.—Naturally, it is impossible to present figures of the mortality of labor in contracted pelvis, and the morbidity will always remain indeterminable. Mild degrees of pelvic contraction may not have much effect on the labor except by the production of malpresentations, etc., which demand interference, and operative measures all carry a certain mortality and morbidity. In general, the prognosis of a given labor depends upon, first, the degree of pelvic contraction; second, the size and hardness of the child, especially of its head; third, the presentation, position, and attitude; fourth, the strength of the pains. If a complication, as eclampsia or placenta prævia, is superadded, the prognosis is, of course, altered, and, finally, much depends on the cleanliness and skill of the attendants.

The mother is exposed to the following dangers: (1) Obstructed and impossible labor, which eventuates in—(*a*) Rupture of the uterus; (*b*) septicemia; (*c*) exhaustion and shock, with or without operation; (2) pressure necrosis of the walls of the genital tract; (3) injuries of the genital tract, for example, spontaneous rupture of the uterus, cervix, vagina, symphysis pubis, and traumatic rupture of the same; (4) infection in labor, with physometra (tympania uteri) or general septicemia; (5) exhaustion and shock.

If the labor is completely obstructed, the head wedges itself into the narrow canal and becomes firmly fixed (paragomphosis), the vagina and vulva become enormously swollen, suggillated, and almost black, sometimes sloughing out entirely. In the less severe cases the constant pressure produces areas of necrosis which later make deforming scars or slough out, leaving fistulas,—rectovaginal, vesicovaginal, uterovaginal, etc.,—depending on the part of the pelvic viscera which underwent the severest compression between the head and the pelvis. Flat pelves cause more fistulas than generally contracted, because in the latter the pressure is more evenly distributed. Pressure necrosis of the posterior cervical wall may cause adhesion of the peritoneum over the uterus and that covering the promontory, retrofixation of the uterus resulting. The fistulas are often not apparent for a few days, that is, it requires this time for the slough to separate and establish communication between the two cavities.

Injuries usually are the result of operative delivery, but sometimes the uterus itself, acting with terrific power, may force the child through its own walls, or through the unprepared cervix or perineum, or may even burst the pubic symphysis. Rarely the sacro-iliac joints are separated. Traumatic injury of the soft parts is due to too early and too forcible attempts at delivery, and even a skilful accoucheur may cause it when the tissues are softened and brittle from disease or long labor. The scars from these injuries may distort the pelvic viscera, causing malpositions of the uterus, chronic pelvic congestion, dislocation of the bladder; they may even open the sphincter vesicæ, causing incontinence, etc.

Infection in labor may come from without,—the usual way,—the physician carrying the bacteria either on undisinfected hands or transferring them from the vulva and vagina into sterile regions, and it may occur spontaneously, the result of the reduction of local and general immunity. Local immunity is destroyed in prolonged labor by the loss of the epithelium, its weakening by imbibition, by the alteration of the secretions of the parturient tract, the clear mucus being replaced by serum and blood, and, third, the local traumatisms. The liquor amnii is very prone to decomposition, and once the interior of the uterus is infected, the generalization is rapid. Tympania uteri is sometimes due to the Bacillus aërogenes capsulatus, but more often to the Bacterium coli commune. General immunity is weakened by the exhaustion and shock of the prolonged labor, the loss of sleep, lack of food, anesthetics, and operations. Tetanus uteri is of grave omen. While it does not favor rupture of the uterus, labor comes to an absolute stop, and unless aid is rendered, mother and child are lost from exhaustion and sepsis.

Exhaustion and shock must not be forgotten as complications of prolonged labor, and too much given the patient to overcome. In women of gracile type, the highly polished output of our finishing schools, with one or several generations of overcivilized ancestors, the shock of hard labor is badly borne, and the nervous system may suffer permanent damage. While contracted pelves are uncommon in this class (perhaps a tendency to general smallness may be noted), the children are usually well grown, and since the uterine action is nearly always deficient, operative interference is frequently required. It is important to watch the effect of labor on the nervous system and interfere before serious inroads have been made on it.

Breech and shoulder presentations, in some respects, are better for the mother than the head, because they do not cause pressure necrosis, and early attention is called to the anomalous pelvis. The passage of the child in delivery is rapid, and experience shows that intense compression of short duration is less dangerous to the tissues than a mild pressure kept up for a long time.

The Child.—In the highest degrees of pelvic contraction the child has the best chances for its life, because the absolute disproportion is usually early recognized and cesarean section performed. In the very slight pelvic contractions the infant mortality is not much higher than usual, but anomalies of the mechanism of labor must be remembered. Many children still are lost in the cases where the pelvis is contracted enough to show in the course of labor, and this is because the accoucheur has not carefully studied his patient. Too many women are blindly allowed to go into labor, and only after the good time for cesarean section or pubiotomy has gone by is the spacial disproportion discovered. Often it is found only after the accoucheur has failed to deliver with forceps.

Asphyxia causes the largest number of fetal deaths, and it is brought about by —(1) Interference with the placental circulation, the result of the frequent and powerful uterine contractions—the blood is forced out of the uterus by the pains; (2) compression of the brain as the head is jammed through the inlet—the pressure irritates the pneumogastric, slows the pulse, and compromises still further the oxygenation of the fetal blood; (3) as the effect of the early rupture of the membranes and the escape of the liquor amnii the uterus retracts, the placental area is diminished, and abruption of the organ is favored; (4) prolapse of the cord is common, especially in flat pelves, and this is always a very serious affair for the child. As long as the bag of waters is intact these dangers hardly exist, but it would be wrong to say they never threaten the child, because I have seen death of the fetus occur by the above mechanisms with an intact amniotic sac.

Injuries of the brain, of the cranium, and of the body of the child are very common. Many children die from cerebral compression without external injury, and not a few die from concussion of the brain from forceps or breech delivery. More often death is due to intracranial hemorrhage from skull fracture. This may be in the form of fissures radiating from the center of ossification of the flat bones toward the sutures of the skull. Many times cephalhematoma is due to such fissures, the clot in these instances being outside the skull, under the periosteum. Tears of the tentorium cerebelli also occur in difficult labors. Depressed skull fractures occur with forceps, but particularly with breech deliveries, and they look as if the bone had been pressed in with a spoon (Fig. 650). They are sometimes attended by intracranial hemorrhage, and are then usually fatal. They are most often located between the parietal bosses and the coronary sutures, but one of my cases showed the depression right behind and above the left ear.

If not primarily fatal, the child may recover and show no signs of permanent damage to the brain, the deformity becoming less with time, but never disappearing. Another form of skull depression, not always a fracture, because the bone is soft and flexible, is the groove (Fig. 651). This deformity is due to the molding of the head by the sharp promontory, and disappears almost entirely in a few months. It is harmless of itself, but may be serious if large, deep, or complicated by fracture or intracranial hemorrhage. These flat depressions usually parallel the coronary suture. They require no treatment. Separation of the flat bones at the basilar sutures is one of the worst of the birth injuries, because the large cerebral blood-sinuses lie in the neighborhood, and if torn, allow fatal intracranial hemorrhage.

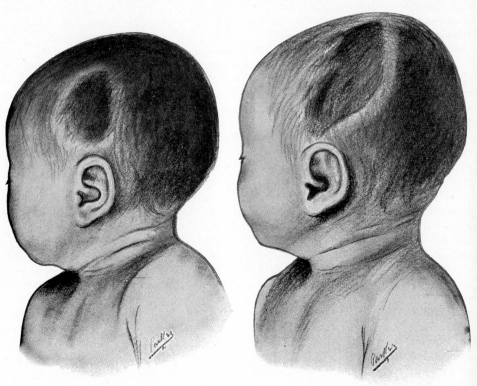

FIG. 650.—SPOON-SHAPED DEPRESSION.   EXTRACTION BY   FIG. 651.—GROOVE DEPRESSION.   FORCEPS CASE.
                         BREECH.
Three successive children had the same injury.

The parietal bone may tear away from the squamous portion of the temporal bone at the anterior lateral fontanel—the sutura squamosa; the occipital plate may separate from the condyles. In the latter instance the plate then may be dislocated directly onto the medulla, causing immediate death.

The morbidity of children delivered through contracted pelves is also very large.

Pressure necrosis of the scalp has been already mentioned. This may be in all degrees from a simple desquamation with redness to actual sloughing of the tissues, with laying bare of the bone and exfoliation of sequestra—in a few instances followed by meningitis. These pressure marks are made by the promontory, but sometimes by an exostosis on the posterior surface of the pubis, and are the external evidence of long labor. Fistulas in the mother usually result at the same time.

Cephalhematoma is a complication of fractures of the skull. The clot lies under the external periosteum, is limited always by the sutures, may be single or multiple, external and internal combined, and may cover a depressed fracture. These hematomata alone are not fatal, but require many months for complete resorption, and leave a ridge of bone at the edges for many weeks more.

Caput succedaneum occurs in its greatest proportions in contracted pelves. It may be visible at the vulva while the head has not yet passed the inlet. Since the caput succedaneum is due to the fact that the pressure inside the uterus is greater than that in the vagina, it indicates strong uterine action. It does not show that the head fits the inlet tightly, and it does not do much to aid in the dilatation of the cervix, as some writers state.

In generally contracted pelves the caput, by lengthening the head wedge, may assist the labor, but little is thus accomplished. Of great clinical importance is the proper estimation of the caput, because if the scalp is visible at the vulva, the accoucheur may hastily conclude that the head is engaged and be misled into unfortunate operating, while in reality the head may be above the inlet. The caput also covers up the landmarks of the head and renders the diagnosis of position very difficult.

Fractures of the clavicle, the humerus, and the femur and disruption of the vertebral column are almost invariably due to brute force, exhibited during operative delivery. The same may be said of tearing of the nerves of the cervical plexus—Erb's paralysis, etc. Fracture of the long bones and of the skull may, however, occur during spontaneous labor.

The author is convinced that many children carry the effects of minor injuries received at birth all their lives. It stands to reason that the innumerable and thickly sown minute hemorrhages found in the brain after forceps and other hard deliveries must leave at least a fibrosis behind. Siegmund has found that cerebral birth trauma causes impairment of the nourishment of adjacent tissues, the resulting degeneration leading to necrosis. These softenings are closely related to the development of cysts, porencephaly, sclerosis, microgyria, etc.

Schwartz found 65 per cent. of all newborns dying within five months presented the evidences of birth trauma, hemorrhages and softening, that could be discerned with the naked eye.

William Sharpe found bloody cerebrospinal fluid in 11 per cent. of 200 normally delivered neonati, and at the Chicago Lying-in Hospital in 12 per cent. of the babies cerebral symptoms were discovered by a thorough routine neurologic examination (Sherman, Sharpe, and Maclaire, Amer. Jour. Obst. and Gyn., 1925, p. 452).

These findings may explain cases of epilepsy, idiocy, paralyses, pareses, chronic headache, tic douloureux, retinal lesions, strabismus, and some other focal nerve diseases in later life. Even abnormal moral and mental conditions might be explained as due to injuries sustained at birth, though at present there is little evidence to support the theory. Such a belief would increase the burden of responsibility, already too heavily laid, on the shoulders of the accoucheur.

The outlook for the child depends, of course, on the degree of pelvic contraction, the severity of the operative delivery, the skill of the accoucheur, and the nature of the operation.

CHAPTER LVIII

TREATMENT OF LABOR IN CONTRACTED PELVIS

No subject in medicine presents greater difficulties in all its aspects than this one, and none demands so much art or practical skill. Science aids comparatively little here. Knowledge of the passages, of the powers, of the passengers, of the mechanism of labor, all help a great deal, but more depends on experience and judgment. Even large experience is fallacious and judgment is difficult—the words of Hippocrates, the truth of which is often proved when the accoucheur finds that a fetus he said could not pass through a certain pelvis is delivered before he can reach the bedside, and another which he confidently predicted would be born easily requires a grave operation. Many factors besides the pelvic contraction enter into the course of the labor, and success in treatment depends on the proper valuation of each and the proper placement of their relations to each other. Some of these factors can be accurately evaluated before or during labor, others partly, and a few not at all. These factors are the attitude, presentation, and position of the child, the size and hardness of its head, the shape of its body, whether there are one or two fetuses, the shape of the pelvis, that is, the distribution of the available space, the height of the promontory, the inclination of the inlet, the movability of the pelvic synchondroses, the state of the soft parts, the character of the uterine contractions (strong pains being able to accomplish wonderful results), the presence or absence of infection in the parturient canal, the nervous temperament of the parturient, and her general health. Outside factors must also often be considered: (1) The environment, whether the parturient is in a squalid tenement, in the country, in a home where every appliance is obtainable, or in a well-equipped maternity; (2) whether in the hands of the general practitioner or a trained specialist; (3) if the patient is a Catholic, all medically indicated procedures not being permitted; (4) the age of the parturient and the probability of her having more children. Even with this enumeration, the possible factors which might influence a labor or our decision regarding the course to pursue have not all been mentioned. *It must always be borne in mind that nature is able to overcome the difficulties of contracted pelves in the majority of cases.* Ludwig and Savor found that 75 per cent. of such cases terminate spontaneously when the conjugata vera is not less than 9.5 cm.; that 58 per cent. with a conjugata vera of 9 cm., 50 per cent. with one of 8.5 cm., and 25 per cent. with one of 8 cm., require no aid from art. A course of watchful expectancy was all that was needed in these labors (Williams and Sun).

Diagnosis of Disproportion.—In all cases the first thing to determine is the existence and degree of disproportion between the child and the pelvis; in other words, the question must be answered, will the child go through the pelvis? The routine measurement of the pelvis of every pregnant woman coming under his care will have directed the accoucheur's attention to the existence of obstruction in the birth canal. Four weeks before labor another examination should be made because it is much easier to obtain the internal measurements at this time. (See p. 252.) Special attention is given the pelvic outlet. The history of previous labors is of great value, but it must be carefully sifted. A woman may have had severe dystocia, even craniotomy or cesarean section, and yet have a normal pelvis which would give no trouble in the present labor. It is possible, with moderate experience and thorough application of our present methods, to obtain a quite accurate knowledge of the actual size of the pelvic lumen.

Not so much may be said of the child. It is harder to form an opinion of its size, and still harder to estimate the ossification and configurability of its head. The intra-uterine length of the child is easily measured (p. 289). With the cephalometer the transverse or the oblique diameters of the head can be obtained, and by deducting $2\frac{1}{2}$ or $1\frac{1}{2}$ cm., the biparietal diameter is approximately estimated—at least, one gains a fairly accurate idea of the size of the head. By grasping the child from the outside and placing the fingers against the head per vaginam, one may balance its body between the two hands and guess its weight and size. This guess is not always trustworthy. One determines the hardness of the fetal head by the general impression of firmness of the bones conveyed to the fingers, the sharpness of the contour of the parietal bosses, the size of the fontanels (if almost obliterated,

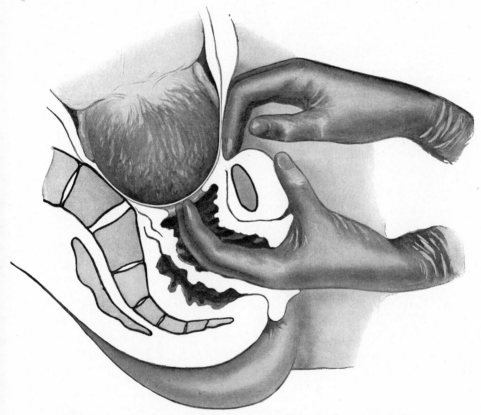

FIG. 652.—PALPATING HEAD AND ITS RELATIONS TO THE POSTERIOR SURFACE OF THE PUBIS.
This head would probably not enter the pelvis. Such an examination may be as well made per rectum.

it shows hyperossification), the extent to which the bones overlap during the pains, and the breadth of the dome of the cranium. If the bones are soft, the dome is acute, while a hard calvarium is more flat. Previous children may have been large or small, with hard or soft heads, and the length of the present pregnancy must also be taken into consideration; also the size of the parents and the shape of their heads. Children that are carried overterm usually have large hard heads.

After getting as good a general idea as possible of the size and consistence of the child, the accoucheur tries to determine, by more direct means, if the head is likely to go through the pelvis. For this purpose it is better if the woman has been in actual labor until the cervix is effaced and pulled up out of the pelvis, thus allowing the fetal head to apply itself more closely to the inlet. However, such conditions are not always met, and one has to form his judgment by allowing duly for disturbing factors. Figure 652 shows the first manœuver. The head is forced down on to the inlet, the fingers inside steadying it, and it is then easy to find if the anterior parietal boss projects in front of the posterior surface of the pubis and how much overriding there is. If the child presents with the occiput posterior, the forehead will be quite prominent in front, and this point must not be forgotten. A full rectum or the placenta will also push the head forward. Müller's procedure consists in having an assistant force the head down into the inlet while the inside fingers determine how far it enters the pelvis. It has value only after the cervix is out of the way, because the soft parts will prevent the head from engaging under the amount of downward pressure it is possible safely to exert by the two hands. The most valuable of all is the determination of the degree of engagement. Reference has already been made to the criteria of engagement of the fetal head (see pp. 310, 311). If the vault of the pelvis is empty, the head being high and floating, in the absence of other causes for nonengagement the pelvis is probably much contracted; if the head enters the region of the inlet with a large segment projecting into the excavation and is more or less fixed, and if, during a pain, the head seems to attempt that mechanism which is best suited to the pelvis the accoucheur may feel fairly sure that the pains will succeed in molding it sufficiently for spontaneous delivery.

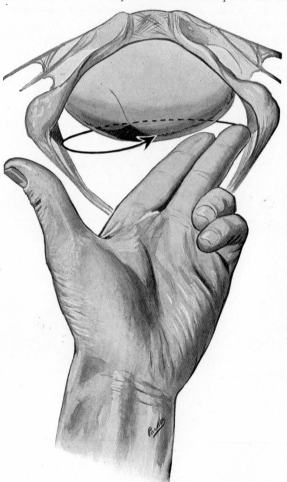

Fig. 653.—Determining the Number of Centimeters the Head Lies Above or Below the Interspinous Line.

The fingers touch the left ischial spine, then swing around pelvis to the right one, then touch the lowest portion of head. This may also be done per rectum.

Passing the fingers around the head and alternately touching the walls of the pelvis it is not hard to form a quite accurate conception of the degree of disproportion. Combined palpation of the head, like that used in estimating the size of the uterus, gives useful information. If the lowest portion of the head has reached the interspinous line (Fig. 653), engagement is usually certain. In flat rachitic pelves the side walls are so low that this sign must be qualified. Here the lowest portion of the head must have passed this line by a little. The other signs—the covering of the sacrum and of the pubis —are also valuable, particularly the former. One must not be misled by the lengthening of the head produced by extreme moulding. One must always determine if the larger portion of the head is not still above the inlet, even though the occiput has reached the interspinous line. Simple pressure of the finger-tips above the pubis in the direction of the sacrum will tell us if and how the head sinks into the pelvis, and the changing level of the chin gives useful information, too.

Now a minute diagnosis of presentation, position, and attitude must be made. If the child presents in a frank O.L.A., the probabilities of a disturbing degree of pelvic contraction are not so strong. If the anterior or posterior parietal bone presents and the attitude does not correct itself under the influence of the pains, usually a badly contracted pelvis exists. The presence of anterior or posterior parietal bone presentation generally must be taken as an indication of grave dystocia, though nature occasionally terminates such cases happily. However, in deciding beforehand whether a given head will pass through a given pelvis these abnormal presentations are very significant, because if they are very marked, the likelihood of a successful spontaneous delivery is remote.

A careful study of the uterine action is now in order. Good regular pains may overcome great resistances. Weak, infrequent, irregular, or cramp-like pains may be unable to terminate a labor otherwise normal. The nervous constitution of the woman will also require some attention. A nervous, impatient, unruly disposition, or even acute nervous prostration, may be the cause for interference when the mechanical disproportion is not great.

Finally, we have the test of labor, but the attendant's decision regarding his conduct of the case must be made before he trusts the case to nature.

For purposes of discussion it is customary to divide contracted pelves into four classes. It must be emphasized, at the very start, that such a division is purely arbitrary, because the size of the child is not considered, nor are any of the above-mentioned factors allowed for, but some common basis for discussion must be had.

I. Pelves with a conjugata vera less than $5\frac{1}{2}$ cm. in the flat, and 6 cm. in the generally contracted, variety. These are absolutely contracted.

II. Pelves with a conjugata vera of $5\frac{1}{2}$ to $7\frac{1}{2}$ cm. in flat, and 6 to 8 cm. in the generally contracted, types. These are relatively contracted.

III. Pelves with a conjugata vera of $7\frac{1}{2}$ to 9 cm. in flat, and 8 to $9\frac{1}{2}$ cm. in the generally contracted. These are moderately contracted.

IV. Pelves with a conjugata vera over 9 and $9\frac{1}{2}$ cm. respectively, and are border-line cases.

I. In the absolutely contracted pelvis no difficulty is met in deciding on treatment. A full-sized child cannot be delivered through it, and for this reason cesarean section is indicated whether or not the child is living. This is the absolute indication for the operation. If the woman is seen early in pregnancy, therapeutic abortion comes up, but the author does not recommend it, preferring cesarean section at term, under the ideal conditions always obtainable when the pelvic contraction is so timely recognized. If the accoucheur is called late in labor, when infection is probably present, Porro cesarean section is indicated or laparotrachelotomy or Latzko's extraperitoneal operation.

II. In the relatively contracted pelvis (conjugata vera, $5\frac{1}{2}$ and 6 to $7\frac{1}{2}$ and 8 cm.) decision also is not very difficult. Nowadays, a pelvis of this degree of contraction is usually discovered early in pregnancy, and, since induction of labor is out of the question, owing to its high fetal mortality, the patient is advised to have an elective cesarean at term. In the event the pelvis is at the upper limit of contraction and the child small, the case falls into Class III, q. v. If called to such a patient after labor has begun, careful consideration is needed. If the child is dead, craniotomy is indicated. A full-sized child cannot be gotten through the pelvis alive, and the question to decide is, Shall the mother be subjected to the risks of the classic cesarean section in order to save the infant? This is the relative indication for cesarean section, and it may be allowed only under certain conditions. If the woman has been in active labor a long time; if the membranes have been ruptured for many hours; if frequent internal examinations have been made, and by hands whose asepsis cannot be assured; if operative delivery has been attempted;

if infection has begun or is suspected—certainly if the woman has fever or fetid discharge, the *classic cesarean section* from the relative indication is prohibited. If bad conditions do not exist, but the case has come early into the hands of a man capable of his task, uninfected, and in suitable surroundings, cesarean section is *the operation of election*. In the first instance craniotomy is not alone justifiable, but demanded, and in the second instance the accoucheur must recommend the abdominal delivery. The facts are to be laid before the patient, the husband, and the family, and they must decide. Naturally, the accoucheur should guide them in the decision, and if they do not agree with him, he should not be constrained to sacrifice the child when the conditions are ideal for cesarean section. Nor should he, when convinced that the disproportion is too great, allow the woman to labor until the right time for the abdominal delivery has gone by. He is at liberty to retire from the case under either circumstance, but must first provide, or see that the family provides, other medical assistance.

These lines were written in 1909, and they are equally true today. However, they do not apply to the man who has learned the new method of abdominal delivery, the low, cervical section, laparotrachelotomy (p. 775). He may extend the indication for abdominal delivery to cases where vaginal examinations have been made, and even where delivery from below has been attempted (in favorable conditions, of course). We must not go too far even with laparotrachelotomy, but in the presence of real genital infection, perform Porro's operation or craniotomy.

An immense mass of literature has been accumulated on the question of the justifiability of craniotomy on the living child. In a paper published in 1901 (American Journal of Obstetrics, vol. xliv, No. 4) the author considered the subject in all its aspects, and has changed his opinions but little since.

Kossmann, Mann, Leopold, Olshausen, Schauta, Chrobak, and Knapp have written exhaustively on it, and reached the same general conclusions. The stand taken by the Catholic Church is well known. Under no circumstances may human life be deliberately taken even when it is done to save another life. In Catholic families, therefore, the accoucheur is in duty bound to consider this aspect of the case, and the author makes it an invariable rule to remind the patient and family of this view of the Church, and to ask that the family priest be summoned to aid in their deliberations.

With few exceptions, all experienced writers are agreed that the sacrifice of the living child is still occasionally justifiable. The cases in which this is necessary are very scarce and becoming scarcer each year, there having been so much improvement in obstetric teaching and practice that severe dystocia is more often recognized early—in time for life-saving operations. Neglected and unrecognized dystocia still occurs, mistaken and unsuccessful operations are still attempted, aseptic care of parturients is still not universal, and infection is still common, so that when the accoucheur finally has to complete the delivery, he is usually glad to be able to save one life. Again, a woman may absolutely refuse to endanger her own life for her child, and this she has a perfect right to do. On the other hand, the necessity of sacrificing a perfectly healthy child never arises. When the patient reaches this point the child has nearly always been injured by long labor, by attempts at delivery, by being infected or, having inspired infected liquor amnii, it very often dies within a few days, even if delivered alive. Furthermore, 30 per cent. of all children die before they are five years old. In comparing the life values of mother and child, these facts must be considered. (See also Coppens, von Oppenrooy, and the late excellent little book of Rev. E. J. Burke.)

Without doubt, in former years too many children were sacrificed and infantile life was held too cheaply. Nowadays we are saving a great many by means of cesarean section and pubiotomy, but there is a tendency to go to the other extreme, and expose the mothers to greater dangers than the end justifies. It is too bad to have to say it, but the author feels it is true—that one of the causes of the present high mortality of the mothers in childbirth in the United States is the exaggerated and often unwarranted valuation put upon the child's life already rendered precarious by complicated labor. As Chrobak observes, "it almost seems we must protect the mothers against the children and that we forget that *salus matris suprema lex*."

Since the vast majority of births occur not in the large cities, where maternities and specialists are obtainable, but in towns, villages, and in the country, it will follow that many children will have to be sacrificed to save the mothers, and the accoucheur will deserve congratulations if, under trying circumstances and amid unfavorable conditions, he saves the mother. All accoucheurs, however, breathe one prayer—speed the day when craniotomy of the living child can be abolished!

If craniotomy has to be performed because of pelvic contraction, the woman, the husband, and the family must be instructed that in the event of a subsequent pregnancy medical aid is to be provided early, and arrangements made for cesarean section under ideal conditions. The accoucheur should not be asked to perform craniotomy a second time on the same woman. Such an operation today is unjustifiable, owing to the perfection of obstetric art.

III. **In the moderately contracted pelves,** those with a conjugata vera of $7\frac{1}{2}$ to 9 cm., and 8 to $9\frac{1}{2}$ cm. (in the flat and generally contracted types respectively), the most delicate questions and the greatest difficulties arise.

Treatment During Pregnancy.—Induction of Premature Labor.—Since a small infant with a soft small head can usually pass through a moderately contracted pelvis and survive, we may make use of this knowledge and induce labor at a period of pregnancy when the child has not yet attained a size sufficient to block the pelvis.

Louise Bourgeois (born 1563, died 1636), midwife to Marie de Médicis, first recommended and practised the induction of premature labor to save the life of the mother, and gave as indication intractable hemorrhage. Roussel de Vauzelme, in 1778, recommended the operation in contracted pelvis, saying that Petit had practised it many years. In the middle of the nineteenth century the operation had a good vogue, and deserved it, because the mortality of cesarean section, symphysiotomy, and craniotomy was so high. As the technic and results of these operations improved the preference went to them, because of the high infant mortality and dangers and troublesome complications of induced labor, but even today the majority of authorities agree that the induction of labor after viability of the child is a valuable operation.

If the contraction of the pelvis is known early in pregnancy, the course of treatment to be pursued must be at once decided upon. Many women consider a previous difficult labor sufficient indication for the induction of abortion, and come to the physician with this request. In the first place, a previous difficult labor may have been due to entirely different causes or even incompetent medical care, and in the class of pelves under consideration this indication will never arise, because, if necessary, labor can be induced after a fetal viability, with no more danger than abortion and with over 60 per cent. chances of saving the infant. The facts are to be laid before the family, but the accoucheur's decision not to do an abortion should be final. Primarily, it must be stated that a large number—perhaps 75 per cent.—of labors in such pelves terminate spontaneously at or near term; second, that cesarean section performed, as it can be, when the need for it is known so far beforehand, has a very low mortality—less than 2 per cent.; third, that should the event prove that labor will not terminate spontaneously, in pubiotomy and laparo-trachelotomy we have operations that will still save the child and not seriously endanger the mother; fourth, that should all our plans fail, craniotomy could be performed as a last resort after the test of labor has been faithfully tried, and we would not lose a larger number of babies than with induced labor.

On the other hand, the operation of induced labor is not absolutely safe. Statistics give the maternal mortality as 1 to 2 per cent., but nowadays, in the hands of a capable accoucheur, there should be no mortality. From 20 to 30 per cent. of the children are lost in labor, and another portion dies within a few weeks, in spite of the incubator, good nursing, etc. Then, too, the uterus is sometimes very sluggish and torpid, requiring much stimulation, instrumentation, frequent examinations, etc., lasting several days to even a week. Although our calculations have been as careful as is humanly possible, and our decisions logical, mistakes often creep in; for example, the child is too large to come through, or it is too small to live after being born. Accidents also complicate the process; for example, the position and presentation are unfavorable, the cord prolapses, the nervous condition of the patient requires interference before the os is open, fever arises, which forces our hand, or, indeed, the child, while large enough, is atelectatic or deformed, so it cannot live. All these conditions have been observed by the author and have much reduced his enthusiasm for the induction of premature labor in contracted pelves, and he very rarely performs it. In marked kyphoscoliosis the growing uterus may so encroach on the chest cavity that respiration is embarrassed—requiring labor before full term.

If the family elects the induction of premature labor as being less dangerous—and in private practice they usually do choose it—the accoucheur has to decide

49

on the right time to begin it. A period must be selected when the child is not too large to pass through the pelvis and yet developed enough for extra-uterine exist-ence. The best time is between the thirty-second and thirty-fourth week. After the thirty-sixth week the child is too large; before the thirtieth week its chances of survival are poor. Added to the difficulties of determining the exact period of pregnancy—and errors of three weeks either way are not uncommon—is the fact that some children develop faster than others, and are as large at eight months as the others are at term. My practice, in cases set aside for premature labor, is as follows: The date of conception is fixed as accurately as possible, using the dates of menstruation, coitus, and quickening as a basis. At the sixth month, and every two weeks thereafter, the child is carefully palpated and measured (p. 283). If, as the thirty-third week approaches, the child is found to be getting too large to pass through the pelvis, labor is started. If possible, the day is selected which would correspond to the time of the menstrual period, because at such periods the uterus is more sensitive and reacts quicker to stimulation. Müller's procedure—pressing the head into the pelvis to see if it can enter—has proved valueless in my hands. The women will not tolerate the small amount of pain thus caused, and, further, the soft parts may prevent the engagement of a head which a few labor pains can force through very easily. The decision as to the right time to begin is one of experience, and everything depends on the judgment of the accoucheur.

J. Aitken in 1790 advised plastics on the pubic bones, and Olliver, about 1858, proposed symphysiotomy in pregnancy, to provide the enlargement of the pelvis for delivery, and Frank and Jellett (1919) practised it shortly before term.

Rotter in 1911 suggested the removal of a piece of the promontory to enlarge the con-jugate, and Schmid in 1913 reported 8 cases in one of which delivery had been successfully accom-plished. Costa in 1921 proposed superior symphysiectomy, i. e., exsection of the upper half of the symphysis pubis, for the permanent enlargement of the inlet. None of these operations has been done in America.

Prochownick's Diet.—A strict diet aiming to restrain fetal growth, of historic interest.

Treatment of Moderately Contracted Pelves During Labor.—In the first stage the question to decide is, shall we interfere at once or shall we await the test of labor?—interference or watchful expectancy? In primiparæ, when the parturient is not quite at term, in cases where the child does not seem very large, or where the pelvic contraction is near the upper limit, with the conjugata vera 9 to $9\frac{1}{2}$ cm., and where the probability of good strong pains seems good, my advice is to wait and see what nature will accomplish. The pains slowly mold the head into the inlet, and disproportion that seemed insuperable is finally overcome, or the head forced so low that it can be easily extracted by the forceps. We can hope for such a termination in 75 per cent. of the cases.

When the conditions are the opposite; when the careful, complete examination shows that the disproportion between the child and the pelvis is one that is not likely to be overcome by the natural forces; if the presentation and position are bad; when the history of previous labors is unfavorable or the general constitution of the woman such that a severe parturition cannot be borne—cesarean section is the operation of choice.

Having decided to give the woman the test, labor should be so conducted as not to spoil the chances for an eventual pubiotomy or cesarean section. Vaginal examination is omitted and but few rectals made. The rupture of the membranes is to be prevented by keeping the patient on her side, forbidding bearing-down efforts, care in internal examinations. When dilatation of the cervix is complete, the membranes may be allowed to rupture in order to permit the head to apply itself snugly to the inlet and complete the molding process. Molding may begin in an intact sac. Should the membranes rupture before the cervix is completely dilated, the colpeurynter—now preferably a Voorhees bag with flat top—is placed inside the cervix. This keeps the head from exerting injurious pressure on the bladder, prevents incarceration of the anterior lip of the cervix between the head and symphysis, preserves the liquor amnii left in the uterus, strengthens the pains, and helps to dilate the cervix. During the first stage an attempt may be made to bring the head into a good position over the inlet. For example, it may be possible, by manually correcting a posterior or anterior parietal bone presentation, to place the head in a way to enter the pelvis easily. By using the crouching position, with one knee up, a head which has slid off the inlet into one iliac fossa may be led back over the inlet (Fig. 654). Hofmeier's impression of the head from the outside may also be tried, but I have never thus succeeded in accomplishing any real results. It is not entirely safe. The hands may bruise the lower uterine segment or compress the cord lying around the neck. Naturally, in such prolonged labors, and with so frequent vaginal manipulations, the dangers of in-

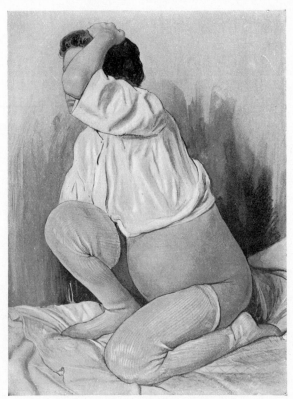

Fig. 654.—Crouching or Indian Attitude.
Only one knee is up.

fection are increased. Special attention must be paid to the bowels, since a full rectum may prevent engagement. The same is to be said of the bladder. Bloody urine and frequent desire to urinate indicate injurious pressure on the bladder, which perhaps will result in gangrene and fistula.

At the end of the first stage, and in the beginning of the second stage, the parturient may be placed in the Walcher position (Fig. 655). Walcher discovered that the conjugata vera could be lengthened by hyperextension of the thighs with the pelvis fixed. The softening of the pelvic joints in pregnancy permits the sacrum to become movable, and by dropping the legs, for example, over the edge of the table on which the sacrum is fixed, the innominate bones rotate downward, enlarging the inlet. Owing to the oblique direction of the articular processes of the sacrum, this motion naturally causes the lower ends of the innominates to approach each other and narrow the outlet.

Mercurio, in 1589, and Melli, in 1738, used this position to facilitate delivery. The true conjugate may be lengthened from 6 to 12 mm., especially in flat pelves. In practice the woman's legs are warmly covered, the pelvis brought to the very edge of the bed, and the feet dropped out straight onto a soft pillow. In a few cases I have gotten the head to enter the pelvis by this procedure, but it is very painful, and few women can be compelled to keep it up over twenty to forty minutes.

My results, curiously, have been better by the use of the exaggerated lithotomy position (Fig. 495, p. 623), which is theoretically contraindicated because it contracts the inlet. The thighs force the uterus up, correcting the pendulous belly so common with contracted pelvis; the uterus and child are straightened out, the former being thus allowed to act with more directness, and the latter being brought into better position over the inlet. It is also possible that an occasional parietal bone or

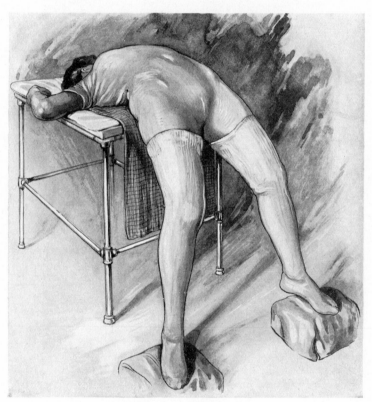

Fig. 655.—The Walcher Position.

ear presentation is corrected. The exaggerated lithotomy position may be kept up for several hours or repeated at intervals. Four dangers must now be watched for —asphyxia of the child, exhaustion of the mother, ascending infection, and rupture of the uterus. The advance signs of these dangers will be described in appropriate chapters. How long the parturient may be allowed to labor depends on the judgment of the accoucheur. Every two or three hours a rectal examination is to be made to measure the progress, and if there is a little, with none of the four dangers impending, it is safe to wait. It is unwise to allow the second stage to continue much over two hours if the pains are strong and the head wedged into the inlet. Fistulas are apt to result, and the child's brain may suffer injury.

If spontaneous labor does not occur, there are five operations that come up for consideration—VERSION, followed by extraction; HIGH FORCEPS; HEBOSTEOTOMY; LOW, OR CERVICAL CESAREAN SECTION; and CRANIOTOMY.

Version is performed only when the head is freely movable, before the lower uterine segment has thinned out enough to invite the danger of rupture during the manipulation and in cases of abnormal presentation, position and attitude; for example, shoulder, face, brow, anterior and posterior parietal bone presentation, and prolapse of the cord. Prophylactic version means version by the breech during or at the end of the first stage of labor in contracted pelves. The term was introduced by Fritsch. Simpson showed that the after-coming head passes through the pelvis easier than when the blunt vertex precedes. The wedge is longer, and the head adapts itself better to the inlet. The accoucheur also has a handle to pull on. Whether the small amount of cerebrospinal fluid which escapes under pressure from the cranium into the spinal canal reduces to any extent the volume of the head is very doubtful. Experience confirms the theory, but the results are not much better, if at all, than leaving the head to mold its way through the pelvis. True, with molding there are the dangers of prolonged cerebral compression, fracture and necrosis of the skull, and vesicovaginal and other fistulas, and peritonitis in the mother. On the other hand, with prophylactic version and extraction the child sometimes suffers severe injury in being dragged quickly and forcibly through a narrow passage, cerebral concussion and fracture of the skull, rupture of the tentorium cerebelli, separation of the occipital plate from the condyles, intracranial hemorrhage, disruption of the cervical vertebræ, fracture of the clavicles and humeri—all these and more have repeatedly occurred.

Paré, in 1585, recommended version in contracted pelvis, but this was before the invention of the forceps, and today, while used occasionally, it is giving way to expectancy followed by pubiotomy, or high forceps and craniotomy. In primiparæ with contracted pelvis, especially the justo-minor, version is rarely elected, the rigidity of the soft parts usually defeating all attempts to save the baby, and deep and dangerous lacerations almost always resulting.

Version may be useful in multiparæ with weak pains, or those who will not work, or when an indication on the part of the mother or child arises which demands immediate delivery. If version is attempted, one must be prepared to perform craniotomy on the after-coming head, because if it does not come through, this is the only alternative. On the other hand, when forceps are applied and fail, we have another operation which may save the child—hebosteotomy. This is an argument against version in contracted pelvis. It has been suggested to place the hebosteotomy saw around the bone, then to perform the version, and, if in the extraction the head is arrested, to cut open the pelvis. An expert might try this.

The Forceps.—When the head has molded so that it seems about ready to slip down into the pelvis and the powers give out, or another indication arises to terminate labor, the forceps may be employed. The instrument is brutal—it overcomes resistance with force, and in all cases either the mother or the babe, or both, suffer. Before beginning the operation the family must be advised, first, that the instrument is applied as a matter of trial, an experiment, and, second, that if it fails they must decide whether hebosteotomy or craniotomy should follow. Pinard, in Paris, Schauta, in Vienna, and Krönig, in Freiburg, insist that the selection of the operation is not the right of the patient or her family, but solely of the accoucheur. In most countries, to perform any operation on another person without his consent, even to save his life, is a tort. Further, the right of a mother to refuse to endanger herself for the child should be self-evident. The physician can and should, in favorable cases, throw the weight of his influence to save the child, and very few families will refuse to follow his advice. Preparations are made for both operations. When the patient is anesthetized, a complete examination will determine if the forceps offer any hope of success. If they do, a few traction efforts, certainly not over three, will demonstrate it. Failing the forceps, hebosteotomy should follow if the child is in prime condition, and craniotomy if it is not. The operation is termed high forceps, and carries with it a fetal mortality ranging from 15 to 40 per cent., and a maternal mortality of 2 to 4 per cent. Much confusion exists as to the exact definition of "high forceps." Most authors apply it to the use of forceps when the largest circumference of the head has not yet passed, but is just about to pass, the region of the inlet, and this seems the best to me. Some writers wish the term "high" to mean the head fully above the inlet, "floating"; some, on the other hand, call the operation high after the head has engaged, but has not yet reached the second parallel plane of Hodge. The difficulty of appraising the values of statistics offered for the operation is thus made apparent, because the dangers of the various operations are vastly different.

In flat pelves, after the head has passed the inlet, delivery is usually easily accomplished, either by the natural powers or by the use of forceps, and the dangers to the mother and babe are very slight. In generally contracted and in funnel pelves the trouble is not over when the head is engaged—it may begin at this point, and if spontaneous delivery does not occur, the worst forms of dystocia may result. The forceps here are equivalent almost to the old-fashioned cephalotribe; the child often dies, is always seriously injured, and the mother never escapes without extensive damage. It is all the more important, therefore, for the accoucheur to determine the nature of the pelvis with which he has to deal, and avoid forceps and version in those with general or funnel contraction. Cesarean section and hebosteotomy come more to the front in these conditions.

As a rule, version and forceps do not compete, but sometimes the conditions for the two operations are evenly balanced and individual preference will decide. In rare cases one may, though it violates traditions, perform version after the forceps have failed.

Symphysiotomy and Hebosteotomy, or Pubiotomy.—By cutting the pelvic girdle it is possible to enlarge the pelvic cavity in all its diameters. If the pelvic joints are loosened more than usual, the enlargement is very marked. Section at or near the pubis allows the bones to separate 2 or 2½ cm., and when the head passes through, they part even 6 or 7 cm.—the latter, however, not without some danger to the sacro-iliac joints. With a separation of 6 cm. the conjugata vera lengthens 1 to 1½ cm., the transversa 2.5 to 3 cm., and obliques about the same. An important gain in space is obtained by the anterior parietal bone fitting into the gap between the divided

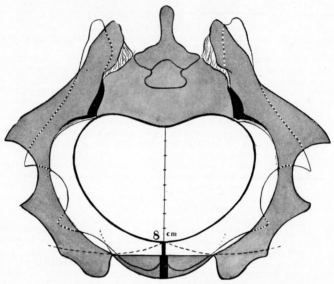

FIG. 656.—ENLARGEMENT OF THE PELVIS IN SYMPHYSIOTOMY (from Farabeuf and Varnier). The area of inlet is augmented about 50 per cent. Note how the head may utilize the gap between the severed bones.

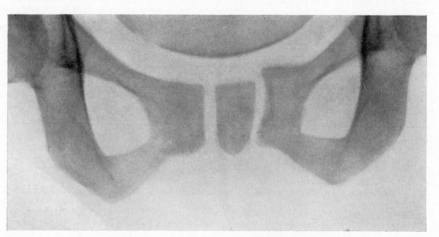

FIG. 657.—X-RAY FOUR YEARS AFTER HEBOSTEOTOMY.

ends of the rami pubis. In flat pelves the greatest gain is obtained (Fig. 656). Section of the symphysis pubis (symphysiotomy) has been replaced almost entirely by the Stolz-Gigli (pronounced "zheelee") operation of pubiotomy, or, more correctly, hebosteotomy, the sawing through of the ramus pubis alongside the joint. The gain in space is the same with the two operations (Cusmano). Symphysiotomy had a mortality varying from 3 to 12 per cent. for the mothers, and 9 to 19 per cent. for the children, and, taking the results of nine of the best operators together, 6.78 per cent. for the mother and 10.6 per cent. for the children. At the operation severe hemorrhage from the wound, particularly when there were varicose veins, extensive injury of the anterior vaginal wall and the perineum, tearing of the levator ani from the rami pubis, the lacerations communicating with the joint, tearing of the bladder and urethra, overstretching of the sacro-iliac joints, with rupture of their anterior ligaments, hematoma around the joint (more with hebosteotomy) were reported with great frequency. In a few cases bony union of the pubis, requiring the saw, and ankylosis of the sacro-iliac joints, necessitating final resort to craniotomy and cesarean section, were met. Convalescence was frequently interrupted and prolonged by infection of the wound and pyemia because of poor drainage, the poor healing qualities of the cartilaginous joint, the proximity of the septic vagina, and the frequent tears communicating with it. Hematomata; thrombosis in the veins and embolism; slow healing of the joint, with prolonged sickness in bed and difficulty of locomotion later (in two of the author's cases locomotion was impaired two and eight months respectively); loss of control of the bladder; descensus and prolapse of the uterus; dislocation and distortion of the base of the bladder and deforming scars of the soft parts; and hernia between the bones were other accidents and sequelæ. The union of the joint was never bony, but after several months a sufficient degree of firmness was attained. It is claimed that most of these disabilities of the operation are removed if one does it by the subcutaneous method of Frank, or Zarate, and that an advantage accrues in subsequent labors from widening of the joint.

Hebosteotomy aims to avoid some of these dangers, and, indeed, the mortality is less for the mother, though about the same for the child, and the morbidity is less. Since the cut in the bony ring is made at the side of the joint, the stuctures around the latter, the urethra, the bladder, the clitoris, the large venous plexuses, etc., are a little less liable to injury. It is said that by making the operation practically subcutaneous, the danger of infection is lessened; tears communicating with the vagina are rarer; severe hemorrhage is rare; the operation requires less skill (?); convalescence is quicker and simpler.

Schläfli, in 1907, reported 700 hebosteotomies with a maternal mortality of 4.96 per cent. and a fetal of 9.18 per cent., but individual operators (Williams, Stoeckel) have had series of 43 and 24 cases without a maternal death (Roemer). Schwarz in 1921 reported 113 cases with a maternal mortality of 2.6 per cent., and fetal, 7 per cent.

	SCHLÄFLI (1908) IN 700 CASES FOUND:	ROEMER (1911) FOUND
Severe hemorrhage	15.00 per cent.	15.40 per cent.
Fatal hemorrhage, two cases	0.00 " "	0.33 " "
Hematoma	17.00 " "	14.00 " "
Vagina tore into wound	15.00 " "	7.00 " "
Deaths of these latter	12.60 " "	3.90 " "
Injury to bladder	12.30 " "	5.20 " "
Fever postpartum	31.70 " "	20.60 " "
Thrombophlebitis	8.00 " "	3.50 " "
Incontinence of urine	4.00 " "	0.00 " "
General (corrected) mortality	4.37 " "	2.66 " "
General (corrected) fetal mortality	9.18 " "	6.66 " "

Neither symphysiotomy nor pubiotomy is often performed today. Cervical cesarean has replaced them. In the rare case of a head arrested at the outlet of a funnel pelvis, after forceps have failed, one might, given favorable conditions, resort to it.

Extraperitoneal Cesarean Section.—This is an operation with an incision just above the pubis, by which access is gained to the lower uterine segment and the child delivered without entering the peritoneal cavity. (See p. 1102 for details.) The reception the new operation got in 1906, 1908, and 1909 was very enthusiastic, because the hope was revived that at last it would be possible to do away with craniotomy on the living child when the conditions were not good for the classic cesarean section. Experience, however, has shown that these dangers beset the new operation: (1) The peritoneum is sometimes opened unintentionally; (2) the bladder is sometimes torn; (3) hemorrhage from the veins may be alarming; (4) the immense space in the connective tissue is liable to hematoma formation or infection, with abscess, which may break into the peritoneal cavity; (5) thrombosis of the immense veins laid bare and embolism; (6) infection and peritonitis, the thin layer of peritoneum not offering an efficient barrier; (7) difficulty of technic; (8) the fetal mortality is high. With proper technic, and this has been much improved of late, most of these dangers are avoided.

Laparotrachelotomy.—This is a simpler method of incision in the neck of the uterus possessing all the advantages of the extraperitoneal operation. It is a transperitoneal approach, but the opening in the abdomen, right above the pubis, is so low that the intestines are not disturbed and the field but slightly soiled by the "spill." Seepage of the lochia is prevented and other advantages follow. This is the operation meant when we speak of the low, or cervical, cesarean, and for which I suggested the name laparotrachelotomy. It is rapidly displacing the old classic section in abdominal delivery, the world over. One may perform it in cases where the former would be too dangerous, i. e., after a prolonged test of labor, after the membranes have ruptured, after vaginal examinations have been done, and even, under favorable circumstances, after minor attempts at delivery have been made. Since it has proved safer under these conditions, naturally it would be safer in clean, elective sections, and, therefore, I use the new operation also in those cases where formerly I did the classic cesarean.

In infected and neglected patients it will show a certain mortality, and for these cases Küstner and Doederlein prefer the purely extraperitoneal method, claiming thus to have almost abolished the necessity for craniotomy on the living child. Most authors prefer Porro's operation or craniotomy.

While I insist that in frankly infected cases (fever, high pulse, foul liquor amnii, gray exudate on vulvar wounds) all forms of abdominal delivery are too dangerous, especially as in such conditions the child's life is already compromised (injury from long labor, from attempts at delivery, from infection), yet experience has shown that the newer operations offer much hope of success where the conditions are not too bad. (See Gottschalk-Portes operation p. 1108.)

Craniotomy.—When the child is dead, craniotomy should be performed as soon as the cervix is large enough to permit it, *i. e.*, 9 cm. across. If the child is dying, or if, in the judgment of the accoucheur, its life has been compromised by prolonged compression in labor, or it has been damaged by attempts with forceps or version, craniotomy should be done. The accoucheur may not plume himself on the success of having delivered the child alive, when it succumbs in a few hours or a few days to the results of labor. The mother has invariably suffered severe injury, and has often been killed by the forced delivery, and these accidents must be charged against the attendant. Craniotomy is much safer, and the end-result for the baby the same. (See Davis.)

With the child in good condition, craniotomy should be the rarest of all operations, but—and practically all authors agree—a few conditions arise where it must be resorted to as the ultimate refuge: (1) If the patient absolutely refuses to incur any danger to herself for the sake of the infant. The operation is, however, not to be repeated in a subsequent labor. (2) If labor has been prolonged and infection is positively or probably present. (3) Where expectancy and high forceps have failed and the conditions are not good for hebosteotomy—for example, an ankylotic pelvis, immense varicosities of the vulva, extreme obesity, nor for the newer cesarean section, see above.

IV. Treatment of Labor in Pelves only Slightly Contracted.—*Pelves Contracted at the Inlet.*

—In pelves with a conjugata vera of $9\frac{1}{2}$ to 11 cm. labor almost always terminates spontaneously, unless the child is very large, in which case the pelvis is thrown back into the class of the "moderately" contracted, just considered. Variations in the mechanism of labor, however, are very common, and the cause for breech, face, brow, and shoulder presentations, for occipitoposterior and other malpositions, and for errors of attitude, as prolapse of the cord, the hand, etc., is often to be found in a slight pelvic contraction which would otherwise pass unnoticed. Operative deliveries, which in normal pelves would be simple, easy, and typical, become, when slight contraction exists, unexpectedly and unexplainedly difficult and complicated. When dystocia arises in such a pelvis the treatment is the same as that just described under Moderately Contracted Pelves.

Pelves Contracted at the Outlet.—As a rule, the obstruction offered by the narrow bony outlet is not recognized until the head has been arrested at this point for several hours, and often the forceps are applied in ignorance of the true conditions. Engagement of the head is the rule, unless, in addition to a narrow outlet, the pelvis is roofed over by a projecting spinal column—*pelvis obtecta*—as in the kyphosis and the spondylolisthetic forms. It is wise, before every forceps operation, to measure the distance between the tuberosities and see how far the sacrum and the coccyx encroach on the anteroposterior diameter of the outlet.

If the anomaly is discovered in pregnancy or early in labor, what was said under the general heading applies here also. If it is found only after dystocia is manifest, the following is suggested: (1) The exaggerated lithotomy position, recommended by the author more than twenty-six years ago (Fig. 495, p. 623). This opens the bony outlet and often produces enough enlargement. Experiments on the cadaver show a gain of $3\frac{1}{2}$ to 5 mm. in the transverse diameter, and also, according to Williams, decided enlargement of the anteroposterior. (2) Jonge's position, the same but with the legs extended, is said to enlarge the outlet still more—even 9 mm. (3) Prolonged expectancy—but during the period of molding the possibility of pressure necrosis of the maternal parts and injury to the brain of the fetus must be borne in mind. (4) The forceps—in mild degrees of contraction this instrument will usually succeed, but a large number of babies are killed by the operation, and the mother almost always suffers severe lacerations, which may extend through the vaginal walls into the ischiorectal fossa and down to the bone. The soft parts may be dragged off their pelvic attachments. Rupture of the symphysis pubis has been frequently reported, and occurs oftener than published. If the child is in good condition when the first real difficulties of the operation are experienced, hebosteotomy is the operation of choice; if it is not in good condition, craniotomy is to be done. Primiparæ suffer the worst from this anomaly. In multiparæ, the resistance of the soft parts being absent, a small amount of outlet contraction may cause little trouble—indeed, may pass unnoticed.

TABLE OF TREATMENT OF MODERATELY CONTRACTED AND BORDERLINE
PELVIS
Induced Labor at 36th week, if preferred.
Usually allowed to go to term,
then

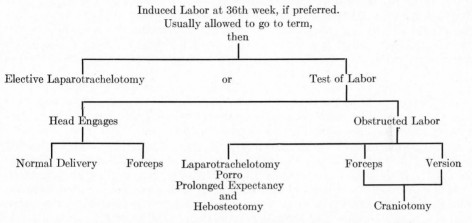

In laying out a course of treatment the above table is very useful. Induced labor being refused (as I believe proper) the woman is allowed to go to term for a "test of labor." Much difference of opinions exists as to what this term means. I feel it is entirely subjective, individual, not definable. Older writers required variable numbers of hours of strong pains after complete dilatation and rupture of the membranes. If the head did not advance the test had failed. A modern obstetrician, grounded in his science and experienced in his art, ought to be able to predict, from a more or less brief study of the parturient at the beginning of her labor what the outcome is likely to be and decide on a definite policy before the lives of two individuals and their health are compromised.

Breech and Other Complications.—Labors complicated by abnormal presentations and attitudes of the child require many modifications in the treatment. In breech, shoulder, brow, and face presentations it is impossible to await the test of labor, and also to fit the head to the pelvis as we do in vertex presentations. It is, therefore, necessary to estimate the degree of spacial disproportion from the pelvic measurements and the adjudged size of the child. The choice of the operation will lie between prophylactic version, cesarean section, and hebosteotomy. Von Franquè suggested applying the hebosteotomy saw provisionally around the joint, to perform extraction, or version and extraction as indicated, and, if the after-coming head is arrested at the inlet, the bone could be immediately sawn through and delivery thus effected in time to save the infant, an ingenious suggestion, but impractical and dangerous. If hebosteotomy is to be done at all, it should be the primary operation. Version is particularly unfavorable to the child, because, unless the narrowing of the passage is very slight, the after-coming head will be stopped at the inlet, the infant will die, and craniotomy will have to be performed. Therefore, in breech, shoulder, and deflexion presentations, unless the accoucheur is convinced that the child will go through the pelvis, cesarean section should be performed as a primary operation—given, of course, good conditions.

Placenta prævia complicating contracted pelvis demands cesarean section if the child is alive. If it is dead, section may still be safer, but one might turn, let nature deliver the trunk—then craniotomy. If to this combination infection is added—Porro. It is doubly dangerous to drag a large child forcibly through the thinned lower uterine segment. Abruptio placentæ demands cesarean section if the cervix is closed. Even rigid soft parts may render the abdominal delivery safest.

Eclampsia seems to be a little more frequent in contracted pelvis. It also makes cesarean section more readily chosen, and the same may be said, speaking broadly, of all other complications requiring rapid delivery.

Hospital versus Home Practice.—The foregoing presentment of the subject gives the treatment of contracted pelvis in the author's own and hospital practice. Without question great differences in treatment must exist between that of the specialist, aided by maternity facilities, and that of the general practitioner, caring for his patient in a flat, or a farm-house, or even a "lean-to," with no help but a nurse or the neighbors. In cities and towns the parturient can and should be transported to a well-equipped maternity, and where this is not practicable, the maternity facilities must be closely imitated in the home, or the accoucheur will have to adapt his treatment to the environment he finds. This is particularly unfortunate for the child, because cesarean section and hebosteotomy are very dangerous performed under such conditions, and, therefore, inadvisable.

Prolonged expectancy is the best treatment for all but the absolutely contracted pelves, followed by a trial with the forceps, failing which craniotomy is the horrible ultimate. If the head is movable, or if the presentation and attitude are abnormal, version is indicated. A high infant mortality is to be expected, but the information gained will warn the attendant to provide ideal arrangements for subsequent labors, and, in the end, a larger number of children will be saved than if the attendant tries to force the conditions in a bad environment. The same statement should apply to prolonged and brutal attempts at delivery with the forceps. A short trial will convince the operator that they are powerless to effect delivery, and if the tractions are persisted in, they can result only in irreparable damage to the mother, and the object sought, a living child, is almost always defeated by the attempt itself. Craniotomy is more humane. A careful study of his pregnancy cases will enable the accoucheur to foresee the above dangers, and, by proper provision, avoid them.

What to Tell the Patient After Labor in Contracted Pelvis.—An inquiry as to the outlook in future pregnancies is the rule after difficult labors, and in order for the accoucheur to be able to express an intelligent opinion he must have carefully observed and noted the character of this labor, the resistances met, the size of the child, etc., etc. He should resist the temptation to magnify the difficulties encountered, either to add to his glory in a successful termination of the case or to excuse his failure. He must carefully distinguish between dystocia from spacial disproportion and that from errors of mechanism—also from errors of art.

In cases of absolutely contracted pelvis the advice is simple—cesarean section every time until it is decided to sterilize the patient. In relatively contracted pelves the patient is advised that cesarean section just as labor begins will probably be the method of election. In moderately contracted pelves the patient may be encouraged by the statement that perhaps, since the soft parts as obstruction have, to a great extent, been eliminated, labor will not be so difficult and may terminate spontaneously. If the child was postmature and large, the induction of labor before term may be recommended for the next pregnancy, and in all events careful supervision must be demanded.

Lacerations in clean cases are always to be repaired at once. In known infected cases the cervical tears, the perineal wounds are left open for drainage, but always a few stitches should be put in to unite a torn sphincter ani. Late repair of lacerations is not to be recommended as a routine. I usually advise the patient to have several children first, and then submit to a complete plastic. The scars from operation would add to the dystocia and they almost always tear again and again. If cesarean section is to follow, of course the plastics may be done.

HISTORICAL NOTE

The ancients believed that the pelvic bones always separated during labor and that dystocia was due to lack of this natural enlargement of the canal. Andreas Vesalius (1543) proved that the pelvic joints are solid, and his disciple, J. C. Arantius (†1589), declared that abnormality of the bones caused difficult labor. Scattered references to contracted pelvis are found in the seventeenth century, e. g., Mauriceau (1668) gave Chamberlen a case of obstructed labor to try his forceps on.

Hendrick van Deventer (1651–1724), sometimes called the father of modern obstetrics, in his book, Oper. Chir. Novum Lumen, exhib. Obstet., 1701, distinguished between flat and generally contracted pelves, which he named pelvis plana and justominor respectively. Huwé (1720) first gave the internal, and John Burton (1751) the external, measurements. Pierre Dionis, de la Motte, and other French accoucheurs of the eighteenth century contributed to our knowledge, but Baudelocque, the elder (1746–1810), did the most and gave us the pelvimeter, named after him. The conjugata externa, to which he ascribed great importance, is called Baudelocque's diameter. Fielding Ould (1742) and Smellie (1751), in England, studied the mechanism of labor, and I have used some of their illustrations as a basis for mine.

In Germany, Roederer, who in 1751 publicly demanded the same honors be accorded obstetrics as were given medicine and surgery, and who introduced the name conjugata; Stein, Sr. (1772), Naegelé (1819), Stein, Jr. (1820), Robert (1842) made important contributions, but Michaëlis' work laid the real scientific foundation to the study. Michaëlis committed suicide by throwing himself under a moving train in an attack of acute remorse (1848). Semmelweis' theory of the causation of puerperal infection was then becoming recognized and Michaëlis had, he was sure, in his ignorance, fatally infected his cousin during delivery. Litzman, his pupil, took up his master's labors, and in 1861 invented the clinical classification of contracted pelves which most authors still find the best. The latest and encyclopedic work on the subject is by Breus and Kolisko. For history see Fasbender and Garrison.

Literature to Chapters LV, LVI, LVII, LVIII

Aitken, J.: Princ. of Midwifery, 3d Ed., 1790, p. 83.—Burke, E. J.: Acute Cases in Moral Medicine, McMillan, 1922. —Coppens, Rev. Charles, S. J.: Moral Principles and Medical Practice, 1905.—Costa: Réforma Med., Naples, August 6, 1921; ibid., Zentb. f. Gynaek., July 9, 1927, p. 1785. 100 cases.—Davis: Amer. Jour. Obst., January, 1915, p. 116.—Eymer: Zentb. für Gyn., January 20, 1923, p. 98.—Fehling: Zentb. für Gyn., 1916, p. 787.— Fitz-Gibbon: Rotunda, Dublin, Contracted Pelvis, 1924.—Frank: Arch. f. Gyn., 1910, vol. lxxxvi, p. 263.— Gauss, C. J.: Zentb. für Gynaek., January 2, 1932, p. 1.—Gellhorn: Jour. Amer. Med. Assoc., January 14, 1915.—Jellett: Surg., Gyn., and Obst., June, 1919.—King: New York Med. Jour., 1909, vol. xc, p. 1054.— —Knapp: "Non Occides," Volkmann's Samml. klin. Vorträge, 1910, N. F., No. 584.—McCormick: Amer. Jour. Obst. and Gyn., June, 1926, p. 794.—Peham: Die Geburtsleitung bei engem Becken, Vienna, 1908.— Pinard: Annales d. Gyn., 1902, vol. ii, p. 165.—Roemer: Zeitschr. f. Geb. u. Gyn., 1911, vol. lxviii, H. 2, p. 319.—Schläfi: Zeitschr. f. Geb. u. Gyn., 1908, vol. lxiv.—Schmid: Zentralbl. für Gyn., 1913, No. 44.—Schwartz: Münchener med. Woch., July 28, 1922. Abst. Jour. Amer. Med. Assoc., October 26, 1922.—Schwarz: Zentb. f. Gyn., 1921, No. 15, p. 525.—Sharpe: Paper read before Chicago Med. Soc., November 14, 1923.— Siegmund: Jour. Amer. Med. Assoc., May 17, 1923. Abst.—Stoeckel: Praktische Ergebnisse der Geb., 1911, vol. iii, H. i; ibid., Jahreskurse für Ærztliche Fortbildung, July, 1917.—van Oppenrooy, Rev. R., S. J.: The Right to Life of the Unborn Child, 1903.—Walcher: Centralbl. f. Gyn., 1889, p. 892.—Williams and Sun: Amer. Jour. Obst. and Gyn., June, 1926.

CHAPTER LIX

THE ACCIDENTS OF LABOR

INJURIES TO THE PARTURIENT CANAL

THE VULVA

ALL primiparæ and many multiparæ suffer from injuries of the parturient canal. These are generally considered normal, but why, the author cannot understand—no other function of the body is always attended by injury. In primiparæ the most frequent lesions are found about the vulvar orifice. Fig. 658 shows the most common vulvar lacerations. They are seldom deep, but if they involve important structures, serious results may follow. If the tear extends through a crus of the clitoris, or even through the organ itself, severe and even fatal hemorrhage may ensue. If a varicose vein is opened, the patient may die from loss of blood. If the duct of the gland of Bartholin is torn across, a cyst may form. If the urethra is involved, a stricture may follow. These wounds often become the seat of puerperal ulcers, and if the infection is virulent or the woman's resistance low, invasion of the connective tissue, even general septicemia, may be the outcome. These lesions are often associated with vaginal tears. Superficial wounds —simply splitting the skin and mucosa—require suturing but seldom, since their edges usually lie in apposition when the legs are brought together. Hemorrhage from clitoris tears and those involving varicose veins is easily stopped temporarily by pressure between the finger and thumb, or by a gauze sponge, and permanently by a draw-string, fine catgut suture through the base of the wound. Often compression is enough. Frenulum tears should be sutured.

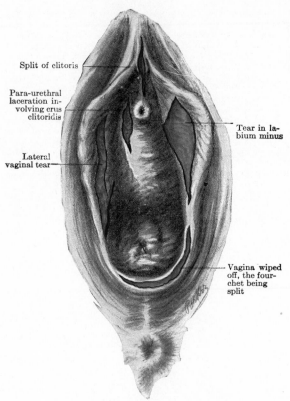

Split of clitoris

Para-urethral laceration involving crus clitoridis

Lateral vaginal tear

Tear in labium minus

Vagina wiped off, the fourchet being split

FIG. 658.—TYPICAL VULVAR INJURIES.

Rupture of the urogenital septum is an inevitable injury in labor, and it cannot be fully repaired. Some relaxation and descensus of the anterior vaginal and urethral wall is an invariable sequence, and it not seldom leads to a slight catarrh at the neck of the bladder—the so-called "irritable bladder" of the older writers. During labor attempts to push the protruding urethra back out of the way of the advancing head always fail, and the urethra is wiped off its pubic attachments.

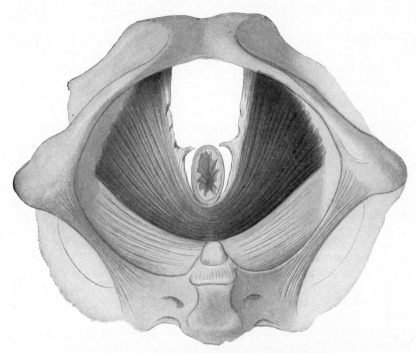

FIG. 659.—SEMIDIAGRAMMATIC. TEARING OF FASCIA OF OUTLET.

Shows the simplest and commonest form of pelvic floor injury. The levator ani pillars are parted and the fascia over them torn, especially in that portion which enwraps the lower rectum. To show the muscle only part of the fascia is drawn—that portion which the author has named "the intercolumnar fascia." Such an injury leads to "diastasis levatoris ani." A few interlacing levator fibers, Luschka's Fibers, are also torn.

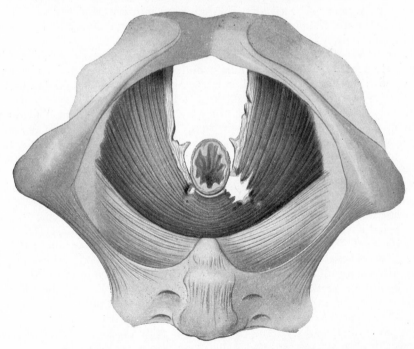

FIG. 660.—SEMIDIAGRAMMATIC. INJURY OF BOTH FASCIA AND MUSCLE.

A much greater injury to the pelvic floor. Not alone is the intercolumnar fascia destroyed, as in Fig. 659, but the muscle is torn at the sides of and behind the rectum, ruining the S-shaped curve of the conjoined levator and thus predisposing to a sliding down of the uterus. (Compare Fig. 662.)

Before reading this subject the student is urged to study the anatomy of the structures as given on page 169.

The Perineum.—If, with the index-finger in the rectum and the thumb in the fourchet, the perineal body be squeezed together, the examiner will be surprised to find how very little tissue there is in it. Indeed, it is composed only of a little fat and connective tissue—the centrum tendineum—with the rudimentary muscles, the constrictores cunni, the musculi bulbi cavernosi, a few levator ani fibers, and the transversi perinei. The fingers will easily outline the sphincter ani, the important closing muscle of the rectum, and, at the sides, the strong rounded masses of the levator ani coming down from the pubis to grasp the rectum from behind. Lacerations of the perineal body occur in the majority of primiparous labors, and while they have considerable importance, it is decidedly less than tears of the pelvic floor —of the levator ani and the fascia in which it is set. When the perineal body is torn, the urogenital septum is destroyed, the anterior wall of the vagina sags, the posterior vaginal wall begins to roll out, and the vulva is permanently open, inviting infection, which almost always results in a vaginal and cervical catarrh. Late effects are descensus uteri and chronic metritis. If the tear is deeper, it may involve part or all the sphincter ani, or even run up the rectal wall more or less. I have seen the rectum torn for a length of 3 inches beyond the sphincter. Complete incontinence of feces is the first effect of such tears, but if they are not so extensive and the levator ani is not seriously injured, the latter muscle assumes vicarious control of the bowel, and the patient may be able to hold the hard feces. Soft feces and gas, however, will usually pass off in spite of the woman's efforts. Rare instances of submucous laceration of the sphincter ani are on record.

The Pelvic Floor.—The levator ani muscle, with its superior and inferior fascia, is almost invariably damaged in labor at term. I believe that the muscle suffers less actual injury than the fasciæ. Owing to destruction of the latter, the muscle bundles fall into new arrangements and also change their point of attachment to the vagina and rectum. The following injuries are easily determinable by careful study of the conditions immediately following delivery and years later, when the evil results become more manifest.

1. *Diastasis of the Levator Ani Pillars.*—As the head comes down, like a blunt wedge it stretches the pelvic floor radially and axially, *i. e.*, the portions in advance of the wedge are forced downward at the same time as they are dilated (see page 178), the fascia being most stretched longitudinally from the cervix to the perineum. The two levator ani pillars are parted, the "intercolumnar" fascia holding them in their relations to the rectum, vagina, perineum, and each other, being destroyed (Fig. 659). Sometimes the skin of the perineum and the vagina do not tear and the accoucheur announces "no laceration," but later on "relaxation of the pelvic floor" shows him his error.

2. *Abruption of the Levator Pillars from the Rectum* (Fig. 660).—This is a continuation of the diastasis of the levator ani pillars. The two puborectal bundles are pushed far asunder, leaving a wide breach. After healing has occurred, instead of a thin, flat sling-like muscle, we find a thick fat one (hypertrophied) forming two pillars at the sides of the gaping introitus, with the rectum pouching up between them. The etiology and pathology remind one of diastasis recti abdominis.

Anatomically we find that, in addition to the destruction of the intercolumnar fascia, the interlacement of the levator ani muscle with the sides of the rectum and sphincter ani is broken and the tear extends more or less deeply into the ischiorectal fossa. The tear may be bilateral, and usually it is deeper on one side. This is always true if this injury results after, and in spite of, episiotomy. The vagina and perineum are always torn and sometimes the sphincter ani too. The rectum, in the bad cases, is exposed for a large part of its circumference and is not only pressed back against the coccyx, but is also pushed downward from its attachments

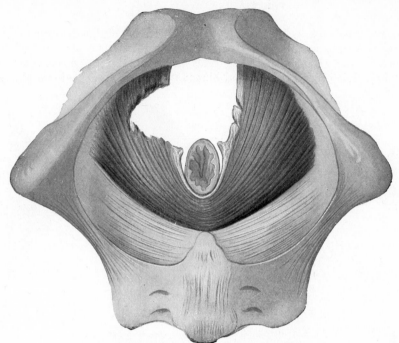

FIG. 661.—SEMIDIAGRAMMATIC. LEVATOR TORN FROM ITS ORIGIN.

An injury to the anterior portions of the levator ani—the puborectal or pillar—due to crushing between the blade of the obstetric forceps and the ramus pubis. Very difficult to repair.

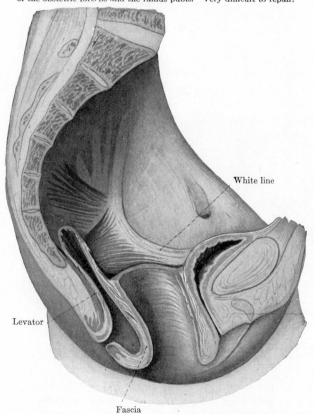

White line

Levator

Fascia

FIG. 662.—SEMIDIAGRAMMATIC. FORMATION OF RECTOCELE.

Shows the destruction of the conjoined portion of the levator ani, the straightening of the S-shaped ledge on which the vagina and uterus rested (cf. Fig. 186, p. 174 and Fig. 664), and the glacier-like sliding of the rectum and vagina downward and outward.

higher up in the pelvis, *i. e.*, it is slid off the superior fascia of the diaphragma pelvis. The vagina accompanies this glacial movement and since its attachment to the rectum is by loose connective tissue it slides off the rectum in the consequent prolapse of the pelvic organs. A clinical hint may be here permitted—in the repair

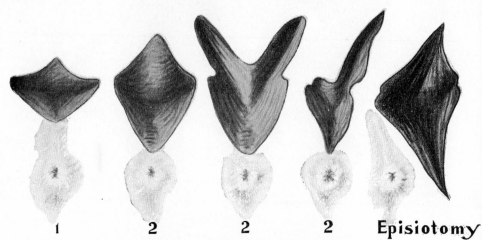

FIG. 663.—DIAGRAMS OF THE TYPICAL PERINEAL INJURIES.
1, First degree tears; 2, 2, 2, second degree tears.

push the rectum and vagina upward into the pelvis and unite them to the fascia high up where they belong.

3. *Subpubic tears* are much rarer and are usually due to rapid operative delivery (Fig. 661). The radicals of the levator may be cut between the forceps and the descending rami pubis if the instrument is bent up too sharply when delivering the head, or they may be twisted off the bone when the head is rotated by means of the forceps. When an injury of this kind is extensive, the bladder lies

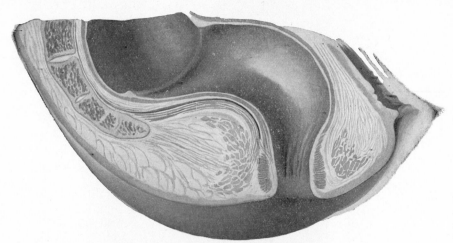

FIG. 664.—THE MINUTE ANATOMY OF THE SPHINCTER ANI EXTERNUS AND LEVATOR ANI (RED) AND THE SPHINCTER ANI INTERNUS. DRAWN FROM A FROZEN SECTION IN VIENNA ANATOMICAL INSTITUTE, 1922.

naked at the top of the wound, the vesicovaginal fascia is usually severed from its rootstock (see Fig. 186) and the angulæ vaginæ are torn from the pubis. The late effects of these injuries, prolapse, etc., may not be discussed here.

Figure 663 shows the various forms of the perineal and pelvic floor injuries as they appear after labor. All the figures were drawn from life.

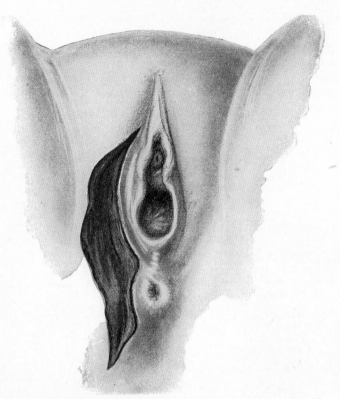

FIG. 665.—CENTRAL RUPTURE OF PERINEUM, ANUS AND VULVA INTACT.
Child emerged through rent.

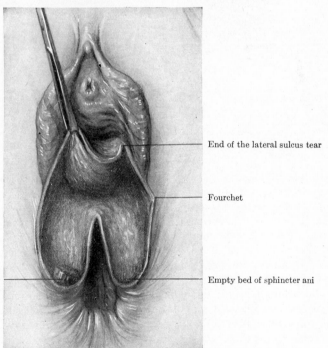

End of the lateral sulcus tear

Fourchet

Sphincter ani torn at posterior
raphé and pulled out of its bed

Empty bed of sphincter ani

FIG. 666.—COMPLETE OR THIRD-DEGREE TEAR. CRITICAL SURVEY OF THE WOUND.
Shows the depth of the wound and how the flap of the vagina may be raised.   The split in the rectum and the sphincter,
torn out of its bed and ruptured at the side (not always in the middle line), are plainly visible.

50

Etiology.—Perineal tears occur with a frequency varying from 9 to 75 per cent., as put by different authors. Forceps labors show 54 to 85 per cent. of tears. In my own experience an anatomically absolutely intact perineum is a great rarity, but extensive lacerations are uncommon, because I use episiotomy often.

The most common cause of perineal lacerations is disproportion between the child and the soft parts—either the head is too large or the canal too small, as occurs

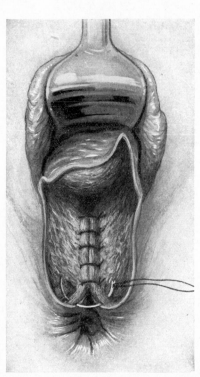

FIG. 667.—SUTURING THE RECTAL MUCOSA.

With a fine needle and No. 0 twenty-day catgut the rectal mucosa is first closed. The needle enters and issues on the wounded surface of the rectum, does not pass through into the gut, and the knots are, therefore, all buried. The needle is putting in the last of the sutures, which are about 0.5 cm. apart and interrupted. If the tear is very extensive, a second row is inserted to reinforce the first.

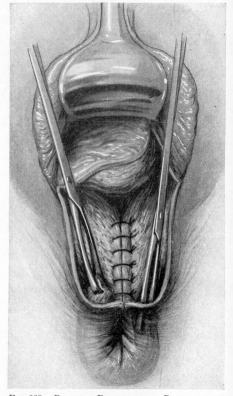

FIG. 668.—REACHING DOWN INTO THE BOTTOM OF THE SPHINCTER PIT.

The finger searches the bottom of the sphincter pit, and with an Allis or tissue forceps the retracted end of the sphincter ani is drawn up. It is usually a part of the retracted torn levator.

with infantile genitalia, or the head presents unfavorable diameters to the passage, as in occipitoposterior positions and brow presentations. Too rapid delivery, either spontaneous or operative, by not giving the parts time to dilate, causes many tears. Therefore we see the most extensive injuries after extraction by the breech or by forceps. Sometimes the forceps directly crush the perineum, or it is torn by introducing the hand alongside the baby's body in breech deliveries, but these are errors of art. Disease of the soft parts must also be mentioned; edema from prolonged labor; excessive rigidity from advanced age (old primiparæ); scars from previous injury; syphilitic infiltration; gonorrhea, with or without condylomata; loss of elasticity from general illness (typhoid, tuberculosis, etc.); status hypoplasticus (Mathes); and sometimes, from no apparent cause, the perineum tears like wet blotting-paper. It occurs to me that such a state of the perineum may be due to a toxemia, since it is usually associated with hemorrhagic tendencies and albuminuria.

An important cause of perineal tears, not generally recognized, is a narrow pubic arch. Unless the head can occupy the space directly under the subpubic ligament, it is forced, by the narrowing rami pubis, downward toward the coccyx, of course thus

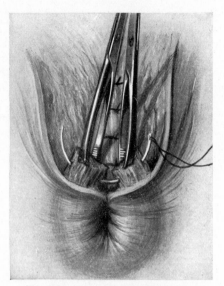

FIG. 669.—UNITING THE SPHINCTER ANI.

To insure broad apposition of the torn ends of the muscle the needle should pass well to the side, and two, even three, sutures may be placed, one of which should unite the fascia surrounding the muscle.   This is the most important part of the operation, and plenty of time should be spent on it.   No. 2 forty-day catgut is used.

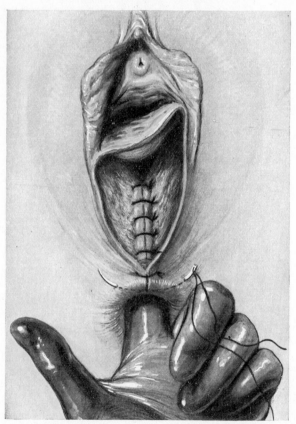

FIG. 670.—REINFORCING SUTURE FOR SPHINCTER ANI.

A rubber glove is drawn on, the index-finger inserted into the rectum, and a suture is now passed through the sphincter ani from the skin surface, using a round pointed needle and silkworm-gut.   This reinforces the catgut suture and brings together the skin fibers of the sphincter ani externus, and the lowest portion of the torn urogenital septum containing the transversus perinei superficialis and some connective tissue of the centrum tendineum.   Sometimes this stitch turns the skin of the anus in a little, hence the edges of the skin where it joins the mucosa are united by a fine catgut suture.

The rest of the operation is like those for incomplete tear.

overstretching the levator ani and perineum. We find, therefore, the most extensive injuries in funnel pelves and those with a narrow pubic arch. In these cases, too, the vagina, around its outlet, being caught between the head and the bones, is forced or dragged, if the delivery is operative, downward and outward, and if, in addition to the other traumatisms, rotatory movements are made with the forceps, the vaginal walls are torn completely off their pelvic attachments and are split in several directions.

The deeper lacerations, involving the muscles of the pelvic floor, take place from within outward, first the muscle tearing, then the vagina, which is first visibly spanned transversely, and, finally, the skin. Sometimes the skin is absolutely intact, but all the deeper structures down to and exposing the rectum are torn

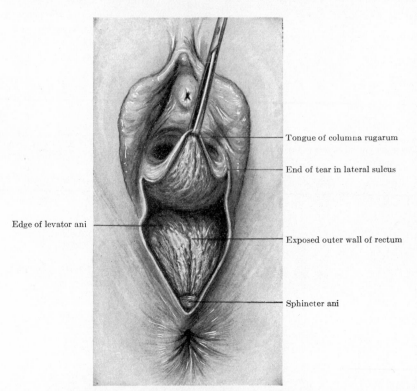

Tongue of columna rugarum

End of tear in lateral sulcus

Edge of levator ani

Exposed outer wall of rectum

Sphincter ani

FIG. 671.—CRITICAL SURVEY OF A SECOND-DEGREE TEAR.

This is a very deep and extensive tear, involving the puborectal portions of the levator ani, separating them from each other and from the rectum in front and at the sides, exposing the rectum and the sphincter ani. The latter can be seen lying at the lower end of the wound, a broad ring of pink muscle. The levator ends lie in the deep recesses at the sides of the rectum. Notice how the anus has dropped toward the coccyx. The sutures must lift it up toward the pubis. The retracted transverse perineal muscles have pulled the walls of the wound to the sides.

apart, and in such instances the superficial observer will fail to discover the extent of the injury, and may even declare that no lacerations exist. In these cases I have found it best to incise the thin bridge of skin medially the whole length of the wound, which gives better access to the deeper structures for suturing. The vagina tears in one or both of the sulci, and the wound may extend up beyond the spine of the ischium, even under the broad ligament.

Perineal tears are divided into three classes or degrees: In the first class are those where the frenulum or posterior commissure is torn to an extent not exceeding ¾ inch toward the anus. The second class includes all other tears excepting those in which the anus and sphincter ani are involved, these being designated as of the third degree or complete lacerations (Fig. 663). This classification is unsatisfactory because it gives no idea of the depth of the injuries of the pelvic floor.

Figure 665 shows a rare form of perineal laceration, and was sketched from a case observed by the author. It is called central rupture of the perineum, and is due to a high and very resistant perineum, narrow pubic arch, or a vulva placed too far forward. The child is delivered through the rent, which may be at the side of the vulvar orifice and anus, as in the figure, or between anus and vulva, or the child may escape through the anus, tearing it in several directions. The sphincter ani and part of the rectovaginal septum may tear without extensive involvement of the perineum. In one case the head appeared at the vulva while an arm protruded

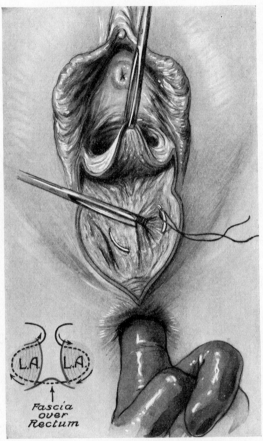

Fig. 672.—Putting in Figure-of-8 Deep Levator Ani Sutures, Inner Loops.

Use silkworm-gut and a large round pointed needle. Oriented by a finger in the rectum (covered by an extra glove) the levator which has retracted to the side is lifted upward and medially. This is aided by pulling the muscle out with an Allis forceps. The needle is passed well to the side, its course describing an ellipse, to get a large bite of muscle and the fasciæ covering it. A tiny bit of the fascia over the rectum is taken and then the needle is put through the levator of the other side, direction reversed.

This is the inner loop of the first figure of 8 and it approximates the puborectal portions of the levator ani which have been stripped off the sides of the rectum; it also unites those few fibers of the levator ani which pass anterior to the rectum to meet in the apex of the centrum tendineum, including the fascia visceralis recti, and it lays the foundation for the suture of higher portions of the puborectalis.

from the anus; in another—a breech—one leg appeared through the anus. In all such cases it is best to perform episiotomy to prevent extensive destruction of the tissues.

Treatment.—*Preventive.*—Protection of the perineum, according to the rules laid down in the Conduct of Labor, will prevent a large number of, but not all, pelvic floor injuries. Even episiotomy does not always suffice to overcome the disproportion between the head and the outlet. (See p. 330, Episiotomy.) Most authors advise incisions in the perineum when it is found too rigid and unelastic, but a few condemn episiotomy, asserting that a tear is better.   I believe that the incision should be often resorted to—that it will save the lives of many children and often preserve the sphincter ani from injury.

Slow delivery is the secret of success in preventing tears in operations.   The tendency to hurry after the forceps are applied is hard to resist, and the head is usually extracted by forcibly overcoming the resistance of the pelvic floor.   If continuous auscultation of the heart-tones shows that the fetus is in good condition,

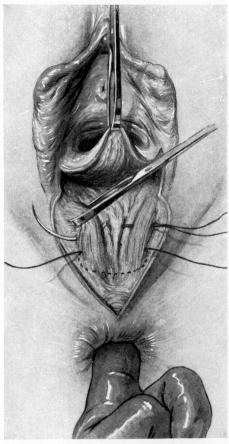

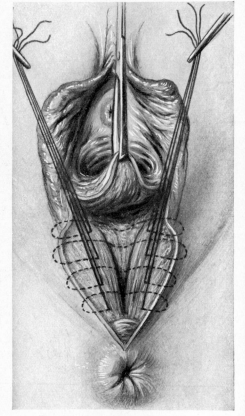

FIG. 673.—THE TWO LEVATOR PILLARS.

The inner loop of the second suture is being laid—again the deep retracted sides of the wound are drawn out.   One seldom sees the levator as plainly as this—it has been too much battered and crushed, and too the wound has been drawn to larger scale.

If examination shows that the levators are not pushed asunder as pictured here, but actually torn through on one side, either near the pubic insertion, as in Fig. 661, or behind and alongside the rectum as in Fig. 660—we repair the damaged muscle on strict anatomical principles—see episiotomy, Fig. 681.

FIG. 674.—READY FOR VAGINAL REPAIR.

The deep loops of four sutures are in place.   Note their elliptic course and how the tissues will be crowded toward the middle line when the knots are tied.   The ends are held out of the way with clamps.   Now the vagina is repaired.

Many operators prefer catgut for this part of the repair.   Then the sutures are put in just as shown and tied.

the forceps extraction may be extended to from twenty to fifty minutes, and in this time the perineum can be dilated safely.   To counteract this desire to hurry it is my custom to place a clock in front of the operating table.   Should threatening fetal or maternal danger demand haste, a deep episiotomy, the colpoperineotomy of Dührssen, should be performed.   Manual dilatation of the upper reaches of the pelvic floor is also useful as an operation preparatory to episiotomy.   In several cases where I had anticipated the necessity for rapid delivery I have used the colpeurynter to dilate the vagina and levator ani.   It is a rather painful expedient,

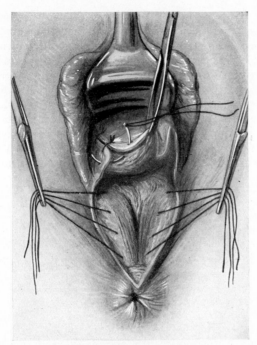

FIG. 675.—CLOSING THE SULCI VAGINÆ.

The vagina is now united. By pulling up the tongue of the columna rugarum the torn edges of the sulcus are straightened and then interrupted No. 2, twenty-day catgut sutures are laid. Be sure to take in the fascia propria of the vagina and,—for the first three stitches,—a tiny bit of the fascia over the rectum, thus anchoring the vagina high on the rectum. Some operators prefer to close the vagina before putting in the levator sutures.

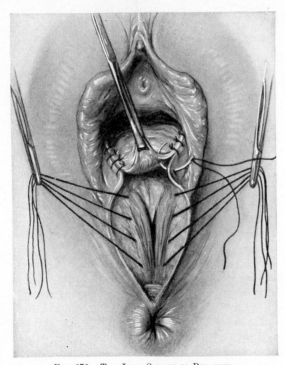

FIG. 676.—THE LEFT SULCUS IS REPAIRED.

Note that the needle takes in only the vagina and its fascia. Later the pelvic floor is brought up under it and the crown suture will hold it in place.

and the results are not uniformly satisfactory. Some operators believe they can manually dilate the lower parturient canal so that the fetus can pass without laceration. Those cases I have seen done by others and my own experience do not confirm this notion. When the child is exceptionally large, or when the head must come through with unfavorable diameters, or very rapidly (intra-uterine asphyxia, etc.), deep episiotomy is indicated (Fig. 663). If, during delivery, spontaneous or operative, the accoucheur notices the vagina on the stretch and beginning to split, episiotomy is indicated to save the sphincter and rectum.

Perineal tears seldom bleed profusely. Occasionally an artery requires a clamp, and always firm compression with a gauze or cotton sponge will arrest the bleeding until the parts may be closed by suture. There is no question but that

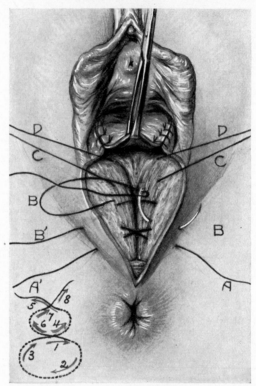

FIG. 677.—COMPLETING FIGURE-OF-8 SUTURES.

The outer loop of the first figure-of-8 suture is in place. The two ends of the silkgut are threaded with spear-pointed needles and crossed. The needle goes from within outward through the urogenital septum, the subcutaneous fat, the skin, again describing an ellipse, emerging 1 cm. from the edge. The process is repeated on the other side, being sure that, when the stitch crosses over, it does not lock itself.

If you are using catgut, you simply make another row of sutures in the urogenital septum, corresponding to the outer loops of the figure 8. For skin closure see Fig. 680, p. 795.

every tear of the perineum requires repair, but it may not be advisable to do it immediately after labor. If the woman is collapsed after delivery or too exhausted for further operation; if there is beginning infection; if the parts are battered and bruised so that necrosis is to be feared; if there is an old laceration which will require extensive dissection for its repair—under such circumstances it may be best to postpone the operation. My own practice in septic cases and those in which the parts are too much torn to hope for a good result is to put one or two catgut sutures in the sphincter ani and one external silkgut stitch to support this muscle, and leave the rest of the wound open for drainage and to allow for eventual sloughing. Several accoucheurs take the opportunity of labor to repair old lacerations, but I do not do this unless the parts are torn anew, or an incision is made. In these

cases the wound may be extended sufficiently to expose the levator ani and a
typical perineoplastic performed.   Hemorrhage is very free, but the technical
difficulties are little greater than are met a year after delivery.   Clean cases, too
exhausted for immediate operation, are allowed to recover and are repaired within
twenty-four hours, never later.   I do not approve of early secondary perineorrhaphy.
If the primary operation cannot be done, the patient is instructed to return after
eight or twelve months for thorough repair.   Hirst performs the secondary suture
on the fifth or eighth day, but my experience has been unsatisfactory.   Capillary
oozing is always troublesome; the tissues are brittle and stiff; it is almost impossible
to work in the connective tissue and to lay bare the levator ani pillars—the crux of

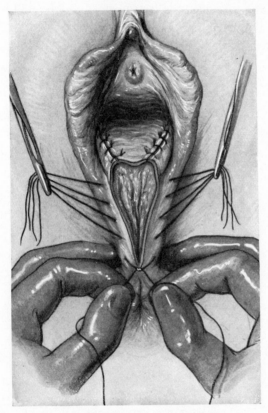

FIG. 678.—CLOSING WOUND.

Bring the deep tissues together by finger pressure as shown, but leave a loop over the skin large enough to lay
your little finger in.   The wound surfaces will lie apposed when the legs are brought together, and the stitches might
even cut a little if there is much edema later.

the operation—and healing is not so satisfactory as is desirable.   Moreover, my
results with primary suture are very gratifying.

It is not advisable to place the sutures before the placenta has been delivered,
because: (1) The edges of the wound cannot be properly coaptated; (2) during
the passage of the placenta blood is forced into the wound; (3) the stitches may
tear out, and, further, should there be a postpartum hemorrhage requiring intra-
uterine manipulation, it may be necessary to remove the sutures to allow the hand
to be inserted.   Then, too, it takes the accoucheur's attention away from the
observation and conduct of the third stage of labor, which may not be done with
impunity.   The parturient needs the undivided attention of the accoucheur during
the placental stage.

Perineorrhaphy.—Anesthesia is not necessary if only one or two sutures are to be inserted, since, owing to the stretching and bruising of the parts, the tissues are not very sensitive. With larger lacerations one should use local anesthesia aided by morphine and scopolamine (see page 320 for technic). Rarely one needs general anesthesia. The patient should lie across the bed, or, better, and to be obtained wherever possible, on a properly prepared table, with the buttocks hanging well over the edge (Fig. 784). The same instruments are needed as for the gynecologic perineorrhaphy—needle-holders, needles, artery forceps, specula, Allis forceps, tissue forceps, scissors, cervix forceps, and uterine packing forceps. It is wrong to be satisfied with less. If one has to operate without trained assistance, which is the rule in general practice, everything—sterile sponges, sterile towels, basins with antiseptic solutions, the instruments, etc.—should be arranged within easy reach of the hand. Abundant light is essential for good work. Where the

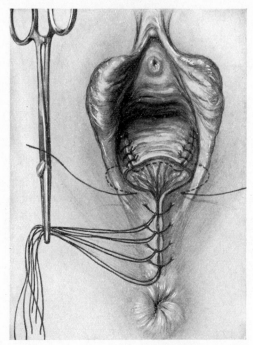

FIG. 679.—THE CROWN SUTURE.

Enter the skin 1 cm. from its edge; swing widely to the side (ellipse again) through the urogenital septum (constrictor cunni); go in the fascia under the vagina (there are two cut edges here); continue in the subvaginal fascia under the tongue of the columna rugarum,—then the same in reverse direction out on the skin.

laceration is complete, the accoucheur should insist on having sufficient help, and should, if necessary, postpone the operation until he can get it. The repair of a complete laceration of the perineum requires great technical skill but can be done in the home though the facilities of a modern operating-room make it easier for the surgeon.

First the wound and adjoining surfaces are to be cleansed, care being taken not to wipe anything not sterile into the freshly broken tissues. If blood comes down from above, obscuring the field, a large gauze sponge is pushed up into the posterior fornix. Do not forget to remove it afterward! A speculum held by an assistant retracts the anterior vaginal wall. A survey of the whole wound is now made, the anatomic structures involved determined, and to what extent and depth. Too often, in a hasty inspection, the fact that the pelvic floor muscles are torn escapes the eye, and a few stitches are put in to close the skin tear. After a few years descensus uteri shows the mistake.

Perineorrhaphy has four stages: (1) Uniting the torn puborectal portions of the levator ani; (2) suture of the vagina; (3) suture of the urogenital septum; (4) closing the skin. In my private practice and in special maternity work I use No. 2, forty-day catgut for the levator ani; No. 2, twenty-day for the vagina and urogenital septum, all interrupted, and a subcutaneous running suture of silkworm-gut for the skin closure. (See Fig. 681.) For general hospitals, for private practice and for young interns the method here described (figure of 8 with silkgut) is, I feel, safer, and will give better results. The only objection, pain in removal, is eliminated by gentleness. To avoid repetition the description of the operation has been put into the legends under the illustrations.

A sutured perineum requires especial care to secure good union. The legs need not be bound together unless the woman is delirious. Even with incomplete

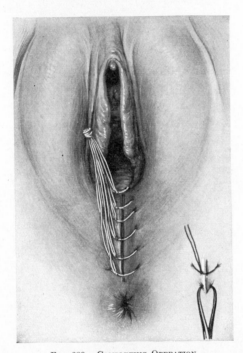

FIG. 680.—COMPLETING OPERATION.

The strands are knotted together smoothly as in the figure. By tying the knot as shown, the ends will not catch in the bed-linen nor drag in the bed-pan, and by cutting close to the knot the sharp points will be covered.
Now the edges of the skin are pinched together with Allis forceps which are left on for three to four minutes. (See inset.) The gauze plug is removed from the vagina and as the last precaution the finger is inserted into the rectum to make sure that none of the sutures has passed through the bowel. If one has, it must be at once removed. After operative deliveries it is my practice to catheterize the bladder to satisfy myself that it has suffered no injury. The parts are drenched with sterile water and a pad applied.

tears one should select the diet, fortify the aseptic treatment of the wound, and provide for an easy first bowel movement with a view of reducing the danger of overstretching the newly united muscles. When the laceration has been complete, special instructions are to be given the nurse regarding the bowels. I do not give opium to bind up the bowels, but order a semisolid diet, free from cellulose, and large quantities of water. After the seventh day liq. petrolatum $\overline{3}$j, A. M. and P. M., is given. On the tenth day a dose of castor oil is ordered, and at the same time the nurse injects, with a soft rectal tube, 8 ounces of sterilized warm olive oil into the bowel, to be retained. The patient is instructed not to strain when the bowels are about to move. After the first movement a daily laxative may be administered unless the liquid petrolatum suffices. If the accoucheur has no trustworthy nurse, he should not risk the success of his operation in incompetent

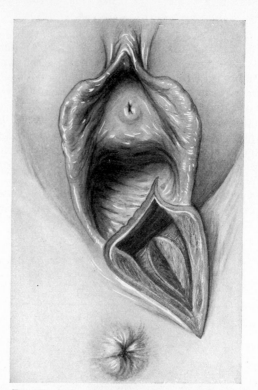

FIG. 681.—REPAIR OF EPISIOTOMY. FIGURE 8 METHOD.

Appearance of episiotomy (somewhat enlarged and idealized) made as in Fig. 323, p. 333. The fascia over the levator ani (intercolumnar fascia) and part of the muscle have been cut.

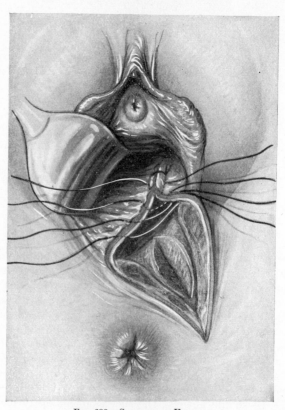

FIG. 682.—SEWING THE VAGINA.

Using No. 2, twenty-day catgut, four or five sutures are laid 1 cm. apart. The first two, the deepest, take in the vagina, the subvaginal fascia and a bit of the fascia over the rectum, high up, *i.e.*, deep in the pelvis. The others pass only through the vagina and its fascia. These are put in but not tied. (Do not pull too hard on them.)

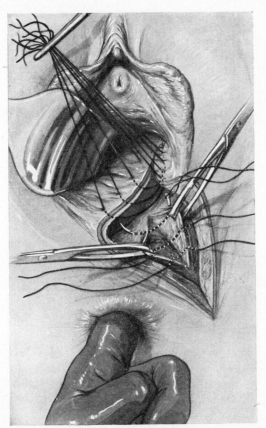

Fig. 683.—Bringing Levator Ani and Intercolumnar Fascia Together.

Three or four silkworm-gut sutures are put in. The cut ends of the levator are raised with Allis forceps, the needle passed far to the side describing an elliptical course, taking in the muscle and the fasciæ above and beneath it. The finger prevents injury of the rectum—also helps to lift up the retracted muscle. These are the first or deep loops of the figure 8.

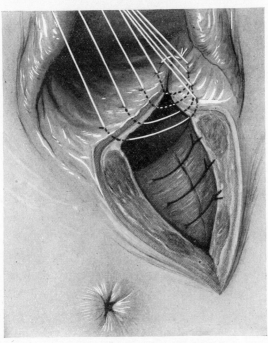

Fig. 683a.—The Sewn Levator Ani.

A magnified "close-up" of the levator suture—but here No. 2, forty-day catgut has been used. Not recommended as routine. See discussion, page 795.

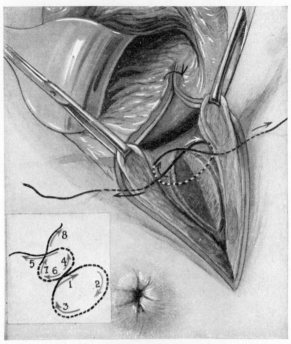

FIG. 683b.—DETAIL OF FIGURE-OF-8 SUTURE.

Close-up. Both ends of the silkworm-gut are armed with needles and the strands crossed. Pull up the two halves of the urogenital septum with Allis forceps. This puts them on the stretch and makes them stand out sharply. Pass the needle from within out, through urogenital septum, fat, skin—emerging 1 cm. from the edge. Repeat on the other side and be careful the thread does not lock. Inset shows the progress,—follow arrows and numbers.

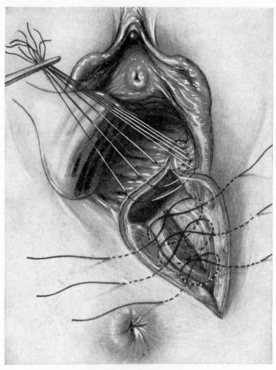

FIG. 683c.—READY TO TIE.
See that all bleeding is stopped. Tie vaginals first.

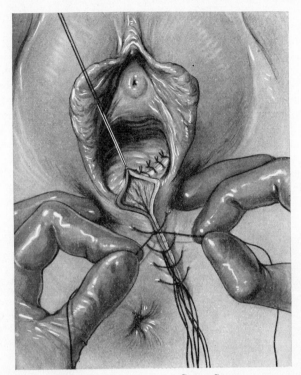

FIG. 683d.—READY FOR THE CROWN SUTURE.

Press the deeper structures together with the middle fingers, but leave a large loop (under which your little finger will pass). This slack will be taken up when you bring the woman's legs together and will allow for some of the swelling. For crown suture see Fig. 679, page 794.

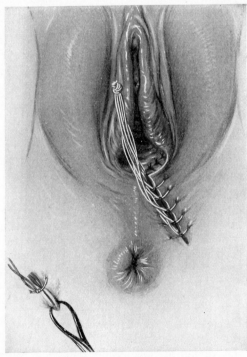

FIG. 683e.—FINISHING TOUCHES.

By twisting all the strands into a cord and pulling them straight up they may be tied into a knot which will stand up—and not drag into the bed-pan. The edges of the wound are pinched with Allis forceps and they stick together. After removing the gauze plug from the vagina, and having passed the finger into the rectum to make sure no stitch has punctured it, the vulva is douched with sterile water, the legs brought together and the Allis forceps taken off. Introitus is exposed to show how posterior vaginal wall lies close to the anterior.

799

hands, but should attend to the above matters himself. With tears of less than the third degree the usual treatment of the bowels is given.

The sutures are inspected daily. A small amount of cutting through may be neglected, or the spots touched with tincture of iodin. Deeply cutting stitches had best be removed. Marked swelling of the vulva usually subsides under a warm moist application of 25 per cent. alcohol in boric acid solution. The vulvar pad should be laid loosely against the vulva, so that feces issuing from the anus may not dam back against the line of sutures. I have known fatal infection to result from this.

The stitches are removed on the tenth to the fourteenth day, being left longer in the larger lacerations. If infection develops, the safest course is to remove the stitches and open up the wound widely for drainage. Occasionally excessive

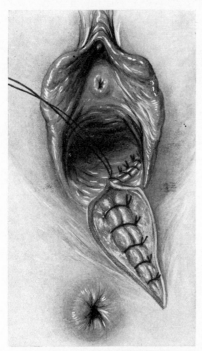

Fig. 683*f*.—Repair with Buried Catgut. The Urogenital Septum.

After the levator wound is closed as in Fig. 683*a*, the vaginal sutures are tied. The halves of the urogenital septum are pulled up as in Fig. 683*b* and the suture passed as described, but each is tied and cut seriatim.

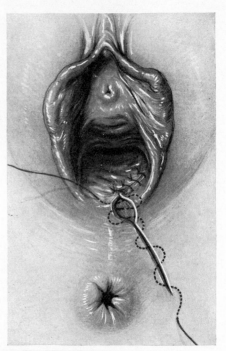

Fig. 683*g*.—The Subcutaneous Closure.

Now a continuous subcutaneous silkworm-gut (some prefer catgut) suture is placed. Begin at the top and make the usual trajectory of the crown suture and bring the end out about 1 cm. from the lower limit of the incision. Make sure (if silkworm-gut) that the thread "runs," then finish as in Fig. 683*e*.

growth of granulation tissue occurs at the margins of the wounds, and after several weeks the patient returns, complaining of pain, burning in urination, and constant irritating discharge. Sometimes, especially after forceps deliveries, there is a periostitis rami pubis, which causes difficulty in locomotion. The granulomata are to be cauterized away with a nitrate of silver stick. Hot applications will help heal the periostitis. The infrared-ray lamp is useful for pain or infection.

LESIONS OF THE VAGINA

Rarely, in spontaneous labor, is the vagina torn, except in association with perineal lacerations, already considered.

Causation.—If the vagina is congenitally too small (infantile) or rigid (old primiparæ), or scarred by disease (gonorrhea, etc.) or previous lacerations or operations, or radium or *x*-ray treatments, it may tear during ordinary labor, and certainly will give way during artificial delivery. Precipitate labors occasionally, but forceps and rapid breech extractions particularly, show vaginal tears. Twisting the head in the pelvis by the forceps—so-called "rotation"—may split the canal the whole length and open up the perivaginal spaces down to the bone. Hemorrhage is such cases is usually very profuse, may tax the best skill, and may even be fatal. Tears of the posterior vaginal wall are usually due to perforation by the tip of the forceps blade, but may be spontaneous and may even go through into the rectum. Perforating tears may be produced by friction of the vagina between the head and prominent bony points, as the spines of the ischia, the promontory of the sacrum, or an exostosis on the posterior surface of the pubis, or from stone in the bladder. The forceps also may be pushed through the vaginal wall. Anterior tears may result from traumatism in delivery, from the operation of hebosteotomy, when the vagina may communicate with the pubic wound, and even the bladder be torn open. During delivery after craniotomy sharp spiculæ of bone, if unprotected, may penetrate the vaginal wall, or even open up the bladder.

Pressure necrosis of the vagina may occur, as was described under Contracted Pelvis, and if large portions of the mucous membrane slough out, lochiocolpos may result and obstruction from stenosis of the passage in a subsequent delivery.

Description.—Usually the tears are longitudinal, and occupy the sulci alongside the anterior or posterior columna. In the former case the bladder, in the latter the rectum, is exposed. Anterior lacerations are often accompanied by a tearing of the levator ani pillars from their pubic attachments. The edges of the tear are usually straight, except when necrosis occurs, and the connective tissue is often widely opened up. In the fornices the tears are generally transverse, unless they communicate with cervix tears. Hemorrhage is free, depending on the location. Sometimes the tear extends more or less circularly around the vagina, near the cervix, and opens up the peritoneal cavity. This is a serious accident, is called colpoporrhexis, is closely akin to rupture of the uterus, and will be considered together with that subject.

Vaginal tears may be the port of entry for infection, with paravaginal abscess or even general septicemia, both of which are rare unless the case is otherwise infected. As a rule, the lacerations of the upper third of the vagina heal without treatment. Lacerations of the lower half of the vagina usually extend into the musculature of the pelvic floor, and should be treated as such, because, if not, prolapsus uteri will follow sooner or later.

LESIONS OF THE PELVIC CONNECTIVE TISSUE

If the reader will call to mind the anatomy of the pelvic fascia and the changes it undergoes during natural labor, as described on page 173, his understanding of what follows will be much easier. Damage to the retinaculum uteri (the connective-tissue web in which the uterus is embedded) and to the fascial planes and seams leading from it to the walls of the pelvis is an almost irreparable injury and sooner or later leads the women into greater or less invalidism. Overstretching of the vagina and the vesicovaginal fascia is responsible for most cystoceles. If at the same time the pubocervical strands of fascia are torn off the cervix, the bladder slides down and off the uterus. If the parametria are overstretched radially and at the same time dragged down, the retinaculum uteri is destroyed. The cervix now begins to slide down toward the hiatus genitalis, the fundus falls backward, and procidentia uteri is soon developed. If the sacro-uterine ligaments suffer traction injury, the cervix will sag downward, with the same sequence of evil results. Destruction of the fascia lying posterior to the cervix and attaching the latter to the rectum causes high rectocele. To resume the simile of page 175, the spokes of the wheel being stretched, broken, or torn out of the hub (the cervix), the hub may be forced into many abnormal positions.

In many cases the urethra and the base of the bladder are pushed down and off their attachments to the posterior wall of the pubis. The vagina may be actually avulsed from its fascial moorings—this occurs invariably when forceps are applied or breech extraction made, before the cervix is completely dilated, and before it, together with the upper fourth of the vagina, is retracted upward out of the pelvis. If the operator wishes to verify these statements let him in a case of undilated cervix pull the head down into the pelvis and he will note what a large pad of tissue is drawn into the inlet in advance of the head. Figures 684 and 685 show the differences between such a condition and one where complete dilatation and retraction of the cervix have been accomplished. Figure 686 is intended to show the destructive action on all the pelvic fasciæ of a forceps delivery performed before the soft parts are prepared for it by the natural powers of labor. It is not exag-

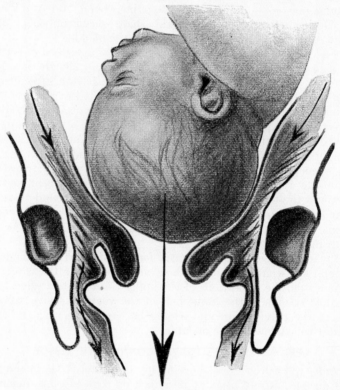

Fig. 684.—Showing how the Head, Dragged Through an Unprepared Parturient Canal, Pulls Down the Soft Parts, Sometimes Actually Avulsing them from their Bony Attachments.
Arrows show direction of the rupture.

gerated. After such destruction of the connective tissue the fat disappears from the pelvis.

Etiology.—While usually these injuries occur with operative delivery, they may result from the action of the natural forces alone. Premature bearing down efforts have the same effects as forced traction from below. Variations in the degree of elasticity of the connective tissue and fascia exist. In old primiparæ they are more likely to tear than to stretch, which explains the clinical experience that procidentia is more common in women who had their first child late in life. Some women are born with so inefficient a pelvic floor that an easy labor destroys it; indeed, prolapse may occur in a virgin. Edema of the pelvic connective tissues invites damage if it does not cause obstruction, and certain toxemic states so alter the tissues that laceration readily occurs in delivery.

Prognosis.—Perineal and vaginal lacerations are not serious if properly treated. Infection is the worst danger. Hemorrhage may be fatal if large veins or arteries are involved, which is especially true of placenta prævia with cervicovaginal tears. The invalidism following destruction of the pelvic connective tissues may not appear for many years. Scar formation may later deform and displace the vagina and neighboring hollow organs, and also cause strictura recti. Incontinence of urine may be thus produced from scars pulling open the neck of the bladder, or in making diverticulæ of the urethra with infection and abscess. The uterus may be dislocated in all directions. In one case I saw the cervix pulled down to the introitus. Subsequent labors may be rendered so difficult by these deforming and obstructive cicatrices that even cesarean section may be required.

Treatment.—*Prevention.*—Nature's own slow methods best preserve the pelvic fascia. Only cesarean section leaves them uninjured. Our practices—manual

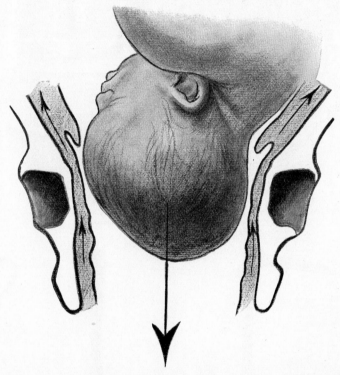

Fig. 685.—Showing how the Head Comes Through a Properly Prepared Parturient Canal. Arrows indicate direction of the tissues retracting above the advancing head.

dilatation, metreurysis, and incisions—are very crude and destructive. Avoid forceps and breech extraction through an ill prepared cervix. Avoid pituitrin. Do not let the woman bear down until the head has passed through the cervix on to the perineum. If the laceration of the anterior and lateral walls of the vagina is unavoidable and the levator ani is endangered, it is better to make a deep incision into this muscle (midway between the pubis and the rectum) than to allow it to be pulled off the ramus pubis.

Tears in the upper third of the vagina require no treatment unless they bleed. A few stitches usually will stop the hemorrhage, but sometimes the flow is so profuse that one cannot see the wound. Here uterovaginal tamponade is indicated instead of the suture. Next day an attempt at repair may be made, or the operation postponed for six months. If free bleeding obstructs the view, rendering the operation technically difficult, it may be possible to tampon that part of the wound from which the hemorrhage comes while the other part is being sutured, or the suture may be passed entirely under the guidance of the finger.   The Sehrt aorta compressor should be useful here.   After suturing, it is best to do a uterovaginal

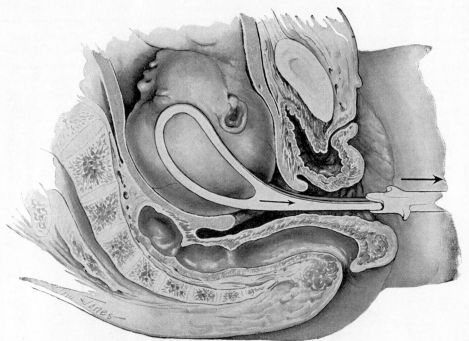

FIG. 686.—SCHEMATIC, TO SHOW THE DISRUPTION OF THE PELVIC FASCIA AND AVULSION OF THE BLADDER CAUSED BY PREMATURE FORCEPS OPERATION.

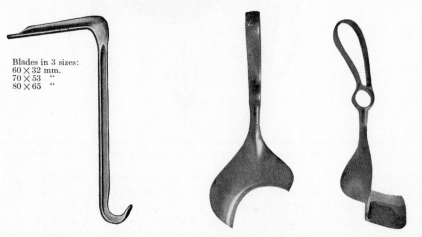

Blades in 3 sizes:
60 × 32 mm.
70 × 53   "
80 × 65   "

FIG. 686a.—AUTHOR'S PORTABLE OBSTETRIC SPECULUM.   FIG. 686b and c.—VAGINAL CORNER RETRACTOR FOR EX-POSING CERVIX.   RIGHT AND LEFT.

tamponade to prevent hematoma formation in the loose paravaginal tissues. Tears around the base of the bladder require accurate repair—even then cysto-cele may not always be prevented.   If the puborectal portions of the levator ani are torn from the posterior surface of the pubis, this fact may be discovered by opening up the rent widely to view. I have tried to reunite the muscle to the obturator fascia, having failed to attach it to the bone, and with fair success.

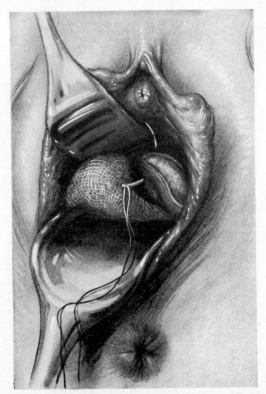

FIG. 687.—REPAIR OF LACERATION AT BASE AND SIDE OF BLADDER.

A broad, short speculum retracts the perineum, a pad holds the cervix out of the way and absorbs the excess blood, a narrow speculum lifts up the bladder. Thus exposed, the wound is visible, but not comfortably accessible. The needle passes through the posterior lip of the wound first, then across the base of the bladder, avoiding the ureters, and out through the upper lip of the wound, the point striking the speculum and sliding over it into the bite of the assistant's artery forceps. If it is possible to pick up the torn levator ani pillar and attach it to the periosteum or obturator fascia, it should be attempted. There are large veins at this point.

A broad speculum, very good light, sharply curved needles, and several assistants are needed for good repair work in the vagina (Fig. 687).

HÆMATOMA VULVÆ ET VAGINÆ

Blood-vessels, particularly the veins, in the pelvis may burst during pregnancy, labor, or postpartum, and a blood tumor or "thrombus" form in the loose connective tissue. Hematomata have been found under the skin of the vulva, around the vagina, under the broad ligaments, in the broad ligaments, and they show a tendency to enlarge, following the lines of cleavage of the connective-tissue layers or fasciæ. If below the levator ani and deep pelvic fascia, they distend the perineum and dislocate the rectum and anus, forming tumors sometimes as large as a cocoanut. If around the vagina, they may fill up the pelvis, forcing the vagina to the side and closing it, causing obstruction to delivery or to the flow of the lochia. They may be pedunculated in the vagina, and may occur in a septum vaginæ. If at the base of the broad ligaments, they may extend up into the false pelvis under Poupart's ligament, or, if behind, they may dissect up to the kidney back of the peritoneum. In the case from which Fig. 688 was taken the blood tumor was so extensive that the woman nearly died of anemia—the vagina was closed, the vulva displaced downward, and the cavity formed by the blood extended up out of the pelvis to a level with the anterior superior spine of the ilium. While the hematoma begins to form at once, it requires a few hours for its presence to become manifest, and usually within ten hours the blood mass is fully developed. Rueff, in 1554, reported the first case of hematoma.

Etiology.—The bursting of the vessel may be caused by injury—the traumatism of spontaneous labor—or by the forceps, etc. Pressure necrosis explains the cases of formation of hematoma late in the puerperium—on the third, eleventh, and twenty-first days, as reported. Varices are said not to favor hematomata.

Rough uterine massage in the treatment of postpartum hemorrhage may cause small hematomata in the subperitoneal connective tissue and in the broad liga-

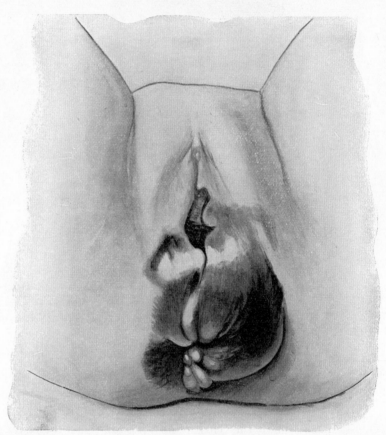

Fig. 688.—Hæmatoma Vulvæ et Vaginæ.
From a photograph, Mrs. F., Mercy Hospital. Case of pregnancy toxemia resembling scurvy.

ments, but perhaps in the fatal cases, where such findings were made, the woman died of a hemophilic diathesis and the latter caused the blood extravasations. In one of my cases, during the treatment of placenta prævia, a tumor developed in the perivaginal connective tissue, extending from the vulva to the uterus, which was taken to be a hematoma, but upon cutting into it with the expectation of turning out a clot, none was found, the tissues being simply infiltrated with blood. Hematomata are rare, about 1 to 4000 labors, but statistics vary. In an experience comprising the pathologic work of over 64,000 routine cases, only 7 cases of large hematomata have come under my notice. Small hematomata are not exceedingly rare, and their formation may sometimes be observed when a vein is pricked while repairing the torn perineum. Toxemia may cause bloody extravasations (Fig. 688).

Symptoms.—Intense pain is the most prominent symptom, and the intelligent patient will describe the tearing open of the tissues and the intolerable pressure on the rectum and bladder. Sometimes the skin or the vagina covering the tumor bursts and the patient may bleed to death. If the hematoma burrows a great distance, signs of anemia from internal hemorrhage appear. Small extravasations, as a rule, are quickly absorbed. Larger ones usually become infected, with abscess formation, or even general septicemia, but sometimes they open spontaneously, the clots are discharged, and the cavity closes (rare). Hematomata which complicate rupture of the uterus are not considered here.

Prognosis.—Nowadays death from this accident is rare, but formerly the mortality was from 12 to 40 per cent. If the tumor does not become infected, recovery is the rule. If it extends up under the peritoneum and infection of the immense blood-masses takes place, peritonitis is the usual outcome. It is wise to make a guarded prognosis until it is determined how far the hematoma is going to burrow, and whether or not infection will occur.

Treatment.—If the hematoma begins to form during labor, its course must at first be carefully watched, and if its growth is rapid, it is to be incised and packed. In cases where delivery of the child may be accomplished this should be effected, and then the whole uterovaginal canal firmly tamponed, together with the hematoma sac. If the tumor begins to form before the placenta is delivered, the latter is manually removed, and then the tamponade made, as in the last instance. If the hematoma is found after labor, at first expectancy and ice applications are to be practised, but if the hemorrhage into the tissues continues, shown by increasing size of the tumor and redoubled pain cries of the woman, the sac must be broadly opened, the clots and fluid blood turned out, bleeding vessels, if found, ligated, and every crevice of the cavity firmly packed with sterile kephalin or mildly antiseptic gauze. Then the uterovaginal canal is packed and a firm abdominal binder applied. To procure a bloodless field while operating an aorta compressor may be used, this only in critical cases. If it is possible to wait twenty-four or forty-eight hours before performing this operation to allow firm thrombosis in the torn vessels, the possibility of secondary hemorrhage at the operation is avoided. Small hematomata may be left to be absorbed, but all are to be opened at the first sign of infection.

LESIONS OF THE CERVIX

Every labor is attended by more or less injury to the cervix, since even a normal uterus cannot stand the enormous radial dilatation required for the passage of the child. Large tears of the cervix result from—(1) Too rapid or too forceful dilatation by the powers of labor (precipitate births) or by the accoucheur, with his operative deliveries before the os is completely dilated; (2) from disease of the cervix, anatomic rigidity, old primiparity, healed ulcers and scars from former deliveries or operations, cancer, syphilitic and gonorrheal induration, etc.; (3) too large child or congenital smallness of the cervix. Most of the tears are of the first class and are due to violence. Every case of accouchement forcè and every manual or instrumental dilatation of the cervix is attended by more or less numerous and deep lacerations. If the operation is performed before the cervix is completely effaced, serious or even fatal injuries may result.

The lesion may be a small nick in the mucosa, or a deep rent extending through the cervix, the vaginal vault, the parametrium, even to the brim of the pelvis, and up under the peritoneum of the broad ligaments, or even into the peritoneal cavity—with all grades between. The large rents are treated under the subject of Rupture of the Uterus. Lateral or bilateral lacerations are most commonly found, owing to the peculiarities of fetal development, but radial tears, from one to five in number, may be observed, and they occupy any part of the cervix. Sometimes a portion of the cervix is dragged off the uterine body at the vagino-uterine junction, or the whole cervix may thus be amputated and cast off as a ring of tissue. The circular amputation of the cervix may be produced by trying to draw a colpeurynter through the unprepared cervix, or the uterus may force the head down, carrying the cervix before it. The resulting scar nearly always closes the uterus. The anterior lip of the cervix may be caught between the head and the pubis and be squeezed off, or suffer so much compression that it becomes necrotic.

Cervix tears are usually not discovered until after the child is delivered, when the hemorrhage begins. Bleeding is not constant. Unless a large branch of the uterine artery or a vein is torn across, there is none of any moment. In placenta prævia cervix tears usually bleed furiously, the immensely dilated veins being opened by even a superficial lesion.

Surgical Anatomy.—Tearing of the cervix follows the lines of its embryonal construction, and the lines of cleavage are modified by disease. At the sides of the cervix there is less muscular and fibrous tissue, and here the structure most often gives way, producing the usual bilateral split (Fig. 689). If only the muscular body of the cervix ruptures, the external and internal mucosæ remaining intact, we find a thin bridge of tissue uniting the anterior and posterior lips (Fig. 689, b). Occasionally muscle at the sides parts the mucous membrane, both stretches and tears, and the wound aligns itself with the rest of the circle of the cervix so that the injury is not apparent at first glance. By separating the two layers of mucosa as in Fig. 689, d, the deep extent of the wound is laid bare. In repairing such a laceration, the thin bridge is to be split, making the wound like the first variety, then the muscular tissue is to be pulled out of the deep recesses at each side. If this is not done, the operation will succeed only in bringing the edges of the mucosa together. There is a third form of laceration which is usually unrecognized. The cervix is stretched radially, and the inner mucosa is slid off its attachment to the muscularis, giving, when exposed by broad specula, the appearance of the everted anus of a horse (Fig. 689, e). This form of injury is often combined with one or both of the previously described varieties. The repair of this damage is not easy—an attempt may be made to suture the mucosa in its place after pushing it up with thumb and fingers (Fig. 689, f).

Prognosis.—Small tears of the cervix, unless infected, heal without trouble, but larger tears always leave deforming scars, leading to ectropion, catarrh, and, some say, to carcinoma. Perforating tears are often fatal. Chronic metritis undoubtedly follows large cervix tears, and, since they are always associated with injury of the pelvic connective tissue, descensus uteri often results.

Treatment.—After spontaneous deliveries in the home, unless there is hemorrhage or collapse, or a probable injury from precipitate birth, the search for and repair of cervical tears are not usually recommended. In maternities with good technic, and where the home facilities permit it, a specular examination, with suture, is routine. It is also the rule after forceps and other operative deliveries, or where injury is expected. If infection is present or probable, the tear is not sutured unless it bleeds and packing will not stop it. Under unfavorable operating-room conditions the woman is safer with the cervix open to drain, and repair may be made later. Hirst and a few others recommend secondary suture on the fifth or sixth day of the puerperium, but the author does not advise it for reasons already given under Perineorrhaphy. Titian Coffey repairs all cervices on the tenth day.

By means of the vulsellum forceps or the cervix forceps shown in Fig. 690 the two lips of the uterus are drawn down to the vulva and become readily accessible for suture, or successive stitches are passed through the most accessible portion of the cervical lips, and pulling on these the higher region—even the base of the broad ligament into which the spurting vessel has retracted—is brought into reach. One must actually encircle the torn vessel, otherwise the bleeding continues retroperitoneally, a hematoma forms which may extend as far as the kidney, and death results. Kerwin advises to tie the uterine artery operating vaginally.

When bleeding is profuse, it is not so easy to sew the cervix, because it is hidden in a pool of blood. A bullet forceps may be clamped on the base of the broad ligament, as advised by Henkel for temporary hemostasis. Another plan is to pass the needle from the inside of the cervix under the guidance of the finger,

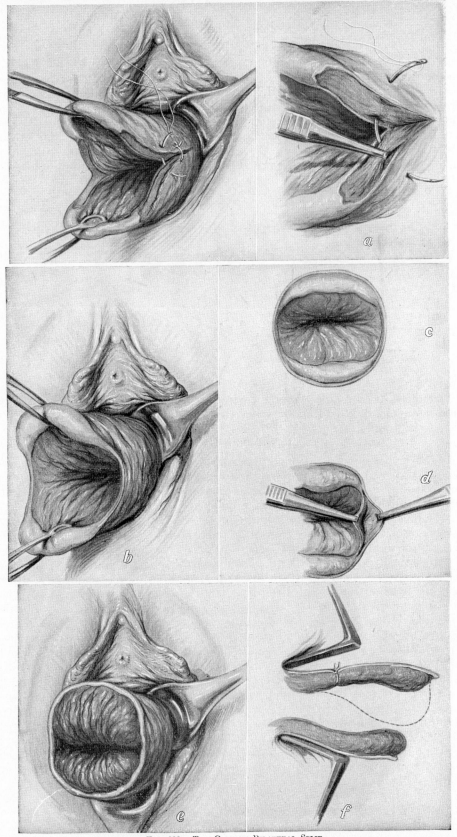

FIG. 689.—THE COMMON BILATERAL SPLIT.

a, Method of suture—lifting out retracted muscle tissue to pass the needle under it. *b*, Occult rupture, submucous. *c*, Appearance before separating mucosal lamellæ. *d*, Exposing the occult tear by pulling the vaginal from the endo-cervical mucosa. *e*, Deep circular overstretching of the muscular and fibrous structure of the cervix with prolapse and eversion of the mucosa. *f*, Suggestion of a method for repair. One tries to push up the swollen prolapsed mucosa and hold it in place by two or three sutures. It does not work well in practice.

and tie the suture inside the uterus. The balance of the stitches are put in from the outside of the cervix, the most important being the uppermost one, near the fornix vaginæ, since it is intended to stop the hemorrhage which comes from the large vessels here. Continued suture is used if haste is demanded, otherwise interrupted No. 2 forty-day catgut. Since the ureter is close by, the needle in the first suture must be passed in a direction nearly parallel to the uterine body. The others are transverse and pass to, but not through, the mucosa. They may be drawn fairly tight, because the cervix rapidly shrinks postpartum. An aorta compressor may be used in urgent cases to stop the bleeding until the wound can be sutured. Should

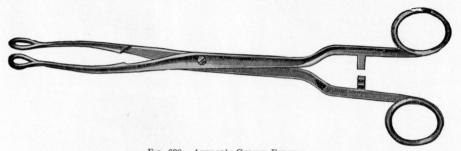

FIG. 690.—AUTHOR'S CERVIX FORCEPS.
Hold tissues securely without tearing them, and present no points to puncture rubber gloves.

infection begin in the puerperium, the stitches are to be at once removed and drainage provided, because otherwise the parametria will be rapidly involved, and even fatal septicemia result. Douches are contraindicated.

RUPTURA UTERI

This fearful accident occurs oftener than is generally believed, and few emergencies in all medicine require so much of what makes a great surgeon as does this one. The uterus may rupture during pregnancy and during labor, and since the latter is more common, it will be first considered.

During Labor.—*Etiology.*—Ruptures of the uterus are divided into two classes —spontaneous and violent or traumatic. Spontaneous ruptures are those which occur as the result of the natural forces of labor, or because the muscle of the uterus is pathologically altered, so that it bursts from the ordinary processes of labor or gestation. Violent or traumatic ruptures are those which result from injury, either from the hand or instrument of the attendant or by external agencies. Often the uterine muscle is so thinned by the action of labor that it bursts with only a little traumatism. The causes of actual rupture may be divided into predisposing and exciting. Predisposing causes are, first, those conditions which produce a weakening of the uterine wall, as fatty or hyaline degeneration of the muscle (Figs. 126 and 126*a*); syphilis; pressure necrosis during prolonged labor; scars from previous operations (cesarean section, salpingectomy with excision of uterine cornu, curetage); scars from previous rupture, from puerperal septic processes, and old inflammations; thinned spots from the removal of adherent placenta in previous labors, fibroids, and other neoplasms; adherent uterus; overdistention of part of uterus; congenitally undeveloped uterus; pregnancy in a horn; interstitial pregnancy; growth of the placenta into the uterine musculature, especially if it happens to be located over a thinned or diseased portion; placenta prævia; edema of the lower uterine segment the result of prolonged labor; polyhydramnion. The second group of predisposing causes comprises all the mechanical factors which stop the advance of the child through the birth-canal, as contracted pelvis of all kinds; overgrown fetus; deformities of the child which increase its size, especially hydrocephalus; malpresentations (shoulder, face, and brow, anterior and posterior parietal bone);

malpositions, as occipitoposteriors; delayed rotation of the head; obstruction of the soft parts, as tumors blocking the pelvis, atresia cervicis or vaginæ, rigid perineum, and incarceration of the cervix between the presenting part and the pelvic brim. Pendulous abdomen, by putting the posterior uterovaginal wall on the stretch, creates a condition favorable to rupture, the resulting lesion being called kolpoporrhexis, or kolporrhexis. Unless the natural powers can overcome these obstructions by a moderate amount of effort, something has to give way, and the weakest point or the most overstretched point is the site of rupture.

Exciting causes of the rupture are the contractions of the uterus and mechanical insult or violence. To understand the mechanism of spontaneous rupture it is

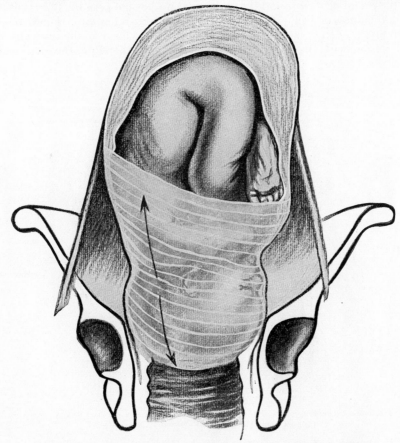

Fig. 691.—Excessive Thinning of Lower Uterine Segment. Brow Presentation. Arrows indicate direction of tension. Note guyrope action of round ligaments.

necessary to refer to the normal mechanism of labor and the formation of the parturient canal. We are indebted to Michaëlis, Bandl, and Freund for the foundation of our knowledge of this subject. Throughout labor the fundus of the uterus contracts, while the isthmus and cervix are dilated from above downward, the muscle being differentiated into an upper zone of contracting, and a lower of dilating, fibers. The fibers of the isthmus uteri and cervix are drawn upward into the body of the uterus, and, at the junction of the contractile with the dilating portions, is a well-defined ring of muscle which Bandl called the *contraction ring*. The sacro-uterine ligaments fix the cervix in the pelvis behind, the bases of the broad ligaments fix it at the sides, and the connective tissue at the base of the bladder anchors it in front, all of which connective tissue and partly muscular support prevent too great upward retraction of the cervix. An additional and important factor in the mechanism of rupture is the fixation of the cervix by the head, squeezing it against the bony pelvis. This is particularly likely to happen if the bag of waters ruptures before the cervix is dilated and retracted above the presenting part. The fundus uteri is held down and prevented from pulling too far up over the child, and away from the pelvis, by the guy-rope-like action of the round ligaments (Fig. 169) and the pressure of the abdominal wall. It is easy to see that if the child may not advance along the birth-canal, the continued action of the uterus will result in the contractile portion having forced nearly the whole child down into the dilating portions, the lower uterine segment and cervix, and itself having retracted above the child as far as the round ligaments and the abdominal wall would permit. The fundus may attain a thickness of 4 cm., the cervix being thinned to a few mm. Figure 691 shows the condition. Sometimes the cervix is more or less fixed at the inlet and cannot wholly retract with the lower uterine segment, and, therefore, the latter is drawn

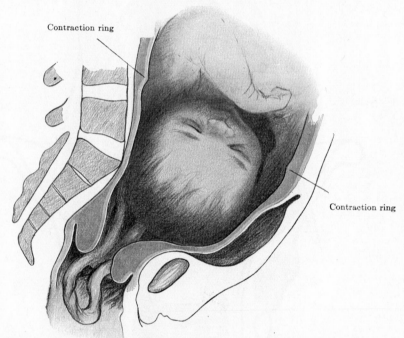

Contraction ring

Contraction ring

FIG. 692.—INCARCERATION OF THE CERVIX BETWEEN HEAD AND PELVIS. CERVIX SWOLLEN.
Rupture would take place just above it. Case of Mrs. G.

out in the length and may tear transversely (Fig. 692). Since the dilatation of the lower uterine segment is never symmetric, owing to the obliquity of the uterus, the irregularity of the body contained therein, pendulous abdomen, etc., some portion of it is stretched more than the rest, and here the rupture occurs. As a rule, first the muscle-fibers separate and tear, then the mucous membrane gives way, and finally the peritoneal covering of the uterus. I have on several occasions felt this occurrence under my hand. If the cervix has already been dilated and fully taken up to form part of the parturient canal, it cannot be fixed below, but retracts upward, with the lower uterine segment, and the full force of this retraction is distributed along the wall of the parturient canal from the contraction ring down the vagina to the attachments of the latter on to the pelvic floor. If the stretching of this canal is too great, the rupture will occur at its weakest spot, and this is usually the posterior fornix of the vagina. Indeed, in cases of shoulder presentation, immense hydrocephalus, pendulous abdomen, where the presenting part cannot imprison the cervix against the pelvis, we find such ruptures of the vagina or kolpoporrhexis (Hugenberger) (Fig. 693).

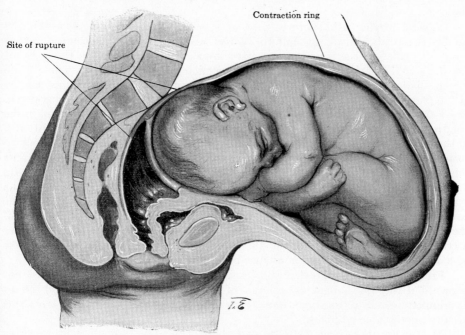

FIG. 693.—KOLPOPORRHEXIS.
Mrs. Y. (Service of Chicago Lying-in Hospital Dispensary.)

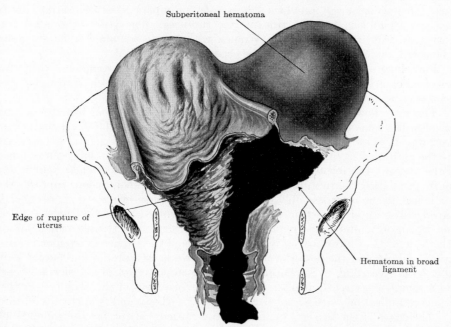

FIG. 694.—DIAGRAM OF UTERINE RUPTURE. BROAD LIGAMENT UNFOLDED AND DISTENDED BY IMMENSE HEMATOMA.

Ruptures in the lower uterine segment are usually longitudinal or oblique; those in the fornix vaginæ usually transverse or even completely circular. The normal contractions of the uterus alone may cause a rupture if the wall is diseased, and in the presence of mechanical obstruction even a normal muscle may burst if the pains are strong. The deadly effects of pituitrin must here be mentioned. In the olden time ergot was the offender.

Violent or traumatic ruptures have no special mechanism, but, as a rule, the fundus is already drawn up, and the lower segment and vagina thinned out as above described at the time the causative injury is inflicted, and on this account the shape and location of the tear are very similar to the spontaneous ones. The forceps blade or the cranioclast may be pushed through the wall, or grasp a portion of the musculature and crush it. Traction with the forceps pulls the cervix down, and a transverse split occurs in the lower uterine segment, already stretched in the length to the point of bursting. The hand introduced alongside the child contained in the ad maxima distended, lower segment may cause the tear; or the attempt to turn the child by bringing the trunk down into the pelvis alongside the head puts too great a strain on this portion of the uterus; or the hand pushes the uterus up away from the vagina, and the rupture occurs at the junction of the latter with the cervix, or finally too rapid delivery through an unprepared cervix simply bursts the narrow canal. Instrumental injuries usually are found in the neighborhood of the fornix vaginae and the cervix; the others usually in the overdistended lower uterine segment, and it is evident that the operator only completed a tear that was already being prepared for or just beginning.

Frequency.—Where good obstetrics is practiced ruptura uteri is almost unknown, but the wide-spread performance of the classic cesarean section, and the indiscriminate use of pituitary extracts serve to keep up a large mortality from this usually preventable accident.

Multiparæ are oftener thus injured than primiparæ,—about eight times as often,—and the danger increases with the number of children. This is due to the structural changes, the weakness of the muscular fibers, the scars and inflammations, the residues from previous labors. In primiparæ the perforating cervix tears are commoner than the true uterine ruptures. The years of greatest frequency are from thirty to forty. Women with loose abdominal walls are more endangered, and fat women seem to be especially predisposed.

Pathology.—Ruptures are divided into two classes—the complete, where the peritoneal cavity is opened, and the incomplete, where the muscle is torn, but the peritoneum remains intact.

Fig. 694 shows an incomplete rupture with a subperitoneal hematoma, and Fig. 694a the same case after the thin peritoneal covering of the blood tumor had given way because of the restless tossing of the patient, and a fatal hemorrhage into the peritoneal cavity had ensued. Note how the peritoneum has been stripped off the uterus. In violent or traumatic ruptures the cervix is oftenest split in the length, or at least the rupture is usually longitudinal; in spontaneous ruptures the tear is usually more or less oblique and often transverse, while it may be L or V shaped. The anterior uterine wall is oftenest involved, then the sides, the left more commonly, and least frequently the posterior wall. Double tears, one on either side of the uterus, are on record. Rupture of the vagina—kolpoporrhexis—is rare, and oftenest the posterior fornix is torn, while the anterior and lateral walls suffer less. According to Stschotkin, there were 36 posterior, 24 anterior, 8 lateral, and 8 completely circular tears in 74 cases. Involvement of the bladder is a very serious complication, with 87 per cent. mortality (Klien), and is, fortunately, rare.

The edges of the tear are suggillated and ragged. If the broad ligaments are opened up, the veins and arteries can be felt traversing the connective-tissue spaces, which are filled with blood, and sometimes with air or gases of decomposition (emphysema). The hemorrhage comes from the large venous plexuses, from the uterine arteries and its large branches, especially the uterovaginal. The hematoma may burrow in the connective tissue, far away from the site of rupture, even to the kidneys. If the tear is behind the broad ligaments, the bleeding may be small, but if it is through the bases of the broad ligaments or involves the site of the placenta, the woman may die in a few minutes from the sudden immense loss of blood. In my cases the loss of blood was greatest in the incomplete ruptures, while the shock was most evident with the complete ones. Urine, meconium, lanugo, vernix caseosa, and liquor amnii may be found in the peritoneal cavity.

Usually, at the height of a pain, the thinned portion of the uterus gives way, but sometimes the separation of the fibers is gradual, and the rupture is completed without producing alarming symptoms (latent rupture). Only after peritonitis sets in or an abscess develops is the condition recognized, or, indeed, at a subsequent labor, when the uterus ruptures again at the site of the previous scar. The point which is most subjected to the strain gives way; then the uterine contractions

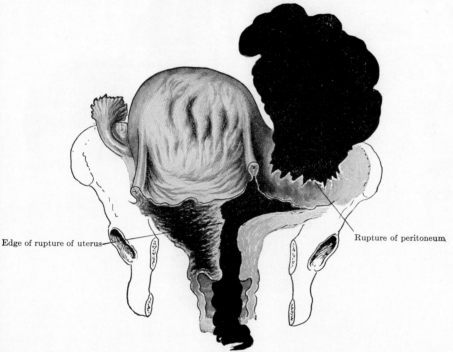

Edge of rupture of uterus

Rupture of peritoneum

Fig. 694a.—Diagram of Uterine Rupture. Hematoma Burst During the Tossing About of the Patient.

force the child through the weak spot thus created. After the child is expelled through this new passage the uterus contracts down beside it and comes to rest. Sometimes the rent is enlarged by the operative delivery. Intestines and omentum may protrude through the opening into the vagina.

Incomplete ruptures occur under the same circumstances, and from the same causes, as the perforating ones, and the tear may involve one or two of the layers of the uterus. That is, the peritoneum only may split, and may give rise to intra-peritoneal hemorrhage, mild or fatal, or the muscle only may part, the mucous membrane and peritoneum being intact, or the peritoneum and muscle break, leaving the mucosa, or the mucous membrane and muscle part, leaving the serous membrane, the last being the commonest variety. Hematoma is the rule in such cases, and the tear is always located at a spot where the peritoneum is loosely attached to the uterus, the sides, and near the bladder. Cervix tears, if extensive, are usually of this type. Bursting of a varix in or on the broad ligament, with subperitoneal or intraperitoneal hemorrhage, tearing of an artery in the broad ligament, have been observed as rare causes of death. Possibly some such accidents occur, but are not discovered.

Symptoms.—If the accoucheur is on the alert, he will almost always be able to detect a threatening rupture of the uterus, and diagnose early a dangerous thinning of the lower uterine segment. In contracted pelves and all cases of mechanical obstruction, and where he knows that the uterine wall is weakened, the attendant will be especially watchful. It must be said, however, that sometimes the tear will occur so gradually that the symptoms will hardly attract notice, or the tissues will suddenly give way without any apparent cause and without any warning. This may occur in the beginning of labor, with few pains and intact membranes, or even during pregnancy, but it is very exceptional.

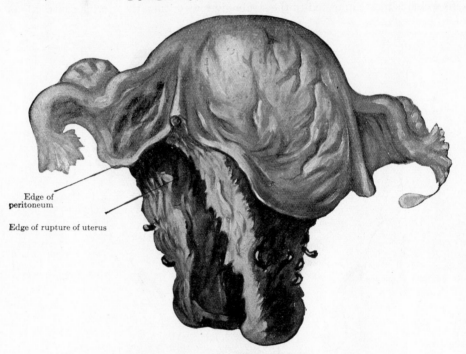

Edge of
peritoneum

Edge of rupture of uterus

Fig. 695.—Rupture of the Uterus (author's specimen).

Fortunately, symptoms are usually present. The parturient is restless, tossing and rolling about the bed; she is anxious about the labor, because there is no progress in spite of her strong pains; she complains of constant soreness and almost continual pain over the hypogastrium, and unconsciously her hands support the lower uterine segment with every uterine contraction; the face is reddened, but the alæ nasi are gray; the mouth and tongue are dry and red; she complains of a desire to urinate frequently, and bears down with the pain in a helpless sort of way, and begs for relief incessantly; the temperature is slightly raised; the respiration is panting; the pulse is fast and usually of high tension. Hoehne says the bearing-down efforts are a protective reflex due to overdistension of the lower uterine segment. If the woman has syncopal attacks, one can infer that slight tearing of the uterus has begun.

The Rupture.—Suddenly, during the acme of a pain, or while the woman is tossing from one side to the other, she complains of a sharp, tearing pain in the lower belly, and may exclaim that something has burst within her. Now the picture rapidly changes from sthenic to asthenic. As a result of the shock and internal hemorrhage the face pales, the lips whiten or become cyanotic, the features sink in, cold sweat appears on the nose and forehead, the temperature drops, the

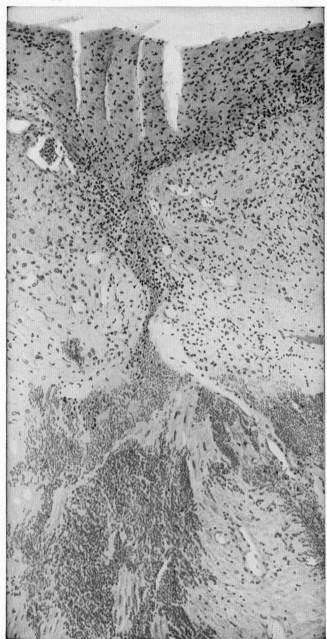

Fig. 696.—Section of the Ruptured Uterus Shown in Figure 695.
Low power. Shows hyaline degenerated muscle. A few decidual cells.

pulse becomes small and running, even filiform, and the respiration sighing; the pains cease and the patient is ominously quiet for a short while. The woman complains of shortness of breath, of precordial oppression, of a feeling of impending death, and soon becomes restless again. Vomiting begins, but usually is not a

52

prominent symptom until later. The pains almost always cease, but if the child
has not been expelled into the abdominal cavity, they may continue, though weaker,
and they may, though rarely, suffice to deliver the child. Hemorrhage from the
genitals now appears, but is usually not profuse. If the blood distends the broad
ligaments pain runs down the leg; if it is free in the abdominal cavity it may seep
under the liver and cause shoulder-pain. The fetal movements for the first few
minutes are very violent, while the child dies, then cease, a phenomenon which
may be observed with special distinctness when the child has escaped from the
rent uterus under the abdominal wall. If the child is delivered and the rupture untreated, the woman may die from primary hemorrhage, from shock, from secondary
hemorrhage (a hematoma bursting), from peritonitis, either early or beginning as
late as the twentieth day, or she may recover unaided if the damage is not great.
The peritoneal edges of the tear adhere, and, in the absence of infection, the wound
granulates.

A few cases are on record where the child, expelled through the rent into the
peritoneal cavity, was changed into a lithopedion, as in ectopic gestation.

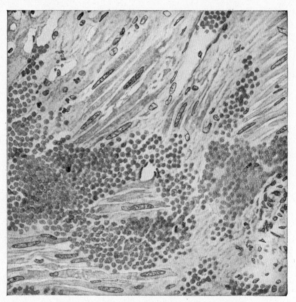

FIG. 696a.—SECTION OF RUPTURED UTERUS.
High power. Shows the torn muscular fibers.

Diagnosis.—(A) *Threatened Rupture.*—It is vitally important that the diagnosis
of dangerous thinning of the uterus be made before the rupture occurs, because if
anything can be done to save the woman, it must be done at once. The findings
on examination are—(1) A restless, excited, anxious patient, high pulse (90 to 110),
irregular respiration, temperature 99.6° to 100.4° F., and, if infection is beginning,
101° to 103° F.; (2) *strong uterine contractions without proportionate advance of the
presenting part;* (3) the uterus hard and drawn up over the child, which lies in the
dilated lower uterine segment (Fig. 697). The fundus is thick and the lower uterine
segment soft; it balloons out during the pains, allowing the fetal body to be outlined with startling distinctness. The latter seems to lie under the skin. This
finding is possible under anesthesia—the exquisite tenderness prevents it otherwise;
(4) a groove is visible and palpable, running obliquely across the belly, higher on
the side of the greatest stretching—the contraction ring (Fig. 697). It may rise
as high as the navel or higher, and the distance from the pubis may be used to

estimate the degree of thinning and stretching of the lower uterine segment; (5) the round ligaments are inserted high on the uterus, are tender, hard, and wiry, and particularly the one on the side which is going to burst may be tense and taut, like a violin string (Fig. 697); (6) the uterus is oblique; (7) the bladder is drawn up high; (8) a general abdominal tenderness is present, but the lower uterine segment is so sensitive that the woman will hardly allow it to be touched; (9) internal examination will reveal the cervix, either imprisoned in the pelvis and swollen, black and blue, or drawn up out of the pelvis with the vagina on the stretch, taut around the presenting part, and hot, reddened, and dry.

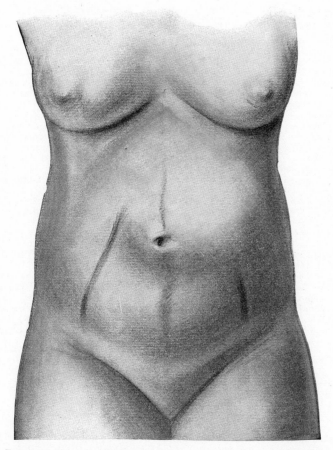

FIG. 697.—ABDOMINAL FINDINGS IN A CASE OF THREATENED RUPTURA UTERI.
Mrs. S., V-para, patient with flat pelvis, obstructed labor. Note the fundus; the ballooned lower uterine segment; the contraction ring; the tense round ligaments. A full bladder may present a picture resembling this.

These findings on the direct examination will enable every accoucheur to discover the danger which threatens the woman in time to institute proper treatment. Unfortunately, in the latent ruptures they may be absent or veiled.

(B) *Actual Rupture.*—The symptoms of the actual tearing of the uterus and of the shock and anemia which follow will almost always be sufficient to make the direct diagnosis, but an examination of the patient must be made to confirm it. The findings in cases of rupture of the uterus vary, of course, with the time in labor when it occurs, and whether or not the child is in the uterus or in the belly when the examination is made. They are: (1) A collapsed patient with all the signs of anemia and of shock; (2) uterine action stopped or very weak; (3) external hemorrhage, mild or severe, rarely absent; (4) abdominally, the child can be felt with surprising distinctness, lying right under the belly-wall, while the empty uterus is pushed to one side, or behind, where it is not palpable. If the child has partly escaped, the uterine tumor is heart shaped. Dulness in the flanks from free blood is very rarely determinable. Tenderness may make the abdominal examination nugatory; (5) externally the hematoma may be felt, or emphysematous crackling; (6) internally, the ragged rent may be palpable, and intestines or omentum may fall into the hand; (7) the presenting part has disappeared from the inlet or has become freely movable.

The author makes it a rule, after every operative delivery, whether or not symptoms are present, to examine the uterus, at least the lower uterine segment, with the whole hand and determine, beyond the suspicion of a doubt, the extent and location of any injury. This practice cannot be too strongly recommended.

Differential Diagnosis.—As a rule, during labor, little difficulty is experienced, but sometimes one has to consider abruptio placentæ, placenta prævia, and extra-uterine pregnancy at term. These have already been discussed under their respective headings. Collapse during or after labor may be due to something else, but rupture of the uterus is first to be thought of.

An important diagnosis to make after delivery is whether the rupture is complete or incomplete, since the principles of the treatment depend on this. Abdominally, little can be found; in rare instances a hematoma may be outlined. Emphysema is not distinctive, nor are signs of peritoneal irritation. Exploratory puncture may help, by showing free blood. Vaginally, the presence of intestines or omentum is, of course, conclusive, but not the discharge of peritoneal fluid, which may be simulated by the serum squeezed out from a blood-clot. The internal examination alone can be relied on to differentiate, and here it may be necessary to use the hand without a rubber glove. This is the only instance where I have had to use the bare hand. The fingers gently pass through the uterine portion of the tear, and come into a space filled with soft clot. Strands of fibrous tissue, nerves, and sometimes vessels span the space, and great care must be exercised to prevent breaking them. I once felt the uterine artery between my fingers pulsating ominously. If the tear is complete, the fingers pass directly into the peritoneal cavity, which may be recognized by—(1) The smooth, slippery surface of the adjacent uterus and of the abdominal wall; (2) the presence of gut and omentum; (3) the great freedom of motion for the fingers; (4) the fingers may lift up the abdominal wall from the inside; (5) outlining the edges of the wound. To recognize the thin, veil-like layer of peritoneum over an incomplete rupture—(1) Note if the fingers are confined to a ragged, walled cavity; (2) try to determine the upper uterine end of the rupture, and find if the peritoneum has been stripped off the uterus here; (3) bimanually, determine if there are any structures between the hands; (4) try to slide the questionable layer of tissue over the fingers, or depress it by the abdominal hand between the two parted internal fingers; (5) note the relation of the gut to it. In the last instance the peritoneum may be so thin and stripped off the underlying structures so extensively that the gut appears to be within the grasp of the fingers, uncovered. Here the differential diagnosis is not so necessary, because in such cases the thin veil of peritoneum will in all likelihood slough off, so that the treatment is the same as for complete tears.

It is sometimes necessary to decide if other organs beside the uterus—the bladder, the rectum and bowels, the omentum—are involved. If there is the least suspicion of such an injury, the case is to be treated as if it really were so. The bladder may be examined with a cystoscope. An x-ray picture may show pneumoperitoneum. The rectum may be explored, but if any injury higher up is suspected, the belly should be opened.

Prognosis.—This is grave in all cases, but, fortunately, the improvement of modern obstetric practice, with asepsis and early recognition and operative treatment of the accident, has effected a substantial reduction of the previous high mortality. Incomplete ruptures are a little less dangerous than complete ones, but the prognosis depends on so many conditions—the site, the extent and method of infliction of the injury, the presence of infection, the environment of the patient (hospital or home), the kind of treatment, etc.—that figures are practically useless. Of the author's 18 cases of complete rupture, 11 died of shock or sepsis; of 19 cases of incomplete tear, 3 died—2 from hemorrhage and 1 from peritonitis. Cholmogarof, in 1894, found mortalities given by different clinics from 21 to 65 per cent., depending on no particular line of treatment, and Koblanck showed 73 per cent. and 78 per cent., Braun, 63 per cent., that for incomplete tears being 25 per cent. For the child, the outlook is still worse. Unless the delivery can be completed at once, the child is surely lost. When the rupture occurs at the end of the second stage, the child may come out alive. If it is forced out into the belly, it usually dies in a few minutes, but three cases are on record where a hasty abdominal section rescued it.

If the mother survives the hemorrhage and shock, her life depends on the presence or absence of infection. Peritonitis is the rule because the cases are usually in the hands of midwives or unclean attendants. Even if she recovers from this labor she is threatened by a worse recurrence of the accident in her next one. Perfect health is never restored; the uterus remains large (chronic metritis), the laceration scars distort and displace it, and the pelvis is permanently the seat of venous congestion.

Treatment.—Prevention of rupture of the uterus is one of the regular duties of the accoucheur, and forms part of the "watchful expectancy" so often spoken of in the treatment of labor. In every case of mechanical disproportion (contracted pelvis, malpresentations, hydrocephalus, etc.) or weak uterus (e. g., previous section), the accoucheur will scan the face of the labor for the first outward expression of threatened rupture. If a diagnosis of ruptura uteri imminens is made, the indication is to empty the uterus as quickly as possible, and, moreover, this must be done with the least possible increase of the intra-uterine tension, i. e., with no further stretching of the already overstretched lower uterine segment, cervix, and vagina. If the cervix is imprisoned in the pelvis, it must first be pushed up, because traction on it from below would stretch it still further in the length and effect the transverse tear which was impending. If all the conditions for forceps are fulfilled, this is the operation of choice, but it may not be forced, since the dragging down of the child may pull the thinned cervix apart. Cranioclasis, followed by cleidotomy and evisceration, is preferable and more humane. It is criminal to attempt version in these cases. In breech presentations the after-coming head must be carefully led through the endangered portion of the parturient canal. In shoulder presentations embryotomy, i. e., evisceration and rachiotomy, is the method of election. Since the child is nearly always dead or dying, the accoucheur should have no compunctions about this operation, especially when version carries so terrible a risk for the mother. In cases where the uterus has only just begun to show evidences of thinning out, an expert accoucheur may, exceptionally, under deep anesthesia and in ideal surroundings, make a gentle trial of version in the hope of saving the infant. Under other circumstances the mother is safest with embryotomy. Cervical cesarean section should always be considered when the child is alive, but the conditions favorable to the mother, too, must be present. Cesarean section must always be done in high degrees of pelvic contraction or obstruction of the soft parts. Pubiotomy rarely comes into the discussion of these cases. Vaginal hysterotomy occasionally does.

To prevent a rupture while preparing for these operations the patient should be instructed to lie quiet. The uterus may be supported by a binder, but the best remedy is a deep ether narcosis to paralyze the uterus until aid is at hand.

It is best not to transport a patient whose uterus is on the point of bursting, because the jolting over rough crossings may tear the thinned wall. Nowadays, by grace of good roads and good ambulances, the risks of the ride may be less than those of inefficient treatment at home. Morphin, $\frac{1}{3}$ to $\frac{1}{2}$ gr., is to be given before starting and the journey rendered as smooth as possible. To prevent the uterine tumor from swaying from side to side and thus putting the endangered lower segment on too great a strain, a well-padded binder should be applied, and sand-bags laid on both sides of the abdomen, or, better still, the accoucheur should accompany his patient and support the uterus with his hands when the ambulance jolts over rough places.

Treatment after Rupture.—Many conditions govern this—the environment (i. e., hospital or home); the state of the patient (shock, anemia, sepsis); the amount of bleeding actually going on; the site of the tear; whether an obstetrician or a general practitioner is at hand. We have to fight hemorrhage and infection.

Hospital.—*Complete Rupture.*—Spontaneous ruptures seldom occur here—they are more frequent in the home, and, fortunately, bleed less than artificial. Traumatic ruptures are commoner in hospitals, during operative delivery, and they bleed furiously. The tear is usually discovered during the removal of the placenta for hemorrhage. Immediate laparotomy is the choice, and is imperative if injury to the pelvic viscera is suspected. If, upon opening the belly, the rent is found to be smooth and the bleeding easily staunched by suture, simple repair may be made, otherwise supravaginal or total hysterectomy is performed; clots, etc., are removed from the peritoneal cavity; hematomata evacuated; the whole extent of the wound explored; perfect hemostasis; wound packed, gauze leading into vagina; peritoneum closed over stump; abdomen closed; hypodermoclysis; blood transfusion (both should be started before operation, if needed). Whether only to amputate or to remove all of the uterus depends on the state of the patient, the skill of the operator as to speed, and the extent and location of the injury, with the possibility of stopping bleeding by the less dangerous method, simple amputation.

In spontaneous ruptures a quick delivery from below, or section might save the child (rare). Delivery per vaginam is never attempted after the child has escaped into the peritoneal cavity, but if it is still in the uterus, the head deeply engaged, forceps or craniotomy is in order, quick tampon or aorta compression, then section. Rupture in transverse and breech presentation—laparotomy at once.

Hospital.—Incomplete Ruptures.—These are usually extensions of cervical tears, and may be repaired from below if not too deep. The wound is exposed by broad specula, the cervix is pulled down by forceps, and deep sutures placed high in the fornices, each suture being drawn upon to make higher portions of the lower uterine segment accessible. It is possible to throw a suture around the uterine artery by pulling down the cervix and holding the anterior wall of the vagina up (Kerwin). Occasionally Henkel's method succeeds, (page 851). If hemorrhage interferes, an aorta compressor may be temporarily applied. It might be well to detach the bladder by an anterior colpotomy to get to the highest angle of the rupture, which must always be secured to prevent hematoma formation in the broad ligament which may extend up to the kidney. Firm uterovaginal tampon after all suturing. If the rupture occurred during extraction in placenta previa—Sehrt aorta compressor, or tight tampon, then abdominal section at once. Everything depends on the severity of the bleeding.

If the tear extends high into the lower uterine segment, or if it is a real rupture of the lower uterine segment, it becomes inaccessible to suture. A skilful operator might perform vaginal hysterectomy, but more often laparotomy is chosen. In practice, if we find suture impractical or unsuccessful, the rent is packed at once. Rarely a single tamponade suffices. If the first tampon is bled through, the vagina is to be filled with cotton while the laparotomy preparations are being hurriedly made. When applying a tampon care is taken not to punch through the thin peritoneum, and to pack lightly, and to handle the patient gently afterward, as the thin veil may tear over the gauze. If the peritoneum is lifted off its attachments for a great extent, as occurs in multiple ruptures, if there is a suspicion of infection, if the wound is complicated, the case is to be treated like a complete rupture.

Once in a great while a lower uterine segment tear does not bleed much. Here a light tamponade, taking care not to push through the peritoneum is all that is required. In a multipara with no need for a uterus, the safest course is hysterectomy, the same as for a complete tear.

Home.—Complete Rupture.—Sad is the plight of the practitioner when this accident occurs in the home. If the child is still in the uterus and readily accessible it should be delivered from below, the rent quickly tamponed, the patient given pituitary, ergot, and morphin, and sent to the nearest hospital, with the precautions of transport above mentioned. If the child is in the belly, no attempt to deliver it may be made, but the tear and the vagina are to be tightly packed and the patient sent to the hospital immediately. Every minute counts. In this my advice agrees with Zweifel's.

If no hospital is available, it may be possible to do a laparotomy at home. Failing this, against his will the accoucheur must deliver the child from below, place a large rubber tube in the peritoneal cavity, and pack gauze lightly around it, or tightly, if necessary, to stop bleeding. It has been recommended to fill the pelvis above the rent with a Mikulicz tampon and make traction on the four corners of the cover so as to pull the plug against all bleeding vessels. Tamponade for bleeding and drainage offers some slight hope for the patient.

Home.—Incomplete Tears.—A skilful practitioner may sew up an extensive cervix-uterine tear at home, even with poor assistance, and his treatment would be as above outlined for the specialist. Most often the bleeding is so profuse that clamping the broad ligaments (Henkel) or tamponade is demanded at once. Whatever is needed must be decided instantly and done quickly —the seriousness of the situation usually brooks no delay.

If called to a case of ruptura uteri, after the bleeding stage has passed, and infection with or without peritonitis has begun, a bad prognosis is to be made, but hope is not abandoned. The usual method is to open the belly, amputate the uterus low, clean out the hematomata, pack their bed in the pelvic connective tissue, drain per vaginam, and close the peritoneum over the stump. Some operators pour ether or mercurochrome into the abdomen and close it, others drain. If the peritonitis is already general, the shock of such a procedure may be fatal, therefore drain above and below.

After-treatment.—Ergot and hydrastis will help to keep the uterus contracted. A firm abdominal binder should be applied, though if it is needed for counterpressure to aid a tampon in stopping hemorrhage not much may be expected. I got good results in one case by sitting by the woman's side and holding the uterus down against the tampon for two hours. The gauze is removed on the third or fourth day. If a tear has been drained it is wise not to let the wound close too rapidly. If signs of infection appear, a vaginal examination is required to determine the presence of an exudate.

Since the site of a healed rupture of the uterus is not strong, the muscular fibers near it being usually atrophied and the scar friable, it is best to instruct the patient that in a subsequent pregnancy she should spend the last four weeks in a maternity. Before labor declares itself cesarean section should be performed. If this advice is unheeded, the accoucheur should, when called during labor, terminate the case with forceps as soon as the conditions are present. Induced labor is slightly less dangerous than labor at term, but if pelvic obstruction is to be overcome it is not, and the abdominal delivery at term is imperative. The induction of abortion for this indication alone is not allowable.

RUPTURE OF THE UTERUS DURING PREGNANCY

This is one of the rarest accidents of pregnancy, if one excludes perforation of the uterus by criminal abortionists. Baisch, in 1903, collected 78 cases. A healthy uterus will tear only under the most violent indirect injury; but if the muscle is diseased, it may give way during the natural growth of pregnancy, or during one of the contractions of the uterus, or from the shock of a fall, a cough, etc. Ruptures of the uterus during pregnancy are to be divided, as in labor, into spontaneous and traumatic. The latter group must be further divided into those due to direct injury applied to the uterus, and those occurring indirectly, as from a fall or straining of any kind. Simple spontaneous rupture may occur from yielding of the scar of a previous cesarean section (very frequent nowadays), or from previous rupture, injury, or from gynecologic operations (fibroid, curetage, etc.); thinning of the uterine wall from manual removal of the placenta, especially if repeated; hypoplastic uteri; malformed uteri, as single or double horned; interstitial pregnancy; actual disease of the wall, carcinoma, hydatid mole, fatty and hyaline degeneration, previous infection, and small-cell infiltration; growth of placental villi into the uterine wall; abruptio placentæ (the uterus may burst over the retroplacental hematoma); displaced and adherent uterus;

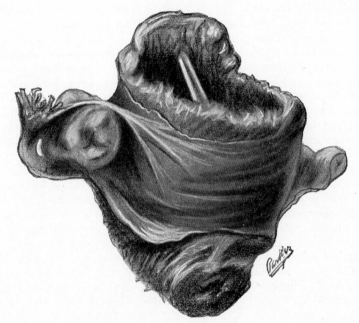

FIG. 698.—TRAUMATIC RUPTURE OF FUNDUS UTERI IN NINTH MONTH OF PREGNANCY.

in short, the same factors which predispose to rupture during labor. There is this difference, however, in labor the lower uterine segment usually gives way; in pregnancy it is the body that is involved.

Examples of direct traumatism are: Puncture of the uterus by sounds, curets, or other implements, used in operations or to produce abortion, by bullet, the horn of a steer, etc. Indirect traumatism is often the cause, but often a disease of the uterus preëxists, because the normal organ can withstand much insult without injury, as witness the case of Hofmeier, where the woman fell from a fourth-story window without rupture, and the one where a drunken man jumped upon the prostrate woman's abdomen without even causing abortion.

Clinical Course.—Baisch found 31 cases of rupture during the first five months of gestation, and in these the uterine wall was diseased. In the later ruptures scar tissue was usually found. The symptoms resemble those of ruptured extra-uterine pregnancy, but the shock is usually more marked, especially when external violence is the causative agent. Pain in the abdomen is the rule, and labor-pains may occur—this when rupture is incomplete. These contractions complete the tear and expel the child from the uterus, after which they subside. When the peritonitis begins, pain recommences, but usually the patient complains of a tender body in the abdomen from the start. Vomiting, hiccup, and other signs of peritoneal irritation are usually present, together with signs of internal hemorrhage.

In Davis', Leopold's, and Henrotin's cases gestation continued, with the child among the bowels, the cord issuing from the hole in the uterus, but these are exceptional, the rule being that the child dies, becomes infected, and peritonitis closes the scene. It is possible that a lithopedion may result. The hemorrhage may be internal, external, or both; sometimes the child tampons the rent, and there is no hemorrhage at all, so that a diagnosis cannot be made until the belly is opened. Hematomata are rare, because the tears are usually fundal. Rupture may sometimes occur in the anterior or posterior wall, and also, but rarely, in the lower part of the uterus. While the labor-pains are forcing the child out through the tear, a bag of waters may form over the os—the child may be even delivered through the vagina before the fundal tear is completed.

Instrumental perforations, if done aseptically and not large, bring on abortion and may heal unnoticed; if done, as usual, without asepsis, they cause decomposition of the uterine contents and peritonitis. (See Septic Abortion.)

Diagnosis.—This is almost always very difficult, but since most of the conditions which simulate the accident require laparotomy anyway, it is not absolutely essential. To be considered here are torsion of a tumor near the uterus, rupture of the liver, gall-bladder, or spleen, ileus, ruptured ectopic gestation, abruptio placentæ, and placenta prævia.

The treatment is laparotomy as soon as the diagnosis is made or becomes even only probable. If a former cesarean scar ruptures—resection of scar and suture in clean cases young women; amputation in suspects (infection) and when mother has a large family (Thomä, Riddell).

INFECTION DURING LABOR

A temperature of 100° to 100.6° F. may frequently be found toward the end of the second stage of labor. It is usually ascribed to the muscular exertion, to absorption of fibrin ferment, excitement, etc., but the author believes it is due to the absorption of toxins and bacteria from the parturient canal. Infection of the uterus during labor may be carried over from the pregnancy, from coitus, self-examinations, etc., or it may result from instrumental interference (colpeurynters, gauze, etc.), or it may be purely endogenic from the blood or from a nearby focus, *e. g.*, appendicitis, salpingitis, ureteropyelitis. If the membranes have been open a long time, bacteria may wander upward. Warnekros has shown that, if the placental circulation is in action, bacteria from the interior of the uterus easily pass into the blood via membranes and placenta. Slemons was the first to show the bacteria had passed through broken amniotic epithelium.

The symptoms of infection during labor are the same as those at any other time. The child is endangered—it, too, may become diseased. I have seen a pneumococcus infection thus conveyed, also gonorrheal ophthalmia. The liquor amnii is usually discolored and odorous, depending on the kind of the bacterium, and the wounds around the introitus and cervix are often covered with grayish exudates. Pus may issue from the genitals. When fever begins, the pains are usually strengthened, but unless delivery is soon accomplished, gas may develop in the uterus and paralysis with distention may result.

The differential diagnosis of the cause of the fever is to be made, *i. e.*, between uterine infection and other diseases—pyelitis, appendicitis, colds, pneumonia, typhoid, etc.

Treatment.—Expectancy gives good results. The accoucheur may well hesitate to force the birth, because of the danger of making extensive injuries, into which the infection will be literally ground. The greatest danger exists in the presence of an invasive streptococcus. It is wiser to wait the spontaneous termination, at least until the head comes down on to the perineum, interfering only when absolutely necessary. Before operation the parts are to be carefully douched with 0.75 per cent. solution of tincture of iodin. It is my practice in such cases not to suture lacerations, but to leave them wide open for drainage. A chill with sharp rise of temperature often follows operation, but the fever usually subsides in twelve hours unless the streptococcus was causative. Bacteria demonstrated in the blood during and directly after labor usually disappear within thirty-six hours. If an imperative indication for terminating labor exists and the conditions are bad for forceps, even if followed by craniotomy, consider Porro cesarean, Sellheim's delivery through an abdominal fistula, Latzko's operation (p. 1102), laparotrachelotomy, Gottschalk-Portes operation (p. 1108) (Wieloch, Ernst). A multipara, needing her uterus no longer, should have a Porro, and fibroids, carcinoma, cervical stricture require the same treatment. The severity of the infection and its location are to be considered also.

DELIVERY OF THE FETUS POSTMORTEM

About 100 cases of spontaneous delivery of the child after death of its mother are on record. The expulsion of the fetus, which may occur within six or more hours, or after days, depending on the cause, is usually produced by the gases of decomposition in the intestines, but it may be accomplished by gases in the uterus itself, or even by contractions of the uterus postmortem. In such cases labor had begun before death, and the parts were thus prepared for delivery. Outside of the scientific interest of these cases, they are important in a medicolegal sense, since the attending accoucheur may be accused of criminal neglect, or even of having permitted the burial of the woman alive (Hellendall, Reiman).

LITERATURE

Davis: Amer. Jour. Obst., January, 1918, p. 136. See also *Bishkow,* Jour. Amer. Med. Assoc., June 7, 1919, p. 1668.—*DeLee:* "Ruptura Uteri," Amer. Jour. Obstet., 1903, No. 3; *ibid.,* Amer. Jour. Obstet., 1906, vol. 1, No. 6. Gives complete literature.—*Dickinson:* Amer. Jour. Obstet., July, 1910.—"Hematoma," Arch. f. Gyn., 1910, vol. xcii, p. 295, H. 2, and *Hill:* New York Med. Jour. and Phila. Med. Jour., April 22, 1905. Gives complete literature up to date.—*Ernst:* Zentb. für Gynaek., 1931, Ergänzh. 11 a., p. 1029.—*Hellendall:* Zeitschr. für Geb. u. Gyn., 1927, xci, p. 103, Lit.—*Hoehne:* Zentb. für Gyn., September 11, 1926.—*Kolaczek:* Inaug Diss., 1903, Breslau.—*Lobenstine:* Amer. Jour. Obstet., November, 1909.—*Mathes:* Constitutional Abnormalities, Halban-Seitz, vol. iii, p. 28, 1924.—*Reimann:* Arch. für Gyn., vol. xi, p. 215.—*Riddell:* Jour. Obst. and Gyn., Brit. Empire, 1926, vol. xxxiii, p. 1.—*Rouvier:* "Kolporrhexis," Amer. Jour. Obstet., July, 1912, p. 116.—*Thomä:* Zentb. für Gyn., March 5, 1917, Literature to date.—*Warnekros:* Centralbl. f. Gyn., 1911, p. 1015; also Arch. für Gyn., 1913, vol. c.—*Wieloch:* Zentb. für Gynaek., 1930, October, p. 2726.

CHAPTER LX

INJURIES TO THE BLADDER, RECTUM, ETC.

THE BLADDER

DURING laborthe bladder is drawn up with the unfolding lower uterine segment, and, when overfilled, forms a rounded tumor above the pubis, extending sometimes even above the navel. It may be mistaken for the dilated lower uterine segment and contraction ring. The full bladder may prevent delivery by weakening uterine action, by making it too painful or impossible for the woman to bear down, and, if it is filled before the head has entered the pelvis, by preventing engagement. Catheterization will make the diagnosis and cure. Tumors of the bladder have caused dystocia, as also have vesical calculi. The head may crush them against the bone and break them, or the vaginovesical wall may be rubbed through, causing fistula. Such obstructions should be pushed up out of the pelvis with the patient in the knee-chest position, and if this is not possible, removed per vaginam. Varices of the bladder may rupture during pregnancy and labor. A kidney may be displaced and become adherent over the inlet, causing dystocia. Horseshoe kidney has thus been observed, but it need not give trouble. Cystocele may come down before the advancing head and delay delivery. It has been punctured for the bag of waters, and torn off as a tumor. The cystocele is not so much to be feared as the abruption of the base of the bladder from its pubic attachments. The duplication of the connective-tissue strands which radiate from the neck and anterior wall of the bladder to the pubis and ligamentum arcuatum—the so-called pubovesical ligaments—are stretched, separated, and torn, allowing a descensus of the bladder. In addition the fibers between the bladder and vagina and those in the base of the broad ligaments which support the bladder are also disrupted, all of which causes cystocele and prolapsus vesicæ. Unfortunately, little can be done during labor to prevent this downward dislocation of the lower half of the bladder. The protruding organ may be gently pushed back above the advancing head, and in a few cases I have done episiotomy to deflect the head from the posterior surface of the pubis and thus relieve the crowding here. For this purpose the operation has not been often enough performed.

FISTULAS

Fistulas are false passages between adjacent hollow organs, and in the pelvis are almost always due to labor, but cancer, etc., may ulcerate, leaving such defects, while foreign bodies, such as pessaries or objects introduced for purposes of masturbation, sometimes do the same. Fistulas due to labor are getting rarer every year by grace of the better practice of obstetrics. In my student days such operations for fistulæ were not uncommon—now they are curiosities.

Pressure necrosis of the bladder results from prolonged compression between the head and the pelvis. This was discussed under Contracted Pelvis. Usually the vaginovesical septum is caught between the two hard objects, and as the result of the prolonged arterial anemia, the area under the compression necroses and is cast off as a slough in the first week of the puerperium, causing incontinence of urine. If the cervix is not dilated, but caught in the zone of compression, the resulting fistula will be cervicovesical, perhaps uterovesical, or ureterocervicovesicovaginal. All sorts of combinations occur (Fig. 699). Without doubt bacteria aid in causing the necrosis.   In their absence the tissues tolerate much more pressure.   Fistulas are caused also by direct traumatism, an instrument being punched through the bladder or cutting the ureter, or from a wound of the uterus extending into the bladder or involving the ureter.   Forceps, the sharp hook, or the cranioclast have thus torn great gashes, and sharp spiculæ of bone in the operation of craniotomy have cut deeply into the soft parts.   Posteriorly, the cervix may be caught between the head and the promontory, or the rectum may be compromised. In the former case adhesion of the uterus to the promontory may result, or, if the tissue necroses, perforation and peritonitis, in the latter case, rectovaginal fistula, which is rare.

The prevention of fistulas has already been considered.   Knowing the causation, and by observing that the portions of the parturient canal below the point of

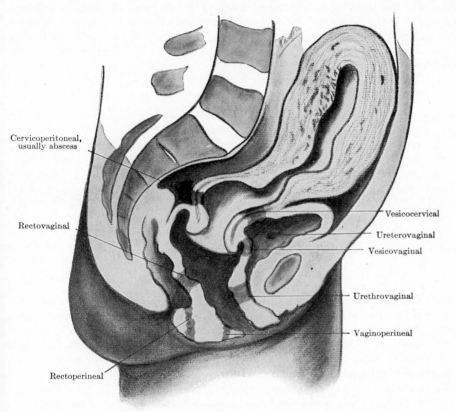

FIG. 699.—SITES OF FISTULAS.

compression are becoming swollen, the suspicion of danger is grounded.   Palpation of the thin portion and bloody urine confirm it.

Immediate delivery as soon as danger is recognized is the treatment, but the delivery itself must be a protective one.   After delivery the bladder is catheterized, and the fact that there is no perforation established; then, if the possibility of too long compression and the fear of a fistula by necrosis are entertained, the woman must be instructed to urinate regularly every four hours, or the bladder must be emptied so often, with a view to avoid further danger of sloughing.   Hexamethylentetramin, in 5-grain doses, is administered four times a day as a prophylactic.

Infection often accompanies such injury, which is unfortunate, because the scars which result from the ulceration radiate to the sides of the pelvis, even to the bone, and, by contracting, pull open the fistula and prevent its closing, also rendering difficult the operations for cure. If sloughing of the compressed area ensues, the administration of urinary antiseptics should be kept up, but bladder irrigations are unnecessary, since there is free drainage. The development of eczema from the continuous dribbling of urine is prevented by proper nursing. A thick salve containing carbonate of zinc, zinc oxid, and vaselin is useful. Later a urinal may be worn. Small fistulas, especially of the traumatic variety,—that is, those perforations not attended with extensive necrosis and radiating scars,—often heal spontaneously. Operation is not to be performed until the parts are thoroughly healed and devascularized, that is, about four months postpartum. Suture at this time, I have found, gives the best results. Although properly belonging here, the operations for the repair of fistulas may not be discussed because of the lack of space.

If a woman whose fistula has been successfully repaired becomes pregnant again, abortion may not be induced, but the advisability of cesarean section at term should be debated with the family. The healing of fistulas is so precarious that this operation should be performed, certainly if the original fistula was a complicated one. Only too often the trauma of the labor reopens the old wound and a new operation may not be at once successful.

INJURIES TO THE RECTUM

Rectovaginal fistulas the result of compression necrosis and direct injury by instruments or spicules of bone have been referred to, as also have been those cases where the rectovaginal septum gives way over the advancing presenting part, head, arm, or breech, and the latter appears at the anus. Splitting of the mucous membrane of the rectum or of the anus is not rare, and results in fissures which may cause painful defecation, bleeding, even local infections. Injury to the rectum may be produced by Ritgen's and Olshausen's manœuvers for delivery of the head. Without doubt much of the pain of delivery is due to stretching and dislocation of the rectum and of the fourth sacral nerve, which supplies the levator ani. The rectum may be implicated in rupture of the uterus.

THE PELVIC JOINTS AND BONES

Softening and relaxation of the pelvic joints have already been discussed, and the value of this factor in the mechanism and treatment of labor pointed out.

Rupture of the pelvic joints during labor, while rare, is not so uncommon as is generally believed. I have treated 10 cases and have learned of 7 others. In 1898 I published 2 cases; in 1901, 2 more, and gave the literature to date (Kehrer).

Rupture of the symphysis pubis is most often found, but sometimes the sacroiliac joints are involved, either alone or with the former. It may be partial or complete. Traumatism causes rupture of the joint, but since it requires the enormous force of from 400 to 2600 pounds to disrupt the pelvic girdle, some inherent weakness of the joint must preëxist. Softening and relaxation of the capsule, caries, rachitis, osteomalacia, chronic rheumatism, trauma during pregnancy, congenital weakness of the ligaments, have all been found in such cases when even the distention of the pelvis during spontaneous labor may cause the joint to give way. Contracted pelvis, especially the justominor and funnel varieties, predispose, because the expansile force acts in the narrow transverse diameter. A large child or especially broad shoulders may act in the same way. In three-fourths of the cases the joint is sprung during operative delivery, and in my collection the forceps caused 67 per cent., and the others, the after-coming head, the shoulder, and the vectis (Boddaert). In one case the rupture occurred postpartum while the woman got out of bed, but probably the separation had been started by the delivery and was thus completed. Improperly directed forceps traction, as by pulling upward too soon or by pulling upward with the patient on a low bed, in both cases the head acting as a wedge between the rami, or using too great force, will produce the rupture, perhaps even in the absence of pathologic softening. These facts are important from a medicolegal point of view, but the physician may not be held responsible, unless it can be shown he employed undue force in delivery. (Reis, Putschar, Haslhofer.)

Symptoms.—The patient may have complained of pains in the pubis and sacroiliac joints, with difficulty of locomotion for several weeks. During spontaneous labor the rupture may be discovered at the moment it occurs, being heard as a dull cracking, or the woman says something has burst. Usually the operator feels and hears the joint open during the operative delivery, and notes that the obstruction to the progress of the child has suddenly disappeared. Later the patient complains of intense pain over the affected joint and radiating down the thighs, and cannot move the legs, which lie everted and abducted. It is a sort of pseudoparalysis, and doubtless has often been mistaken for acute paraplegia due to injury of the nerves in the pelvis or an acute infectious myelitis. Overstretching of the joints without actual rupture sometimes occurs in difficult forceps cases, and makes the woman bedridden for months. Bladder and rectal symptoms are absent unless the viscera are injured at the same time, which is not rare.

When spontaneous cure results, fibrous union takes place between the ends of the bones, but excessive play at the joint may render the patient invalid for years. In general the results correspond with those after symphysiotomy. If the vagina communicates with the wound, suppuration is the rule. Sometimes infection of the joint occurs through the blood or by contiguity, especially if infection of the parturient canal exists. In pubic arthritis complicating general sepsis it is hard to decide if the joint was primarily or secondarily involved. Chills and high fever betoken the advent of infection to the joint; pus forms rapidly, burrows far, and makes a big abscess unless evacuated early, and may even cause fatal pyemia. Gangrene of the feet, pulmonary embolism, cartilage sequestration have occurred.

The *diagnosis* is usually easy if the condition is at all considered. The history of difficult delivery, the position of the patient in bed, the pain and tenderness of the pubis, the palpation of a groove over the joint, with movability of the pubes on each other, enable one to make the diagnosis on the direct examination. In the differential diagnosis paraplegia is excluded by finding the reflexes normal, the individual muscle groups functionating, normal sensation, and the x-ray picture positive.

Later, after fever has developed, in their order must be considered acute sepsis, pelvic inflammations and pressure on the nerves by the pelvic exudates, acute toxic neuritis, myelitis, cystitis, or even only full bladder and hysteria. When an abscess has formed around the joint, one must determine if the suppuration is primary or secondary—that is, part of a general infection, the latter mainly for the prognosis. Even recognized early, this accident is very dangerous, although often recovery and later restoration of function occurs, the latter requiring from three to eight weeks, like symphysiotomy. Injuries to adjacent viscera, primary hemorrhage, shock, and later sepsis, bring the mortality of reported cases up to 35 per cent. Infection of the joint is serious, and very serious if more than one is involved, because the abscesses burrow far and wide. Permanent wide separation of the ends of the pubis may require a bone operation, wiring or nailing, to restore function. The treatment is the same as after symphysiotomy (q. v.).

Loosening of the sacrum from the innominates may result from labor, and, without doubt, explains many of the cases of backache after normal as well as operative delivery. Pain and tenderness over the joints, abnormal mobility, the two latter determinable best by intrapelvic exploration, the pelvic organs being free of disease, will make the diagnosis. The treatment is along orthopedic lines.

Injury to the Coccyx.—During delivery the coccyx is forced backward an inch or more, this excursion of the bone being permitted by a healthy sacrococcygeal joint. If the joint is ankylotic, the bone itself may be fractured, or the joint may break open, a chronic arthritis resulting.

Dislocations of the bone on to the anterior or posterior surface of the sacrum occur, and also a pericoccygeal cellulitis, which is chronic and very painful. Without doubt many, if not most, of the cases of so-called coccygodynia are referable to the above conditions. After injury to the bone the ends may unite at a right angle, or such deformity may occur at the joint, though oftener, because the bone is moved so frequently (walking, defecation, sitting), a pseudarthrosis is formed.

Even while the woman is in bed there are symptoms referable to the injury, as pain in defecation, and tenderness, but usually the first sitting-up attracts the attention of the accoucheur. Inability to sit with comfort, the patient often resting her body on either trochanter, pain radiating up the back and down the thighs, difficulty of locomotion because of pain, painful defecation, and intense nervousness—often a real neurasthenia—are the main symptoms. The diagnosis is easy, since the history will draw attention to the location of the trouble, and an examination with the finger in the rectum and the thumb over the coccyx will show dislocation of the bone, fracture (crepitus), or excessive tenderness in or around the joints (Fig. 700). The x-ray also is helpful.

Spontaneous recovery is the rule, but sometimes it requires many months. (See Hirst.)

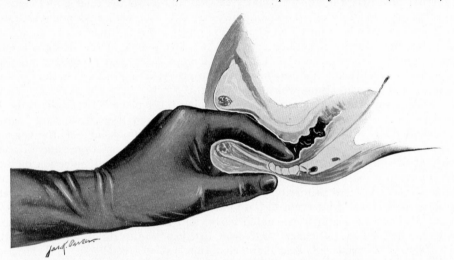

FIG. 700.—PALPATING THE COCCYX WITH A FINGER IN THE RECTUM.

Treatment.- Local applications give very little relief. In cases of cellulitis a gentle massage, after the acuteness has subsided, will help. For fracture and dislocations a period of at least six months should be allowed for spontaneous cure, and then, in the absence of improvement, the bone is to be excised. For three days before the operation the bowels are to be kept free, then bound up with bismuth and a few doses of opium, as before operations for fistulas. Sim's position is used. A 2-inch incision is made over the joint, and the firm fibrous tissue is cut down to the bone. This is bared and lifted up with a bullet forceps. With a sharp knife it is detached from the coccygeus on each side and the lower fibers of the sacrosciatic ligament, taking care to avoid tearing the fascia on its anterior surface. The joint is severed last, or, if the fracture had not united, the distal portion of the bone is excised and the proximal portion smoothed with the bone forceps. The whole coccyx had best be removed. The rectum is attached to the end of the sacrum by a few firm strands of connective tissue; care is required to prevent tearing this organ. Hemorrhage is stopped by packing with hot iodoform gauze for a few minutes. Then the two edges of the coccygeus muscle are united in the median line by interrupted catgut sutures; next the fascia which was over the bone, then three or four deep silkworm-gut sutures close the skin. Accurate coaptation of the edges of the skin should be obtained, and the wound painted with collodion. The patient should keep the side position for three days. Two ounces of liq. petrolatum are given daily, and on the tenth day castor oil. It is highly important that feces and urine do not contaminate the wound, and the patient should sit up straight or bend forward when the bowels move.

Other Injuries.—As the result of overpowerful bearing-down efforts the woman may fracture her sternum or dislocate one or more ribs upon it. The severe straining may rupture the vesicles of the lung and give rise to emphysema of the neck, chest, even of the entire body. Kosmak, in 1907, collected 77 cases in the literature since 1791. I have seen three. Primiparæ are usually affected. Tenderness and dyspnea are prominent; the prognosis is good, the swelling disappearing in a few days without treatment.

LITERATURE

DeLee: "Ruptura Symphysis Pubis," Amer. Jour. Obstet., 1901, vol. xliii.—*Devraigne:* L'Obstetrique, February, 1910. —*Eisenberger:* Zentb. für Gyn., 1926, No. 43, p. 2771.—*Haslhofer, L.:* Arch. für Gyn., 1931, vol. 147, H. 2, S. 229.—*Hirst:* Amer. Jour. Obst. and Gyn., February, 1924.—*Kayser:* Arch. f. Gyn., 1903, vol. lxx, p. 50; also *Kehrer,* Monatsschr. für Geb. u. Gyn., October, 1915. Literature.—*Kosmak:* Bulletin of New York Lying-in Hospital, March, 1907.—*Putschar:* Entwickelung etc. der Beckenverbindungen des Menschen, G. Fischer, Jena, 1931, Lit.—*Reis, Baer, Arens, and Stewart:* Surg., Gyn. and Obst., September, 1932, p. 336.

CHAPTER LXI

PATHOLOGY OF THIRD STAGE

DURING the third stage of labor, using the classification previously adopted, we must consider anomalies of the powers, of the passages, and of the passenger, superadded on which we sometimes find complications, especially on the part of the mother, some occurring during the third stage, but mostly carried over from the first two stages.

(1) Under anomalies of the powers we have, too strong uterine contractions (rare); too weak contractions (atonia uteri) more common; hour-glass contraction (constrictio uteri); insufficient retraction of the uterus, general and local, the latter

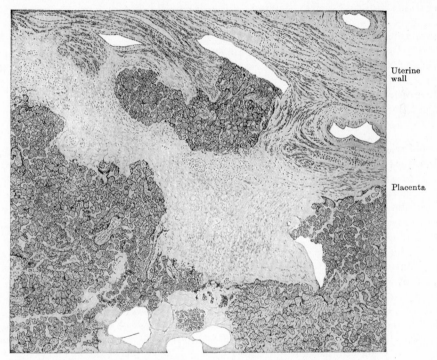

FIG. 701.—PLACENTA INCRETA (from Schauta and Hitschmann).

either at the placental site in the fundus (Fig. 704) or in the lower uterine segment (placenta previa). In practice it is not always possible to distinguish anomalies of contraction from those of retraction. A combination of both exists in Inversio Uteri, and a special chapter is to be devoted to this particular complication.

(2) Under anomalies of the passages we would place those conditions produced by spasm of the cervix or by tumors. Retentio placentæ separatæ comes in this class.

(3) Anomalies of the passenger are well known and feared; tumors of the placenta almost never cause dystocia, but we find abnormal adherence to the uterus (placenta accreta), or ingrowth of villi deep into the muscle (placenta increta) total, rarely partial, with the leaving of a piece attached to the uterine wall, not so seldom (Heidler).

Placenta Accreta or Increta.—Figure 701 shows a not very rare anomaly, a placenta which grows, in part usually, or rarely all over, into the uterine wall itself. The villi burrow into the uterine muscle, which is degenerated, and one sees irregular infiltrations of syncitium and Langhan's cells. This anomaly is due to a primary atrophy of the endometrium, the decidua serotina being absent. Endometritis, previous injury of the endometrium (curettage, cautery, manual removal of the placenta) are causative. Hemorrhage postpartum is the main symptom. Manual removal of the placenta is the treatment. Care is needed not to puncture the uterus with the finger—better leave a piece of placenta that is too deeply embedded, and tampon, with the hope the remnants will come away with the gauze. If the whole placenta is "increta," uterine extirpation should be considered—this certainly if the patient is already infected (Dietrich, Lit.).

Broad, thin placentæ separate from the uterus with more difficulty than thick ones, and the same may be said of soft and hard placentæ; those situated in the tubal corners seem to stick harder than those in the lower uterine segment, which not seldom are loosened from their beds during the passage of the child, and are extruded right after the feet of the latter escape from the vulva.

(4) The complications which disturb the third stage are usually due to lacerations (uterus, cervix, vagina, vulva), causing hemorrhage, but many other dangers threaten the parturient—syncope and shock, embolism, toxemia, to mention only a few.

Inasmuch as bleeding is the main symptom of all the anomalies of the placental stage (excepting some of those in the fourth class) it is clinically more useful to present the subject from this point of view. I shall, therefore, adhere to the practice of most authors, and group the conditions presented to the accoucheur under the title:

POSTPARTUM HEMORRHAGE

Strictly speaking, postpartum hemorrhage means bleeding after labor, that is, after the placenta is delivered, but for purpose of study it is best to consider under this heading all hemorrhages occurring from the time the child is delivered until the puerperium is completed. Those which occur after the first twenty-four hours are called late hemorrhages, and will be considered separately. At present we are concerned only with those attending the delivery of the placenta and immediately thereafter.

The reproductive function is the only one normally attended by hemorrhage, and nature, by wise provision, fortifies the woman against the inevitable loss, and even overprovides, so that she may survive a drain that would prove fatal in a nonpregnant female or a male. During pregnancy the total quantity of blood is increased, and the fibrin is also greater in amount, these changes beginning after the fifth month. There is a slight leukocytosis which becomes marked (16,000) during labor. In healthy gravidæ these are the changes, while in a sickly or anemic woman, pregnancy may induce a condition of chloranemia. The point has a strong clinical bearing.

In healthy gravidæ a loss of blood up to one pint (500 gm.) is usually borne without any symptoms, and it is generally believed that the woman has gained about this amount during pregnancy. The average loss during labor is about 300 gm.—8 to 10 ounces. It is best to consider a loss above a pint as pathologic. Bloodless labors are very rare, and are usually found where the fetus has been dead a long time and firm thrombosis has occurred in the placental site. Leukemics also are said to have bloodless labors, which is fortunate, if generally true, because leukemics stand bleeding badly. Before the expulsion of the placenta the oozing should be very slight, if any, and after it the puerpera should not lose over 3 ounces of fresh blood in the first two hours. Inclosed in the placenta will be found the bulk of the blood. If the blood gushes from the genitals or oozes steadily in larger amounts than here indicated, the case is pathologic.

ETIOLOGY

During the separation and expulsion of the placenta hemorrhage is prevented by the retraction and contraction of the uterine muscle and by thrombosis of the uterine sinuses. The more important factor in securing hemostasis is the uterine action, since thrombosis may be absent and no hemorrhage occur; and, conversely, thrombosis alone, unaided by the contraction and retraction of the uterus, will not check a hemorrhage.

The sinuses in the uterine wall are simply blood-spaces, lying between the muscular lamellæ and muscle-bundles, and lined with a single layer of endothelium. As the uterus empties the muscular lamellæ become superimposed, the muscle-bundles crowd closer together, the several layers sliding over each other. As a result, the blood sinuses are bent and twisted on themselves, the muscle effectually choking off the current of blood that flowed through them. There is even some influence on the larger vessels at the sides of the uterus after they enter its wall. The retraction of the uterine muscle does the actual work in this operation. The regularly recurring uterine contractions aid and support the permanent retraction.

Postpartum hemorrhage, therefore, will be most often found to be due to some anomaly of this physiologic mechanism, and such anomalies are usually due to weakness or abnormal contraction and retraction of the uterus. In practice we find two additional factors—lacerations of the parturient canal and disease of the blood or blood-vessels.

(A) *Lacerations* of the genital tract play a much more important rôle in the production of hemorrhage postpartum than is generally believed. Many hemorrhages called atonic are due to tears in the genitalia.

Lacerations of the clitoris and of the bulbi may give rise to even fatal hemorrhage, as may also a ruptured varix of the vulva or vagina, though both are rare. Perineal tears seldom bleed enough to require immediate suture, and vaginal tears are also rarely attended by much hemorrhage. They may, however, require suture or packing, and when they do, packing is the best method, because the field is so inundated with blood that it is impossible to see where to place the sutures. High vaginal tears, extending into the fornices, may lay open the bases of the broad ligaments and may bleed furiously. They are usually combined with cervix tears and may occur in spontaneous deliveries.

A laceration of the cervix extending into the broad ligament may not bleed if the tearing is gradual and not forced. Such findings are occasionally made after spontaneous labors or dilatation with one of the crushing dilators (the Bossi, de Seigneux) or the hands (Bonnaire, Harris). Usually, however, a deep cervical tear gives rise to serious hemorrhage. Deep cervical tears are most likely to occur if a rapid delivery is made before the cervix is completely effaced or shortened, that is, drawn up into the body of the uterus. Even after the cervix is completely dilated a laceration of the upper fibers may result if the extraction of the child is forced during a spasmodic contraction of the lower uterus and upper cervix. Sometimes the head passes through the cervix and the contraction ring closes down around the neck of the child. Forcing the delivery in such a case may cause the shoulders to tear the edge of the contraction ring. In the last three varieties of cervical laceration the tear is more likely to be a longitudinal split of the cervical wall, usually lateral, extending more or less deeply into the broad ligament, and indicating that if it went much further it would have to be called a rupture of the uterus, incomplete or complete, depending on whether or not the peritoneal cavity was opened. Without doubt many cases of so-called postpartum hemorrhage are, in reality, ruptures of the uterus, as likewise are many cases of "shock" after labor.

When the cervix is torn after complete effacement, but before complete dilatation, few large blood-vessels are opened unless the tear extends into the bases of the broad ligaments.

53

Special emphasis must be placed on the lacerations of the cervix and lower uterine segment occurring in placenta prævia. It is usually thought that the frequency of postpartum hemorrhage in placenta prævia cases is due to uterine atony, while as a matter of fact atony is rare, there being often too strong uterine action. The branches of the uterine artery supplying the lower uterine segment are given off above the contraction ring, and therefore are somewhat compressed by the contracting uterus before entering the relaxed lower uterine segment. While one would expect a placental site, located out of the active contracting zone, to permit free oozing, this is, to a large extent, prevented by the peculiar situation of the blood-supply. Hemorrhage, therefore, is due to some other cause, and this will usually be found to be a laceration. The extreme vascularization of the lower

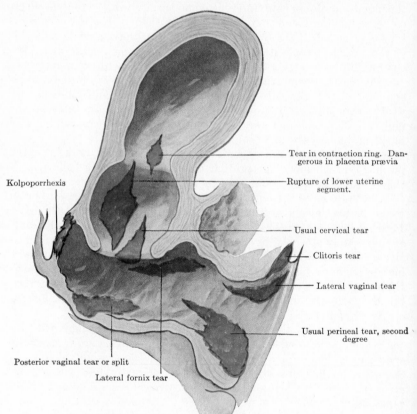

Kolpoporrhexis

Tear in contraction ring. Dangerous in placenta prævia

Rupture of lower uterine segment.

Usual cervical tear

Clitoris tear

Lateral vaginal tear

Usual perineal tear, second degree

Posterior vaginal tear or split

Lateral fornix tear

FIG. 702.—DIAGRAM OF TEARS OF PARTURIENT CANAL.

uterine segment and cervix, due to the placental implantation, permits every tear to bleed profusely. Since the veins and sinuses are situated close to the surface, a laceration one-eighth inch deep may cause uncontrollable hemorrhage and may be discovered only at the autopsy.

(B) *Insufficient retraction and contraction* of the uterus, or anomalies of the same, cause few of the fatal postpartum hemorrhages. They may be associated with any of the lacerations previously described, and when the tear is situated in the lower uterine segment, the absence of a firm restraining action of the uterus is apparent.

It is not feasible to try to separate anomalies of retraction from those of contraction. Normally, the two functions coöperate, and in practice we find that where the uterus does not contract well, it does not retract well. We will call a uterus atonic when the contraction and retraction of its muscles are insufficient or irregular, though etiologically and strictly other terms should be used. "Uterine atony" is a favorite term for these conditions, but it does not always apply to the case.

The causes of atonic hemorrhages are general and local. Generally weak women—those of excessive cultivation, who often have poorly developed genitalia and generally poor innervation—have slow labors and a greater tendency to atony in the third stage. Exhaustion from prolonged labor, especially if the parturient takes no food, may lead to atony. In some families a tendency to postpartum hemorrhage is transmitted. This is an entirely different condition from hemophilia, which is to be considered later. Some women have atony of the uterus in successive labors. This may be due to a persistence of a local cause. Blonds and red-haired women, in the author's experience, are likely to have hemorrhage postpartum, but how much is dependent on the constitution of the blood it is impossible to say. Myocarditis, valvular disease, and pulmonary affections are said to favor atonia uteri, but the writer has had little trouble with it in such cases. Chronic nephritis has been given as a cause of atony, a hyaline degeneration of the uterine muscle and disease of the blood-vessels being directly active. Hypo-epinephrinemia is a cause of atony of the uterus, and if associated with the status hypoplasticus, death from even a slight bleeding may result.

The use of chloroform during labor undoubtedly increases the tendency to hemorrhage, though this action is not constant.

Of local causes there are many: Overdistention of the uterus by twins—polyhydramnion; a large or diseased fetus, or an accumulation of blood (abruptio placentæ). The elongated muscle-fibers need time to accommodate themselves to the rapidly diminishing uterine cavity, so that sudden emptying of such a distended uterus nearly always predisposes to hemorrhage. Abnormal shape of the uterus, bihorned uteri, uterus arcuatus, septus, etc.; distortion of the uterus by adhesions (rarely); distortion by tumors, as fibroids (commonly); old scars in the uterus, after cesarean section, or ruptures—all these interfere with the contraction and retraction of the organ and allow the sinuses to remain open, and from these more or less profuse hemorrhage occurs.

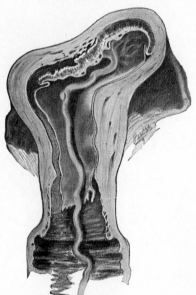

FIG. 703.—TUBAL CORNER PLACENTA, WITH IMPERFECT SEPARATION AND HEMORRHAGE.

Metritis is given by J. Veit as a cause of atony. Labhardt found an anatomic basis for such hemorrhages in an increase of the uterine fibrous tissue around the blood-vessels. This may have preëxisted or have developed during pregnancy, and explains the frequency of hemorrhage in old multiparæ, in cases of subinvolution, and after puerperal infection. After "missed labor" atony is the rule.

Endometritis is a cause, since retention of pieces or all the placenta is favored. A retained piece of placenta, or what acts the same way, a thick layer of decidua with clots deposited on it, prevents proper retraction of the uterus and the latter fills with blood. Retained membranes, sometimes mixed with a clot, or a large hard clot itself, may act like pieces of placenta. They cause persistent oozing after labor, which may be enough to demand interference. If the primary hemorrhage ceases, the foreign body may dissolve and come away in the lochia, which are profuse and fetid, or it may be discharged *en masse*, more or less decomposed, or there may be repeated hemorrhages which require interference, or a placental polyp forms. Tubal corner placentæ (Fig. 703) separate poorly because of the bad uterine action. Atony of the placental site (Fig. 704) is more frequent than is generally thought. It may be the beginning of inversion.

Irregular action of the uterus itself, the formation of contraction rings (see p. 626, Strictura Uteri), the best known of which is the "hour-glass contraction" (Fig. 705), an exhausted uterus, one displaced by a full bladder or rectum—all these may be attended by bleeding. The full bladder as a cause must be emphasized.

Improper conduct of labor, too rapid delivery of the child, which is dragged out of the uterus without allowing time for the latter to adapt its walls to its diminishing contents; too much massage of the fundus in the third stage, with premature attempts to expel the placenta by Credé expression, traction on the cord, giving

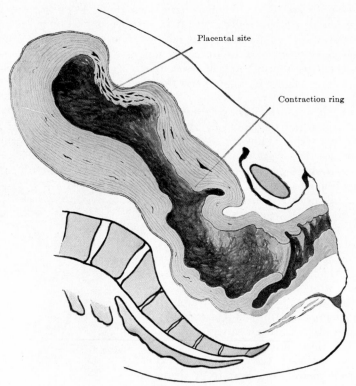

Placental site

Contraction ring

FIG. 704,—ATONY OF PLACENTAL SITE.
Its spongy nature is shown and the ease of perforation is made plain.

ergot too soon—all these disturb the normal mechanism of the third stage by producing anomalous uterine action, breaking the retroplacental hematoma, separating the placenta partially, bruising the uterus, and crushing the placenta, which favors retention of pieces of it, and all cause bleeding.

(C) *Abnormal blood states* or diseases of the blood-vessels may cause severe and even fatal postpartum hemorrhage. Hemophilia is unproven, but thrombopenia may cause severe hemorrhage and death may result. Ahlfeld reported a fatal case; the author has had two fatal, and two other severe, hemophilic bleedings; Wells reports one. Scurvy, Werlhoff's disease, syphilis, certain chronic anemias, toxemias, and sepsis may all lead to profuse hemorrhages. Without doubt such hemophilic tendencies may develop during pregnancy, and they may be related to a diseased ovum, see Abruptio Placentæ. Theories are many, facts scarce (Kraul).

SYMPTOMS

General.—The symptoms are those of loss of blood, and vary in intensity with the rapidity of flow, the amount, the condition of the patient, and idiosyncrasy. A sudden large loss is attended by shock, which, being overcome, the patient rapidly improves. A slow prolonged bleeding is more often fatal. Previous repeated hemorrhages, as from placenta prævia, exhaust the blood-making organs, so that even a small loss in labor is badly borne. Hypoplastic individuals, anemics, sufferers from malarial and certain cachexias, diabetics, and typhoids are bad subjects.

The symptoms of hemorrhage in the usual order of their appearance are: Faintness, dizziness, air-hunger, yawning, nausea, restlessness, thirst, precordial anxiety, smothering fear of impending dissolution, vomiting, fainting, collapse, convulsive twitchings, and, as death nears, involuntary bowel movements and coma. These symptoms in a person already anemic come on sooner and more pronouncedly. Examination will show the face pallid, the lips bluish white, the nose and forehead cold, and sometimes covered with sweat, the eyes sunken, the conjunctivæ pearly, respiration rapid and shallow, low blood-pressure, the pulse small and fast, filiform, and finally gone from the wrist. Sometimes the pulse holds up well for a while, then suddenly disappears. These cases give a false sense of security, because the pulse is slow. By determining the fullness of the vessel and the diastolic pressure an error of judgment may be avoided.

It is astonishing how much blood a woman can lose and survive. Ahlfeld confined several thousand women on a bed with a hole through the center, underneath which was placed a glass graduated pail. He found that in a normal labor the loss of blood would average 435 c.c.; that pathologic labors show an average of 677 c.c., the average blood-loss of all labors being 505 c.c. Ahlfeld, therefore, concludes that a loss up to 800 c.c. is normal, and that a healthy woman of average weight may safely lose a liter, which is a little more than a quart. Ahlfeld found that the first symptoms following loss of one liter were pallor and rapid pulse; as the flow continued up to 1600 or 1800 c.c., the surface of the patient grew cold, sweat appeared, and thirst, dyspnea, yawning, dizziness, and faintness were to be noted. *Occasionally, death occurred with a loss of less than two liters.* In 6000 labors there were 14 hemorrhages over 2500 c.c. (5 pints), one of which was over 3000 c.c. All the patients recovered. A loss of 3800 to 4000 c.c. (a gallon) is considered absolutely fatal. No doubt the danger to life of severe blood-loss postpartum appears greater than it really is, but since one cannot predict the woman's ability to withstand bleeding, it is prudent to take alarm at small hemorrhages and quickly institute means to check them. Ahlfeld's cases were hardy peasant women. Our highly bred American women would show more serious results and many would die from such excessive losses of blood.

Local.—The bleeding may be internal or external or both. If the cervix is occluded by a clot, membranes, or the placenta, or if the vulva is held closed by apposition of the thighs, an enormous amount of blood may be dammed back, distending the vagina and the uterus. When the hand is borne on the belly or the uterus, blood gushes out. Sometimes there is a terrific rush of blood following the child, and it may be fatal in a few minutes. Only a man who has seen one would believe such a flooding could occur. Usually there is a steady oozing or more copious flow, necessitating frequent changing of the sheets. A wise accoucheur will make note of the number of changes. Sometimes the flow is interrupted, the uterus filling and emptying several times, or there may be one gush and that be all, the uterus having obtained a firm grasp of itself. The first blood is thick and deep red; later it grows paler, and it appears to me it has lost its clotting power. Sometimes the blood is dark, like port wine, and the clots are black, or it seems to be lake colored—translucent; this an evidence of hemolysis. If the placenta is totally adherent the bleeding is minimal, the worst hemorrhages coming from the sinuses opened by partial separation, the attached portion of the placenta preventing closure of the gaping vessels.

The local findings vary with the cause of the hemorrhage. If from laceration, the uterus is usually hard, but sometimes it fills up with blood and becomes atonic. In real atonia uteri it is difficult to locate the flabby fundus; the whole abdomen feels boggy. If the placenta is separated but incarcerated, the uterus is firm and globular, but balloons out between pains, and each contraction is attended by a gush of blood from the vagina (Fig. 705).

DIAGNOSIS

Ideal obstetrics demands that no woman should lose enough blood to give rise to symptoms of anemia. If such are present, the accoucheur must quickly determine their cause, and shock, rupture of the uterus, inversion, rupture of an abdominal viscus, pulmonary embolism, pituitary shock, and uremic collapse are to be considered. When the amount of blood known to have been lost is small and the uterus is well contracted, probably some other cause is acting, but the idiosyncrasy of the patient must be remembered. Almost always the question to decide is the source of the bleeding. Broadly speaking, a bleeding with a hard uterus comes from laceration, and when the organ is large, boggy, or even too soft to outline, atony is the cause. The history of the labor will give valuable data; if the uterine action was torpid in the first two stages, inertia may be expected in the third. (See Etiology.)

After forceps or other operations, lacerations are to be looked for, and they will be found in the operative field. Before the placenta is out it may be impossible to decide between atony and injury. As a rule, diagnosis and treatment go together, and this is the usual procedure: A brisk massage is given the uterus, and at the same time the vulva and introitus are sponged free of blood and inspected carefully for tears. If firm contraction of the uterus ensues, the hemorrhage ceasing, atony was probably the cause, and nothing further is done. If not, the placenta is removed. Now if the bleeding continues with a hard uterus, laceration is probably the cause. A vaginal examination will settle the doubt. Venosity of the blood is no criterion of atony. Concealed hemorrhage may be due to a tear as well as atony, and the blood may not appear for from five to fifteen minutes after delivery. It is ofttimes necessary to decide whether or not a piece of placenta or a clot is still in the uterus. In the first place, a careful inspection of the placenta should invariably be made immediately after its delivery, while it and the accoucheur's hands are still aseptic, because it may be necessary to at once enter the uterus.

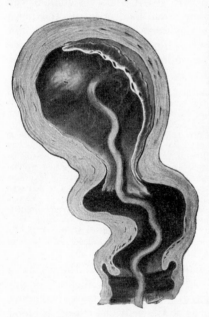

FIG. 705.—HOUR-GLASS CONTRACTION. IMPRISONS PLACENTA.

If the placenta is too much torn to guarantee certainty that nothing has been retained, and bleeding continues, it is best to revise the uterus with the hand. A large elastic, globular uterus, issuing occasional gushes of blood, almost always has something inside it. If a clot is seen or felt in the vagina, probably another lies in the uterine cavity. If the attendant notes the discharge of blood-serum from the vagina, he may be sure that there is a clot in the parturient canal.

Incarceration of the placenta is diagnosed from—(1) The large globular uterus, whose contractions are irregular as to time, strength, and location; (2) the intermittent gushes of blood; (3) the cord advances and recedes when pressure is made on the fundus; (4) the vein in the umbilical cord becomes tense when the uterus is compressed; (5) internal examination discloses the tight contraction ring with the placenta above (Fig. 705).

PROGNOSIS

Nowadays few women die from postpartum hemorrhage. In over 55,000 consecutive cases in the Chicago Lying-in Hospital Dispensary service only five women died from it, but there were 28 more who came very near death. Statistics are hard to get. In the United States about 1100 deaths from puerperal hemorrhage (all kinds) are annually recorded. Dührssen said that in Germany a woman dies every day from postpartum hemorrhage. In general, it may be said that severe hemorrhage occurs in about 2 per cent. of labors, but that a death in experienced hands is rare—probably not oftener than once in 11,000 deliveries. Cases of true atony are rare, and often fatal, but not more often fatal than cervix tears in placenta prævia. Simple cervix tears offer a better prognosis than atony, especially if the latter is due to disease of the uterine structure. Tears of the clitoris and of varices in the vagina may be fatal unless recognized early.

In individual cases the expressed prognosis as to life will depend on the physician's examination and his estimate of the proportion of the woman's blood that is lost. One should remember that one-eleventh of the body weight is blood, and that death ensues when the loss approaches one-half of the total. The pulse, while a good one, is not always a reliable guide. I have felt a fairly good *slow* pulse with a serious hemorrhage. It seems as if the arteries can keep their grasp on the circulation up to a certain point, which, being passed, they lose their grip and collapse occurs. The quality of the pulse-beat gives more information than its rapidity. Blood-pressure below 90 indicates great danger. Hurried respiration, extreme dyspnea, and air-hunger are very ominous but not necessarily fatal symptoms. Extreme restlessness and repeated vomiting indicate a very serious condition. The degree of pallor aids in prognosis.

At the beginning it is impossible to foretell how dangerous a certain bleeding will become. Slight oozing may baffle the accoucheur entirely, while a furious cascade of blood may suddenly cease. It is advisable to stop all hemorrhages as soon as possible, because the constitution of the patient is an unknown quantity and the blood loses its clotting power when thinned.

There are remote dangers in these cases. Thrombosis and embolism are commoner after severe losses, and infection, too, the latter because the resisting power of the woman has been lowered, and, secondly, because the accoucheur, in his haste, has forgotten the principles of asepsis. Hemorrhage into the retina and edema with blindness, chronic diarrhea, gastric ulcer, and permanent debilitation of the blood and neurasthenia have been noted as sequels. Even in cases where the blood-loss did not exceed 800 gm. the patients made slower recoveries, lactation was interfered with, subinvolution was commoner—altogether the convalescence was not so satisfactory as in those women where the bleeding was strictly limited.

TREATMENT

Prevention should begin during pregnancy, and the patient's family and personal history will be the guide. If such a history should discover any of the causes of postpartum hemorrhage mentioned under Etiology, appropriate treatment during gestation may prevent trouble, at least, the warning will have been sounded in time to have everything in readiness. Forewarned is forearmed. Calcium chlorid and thyroid during pregnancy, and 50 per cent. glucose (50 c.c.) during labor may fortify the blood against bleeder tendencies. During labor the possibility of postpartum hemorrhage must be borne in mind, particularly when the action of the uterus is sluggish, and in cases of overdistention, twins, polyhydramnion, etc. By supporting the parturient with food, rest, and help at the proper time much can be done. Too early operative interference causes lacerations and hemorrhage. In delivery the uterus must be slowly emptied, and especially must the rules of the conduct of the third stage be closely observed. If labor has dragged on a long time, with or without infection (which may cause atony), a prophylactic dose of pituitary should be given as soon as the baby's head is born and a hypo of gynergen after the placenta is delivered.

Preparations.—Every obstetric kit should contain the apparatus for coping with this complication: (1) Instruments for the repair of lacerations; (2) for packing the uterus, uterine packing forceps (Fig. 706) and specially prepared gauze; (3) for the treatment of anemia, salt solution apparatus, cannulæ, sodium citrate solution in ampules for transfusion, ampules of glucose, gum acacia, hypodermic syringe with stimulants, gynergen, pituitary extract, etc. Forearmed is forewarned.

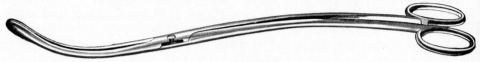

Fig. 706.—Author's Packing Forceps.
It is 11½ inches long and rounded end is ½½ inch across.

Treatment of Hemorrhage During the Third Stage.—When a severe bleeding follows the delivery of the child, the first move is to grasp the uterus and massage it vigorously, an operation first recommended by Dussè in 1722. As a rule, as soon as the uterus contracts the hemorrhage ceases. At the same time the attendant inspects the genitals to find the laceration that may be bleeding. If the uterus

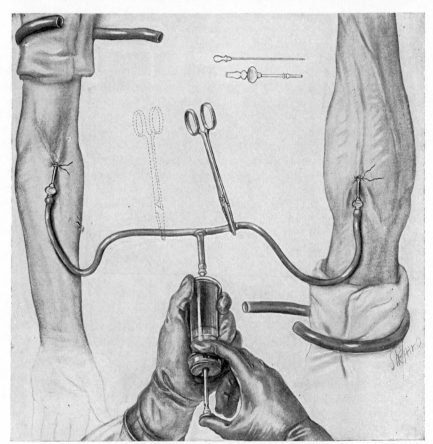

Fig. 707.—Author's Transfusion Apparatus (Available Everywhere).
Direct method. Above, detail of trocar.

contracts and the hemorrhage continues, an internal examination should be made to see if there is a cervix tear. Should the bleeding continue, it is necessary to remove the placenta whether or not a tear is found. Massage the womb vigorously, and in the moment of contraction perform Credé expression. This maneuver may stop the flow; if not, it will be needful to remove the placenta manually. Before attempting the Credé one must empty the bladder by catheter and bring

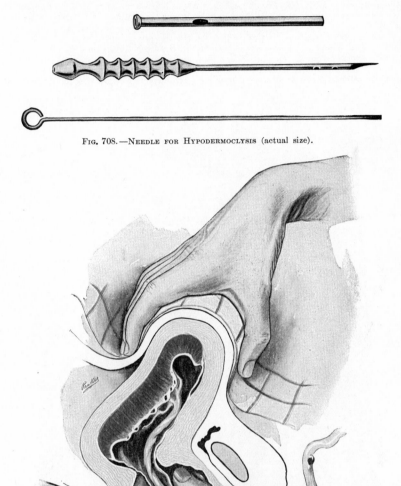

FIG. 708.—NEEDLE FOR HYPODERMOCLYSIS (actual size).

FIG. 709.—MANUAL REMOVAL OF PLACENTA. HAND, CONE SHAPED, GOING THROUGH CONTRACTION RING. For artistic effect the rubber gloves are not shown.

the uterus to the median line. Squeeze only when the organ is contracting and hard. If is useless and very dangerous to squeeze a soft uterus.

Manual Removal of Placenta.—Having decided that it is necessary to remove the placenta manually, the patient is brought across the bed, with the buttocks well over its edge; the assistant, either a physician, a nurse, or, if absolutely necessary, the husband or a courageous neighbor, holds the legs in the lithotomy position, and the accoucheur sees that his instruments, basins with antiseptic solutions, gauze for packing the uterus, and a hot douche are all prepared and within easy reach. If the accoucheur has his obstetric technic well developed, and his assistants and, most important of all, his clientèle, properly trained, it is possible to be so prepared for labor cases that a change from the bed to the kitchen-table may be made in a minute. Usually, however, the exigencies of the case will force the physician to operate with the patient across the bed, but whenever it is possible one should do these things on a table. Removal of a placenta only incarcerated in the uterus is a simple procedure, but excochleation of a *placenta increta* is one of the most dangerous operations in obstetric practice, because of the likelihood of infection of the naked placental site. Its mortality is placed by Bumm at 10 per cent.

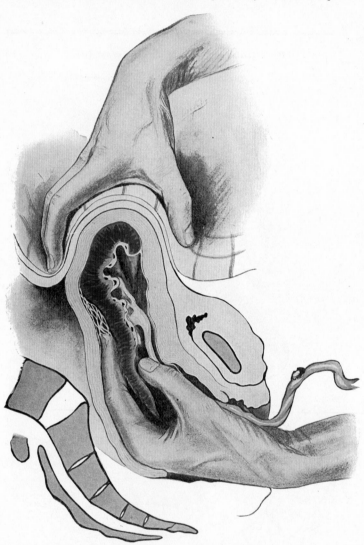

Fig. 710.—Manual Removal of Placenta. Separating it from Uterus.

A careful disinfection of the external genitals and the lower vagina should now be made. No hemorrhage is so dangerous that such preparations may be neglected. The danger of sepsis would thus replace that of hemorrhage. Catheterize. The parts have already been shaved, and they have been well washed with antiseptic solutions during the delivery. Before inserting the hand the externals should again be liberally sponged with 1 : 1500 bichlorid and then with 1 per cent. lysol solution. The vagina should be well flushed out with 1 per cent. lysol solution, squeezing the solution from large cotton or gauze sponges. The use of rubber gloves cannot be too warmly recommended for obstetric practice, and, especially for this dangerous operation of invading the uterine cavity, they are almost indispensable. The gloves should be long, should fit well, and they should be drawn on dry, over sterile hands. A sterile towel is laid on the abdomen, and the hand put into the vagina, avoiding the anus and perineum. The left hand is usually found to be most adapted for internal work. The fingers spread out in the cervix so that the membranes and cord fall into their grasp, then the tips of the fingers are brought together to form a cone for passage of the contraction ring (Fig. 709). It is seldom necessary to use force in passing this point. If ergot has been administered or if the contraction ring has closed down, it may be necessary to

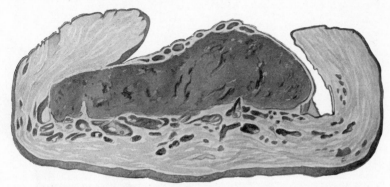

Fig. 711.—Section through Uterus and Placenta (Still Attached), Showing Large Venous Sinuses at Placental Site and how Easily Finger may Perforate Wall (Barbour).

press the fingers firmly through the constriction. Profound anesthesia aids much, but in exsanguinated women it is better to operate without it if possible. The fingers seek the edge of the placenta, and the hand on the belly forces the uterus down over the inside fingers (Fig. 710). With a gentle combined movement the placenta is separated from its bed. It is usually very easy to separate the organ; but if it is pathologically adherent, tough strands will have to be sawn through by the fingers supported by the outside hand. A warning not to bore into or through the uterus

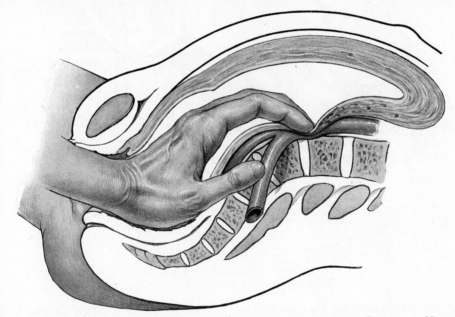

Fig. 712.—Compression of the Aorta from Within the Uterus. Useful as a Temporary Blood-saving Measure Until the Uterus Can be Stimulated to Control Itself or Can be Packed.

must be given, because this is sometimes surprisingly easy (Fig. 711). Oswald reported 38 cases of it in 1903. The gut has been brought down; indeed, almost unbelievable as it seems, the spleen has been pulled out for the placenta (Kockel). After the placenta has been cleanly separated the two hands give the uterus a brisk massage, and a contraction will expel the hand containing the placenta. It is better to let the uterus expel the hand with the placenta than to drag the latter out. After washing the blood off the hand, and again sponging the parts with antiseptic solution, the hand is once more inserted, and the whole interior of the uterus carefully inspected. One must be absolutely certain that the uterus is perfectly empty. Care should be taken to remove all the membranes and thickened decidua. The rubber gloves are so slippery that shreds of decidua cannot be grasped. One misses the sharp finger-nail in such cases. The author covers the fingers with gauze for the purpose of cleaning off the decidua and membranes. One may now give a hot 0.5 per cent. lysol intra-uterine douche, which usually causes firm contraction and retraction. A hypodermic of gynergen or aseptic ergot is also administered, also one of hypophysin.

If it is impossible to remove the placenta, or if pieces of cotyledons or shreds of membrane are unavoidably left adherent on the uterine wall, a firm uterovaginal tamponade is made and the gauze removed in forty-eight hours. Missing portions often come away with the gauze. Infection combined with adherent placenta indicates hysterectomy.

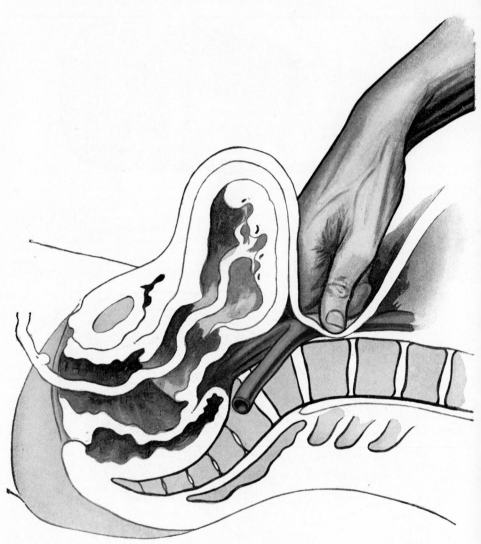

FIG. 713.—COMPRESSION OF AORTA.
This method may be used in cesarean section also.

Treatment after the Placenta is Out.—In all labor cases, as soon as the placenta has been delivered, inspect it carefully before throwing it in the drainage-jar. This is done at once, because if a piece of it is missing, one may adopt appropriate measures, and will not be surprised by a hemorrhage after the patient has been prepared for bed, or, indeed, after the physician is ready to leave the house. If convinced that a piece of the placenta has been retained, it must be removed.

If the membranes are missing or incomplete, should you enter the uterus for their removal? Opinions of authorities differ. In maternity hospital practice, with the protection of sterile rubber gloves and an aseptic confinement room, the author removes such retained membranes. If only a third or a half of the membranes is left, providing there is no hemorrhage, the removal of the missing portion may be trusted to nature. In private practice, under usual conditions, it is safer to trust the expulsion of the membranes to the uterus. Ergot and hydrastis are given for two weeks, and usually the uterus gets rid of the membranes in the first eight days. Sapremic fever is not rare, but usually subsides safely.

Routine.—In all cases of postpartum hemorrhage a *brisk uterine massage* is the first action. Uterine contraction has a deterrant effect even on the flow from cervical laceration. The first motions should be slow and even, but unless the uterus responds promptly, they should be rapid, and spread all over the fundus and also at

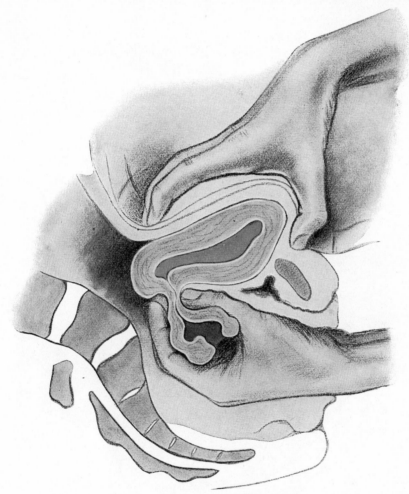

Fig. 714.—Bimanual Compression of the Uterus in Anteflexion.

the sides, near the tubes and ovaries, *an attempt being made to felt the uterine muscle together.* Another method, recommended by Kumpf, is compression vibratory massage. The uterus is grasped by the right hand, pressed down into the inlet; the arm is held rigid, and then a rapid vibratory massage is administered, the excursions of the muscles being very small. If the other hand happens to be in the uterus, a combined massage may be thus given. If a mechanical vibrator is available, it may be used. As an aid to uterine massage the accoucheur may irritate the sympathetic ganglia around the bifurcation of the aorta. The hand very gently rubs over this region, and uterine contractions often result. If the hemorrhage is very profuse, threatening the woman's life, the same hand should compress the aorta firmly against the spine (Fig. 713), as recommended by Saxtorph in 1774. This will check the flow until the uterus by its retraction has obtained control of itself, or until the attendant can put on sterile gloves, prepare the patient, his instruments, gauze, etc., for effective hemostasis.

Second, 10 units of pituitary are given hypo, followed by 1 ampule of gynergen. If the uterus does not respond to the action of the pituitary fast enough to meet

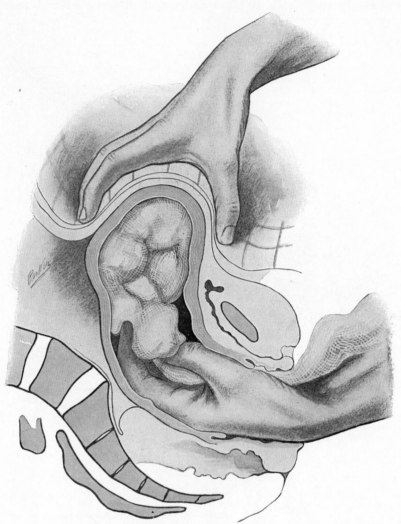

FIG. 715.—PACKING THE UTERUS WITH THE HANDS ALONE.
The thumb pushes up the gauze for the fingers to pack.

the demands, another dose is given—this time directly into the uterine muscle through the abdominal wall—or intravenously in one-half the dose. Experience has proved that it is not wise to give ergot until the placenta has left the contracting portion of the uterus. The author uses pituitary as routine after the child is born, but is not yet certain if it may be safely recommended for general practice.

Third.—One does not wait for the sometimes delayed action of pituitrin and ergot, if the bleeding continues, and the discharge of blood is narrowly scrutinized. Fresh sterile gloves are quickly put on, the vulva and introitus are drenched with antiseptic solutions, the hand is inserted, and the uterine cavity is cleared of clots of membrane, placental, and decidual débris.

In the great majority of cases the above treatment will suffice to stop the hemorrhage completely. If it does not, one has to do with an extensive laceration or a bad case of atony of the uterus. A laceration, of course, will have been discovered when the hand was inserted either for removal of the placenta or of the clots. Treatment of lacerations naturally occurs at this point, but we will leave the discussion until later. Should the diagnosis of severe inertia be made, one has to

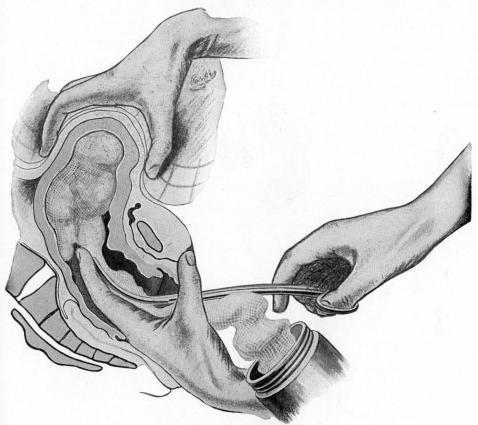

FIG. 716.—PACKING UTERUS WITH LONG FORCEPS.
Hand as a directing speculum; assistant outside steadies fundus.

adopt other measures. Time is an element in such cases. Give the uterus a little time and it will retract, but one must not allow the bleeding to continue all the while. To stop the hemorrhage and to give the uterus this opportunity (*fourth*), *compress the uterus between the two hands,* as in Fig. 714. The cervix is grasped by the whole hand and folded together, while the outside hand forces the uterus down firmly against the pubis and inside hand. One may feel the uterus gradually assuming its normal shape and consistence, and when, after two to five minutes, the pressure is relaxed, the physician finds that the flow has ceased, he may remove his hands. Should the flow continue in spite of this maneuver, or should it recommence after he has removed his hands, no further time and blood should be wasted, *but the uterovaginal tract should be packed (fifth).*

Uterine Tamponade.—One may tampon the uterus with gauze, using the hands alone, or with the single aid of the uterine packing forceps, or by sight, having drawn the uterus down with the vulsellum forceps and spread the genitals by specula. The kind of gauze is very important and the author recommends a ½ per cent. moist lysol gauze, whose method of preparation is described in his Obstetrics for Nurses.

Most often it will be necessary to operate with insufficient help, and then the second method is employed (Fig. 716). The operator puts the left hand into the vagina, the fingers inside the uterus as high as possible. Anesthesia is not usually required, but is better.

With long uterine packing forceps the end of the strip is carried up to the top of the uterus, taking care that the tip of the forceps does not catch on the contraction ring or in a fold of the relaxed uterine wall. A sterile towel is laid on the belly, and with his right hand the operator

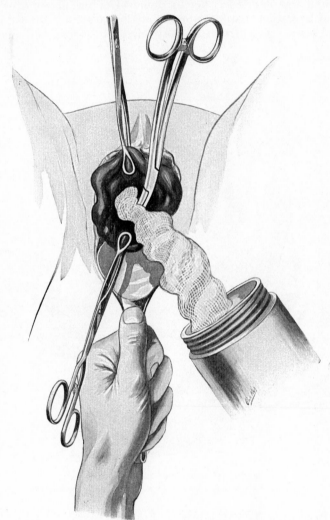

FIG. 717.—PACKING UTERUS—INSTRUMENTAL.
Two cervix forceps pull the uterus down and straighten it. The assistant's hand should control the fundus to make sure that the gauze enters it.

determines that the tip of the forceps carrying the gauze is really in the highest point of the uterus. The gauze is then evenly packed into the uterine cavity, from side to side, and from above downward. An assistant steadies the fundus, or the operator from time to time assures himself that the uterus is being evenly filled. The inside hand acts as a grooved channel along which the gauze and forceps find easy direction. The first part must be most firmly placed. When the uterus is full, the forceps are laid temporarily in the basin; two fingers of the left hand are placed against the tampon; the right hand grasps the uterus through the sterile towel, and the fingers force the gauze upward more firmly into the fundus, thus leaving room in the cervix for more gauze. This manœuver must be performed carefully and gently, and one must leave a vent for the escape of air, otherwise there is danger of air-embolism. It is well to have the trunk a little higher than the pelvis. The nurse holds the gauze jar near the vulva, exactly as in the illustration (Fig. 716). In the absence of a nurse or other person to hold the jar of gauze it may be held between the accoucheur's knees, as he sits before the patient, with his heels caught on a rung of the chair.

The writer, in several cases of great urgency, applied the gauze successfully with the hands, the left hand forcing the strip up into the uterus as it was fed into it by the right hand (Fig. 715).

If the operator prefers the third method, a table, good light, and several assistants are required. A broad speculum retracts the perineum; one cervix forceps is placed on the anterior lip of the cervix, and, if necessary, one on the posterior lip, the operator holding one, the assistant, the other. The right hand, armed with the long forceps, inserts the gauze, while the hand outside controls the fundus uteri and guards against false movements (Fig. 717).

In all cases, after the uterus is firmly plugged, the vagina is firmly tamponed with the remaining portion of the strip. Dührssen advised tamponing the vagina with cotton, which is better in some respects, but gives more pain and trouble in removal. Wendelstaedt invented uterine tamponade in 1806, but Dührssen popularized it.

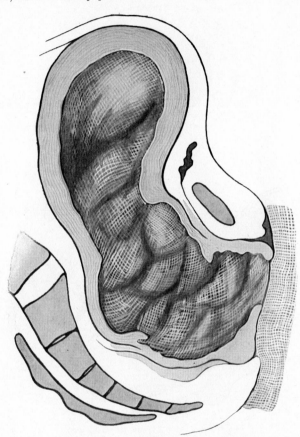

Fig. 718.—A Uterus Correctly Plugged.

In all but a very few cases packing will stop the bleeding. Chrobak, Ahlfeld, Bumm, von Braun report 10 failures in 120 cases, but an exact study of the histories shows that too much was expected of the operation. The author has plugged the uterus over four hundred times for conditions not due to lacerations. Only twice was it necessary to replace the pack with a second one. In two cases of laceration of the cervix with hemophilic diathesis the women died of hemorrhage. In two cases of atony of the uterus with hemophilic diathesis it was necessary to repack with gelatinized gauze. After abruptio placentæ packing is uncertain.

Without doubt most of the reported failures are due to poor technic: the gauze is not put in correctly. Figure 718 shows the parturient canal correctly packed; Fig. 719, a case where the operator has failed to grasp the situation. If the first tampon

54

is unsuccessful, the vaginal portion should be removed, the balance tamped more snugly into the uterus, then the rest of the parturient canal packed tightly with dry, *non-absorbent* sterile cotton. After the tamponade ergot and pituitrin are given as usual, and the hand should guard the uterus, massaging it lightly, or rubbing the aorta gently, if there be any tendency to further atony, for several hours. A tight abdominal binder or an adhesive strap may be employed, but the author has not seen any real value in either. It is better to hold the uterus down from the outside, while the balled fist exerts counterpressure from the perineum. The gauze

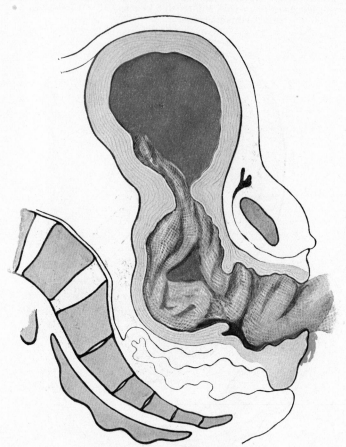

Fig. 719.—A Uterus Incorrectly Plugged.

is removed in twenty-four to twenty-six hours, and must be withdrawn very slowly, twenty to thirty minutes being consumed in the operation.

If the tampon fails to stop the bleeding, *i. e.*, if the uterus balloons out or oozing recurs through the pack, more action is demanded. Remove the gauze quickly and either clamp the bases of the broad ligaments, including the uterine arteries (Henkel's method, Fig. 720), or ligate the uterine arteries (Kerwin's method, Fig. 721a) or sew up the cervix tight (author's, Fig. 722) or extirpate the uterus.

Many other methods have been proposed, and occasionally they will prove useful. Compression of the abdominal aorta may be employed as a temporary expedient until one can prepare for more permanent measures. Packing the vagina with a ball of gauze, a towel, or anything sterile that is near at hand, and pressing the uterus against this from the outside, may limit the flow until the accoucheur can procure gauze for packing.

Fritsch recommended pulling the fundus forward over the pubis and filling up the space between it and the promontory with towels, after which one was to put on a very tight abdominal

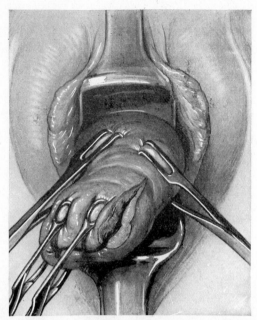

FIG. 720.—HENKEL'S METHOD. COMPRESSION OF UTERINE ARTERIES.

The cervix is gently drawn down and to the side; the anterior vaginal wall and bladder lifted up and out of danger; a strong vulsella is placed on the base of the broad ligament, pinching the side of the uterus and the large vessels here; shanks are surrounded with gauze; removal in eight to twenty-four hours, after leaving unlocked for one hour. Squeeze tightly enough to stop bleeding—both sides.

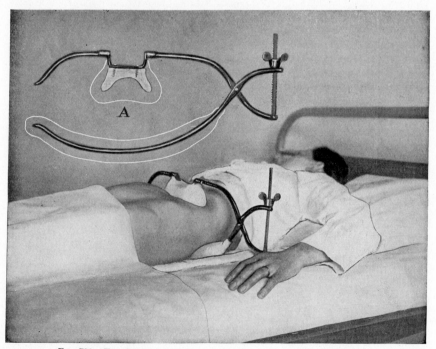

FIG. 721.—THE SEHRT AORTA COMPRESSOR APPLIED. A, ENLARGED DETAIL.

binder. The uterus has been folded together from the side, twisted on its axis, turned inside out, ligated, etc. A very hot uterine douche may cause firm contraction, and sterile vinegar or lemon juice may be added to fortify its action.

Parsenow recommended pulling the cervix down to the vulva with vulsellum forceps, thus stretching and kinking the uterine vessels, and Henkel advised placing a vulsellum temporarily

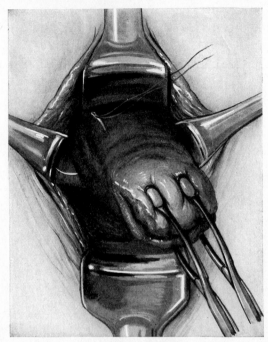

FIG. 721a.—KERWIN'S RECOMMENDATION.
Tying the uterine arteries for inveterate postpartum hemorrhage.

on the uterine vessels at the sides of the uterus through the lateral fornices. The latter has proved safe and effectual (Fig. 720).

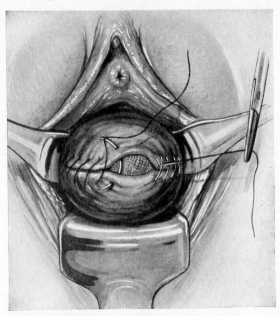

FIG. 722.—UTERUS BEING CLOSED OVER A PLUG.
After packing the uterus the cervix is quickly closed by a continuous suture. Removed in twenty-four to thirty-six hours.

Momburg proposed circular constriction of the waist with a rubber tube, to cut off the circulation in the lower half of the body, which he had used successfully in surgery. La Torre had mentioned this as early as 1875. Rissmann and Sehrt invented aortic clamps, embodying the century old principle of the mechanical tourniquet (Fig. 721).

To sum up briefly the treatment of atonic postpartum hemorrhage: First, if the placenta is in the uterus, massage; failing this, expression of the placenta; failing this, manual removal. Second, after placenta is out, massage, ergot, hypophysin, cleansing of uterine cavity, compression of the uterus in anteflexion; failing all these, uterine tamponade, elevation of foot of bed, aorta compressor, or some method of controlling the uterine arteries.

Operating in Shock.—The consultant sometimes finds a woman in deep shock after delivery, a history of hemorrhage being given. Here delicate points at once present themselves for decision: (1) Is it a postpartum hemorrhage or something else? (2) Is the bleeding actually going on internally? (3) Will the slight oozing cease of itself, and, if so, before the state of the patient becomes precarious? (4) Will the necessary blood loss attending the manipulations required turn the delicate scale against the woman? (5) Which is more dangerous, expectancy or interference? (6) Is the state of shock due solely to loss of blood? (7) Could the patient stand an anesthetic? (8) Would stimulation start the bleeding anew? (9) Has the bleeding stopped at the source? Lack of space forbids a full consideration of these critical situations, the solution of which depends on individual experience and judgment. A few bits of general advice may be helpful:

It is best not to operate in shock, but if the bleeding continues, operation is the lesser danger.

Avoid anesthetics if at all possible. Give ⅓ grain morphin hypo. If necessary use ether.

Operate in the exaggerated Trendelenburg position, or have two assistants hold the patient inverted.

Have everything ready for rapid work, gauze for packing, the needles threaded, etc.

Start the salt solution or the blood transfusion at once, letting it continue while the operation is being finished. In absence of diabetes, give 800 c.c. of 20 per cent. glucose solution intravenously. When bleeding is controlled—ephedrin gr. ⅜ hypo.

Be very deliberate in deciding to operate, but have preparations started while deliberating, and, if operation is decided upon, do things quickly and thoroughly.

Remember the Sehrt aorta compressor, or compression by the hand may stop bleeding while preparations are being made.

TREATMENT OF LACERATIONS

When a tear of the parturient canal has been discovered, the treatment of the case must be modified somewhat. If you compress a clitoris, vulvar or lower vaginal tear for a few minutes, very often the bleeding will cease and the regular conduct of the third stage will not need to be altered. If compression does not suffice, a few sutures will always do so.

Higher vaginal tears and cervix tears, especially in placenta prævia, may cause most serious hemorrhage. It is important to get rid of the placenta at once and get contraction and retraction of the uterus. This part of the treatment is the same as for atony. If the bleeding continues, two courses are open—one, uterovaginal tamponade, the other, suture of the laceration. One may combine the two procedures. Without doubt the best way to stop hemorrhage from a laceration is to sew up the tear, but it may be impossible to do this because of lack of proper preparations, of assistants, light, or skill. Then, too, sometimes the bleeding is so profuse that you cannot see where to place the stitches, the whole field being a lake of blood. It may also be inadvisable to sew up the tear because of sepsis, or because the facilities are not at hand for aseptic work. It may thus be safer to leave the wound open for drainage. In such cases the tampon will be indicated, but it is not so certain a remedy as in atony of the uterus.

When plugging a uterus and tear, the operator must be careful not to enlarge the latter by pushing in too much gauze, and the whole parturient canal must always be snugly and smoothly filled, never the vagina alone.

Lacerations are sewed as shown in Fig. 689 and Fig. 687, p. 805. Free, perhaps torrential, bleeding may render such operations difficult, and I have found the following measures useful, to enable me to see the field. Compression of the aorta (now, perhaps, Sehrt's compressor); traction on the lips of the cervix with cervix forceps; packing one side of the cervix tear while the other is sutured; compression of the bleeding surface with a large wad of dry cotton or the hand for twenty minutes; Henkel's method of clamping the bases of the broad ligament with bullet forceps; filling the uterus tight full of gauze, and sewing the cervix together over the plug (Fig. 722). Occasionally a spurting vessel may be clamped and ligated.

After-treatment.—All danger is not past when the hemorrhage has been stopped. The patient may die from the loss of blood. Unless one has plenty of medical assistants, this part of the treatment will have to be left until the accoucheur has stopped the active hemorrhage. This is the advantage of doing obstetrics in a maternity—while stopping the loss of blood an interne may be filling the patient's blood-vessels with salt solution or blood transfusion may be done.

During obstetric operations in general, and the treatment of hemorrhage in particular, the patient should be kept covered and warm. After a hemorrhage has been checked the patient should be warmly covered in bed and surrounded by hot-water bottles. In all cases the foot of the bed should be elevated at least two feet. To tide the patient over a fainting spell give a hypodermic of 1/1000 adrenalin, and let her sniff some smelling salts. While doing these things saline solution for subcutaneous administration should be prepared. Sterile tablets (Ringer) should be carried in the obstetric satchel. A douche-bag, a bath-thermometer, and salt solution needle should be boiled. Two drams of sterile salt are placed in the bag; the end of the tube, armed with the needle, is also put in the bag; then one quart of boiling water is poured on the salt. The mouth of the bag is stoppered with a large wad of sterile cotton, and the bag is held under the cold-water tap or in a dish-pan of cold water until the thermometer registers 115° F.

The solution is absorbed quickest from the broad connective spaces under the mammary glands and the needle is directed here. A liter may be injected on each side. It is advisable to lower the bag occasionally to prevent overstretching and too rapid opening up of the lymph-spaces. If the case is critical, the other side, as well as the two flanks, may be injected. In one patient I injected 116 ounces of saline solution in one sitting, using the 4 points named. The patient recovered. This patient also absorbed 2 quarts from the rectum. Such immense quantities are rarely needed. It is good to give also 20 per cent. glucose solution intravenously up to 1 liter. Gum (acacia) glucose solution is still better but seldom available. Shall you inject these solutions while the hemorrhage is still going on? Yes, subcutaneously and intravenously. The blood lost then will not be pure, but mixed with substitutes, and it is not so precious. By the time a quart has been absorbed the accoucheur must have the hemorrhage in his control, or the patient will have died. Some authors advise against these injections until after the flow has ceased. This is a relic of the times when we waited for fainting to occur and the resulting thrombosis in the open vessels stopped the bleeding. Nowadays we can act promptly and expeditiously but we must keep the patient alive until we can shut off the flow.

Per rectum, salt solution, with perhaps 3 ounces of coffee, is quickly taken up, and a quart may be administered every three hours.

If one can collect the lost blood cleanly it may be given per rectum, mixed with saline solution (Lindeman). I have also given the blood contained in the placenta from another woman (with negative Wassermann, of course). All but the corpuscles is absorbed. It is not wise to administer anything per rectum until the hemorrhage has been permanently stopped, because if any local treatment is to be carried out, the discharge from the bowel may infect the field, the hands, instruments, gauze, etc.

By mouth the patient may have hot coffee, water, or a hot oyster-stew. If vomiting occurs, she usually feels relieved, after which liquids may again be allowed, using care not to overload the stomach. Finally, a hypodermic of morphin may be given to quiet and sustain the patient.

Transfusion.—To transfuse blood from another person is now a daily practice and is especially successful in hemorrhage cases. Therefore the accoucheur should command the technic of at least one method. Although direct transfusion is safest and best, owing to the exigencies of obstetric practice, the sodium citrate, or indirect method will be most often used. The blood is collected in a graduate containing sodium citrate solution (Lewisohn) diluted to 0.2 per cent. citrate (*i. e.*, 1 gm. of sodium citrate in every 500 c.c. of blood), and then slowly injected into the vein. For direct transfusion the author's instrument may be used (Fig. 711).

Timothy Clark in 1657 first transfused animals, then Denis and Lower, the human in 1666. Complete history, and lit., Scholten.

During the first week nourishment must be given freely. The bed is lowered in two or three days or sooner, depending on the condition of the patient. It is lowered a few inches at a time to avoid syncope. Not seldom, after severe hemorrhages, the puerpera will have a rise of temperature to 102° F. within the first twenty-four hours. This is reaction fever, and will go down without treatment. But occasionally sepsis follows in the wake of a severe loss, first, because the resistance of the patient is so much lowered that infection finds easy access, and, second, because, in the excitement and unpreparedness attending most of such cases, the rules of asepsis are forgotten or are impossible of being carried out in detail. Sepsis under these conditions is likely to follow a severe course.

The milk secretion is diminished, Ahlfeld's statistics to the contrary notwithstanding. Ahlfeld had strong peasant women to deal with. The high-strung American mother cannot stand the drain of lactation after severe loss of blood. My experience has been unequivocal on this point, and I notice that von Braun warns against forcing the nursing of the infant on neurasthenic women. One may permit a partial breast-feeding until the woman has completely recovered from the exhaustion of the hemorrhage. Some women recover very slowly from the spanemia and require blood-tonics for long periods. The best treatment the writer knows for such cases of severe hemorrhage is living at the seashore, and the woman should be sent there as soon as she can bear the journey. Liver, spleen, etc., in the diet.

INVERSION OF THE UTERUS

Figure 723 shows a complete inversion or turning inside out of the uterus, together with prolapse, *i. e.*, prolapsus uteri inversi. Lesser degrees occur, and only the placental site may be depressed, as in Fig. 704, p. 836—the so-called atony of the placental site. All grades between these two extremes are observed, and are called incomplete or partial inversions, the most common of which are those in which the fundus comes to lie in the vagina just within the introitus, and feels like a soft, large, globular, fibroid polyp. The placenta may still be attached, or only partially adherent. If the inversion occurs after the third stage, the naked uterus lies in the vagina or may be expelled outside, in which case the open sinuses and tubal ostia are visible. In the "inversion funnel" from the abdominal side, the tubes, ovaries, the round and broad ligaments, sometimes the gut and omentum, may be seen.

Etiology.—In one of the author's cases, during the removal of the placenta, the uterus was felt to contract, the contraction ring opened outward, a condition shown in Fig. 724 appearing for a few moments. The view that an inversion could be thus produced by contraction of the fundus, with relaxation of the lower portions of the uterus, was held by Rokitansky, Duncan, Reusch, and others, but Schauta strongly asserted the contrary—that it was atony of the uterus which caused the accident. While atony of the organ may cause the majority, I am convinced that the view of Rokitansky is correct in some cases. Contraction of a part of the uterus before retraction has been fully established may explain the mechanism. An atonic uterus may become inverted by a sudden action of the abdominal muscles, increasing intra-abdominal pressure, such as bearing down to express the placenta, turning in bed, sitting up, coughing, raising the hips to allow a clean sheet to be placed. Inversion from such causes is called *spontaneous*. *Violent* inversion may be due to traction on the umbilical cord in the effort to remove the placenta (24 of 47 cases of Vogel), traction on part of the placenta or on the membranes, and too powerful Credé expression of the placenta, or even the squeezing out of a blood-clot. Spontaneous inversion may result from pulling on the too short cord by the child during natural delivery. While many cases are reported as spontaneous, probably most of them are the result of errors of art.

Lack of general tonus, hypo-adrenalinemia, and chronic metritis with resulting fibrosis have been suggested by Mansfeld as predisposing causes.

Inversion of the uterus is rare in hospitals. Braun, in 250,000 labors, did not see one, and in Dublin only one was observed in 190,000 consecutive labors. Most of the cases occur in private practice, but the accident is exceedingly rare. It may occur in abortion as early as the fourth month, Holmes having had a case at the fifth month, and it may appear on the second, sixth, even the fifteenth, day after delivery.

Symptoms.—As a rule, the inversion is gradual, beginning as a little depression, and then suddenly the fundus drops into the vagina (Fig. 725).   If traction on the cord has been made, the move-

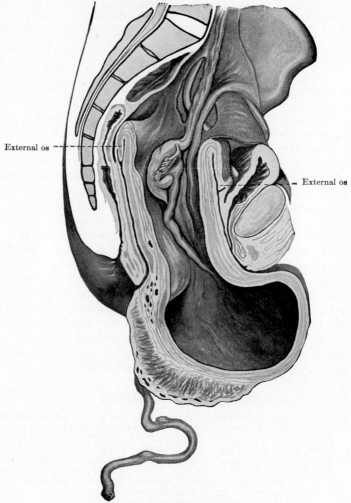

External os

External os

FIG. 723.—INVERSIO UTERI TOTALIS (adapted from Tandler).

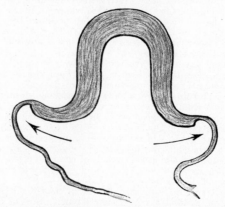

FIG. 724.—DIAGRAM TO SHOW HOW A UTERUS CAN INVERT ITSELF BY CONTRACTION.

ment is more abrupt. The patient utters a sharp cry and bears down, the latter having a tendency to increase the prolapse. Shock is almost always present, certainly if the uterus turned inside out suddenly, and is due to the stretching of the peritoneum and the nerves of the broad ligaments, perhaps also from the reduction in intra-abdominal tension and consequent downward

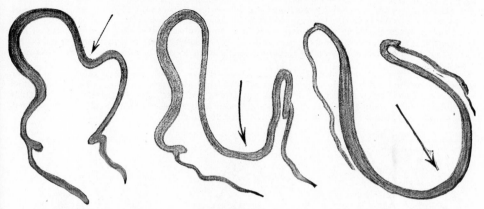

Fig. 725.—Diagrams to Show how an Atonic Uterus may be Inverted.
Arrows show placental site.

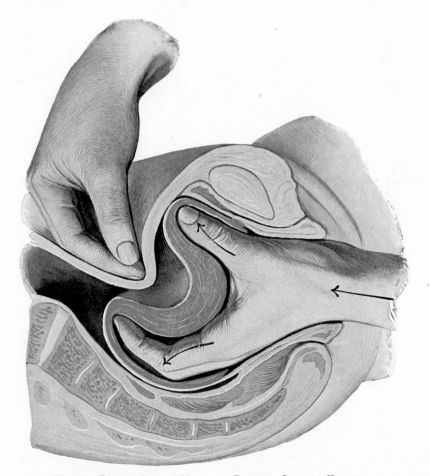

Fig. 726.—Diagram Showing Method of Replacing Inverted Uterus.
After the whole hand, grasping the uterine body, has replaced same in vagina, the constricting cervical ring is spread by means of the fingers and thumb, while the palm of the hand forces up the fundus in the directions indicated by arrows. The outside hand aids to dilate the funnel.

displacement of the diaphragm, the heart, etc. Profuse hemorrhage is the rule, because the placenta has almost always been either partly or completely detached, but it may be absent if the

organ is still adherent to the inverted uterus. Shock is disproportionate to blood loss. If the
uterus contracts, especially if the cervix snaps together around the extruded fundus, the bleeding
may be slight, but this is the exception. In rare instances both collapse and severe bleeding are
absent, and the condition is discovered only at a subsequent examination. If the woman does not
die from shock or hemorrhage, the inverted fundus may slough off, resulting in death or recovery;
it may be infected, resulting in septicopyemia, or it may undergo involution and come under late
treatment, or it may, spontaneously, and without explainable cause, be reinverted. Such cures
have been observed a few hours after the occurrence and as late as five and eight years (Meigs and
Baudelocque).

Ileus, from incarceration of the gut in the inversion funnel, has been observed. In the
chronic cases the fundus in the vagina atrophies and becomes covered with dry, slightly hornified
epithelium, and is often the seat of erosions and ulcers. Menorrhagia, leukorrhea, and irregular
bleeding are often complained of, with dragging pains in the back and a feeling of bearing down,
but, remarkably, one or all of these symptoms may be wanting.

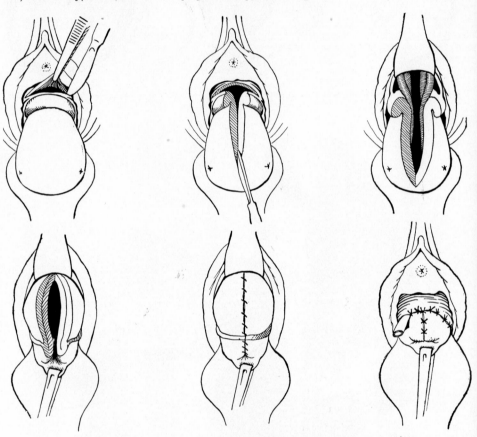

Fig. 726a.—Spinelli's Operation. Anterior Hysterocolpotomy (Chronic Cases).

Diagnosis.—If only the attendant would bear this accident in mind, there need be no difficulty in making the diagnosis on the direct examination. A large, roundish tumor in the vagina,
with absence of the fundus uteri from its proper place, in the presence of shock and hemorrhage,
will clear up the situation at once. It may be possible to feel the inversion funnel from the abdomen after the bladder is emptied. In the differential diagnosis fibroid polyp, adherent placenta,
and total atony of the uterus are to be considered, and a careful bimanual examination will easily
decide between them. The inverted fundus has been torn off under the notion that it was the
placenta alone; it has been cut off as a tumor, and the whole uterus has been pulled out as a
second twin! If the fundus is prolapsed, the bright red, rough, bleeding endometrium, or the
placenta, cannot fail to tell what has happened. In debating the causes of postpartum shock
inversio uteri must be considered with rupture of the uterus, hemorrhage, etc.

Prognosis.—This is better now than formerly, by grace of asepsis and better obstetric practice in general. Crosse, in 1843, found that 80 of 109 reported cases died; Vogel, in 1900, reported
only 22 per cent. mortality; Zangemeister, in 1913, 23 per cent. Even some of the cases where the
uterus has been torn off recover if infection is absent. Reposition improves the outlook. It may
be possible even after twenty years. (Miller, 1927, Naujoks, 1932, Lit.)

Treatment.—Although inversion of the uterus is rare, the accoucheur's routine technic in handling labor cases should comprise means for its prevention. Traction on the cord must be avoided, and, while drawing the membranes off the uterine wall, the outside hand must lie on the fundus and assure its contraction. Atony of the uterus postpartum is to be rectified as soon as possible. In turning the newly delivered woman from side to side, or when she raises her hips for the removal of soiled bed-clothes, the bed-pan, the rubber pad, etc., the attendant must lay a hand on the uterus and be sure that it is firmly contracted. During the manual removal of the placenta the first beginnings of inversion are to be corrected.

What to do in acute cases requires deliberation, because if the attempt is made to put the uterus back while the woman is in deep shock, the delicate balance will be turned against her. Zangemeister showed that 23 per cent. died when operated during shock, while none died when reaction was awaited. Here it is better to replace the fundus in the vagina, pack the latter firmly with antiseptic gauze, and let the parturient rally, aiding her by morphin, saline solution, or transfusion. If bleeding is going on, however, it may be necessary to risk the added shock in order to stop it. If an aorta compressor is available, by it one can prevent further blood loss while the woman is being treated for shock. Ether is the anesthetic of choice, but sometimes only a little encouragement is required to enable the woman to stand the operation. The shoulders should be raised a little to avoid air embolism. It is best to remove the placenta cleanly before reposition is attempted, but if the case seems favorable the removal of the placenta may be done after the uterus is returned. If the attendant feels that the surroundings and his assistance do not justify his interference, the external portion of the mass may be returned to the vagina and the latter packed, to await the arrival of help or during transportation of the patient to a maternity. Spontaneous reinversion may thus occur.

The technic of the operation in acute cases is simple (Fig. 726). While the whole mass lies in the grasp of the hand, the fingers spread out the constricting portion of the uterus, and the palm pushes up on the inverted fundus—all this in the direction of the axis of the pelvis, well forward, to avoid the sacrum. The maneuver may be aided by the outside hand dilating the funnel. It is helpful to reduce the size of the swollen fundus by continuous, even, firm compression with the hands, before attempting the reduction—a maneuver invented by Charles White in 1773. It may be best to push up one side of the uterus first—a sort of taxis—replacing first the part which came down last. Great care is to be exercised to avoid puncturing the soft atonic uterine wall. It occurs surprisingly easily. Deep anesthesia must be induced if there is a tendency to spasm of the constricting portion and the operation may be neither prolonged nor forced. Irving and Foster recommend, after a gentle attempt at reposition has failed, to pack the vagina firmly, restore the patient's vitality with transfusion, saline, glucose, perform laparotomy and draw the fundus out of its inversion with Allis forceps, beginning at one round ligament.

In more chronic cases one may use colpeurysis. Sometimes several—as high as twenty—applications may be needed. The colpeurynter is left from twelve to thirty hours, and the foot of the bed is elevated. Gentleness, asepsis, and patience are the watchwords. After reposition it is wise in all cases to tampon the uterovaginal tract. If reinversion fails it may be necessary to employ the knife, and then Küstner's operation or one of its modifications, Spinelli's, may be used. Failing this operation, vaginal extirpation of the uterus may be required. In acute cases such operations are almost never needed, sepsis, gangrene, or intractable bleeding giving the few rare indications. When extirpation is done it is best to split the fundus to avoid injury to structures which may have fallen into the funnel, and to obtain easier access to the broad ligaments. (For discussion of labor after operative reinversion see Milander.)

LATE PUERPERAL HEMORRHAGES

Even after delivery the woman is not safe from the dangers of bleeding, since such may occur as late as the fifth week postpartum. A hemorrhage which begins after the first day after labor is called late, though some authors distinguish between those which occur in the early puerperium and those of the late puerperium. Sometimes, without apparent cause, the puerpera begins to flow, and the amount of blood lost may be so great that a serious anemia or even death results.

Etiology.—Among the commonest causes may be noted retention of placental fragments, of thick membranes, of decidua compacta (especially in abortions), and sometimes simply a hard blood-clot. A large piece of placenta may come away, more or less, or not at all, decomposed, as late as the twelfth day, and usually there is not much bleeding. Cases are on record of the retention of pieces of placenta for as long as eleven months, and Ries found placental villi in the uterine vessels eighteen years after the last delivery. Ramsbotham records a case where the whole placenta was retained, and, as far as the woman knew, never came away. Small and thin pieces of placenta may dissolve in the lochia, which are then profuse, prolonged, bloody, and perhaps fetid. The same may be said of membranes and decidua. If bits of placenta or decidua do not become infected, blood is deposited on them in successive layers, and a fibrinous or placental polypus results (Figs. 726 b and 726 c). These keep up irregular hemorrhage until they are removed, or

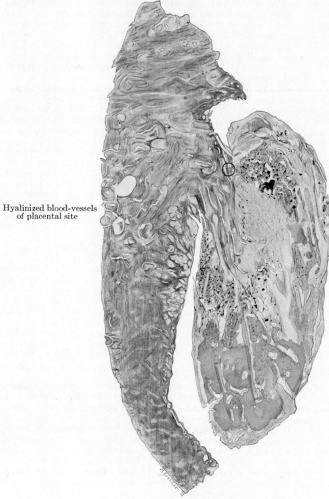

Hyalinized blood-vessels of placental site

Degenerated villi

FIG. 726b.

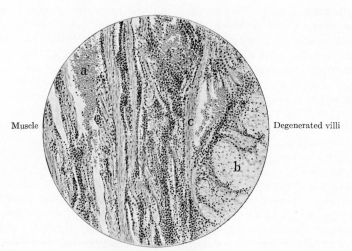

Muscle

Degenerated villi

Inflammatory reaction

FIG. 726c.

they become infected, break down, and are discharged piecemeal, with fetid discharge and fever, sometimes with hemorrhages, or a pyemia may ensue.

Subinvolution stands next in frequency, the large boggy uterus bleeding on the slightest provocation. Frankl mentions subinvolution of the blood-vessels, Kermauner, hyaline degeneration of these as well as the uterus. Low-grade infection, with large thrombi in the placental site, plays a large rôle. Displacements of the uterus are usually part of the same process, and in retroflexion of the puerperal uterus hemorrhages are not infrequent and prolonged, and bloody lochia—in some cases for six or eight weeks—are very common. Favored by subinvolution and displaced by a full bladder or rectum, the uterus may bleed, and a disquieting degree of anemia may result.

Nervous influences unquestionably play a rôle. I saw a very serious hemorrhage result from relaxation of the uterus on the eleventh day when the puerpera had been frightened by a domestic quarrel. We know that the menses may cease, and that metrorrhagia may ensue, upon a nervous shock. Precocious ovulation may also be thought of, i. e., an abnormal menstruation.

Sudden physical strain often causes a reappearance of the bloody lochia, as is so often observed when the puerpera gets up for the first time. Severe hemorrhages at this time are rare, but do occur (subinvolution).

As occasional factors may be mentioned myomata, especially the mural and submucous varieties, carcinomata, cervical erosions, ulceration of a cervical vessel (phlebectasia), rupture of a small uterine or cervical hematoma, unrecognized rupture of the uterus, traumatic aneurysm of the uterine artery, inversion of the uterus, deciduomata, chorio-epithelioma, secondary hemorrhages after suture of a cervix tear, as occurs sometimes after gynecologic operations, traumatism from coitus, sometimes with rupture of the vagina, and puerperal septicemia with softening of the thrombi of the placental site. The last form of hemorrhage is very fatal.

A reconsideration of the occurrences during the labor may discover a probable cause for the hemorrhage. By recto-abdominal examination malpositions, subinvolution, inversion of the uterus can be determined. A large boggy uterus with a patulous os usually has something in it. Because of the bacterial content it is not safe to invade the uterine cavity with the finger until after the fourteenth day, but if the hemorrhage is alarming one may have to do so to make a diagnosis. The worst bleedings come from the uterine artery. It probably was torn during labor and a traumatic aneurysm formed around its ends, or it may have been temporarily compressed by a tampon or suture. A little overstrain late in the puerperium bursts the aneurysm and a flooding results. Only a digital and specular examination will clear up the etiology and indicate the method of procedure. A positive Aschheim-Zondek test indicates the retention of placental tissue or chorio-epithelioma.

Prognosis.—Even though severe, the hemorrhage is seldom fatal, and it responds quickly to treatment. The most dangerous are the cases of placental polyp, the frequently repeated hemorrhages depressing the puerpera a great deal, and especially critical are the infected placental fragments, because if it is necessary to remove them, the unavoidable manipulations grind the infection into the placental site, into the open veins, and into the thrombi here, pyemia easily resulting. Rupture of a traumatic aneurysm of the uterine artery may also be fatal.

Treatment.—Early in the puerperium it is dangerous to submit the patient to active local treatment, especially if she has fever. A mild infection may thus be changed to a fatal one. Therefore external remedies are to be tried at first. Ergot and hydrastis internally, pituitrin, hypodermically $\frac{1}{2}$ c.c. every four hours, massage of the uterus, and the ice-bag or a hot vaginal douche may be ordered. If the hemorrhage persists, the uterovaginal tract may be packed with slightly antiseptic gauze. This will care for a hemorrhage from atony as well as one from the retention of a piece of placenta—indeed, it favors the separation and expulsion of the latter. Manual or instrumental curetage is not to be performed in the early puerperium. It is best to temporize, if possible, using occasional tamponade, rest, medicine, etc., until the fifth or sixth week of the puerperium, by which time the uterus has cleansed itself, involution is so well along that the uterine muscle will not be easily perforated, and the blood-vessels so tightly organized that the finger or the curet will not be able to carry infection into them. During the period of expectancy the woman should be supported by a roborant diet, by blood transfusions, etc. An aorta compressor is to be kept nearby, ready for emergencies. Should the indication to remove the mass be positive, the placental forceps and the finger are to be used, not the curet; an antiseptic uterine douche precedes, and a weakly antiseptic, firm, uterine pack completes, the operation because the bleeding may be dangerous.

Subinvolution is treated by ergot, hydrastis, pituitrin, hot douches, and uterine massage.

Rupture of an aneurysm requires prompt action. While preparing for operation hemorrhage may be controlled by compressing the aorta. Under full exposure of the field the bleeding vessel is tied or the uterus extirpated. Transfusion may be needed before or after operation. Myomata, cancer, erosions, etc., are treated on general principles. Temporary tamponade of the vagina may tide the patient along until the best time for operating arrives. (See Anderodias et Péry.)

SYNCOPE AND SUDDEN DEATH

A gravida, a parturient, or a puerpera may collapse and die suddenly, the cause being sometimes determinable only at the autopsy. Often, however, the complication may be expected, knowing previous disease to exist. Only a partial enumeration of the causes may here be attempted, otherwise we would have to cover the entire field of medicine. The causes may be divided into—(a) Those which may be properly said to accompany the puerperal state; and (b) those which are extragenital, but in which the performance of the reproductive function is the exciting factor. (See E. P. Davis.)

A. (1) Sudden collapse and death may be due to hemorrhage and shock from any of the obstetric accidents already discussed, for example, ruptured ectopic gestation, uterus perforated by hydatids, placenta prævia, abruptio placentæ, rupture of the uterus, postpartum hemorrhage, inversio uteri, rupture of the pelvic joints, rupture of a varix in the broad ligament.

(2) The acute toxemias which go with the pregnant state, the prostration and collapse of hyperemesis gravidarum, the toxemia of eclampsia, of pernicious anemia, uremia (Strümpell, Bartles), and those of sepsis. Almost fatal syncope from acute uremia or from acute pregnancy toxemia, with characteristic urinary findings, I have observed twice. Zweifel reported such a case, confirmed at autopsy, and Norris another. Eclamptic toxemia may cause sudden death by cerebral hemorrhage, and this may occur when the convulsions and other signs of the disease are absent. Syncopal attacks in severe sepsis, due to passing cardiac weakness, are common, and the end in such cases is often due to paralysis of the heart, which may come on suddenly. Acute pulmonary edema, with or without high blood-pressure, may be fatal.

(3) Pulmonary embolism is an often mentioned cause, the clot usually being found plugging one or more of the pulmonary arteries. The embolus almost always comes from the thrombosed veins in the pelvis or thigh. Slowing of the circulation in the veins allows the blood-platelets to accumulate on the wall and build a white thrombus, on which the red clot will always be found. Alteration of the blood may predispose to thrombus formation, especially if the vessel-wall is injured. It is possible that clots may form in the large veins of the thigh if the limbs are held in a cramped position for a long time, as in protracted operations with the patient in the exaggerated lithotomy or Trendelenburg positions. Puerperal infection acts in

two ways, first, by an alteration of the blood, predisposing to thrombi distant from the site of the disease, and second the infection may spread along the veins or to the veins, directly causing thrombosis. Although most authors emphasize the mechanical factors, the precipitation, the agglutination, etc., I have never seen a thrombosis where infection, either endogenic or exogenic, could be ruled out. Veit believes the same. Angus McLean experimentally proved that thrombosis and embolism could not be produced in animals without infection. Thrombosis may follow as the direct result of an intestinal infection. In cases of severe anemia or profound shock, the circulation in the heart being almost in abeyance, a clot may form, and, after a few days of only partial recovery, sudden death from cardiac paralysis may occur. Pus from a pelvic abscess may break into a vein and reach the heart. In 1929–31 a marked increase in the incidence of thrombosis and embolism—both medical and surgical—was noted all over the world and this evoked numerous studies of the subject—without much gain of knowledge however (Dietrich, Bancroft and Brown). After all I believe, *no infection, no embolism!*—an opinion shared by Gideon Wells.

Air-embolism has frequently been given as a cause of sudden death in pregnancy and labor. A colleague of the author told of a woman, pregnant four months, who, while taking a douche with a bulb syringe, died suddenly from this cause. Such deaths have been reported from attempts to produce abortion by injecting air into the uterus. During obstetric operations, especially with placenta prævia, the accident has time and again occurred. Curiously enough, experiments on animals have shown that enormous quantities of air can be injected into the veins leading directly to the heart, without any, or quickly passing, bad symptoms (Fitzpatrick). In the human, however, the danger of the admission of air into the veins through the uterine sinuses is a well-established fact. During the operation of uterine tamponade in placenta prævia the author had one case of collapse from air-embolism (recovery). In personal communications Dr. Skeel and Dr. Bogardus report two others, one of which was fatal. Gough reports a fatal one. Gases of decomposition which accumulate in the uterus may gain entrance to the veins. The Bacterium aërogenes capsulatus has been found in these cases, and the presence of such gases may bring the diagnosis into question.

(4) The nervous shock of labor may cause syncope and even death, and a psychic shock at the time of labor may be fatal. In the First Book of Samuel, Ch. iv:19, 20, it is said that Eli's daughter, learning that her husband and father-in-law were killed and the ark of God taken, went into labor and died. Hirst tells of a widow, illegitimately pregnant, who, on being shown the child, went into delirium and died. Sue (Histoire des Accouchements) relates that a pregnant woman was told by a gypsy that she would die in labor. She made her will and expired. Williams had a similar experience, but, by giving morphin, he put the woman asleep, during which time she forgot her obsession. That profound nervous influences can produce postpartum hemorrhage I am convinced from actual experience. Acute delirium in labor, the result of excessive pain in a nervously disposed individual, may be an indication for the termination of labor. Loss of consciousness may occur during the second stage, the result of intense pain, and the child may be delivered without the knowledge of the mother. I have observed this myself, and agree with Freyer that in medicolegal cases cognizance should be taken of it as a fact—for example, in cases where a mother, bearing alone, is accused of infanticide. Syncope after delivery, in the absence of hemorrhage, rupture of the uterus, etc., is very rare. I have seen it follow the delivery of the child in a case where the woman had been enforced to breathe very rapidly and deeply with a view of preventing her making bearing-down efforts, the object of the same being to keep the child back until the accoucheur could get to the bedside. This phenomenon is probably an acapnia. Traction on the uterine ligaments by forced delivery through an unpre-

pared parturient canal may produce peritoneal shock. I have seen the same during the removal of gauze used for packing. Pituitrin sometimes causes stenocardial attacks.

Anderson and Rosenau try to find a connection between the admixture of fetal to maternal blood and eclampsia, a sort of anaphylaxis. While the idea is not proved for eclampsia, some cases of collapse and sudden death postpartum resemble certain forms of anaphylaxis. The status thymicus has not been sufficiently studied in this connection. Disturbances of the pluriglandular system—hypo-epinephrinemia—may explain some cases, then this disturbance must be explained. I have seen syncope from acute dilatation of the stomach and death from the status hypoplasticus after labor. Acute dilatation of even a normal heart may occur at the end of a protracted second stage, with exhaustive bearing-down efforts.

Some of these cases ought to be called "obstetric shock," and may be explained by a sudden disequilibrium in the vagosympathetic system, the result of rapid emptying of the uterus, etc. (Rivière); others are similar to the familiar surgical shock in which Baruch has demonstrated a diminution of hematopoietic capacity (with red venous blood).

Faintness or even real syncope may occur when a puerpera gets out of bed for the first time. Formerly, when puerperæ were kept in the horizontal position for many days, such accidents were commoner than now, when more activity in the lying-in period is allowed.

B. Sudden death may be due to causes which have indirect connection with the parturient function—for example, heart disease, especially mitral stenosis and myocarditis, hydropericardium, adhesive pericarditis, hydrothorax, displacement of the heart and lungs in kyphoscoliosis, struma with acute strumitis, etc. The straining of labor may rupture the heart, the spleen, the aorta, the splenic or mesenteric veins, the gut, the gall-bladder (Ries), peritoneal adhesions, or a walled-off abscess (appendix or tube), and cause collapse and speedy death. The same may be said of rupture of a blood-vessel in the brain, of the bronchioles of the lung with emphysema (very exceptional as a cause of death alone), of hemoptysis, of hemorrhage into the stomach from gastric ulcer, of rupture of the pancreas and of the splenic artery. Brain diseases, tumor, abscess, thrombosis of the sinuses, and, finally, poisoning by drugs or antiseptics—*chloroform*, morphin, scopolamin, bichlorid, iodoform, carbolic acid, lysol—must be mentioned.

Symptoms.—These depend on whether the death is cerebral, pulmonary, or cardiac, and the underlying cause will determine which one occurs. Pulmonary embolism with cardiac death is the most frequent form. The patient falls as if struck, cries once with pain over the heart, gasps for air, becomes cyanotic, develops edema of the lungs with bloody expectoration, and dies in a few minutes. Sometimes one attack passes over, or the woman may have several mild ones, but usually the second or third is fatal. Between attacks cyanosis, dyspnea, fast heart, dilatation of pupils, nervous excitation, with fear of impending dissolution, are more or less marked. If the embolus is small, it may pass on into the lungs and the patient may recover. Mild symptoms of shock, with pain on the affected side, bloody expectoration, and, locally, perhaps, a friction-sound, will enable one to make the diagnosis. The embolus may pass through an open foramen ovale into the general circulation. Fever of a mild type almost always precedes the occurrence of the embolism, and experience shows that women with varicosities, with myomata, and those on whom operations near the veins have been performed, are oftenest stricken. Infection, however, is accountable for the majority of cases. Mahler believed to have proved that a regularly increasing frequency of the pulse indicates thrombosis in the veins. I cannot confirm it. In air embolism, on the occasion of local interference, the patient goes into collapse, breathing becomes difficult, she has sharp precordial pain, coma, and in three to ten minutes expires. In one case I observed a severe chill with the pulmonary and cardiac symptoms, followed by profuse sweating. Skeel, in his case, heard "typical churning noises" over the heart, and J. Y. Simpson refers to a reddish suffusion of the cheeks, and petechial spots in the skin and retina may be found. At autopsy in such cases the heart and pulmonary vessels are filled with frothy blood, and death is due to heart paralysis—it cannot pump such a mixture. Perhaps the coronary vessels are sometimes plugged with an air-embolus which acts just like any other, the clinical picture resembling angina pectoris (Gough).

Diagnosis.—When a woman faints or collapses after delivery, the accoucheur should rapidly review the course of the labor for signs of any of the following conditions: Postpartum hemorrhage, rupture of the uterus, inversion of the uterus, intraperitoneal hemorrhage, excessive operative traumatism. Next, uremia and toxemia must be considered, then heart and lung diseases. Emboli are commoner in the puerperium. True syncope and shock can be diagnosed only by exclusion. Postanesthetic collapse must always be borne in mind. Chloroform is the most dangerous in this regard, and the amount administered need not be large, especially if the woman had any slight latent kidney, heart, or liver disease. Late chloroform death, due to fatty degeneration and cytolysis of the liver, kidneys, and heart, may occur from a few hours to twelve days after delivery. It resembles acute yellow atrophy of the liver, with delirium, coma, jaundice, and cardiac paralysis. It may be very acute, terminating fatally within twelve hours (author's case).

Treatment is on general lines, depends on the diagnosis, and a quick but thorough general physical examination may reveal something that may be operated upon.

Trendelenburg for pulmonary embolism, advised exposure of the vena pulmonalis, and extraction of the clot. Twenty-four cases are on record with 5 recoveries (Nyström's, Meyer's, Kirschner's), and two which might have been saved (Klein, Fehling).

An attempt should be made to prevent air-embolism when operating or moving the patient. While packing the uterus a large vent should be left alongside the hand. Sometimes the chance must be taken. For prevention of embolism in phlebitis, see page 935.

Literature

Adair: Surg., Gyn., and Obst., February, 1912.—*Ahlfeld:* Zeitschr. f. Geb. u. Gyn., vol. li, H. 2; *ibid.*, vol. lxvii, p. 224. *Anderodias et Péry:* Gyn. et Obst., Paris, September, 1931, p. 381.—*Aschoff:* "Thrombosis," Centralbl. f. Gyn., 1911, No. 45.—*Bancroft and Brown:* Surg., Gyn. and Obst., June, 1932.—*Baruch:* Jour. Amer. Med. Assoc., Belgium Letter, October 1, 1923.—*Curtis and David:* Jour. Amer. Med. Assoc., October 28, 1911.—*Davis:* "Sudden Death, etc.," Trans. Amer. Gyn. Soc., 1905, vol. xxx, p. 345. Gives literature.—*DeLee:* Uterine Tamponade, Amer. Jour. Obstetrics, 1903, vol. xlvii, No. 4.—*Dietrich:* Placenta Accreta, Zeitschr. f. Geb. u. Gyn., 1922, vol. lxxxiv, Band iii, p. 580.—*Dietrich, A.:* Thrombose, Grundlage u. Bedeutung, Springer, Berlin, 1932.—*Fehling:* Monograph, Thrombosis and Embolism, Enke, Stuttgart, 1920. Literature.—*Fitzpatrick:* New York Med. Jour., November 26, 1910.—*Foges:* Centralbl. f. Gyn., 1910, p. 1502; also 1911, No. 4.—*Frankl:* Arch. für Gynaek., June, 1926, vol. 129, i, p. 87.—*Gough:* Surg., Gyn., and Obst., March, 1924.—*Heidler:* Monograph, Die Manuelle Plazentalösung, Kabitsch, Leipzig, 1927.—*Irving and Foster:* Amer. Jour. Obst. and Gyn., 1931, September, p. 440.—*Jones:* Surg., Gyn., and Obst., June, 1913. Full literature on Inversio uteri; also *Thorn:* Volk. Samml., No. 625.—*Klein:* Arch. f. Gyn., 1911, vol. xciv, Heft 1.—*Kockel:* Handb. der Geb. Doederlein, 1916, Band ii, p. 561.—*Kraul:* Arch. für Gynaek., 1925, Band 124, H. 1, p. 241. Literature.— *Kumpf:* Centralbl. f. Gyn., 1897, p. 289.—*Labhardt:* Zeitschr. f. Geb. u. Gyn., 1910, vol. lxvi, p. 407.— *Lespinasse:* "Transfusion of Human Blood in Infants," Surg., Gyn., and Obstet., 1912, vol. ii.—*Lindemann et al.:* Amer. Jour. Obstet. and Gyn., November, 1921, p. 579.—*McLean:* Paper read before Chicago Med. Soc., January 13, 1915.—*Mansfeld:* Zentralbl. für Gyn., December, 1913, No. 52.—*Meyer:* Surg., Gyn., and Obst., May, 1930 (3 recoveries).—*Milander:* Zentb. für Gyn., 1927, July 16.—*Miller:* Amer. Jour. Obst. and Gyn., March, 1927, p. 307, and Lit.—*Momburg:* Centralbl. f. Chir., 1908, No. 23. Also L'Obstetrique, January, 1911. Literature.—*Naujoks:* Arch. für Gyn., 1932, vol. cxlviii, H. 3.—*Neu:* Arch. Gyn., 1908.—*Norris:* Amer. Jour. Obstet., July, 1903.—*Nyström:* Jour. Amer. Med. Assoc., December 15, 1928, p. 1936.—*Opitz:* Centralbl. f. Gyn., 1908, p. 1503.—*Oswald:* Beit. u. Geb. u. Gyn., Band vii, H. 1.—*Peterson:* "Inversion of the Uterus," Amer. Gyn., June, 1903.—*Reusch:* Zentb. für Gyn., 1916, p. 35.—*Ries:* Personal communication, July, 1912.— *Rivière:* Bull. de la Soc. d'Obs. et de Gyn., Paris, March, 1927.—*Saxthorph:* Arch. Mens. d'Obst. et de Gyn., February, 1914, p. 211.—*Scholten:* Ergebnisse d. Praktische Geburtsh., 1922, Heft 1. Literature.—*Sehrt:* Zentr. f. Gyn., January, 1920.—*Siegel:* Doederlein's Handb. der Geb., vol. iii, p. 642.—*Sigwart:* Arch. f. Gyn., 1909, vol. l, p. 47.—*Thorn:* "521 Inversions," Volkmann's Samml. klin. Vörträge, 1911, No. 299. Literature.—*Veit:* Prakt. Ergebnisse, 5th year, H. I., p. 87.—*Vogel:* "Inversion," Zeitschr. f. Geb. u. Gyn., 1900, vol. xliii, p. 490.—*Wells:* Therapeutic Gazette, October 15, 1910.—*Zangemeister:* Deutsche med. Woch., April 17, 1913.

CHAPTER LXII

ACCIDENTS TO THE CHILD

IDEAL obstetrics demands that every child not congenitally deformed be delivered alive and absolutely uninjured. This ideal is far from being realized. Statistics show that over 4 per cent. of the children die during birth. Schultze, in 1877, estimated that 5 per cent. of children are still-born, and 1.5 per cent. die very shortly after birth, the result of the trauma of labor (Thomas). Holt, and Babbitt found 4.4 per cent. of still-births in 9747 viable children at Sloane Maternity, New York, and Kerness, 5.2 per cent. at the Munich Frauenklinik. Harries found 2.08 per cent. in the last 35,179 births at the Chicago Lying-in Hospital. Some confusion exists regarding the definition of "still-births." Ballantyne suggests that the term be applied to a child born "still," but with discoverable signs of life, and that "dead-born" be applied to those in whom life is actually extinct. According to Ballantyne some still-born children may be saved. The majority of authors hold still-born and dead-born to be identical, which appears to me the simplest way. A large percentage—how large it is impossible to say—is more or less injured, and this, too, in so-called normal delivery. Any one performing autopsies on new-born children will be struck by the frequency of hemorrhages, punctate and larger, in the brain, in the larger ganglia, along the sinuses and the sutures. It is certain that such extravasations leave scars, perhaps minute, in the cerebral structures, which may explain some cerebral symptoms later in life (Cohen. Lit.).

The greatest danger which besets the child on its way into the world is the interruption of its respiratory function. It often comes in a condition of partial or complete anaërosis. The old and universally used term to express this state is "asphyxia," but this is etymologically incorrect, because it means "without pulse" (from a- σφύξις), and the children are not so at all—the pulse being the last to disappear. Numerous terms have been suggested to take the place of the generally and long-recognized inappropriate "asphyxia," such as dysapnea, euapnea, ecchysis pneumocardia, anhematosis, anoxemia. The one here suggested by the author, anaërosis, from a, privative, αηρ, air, and -osis, the condition of, expresses the state of the child and covers practically all the causes. In the succeeding pages the two terms, anaërosis and asphyxia, and their derivatives, will be used synonymously, or as indicating that the former leads to the latter.

ASPHYXIA NEONATORUM

As pregnancy nears the end the fetus' blood becomes more and more venous, which is due to the gradual narrowing of the ductus Botalli and ductus Arantii. It is generally said that the fetus cannot stand a sudden increase of this venosity as well at term as earlier in pregnancy, but my own experience does not confirm such a statement. From Hippocrates' time a popular notion has prevailed that seventh month babies are more likely to live than those of the eighth month, and probably this idea is founded on the possible greater tolerance of asphyxia by fetuses of the earlier months of pregnancy.

The child exists in a state of apnea, that is, without respiration, because it has enough oxygen for its wants. Observation of the fetus at cesarean sections, and of the foot or arm in the intact bag of waters, shows a slight bluish tint of the skin, which would indicate that there is a slight increase of CO_2 over that of the delivered child. The fetus, therefore, is not in a state of acapnia. During labor the fetus suffers physical and chemical changes which reach an acme at the point of delivery. Since these are controversial I can present only the most plausible theories here. With each pain there is a slight retardation of the maternal blood-current through the placenta, and at the same time a very slight increase of pressure on the fetal head, if the latter has already entered the pelvis. After the bag of waters has ruptured both conditions are more marked, and as the head passes the vulva the greatest change takes place, that is, the head suffers the greatest pressure, the uterus contracts the hardest, forcing the maternal blood out of its meshes, and this may also slacken the flow of fetal blood through the placenta. All these factors have a positive, sometimes marked, influence on the child. In the first stage of labor they usually cause a slight slowing of the fetal pulse. Seitz finds the opposite—a slight increase of rapidity. In the second stage the slowing is the rule, and at the very end it is invariable, a fact easily proved by listening with the head stethoscope or feeling the cord directly after birth.

There is an increase of the fetal blood-pressure during the pains but only after the membranes are ruptured (Guttner). Although Haselhorst found that the O and CO_2 content of the cord blood changed little from the beginning to the end of labor there can be little doubt that the blood in the brain is markedly venous in the second stage of labor. One can see this on the baby's face. Whether there is a fetal acidosis or whether the child's blood reacts to the changes in the mother's as described by Siedentopf, remains to be learned. One can safely assume that the blood in the brain under higher arterial pressure and obstructed venous return is both deoxygenated and hypercarbonated, but whether the one or the other causes the slowing of the heart via the vagus center is unsettled. Rech says neither. That cerebral compression acting on this center slows the heart seems proved as is also that prolonged anoxemia and increasing CO_2 depress and finally paralyze the cardiac mechanism.

The accumulation of CO_2 stimulates the respiratory center and elicits spasmodic contraction of the muscles of respiration. The fetus gasps, and whatever lies near its mouth is sucked into the lungs—liquor amnii, vernix caseosa, meconium, blood, vaginal mucus, feces, etc. This inspiration also dilates the capillaries of the lungs, and unless there is something in the alveoli (air) to exert counterpressure, some of the capillaries may burst. As a fact, smaller and larger hemorrhages in the lungs and pleuræ are the rule in cases of asphyxiation. If the loss of oxygen and increase of CO_2 are very slow, the respiratory center may be benumbed and the fetus may die without having made any attempt at respiration. These cases offer a bad prognosis, even if the child is delivered with the heart still beating. The continued stimulation of the vagus center results finally in its paralysis, its inhibitory action is gone, the pulse jumps to 180 to 200 or more. Sometimes the fetal heart becomes irregular, both as to rhythm and quality of the beats. In other cases of threatened intra-uterine asphyxia the fetal heart-tones are very rapid from the start—180 to 210. It is possible that such frequencies are preceded by slowing of the pulse, though in several cases in which the heart-tones were carefully noted the latter was not observed. It is hard to explain the primary acceleration of the pulse, though perhaps cerebral compression may do it (Schröder). Why compression of the brain should slow the heart in one instance and hurry it in another is not understood. Direct irritation of the cortex can stimulate the cardiac and respiratory centers, and peripheral irritants may act likewise. It is possible that some of the irregular phenomena observed during labor may be explained in this way.

Etiology.—Death of the fetus *during pregnancy* may be due to a great variety of causes, though interference with the function of respiration is found in the last analysis of nearly all of them. All the acute infectious diseases, especially if combined with high fever; chronic infections, syphilis, tuberculosis; poisoning by eclamptic, uremic, or other toxemic poisons, by chemicals, morphin, phosphorus, etc., asphyxia and anemia of the mother; injuries to the fetus by stab or blow, congenital deformities; diseases of the fetus itself, as infection, leukemia, sarcomatosis, Buhl's disease, heart and abdominal affections; all these and more like them may be found. Sudden nervous shock to the mother may kill the child in a manner not yet explained.

During labor the causes of fetal anaërosis may be divided into two classes: (1) Those which directly cut off the supply of oxygen (suffocative), (2) those which cause compression of the brain (paralytic).

1. *Those Cutting Off Oxygen Supply—Suffocative Asphyxia.*—(a) Prolonged and hard labor pains, recurring so frequently that the blood in the placental sinuses cannot be renewed, are the most common factor. This is observed at the end of the second stage, with rigid pelvic floor, in contracted pelvis, with tetanus uteri, and, but rarely nowadays, with the use of ergot. Pituitrin occasionally acts this way. The general mortality of the children in protracted labor increases in proportion to the length of labor; (b) excessive retraction of the uterus away from the child, with diminution of the placental area, and perhaps with some partial separation of the placenta, for example, neglected shoulder presentation, threatened ruptura uteri; (c) compression of the placenta when it is low in the uterus, or of the insertion of the cord, either by the head or trunk, or sometimes by the colpeurynter; or compression of the placenta by the head when the child presents by its breech; (d) compression of the umbilical cord, either with prolapse of same or while it still lies in the uterus; coiling of cord around the neck of the child may cause anaërosis, and here, too, it is especially exposed to injurious pressure from the tip of the forceps blade; knots, rupture, hematoma of the cord; (e) partial and complete abruption of the placenta, either normally or abnormally implanted, in either head or breech presentations; (f) anemia of the child from rupture of the placental vessels (placenta prævia) or tearing of a velamentous vessel; (g) narcosis (morphin), asphyxia, anemia of the mother, the child dying first, since it gives back oxygen to its mother.

During the first few minutes after birth the child may be asphyxiated by its air-passages being blocked. A tight caul; the aspiration of vaginal mucus, blood, meconium, or the mucus which often lies in the child's own glottis and is drawn down by the first breath; edema of the glottis and throat consecutive to face presentation; congenital atelectasis (syphilis, etc.); heart and other diseases; gross and microscopic deformities—all these have been found more or less often.

2. *Compression of the brain* brings about asphyxia in several ways, depending partly on the manner of compression, whether internal or external. This is *paralytic asphyxia.* Internal compression from hemorrhage or fracture, as well as external pressure from a contracted pelvis or a rigid perineum, may slow the pulse and cause anaërosis, because the blood is hindered from reaching the placenta. Internal local compression of the cardiac and respiratory centers may cause asphyxia by directly paralyzing the vagus or stimulating respiratory action. The slowing of the heart from cerebral compression can be easily demonstrated during forceps operations if the accoucheur will but listen while he closes the blades of the instrument. In some cases the effect is not immediate, but it is always present if the pressure is kept up a few seconds or if it is made quite strong. Sudden and marked slowing of the beat is proof that the cord has been caught in the grasp of the blades. It is probable that in cases of cerebral compression without hemorrhage there is also an additional external cause which reduces the amount of oxygen in the fetal blood which may be found under Class 1.

Finally may be mentioned the premature respirations made by the child, the result of external stimuli, version, forceps, pulling on the leg in breech extraction, and the presence of air in the uterus. Compression of the vessels in the neck (face presentation, coiling of the cord) produces a local venous congestion of the brain.

Pathology.—Postmortem findings vary, of course, with the cause and the rapidity of the asphyxia. In general one finds the effects of an intense venous congestion combined with that of localized spasm of the arterioles. The auricles of the heart, the pulmonary system, the liver, and the spleen are engorged with blood. The back pressure in the veins of the lungs, pleuræ, pericardium, peritoneum, brain, kidneys, and suprarenals causes extravasations of blood, varying in size from a pinhead to one inch, and, particularly in the brain, immense hematomata may form. Minute hemorrhages in the retina, the ear, and in the ganglia at the base of the brain may cause serious disturbance of function if the child withstands the primary asphyxia. Serosanguineous transudations may be found in the pericardium, pleuræ, peritoneum, and in the brain; also edema cerebri. If respiratory movements had been made, liquor amnii, meconium, blood, etc., may be found in the lungs, parts of which are atelectatic and parts full of air. Seitz emphasizes the importance and frequency of edema of the prevesical connective tissue around the hypogastric arteries, and edema of the genitals, particularly of the scrotum. Edema of the vulva and scrotum is not rarely observed after natural labors, and Seitz says it is likewise due to asphyxia. When the umbilical cord is compressed, the back pressure is felt first in the vein and then in the arteries near the navel. I have seen 3 cases of "traumatic asphyxia" in the newborn. The condition is identical with that occurring in the adult from crushing of the thorax (Heuer, Lit.).

Symptoms and Diagnosis.—*Before Delivery of the Child.*—1. The most important, because the most reliable, external evidence of danger besetting the child in utero is a change in the fetal heart-sounds. These may be altered as to frequency, regularity, strength, and rhythm. A persistent slowing of the fetal heart to 100 beats a minute is always significant of danger, and if, during the uterine contraction, the rate goes down to 80 or less, there is no doubt about it, and delivery is demanded forthwith. As the rate sinks from the usual 140–136 to 124–112, then to 112–100, the two rates given as those between and during the pains, respectively, the accoucheur becomes more and more certain that there is some factor causing a stimulation of the vagus. At the same time the tone becomes stronger, and occasionally a little accentuation of the second sound may be distinguished. Primarily increased rapidity of the heart-tones is not so good a sign, but if the heart-tones are continuously above 175 (Winckel says 160), without fever of the mother, danger to the life of the child may be apprehended. The sudden change from slowed heart-tones to excessive rapidity denotes paralysis of the vagus center and is of very bad omen. As a rule, at this time the respiratory center awakens and elicits inspirations. Irregularity of the fetal heart is also significant. A few strong beats are followed by a run of light, short taps, and sometimes the heart may run and stumble along in a most erratic manner. This irregularity is very ominous if it follows a period of slowed action. Sometimes the rate of the heart will run from 140 to 170 without definable cause and without relation to the uterine contractions. In one otherwise normal case I counted 240 beats per minute. It is wise to distrust such cases. The strength of the tone gives additional information, a slow, strong sound indicating vagus stimulation, a rapid, weak one, paralysis or general fetal weakness. If the first sound of the heart is booming, a healthy muscle may be diagnosed; if it is weak and valvular, gallop-rhythmus being present, danger exists. In general, the above findings are positive of threatening danger, but in rare instances most of them may be present and the child is born alive and well, while still more rarely the heart may show no evidences of distress and yet the infant is still-born or asphyctic. Cerebral hemorrhage may sometimes do this. Other signs of intra-uterine anaërosis will aid the accoucheur here, but he will not be much amiss if he interferes in the labor on the indication given by a study of the fetal heart-tones. (See Sachs.)

(2) The passage of liquor amnii stained with fresh meconium is a valuable sign of impending intra-uterine asphyxia. It was the only one the ancients had. The sign is of no value if the presentation is a breech, unless the latter has not neared the inlet. The passage of meconium is due to an active peristalsis set up by the anaë-rotic blood, and finds its analogy in the bowel movements of drowned or otherwise asphyxiated persons. It is true that the use of quinin will cause the discharge of meconium, and that in a certain percentage of natural deliveries meconium will come away in the liquor amnii and the child will show no evidences of distress when born. My experience and Rossa's agree, that the character of the labor in these cases was such that anaërosis would be very likely to occur. While I am willing to agree that the sign does not have the absolute significance that some writers ascribe to it (Küstner), I am inclined to give it more value than does Seitz in his monograph.

Liquor amnii stained with old meconium is olive-green in color and the meconium is thoroughly mixed with it. Fresh meconium is dark sea-green and is lumpy. If such a mixture is expelled, the accoucheur should study the fetal heart-tones and the nature of the labor, and if any cause for anaërosis or any irregularity of the heart-tones is discovered, the sign becomes of positive value. In obstructed labors the passage of meconium may long precede the slowing of the heart.

If the asphyxia is fairly well established, the child makes respiratory movements and these may be seen, felt, or heard by the attendant. (3) During breech deliveries one may see and feel the diaphragm come down; during forceps operations it is often possible to feel and see the gasps of the child as jerks of the forceps or as a jarring of the lower abdomen. It may be impossible to distinguish these jerky gasps from fetal hiccup. The fetal heart-tones, the nature of the labor, and the meconium must aid in the differentiation. Unless the child can be extracted within a few minutes after it gasps it is lost, and even if delivered alive, it will very likely die within a few days from atelectasis pulmonum or cerebral hemorrhage.

Vagitus Uterinus.—This term has been applied to the crying of the child in utero—before it is born. Many authentic cases are on record. It is said that Mahomet and St. Bartholomew made themselves heard while in the uterus, but these probably are fables. If air is introduced into the uterine cavity alongside the hand, as in version, or with instruments, or by a simple examination, or if gases develop there, the child may inspire, and on expiration may produce a cry. Sometimes this may occur without evidences of dyspnea, and the child may be delivered in good condition, sometimes hours or days afterward. In Kristeller's case the child cried eight different times when the forceps were closed on its head. If the heart-tones show the least indication of trouble delivery is to be effected at once (Fuchs, Lit.). From a medicolegal point of view the cases of vagitus uterinus are very important, since the lungs may be partly inflated and the child die before birth. Finding air in the child's lungs would be no evidence against the individual accused of infanticide. Reidy reports 3 cases (v. Klein).

Other signs of threatening intra-uterine asphyxia are: (4) Very active fetal movements, felt by the mother or by the attendant, a phenomenon which occurs especially if the anaërosis is sudden, and may indicate a death-struggle or attempts to respire; (5) the persistence of a loud umbilical souffle; (6) the loss of tonus of the anus in breech cases; (7) the weakening and disappearance of the pulse in a foot or hand which may be brought down, or from the cord, which may have prolapsed. In many cases I have passed the hand into the uterus to feel the heart. (8) Pulsation of the fontanel is not discoverable, but in one case I could feel the child's heart through the thin abdominal wall.

After Delivery.—Cazeaux defined two degrees of asphyxia in the new-born child—*asphyxia livida* and *asphyxia pallida*. The symptoms, of course, depend on the degree of the anaërosis, and between the two states mentioned there are many gradations.

In asphyxia livida the child is dark blue, sometimes purplish and mottled, the face swollen and congested, the eyes somewhat prominent, and the conjunctivæ injected; the skin around the nose and mouth may be slightly pale, but the lips are deep blue. Tonus of the muscles is not lost; the arms are held up; the body is fairly rigid; the mouth closes on the finger; the throat reacts. If the face is blown upon or wet with cold water, the muscles twitch. The heart and cord pulsate slowly and strongly; there is an occasional gasp, accompanied by a gurgling sound, the mouth and bronchi being full of mucus. These are the mild cases, and they respond quickly to treatment.

In asphyxia pallida an entirely different aspect is presented. The child is pale and waxy, but the lips alone are blue. The body is limp, the extremities hang-

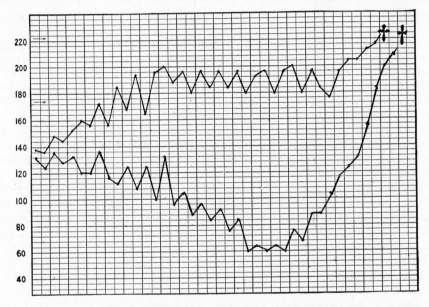

<small>Fig. 727.—Tracings of the Two Types of Heart-tones in Asphyxia in Utero. Lower Curve the Usual Type.</small>

ing down without any tonus at all; the jaw drops relaxed—the throat does not react. There are no respiratory movements, or a rare gasp which is very superficial and may be simply a movement of the jaw. The only evidence of life is a weak and slow, or perhaps very rapid, heart-beat. This may not be palpable, but will be audible with the stethoscope. The cord is limp and collapsed; the baby looks like a corpse. The criteria of this severe form of asphyxia are the absence of muscular tonus and the loss of reflex excitability. This condition is of much worse prognosis, and even if the infant is revived, it may die later of secondary asphyxia. The lung is not fully inflated; areas of atelectasis exist which offer great resistance to the flow of blood. The heart soon fails. Hypercarbonization and deoxidation of the blood cause acidosis. This and the anoxemia affect the nerve centers and the child sinks into coma, rarely there are convulsions. The respiration, which never was adequate and was attended by a grunt or whine, becomes more and more superficial and rapid, finally ceasing. The heart continues to act for a while through its own automaticity, but soon this disappears. At the autopsy hypostatic edema is determined in addition to the other findings.

Diagnosis.—Not all children that are born in an apparently moribund state are asphyxiated. Other conditions are pressure on the brain, anemia, apnea, and morphin-poisoning. Brain compression may be both the cause and the result of asphyxia. We have seen how it can cause asphyxia. In cases of asphyxia there are great cerebral congestion and sometimes spasm of the arterioles. The thin-walled vessels of the brain may burst, causing hemorrhage, which may be subdural, subarachnoid, or intraventricular. This in turn causes anaërosis.

The diagnosis of cerebral compression is not easy, and the character of the labor must be the guide, e. g., a hard forceps or extraction, in which it is known that injuries to the skull have been made. Focal symptoms are usually absent in the very early stages. In some cases of cerebral hemorrhage it is possible to keep the heart going for many hours with artificial respiration, but the infant cannot be made to breathe. The treatment must be like that of asphyxia. An anemic fetus resembles one with pale asphyxia, and the diagnosis may be made only if it is known that the infant suffered a loss of blood, as from tearing of the placenta when it is prævia, or rupture of a velamentous vessel.

An apneic or oligopneic child is often called an anaërotic one, and frantic efforts are made to get it to breathe when only a few minutes' patient waiting is all that is required. Such an occurrence is frequent at cesarean section. In apnea the child looks natural, the lips are slightly cyanotic, the features are not distorted, the color is light grayish blue, the heart-beat is strong and not much slowed at first. Gradually the cyanosis deepens, the pulse slows, the child becomes anaërotic, which stimulates the respiratory center or prepares the center for the reception of the stimulus from the outside air, and the first gasp occurs, or a sneeze which removes the mucus from the air-passages. A few tiny respirations precede the gasp, and a vigorous cry follows it.

Morphin-poisoning is not rare under the use of scopolamin-morphin anesthesia and when the latter drug is given in eclampsia. The child is very quiet and limp, cyanotic, the pupils contracted, the conjunctivæ insensible, but the heart-beat is usually strong, regular, and not very slow, unless, in addition, the infant is asphyxiated. If spanked, the child opens its eyes or grimaces with pain, but does not cry nor breathe. Usually there is no mucus in the air-passages. Resuscitation is at first successful: the child may be brought to cry or even to open its eyes, but it soon relaxes into somnolence and coma. I kept such an infant alive for six hours until the heart gave out. Lung and heart diseases cause asphyxia.

Prognosis.—It is naturally impossible to form a true estimate of the frequency and of the mortality of asphyxia neonatorum, since there is no standard by which the severity of such cases may be measured. In general it may be said that the milder and shorter the asphyxia is, the better the chances of immediate and permanent recovery are, and the severer and more prolonged it is, the more dark the prognosis. It has been found that many children die from the effects of asphyxia as late as the fourteenth day, though the greatest secondary mortality occurs within forty-eight hours. Children that have been for a long time in a state of partial anaërosis in utero,—two to six hours,—even though delivered alive, often die immediately or shortly after birth. This fact must be taken into consideration when selecting obstetric operations. Children on whom efforts of resuscitation had to be prolonged to bring them back to life also die in large numbers within a few hours or days, simply because the asphyxia was very deep and fatally damaged vital structures.

Asphyxiated children are more liable to infection, to bronchopneumonia, intestinal inflammation, melæna neonatorum, icterus, hemorrhage into the parathyroids, with spasmophilia (Graham), meningitis, acute and chronic atelectasis pulmonum, and they often suffer from the effects of the anaërosis—cerebral and other hemorrhages, as well as from the injuries which sometimes are inflicted on them with too violent methods of resuscitation. These are bruises, burns, fracture of the ribs and sternum, blowing foreign matter into the lungs, rupture of viscera, etc.

Boys die from asphyxia in a greater number than girls, because they are larger and harder, causing dystocia more often. Children of primiparæ suffer from it oftener than those of multiparæ. Rigid pelvic floor causes a high infant mortality. Asphyxia, directly due to operative deliveries, and also the shock to the fetus attending the same, must always be considered. Of great interest and importance is the well-established fact that children that were asphyxiated or brain-injured during birth often suffer from severe psychic and nervous diseases later in life. Prolonged labor and operative deliveries with asphyxia, combined or singly, produce the untoward results—for example, spastic cerebral and spinal paralysis, porencephalus with idiocy, syringomyelia, congenital athetosis, chorea, epilepsy, backwardness, stuttering, and, the author would like to add, retinal atrophy, strabismus,

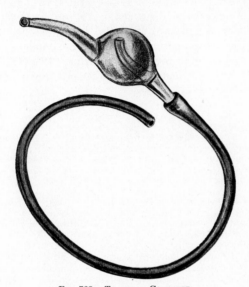

FIG. 728.—TRACHEAL CATHETER.

This is a woven catheter, open at the end, size 14 or 15, French scale. For premature infants, size 10 or 11 is used. These catheters may not be boiled, but are sterilized chemically or in formaldehyd vapor.

and mental aberration. Yet, N. B., all these conditions have frequently been found in children after easy natural deliveries. Jacobi and Kerley also emphasize the injurious effects of asphyxia. We know that in adults concussion of the brain is often followed by weakness of memory, lack of concentration, easy fatigue, emotionalism, susceptibility to alcohol, traumatic neuroses, etc., and it is not illogic to assume that the tender brain of the newborn, in the formative state, could be similarly affected by the concussion of a violent delivery. On the other hand, even the severest cerebral compression and prolonged asphyxia may leave no traces discoverable in after life. Beach, in 810 idiots, found a history of hard forceps in 4 per cent., and in 26.6 per cent. spontaneous but difficult labor. Porter states that 17 per cent. of the epileptics in the Indiana School for Feeble-minded had a history of difficult labors. Dayton, using the Massachusetts psychiatric examination in 20,473 cases, demonstrated a relationship between abnormal labor and physical and emotional states. (See Stein, Hannes, Meyer, and Sharpe.)

Treatment Before Birth.—The prevention of asphyxia of the child *in utero* comprises the recognition of the causes, and a studied avoidance of them, which means, in short, that the accoucheur should direct the course of labor into normal channels and interfere only when really necessary. In every labor, and especially if it is foreseen that the child may be anaërotic, preparations for treatment must be made. A suitable table or a place on the bed is arranged, with a supply of warm towels, a hot-water bag, and two tracheal catheters (Fig. 728). These are No. 14 and No. 15 (Fr.) linen catheters. They may not be boiled, but are thoroughly washed inside and out after using, then immersed in 1 : 1000 bichlorid, flushed with alcohol, and dried. In maternities they may be sterilized in a tall jar in formaldehyd gas. No obstetric satchel is complete without tracheal catheters. The glass bulb shown in the illustration is a saliva trap, and at the same time prevents mucus, meconium, etc., from being drawn into the operator's mouth.

At an interval of a half-hour or oftener in the first stage, and at least five to two minutes in the second stage, or even every half-minute if the delivery is laborious, the fetal heart-tones should be auscultated, which is rendered easy by the head stethoscope shown on page 283. At the first sign of fetal distress redoubled watchfulness is practised, the fetal heart listened to almost continuously, and preparations for operative delivery are made.

As soon as the fact of fetal danger is established, two courses of treatment are indicated—either the cause of the anaërosis must be removed or the child be gotten out where it can get air.

The most common causes of asphyxia in utero are: interference with the circulation in the cord, tumultuous pains preventing the change of blood in the uterus, and abruptio placentæ. Occult prolapse of the cord is usually the first thought when the fetal heart shows signs of agitation, and an attempt may be made to relieve it from the supposed pressure. If the cord is palpable above the pubis one may stroke it upward. Change of position—the parturient turning on either side, or adopting alternately the Sims, Trendelenburg, or knee-chest posture—often helps by relieving the funis of tension or compression. (See Treatment of Prolapsus Funis, page 683.)

Tumultuous pains are calmed by ether, which may be kept up for an hour or more. If a diagnosis of abruptio placentæ with a living child is made, cesarean section is indicated.

Rapid delivery offers the best hope, but it may not always be possible, and, further, often the operative trauma itself kills the infant. Delicate questions are here involved, and the principle of *primum non nocere* should not be violated. Broadly speaking, in cases of threatened asphyxia *in utero* the child should be delivered as soon as possible, having due regard—(1) To the state of the child and the probability of its being gotten out alive and of living afterward; (2) to the amount of injury which the interference will inflict on the mother; and (3) to the actual danger to her life which it will incur.

If the distress of the child is discovered when the cervix is fully opened, immediate delivery is performed, by forceps if the head is engaged, by version and consecutive extraction if it is not. If the cervix is effaced but only partly dilated, a bag may be put in and the needful enlargement thus obtained or Dührssen's incisions may be made and extraction performed at once. Only a skilful obstetric surgeon may attempt the latter procedure. If the cervix is uneffaced two courses are open—bag dilatation and cesarean section. Usually the conditions are such that the former must be chosen, and the results are much better than one would expect. The bag displaces the head (relieving a possible compression of the cord), stimulates the pains, and opens the cervix. In cases where the life of the child possesses a higher evaluation than usual, *e. g.*, in an aged primipara, or where some adjuvant factor exists, such as contracted pelvis, rigid cervix, heart disease, etc., the abdominal delivery may be selected—here, preferably, laparotrachelotomy.

Treatment After Delivery.—When a child is born apparently dead it is of instant importance to determine if the asphyxia is mild or severe, because in the last condition no time may be wasted on inefficient measures, while in the former the simplest remedies are usually successful. The heart-beat, the presence of reaction in the skin and throat, and the degree of body tone will enable a quick diagnosis. Three grand principles govern the treatment: (1) Clear the air-passages from obstructions; (2) maintain body heat; (3) supply oxygen to the blood.

The importance of keeping the baby warm is not generally appreciated. The infant is wet; exposure is often prolonged; evaporation is rapid; the body temper-

ature sinks rapidly. This is very depressing, and the *shock* of delivery is thus augmented—indeed, it has occasionally happened that the infant, wrapped up and put away as dead, has recovered through the influence of warmth alone. Therefore the baby should be received in warm towels, and kept covered as much
as possible during the subsequent manipulations. Some of these may be carried out while the child is in a warm bath.

The first duty is to clear the air-passages. It is dangerous to perform artificial respiration when the trachea, bronchi, and sometimes the alveoli are full of amniotic fluid, meconium, blood, or vaginal secretions. These must be removed before any attempt is made to bring air into the lungs, otherwise the foreign substances would be forced still further down and give rise to atelectasis, pneumonia, and sepsis.

During the delivery, as soon as the child's nose and mouth appear, they are wiped with pledgets of lintine or soft linen. In breech labors one of the fingers introduced for the performance of the Veit-Smellie manœuver should block the glottis to prevent the gasping infant from aspirating

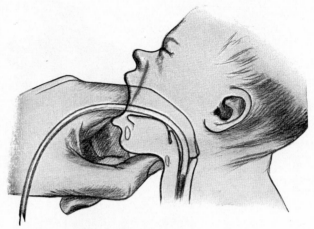

Fig. 729.—Introducing the Tracheal Catheter.

The index-finger of the left hand pulls the epiglottis forward and comes to touch the arytenoid cartilages. At the same time the catheter is passed along this finger until it lies over the rima, just behind the epiglottis. Now the inside index-finger pulls the very tip of the catheter sharply forward, while the right hand, giving the tube a slight twisting motion, pushes it down into the trachea. The lips are applied to the glass mouth-piece, and a light suck draws the contents of the trachea into the catheter, which is then removed and its contents forcibly blown out on a towel for inspection. Sometimes the sucking on the catheter is continued as it is withdrawn to clear the whole tract. It may be necessary to repeat this procedure several times. It is wise also to compress the chest between the thumb and four fingers to force the material out of the smaller bronchi, to gain the advantages claimed for Schultze's swingings. By pushing the catheter deeply into the chest and turning the head and neck of the child sharply to either side, the right and then the left bronchus may be emptied.

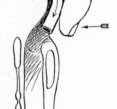

mucus, blood, etc. In head labors, after delivery of the head, while clearing the pharynx, two fingers gently strip the neck toward the jaw in an effort thus to bring inspired matter into the throat. *It is important to clear the uppermost air-passages before the child makes the first gasp.* In the mildest cases this is all that is required, because the irritation of the throat excites cough and respiration. When the child is fully delivered, it is held up by the ankles, while the head rests on some flat surface, and in this position the throat is cleared.

In the more severe cases—real asphyxia livida—the child usually has drawn foreign matter deeply into the lungs, and this must be removed—best, in my experience, by means of the tracheal catheter (Fig. 729). With a little practice the use of this instrument becomes easy. This method was recommended by Scheel in 1780.

When the air-passages are free, it is time for external stimulation. As a rule, the catheterization of the trachea has stimulated the respiratory center, and respiratory movements, in the form of gasps, usually follow this operation. If the reaction is too slow, the buttocks may be spanked, the back rubbed vigorously, or gentle traction made on the tongue (Laborde, 1892). Grasping the tongue between the thumb and index-finger, it is gently drawn out and let go back 30 to 40 times a minute.

Among the host of external irritants employed for this purpose may be mentioned the hot bath, with or without mustard, wine, etc., the hot and cold plunge, cold bath, tickling the nares,

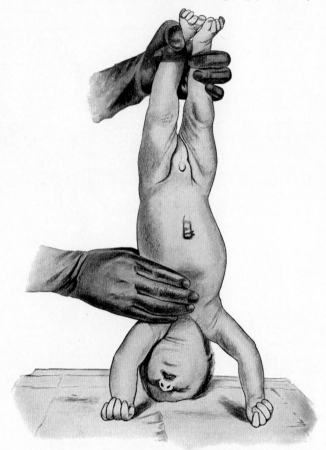

FIG. 730.—PROCHOWNICK'S METHOD OF RESUSCITATION.

The child is suspended by the feet, the forehead resting lightly on the table so as to deflex the chin and straighten out the trachea. The body is gently shaken, and the chest compressed between the thumb and four fingers so as to squeeze out foreign matter from the bronchi. Now an assistant wipes out the throat, and the pressure on the chest is suddenly relaxed. Air may be heard rushing in. The compression and sudden release may be repeated 16 to 20 times a minute. This method gives even better results if the tracheal catheter is in place.

snuff, dilatation of the sphincter ani, hypodermic injections, adrenalin, electricity, etc. The warm bath may not be prolonged over five minutes. A better method is to wrap the infant in warm towels and lay it on a warm-water bag. The alternating cold and hot plunges are distinctly shocking to the tender infant and, in my opinion, dangerous, as well as unnecessary.

Where the respiratory center is still responsive, no more need usually be done —indeed, more may be harmful. The accoucheur simply keeps the infant covered. If the child is improving, the gasps recur with increasing frequency, or tiny respiratory motions of the chest become visible and the heart impulse grows stronger and regular. Soon the gasps become double, and end with a long inspiration, expiration being attended by a light moan. Now, between the gasps, the tiny respiratory movements of the chest become more pronounced, while at the same time the cyanosis begins to lighten and give way to redness, soon after which the child gives a lusty cry. It is best to leave the infant alone as long as it improves,

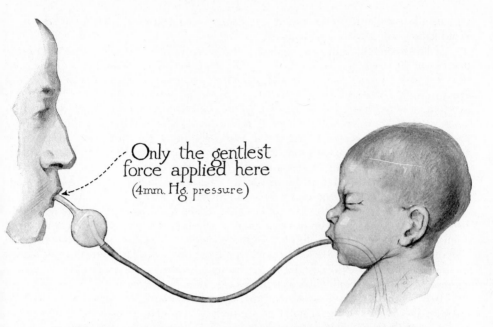

FIG. 731.—MOUTH-TO-LUNG INSUFFLATION WITH THE TRACHEAL CATHETER (Elisha-Smellie).

After inserting the catheter, as was done for the removal of mucus, the operator fills his lungs and *mouth* with fresh air, then applies his lips to the mouth-piece, *with his glottis closed*, and simply, under the gentle action of the cheeks (like a glass-blower), forces pure warm air into the child's lungs. Only as much as can be held in the mouth may be forced in. Compression of the chest causes the air to escape, and this procedure may be repeated fifteen times a minute. Use very little pressure, not more than 4 mm. Hg. Chaussier, in June, 1806, recommended oxygen for this purpose. Henderson says oxygen with 5 per cent. CO_2 is better, but Eastman prefers oxygen or air.

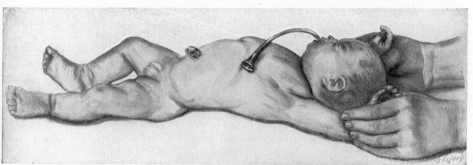

FIG. 732.—SYLVESTER'S METHOD OF RESUSCITATION, WITH THE TRACHEAL CATHETER. INSPIRATION.
The child is kept covered with a warm receiver and the catheter held in position by means of a safety-pin.

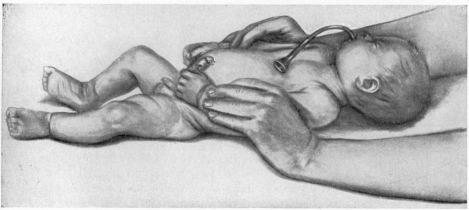

FIG. 732a.—SYLVESTER'S METHOD OF RESUSCITATION. EXPIRATION.

and in all cases precipitate and frantic haste with trials of different methods in rapid succession is to be condemned.

If improvement is not immediate, and if, from the start, the case impresses one as one of asphyxia pallida, this simple treatment does not suffice. Time may not be wasted trying the various skin reflexes, but two serious purposes must be accomplished—first, oxygen is to be got into the fetus' blood by artificial respiration; second, the circulation, which is almost in abeyance, must be started again. Of the numerous methods of resuscitation the author has found the following safe and successful: rhythmic compression of the heart and lungs with the child in inverted suspension, with and without the tracheal catheter in place (Fig. 730); mouth-to-lung sufflation with the tracheal catheter (Fig. 731), and the application of heat and general massage. The once famous Schultze swingings are declassé. They are too dangerous and are unnecessary.

Authorities are divided as to the value of tracheal insufflation. It is said to be dangerous because of the possible production of emphysema and pneumothorax from rupture of the alveoli, and it requires considerable skill in intubation to avoid making a false passage. Bichat proved that it is possible to blow air into the vessels of the heart and general circulation if too much force is used. Performed gently as here described, I believe these dangers can be avoided.

In a few cases I have successfully stimulated the heart by rapid vibratory percussion, and to hasten the circulation through it have compressed the heart against the chest wall from below, through the relaxed abdominal wall, a sort of cardiac massage. Adrenalin, 7 ♍ of a 1 : 10,000 solution, i. e., 0.06 to 0.05 mg. may be injected into the umbilical vein or even the heart (Hoffmann). If the child is anemic from blood loss, salt solution or blood may be supplied.

My routine practice in cases of *asphyxia pallida* is as follows: As soon as the child is delivered it is laid on a sterile platter, which lies on the lap; the air-passages are cleared by the catheter; the cord is tied and cut; the chest is gently, rhythmically, compressed for thirty seconds, during which time the cardiac pulsations and any respiratory action are determined; the tracheal catheter is inserted, and the lungs are filled with air systematically for two or three minutes, either by squeezing and relaxing the chest or by blowing with the mouth, the child being well wrapped up; the tracheal catheter is removed, cleared, and again inserted; the infant is placed on a hot-water bag, the operator arranges things conveniently and keeps up artificial breathing until the child recovers or its condition shows that further effort is useless. Several instruments—the lungmotor, the pulmotor—have been recommended for artificial respiration (Engelman). No instrument can surpass in efficiency and safety the simple tracheal catheter. A valuable addition to our remedies is lobelin—a small ampule into the deltoid or if possible into the umbilical vein, in one-half dose, repeated in fifteen minutes if needed. Its action is sometimes dramatic.

How long to keep up efforts at revival depends on the case. Usually an hour suffices to show if there is any hope at all of saving the infant, and the remedial measures should be kept up for two or even three hours if the heart beats. Smith has shown with the electrocardiograph that the heart activity may continue for three hours after apparent still-birth. Cases are on record of recovery after two, three, and even four hours' effort. With a cerebral hemorrhage or a fracture at the base, the heart may beat as long as the blood is kept supplied with oxygen. In one such case I kept up mouth-to-lung insufflation for nine hours steadily, the heart beating strongly and the child's color being good until I stopped, when the circulation gradually ceased, there not having been a single gasp to reward the prolonged effort.

After-treatment.—Asphyxiated and premature children and children delivered by severe operative procedures should always be watched for the first hours and days after labor. Not seldom they develop, in a few minutes to a few hours, a secondary asphyxia. This is due, usually, to atelectasis pulmonum, but the author has reason to believe that there is some pulmonary circulatory trouble in addition, and occasionally the x-ray discloses a large thymus. In other cases a small hemorrhage occurs in the medulla. The child may be found dead in its crib, or it may turn pale, cyanotic, with a reddish line at the skin margin on the lips; it whines or grunts at each expiration; soon it becomes unconscious, will not cry on being hurt, and dies under a slow asphyxia. These children are also more subject to icterus, to hemorrhagic disease, melena, to sepsis, especially the bronchial and intestinal forms, and if they grow up are not likely to be so strong as other children—chronic atelectasis. The treatment of secondary asphyxia with atelectasis is not at all satisfying. I have tried all known methods of distending the lungs and have failed. The lung is solid with exudate or pneumonia (F. J. Browne). Often cerebral hemorrhage is the cause of the secondary asphyxia. Attacks of syncope are treated with the warm bath, the incubator, oxygen insufflation, the oxygen tent and artificial respiration.

INJURIES TO THE CHILD IN BIRTH

Manifestly, it is impossible to consider all the injuries which the infant may suffer during birth. Only a few of the most common and most important will be described, and as many of the others as possible named. A glance at the list will show the reader what a gantlet of perils the infant runs on its way into the world. Since a great many of them are preventable, the list will also show what a heavy responsibility rests on the shoulders of the modern accoucheur.

The Head.—Caput succedaneum, the soft, boggy tumor which forms on the presenting part in prolonged labor, was discussed on p. 154. It must be distinguished from cephalhematoma, which is a hemorrhage under the periosteum of the skull (Fig. 733). Cephalhematomata are always due to injury, which may be made by the accoucheur in forceps or breech extraction, especially in cases of spacial disproportion, or by the natural forces, even during delivery over a tight perineum. I have seen 4 cases after spontaneous breech deliveries. Fissure of the bones, that is, linear fractures, often accompany the blood extravasation. They may be single or multiple, are always limited by the sutures (unless the latter are ossified), and are absorbed in from two weeks to three months, depending on their size. At the edge, where the periosteum is lifted up, a ridge of bone develops, and this requires still longer time to disappear. Bone salts are sometimes deposited in the elevated periosteum. The diagnosis is easy; there is a soft, non-pulsating, fluctuating, elastic tumor over one of the flat cranial bones. In the differential diagnosis caput succedaneum, hernia cerebri, and neoplasm are to be considered.

CAPUT SUCCEDANEUM.	CEPHALHEMATOMA.
1. Is present at birth.	1. May not appear for a few hours or days after birth.
2. Soft, boggy, and pits on pressure.	2. Soft, elastic, no pitting.
3. Not well circumscribed.	3. Sharply circumscribed, and with a distinct, sometimes hard, edge.
4. Dark red, mottled, sometimes purple and ecchymotic.	4. Unless under a caput, normal skin.
5. Lies over sutures.	5. Limited by sutures to individual bones.
6. Movable on skull and seeks dependent portions.	6. Fixed to site originally taken.
7. Is largest at birth and grows smaller, disappearing in a few hours.	7. Appears after a few hours, grows larger for a time, and disappears only after weeks or months.

In hernia cerebri the location of the tumor, the more or less marked pedunculation, the translucency, the impulse when the child cries, the meningeal symptoms, will make the diagnosis easy.

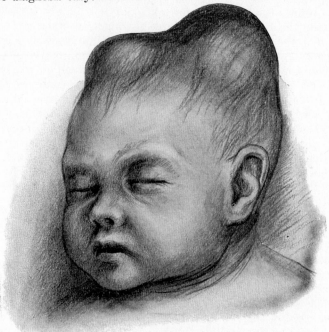

FIG. 733.—DOUBLE CEPHALHEMATOMA.
This followed a spontaneous and relatively easy delivery.

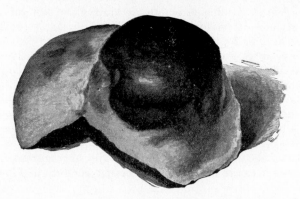

FIG. 733a.—CEPHALHEMATOMA (from the collection of Dr. W. W. Jaggard).

Direct injuries to the scalp; cutting by forceps; pressure necrosis from contracted pelves and exostoses; punctures and tears with instruments under the mistaken idea that the scalp was the membranes; tearing off of an ear, crushing of the nose (later deflected septum and ethmoid troubles); subcutaneous hematomata in the cheeks and neck from forceps; fracture and dislocation of the jaw (breech extractions); tearing off of an eyelid; complete enucleation of the eyeball; conjunctival hemorrhages, corneal opacities—all these I have seen either in my own or in consultation practice. Wolff and Paul have found retinal hemorrhages and detachment in a large percentage of normal labors, and almost always after operative delivery with more or less asphyxia. Fracture of the orbital plates; hemorrhages into the chambers of the eye and around the eye (exophthalmos), in the optic nerve; dislocation of the lens; paralysis of the eye muscles (from intracranial as well as extracranial trauma); congestion of the optic nerve vessels and secondary atrophy of the bulb—have all been reported, and should lead to care in operations (Wolff, Lequeux). Similar hemorrhages occur in the ears, and may cause deafness. It would be interesting to learn how many deaf-mutes had difficult births (Voss).

Other Injuries.—Fractures of the skull have already been considered. The spoon-shaped and grooved depressions of the bone which need not always be complicated with fracture or fissure are the commonest, but fracture at the base, abruption of the occipital plate from the condyles (with breech extraction); laceration of the capsular ligament between axis and atlas, and rupture of the sutures have been observed. Tearing of the tentorium cerebelli deserves special mention as a cause of cerebral hemorrhage (Beneke, Holland). Vischer reports 51 cases of it in 186 children stillborn or dying shortly after birth. One occurred during cesarean section, others in natural birth. Hedren found 50 of 65 cases of cerebral hemorrhage followed spontaneous delivery. (See Spencer, Schaefer, Fig. 734.)

Hemorrhage into or on the brain may accompany a fracture, a fissure, or come from rupture of a cerebral or meningeal vessel sometimes caused by extreme overlapping of the cranial bones in cases of marked molding of the head, the sinuses being compressed; it may be the result of asphyxia—indeed, from no apparent cause, as in one of my cases after a spontaneous labor attended with no compression of the head and no anaërosis. The child may have hemophilic tendencies and a slight trauma causes hemorrhage not alone into the brain but in other parts of the body. In many cases a constitutional inferiority is evident. Syphilitic children are predisposed to brain hemorrhages (Osler), also those from toxemic mothers. Bleeding may take place

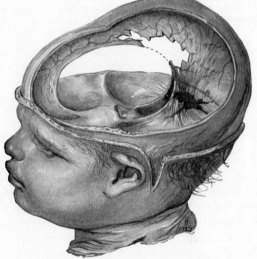

Fig. 734.—Tears in Falx and Tentorium.
Drawn from a Specimen in the University of Munich. Courtesy of Prof. A. Doederlein.

in the spinal canal also, and be limited here. Crothers, Schwartz, Gurewitch, Chase, *et al.* emphasize the bad effects of prolonged compression and trauma on the whole brain and basal ganglia, and Hemrath and Canavan proved the frequent occurrence of microscopic hemorrhages.

The symptoms come on within three or four days—usually the second day—and if the bleeding is a slow one, may last a week or more. They are restlessness, crying, refusal of food, inability to swallow, twitchings of groups of muscles, of one whole side, or general tremors, especially of the lower jaw, signs of local irritation, for example, chewing or sucking movements, irregular pupils, nystagmus, sharp, high-pitched, cramp-like cry, coma, cyanosis of the lips, often fever, even 103° F., pallor of the skin with dermographism, rapid and irregular respiration, sometimes Cheyne-Stokes', rapid pulse, 160 to 180, prominent tense fontanels, convulsions, rigidity of the body, then paralysis with cyanosis, cessation of respiration, and finally of the heart. Edema of the retina shows the increased intracranial pressure (Kearney), and the spinal manometer at lumbar puncture may measure it.

The prognosis of cerebral hemorrhage is not absolutely bad. A few of the

56

children presenting even positive signs may recover, but usually the later history is unfavorable—epilepsy, idiocy, spastic paralyses, etc.

Mild symptoms of "meningisme" are not seldom observed after operative deliveries. They are probably due to acute cerebral congestion, possibly with tiny hemorrhages, and subside in a few days. The treatment of cerebral hemorrhage in infants is symptomatic. It consists of the administration of sodium bromid and chloral, of each 2 grains per rectum every six hours; mother's milk, and quiet; ice-cap. Human blood or horse-serum should be administered as an attempt to arrest the bleeding. Lumbar puncture may be used for diagnosis; sometimes it is a curative measure (Sharpe). The same is true of puncture of the fontanels, and in appropriate cases this should be tried. If the symptoms point to cortical pressure, that is, if they are localized, trephining should be considered. More is to be hoped from a decompression operation than we have heretofore expected (Commandeur, Seitz, Cushing). Henschel collected 16 cases; 7 recovered. (See Blanco, Meyer).

The differential diagnosis between subtentorial and pretentorial or cerebral hemorrhage can sometimes be made. Spasm, convulsions, twitchings of face and extremities, increased reflexes, slow pulse and respiration, bulging of the fontanels, irregular pupils, paralysis of cerebral nerves, exophthalmos, conjunctival hemorrhages—these symptoms point to hemorrhage over the hemispheres. The child cries much in a loud high-pitched tone. Spinal puncture is negative, but aspiration of the subdural space will often help in the diagnosis. The needle is inserted at the outer angle of the large fontanel, being directed backward under the parietal bone. Both sides are punctured, and if necessary the posterior fontanel also.

In subtentorial or peribulbar hemorrhage the breathing is irregular, convulsions less marked, the cyanosis greater, the child is quieter, the symptoms come on earlier and follow more immediately the asphyxia after delivery. Spinal puncture gives bloody fluid. If the blood is too firmly clotted all punctures may be negative.

Crothers calls attention to the injuries of the spinal cord from excessive traction and Foederl shows that death may be due to crushing of the cervical cord by overflexion and overextension during delivery.

Facial paralysis frequently results from injury to branches of the nerve as they pass through the parotid gland (Rossenbeck). Forceps are usually to blame, but abnormal attitude of the child, for example, sharp flexion of the neck on the shoulder, may cause it (Dahlman). It may be due to primary agenesis of the ear vesicle (Carlsson). Central lesions of the nerve are due to cerebral trauma and hemorrhage. Here the paralysis comes on after the first day, and in the peripheral forms it appears right after delivery. Usually in a few hours to a few days the facial deformity is gone, but it may last three months or longer. In central types, and if there is a fracture of the temporal bone, it may be permanent. The paralysis may be only part of a congenital facial hemiatrophy. The differential diagnosis between the two types is made on the usual lines; peripheral paralysis, when there is extensive involvement of the distribution of the nerve, lagophthalmus, absent reflexes, etc., and central, when the eye is not involved, the reflexes present, and there are other cerebral symptoms, etc. No treatment is required. In the chronic cases muscular atrophy should be prevented by massage and electricity.

The Trunk.—Fractures of the spine, disruption of the vertebræ, separation of the condyles from the occipital plate, dislocation of the atlas on the axis, occur in violent breech deliveries and cause instant or rapid death. In nearly all cases they are errors of art. Palpation of the spine from the outside or through the pharynx will enable the diagnosis to be made. Complete avulsion of the trunk from the head is rare; the head may be torn off the body, or the body from the head, leaving the latter in the uterus, 2 cases of which have come to my knowledge. Unless the tissues are pathologically soft, macerated, or actually brittle, such an occurrence is the result of *delirium operatorium*, an acute lapse of operative reason which may affect the accoucheur after much loss of sleep, the nervous wear of a prolonged labor, the exactions of the family, combined with the sudden appearance of extraordinary difficulties. The head in these cases is usually easily removed, but it has been left, to come away finally by prolonged suppuration, with fistulas, lasting months or years, or the woman may die of sepsis.

Traumatism of the skin (face by forceps, arms in delivery of the shoulders) may cause indurations more or less deep. They are usually absorbed in one to six weeks, but may suppurate (Ehrenfest, Monograph, Birth Injuries).

Injury of the sternocleidomastoid muscle is not so rare an accident as statistics would show it to be. It is often overlooked or intentionally secreted for fear of the legal responsibility which older authors erroneously attached to it. Rupture of a healthy sternomastoid can be brought about only by very violent traction, combined with extreme torsion of the head. I have often demonstrated the possibility of turning the head of a newborn infant through an arc of 200 degrees or more without even making it cry. The blade of the forceps may directly crush the muscle, but even this injury, in the absence of antecedent disease, in my opinion is not likely to cause permanent caput obstipum.

Sippel found atrophy of the muscle, hematomata in various stages, and fibrous changes, degeneration and scar formation, which even extended to neighboring fasciæ and muscles. Without doubt—and in this the author is sustained by Pincus, Sippel, and Petersen—the muscle was already shortened and pathologically altered while the child was still *in utero*. Caput obstipum is a congenital disease and may follow normal and easy labors, with and without injury to the muscle produced at birth, all of which is important from a medicolegal point of view. Indeed, the frequent concomitant facial hemiatrophy points to a central origin of the disease. Shortening or rigidity of the muscles will be found not infrequently in newborn children which have lain in the uterus in a cramped attitude for longer periods, and especially if the liquor amnii is scanty. This has been demonstrated by the x-ray as early as the seventh month. Indeed, the head of the child may be flattened or twisted. For example, in breech cases, in primiparæ, the posterior sternomastoid is shortened and the anterior parietal bone flattened; in multiparæ, owing to the pendulous belly, the posterior parietal is flattened and the anterior sternomastoid shortened. Sometimes the arms or legs of the child are fixed in bizarre attitudes by shortened muscles, and it requires some force to straighten them.

If the healthy muscle is crushed or torn, whether or not a hematoma forms, spontaneous recovery is the rule, and *shortening is absent*, a fact which experience in general surgery will confirm. If the injured muscle becomes infected, by way of the blood, from the bowel, the navel, or the lungs (Mikulicz), a myositis may occur and shortening will follow. Hematomata which usually call attention to the disease are observed shortly after birth as a hard knot in the muscle, which is only slightly tender. Myositis is found later—fourth to twenty-first day—as a hard, fusiform swelling of the whole muscle, exceedingly tender, together with febrile symptoms. Myositis causes the child to cry much, especially when handled; indeed, these symptoms may attract attention to the trouble. The early diagnosis is easy—one finds the head inclined to the affected side, the tenderness, and the tumor. In paralysis of the nervus accessorius the head is turned to the well side. This latter is similar in cause to facial paralysis, and usually heals quickly. In later life dislocation of the vertebræ and facial hemiatrophy come up for consideration.

Treatment of injury to the sternomastoid and of the other cervical muscles consists of prevention, in the first place, and rest of the muscle after it occurs. During breech deliveries the possibility of injury must be borne in mind, but during forceps operations it is usually impossible directly to protect the muscles, except by a strict observance of the indications and proper technic. After delivery the child is to be handled as little and as carefully as possible, the nurse being properly instructed. In several cases I had the infant strapped to a well-padded board like a papoose for a week, and bathing omitted (Couvelaire, Behm, Fitzsimmons). Operation in the early weeks is sometimes advisable.

Injuries to every one of the viscera of the chest and abdomen have been reported, rupture with hemorrhage being the usual finding. Fractures of the ribs and sternum in version and breech extraction have occurred. In one case I found that the attending accoucheur had dilated and ruptured the anus, thinking it was the tightly closed cervix, and in another the child's perineum and rectovaginal septum had been torn through under the same erroneous impression. The swollen scrotum has been held for the membranes and punctured. Spontaneous rupture of the umbilical cord occurred in 2 cases in the service of the Chicago Lying-in Hospital Dispensary, in one of which the child died. The cord in one case was very brittle. During a forceps operation I inadvertently cut the cord clean across with the very tip of the blade. Tearing of the cord off the placenta, off the belly, once with stripping up of the abdominal wall, rupture of the veins, rupture of a large varicosity,

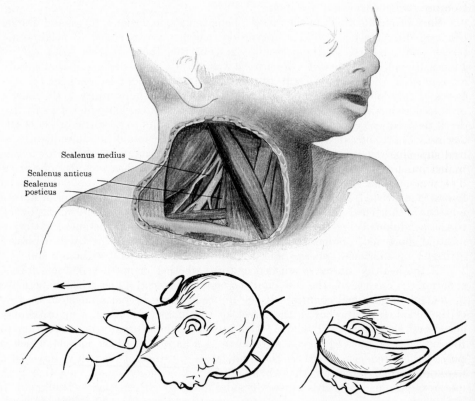

Scalenus medius
Scalenus anticus
Scalenus
posticus

FIG. 735.—SEMIDIAGRAMMATIC, TO SHOW THE PART OF CERVICAL PLEXUS INJURED BY FORCED DELIVERY. This is the so-called Erb's point. Sketches below show usual mechanisms of injury, traction, and compression.

have all been observed, either with or without the action of external trauma (important medicolegally). A too brittle cord, coiling, or a knot is usually responsible for the spontaneous injuries. Rupture of the liver, of the spleen, of the gut has occurred in natural birth (Hedren, Genell).

Paralysis of the muscles of the extremities is not an infrequent result of severe operative deliveries. Central cerebral or spinal cord lesions result usually in extensive paralysis, often with rigidity and athetosis, for example, cerebral spastic paralysis (Little), diplegia, hemiplegia, paraplegia. Of the local paralysis, Duchenne-Erb's is clinically the most important, though isolated paralyses and pareses occur—for example, one whole arm, the forearm and elbow, from brachial nerve injury or callus. Erb's paralysis is due to injury of the fifth and sixth motor roots of the brachial plexus—the upper arm type. Klumpke's paralysis is due to damage of the seventh and eighth cervical, sometimes the first thoracic root—the lower arm type. Sever found 25 per cent. of 1100 cases had whole arm paralysis.

The pathology of the injury has been much discussed. The older notions were that the nerves were compressed as they issue from between the scaleni muscles; that they were caught between the clavicle and the first rib; that a broken clavicle tore into the cervicobrachial plexus; that the roots were torn out of the spinal cord. Adson found that great force applied in an especially unfavorable direction was required to tear the nerves, and believed that destruction of the deep cervical fascia with injury of the perineurium causes the paralysis. Thomas believes that these palsies are only part of a more extensive shoulder injury, that there is a subluxation of the head of the humerus, and extravasation of blood in the plexus with scar formation. This paralysis may follow normal labor.

The paralysis is usually a traction lesion and may be unilateral or bilateral. Compression by the blade of the forceps and by callus formation is also to be mentioned, and in these cases the paralysis is a little more likely to disappear. The muscles involved are the deltoid, the supraspinatus and infraspinatus, the coraco-brachialis, brachialis internus, the biceps, and in some cases the supinators longus and brevis. A characteristic position is assumed by the arm. It hangs flaccid at the side of the chest, with the hand rotated inward, the thumb pointing back. Flexion of the forearm on the arm and supination are impossible. Sensibility remains intact, but muscular atrophy is rapid. The prognosis is fair, most cases recovering, a few with some weakness of the arm, and rarely complete palsy. Babies in whom the signs are mild, and perhaps due to bruising, with exudate around the nerve-roots, may recover, but if the paralysis shows no improvement in a month, or if pupillary inequality or neuritis exists, the outlook is gloomy.

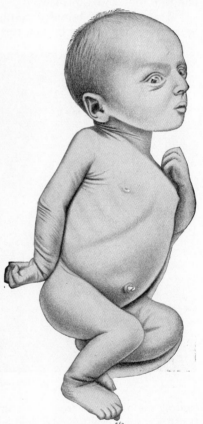

The greatest field lies in prevention. In ordinary labor, during the delivery of the shoulders, care must be taken not to lift the head up nor to pull it down from behind the pubis too sharply, and in breech cases the neck may not be stretched too much, nor the fingers allowed to draw directly upon the cervical muscles and nerves. The head may not be twisted on the shoulders, particular care being required when the neck is already on the stretch. An x-ray picture should be taken to determine if a broken bone is the cause, or a subluxation of the head of the humerus, or a fracture of the

FIG. 736.—CASE OF ERB'S PARALYSIS.

neck. In the differential diagnosis central lesions, syphilis, etc., are to be considered. Treatment is on general neurologic lines. The affected arm is held quiet in a comfortable position for ten days, then gentle massage and passive motions are given. Lately, nerve transplantation operations are being done on such cases (Taylor, Sharpe). If the roentgenogram shows the shaft of the humerus broken from the epiphysis, an osteoplastic operation should be performed.

Fracture of the bones of the extremities, especially of the clavicle, is quite common. A critical examination of newborn children, as Riether has done, will show that this occurs much oftener than is expected. It may be the hard lump on the bone (the callus) which first draws attention. Clavicle fractures occur from direct trauma, as by pulling on the bone in breech presentation, or indirectly by pulling on the arm or the head, the bone being caught between the source of the power and the pelvis. Bringing down the arms in either head or breech presentations, pulling up or down on the head to deliver the trunk, pulling with the finger in the axilla, and even the power of natural labor when the shoulder stems against the pelvis, may break the bone. I observed one fracture of the clavicle in a spontaneous labor with very strong expulsive pains, and heard the bone crack. If, after every operative delivery, the child be carefully inspected for injuries, such a fracture will not escape notice—mobility, crepitus, and deformity being present. Greenstick fracture may occur. The favorite site is the outer third, but the middle may break under direct pressure, and the bone may break at, or be torn from its attachment to the sternum or scapula. The treatment is simple. A small pad of absorbent cotton is placed in the axilla, the arm bandaged to the side, and the bandage well sewed in place.

Fracture of the humerus results from direct trauma in delivering the arms. I have twice deliberately broken this bone to save the child and succeeded. Separa-

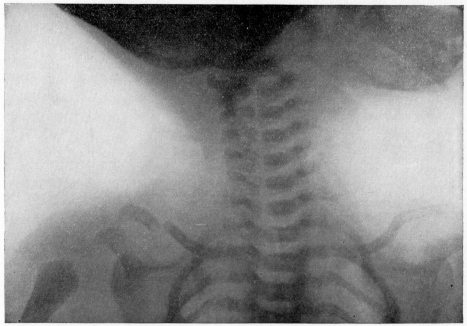

Fig. 737.—Fracture of Right Clavicle.

tion of the diaphysis from the epiphysis is much more common, and more serious because it may easily be overlooked. The epiphysis is rolled out, the arm rolled in (like an Erb's paralysis), and if healing is thus allowed, permanent disability and shortening result. To prevent such injuries, the proper technic should be practised in an arm and shoulder delivery. Dislocation of the humerus is very rare—usually a fracture is mistaken for it.

Fracture of the femur is almost always an error of art, too much force, or force applied in a wrong direction, being the cause. Bringing down the leg with bad technic, grasping it improperly, and pulling out of the axis of the pelvis are usually responsible. Nowadays few accoucheurs put the forceps on the breech, or use the blunt hook or slings. Even the fingers in the groin may break the bone. Dislocation of the femur is rarer than fracture, but separation of the epiphysis is commoner. It may be impossible to distinguish between congenital and acquired dislocation of the femur—indeed, a traumatic dislocation can hardly occur, fracture of the epiphysis usually being the result of force exerted on the joint.

Spontaneous fracture of any of the long bones may occur in labor. In one of my cases 2 children of one mother had broken clavicles because of fragility of the bones. Besides fractures, the extremities may be torn or bruised or infected by the attendant, or they may suffer pressure and gangrene by being imprisoned between the head and the pelvis.

A very important consideration is the medicolegal aspect of all these injuries, since too often the physician has to defend himself against damage suits because of them. While it is true that most of these traumatisms can be prevented by proper application of our art, it is equally true that, with few manifest exceptions, they can be brought about by the forces of natural labor alone. Since this is a fact, in any given medicolegal case it will be necessary to prove that the particular injury was plainly due to carelessness, ignorance, or lack of skill on the part of the accoucheur. In passing judgment, also, these things must be borne in mind: Our medical schools do not as yet furnish enough material so that the general practitioner can get the proper training to meet all the emergencies that may arise; the surroundings of the labor case in a home; a low bed and inefficient assistance or none; the loss of sleep; the nervous wear and tear of a confinement case, and the state of mental fatigue in which the accoucheur often has to undertake the most dangerous and delicate operations, involving two lives; and, finally, many of the accidents named have occurred in the hands of the best obstetricians the world has known.

LITERATURE

Adson: Surg., Gyn., and Obst., March, 1922, p. 352. Literature.—*Ballantyne:* Jour. Obst. and Gyn., British Empire, March, 1914, p. 140.—*Blanco and Paperini:* Jour. Amer. Med. Assoc., 1926, vol. 87, p. 1261.—*Boehm:* "Torticollis," Jour. Amer. Med. Assoc., September 18, 1909.—*Bonnaire:* "Hemorrhages of Newborn," L'Obstetrique, October, 1911. Literature.—*Browne, F. J.:* Brit. Med. Jour., September 30, 1922.—*Cohen:* Zentb. für Gynaek., February 19, 1927, p. 505.—*Commandeur:* L'Obstetrique, July, 1910.—*Couvelaire:* Annal. de Gyn. et d'Obst., January, 1911; also Surg., Gyn., and Obst., June, 1911.—*Crothers, B.:* Amer. Jour. Obst. and Gyn., April, 1931.—*Dahlman:* Charitè Annalen, Jg. 37, 1913, p. 376.—*Dayton:* New England Medical Journal, July, 1930. —*Dorman:* "Fetal Death," Amer. Jour. Obstet., February, 1909, p. 332.—*Eastman:* Johns Hopkins Hosp. Bull., January, 1932, p. 1.—*Engelman:* Zentralbl. f. Gyn., 1911, p. 7; also L'Obstetrique, May, 1909, p. 362.— *Ewarts Graham:* Jour. Exper. Med., April, 1912.—*Fitzsimmons:* Jour. Amer. Med. Assoc., February 20, 1915.— *Foederl:* Arch. für Gynaek., 1931, Bd. 143, iii, p. 598.—*Fuchs:* Zentb. für Gyn., November 13, 1920, p. 1313. Literature.—*Genell:* Acta Obstet. et Gyn., 1930, vol. ix, fasc. 1–4.—*Guttner:* Arch. für Gyn., April, 1932, Band 149, H. 1, p. 70.—*Hannes:* Zentb. f. Gyn., July 23, 1921.—*Haselhorst and Stromberger:* Zeitschr. für Geb. u. Gyn., 1932, Band 132, H. 1, p. 16.—*Haskovec:* Wien. med. Blätter, 1899, "Cerebral Injuries," No. 37. Literature.—*Hedren:* Ref., Jour. Amer. Med. Assoc., June 22, 1928, p. 1988.—*Hemsath and Canavan:* Amer. Jour. Obst. and Gyn., April, 1932, p. 471.—*Henschel:* Zentralbl. f. Gyn., 1913, p. 929; also *Frazier:* Virginia Med. Semimonthly, December 26, 1913.—*Hofmann:* Zentb. für Gyn., June 20, 1931.—*Holland:* Quoted by Bourne, Recent Advances in Obstetrics and Gyn., 1926, Blakiston.—*Holt and Babbitt:* Jour. Amer. Med. Assoc., January 23, 1915.—*Heuer:* Surg., Gyn., and Obst., May, 1923, p. 686.—*Kearney:* "Fundus Oculi in Intracranial Conditions," Amer. Jour. Obst., December, 1917, p. 904.—*Kerness:* Quoted by Holt.—*von Klein:* Monatsschr. für Geb. u. Gyn., October, 1922, vol. 60, 154.—*Knapp, L.:* Der Scheintod der Neugeborenen. Complete monograph. Literature.—*Lequeux:* "Ocular Lesions," L'Obstetrique, February, 1912.—*Meyer:* Zentb. f. Gyn., November 13, 1915. Full Literature. "Intracranial Hemorrhages of Newborn."—*Rech:* Arch. für Gyn., October, 1931, Band 147, H. 1, p. 82.—*Reidy:* British Med. Jour., October 29, 1912.—*Reuben:* Med. Record, vol. lxxxiv, p. 236.—*Rodda:* Jour. Amer. Med. Assoc., August 14, 1920.—*Rossa:* Arch. f. Gyn., vol. xlvi.—*Rossenbeck:* Zentb. f. Gyn., July 16, 1921, p. 983.—*Sachs:* Zeitschr. f. Geb. u. Gyn., 1920, Band 82, H. 2, p. 313.—*Schaefer:* Zeitschr. für Geb. u. Gyn., 1922, vol. lxxxiv, p. 240.—*Schwartz:* Zent. für Gyn., 1926, December 22, p. 3353.—*Schwartz, Gurewitch, et al.:* Monatsschr. für Geb. u. Gyn., September, 1931, p. 88, Lit.— *Seitz:* Die fötalen Herztöne während der Geburt, Munich, 1903. Literature; also Zentb. für Gyn., 1916, No. 26.—*Sever:* Jour. Amer. Med. Assoc., December 12, 1925.—*Sharpe and Maclaire:* Jour. Amer. Med. Assoc., January 30, 1926, p. 332. Literature.—*Sippel:* Zeitschr. f. Geb. u. Gyn., 1922, Band 84, p. 226.—*Smith:* Jour. Amer. Med. Assoc., July 1, 1922, p. 4.—*Spencer:* London, Obstetrical Transactions, 1891–92, vol. 33, p. 203.— —*Stein:* Jour. Amer. Med. Assoc., August 4, 1917, p. 334.—*Taylor and Clark:* Jour. Amer. Med. Sci., 1906; also 1913, p. 836.—*Thomas:* Amer. Jour. Med. Sci., 1920, clix, 207; *Ibid.,* "Still-births," New York Med. Jour., 1913, vol. xlviii, p. 413.—*Vischer:* Corr. Blatt für Schweizer Ärzte, February 22, 1919.—*Voss:* Zentb. für Gyn., 1926, December 22, p. 3357.—*Wolff:* Beiträge f. Augenheilkunde, 1905. Literature.

PATHOLOGY OF THE PUERPERIUM

NOWADAYS the puerperium, aside from after-pains and minor disturbances of urination and of lactation, is usually an uneventful convalescence. When the soreness is gone from the muscles and joints and the body functions are ordered, which requires about seventy-two hours, the puerpera should feel as well as, if not better than, she ever did. Two dangers, however, beset her: infection of the genitalia and infection of the breasts. Naturally, a woman at this time may be seized with any general or local disease, as typhoid, pneumonia, the exanthemata, erysipelas, etc., and such affections are usually aggravated by the puerperal state. In importance, however, puerperal infection overshadows everything else.

CHAPTER LXIII

PUERPERAL INFECTION

PUERPERAL fever is a term introduced by Richard Morton in 1692 to apply to an acute febrile disease which seized lying-in women and exhibited a high degree of fatality. Willis (about 1662) wrote of "febris puerperarum."

History.—In the primitive practices of savages untouched by civilization are found many evidences that puerperal fever existed among them, and that means of prevention were adopted —for example, the isolation of the parturient and puerperal members of the tribe, the cleansing bath in a stream after labor, the fumigations of the vulva with aromatic herbs, fumigation of the apartment after the puerpera left it, washing the belly with banana wine, etc. In the Ayur Veda of Susruta, a thousand years before Christ, it is mentioned. Hippocrates (400 B. C.) describes cases of it so accurately that the words could well be read in a modern class-room. He mentions epidemics of the fever. Celsus and Galen describe it, and historic references to it throughout the middle ages are numerous. The first authentic report of an epidemic of the disease is given by Hervieux, and is said to have occurred in Leipzig in 1652 to 1665. The first lying-in ward was established in Paris at the Hôtel-Dieu, and here the great obstetricians, Mauriceau, de la Motte, Portal, and Peu, obtained their experience. Mauriceau states that, in 1660, an epidemic of puerperal fever broke out in the city of Paris and in the Hôtel-Dieu, and here two-thirds of the women delivered died of it! Even in 1831 the mortality still was 9 per cent. in the Paris Maternité. In 1750 and 1761 epidemics occurred in London; in 1772, in Edinburgh; in Berlin in 1778—to mention only a very few of those reported. Since the maternities were opened to students at the same time the states placed dead bodies at the disposal of the universities for study and instruction, it is easy—for us—to see why the scourge increased. In Vienna, where the postmortems of the great Rokitansky were so assiduously visited by the students, the disease raged fearfully. In 1842 the mortality of the women varied, with the months, from 18 to 31 per cent. Every day there were two or three autopsies on such cases, and the students went directly from the morgue to the lying-in room. In England the disease was very well known, and it was there considered contagious, like smallpox. (Hirsch, Fasbender, Mauriceau, Semmelweis, Holmes, Sinclair.)

Definition.—Puerperal fever, or puerperal infection, is a general term embracing all the conditions, usually of a febrile nature, but sometimes non-febrile, affecting puerperæ, originating from infection of the genital tract at any point of its extent.

It matters not whether the symptoms be mild, lasting but a few hours or many days, whether there be a vulvitis, an endometritis, or a septicemia, whether one of the milder forms of saprophytic bacteria or the most virulent streptococcus be causative, whether the patient has fever or rapid pulse—if the complexus of symptoms points to a genital infection, the woman suffers from puerperal fever. Custom has omitted from this definition post-cesarean peritonitis and, by some, that following rupture of the uterus. It also shuts out small-pox, malaria, the essential infectious fevers, for example, typhoid, diphtheria of the throat, erysipelas of all other portions of the body but the genitals, etc., and since the definition includes many and widely differing clinical forms of disease, a careful classification of these forms is necessary. This is not easy. The exact nature of puerperal infection has been discovered through the science of bacteriology.

Up to the seventeenth century the theory of Hippocrates was the generally accepted one. He ascribed the disease to suppression of the lochia, taking the effect for the cause. Celsus and Galen, Avicenna, Mauriceau, Sydenham, and Michaëlis accepted this theory. If, as the presumable result of fright, of taking cold, etc., the lochia ceased, they were absorbed into the blood and caused puerperal fever. Mercurialis, and especially Puzos, of Paris, taught the *milk theory*. During pregnancy the milk secretion begins, but it is all determined to the uterus, where the fetus uses it for nourishment. After labor it is excreted by the breasts. If by catching a cold, etc., the secretion should be checked, so-called milk metastases occur and cause fever—again mixing cause and effect. Then the milk appears in the lochia (the purulent lochia of sepsis), in the peritoneal cavity (the pus of puerperal peritonitis), in the pleural cavities (pus from pleuritis), or in the joints (pyemic arthritis). Chemists even claimed to have made butter from the exudate in the peritoneal cavity, one saying he had found sour milk and butter under the skin of a woman dead of puerperal fever.

There was no lack of other notions. Plater, in 1602, said it was a metritis; Hunter, in 1780, a peritonitis; Tonnelè, in 1830, a lymphangitis, etc. Mauriceau called it malignant fever, others a gastric or bilious fever, puerperal erysipelas, typhus, omentitis, putrid fever, etc.

Cruveilhier said it was somewhat like typhoid, while the "essentialistes," as they were called in France, among whom are the names of Dubois, Depaul, Litzman, and Michaëlis, said it was due to a miasm and was a specific contagious process, propagable through the air, and governed by telluric, cosmic, and atmospheric influences, etc., a view later held by Fordyce Barker in America.

Ideas of the indirect transmissibility of the disease had long been held. Levret (Paris, 1770), in speaking of Smellie's leather-covered forceps, asks if contagion could not be carried in the blood which decomposes in the meshes of the leather. In England, Charles White, in 1772, said that other persons could be infected by the discharges of a septic puerpera; in 1795 Gordon referred to the contagiousness of the disease, and Denman, in 1768, declared it was carried by physicians and midwives from one puerpera to another. One quotation, whose origin I cannot find, states that the disease may be carried on sponges used on several puerpera. Thomas Watson, in London, in 1842, taught that doctors carried infection on their hands from diseased puerperæ, from phlegmons, etc., and recommended chlorin-water ablutions. Dr. Blackman, in Edinburgh, in 1845, said that puerperal fever was conveyed by the dirt under the finger-nails. Abstention from obstetric practice was enforced on physicians who had a succession of puerperal fever cases, even the use of impervious gloves was recommended by Steinau in 1855 and Watson in 1858.

In 1842 our own Oliver Wendell Holmes heard a report of the case of a physician who, inoculated at a postmortem, died of septicemia, but before this had attended several women in labor who also died of the same disease. Struck with this association of fatalities, he studied published articles on the subject, and in 1843 presented his results in a paper entitled "The Contagiousness of Puerperal Fever." He proved, by an array of clinical reports, that it was carried from one patient to another *as a contagium*, and that, also, it was caused by *inoculation* of the puerpera, and that the sources of infection could be erysipelatous processes as well as cadaveric poisons. He suggested these rules of prophylaxis:

"1. A physician holding himself in readiness to attend cases of midwifery should never take any active part in the postmortem examination of puerperal fever cases.
"2. A physician present at such postmortems should use thorough ablution, change every article of dress, and allow twenty-four hours or more to elapse before attending a case of midwifery.
"3. Similar precautions should be taken after the autopsy or surgical treatment of cases of erysipelas if the doctor is obliged to unite such duties with his obstetrical work, which is in the highest degree inexpedient."

Holmes' views met violent and bitter opposition from the two foremost obstetricians of the time, Hodge and Meigs, and made very little impress on the profession. In 1855 he again took up the subject, but, unfortunately, for the last time.

In 1847 Semmelweis, a young assistant in the clinic in Vienna, which was later occupied by Carl Braun, announced that puerperal fever is caused by the absorption into the blood, from the genitals, of *decomposed animal matter* from any source; that the hands, or any article brought into the genitals, may be the carriers of same. He did not come upon this by accident, but it was the result of years of hard work and study. He noticed that the division of the clinic which was used for the instruction of midwives had a 2.7 per cent. mortality from puerperal fever, while that for doctors had 11.4 per cent., and that the children were affected with sepsis proportionately also.

The discrepancy between the two clinics was public knowledge—it was the subject of municipal investigation; the midwives taunted the physicians with the facts, and the patients, when they learned they were to be assigned to the doctors' clinic, on their knees would beg to be sent home.

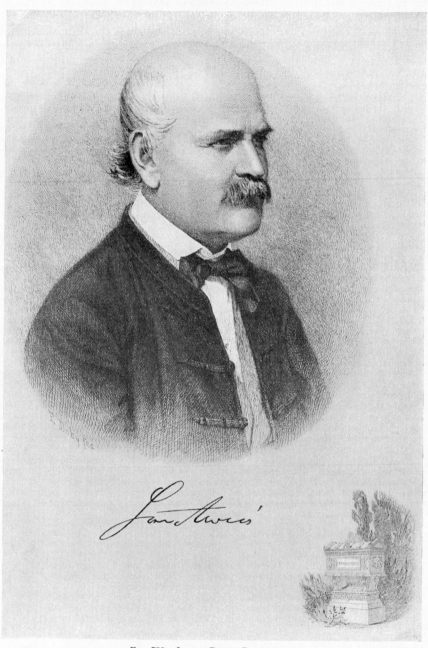

Fig. 738.—Ignatz Philip Semmelweis.
Below is the monument marking his grave in Buda-Pest, Hungary.

Semmelweis noted that the disease prevailed with irregular, unassignable fluctuations, year in and year out, in the hospital, but not in the homes; that women who were delivered on the way to the hospital seldom sickened; that parturients who had long, hard, or instrumental labors were nearly always affected; that one or the other assistant had the most cases; the maternities where students were not taught showed the best results (except the Paris Maternité, where the midwives made autopsies); that overcrowding of the hospital had no influence; that fright and nervous influences had no effect; that the disease affected the married as well as the single; that the new-born children died of the same disease as their mothers; that no alteration of the diet, of the ventilation, of the methods of treatment, produced a change for the better—and all the time the difference in the conditions of his clinic from that of the midwives mystified and oppressed him. He said: "Everything was in question; everything was unexplained; everything was doubtful—only the large number of deaths was a positive fact." Finally, the death of his friend, Professor Kolletschka, gave him the inspiration. A student had pricked Kolletschka's finger at an autopsy, and the professor died of septicemia. The postmortem of Kolletschka struck Semmelweis by its similarity with those he had made on puerperal fever cases. The explanation of puerperal fever was then clear. The hands carried particles of cadaveric decomposition into the puerperal wounds, and these caused puerperal fever.

With the cause he sought the remedy. He instituted washing of the hands, cleaning of the finger-nails (!), and the use of chlorin water; later, chlorid of lime solution. The result was dazzling. The mortality sank to 1.27 per cent. in 1848, even lower than it was in the midwives' clinic. Later an incident—rather, a calamity—showed him that any decomposing animal matter can be causative. Thirteen women lying in adjacent beds were examined in succession by the assistant and staff. The first was a case of gangrenous carcinoma of the cervix of the uterus; the rest were normal cases—11 of the 12 women died of puerperal fever. Later a woman with caries of the left knee became the origin of a run of 19 fatal cases of infection. Experimentally, he proved that the introduction of pus and ichor from these women was fatal to puerperal animals.

At the same time that the mothers' mortality improved the infections of the new-born were substantially reduced.

Semmelweis' theory, then, reads that puerperal fever is a resorption fever, brought about by the introduction of decomposed animal matter into the genitals. He said that this matter could come from cadavers, from infected wounds of all kinds, and was carried into the genital wounds, the uterus, the cervix, and the perineum by the finger of the accoucheur, the instruments, the douche-nozzle, the sponges, infected air, the bed-linen, the bed-pans—indeed, everything which could transport the *decomposed animal matter* from its source to the parturient canal. He said that the disease was only one form of pyemia, that it also occurred in surgical cases, and he recommended his methods of prevention to the surgeons! But, sad to relate, his words fell on deaf ears. If the term "bacteria" is substituted for the words "decomposed animal matter," the definition of puerperal infection is perfect as we believe it today. Semmelweis' theory, like most great truths, was not accepted; he struggled with his opponents for fifteen years, when signs of dementia appeared. He died without the recognition he deserved, in an insane asylum, and, curiously, of pyemia.

With Bretonneau, Pasteur, and Koch, the germ theory of disease was born, and when Lister came in the seventies, the true worth of Semmelweis' work was appreciated. To an obstetrician, then, is due the credit of pointing the correct way to modern antisepsis and asepsis.

While Holmes proved that the propagation of puerperal fever took place by contagion or inoculation in a general way, to Semmelweis the credit must be given for having, with unerring aim, struck the exact cause of the disease, for having shown unequivocally that it is an infection of the genital wounds, and for having indicated the correct manner of prevention. Holmes dropped the subject after a few efforts; Semmelweis fought for his doctrine and the lives of myriads of women with all his powers, and quit the struggle, as Sinclair says, only to descend into the tomb. (Sir W. J. Sinclair: Semmelweis, His Life and His Doctrine.) (See Adami.)

Since 1870 the history of puerperal fever has been that of Listerism. Whereas at first the women were delivered under a carbolic acid spray, and the air, which Lister believed was the dangerous element, excluded,—one Russian author even wishing the women delivered in an antiseptic bath,—later the hands and instruments were recognized as the materia peccans, and rigid antisepsis, both objective and subjective, practised. In the eighties and early nineties the women were given carbolic and bichlorid douches before, during, and after labor. This was found harmful, and now a more aseptic technic is practised, identical in principles with that suggested by Semmelweis in 1847.

Etiology.—Puerperal fever is nothing more nor less than an infectious wound disease. Cruveilhier, in 1831, said that the puerpera was a wounded person, and Mauriceau, in 1668, called the lochia a wound secretion, likening it to that of an amputation.

Since puerperal infection is a surgical wound infection, it follows that the germs which attack surgical wounds will also be found attacking the puerpera. This is true. The pathology of puerperal infection is the same as that of surgical infections, but, because of the anatomic structure of the parts, the physiologic changes of pregnancy, of labor, and the puerperium, with the peculiar chemisms of these functions, many variations exist which demand special consideration.

The following bacteria have been found as positive and probable causes of puerperal infection. In collecting these the author has made use of the exhaustive articles of Walthard, Schottmüller, Harris, Werner, and Wegelius:

Streptococci, hemolytic and non-hemolytic, aërobic, anaërobic, many strains, facultative, obligate; S. viridans; S. putrificus (Schottmüller, Schwarz), etc.
Diplostreptococcus puerperalis.
Staphylococcus aureus and albus, some hemolytic.
Diplococcus lanceolatus pneumoniæ.
Bacillus coli.
Gonococcus of Neisser.
Bacillus pneumoniæ of Friedländer.

Bacillus pyocyaneus.
Bacillus proteus.
Bacillus aërogenes capsulatus (Welchii).
Bacillus fusiformis and spirilla (often found in hospital gangrene).
Bacillus typhosus.
Bacillus tetani.
Bacillus anthracis.
Bacillus diphtheriæ.
Bacillus influenzæ.

A host of other bacteria causing putrefaction and decomposition have been found, a few of which may be mentioned: Micrococcus fœtidus, Bacillus funduliformis, Bacillus racemosus, Bacillus radiiformis, Bacillus pseudotetani, Bacillus nebulosus, Bacillus caducus, Staphylococcus parvulus, and many more, named and unnamed, and some bearing several names or in pleomorphic states.

It is rare to find one of this number the sole cause of the disease. Usually two or more, even to the number of 15, have been found. The streptococcus combines with the staphylococcus, or the Bacterium coli or pyocyaneus, the latter increasing the virulence of the former. Symbiosis usually seems to enhance virulence, and sometimes the opposite is true. The proteus and the colon bacillus group, or the proteus with the staphylococcus group, may cause bad infections, as do the combinations of coli and Bacillus aërogenes capsulatus.

Neither the symptoms nor the bacteriologic examination nor the autopsy findings will invariably permit us to decide which organism was the causative one. A presumptive diagnosis may often be made.

Sources of the Infection.—These bacteria are to be found in decomposing animal and vegetable matter, cadavers, in diseased animals and human beings, their excreta, in the air, and in dust. The most important ultimate source, so far as our subject is concerned, is the *diseased human being*. The infectious organisms are carried from suppurations, gangrene, ulceration, infections which are excreted, as diphtheria, scarlet fever, pneumonia, nasal catarrhs, etc., erysipelas, necrotic cancers, lochia (even of normal puerperæ), the menstrual blood, and from objects soiled with such discharges. In hospitals the medical and surgical wards are prolific breeding grounds for dangerous bacteria, and a case of septic abortion or mild puerperal infection may easily be the starting point for an epidemic.

Modes of Transmission to the Genital Tract.—Semmelweis distinguished two modes of inoculation—one from without, *exogenous* infection; and one from within, *endogenous*, which he called auto-infection.

Autoinfection.—As our knowledge of the subject grew and our preventive measures became more and more successful, there appeared those who declared that all cases of puerperal infection were exogenous in origin (for example, Jaggard), and that, therefore, when a woman took sick with a puerperal process, some one was to blame for it. The results of this teaching are still wide-spread and still cause a great deal of injustice, because it is not true. Ahlfeld, since 1885, and a few others—Winckel, Koch, Tarnier, Doléris—had always maintained that, in addition to the inoculation from without (hetero-infection), the woman occasionally became infected from bacteria which she carried in her own person—autoinfection. Leopold, Döderlein, Krönig, Fochier, Pestalozza, and Williams denied the possibility. Some of these authors have changed their minds. Ahlfeld distinguished three kinds of autoinfection—first, that from bacteria in the genital tract, including the vulva (*e. g.*, gonorrhea), whether they entered the tissues themselves or were introduced by absolutely sterile fingers or instruments; second, that transported to the genital canal via the blood from a distant site of suppuration, such as the tonsil, the lungs, a mastitis; and, third, the infection of the genital canal from contiguous disease, for example, appendicular abscesses, pyosalpinx, pyelo-ureteritis, thrombophlebitis. To this might be added a fourth, the inoculation of the patient by herself with bacteria, either present on her hands, or carried by her from a focus of suppuration, for example, ulcus cruris, tonsillitis, a sinus disease, otitis, abscess of the breast, an intertrigo, etc. Some forms of anemia are the expression of a larvated infection which may become fatally virulent after delivery. It is hard to differentiate these forms from Ahlfeld's second form. With Wegelius, Winter, and Walthard I would prefer to limit the term "auto-infection" to those rare cases where the bacteria of the genital tract, including the vulva, develop virulence and invade the tissues. It is better to exclude from this definition all reference to the transference of infection from distant foci in the body, as well as the admission that even the aseptic hand may inoculate the bacteria which were present in the vagina into the puerperal wounds. (See Benthin.)

The studies by Bumm, Natvig, Wegelius, Krönig and Pankow (1909), Seligman, and Walthard (1930), employing very favorable culture-media (grape-sugar bouillon and blood-agar), seem to prove that the vaginas of apparently healthy women in the last weeks of pregnancy contain streptococci and staphylococci in from 15 to 75 per cent. of the cases examined, and that these bacteria, while usually living a saprophytic existence, may wander from the vulva, the vestibule, the vagina, up into the uterus or into the wounds during the puerperium and cause puerperal fever. From general practice we have analogies of auto-infection to draw upon, to mention only two examples, the acute pelvic peritonitis of virgins, the result of "catching cold" or refrigeration during the menses, and osteomyelitis in children after severe exposure. It must also be remembered that cats, pigs, and other domestic animals have puerperal fever.

On the vulva, as was to be expected, streptococci, staphylococci, Bacillus coli, Bacillus pseudodiphtheriæ, and many saprophytes are to be found, and especially if there are pustular or eczematous eruptions near by, and in slovenly women. In the urethra the same germs vegetate. In cystitic urine the same, and Proteus vulgaris, with others still. Ascending ureteropyelitis has already been discussed, and germs here present may be dangerous to the parturient canal. Even in apparently normal women bacteriuria occurs, and the streptococcus (author), the colon bacillus, and typhoid bacilli have been demonstrated.

In the vagina, under apparently normal conditions, the following bacteria have been demonstrated (Walthard, Bar, Permar, Harris, and Wegelius):
(1) Facultative anaërobic streptococci of the type of the Streptococcus pyogenes puerperalis. (2) Facultative anaërobic streptococci of the type of the Diplostreptococcus puerperalis. (3) Obligate anaërobic streptococci of the type of the Streptococcus anaërobius. (4) Aërobic streptococci, hemolytic and anhemolytic. (5) Staphylococci pyogenes albus, aureus, and citreus. (6) Bacillus coli. (7) Gonococcus. (8) Bacillus funduliformis. (9) Pseudotetanus bacillus. (10) Bacillus aërogenes capsulatus (Welchii). (11) Bacillus vaginalis (Döderlein) said by Joetten to be identical with the Bacillus acidophilus or B. lacticus. (12) Bacterium pseudodiphtheriæ. (13) Micrococcus tetragenus. (14) Saccharomyces. (15) Bacillus of Weeks. (16) Bacillus bifidus. (17) Gram-positive cocci, diplococci, bacilli, and diplobacilli, and numerous other anaërobic and aërophilic cocci and bacilli and streptobacilli and spirochetes (Lash).

Döderlein distinguishes two forms of vaginal secretion—*normal*, which is white, like curdled milk, acid, contains no mucus, and is small in amount; and *pathologic*, which is thick, yellowish or greenish mucus, sometimes foamy, usually alkaline, but not necessarily so, and contains numerous pathogenic and non-pathogenic microörganisms, and the Trichomonas vaginalis (Hoehne), whereas the normal vaginal secretion contains only the Bacillus vaginæ, a harmless organism. It is certain that the pathologic discharges contain more of the mentioned organisms than do the normal, but it is not easy to divide the cases sharply into two classes either clinically or bacteriologically.

The closed cervix is infected in its lower third, the mucous plug here being cloudy yellow, showing the presence of pus and bacteria. It is white in the next zone and clear in the upper part, being here sterile. (See Fig. 295, p. 296.) Under normal conditions, according to the recent researches of Winter, Menge, and Walthard, the uterine cavity is sterile, but it may harbor bacteria, and they then live in the decidua and fetal membranes.

Since the bacteria mentioned exist in the genital tract of the gravida, and are there even during labor, why does not every woman become infected? First, they live as saprophytes, requiring special conditions to develop invasive qualities or virulence. We have several analogies. In the mouth and nose the streptococcus, the pneumococcus, the diphtheria bacillus, and the staphylococcus may live harmlessly, and only under extraneous influence cause sickness, but they may be infectious for others. In the horse the tetanus bacillus, very fatal if inoculated into a wound, lives as a harmless parasite. Second, the vagina has some power of purification, at least it has qualities which ordinarily keep the activities of its flora within safe bounds for the particular woman. Döderlein ascribed this power to the lactic acid produced by the Bacillus vaginæ, which makes the vaginal secretion unsuitable for the growth of other bacteria or the bacilli use up the nourishment or the oxygen, needed by other harmful bacteria. Menge believed that phagocytosis going on in the cervix and vagina had something to do with it. Perhaps other immunizing forces are at work to produce local cell immunity, and the process will be explained when the biochemical studies in immunity of Metchinkoff, v. Behring, Ehrlich, and others are carried to completion. Third, during labor there are the mechanical scouring-out of the bacteria, the flow of the liquor amnii, and the outpouring of mucus and blood, and the passage of the child and placenta, which remove large numbers of bacteria. Fourth, newly let blood has antiseptic properties for a short time. The lochia (vide infra) in the first forty-eight hours show very few bacteria, while on the third day the increase is marked, but by this time the wounds have closed, a bank of granulations has been thrown up, through which the bacteria may not easily break, excepting the virulent streptococcus and the staphylococcus, and the cervix has closed, shutting off the uterine cavity more or less. Fifth, the downward and outward current of the lochia and the mucus covering the surface must also be considered. Sixth, Hofbauer has shown that the reticulo-endothelial system of the pelvis is a powerful factor in local immunity.

During labor, owing to change in acidity (alkaline liquor amnii) and the addition of blood and serum from tiny wounds, the streptococci, staphylococci, Bacillus coli, and gas producers from the intestine increase, all this spontaneously, but of course extremely favored by vaginal examinations, etc.

Natvig and Wegelius have shown that the flora of the vagina in the puerperium is the same as, or at least very similar to that of the vulva, vestibule, and vagina before labor, and many of the bacteria mentioned on p. 892 have been demonstrated in the lochia of fever-free puerperæ. Therefore the bacteria have the power to wander into and up the genital tract. In three-fourths of the cases examined the bacteria were found in the uterus itself on the fourth day. They were few in number, and almost always all obligate anaërobes, the facultatives being lightly represented. On the ninth day 90 per cent. of the cases showed bacteria in considerable number, but they were almost entirely obligate anaërobes, only once in 10 cases a facultative anaërobic streptococcus being met. In spite of all this, if the woman is not molested by meddling accoucheurs, she will almost always recover from her labor by grace of the immunities provided by nature, *and while mild cases of auto-infection may occur occasionally, fatal cases are exceedingly rare*. The practical lesson to be learned from these investigations is that the accoucheur should studiously and consistently avoid those conditions which render these bacteria virulent and invasive, and which carry them to regions of the parturient canal where they may unfold their latent powers. Conditions favoring autoinfection are excessive bruising of the parts from prolonged labor, great delay in delivery after rupture of the membranes, the retention of pieces of placenta in the uterus, or membranes which hang down into the vagina and form a bridge on which the bacteria may mount into the uterus, or blood-clots in the vagina, lochiometra, and lochiocolpos.

Hetero-infection.—Infection from without—exogenous infection—is by far the most common, and is always first to be thought of when a puerpera develops fever. Infection may be brought to the genital tract from the outside in many ways:

(1) *The most common carrier is the physician or midwife, rarely the nurse.* The finger, or an instrument insufficiently sterilized, introduced into the genitalia, deposits virulent germs in the tissues. These germs have been brought from a case of puerperal sepsis, from the dressing of an ulcer, or any suppurating or infected wound, from a postmortem, an erysipelas case, a cancer, pneumonia, typhoid, scarlet fever, diphtheria, from a baby with infected umbilicus or enteritis, etc., from the lochia of even normal puerperæ, or even the ordinary filth under the finger-nails. The bacteria attain great virulence by "passage" through a human being. The attendant may have the focus of infection on his own person—a felon on the finger, furunculosis, a wet eczema (they often contain streptococci), tuberculosis, ozena (as the famous case of Dr. Rutter, of Philadelphia, in the forties), an acute rhinitis, or a pharyngitis. A small epidemic in the dispensary service of the Chicago Lying-in Hospital originated from the throat of an intern. In the discharges from the nose a hemolytic aërobic streptococcus was found in almost pure culture. Some years ago a local hospital suffered an epidemic of fatal post-operative peritonitis, and a virulent streptococcus was isolated from the throats of many of the nurses and interns, as well as from the dust in the wards and operating-rooms. Schatz and Benthin observed puerperal fever epidemics of similar origin. In these cases the bacteria get on the hands, instruments, or sponges, and are thus carried into the genitals, or they are expectorated directly on and into the vulva and puerperal wounds, or they settle on them from their suspension in the air as droplets or as dust.

(2) *The environment has much to do with the causation* of puerperal infection, and the author must here express a change of opinion from that held in 1898. In my mind there is now no doubt but that many cases of puerperal fever are due to the infected dust and air of hospitals and other places where the birth occurs. Bacteria from puerperal cases, from the dried pus of suppurations, from the autopsy room, the pathologic laboratory, and from the innumerable sources of infection of a general hospital, get into the air and the dust, and are carried by air-currents *or persons* to all parts of the institution, including the delivery-room and the lying-in chambers. The infection-laden dust settles on the sterilized tables, the towels, the hand solutions, and on the vulva. From here the bacteria are carried into the vagina by sterilized and gloved fingers, the instruments, catgut, gauzes, etc. Or they settle on the bed-clothing of the puerpera and thus come in direct contact with the patulous vulva, whence they wander up into the uterus. The staphylococcus is almost always found in the air of closed rooms where people congregate, but in hospitals other bacteria also are found. Flies carry pyogenic cocci (Scott).

The environment is a further source of danger in that the interns, nurses, servants, even the patients themselves become carriers of infection, usually in the throat and nose, as was already mentioned. Weaver found that the incidence of cross-infections and carriers in the Durand Contagious Disease Hospital was very much reduced when the attendants used gauze covers for the mouth and nose. He also admits the possibility of air-borne infection

Air-borne infection is at present the subject of much controversy, and, notwithstanding the published experiences of several pediatricians regarding diphtheria and scarlatina, the author is convinced that pus and other infections may be carried to the parturient, the puerpera, and the infant in this indirect manner. I have done obstetric work in five general hospitals having more or less isolated maternity wards, and in one special maternity hospital which for fifteen years accepted no infected cases, and in a maternity hospital which kept such cases under the same roof with clean cases, also during the same period in a large dispensary service in the homes of the poor, and, finally, in private practice in the homes of the well-to-do. The technic employed in all these places is practically identical, and in the general hospitals I use my own sterilized gloves and gauzes for packing. The least number of fevers postpartum, suppurating stitches, of breast abscesses, of infected babies I found in cases I delivered at home. The next best results were obtained in the maternity hospital, and I noticed a change after infected cases were cared for in the building. The largest number of infectious complications occurred in the general hospitals, and here the percentage varied with the thoroughness of isolation of the maternity ward. The surgical technic of these hospitals is excellent, and it would be difficult to prove direct contact infection. In one case an almost fatal staphylococcus puerperal infection occurred in a patient occupying a room just vacated by a man suffering from a suppurating knee. In this hospital I had three streptococcus puerperal infections, two of which were fatal. In one of the maternities a small endemic of mastitis occurred in spite of painfully rigorous precautions.

The children also showed the effect of the prevalence of infectious material. In the general hospitals marked rises of temperature on the third to the sixth day were observed in a proportion reaching at times as high as 40 per cent. of the infants. In one hospital, indeed, high fever was so common that it was considered physiologic, while at home and in the maternity free from infected cases a rise of temperature in a new-born was a rarity. In one of the general hospitals two epidemics of sepsis carried away 15 infants, in another 3 died from sepsis apparently pharyngeal in origin; in all of them intestinal infections with unusual enteric flora were frequent. When discussing the mortality and morbidity of obstetric institutions, the children should be given more consideration—the newborn child is a sterile medium, and much more sensitive to infection than gelatin and agar. Epidemics of otitis media are not uncommon in children's hospitals.

A maternity in a neighboring town suffered an epidemic of puerperal infection, which resisted all attempts at eradication. The technic of this institution is well-nigh perfect. It also had to be closed temporarily—in 1927. Werth and Schroeder, in Kiel, noticed an increase in fever cases of women *not examined in labor*, during the prevalence of a puerperal fever epidemic in the institution. Winter (1916) regards as dangerous an apparently healthy gravida who has hemolytic streptococci in the vagina, and isolates her as a "carrier." Zweifel, in 1911, reported a series of deaths following and due to the opening of a stinking abscess in his operating room. Bumm (1912) reports a four months' streptococcus endemic originating from a parturient believed to have fever from eclampsia, but really septic. In spite of rigorous antiseptic measures the endemic continued, and it did not abate until after the whole confinement suite and all the furniture had been painted. Schauta, Chrobak, Leopold, Bumm (1916), Tarnier, Pinard, Florence Nightingale, Walthard, Zweifel, Mackenrodt, and others demand separate confinement rooms and lying-in wards for septic cases.

Epidemics of pemphigus (impetigo) are the bane of present-day hospitals as they occur in spite of the most meticulous technic.

Hektoen and Kirschsteiner have shown that the streptococcus and staphylococcus will live dried in the air, exposed to diffuse daylight, from eighteen hours to ten days, and in dark cellars over a month. In the Prague maternity during an epidemic of tetanus, Nicolaier's bacillus was found in the dust of the wards occupied by infected cases. v. Eiselsberg proved the tetanus spores to be virulent after two and one-half years' drying on a wood splinter. Benthin, in an epidemic of puerperal streptococcus sepsis, found this bacterium on the beds and furniture in the puerperal wards. One woman never examined, two hours' labor, died of streptococcus septicemia. Flexner (1916) found active virus in the sweepings from rooms where cases of poliomyelitis were lying. The dried secretions of the nose were thus disseminated through dust. In veterinary practice the bacterium of infectious abortion is known to be transmitted via the respiratory and digestive tracts as well as by the phallus of the bull. It also occurs in milk supplied for consumption (Mohler). Trillat (1918) proved how readily bacteria may be transported by air-currents in droplets of moisture, some of these becoming "veritable culture-media." Friedewald and Deicher (1926) using Dick's methods, proved that the Streptococcus scarlatinæ can float about in the air of the sick-room, and lodge in the throat, possibly keeping up the infectivity of a carrier.

Air-borne infection is a reasonable assumption but hospital administrators are very loath to believe it, because acceptance of such a principle would create a moral necessity to build the maternity in absolute isolation and maintain a completely separate personnel—both very expensive.

(3) *The preparatory bath before delivery may be a source of danger.* In a general way the water is not infectious. In Philadelphia, some years ago, an epidemic of tetanus was probably due to the use of unboiled Schuylkill water.

Stroganoff proved that the bath-water obtained access to the vagina when, as in multiparæ, the vulva gapes more or less, and other laborious investigations have been made. The question can be very simply decided by asking multiparous women whether the bath-water enters the vagina. Most of them answer in the affirmative; therefore, the scales of epithelium and soil from the whole body, mixed with the water, and some of the bacteria, must gain entrance to the vagina. If a woman has an ulcer or other suppuration on her body, the danger is greatest. In such cases the general bath should be forbidden. Bumm, when in Halle, reported two cases of severe vulvar streptococcus infection occurring from baths in a tub in which old culture-tubes of the streptococcus had been washed. During the process of shaving and vulvar disinfection preparatory to labor, infected hairs, scurf, suds, etc., may be carried into the gaping vulva. That puerperal infection can be carried from one patient to another on the bed-pan, douche-points, etc., is a fact known since before Semmelweis emphasized it.

(4) *The husband is a source of infection.* Among the lowest classes coitus in the latter weeks of gestation is by no means rare, and it has been performed even during labor. Kisch refers to the practice of certain midwives who ask the husband to have intercourse with the parturient to stimulate the labor-pains. In one of the fatal cases of sepsis in the dispensary service of the Chicago Lying-in Hospital the bag of waters was ruptured by the act, and the child was born before the arrival of the physician. In another coitus was performed thrice during the night, pains beginning at 3 A. M. and delivery being completed at 11 A. M. Lustgarten, Wassermann, and others have shown that the streptococcus vegetates in the urethra of healthy men, Asacura finding it in 12.5 per cent. of 112 cases, and, further, the staphylococcus group and pseudodiphtheria bacilli are often found. In the diseased urethra streptococci, pyococci, diplococci (Gram-negative), gonococci, Bacterium coli, and cocci which resemble the Diplostreptococcus puerperalis have been found. The penis is never sterile, and, if it were, it would carry in bacteria from the vulva, as Zangemeister and Batisweiler have shown.

(5) *The patient herself may carry infection to the genitalia* on her fingers. I have seen severe and even fatal puerperal disease result from a carbuncle on the neck (a precipitate labor), a running ear (a streptococcus infection following influenza), ulcus cruris, a paronychia, and there are on record authentic instances of the transportation by the patient of virulent organisms from other distant parts of the body to the genitals, for example, from the purulent cavity of an artificial eye, from a weeping ezcema, a mastitis, an intertrigo. But in such cases the blood may transfer the bacteria, as we know it sometimes does in tonsillitis, pneumonia, pyelitis, erysipelas, etc.

A suppurating or inflammatory focus in or near the genital tract is often a source of danger. In my own experience a vaginal abscess which ruptured during delivery caused an extensive bilateral parametritis; a cervical erosion, a septicemia; an appendix adherent to the tube caused a fatal endometritis and bacteremia; a gonorrheal vaginitis, late infection and pyosalpinx; a non-gonorrheal vaginitis, an endometritis saprophytica with toxinemia; a recto-uterine fistula, fatal peritonitis; a gangrenous myoma, a severe toxinemia; infected urine (streptococcus), septicemia, and double phlegmasia alba dolens. Cases are reported of puerperal fever from ruptured appendical abscesses, from cystitis, from bartholinitis (gonococcus and streptococcus), from cancer of the uterus, from eczema and intertrigo pudendi, from enterocolitis (streptococcus and Bacterium coli). It must be added that many women affected with the diseases mentioned go through labor *without* the development of infection, the local and general immunities having been sufficiently developed to repel the invading microörganisms.

Predisposing Causes.—(1) Pregnancy itself favors the attack of bacteria, which is perhaps explained by the changes in the liver, in the kidneys, and the demineralization of the tissues. Animals are more sensitive to infection at this time. (2) The shock of labor, which is really a surgical operation, comprising the making of wounds, many of which are contused, and the bruising of the peritoneum, lowers the vital resistance. (3) All conditions which reduce the vitality, as profuse hemorrhages, eclamptic toxemia, coincident affections, as typhoid, pneumonia, grip, syphilis, cardiopathies, alcoholism, overwork, hunger, malnutrition, etc. (4) Lack of thyroid or action of other blood-forming glands may be operative. (5) Prolonged labor, especially after the rupture of the bag of waters, because of the frequent vaginal explorations, and the greater time and opportunity for bacteria to wander upward, increases both the frequency and the severity of the infections. Demelin, in 513 cases, has shown that, as the time elapsing increased from twelve hours to five days, the percentage of infections increased from 0.8 to 11.26 per cent. The bad influence of exhaustion deserves repetition here. (6) Operative interference, because of the wounds, contusions, and the bacteria introduced from without, increases both morbidity and mortality. Too early rupture of the bag of waters acts in this way; the hard head tears the cervix instead of dilating it softly, and, besides, dry labors often have to be terminated instrumentally. (7) Retention of pieces of placenta, of membranes, and of blood-clots favors infection, the most dangerous being the placental remnants. The glycogen and peptones of the involuting uterus produce favoring cultural conditions. Lochial retention causes fever, but is seldom continued long enough to cause real sickness. Uhlenhuth has proved that anaphylatoxin is absorbed from normal vaginæ. (8) Relaxed uterus with clots filling the placental sinuses, following twins, polyhydramnion, etc.

Reaction of the Organism Against Infection.—Very properly the whole parturient canal is regarded as a wounded surface after delivery, and healing takes place in the manner of ordinary surgical wounds. The endometrium is more or less covered by a layer of necrosing decidua, but the ends of the septa between the glands are partly exposed, and when the decidua falls, they are fully exposed, but, fortunately, at this time they are protected by the bank of leukocytes beneath the surface. Under the necrosing decidua an active leukocytosis occurs, the connective-tissue cells increase in numbers, plasma cells are thrown out, all of which prevents the invasion of all but the most virulent bacteria, and, at the same time, aids in the casting off of the dead decidua. By the sixth day, in normal cases, epithelization is usually complete, except at the placental site. Here the thrombi in the open vessels require more time and different methods. The placental site is rough and raised; often is covered with irregular masses of thick decidua, tough fibrin, and sometimes even shreds of placenta or bits of villi. Organization occurs in the thrombotic sinuses; the bank of granulations thickens and causes the exfoliation of the superimposed foreign masses. This may require two weeks (Figs. 251–253).

The effect of bacteria on these healing processes varies with the nature of the microörganism and the manner in which it is introduced.

If the germs are saprophytic—that is, without invasive qualities—they may not disturb the healing process at all; at most, if they produce caustic toxins, superficial necrosis results. Blood-clots, decomposing bits of membrane and of placenta, and dead or injured tissues harbor saprophytic bacteria. Without doubt the toxins they develop can produce cloudy swelling, even necrosis of the uppermost layers of cells. Since the vagina and the uterus postpartum are actively resorptive, the diffusible poisons and other physiologically active products made by the bacteria may be absorbed into the blood. Under the necrotic layer a bank of leukocytes limits the further advance of bacteria. All this is very superficial, and even sutured wounds heal in the depths—just the edges, being exposed to the noxa, may be slightly affected. More or less pus is formed on the surface, and its discharge continues until all the dead tissue is removed. Symptoms, if there are any, are due to the toxins—and few bacteria—absorbed, and the condition is called *toxinemia.* Duncan named it *sapremia.*

If the bacteria are pyogenic, but without marked invasive qualities, they go a little deeper into the tissues and the wound reaction is greater. Owing to the favoring conditions of the puerperal tissues, the succulence, the bruising, with lowered vitality, and the presence of peptone and glycogen from the involuting uterus, the bacteria rapidly multiply. Their presence and their toxins cause a dilatation of the local blood-vessels, and by a positive chemotaxis phagocytes and leukocytes are crowded into the neighborhood of the invaders, and exudations rich in polymorphonuclears and eosinophiles, plasma cells, and lymphocytes are thrown out. Gradually the fixed connective-tissue cells and the leukocytes form a firm bank or granulation wall, which resists the further advance of the bacteria and prevents the absorption of their posions. This granulation wall is composed of polynuclear and mononuclear leukocytes, eosinophiles, fibroblasts, and polyblasts, and is accompanied by an outpouring of lymph. Absence or paucity of the multinuclear neutrophiles and the eosinophiles, with increase of the mononuclears, indicates poor tissue reaction (Adami).

This inflammatory reaction of the tissues against the invasion of the noxious elements is nature's attempt at defense and repair. If the tissues and leukocytes are much injured by the toxins of the bacteria, or if their nutrition is cut off by the plugging of the capillaries, local necrosis—pus formation—occurs. If not, the poisons are neutralized, the exudates are reabsorbed, the bacteria dissolved or removed by the leukocytes, which also help remove the phagocytes killed in battle, and the fixed connective-tissue cells organize into more or less permanent fibrous tissue, leaving scars. During all this process toxins—and a few bacteria—get into the blood, producing general symptoms—fever, rapid heart, prostration, etc. This process is, however, quite local, and the condition is still called toxinemia.

If the invasive power of the bacteria is very great, a quality of certain strains of streptococcus, even the intact vagina may not be able to withstand the attack. The streptococci drive away the leukocytes, and quickly invade the lymph-vessels, and the subcutaneous and submucous tissues, multiplying rapidly. Within an hour after inoculation (some say a few minutes) they are beyond the reach of the most powerful antiseptic, and the result to the patient depends on her power of resistance. The battle between the streptococcus and its toxins—streptocolysin, leukocidin, etc., with the patient's leukocytes, and immune bodies, alexins, etc.—is soon transferred to the blood itself, and a real *bacteremia* occurs. (See Vaughan.)

That metabolism is profoundly affected by infection is well known but of its mode of action—very little, which is not surprising when the complicity of the process is remembered. Aschoff and Landau very recently called attention to peculiar cells, of mesoblastic origin, found singly and in groups in the liver, lungs, spleen, lymph-glands, bone-marrow, and in all the connective tissues including the precapillary blood- and lymph-vessels. They named these cells histiocytes and called the system they formed the reticulo-endothelial system. Louros among others proved that these cells play a strong rôle in metabolism and in the destruction and removal of bacteria and their products, in which work the leukocytes help. It is evident therefore that the reception given the bacteria, *i. e.*, the soil, has a great deal to do with the reaction of the patient. The reader is referred to more appropriate text-books for further information.

The *Streptococcus pyogenes*, discovered by Mayerhofer in 1865, cultivated by Pasteur in 1879 from the blood of women dying from puerperal fever, and isolated in pure culture by Ogsten in 1883, is the cause of the majority of the cases of infection after childbirth. It gains entrance at any point of the parturient canal, passes at once into the lymph-spaces and along the capillaries into the blood-stream, without producing much local reaction. Serous and seropurulent exudate may be slight or much, depending on the virulence of the invader. There are many kinds of streptococci, but those mostly concerned in producing puerperal infection are the ones listed on p. 892. Hemolysis is not a constant characteristic, and does not indicate excessive virulence, nor does the length of the chains, although usually the long chains are the most dangerous. As was already stated, the streptococcus may be found in the vagina of many apparently healthy women. It exists in a state of very low virulence. By proper cultural treatment it may be made very active and extremely pathogenic for animals. We have an analogon in the case of the human, when streptococci, made virulent by "passage" through one puerpera, are introduced into the genitals of another, there causing a violent infection, or when they are carried from the inflamed nose or throat of an attendant to the puerperal wounds. All forms of puerperal infection, from a simple toxinemia from retained lochia to the bacteremias which may be fatal in a few hours, may be produced by the streptococcus. Which it shall be depends on the natural strength of the inoculated coccus, the natural resistance of the patient, the number of the bacteria introduced, the concomitant injury of the tissues, the location of the point of entrance, and the time of the infection. Severe disease will result if only a few chains of a highly invasive organism are introduced, or if the woman's resistance happens to be very low at the time, as by hemorrhage, shock, renal or hepatic disease, etc. If the tissues are much bruised by labor they are not in condition to resist invasion by even a mild streptococcus. If the germs are deposited near the peritoneal cavity, for example in a deep cervix tear or on the thrombi of the placental site, dangerous infections, peritonitis, and metrophlebitis are more apt to follow than if they were inoculated into a perineal laceration. If the inoculation occurs late in the puerperium, the lymph-vessels are quite closed, the blood-vessels sealed, the local immunities well developed, and the surface well protected by a granulation wall—all of which preserves the patient from invasion. The severest fevers result from direct inoculation of the endometrium and placental site during labor itself. Then, too, as Rosenow has shown, there are many strains of streptococci, each one capable of producing a peculiar localization of infection. I believe this is true also of the staphylococcus, as I saw one epidemic of mastitis caused by a staphylococcus which apparently had an affinity for breast tissue only. Gordon isolated 90 strains of streptococci from many sources, and by serum agglutination tests grouped them into three types. His work may lead to conclusions of therapeutic value. Finally, and this is true of many bacteria, pleomorphism may explain variations of virulence. (See Hadley.)

The *staphylococcus* was separated from the streptococcus by Ogsten in 1883 in purulent affections. Doléris found it in 1880, and Brieger, in 1888, demonstrated the Staphylococcus aureus in 5 fatal cases of puerperal infection. All the staphylococcus group—Staphylococcus aureus, albus, flavus, and citreus—have been found in these cases, and occasionally one or the other is associated with the streptococcus (Bar, Tissier, the author). Members of the staphylococcus group are less invasive than the streptococcus. Local and general leukocytosis characterizes infections with this bacterium, and, contrary to a general belief, severe and fatal puerperal fever can be caused by it.

Staphylococci are found on every vulva and in most vaginas before and during the puerperium, but they live as harmless parasites unless their virulence is exalted by accidental conditions. They may cause suppuration in perineorrhaphies, non-union of cervix tears, and are responsible for many cases of parametric abscesses and of slow pyemia, but, as was said, they may cause any and all the forms of puerperal fever which the streptococcus can produce.

Bacillus coli, or the colon bacillus, is the exponent of a group of organisms inhabiting the intestinal tract, and has been repeatedly found in fatal cases of puerperal infection. In one case it was introduced by the gauze used for the packing of the uterus, the patient having a diarrheal evacuation at the time, unobserved by the operator. Gebhard demonstrated the Bacillus coli in a case of tympania uteri which I had the privilege of observing, and Widal, Bar, Durante, and von Franquè have proved it causative of puerperal infections. Bar called attention to the "colibacillose gravidique," which manifests itself as appendicitis, cholecystitis, or uteropyelonephritis. It may cause general septicemia, with or without metastases, endocarditis (Rendu), meningitis, otitis, peritonitis (but the local symptoms are minimal), and phlegmasia alba dolens (Jeannin). Usually the infection is local, causing decomposition and suppuration, with fetid lochia and toxinemia. It is often associated with the streptococcus, and the symbiosis exalts the virulence of the latter decidedly (Bar and Tissier).

The *gonococcus* was proved by Krönig, in 1894, to be responsible for many cases of puerperal infection. It acts in two ways—first, by preparing the tissues for the invasion of other organisms, and by symbiosis exalting their virulence, as well as its own, or it takes a leading rôle itself. In a fatal puerperal infection I demonstrated the gonococcus and the streptococcus in the peritoneal exudate, and in another a pure culture of gonococcus was found. Hallè and Rendu, Harris, and Dabney have shown that it can cause general septicemia with endocarditis. Metastases may occur in the joints, resembling those of pyococcal and streptococcal infections, and in the eye, brain, skin, bones, pleuræ, etc., but usually the processes are local, that is, acute urethritis, endometritis, salpingitis, pelveoperitonitis, parametritis, and ovarian abscess. A latent, apparently cured gonorrhea, may, as the result of the traumatism of labor and the favorable cultural conditions of the puerperium, become acute and progredient. Infections with the gonoccocus develop pus and purulent exudates, the general toxinemia being mild and the course of the disease usually favorable, though protracted. Owing to the slow growth of the organism the morbid manifestations usually appear late in the puerperium.

The above-mentioned organisms, streptococcus, staphylococcus, Bacillus coli, gonococcus, all pus producers, are the most common causes, but other well-known bacteria have been found as the agent of more or less severe puerperal infections. Bacillus pyocyaneus, a dangerous organism for children, rarely causes trouble with the mother, but when it does, the reaction is usually severe, with high fever, much prostration, hemorrhagic diathesis (pyocyaneus hematoxin), and splenic tumor.

Bacillus typhosus.—In 1898 I found, in the uterine lochia of a puerpera who was ill, apparently with typhoid, a culture of the Bacillus typhosus. The Grünbaum-Widal reaction was very marked in her blood. An internist, on the general symptoms, would not make a positive diagnosis of *entero*-typhoid, while the local findings—large, tender uterus—pointed to an infection. The disease terminated by lysis. Blumer and Williams reported similar cases.

The *bacillus of tetanus* has repeatedly been demonstrated in puerperal tetanus (*vide infra*), and the Klebs-Löffler bacillus of diphtheria has been found in true diphtheric exudates on the puerperal wounds. Over 42 cases of true diphtheric infection in the puerperium are on record (Bourret). The streptococcus and the staphylococcus, especially in association with bacilli of the colon group, may produce grayish, greenish, or yellowish pellicles on the vulva and vagina, but these are not so thick as those due to true diphtheria, and they are more adherent to their base. Bacteriologically, they are easily differentiated.

Bacteria of decomposition and putrefaction, of which there is an immense host, may, if given proper conditions—large amount of dead material to feed on, insufficient drainage—produce serious, even fatal toxinemias. They produce poisons, and these, with the by-products of their action on protein being absorbed, cause chills, fever, vomiting, stinking diarrhea, prostration, delirium, etc. Duncan gave the name "sapremia" to this condition, and if thus restricted, it is a term which ought to be retained. Many authors use the term as synonymous with toxinemia from all *local* causes. These putrefactive bacteria are legion, anaërobic and aërophile. As a rule, they possess no invasive power, but under favorable conditions some may break through the leukocyte wall into the lymphatics and the blood. If there is much dead or deeply injured tissue about, they may produce putrid gangrene, as in putrid endometritis, and the absorbed toxins may be fatal. Sometimes living tissue will succumb to the gangrene-producing bacteria and slough off—metritis dissecans.

Gas-forming organisms are often found in cases of fetid and frothy lochia. Dangerous gas builders are the Bacillus coli, the Bacillus aërogenes capsulatus, Bacillus œdematis maligni, which is perhaps identical with the "vibrion septique" of Pasteur and Dolèris, and the pseudobacillus of malignant edema. Of these, the best known, through the labors of Welch, is the Bacillus aërogenes capsulatus. If it invades the tissues, these become emphysematous and gangrenous; if the blood, the vessels are full of frothy blood, and the liver and the spleen become spongy with gas. The body swells up with general emphysema, and there are hemorrhages and icterus. Some cases of so-called air embolism are really infections of this sort. It is rare to find this organism alone—usually the pyocyaneus, the proteus, the colon group, other gas-forming bacilli, and especially the Streptococcus pyogenes, are found in association. If these gas-builders once get beyond the confines of the surface of the genital tract, they usually evince terribly invasive qualities, leukocytosis is scant, and toxinemia rapid and prostrating. The heart is quickly depressed, hemolysis occurs, with jaundice and bleeding into vital organs, the serous surfaces, and the skin. (See Toombs.)

Finally, in many cases of puerperal fever, bacteria have been found which cannot be placed in our present nosology, and many occur which cannot be grown on our known media.

Mention, at least, must be made of the recent work of Kendall, Calmette, *et al.* in the study of an ultra- or filtrable virus stage of well-known bacteria. Soon we may have to remodel all our notions of infection.

Classification of the Forms of Puerperal Infection.—Puerperal fever is a protean disease. As may be seen from the above, many bacteria, single and in combination, may be operative, and these may produce local and general infections, both mild and severe. Women react differently to these various agents—some possess immunity, other a weakness against particular bacteria. Some possess idiosyncracies for the toxins produced by certain bacteria. Diseases of the vital organs alter the general reactions of the system against invasion, and there are many other conditions which make the clinical pictures exceedingly complex, so that a perfect anatomic and pathologic diagnosis may rarely be made. For the same reasons no classification of them so far offered is entirely satisfactory. We may now appreciate the achievement of Semmelweis, since he saw, through the maze of apparently divergent pathologic processes, that they all were due to one underlying cause—wound infection and resorption.

A classification founded on the bacteriology, a botanic or biologic classification, would be the most scientific, but, clinically, this is impractical because—(1) Several (from 1 to 15) different organisms may combine in producing the symptoms; (2) one organism can produce several different forms of puerperal disease and differing degrees of severity; (3) that organism which may be isolated from the lochia or the blood, though it often is, may not be, the cause of the morbid process; (4) it may not be possible to identify the germ which is causing the worst symptoms, or even to discover it at all.

Another classification is that based on anatomic pathologic findings, and which divides the cases strictly according to the parts involved. Thus there are vulvitis, vaginitis, endometritis, parametritis, perimetritis, metrophlebitis, etc. Clinically, this is better, but not all the forms of puerperal fever are localized to the sites at which the infection enters—a general sepsis may occur from a frenulum tear, and any of the germs mentioned may gain entrance at any place in the genitals and produce various and complicated symptom-complexes, and, further, the simple knowledge of the site of the disease is not a sufficient guide to a rational treatment. To say, for example, that a woman has endometritis is by no means enough.

Credè divided the cases into local and general infections, a plan which Olshausen and Bumm, to a certain extent, have followed. Bumm first describes the cases of "wound intoxication," or toxinemia, which is similar to the sapremia previously defined, and then mentions "wound infection," which he divides into—(1) The local processes in the perineum, the cervix, and the endometrium; (2) the spreading of the infection beyond the wound—(*a*) through the blood-vessels, causing septicemia, thrombophlebitis, pyemia; (*b*) through the lymph-vessels, causing perimetritis, parametritis, metritis dissecans, etc. To these should be added surface extension of the infection, *e. g.*, gonorrheal endometritis, salpingitis, etc.

The division of the cases into three forms—*sapremia, septicemia*, and *pyemia*—is an old one, and inappropriate. Sapremia has already been defined. It had better be replaced by the term "toxinemia" or "septic intoxication." Septicemia or sepsis means the invasion of the blood by living ferments—bacteria, which, multiplying there and in the fine capillaries, produce intense morbid changes, either by the toxins or by capillary embolism and thrombosis. A better term is "bacteremia," septicemia being etymologically incorrect. Pyemia literally means pus in the blood, and in some cases it may be appropriate, and if it is understood to apply only to those cases where suppurating emboli break loose from an infected thrombus in a vein, producing distant purulent metastases, it may be retained. It were better, however, to replace it with the term "metastatic bacteremia," because this describes those cases where the bacteria themselves are transported from the infected thrombus. These three clinical forms almost never exist alone, but are combined. It cannot be doubted that in all local infectious processes many bacteria get into and are killed in the blood-stream. The culture of the germs from the blood, therefore, is not positive evidence of progressive bacteremia. In all bacteremias there is also toxinemia, from toxins both developed in the blood and absorbed from the site of entrance of the germ—the wound infection. As was shown above, the streptococcus, the staphylococcus, the colon bacillus, the capsulated gas bacillus, and many others may play the rôle of a saprophyte, or may, as the most invasive infectious agent, cause a mild toxinemia, a deadly bacteremia, or a metastatic bacteremia. It is evident now that a generally applicable single classification is impossible, and for the purposes of nosology in practice it will be necessary to state—(1) The site of the entrance of the infection and its course; (2) the extent of the infection, whether mainly local or already generalized; (3) the kind and degree of virulence of the germ which is causative; (4) the mode of extension of the infection, lymphatic, vascular, surface, or combinations. It may not always be possible to get all this information. Our diagnoses will read like the following examples: Toxinemia from vulvitis caused by Staphylococcus aureus; toxinemia from placental fragments decomposed by saprophytic organisms; toxinemia—and perhaps slight bacteremia—from parametritis—streptococcus; bacteremia from endometritis—streptococcus, virulent; metastatic bacteremia from metrophlebitis—Staphylococcus aureus, mild; septic pneumonia following endometritis, streptococcus, and so on.

LITERATURE

Adami: Principles of Pathology, 1908, vol. i, Inflammation; Charles White and Puerperal Fever, Univ. Press, Liverpool, 1922.—*Ahlfeld:* Zeitschr. für Geb. u. Gyn., 1913, Bd. 73, i, p. 17.—*Aschoff, Louros:* Quoted by Stoeckel Geburtshilfe, 1930, p. 781.—*Batisweiler, J.:* Zentb. für Gynaek., September 26, 1931, p. 2858.—*Benthin:* Zentb. f. Gyn., 1915, No. 34, p. 594; also March 10, 1916, p. 193.—*Blumer:* Amer. Jour. Obst., 1899, vol. xxxix, p. 42.—*Bumm and Sigwart:* Arch. f. Gyn., July, 1912, vol. xcvii, Bd. iii, p. 628.—*Fasbender:* Geschichte der Geburtshilfe, p. 804.   Literature.—*Flexner:* Jour. Amer. Med. Assoc., July 22, 1916.—*Gordon:* Editorial, Jour. Amer. Med. Assoc., June 25, 1921, p. 1843.—*Hadley, P.:* The L. Hektoen Lecture of the Frank Billings Foundation, March 25, 1932.—*Hirsch:* Histor. und Path. Untersuch. über Puer. Fieber, Erlangen, 1864.—*Hoehne:* Zentb. f. Gyn., 1916, No. 1, p. 11.—*Holmes, Oliver Wendell:* "Puerperal Fever a Private Pestilence," Medical Essays.—*Hüssy:* Jour. Amer. Med. Assoc., May 15, 1915, p. 1691, ref.—*Joetten:* Zentb. f. Gyn., 1923,

p. 1200.—*Krönig and Pankow:* Zentralbl. f. Gyn., 1909, p. 161.—*Lash:* Amer. Jour. Obst. and Gyn., September, 1930.—*Lea, A. W. W.:* Puerperal Infection, 1910. Oxford Medical Publications. Gives literature.—*Mauriceau:* Chamberlain's Translation, 1668.—*Mohler:* Circular 198, Bureau Animal Industry, U. S. Dept. Agric., March 2, 1912.—*Permar:* Amer. Jour. Obst., April, 1917.—*Ricketts:* Infection and Immunity, Chicago, 1908.—*Rosenow:* Chicago Surgical Society, January 9, 1915.—*Salomon:* Endogenous Microbism, Monatsschr. für Geb. u. Gyn., October, 1921, vol. lv.—*Schwarz:* Amer. Jour. Obst. and Gyn., April, 1927, p. 467.—*Scott:* Edit., Jour. Amer. Med. Assoc., April 20, 1918, p. 1162.—*Semmelweis:* Gesammelte Werke, 1905.—*Steinau:* See History of Gloves by Ebstein, Monatsschr. f. Geb. u. Gyn., lxxvi, 1927, Heft 1. Literature.—*Toombs:* Amer. Jour. Obst. and Gyn., 1928, 15, 379.—*Trillat:* Jour. Amer. Med. Assoc., January 2, 1915; also Bullet de l'Acad. de Med. Paris, October 22, 1918, p. 369.—*Uhlenhuth:* Zentb. f. Gyn., 1915, p. 47 (ref. Hamm).—*Vaughan:* Jour. Amer. Med. Assoc., February 21, 1914.—*Walthard:* Handbuch der Geb., v. Winckel, vol. iii, 2.—*Ibid.*, Stoeckel's Geburtshilfe, 1930, p. 87.—*Watson, T.:* Lectures on the Principles and Practice of Physic, London Med. Gazette, 1840, 42.—*Weaver:* Jour. Amer. Med. Assoc., January 12, 1918.—*Wegelius:* Arch. f. Gyn., 1909, vol. lxxxviii, H. 2, p. 360. Literature.—*Werner:* Zeitschr. für Geb. u. Gyn., 1914, Bd. 75, iii, p. 521.—*Williams, J. Whitridge:* In Jewett's Practice of Obstetrics, gives literature to 1899; Von Winckel's Handbuch, up to 1906; Zeitschr. f. Geb. u. Gyn., vol. lxix, p. 634, up to 1912.—*Winter:* Zentralbl. f. Gyn., 1911, p. 1501.—*Zangemeister:* Arch. für Gyn., vol. civ, 1917.—*Zweifel:* Doederlein's Handbuch der Geburtshilfe, 1920, Band iii. Literature to date.

CHAPTER LXIV

CLINICAL TYPES OF PUERPERAL INFECTION

EVEN though it is usually impossible clearly to distinguish between a retention toxinemia and an infection or bacteremia, and even though in practice the various forms of puerperal infection to be mentioned may merge into each other, still they often present clinical pictures which are fairly characteristic and typical, and sufficiently sharp for diagnosis, prognosis, and treatment. The following are the forms of puerperal infection most commonly met, being placed about in the order of their frequency: vulvitis and colpitis; endometritis, mild and malignant; retention intoxication (the sapremia of Duncan, or toxinemia, from material pent up in the genitalia); parametritis; peritonitis, pelvic or general; true bacteremia or septicemia; metastatic bacteremia or septicopyemia; phlegmasia alba dolens; endocarditis; tetanus genitaliæ; diphtheria genitaliæ.

Vulvitis.—Causes are traumatism during labor plus infection. Previous disease predisposes—for example, bartholinitis, abscess, fistulas, etc. As a rule, after operative deliveries there are more or less contusion of the parts and many little wounds and abrasions. If a perineorrhaphy has been done, the possibility of wound infection is greater. The alkaline blood and serum permit the saprophytic streptococci and other bacteria to regain some of their virulence, and it is not unusual to find these wounds covered with grayish or greenish exudates, and even superficial ulceration may occur. These are called "puerperal ulcers," and are often accompanied by pronounced swelling of the whole vulva. In from six to eight days the swelling subsides, the superficial sloughs are cast off, pink granulations pushing up to the surface, and epithelization rapidly takes place, scar formation being slight. If the perineorrhaphy wound becomes infected, the parts are swollen, with a brawny exudate; the edges of the wound are red, their line of apposition not united, but separated by pus and sloughing tissue, serum and pus oozing out of the stitch-holes.

Symptoms.—If the drainage is free, there are no marked symptoms. The patient complains of burning on urination, more or less inability to urinate, pain and discomfort from the swelling, with a sense of local heat. The temperature is seldom raised above 101° F., the pulse above 100. If suturing prevents the exit of the infected exudations, or if the infective agent was an alien streptococcus, a sharp chill and fever, even of 104° F., may usher in the disease; the pulse may go above 120, and this may be the starting-point of a general bacteremia.

Vaginitis.—The causes are the same—too much traumatism during labor plus infection. Too prolonged labor, too frequent examinations, the use of very hot douches or of too caustic antiseptics, prolonged application of the colpeurynter, of gauze packing, bruising from brutal operating, cutting by the forceps, by spiculæ of bone in craniotomy, the retention in the vagina of blood-clots, membranes, gauze sponges, etc.—all these favor infection by producing conditions which develop the virulence of the germs normally present in the vagina (for example, the streptococcus and the staphylococcus). If, in addition, alien bacteria are introduced, the woman seldom escapes a dangerous malady, because they find ideal conditions for their growth in the contused tissues bathed in an alkaline blood-mixture containing much dead material, that is, the lochia. Astonishing are the recuperative powers of the vagina in the absence of hetero-infection.

If the vagina were opened to view by specula (which is contraindicated), the usual signs of inflammation would come into view, with many puerperal ulcers discharging purulent secretions. If many injuries had been laid, the wounds will be seen, their edges covered with sloughs, and an infiltration extending around the vagina, even to the walls of the pelvis, and a lymphangitis may also be found. These wounds heal by granulation, with the free discharge of sometimes foul-smelling pus, and leave cicatrices which may extend to the base of the broad ligaments, to the periosteum, or under the base of the bladder, causing fixation and distortion of the pelvic viscera. Alien bacteria, especially the streptococcus, may cause pericolpitis, peritonitis, and even bacteremia. The symptoms are severer than those of vulvitis, especially if the causative bacteria are invasive or produce much toxin. If drainage is free, the general reaction is usually mild; if the discharges are retained (a condition called *lochiocolpos*), severe toxinemic manifestations arise (*vide infra*).

The *diagnosis* of vulvitis is easily made by inspection of the vulva. This is a good place to call attention to the value of the signs present on the vulva indicating infection higher up. Early in the disease the presence of puerperal ulcers may be very significant of grave infections involving the uterus. The infectious lochia washing over the vulvar wounds almost always cause superficial necrosis. As the disease heals the local signs disappear. Again, the vulva heals while the disease spreads above. Vaginitis is never present without vulvitis.

Treatment.—Douches, internal examinations by the finger or with specula, are contraindicated. If the retention of a gauze sponge is suspected, a rectal examination will disclose it. If there are sutures in the perineum, they are to be removed on the first suspicion of an infection. To leave them in the hope of getting a union in spite of the infection is to trifle with an unknown foe, and usually be defeated in the end. If the confined infective exudates do not cause paracolpitis, parametritis, or even general infection, the tissues break down into pus which escapes into the vagina, and the skin only uniting, prolapsus vaginæ and descensus uteri follow, nevertheless. After removal of the sutures and opening up the recesses of the wound widely the latter may be flushed with tincture of iodin, and a thin strip of gauze laid between its edges to keep up drainage. External flushings with a weak antiseptic are frequently practised, but no vaginal douches, since these may carry the infection higher. Ergot and hydrastis, 15 minims of the fluidextract of each, are given four times daily, the bowels are kept free, and hexamethylentetramin, 5 grains four times a day, exhibited, if there is the least indication on the part of the bladder. I often use the latter as a preventive. For the relief of local pain and discomfort a warm 30 per cent. alcohol or lead-water dressing may be used.

Goodall draws attention to mild and severer infectious processes occurring in and around the cervix. These areas he calls "silent" because the sensory nerve-supply is scanty, and therefore local symptoms are missing.

Endometritis.—Very few puerperal infections occur without involvement of the endometrium. Indeed, the cervix and endometrium are the ports of entry to the parametrium, the perimetrium, the tubes, and the shortest way to the blood itself. The reasons for the frequent involvement of the endometrium are: (1) The cervix and the lower uterine segment are particularly exposed to the traumatisms of labor and of operative delivery; (2) the mucous membrane is very delicate in structure as compared with that of the vagina, and it is covered with a layer of dying decidua, favorable to the growth of bacteria; (3) blood-clots, membrane, even placental fragments, may be retained; (4) the infection may have been present in the endometrium during pregnancy (see Microbic Endometritis, also Curtis), or brought there directly by colpeurynter, bougie, or decomposed liquor amnii; (5) shreds of membrane hanging down in the vagina act as a bridge on which the bacteria mount into the uterus; (6) the open vessels of the placental site are particularly favorable to the nidation of germs; (7) if the uterus is flabby and relaxed, stasis of the lochia may occur, a condition particularly favorable to bacterial growth.

It must not be supposed that the presence of decidua or even a piece of placenta in utero means that it will cause an endometritis. The infection must also be present. Pieces of placenta can remain in the uterus for weeks without decomposing, until, after a careless examination, the infection begins.

The importance of a well-contracted uterus was recognized even in the olden time. A uterus that is relaxed absorbs very actively toxins produced in its interior, and again it allows them to accumulate here. A well-contracted uterus expels decomposing clots, secretions, etc., and, in addition, has less absorptive power, since both blood-vessels and lymphatics are held closed. If the uterus becomes bent on itself at the cervix, especially after the sixth day, when the uterus, being strongly anteverted, may catch behind the symphysis, or if retroflexed, under the promontory, the lochia may be pent up, and a condition analogous to lochiocolpos results.

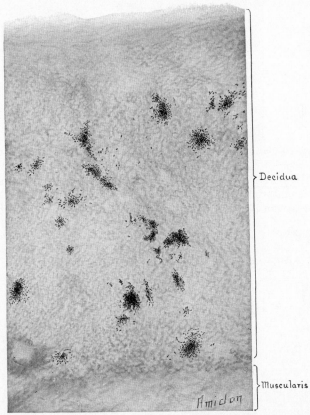

Decidua

Muscularis

Amidon

Fig. 739.—Decidua in Six-weeks' Abortion. Decidua Only Infected. Eosin and Methylene-blue Stain (specimen presented by Dr. Reinhart). See detail in Fig. 740.

It is more common than this, and is called *lochiometra*. It usually causes a severe chill and rise in temperature, which go down just as quickly if the cause is removed.

Pathology.—To avoid repetition, the reader is referred to p. 221 for a description of the puerperal changes in the normal uterus. In endometritis the mucous membrane is swollen, rough, covered with thickened decidua in a state of necrosis, and the surface is moist, with a mucopurulent, sometimes hemorrhagic, smeary material. The cervix is almost always involved in the same way; it is swollen and eroded, and, in addition, the wounds are covered with puerperal ulcers. Involution becomes slower, and the uterus becomes edematous and relaxed, giving the germs ready access to the blood. Bumm distinguished two forms of endometritis—first, that due to putrid or bacillary infection, in which the bacteria were limited to the surface and to the necrotic material there by a protecting bank of white cells and granulations, and, second, a coccal or septic infective form, where the bacteria, usually strepto-cocci and staphylococci, invade the lymphatics and blood-vessels after overcoming the bank of leukocytes and granulations. After examining many specimens I was able to find only one where the bacteria were limited to the surface (Figs. 739 and

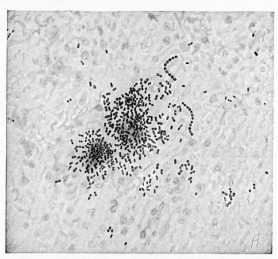

FIG. 740.—BACTERIA IN INFECTED DECIDUA. HIGH POWER. EOSIN AND METHYLENE-BLUE STAIN.

740). In the putrid endometritis the surface of the endometrium is covered with a thick, fetid material, often containing gas-bubbles, and of a grayish or yellowish-green color—even black from decomposed blood. It is impossible to wipe the sur-

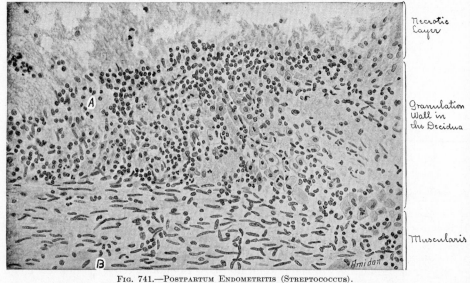

FIG. 741.—POSTPARTUM ENDOMETRITIS (STREPTOCOCCUS).
Granulation wall in endometrium. Hematoxylin and eosin stain. Bacteria have passed through this protecting wall. See Figs. 742 and 743, which were taken from the places here indicated by A and B.

face smooth, as in the normal uterus. If the bacteria are more virulent, they cause actual sloughing of the endometrium, with many superficially ulcerated areas, covered with a diphtheroid (not diphtheric) exudate, and the whole interior of the uterus has a putrescent appearance and odor—putrescentia uteri. Usually the pus cocci and the bacteria of decomposition are here associated. If the gangrene goes deeper into the wall of the uterus, an evidence of still greater virulence of the bacteria (streptococci anaërobes), larger or smaller portions of the lining of the uterus, or even of the muscle itself, may slough off—the metritis dissecans of Garrigues. Schottmüller showed that the majority of cases of endometritis putrida were due

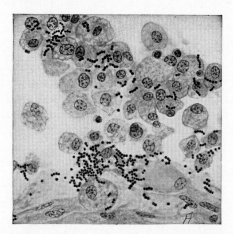

FIG. 742.—STREPTOCOCCI AMONG DECIDUAL CELLS. ENDOMETRITIS POSTPARTUM, GRAM STAIN.
From point A in Fig. 741.

to an obligate anaërobic streptococcus, S. putrificus. He demonstrated this coccus in parametritis and perimetritis, in pyosalpinx, and in the blood of cases which formerly were called toxinemia.

Infections due to Streptococcus pyogenes and the pyococci alone do not give rise to fetor, and the surface of the uterus is usually smooth and not deeply

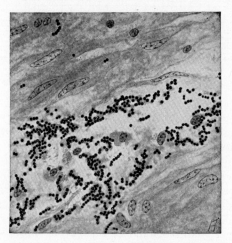

FIG. 743.—STREPTOCOCCI IN UTERINE MUSCLE. ENDOMETRITIS POSTPARTUM, GRAM STAIN.
From point B in Fig. 741.

necrotic. In rare instances the infection is limited to the placental site, being usually mild, due to a pyococcus of attenuated virulence, and producing little local inflammation, but often protracted forms of metastatic bacteremia. (See Pyemia.)

As a general rule, the bank of granulations suffices to limit the infection to the uterus, unless nature's beneficent processes are disturbed by the meddling accoucheur; but sometimes the bacteria, especially the streptococcus, pass on into the lymphatics, causing parametritis and perimetritis, even general peritonitis, or bacteremia, or, through the veins via the thrombi, causing metastatic bacteremia of an acute type. To these forms reference again will be made.

Symptoms.—For the first two or three days the puerpera is fairly well, but an

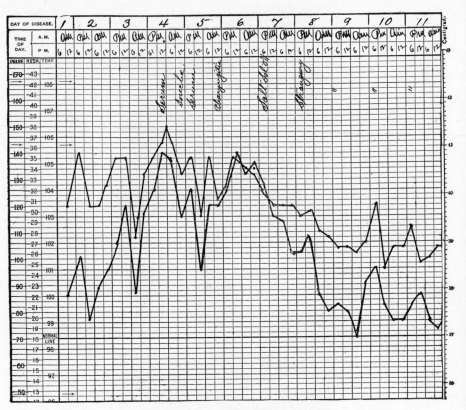

FIG. 744.—ENDOMETRITIS IN PUERPERIO.
A streptodiplococcus was found in the lochia.   Recovery.   Upper line is the pulse.

acute observer will find that there are vague indications of brewing trouble.   Slight malaise, unrest at night, pain in the uterus, prolonged after-pains, or their recurrence after having subsided, will attract the accoucheur's attention.   On the third, fourth, or fifth day there is a slight chill or chilly sensation, with rise of temperature, and all the usual febrile symptoms—feeling of heat, anorexia, insomnia (except in the very mild cases), headache.   Objectively, the accoucheur will find the pulse 100 to 140, and the temperature 101° to 104° F., depending on the severity of the infection.   The abdomen is perhaps a trifle distended, but there is no tenderness; the uterus is usually larger than it should be on the day in question, and softer than normal—that is, in a state of retarded involution.   Rarely is tenderness absent, and the sides are often sensitive to even light palpation.   The lochia at the very first are unaltered, but within forty-eight hours have lost their characteristic qualities and become serous, flesh-water colored, or seropurulent.   Unless saprophytes have developed in large numbers, the lochia are not foul, but they have an insipid or purulent odor.   The lochia have caustic and infective qualities, and soon the wounds about the vulva are covered with a diphtheroid exudate, forming the puerperal ulcers already mentioned.

Unless the infection is very virulent, the symptoms and objective signs are no more threatening than described; the temperature, after pursuing a remittent (1° to 2° F.) course for four or five days (Fig. 744), subsides by lysis, the pulse slows, and in six to ten days recovery is established. If the infecting bacteria are strong enough to overcome the protecting wall of leukocytes, the blood is involved and the general symptoms are marked, the case having become a bacteremia (see below).

Diagnosis.—Endometritis has no characteristic symptoms. With the usual manifestations of infection one finds a large, sensitive uterus, evidences of slight peritoneal irritation, and altered lochia. The vulvar wounds have an unhealthy aspect, except when the endometritis is due to non-virulent saprophytes, in which case these wounds may heal under healthy granulations. If a specular examination is made, the condition of the cervix will be a criterion of the condition of the endometrium. The lochia in the putrid infections are profuse, thick, and foul, while in the streptococcic kinds they are diminished, thin, sanious, with an acrid odor. The absence of signs of peritonitis and of tumor eliminates localization outside the uterus. Prognosis and treatment will be discussed later.

Sapremia, Retention Fever, Toxinemia.—Clinically, a not small group of cases exists with fever and often very threatening symptoms, due to the absorption of toxins from decomposing material in the genital tract. Lochiocolpos and lochiometra have already been referred to. If the toxins were always the result of the action of saprophytic bacteria, the organisms of putrefaction, the term sapremia, proposed by Duncan, would apply. But the streptococcus and other cocci and bacteria may grow in the dead tissue and produce toxins, which are absorbed, and, further, the author would rather agree with Schottmüller, Latzko, and Zangemeister, as opposed to Döderlein, Bumm, and others, that in all these cases many bacteria get into and are killed in the blood. The distinction, therefore, between toxinemia and bacteremia is mainly one of degree, and the term sapremia must be limited to those infections where only putrefactive organisms are present. We use the terms septicemia and sepsis in a very loose way to mean a bacteremia by the pus-cocci, when the Greek original means putridity. We might also thus use the term sapremia, but it would be better to discard all three, which, however, at present is impractical.

When a puerpera develops fever, which by exclusion is found to come from the genitals, the first question that arises is, Is there anything in the uterus? If there is a piece of placenta, a clot, or a mass of membranes in the uterus, the same may not become infected if the uterus is firmly contracted and if no alien bacteria are carried in from the outside. Should it become infected, the symptoms are those of endometritis, and there is always more or less reaction in the endometrium.

Another danger of these infected, necrosing bodies lies in their providing a favorable nidus for the virulent streptococcus, in developing the virulence of weakened cocci, or native bacteria, or in altering the subjacent mucosa, so that it offers less resistance to the microörganisms normally present in the vagina, cervix, and uterus. Bacteremia has often followed, but in most cases the disease remains local, and there is no marked invasion of the lymph- and blood-streams.

Symptoms.—It is impossible to distinguish this condition from an endometritis, since the symptoms are nearly identical. Lochiometra and lochiocolpos are characterized by absence of the lochia. If a piece of membrane or placenta has been retained, the after-pains often continue until it is expelled, after which also the fever and rapid pulse subside. Profuse and very bloody lochia are the rule if portions of the placenta are retained, and repeated hemorrhages or the passage of clots are almost pathognomonic. The uterus is large and soft in such cases. As an aid to the diagnosis the history of the labor is useful, since the placenta may have shown defects, or the prolonged oozing postpartum may have led the accoucheur to believe that there was a clot in the uterus. Since uterovaginal examinations are not permitted, the state of the uterine cavity can only be guessed at. A rectal exploration might reveal a mass in the vagina, or a retroflexed or anteflexed uterus, causing lochiostasis, and the protrusion from the vulva of a shred of membrane or a bit of placenta might indicate that there may be more higher up. Treatment will be considered later.

Parametritis.—Mauriceau, about 1760, first described inflammations of the

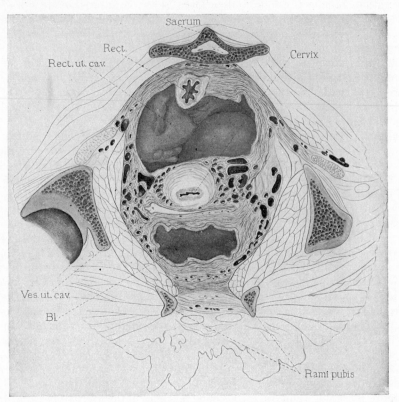

FIG. 745.—THE PARAMETRIUM (VON ROSTHORN).
Section of pelvis. Note immense veins and large meshes of connective tissue surrounding the organs.

pelvic connective tissue, and Velpeau associated them with the genital organs, which Doherty proved in 1843. Virchow applied the term *parametritis* to these pelvic phlegmons, but *pelvic cellulitis* is a better one, because the disease is very seldom limited to the neighborhood of the uterus, but may involve the connective tissue from the vulva to the kidney and, further, it does not always begin around the uterus. Through the researches of Matthews Duncan, W. A. Freund, and A. von Rosthorn, our knowledge of pelvic cellulitis has been placed on firm foundation.

Causation.—As in the other puerperal infections, pelvic cellulitis is caused by bacteria, and these gain entrance to the connective tissue in various ways (Fig. 746). In most cases the atrium of infection is a wound of the cervix or lower uterine segment, but the injury may have been in the vagina or even the perineum. Bacteria may break through the granulation bank in the endometrium, and, passing through the uterine wall by way of either the lymphatics or the blood-vessels, reach the parametrium, and, finally, they may wander into the subjacent tissues from the peritoneum or the tubes, which may be infected.

Nearly always it is the Streptococcus pyogenes which is the causative organism, but the staphylococcus has been found, also the colon bacillus, though usually as a concomitant infection, and even the gonococcus (Menge and Döderlein). Many factors favor infection of the connective tissue in the pelvis after labor. Besides the general softening, the edematous imbibition of the tissues, the enlargement of the connective-tissue spaces, and the increased vascularity due to pregnancy, there is the direct bruising of the parts, with the bloody and serofibrinous extravasations. To these must be added the immediate introduction of alien and native bacteria through lacerations into the opened spaces, by means of the hands, instruments, gauze, etc.

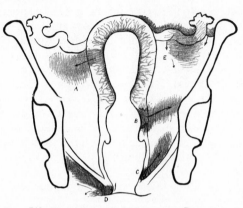

Fig. 746.—Directions Taken by the Bacteria to Reach the Pelvic Connective Tissue.

A, From endometritis through uterine wall; B, from cervix tear; C, from vaginal tear above levator ani; D, from perineal tear; E, downward from peritonitis.

Pathology.—Cellulitis in the pelvis differs very little from cellulitis under the skin or elsewhere. The bacteria, by their presence and the toxins they produce, irritate the tissues, a protective serum is thrown out (inflammatory edema), leukocytes hurry to the scene, the binding cells proliferate and form fibrin, all of which compose an exudate in the infected area. The bacteria pass along the lines of least resistance, and these are the natural planes of cleavage of the pelvic connective tissue, and are limited by firm layers of fascia and by the organs in the pelvis. The inflammatory exudates, therefore, following the infection will extend in certain directions, passing along the planes of fascia, and surrounding and embedding the hollow pelvic organs. Since the inflammatory reaction is sometimes excessive, the amount of serum and fibrin and cellular infiltration may overfill the tissue-spaces, and the exudate itself may wander. On the other hand, the bacteria may select an unanatomic course, for example, through a fascia or muscle, and then the inflammatory exudate will be found where it was not expected. Von Rosthorn's classification of pelvic exudates is the most practical: (1) Lateral horizontal exudates located in the bases of the broad ligaments, with a tendency to spread to the side walls of

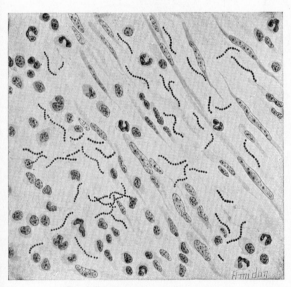

Fig. 747.—Parametritis Puerperalis.
Drawn from a specimen of Dr. Ries'. Streptococci in the tissues.

58

the pelvis and around the cervix; these usually come from cervix tears; (2) high intraligamentous infiltrations beginning near the cornua uteri, forming tumors, rounded above, with a tendency to unfold the broad ligaments and climb up into the iliac fossæ; these usually come from endometritis; (3) exudates in the retrocervical connective tissue, with a tendency to spread either posteriorly along the uterosacral ligaments or sink in the rectovaginal septum; (4) exudates in the precervical tissues, and spreading toward the sides, around the ureters; (5) exudates anterior to the bladder, behind the pubis, with the tendency to rise behind the recti muscles, even to the navel—"plastron abdominal" of the French. Several of these forms may be combined. The most common is the lateral, extending from the side of the uterus to the bony pelvic wall, then anteriorly around the ureter, raising the peritoneum up and appearing above Poupart's ligament. Rarer distributions are: Posteriorly, to the sacrum and up to the kidney, or even to the diaphragm and through it; laterally, out through the sciatic foramen into the thigh; or inside the infundibulopelvic ligament along the psoas, involving the tissues around the lumbar plexus of nerves.

The exudation varies in extent and consistence, depending on the virulence

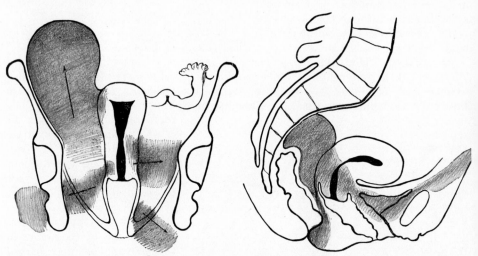

Fig. 748.—Diagram of Course of Infections of Pelvic Connective Tissue.

Fig. 749.—Course of Infections of Pelvic Connective Tissue.

of the germ and the resistance of the patient. In mild cases there is only a simple inflammatory edema, and in the severest cases also the process is limited to a serous and poorly cellular infiltration, the bacteria passing quickly through the lymphatics into the blood. Most often there is adequate reaction, with the formation of large exudates. If a section is made through the inflamed tissues at the side of the uterus, the lymph-vessels will be found thickened, tortuous, and beaded, and a yellowish or whitish pus exudes from numerous fine openings. Around them the exudate lies, and it gives the surface a glistening, glassy, moist appearance. Later, white-cell infiltration and fibrin exudation solidify the tissue and make it opaque. The veins are often thrombotic, and if they were primarily infected, or even if they become so secondarily, the thrombi may undergo puriform degeneration, the débris breaking up and often getting into the circulating blood as infected emboli. The arteries are usually not affected. Later, when shrinking of the scars occurs, the arteries may be kinked, the same being true of the veins, and varicosities may develop, or chronic venous congestion, with its noxious results. Implication of the ganglia and the nerves in the pelvis results in their partial destruction, but more often in neuritis and perineuritis, with recovery or compromise of function.

The peritoneum of the pelvis always takes part in the inflammation; the tubes and ovaries are matted to the broad ligaments or the uterus, and the intestines are adherent to the pelvic masses of exudate. It may be difficult to say whether the parametritis or the perimetritis is of greater moment.

Nature cures these cases in two ways: Either the exudates are reabsorbed or they suppurate. In the latter instance the pus is discharged externally or encapsulated, or complete resorption occurs. If resolution takes place, the exuded fluids are absorbed, phagocytes attack the fibrin and detritus (the dead leukocytes and dead bacteria), and digest them or carry them off. The new-formed connective-tissue cells make the scar tissue, and fibrous bands, and cicatricial thickenings which mark the site of the inflammation. These cicatrices distort the pelvic organs, as regards position, shape, and function. The uterus is sometimes found drawn over to one side of the pelvis, and moored here immovably; or it may be drawn up toward the sacrum by the shortening of the uterosacral ligaments—Schultze's anteflexion,—or it may be twisted on itself. Sometimes the neck of the bladder is pulled open by the retracting scars, causing incontinence or "irritable bladder." Stricture of the rectum may result. Thickenings in the fornices, in the uterine ligaments, with displacements of the uterus, are very common in daily practice and indicate the frequency of mild forms of pelvic cellulitis (Emmett).

If the process ends by suppuration, necrotic areas appear in various parts of the exudate, which become converted into pus. The whole exudate may become one abscess or several, separated by septa. Thus the entire pelvis may be riddled with abscesses. Depending on the location of the exudate and its proximity to one of the hollow organs of the pelvis, pointing will occur, and unless there is operative interference, in the course of from twenty to seventy days the abscess will break into the rectum, vagina, bladder, ureter, skin, or general peritoneal cavity. Then, if there is no other focus of suppuration, the cavity closes rapidly. If there are other foci, these may undergo the same process, and thus the patient may be ill with suppurating cavities for months and even years.

These latter cases and the immense exudates extending to the navel or kidney are very rare nowadays, but in the preantiseptic time they were common. Sometimes the abscess does not open, and nature cures by encapsulating the pus. The wall of the abscess thickens and gets firm with fibrous tissue; the more fluid part of the pus is absorbed, and such a tumor may persist in the pelvis for years, gradually shrinking in size. I watched one such case eight years, and the condition had existed for six years before. A clinically important fact is that the germs do not always lose their virulence, but may, on the occasion of traumatism, exposure, ill health, etc., break out with renewed fury and establish a general bacteremia. Even in the scars from exudates which supposedly had been reabsorbed tiny pus cavities containing virulent bacteria may later be found, a point of immense clinical and medicolegal importance.

Symptoms.—In the mildest forms, traces of which are found during a gynecologic examination as a thickening in one of the fornices, or a displaced uterus, the symptoms during the puerperium are hardly noticeable. A slight rise of temperature, a little local tenderness, and mild febrile symptoms, which are usually referred to something else or to "*milk fever*," may not even call the attention of the accoucheur to the pelvis at the time.

With the severer grades, however, there are marked signs of disease. The symptoms usually begin on the third or fourth day. If the fifth day has passed without symptoms, according to Olshausen, there is little danger. Still, I have seen parametritis begin on the eighth and ninth day. These cases are called *late fever*, and are sometimes due to too early getting up, which starts up anew an unnoticed parametritis, or the movements tear open some small wound in the cervix, or, after some local treatment or examination, these wounds are reopened and infection enters.

Nearly always the symptoms of an endometritis precede those of parametritis, and an acute observer may be able to determine the time when the infection passes the bounds of the uterus and strikes into the broad ligaments. A chill or chilliness, fever of 103° or 104° F., pulse-rate 100 to 110, and marked local pain are constant, together with the general manifestations of the febrile state—headache, anorexia, restlessness, sleeplessness, soreness of the body. All movements, coughing, sneezing, etc., are painful. Nausea and vomiting are unusual, but do occur, and generally indicate that the peritoneum is involved to some extent. They do not persist as in peritonitis. The general impression the attendant gets is that the patient is not seriously ill. Sometimes the parametritis is hidden under the symptoms of a general sepsis. The fever is at first quite continuous, but soon becomes remittent, and later, when pus has formed, it may be intermittent. Now, repeated chills occur, and sweats accompany the defervescence. Unless the pus cavities are freely evacuated, the patient may pass into a condition called by the older writers "hectic," and may die of exhaustion, having wasted to a skeleton. Rapid disappearance of the symptoms follows on proper drainage of the abscesses.

If absorption of the exudate takes place, the temperature gradually subsides, the local symptoms disappear for the time, but later symptoms referable to some pelvic displacement make themselves apparent, and often the patient becomes an invalid for life.

Resolution may require only ten days, while sometimes it may be sixty days before the patient can safely get up. The severity of the local process can usually be determined by the general symptoms, e. g., temperature and pulse, but not always, as sometimes a moderate amount of exudation causes severe symptoms, while again a large exudate will exist with only mild manifestations of disease.

Locally in the early period will be found the large, soft, tender uterus of infection, subinvolution, and at either side of the uterus, deep in the flanks, marked tenderness on pressure, but, relatively to peritonitis, little rigidity. It is not best to make a vaginal examination. When I have done so at this time I found the whole pelvis hot and soft, with one spot, usually the lateral fornix, very sensitive, and an ill-defined thickening present in this region. The lochia may have the appearance of the lochia from endometritis. If the infection entered at the site of a cervical tear, the puerperal discharges may not be much altered. Later the exudate may be palpated as a firm, sometimes almost wood-like, tumor, at the side of the uterus or filling the pelvis more or less, embedding the pelvic organs as one might do with paraffin. If suppuration occurs in the mass, the numerous tiny abscesses fuse together into a large one, palpable to the finger, and pointing occurs. Vaginally, the soft abscess may be felt bulging down one of the fornices, or it may better be felt per rectum. Abdominally, the tumor causes a prominence above one or the other Poupart's ligament, the skin becomes slightly edematous, reddens, and, unless the accoucheur anticipates it, the tissues break down over the abscess and the pus escapes externally. Spontaneous rupture of the pus-sac into the rectum, the bladder, or the vagina seldom occurs before the third week, and, through the abdominal wall, still later. If resorption occurs, the tumor hardens and shrinks, at first rapidly, later slowly, requiring three to twelve weeks, and rarely several years, to disappear.

Pressure of the exudate on the various hollow viscera in the pelvis, and communication of the infection to them, are accompanied by symptoms appropriate to each organ. Cystitis, ureteropyelitis, even hydronephrosis from ureteral obstruction, with uremia and death, have been noted. Œdema bullosum precedes the opening of the abscess into the bladder. Proctitis, with mucous and bloody diarrhea, often precedes the discharge of the pus per rectum. Involvement of the nerves in the pelvis causes neuralgias, and even paralyses of the muscles in the legs. If the infection takes the path along the blood-vessels to the thigh, one of the forms of phlegmasia alba dolens may result (*q. v.*).

Diagnosis.—At first it may not be easy to differentiate this inflammation from others in the pelvis, though the history of cervical injury, the pain and tenderness at the sides of the uterus, with absence of peritonitic symptoms and signs, will render such a suspicion well grounded. When the tumor develops, the diagnosis is usually easy and its discussion will be taken up later.

The *prognosis* is usually good. With proper treatment the patient has a mild course of fever, and absorption of the exudate takes place. Even after the formation of abscesses the prognosis as to life is good, as they either break or are incised and then heal. In the larger abscesses the prognosis is to be guarded, as they sometimes suppurate for months, the pelvis becoming riddled with sinuses, and the patient finally dying of hectic fever and exhaustion.

The prognosis as to health is not so good, because only too often the women have permanent backache, leukorrhea, or disturbed pelvic circulation—dysmenorrhea—and symptoms of uterine displacements. The scars may contract and cause pressure on the nerves (neuralgias and paralysis) or on the ureters, producing hydronephrosis,—which the exudate may also do,—or traction on the bladder, and cause tenesmus and incontinence, or on the rectum, making a stricture. The uterus is sometimes drawn to different parts of the pelvis and fixed, or it is walled up in thick connective tissue and atrophies.

Treatment of Pelvic Cellulitis.—Besides the treatment applicable to all puerperal infected cases, attention is to be directed to the prevention of the spread of the infection and to the evacuation of pelvic abscess, or to means to hasten the absorption of large exudates. Since sitting up and getting out of bed are known to cause extension of the disease, manifested by chill, increased pain, and fever, the patient must lie quietly on her back during the acute stages. Vaginal and intra-uterine manipulations are unwise and harmful. An ice-bag, a hot-water bag, or warm, moist heat may be applied. Cathartics are sparingly used, and if enemata are required, they may not exceed six ounces in amount. Operation is contraindicated in the acute stages, even if the exudates are immense—reaching above the navel. If the symptoms—irregular fever, chills, emaciation—point to suppuration in the mass, or if fluctuation is demonstrated, the abscess is to be opened. As a rule, there need be no precipitation in this matter, experience having shown that it is best to wait until the attack on the pus cavity has become easy and simple. If the mass points above Poupart's ligament, one may wait until the adhesion of the dome of the abscess to the abdominal wall is firm and extensive, thus making certain that the general peritoneal cavity will not be opened. By careful dissection, layer by layer, the tissues are reflected until the infiltrated wall of the abscess is reached. A small opening is made here, part of the pus evacuated, and the finger inserted. A gentle exploration is made to determine the extent of the cavity, and also whether it will be better to drain per vaginam also. If the lowest part of the abscess lies beneath the level of the cervix, the vagina may also be opened from below, guided by the finger in the pus-pocket. It is well to avoid manipulation at the sides of the uterus at the bases of the broad ligaments, because of the large vessels here, and in general to move the fingers about as little as possible to preserve the peritoneum. Tubular drainage through one or both openings is employed. Healing is remarkably quick, unless the operation was done too early, when time may be required for an undiscovered pus-pocket to break into the operative sinus. Cullen recommends to open the abdominal abscesses just above Poupart's ligament, extraperitoneally. If the abscess bulges in the posterior culdesac, it is attacked here. If the abscess bulges down one of the lateral fornices, it should be attacked behind, as near in the middle line as possible, to avoid injuring the ureter or uterine vessels (*vide infra*). Since most cases of pelvic cellulitis heal by absorption, prolonged expectancy is required. When amelioration of the general symptoms indicates that the acuteness of the local process has subsided, the attendant may try to hasten the absorption of the exudates. Hot prolonged vaginal douches, repeated thrice daily, are useful, also the hot-air bath of the pelvic region, recommended by Bier and Polano. Such an apparatus is easily improvised by mounting 8 to 10 electric lights on the inside of a cradle lined with asbestos paper. Gellhorn describes the details of the treatment, which can be heartily recommended. The patient may not leave her bed until the masses have almost disappeared. General muscular tone is to be maintained by massage, but no massage is given the pelvic structures until several months after the patient is up and about. Then massage, gentle at first, watching the effect, may be used to mobilize the uterus and tubes; later, diathermia.

Perimetritis.—Pelvic peritonitis accompanies many forms of local puerperal infection, as parametritis, endometritis, uterine abscess, salpingitis. Since the inflammation is limited to the pelvic peritoneum, we may conclude that the infecting bacteria are of low virulence, and the staphylococcus, the gonococcus, and saprophytes are usually found. Diplostreptococci and pneumococci have been

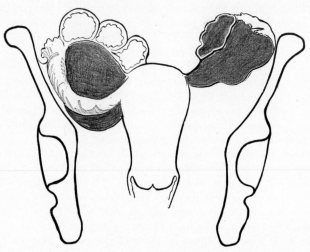

Fig. 751.—Diagram to Show Locations of Peritonitic Effusions. Pus-tube and Ovarian Abscess on Left. Peritubal Effusion on Right. Intestines Form Part of Wall of Abscess.

present, and the Bacterium coli also, either alone or in symbiosis with the others, less often the Bacillus aërogenes capsulatus, the pyocyaneus, and anaërobes. Streptococci of low virulence may cause a mild peritonitis. If of high virulence,

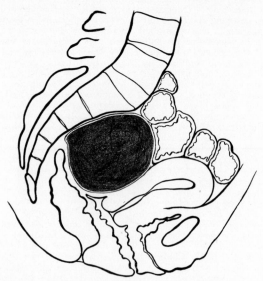

Fig. 752.—Diagram to Show Location of Peritonitic Effusion. Abscess in Douglas' Culdesac. Intestines Form Part of Wall of Abscess.

they quickly invade the whole peritoneum, and may be more quickly fatal than even a bacteremia. The immense surface of the peritoneum absorbs the toxins of the streptococci so rapidly that the heart and nervous system are overcome within a few days or even a few hours after inoculation.

Causation.—(1) Traumatism, as where the uterus is much squeezed or torn, may have a mild plastic peritonitis as a sequel, and the most dangerous infections are likely to follow the introduction of even weak bacteria under such circumstances. In cases of pressure necrosis of the soft parts between the head and the bony pelvis a reactive inflammation usually prevents the spread of the inevitable infection. If a careless examiner should tear the surfaces asunder, or if alien bacteria are introduced, a rapidly fatal process may ensue. (2) Endometritis, uterine lymphangitis, pelvic peritonitis, a sequence demonstrated by Tonnelè, explain most of the cases, and sometimes the bacteria (streptococci) may be demonstrated on their way in the lymph-spaces through the uterus; (3) a parametritis may develop from a torn cervix or vagina, and the bacteria, without meeting a reactive inflammation in the broad ligaments, may reach the peritoneum; (4) gonorrhea may cause, in succession, by surface extension, endometritis, salpingitis, ovaritis, pelvic peritonitis, or a gonorrheal pus-tube may burst during or after labor; unless the streptococcus is also present, such infections are usually mild, with a strong tendency to localize; (5) rupture of an appendical abscess, extension of a perityphlitis to the pelvis, or the bursting of a collection of pus anywhere near the pelvis, may cause a peritonitis localized to this region, or even spreading over the whole serous surface; (6) the bacteria may reach the peritoneum from the veins in the broad ligaments in cases of streptococcus thrombophlebitis. It is clear, therefore, that infection may spread to the pelvic peritoneal cavity in several ways—via the lymph-vessels—the most common,—by surface extension along the tubes, and via the blood, in addition to the inoculation of the serous sac by direct means, the introduction of the bacteria by the hand or instruments, or the rupture of infected pus-sacs.

Pathology.—The pathologic findings are the same as are usual in surgical peritonitis. The peritoneum is reddened, the surface lusterless, the bowels distended, adherent to each other, with deep-red streaks on them where the surfaces do not lie directly apposed, and covered with long strings of fibrino-pus and serous exudate. Between the matted intestines a seropus is found in which float whitish-yellow flakes of fibrin, or the exudate may be all fibrin and pus.

In streptococcic infections the serous membrane may be only reddened, there being little exudate and only few shreds of fibrin. The tendency to localize is not marked. Subperitoneal cellulitis also marks the streptococcic infections, and since it is impossible to drain these spaces, opening the peritoneal cavity offers little hope of cure. Blood may tinge the exudate, which may have an acrid, penetrating odor, stinging the hand immersed in it. If the infection is mild, the reaction of the serosa may limit its progress, which nature accomplishes by throwing out a coating of lymph which binds the viscera together. The tubal ostia are closed, the fimbriæ being matted together. The exudates are thus confined in pockets bounded by adhesions, and take on the character of pus. They may break into neighboring organs,—the bladder, vagina, or rectum, —and they may creep up out of the pelvis, usually on its posterior surface, toward the diaphragm, the way being laid out by an advancing line of fresh adhesions which prevent the spread of the infection over the whole peritoneum. Great care must be exercised in palpating such cases, because rough pressure may rupture the adhesions, flooding the peritoneal cavity with pus, and causing death.

The usual locations for these collections of pus are in Douglas' culdesac, and high up at each side of the uterus, in the fold between the infundibulopelvic and broad ligaments. As they form when the uterus is in the abdomen, and become adherent at the level at which they form, they do not sink with the uterus, and, therefore, are found high up. This distinguishes them from parametritic exudates, which are low, nearer the vagina. The course of these exudates is the same as in parametritis—resolution, absorption, suppuration, and abscess. The latter is more common than in parametritis. The former takes longer than in parametritis, and the organs are left more deformed, bound down, and matted together. Frequently the women are left gynecologic invalids, and are almost always incurably sterile, from closure of the tubes.

If the infection is virulent, the streptococcus, alone or in symbiosis, being the

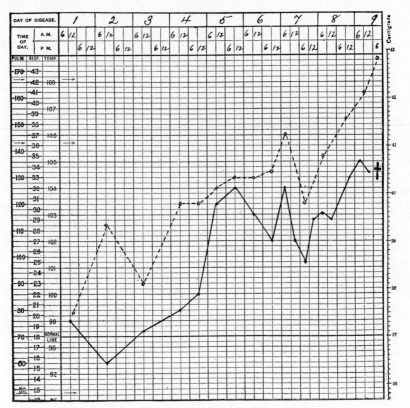

Fig. 753.—Chart of Case of Peritonitis.
Dotted line is the pulse.

cause, its spread is very rapid, involving the whole lower abdomen within a few days or even only a few hours. Seldom is there time for the peritonitis to become universal, because the patient dies from the inundation of the system by toxins rapidly formed, and absorbed so readily from the immense area of surface of the peritoneum. The exudate in cases of general peritonitis may be small or measure several quarts in amount.

If the infection reached the peritoneum from the endometrium, it may be possible, microscopically, to trace the bacteria along the lymph-spaces. At the sides of the uterus, in the larger lymph-vessels, droplets of pus may be found on section, and the peritoneum over the uterus shows the intensest inflammation, redness, and fibrinopurulent exudate.

If the peritoneum was infected by way of the tubes, these are usually dilated, forming pus-sacs; often the ovary is involved, an ovarian abscess resulting, and nearly always the process is mild, being limited to the pelvis, unless improper treatment transports the infection higher up.

Symptoms.—Both local and general symptoms and signs depend on the mode in which the infection reaches the peritoneum. The bursting of a pus-sac is almost always attended by stormy symptoms, which resemble those of ruptured ectopic pregnancy: sharp, severe pain at the site of the abscess, with tenderness, both rapidly spreading over the abdomen, collapse, followed by febrile reaction and the evidences of peritonitis mentioned below. If the peritonitis follows a rupture of the uterus, it resembles in all respects that following a severe operation. Usually the mode of entry is via the lymphatics from the endometrium, and, therefore, the symptoms and signs of endometritis precede those of peritonitis. (See Endometritis.) As soon as the peritoneum becomes involved pain becomes a prominent symptom, localized at first in the uterus and lower abdomen, spreading, in the bad cases, all over the belly. Vomiting is almost a constant occurrence, preceded and accompanied by continuous nausea and sometimes by singultus. The vomit is at first watery, then bilious, and at last stercoral in character, and the action is sudden and expulsive, so that sometimes the bed may be soiled before the nurse can hand the basin. It brings no relief from the intense nausea. Constipation is the rule at first, and flatus is not passed, peristalsis being paralyzed. This paralytic ileus leads to immense abdominal distention and dechloridization. The decomposition of the intestinal contents (by the Bacillus coli, the perfringens, pseudotetanus, and others) leads to an auto-intoxication, which contributes much to the fatal ending. Later in the disease the bowels sometimes loosen, and exhausting, foul diarrheas are observed. Thirst is excessive, restlessness is distressing, but usually the mind is clear until near the end, when either delirium or coma supervenes, or—and this is most ominous—a state of well-being—euphoria—begins.

Examination shows the patient on her back, with the knees drawn up, both to relax the muscles and to take the weight of the bed-clothes off the belly. Her expression is anxious, her color at first reddened, later pale and gray or subicteric. The face at first presents a febrile aspect, but later this is replaced by one of collapse—sunken eyes, cold, pointed nose, cool forehead bedewed with clammy sweat —in short, the typical "facies Hippocratica." Owing to the constant loss of body fluids and the inability to replace them, the tongue soon becomes dry and brown, with fetor ex ore and fuliginous gums; the urine is reduced in amount and contains albumin, casts, indican, and often the bacterium causing the peritonitis. This finding shows that most fatal cases are really septicemias. The temperature during and after the usual initial chill is raised,—often as high as 105° F.,—the pulse becomes very rapid, and, at the same time, of a peculiar snappy character, and later, when the toxins paralyze the vagus and heart muscle, uncountable or filiform. Respiration is quickened and costal, first because of the toxinemia, and, second, because of the immense tympany which anchors the diaphragm high, and, third, because of the pain in the belly. Dilatation of the veins in the splanchnic area causes symptoms of shock.

Râles are usually heard over the lower part of the lungs, and friction-sounds, if the patient lives long enough to develop a pleuritis also. The first sound of the heart early loses its booming quality, the toxins affecting the muscle. Friction may be heard over the liver, but hardly ever over the lower abdomen. Gurgling is absent (aperistalsis), but metallic tinkling may be found. The belly is tympanitic over its lower part at first, and, as the infection spreads, it may be immensely distended. The walls are usually very rigid (defense musculaire) and markedly tender. Deep pressure may sometimes be borne without complaint, but sudden lifting of the hand causes pain. Remarkably, but true, some cases of peritonitis— and these are usually due to pure streptococcous infection—show very little tenderness, hardly any rigidity, and are attended by little pain. It seems that the toxins produced are so caustic that they benumb the nerve-endings, or they quickly bring about general toxinemia and bacteremia, with insignificant local reaction. In such cases of latent peritonitis a diagnosis of peritonitis may not be possible during life.

If the infection is virulent, the symptoms grow worse rapidly, the temperature keeps high until shortly before death, when it drops, the pulse mounting in frequency, the two curves crossing on the chart—the "cross of death"; collapse follows, and edema of the lungs or exhaustion closes the scene.

If the patient is able to withstand the onslaught of the infection, the symptoms and signs are all milder from the very first and are limited to the pelvis. Very soon signs of localization become apparent—the pain begins to subside, the vomiting ceases, the bowels begin to act, the movements having natural color and odor, the general findings improve—the pulse particularly, by slowing, indicating the turn for the better. It is not safe to examine these cases bimanually for several weeks, that is, until the exudates are bound off by firm adhesions and resolution in them is begun. It may now be possible to find a fluctuating tumor in the culdesac or high up, at either or both sides of the uterus. Great care must be exercised in palpating these peritonitic collections. I have seen two deaths result directly from the bursting of such abscesses into the hitherto protected general peritoneal cavity. Should such an accident occur, the belly must at once be opened and drainage above and below established. Prognosis bad.

If the patient recovers, the pelvic organs and intestines are matted together, the uterus distorted and displaced, the tubes kinked or occluded, the ovaries are involved in a mesh of adhesions and develop a tendency to become cystic, and the pelvic circulation, as in parametritis, is disturbed. If a pyosalpinx or ovarian abscess is the residuum, the recovery is never complete. As a result of all these changes the woman usually dates life-long invalidism from her confinement, her symptoms being pain in the pelvis and back, bearing down, inability to do her duties, neurasthenia, sterility, dyspareunia, dysmenorrhea, menorrhagia, leukorrhea, and the signs of pelvic congestion. Mild cases of perimetritis—so mild as to escape the notice of all but the acute observer—may leave such traces, and a goodly proportion of the gynecologist's clientèle is of this class.

Diagnosis.—It is not always possible to differentiate between a parametritis and a perimetritis in the early stages—indeed, they often occur together. Chill and high fever are common to both, but the chill is usually more pronounced in the cellulitis, but the general impression is of a less severe illness. Nausea, singultus, and vomiting, with prostration, rapid pulse, excessive local pain and tenderness, with increasing and spreading abdominal rigidity, point to peritonitis. The exudate in parametritis is usually low down and unilateral; that of peritonitis is higher up and more often posteriorly than at the side; the cellulitis shows a brawny, hard infiltrate, which softens late; the perimetritic exudation is soft from the start. The shape of the pelvic tumor gives useful indications. In cellulitis the infiltrations follow the layers of fascia and the ligaments; in peritonitis, the peritoneal pockets are first filled with the exudates, Douglas' culdesac, and the regions of the ovaries. Pyosalpinx and ovarian abscess usually cannot be palpated out of the pelvic inflammatory masses in the early stages. After a few weeks the parametritic infiltrates are absorbed, and then one may be able to outline the structures. The aspirating needle may be used to discover the nature of fluid in the peritoneal cavity. Don't forget appendicitis in the differential diagnosis.

Prognosis.—This should always be withheld in the early part of the illness, because we are usually in ignorance of the nature of the infecting bacterium and of the road it takes to the peritoneum. Streptococcic infections are particularly fatal: they seldom localize, and the absorption of the toxins is so rapid that the heart muscle and nervous system are quickly overcome. Staphylococcic, gonococcic, and colon infections are much more favorable. All depends on the ability of the peritoneum to wall off the advancing bacteria by the layer of leukocytes, the throwing out of lymph, and matting of the pelvic viscera together. Symptoms and signs which indicate such a process justify us in giving a favorable prognosis. The pulse gives us the most reliable information of what is going on in the peritoneum; next, the general condition of the patient. Low blood-pressure is of bad omen. Slowing of the pulse is a good sign.

Treatment of Peritonitis.—At the beginning it may not be possible to differentiate a peritonitis from a cellulitis, and the treatment, therefore, will be the same for both. If the case starts out as a violent, acute puerperal peritonitis, very little can be expected from any treatment. Simply opening the abdomen in the midline above the pubis, or posterior colpotomy, will not do much harm. If such an incision reveals a ruptured uterus or a burst pus-sac (pus-tube, appendicitis, etc.), appropriate treatment is made; otherwise several rubber gloves for drainage are placed

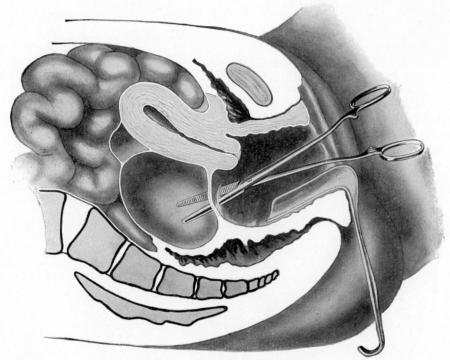

Fig. 754.—Opening Abscess in Culdesac.

radially in the abdomen, one reaching to the culdesac, and a large moist dressing is applied. Some operators irrigate the peritoneal cavity with normal salt solution, but most men are opposed to this, as well as to eventration, because it shocks the patient too much. There is more reason to hope for good from simple drainage and instillation of ether (Benthin). If the course of the disease is milder—more chronic—more may be expected of operation, and it is these cases which give the better statistics—for example, Bumm, 50 per cent.; Leopold, 23 per cent.; Jeannin, 50 per cent. mortality. The gonococcus, the staphylococcus, or a mild streptococcus are usually found here. My own experience with operation in acute diffusing puerperal peritonitis shows only one recovery in 12 women drained, but postoperative cases show much better results. When there is a tendency to localization, it is safer to wait until the abscess has formed and then drain it, usually from below. At present we are experimenting with bacteriophage.

The vagina is exposed by short, broad specula, the cervix steadied, but not pulled down with a vulsellum forceps, and the posterior fornix is incised cleanly with a sharp scissors or scalpel, the tissue to be cut being held by long tissue forceps, and the opening enlarged by stretching with an 8-inch artery clamp. The sac *may not be punched into*—every effort must be taken to avoid increasing its tension, because a delicate adhesion in its roof may give way and pus will escape above into the general peritoneum, an accident which even the immediate laparotomy may not prevent being fatal. After the pus is evacuated one or two fingers may be passed into the cavity, and gentle palpation of the walls made, but it is unwise to try to isolate a pus-tube unless it is within easy reach, when it may be drained through the same opening. An ovarian abscess is treated similarly. The drainage-tube should be left in place for a day after it has ceased to drain, and the opening kept open a few days longer with a bit of gauze. Irrigations are unnecessary and harmful. The patient is kept in the Fowler position for a few days. In the very chronic pelvis sinuses vaccine therapy may be useful. Vaginal douches to hasten the absorption of exudates and the hot-air bath may be used in chronic cases, but are not so successful as in parametritis. Massage may be employed in the latest stages. It is hazardous to remove pus sacs in the acute stages. It is better to use expectancy until the inflammation has quite subsided, relieving immediate danger, if very necessary, by drainage or puncture. If the temperature rises after an examination or a hot douche, the process is still too acute for operation. The blood sedimentation test will also help to decide on the proper time for operation.

Bacteremia is an acute infectious disease, due to the entrance into the blood of microbes, usually the Streptococcus pyogenes, but sometimes of other cocci and

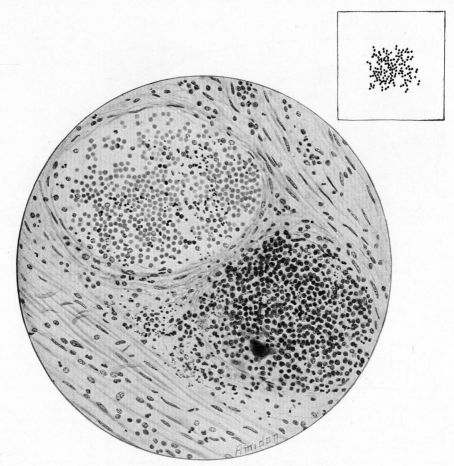

FIG. 755 —UTERINE LYMPHANGITIS.
Above is a clump of streptococci taken from the lymphatic.

bacteria, and their toxins, which produce a dissolution of the blood, degenerative changes in the organs, and the symptoms of a rapid intoxication. The terms "septicemia" and "sepsis," from the Greek σῆψις, meaning decay, have gained such general usage as applied to all forms of severe infection that they will probably be retained. Septicemia is synonymous with bacteremia, which term should replace it. The essential quality of these infections is the invasion of the blood-stream by the bacteria. Most often the streptococcus is causative, but the pneumococcus, the staphylococcus, the Bacillus pyocyaneus, the gonococcus, the Bacillus aërogenes capsulatus, and several anaërobes have been found. Entrance to the blood is

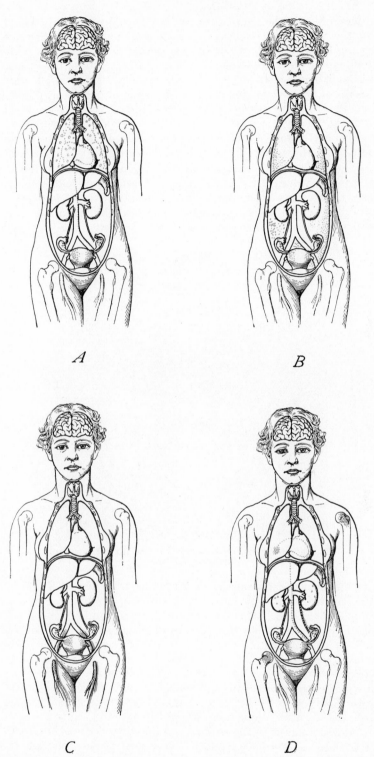

A

B

C

D

Fig. 756.—*A*, Metrophlebitis, Septic Pneumonia, Bacteremia. *B*, Diffuse Puerperal Peritonitis, Pleuritis. *C*, Thrombophlebitis. Double Phlegmasia Alba Dolens. *D*, Metastatic Bacteremia. Septic Emboli in Lung, Kidneys, Thyroid (Rare), Eye (Rare), Joints, etc.

gained in two ways—via the lymphatics, the most usual, and via the blood-vessels, particularly the veins, and *sometimes in both ways at the same time.* Differing clinical pictures are produced, depending on the mode of invasion, and it is often possible to designate the symptoms appertaining to each form. Just as often the pictures are indistinct, partaking of the characters of the two affections. The lymphatic form of bacteremia usually develops from an endometritis, the bacteria passing along the lymph-spaces of the uterus and broad ligaments into the blood, or out on to the surface of the peritoneum, causing peritonitis, pleuritis, etc. The vascular form of bacteremia begins as a metrophlebitis, usually at the placental site, with thromboses in the veins. From these infected thrombi the bacteria get into and multiply in the blood, locating in distant organs—the lungs, the brain, the cord, the joints, the valves of the heart, etc.—in short, a true bacteremia develops. In such cases the local symptoms may be insignificant. A slower form of general infection occurs in the metrophlebitic cases. The thrombi suppurate—a condition not common with the streptococcus—and bits of infected fibrin or microscopic

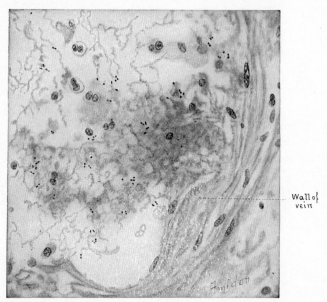

FIG. 757.—INFECTED THROMBUS FROM CASE OF TUBAL PREGNANCY.
Methylene-blue stain.

droplets of pus, or even larger pieces of thrombus, may break off and be swirled away by the blood-stream to the lungs, the kidneys, the brain, etc., where they set up new foci of suppuration. This last disease has been named pyemia, but there is almost never any "pus in the blood." Von Herff has suggested the term "metastatic bacteremia" for this affection. Often it begins as a septicemia, developing the characters of a pyemia later.

Pathology of Septicemia.—A bacteremia may follow an insignificant lesion located at any part of the genital tract. Even a frenulum tear may allow the virulent streptococcus rapid access to the blood. Again, the resistance of the patient may be broken down only after a long fight or after ill-advised local treatment—that is, a process that was limited to the surface is allowed to become invasive. An example of this is the severe bacteremia which usually follows curetage in cases of streptococcic endometritis.

In the lymphatic varieties of septicemia the findings at autopsy are quite typical: (1) Endometritis gangrenosa, or metritis dissecans, often the whole tract being covered by a grayish, sloughing, diphtheroid exudate. (2) Parametritis and lymphangitis, the lymph-vessels at the sides of the uterus being filled with purulent fluid which exudes from the cut surface; the connective tissue may be infiltrated and edematous, and this cellulitis may spread so fast and far as to justify the name Virchow gave it—erysipelas puerperalis malignum internum. The changes in the parametria may be simply a serous infectious edema, or necrosis may occur—a real phlegmon. (3) Pelvic peritonitis, then general peritonitis (Fig. 759.) (4) If the patient lasts long enough, pleuritis and pericarditis. (5) Gastritis submucosa—gastritis, enteritis, and colitis. (6) General pathology of acute infectious disease—swollen spleen, fatty degeneration and cloudy swelling of muscles, and especially of the heart (tiger-heart), liver, and kidneys. Bacteria in immense numbers are found in the minute capillaries and lymphatics of these organs (Fig. 759a). (7) The findings of the metastases in the lungs, heart, brain, joints, connective tissue, and so on.

Even in the vascular forms the lymphatics are usually more or less involved, a periphlebitis either preceding or succeeding the thrombophlebitis. The veins of the placental site are filled with large thrombi, which are swarming with bacteria. The bacteria erode the endothelium of the vessel; fibrin is deposited on the surfaces; the lumen is occluded, and the process advances through the venous plexuses of the broad ligament into the spermatic and iliac veins, even to the cava. From the surface of these thrombi bacteria are liberated in the blood-stream, and if they are strong enough to multiply in it, a fatal bacteremia will result or the lungs are showered with them, a pneumonia developing which may dominate the clinical picture. If the bacteria are less virulent or of a more pyogenic character, the process is more chronic, the thrombi undergo puriform softening, and solid bits or droplets of pus break loose, and, floated by the blood-stream, lodge in distant portions of the body, setting up new foci of suppuration. This condition has been called pyemia, and will be considered directly.

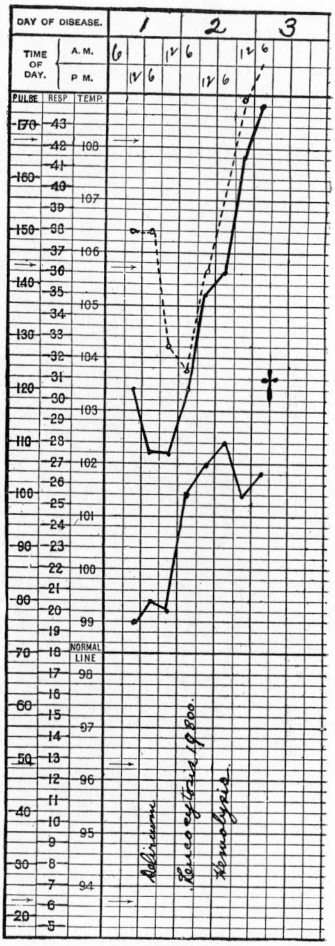

Symptoms.—A period of incubation of from one to three days usually precedes the outbreak of the severe symptoms. In rare cases threatening prodromes appear within a few hours after the inoculation, and the woman gets very sick and may die

FIG. 758.—ACUTE BACTEREMIA. Forehead presentation. Forceps, etc. Lowest line is temperature, dotted, the pulse.

before thirty-six hours have passed (Fig. 758). Ordinarily, the prodromal stage is manifested by the signs and symptoms of the local process from the site of which the bacteria gained access to the blood. The reader is referred to the chapters on Endometritis, Parametritis, etc., for these symptoms. It is often—indeed, usually—impossible to determine when and how the germs get into the blood. Schottmüller, using anaërobic methods, has been able to cultivate the streptococcus from the blood in many cases where the diagnosis of a purely local process had been made. That a serious bacteremia exists will be apparent from the following syndrome, though it must be admitted that the absorption of toxins in large amounts will produce the same conditions.

A severe chill, lasting from five to thirty minutes, ushers in the affection. During the rigor the skin is pale, the lips and fingers cyanotic. There is some resemblance to anaphylaxis; the temperature rises rapidly to 103° or 104° F., and the pulse jumps at once above 120, soon attaining a frequency between this and 160. At first bounding, it soon becomes soft and compressible, the toxins weakening the heart muscle. Owing to the destruction of the red blood-corpuscles the oxygen-carrying power of the blood is diminished, the patient exhibits a marked pallor, and the respirations are hurried. Tympany and peritonitis still further compromise the breathing. Very early in the attack malaise is decided—the woman appears as if stricken down, is apprehensive of a dangerous illness, even of impending death, the change being sudden and significant. Headache and sleeplessness are constantly complained of—the latter, in the absence of sufficient cause, being particularly ominous. While the mind may remain clear until near the end, this is unusual—mild delirium, delirium in somnolence, and often maniacal outbursts characterize the last days. Acute endocarditis is almost always marked by delirium.

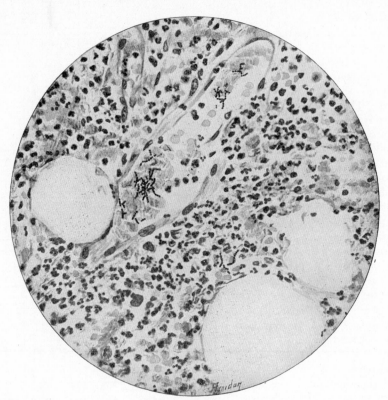

FIG. 759.—PERITONEUM INFECTED WITH STREPTOCOCCI FROM CASE OF PUERPERAL INFECTION. HEMORRHAGIC SEPTICEMIA.

Symptoms of peritonitis—nausea, vomiting, pain, etc.—very soon begin, and the facies Hippocratica shows that the fatal termination is not distant. The lochia are usually profuse and putrid, the result of a gangrenous endometritis, though sometimes the lochia are scant. The odor is not marked, being pungent to the nostril. The puerperal wounds become necrotic. Signs of peritonitis—tenderness, tympany, spreading rigidity, ileus, etc.—begin, and if the patient lives, become marked, and the picture becomes one of virulent peritonitis. While the temperature goes down, the pulse rises higher, and the tongue becomes dry and fuliginous. A peculiar fruity odor—sweet, sickening—may be noticed about the patient. After three or four days the patient feels easier, but the objective signs are worse. Her body is cold, sometimes even the trunk, and bedewed with a cold sweat; she is of a yellowish color, while the translucent parts, for example, nose and ears, are a leaden gray. Consciousness is sometimes retained until a few hours before death, which usually occurs in coma, preceded by edema of the lungs. Oftener, the course is marked by delirium, and in cases where the liver is much involved, the symptoms may resemble those of acute yellow atrophy of the liver (*q. v.*). If the patient lives long enough, a pleuritis develops.

The disease lasts for from two to ten days. It is especially virulent if it begins during labor, when the course is usually short and violent—"foudroyante," as the French say. Eruptions on the skin resembling measles or scarlatina occasionally occur. This has nothing in common with true scarlatina, though the puerpera, like every one, may contract this disease. It may be difficult to make the differential diagnosis. Pustular and vesicular eruptions (containing the infecting organism) are very rare, as also are petechiæ and hemorrhages in the skin, all of which

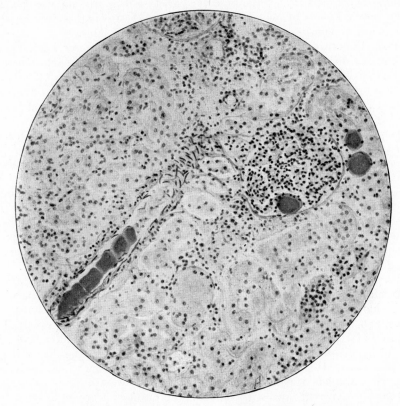

Fig. 759a.—Bacterial Emboli (Blue) in Kidney. Case of Septicemia.

denote a very dangerous form of the malady. A marbling of the skin which shows the course of the superficial veins is of bad omen—it indicates general hemolysis. An erysipelatous inflammation may begin at the vulva and invade a large part of the trunk and legs. Albuminuria is the rule, with casts, kidney epithelium, and sometimes the causative bacterium. Severe diarrheas, fetid and acrid, may still further reduce the strength of the patient. Thyroiditis is not a rare complication. Examination of the blood reveals the streptococcus or other organism in the majority of the cases, especially if the bacteremia is of vascular origin. In the lymphatic forms the toxins from the parametrium and peritoneum may kill the patient, with little invasion of bacteria in the blood. Leukocytosis is usually present, but its absence does not signify much (*vide infra*). There is a hemoglobinemia and an increase of the polynuclears and mononuclears, with a decrease of the

59

eosinophiles and of the reds. The spleen is large (at autopsy it and the bone-marrow show a raspberry color), and, indeed, the clinical picture may resemble acute pernicious anemia or leukemia. There are profound changes in the metabolism.

If the patient is able to overcome the attack of the bacteria, it is evidenced by a degree of mildness of the symptoms and a protracted course of the disease. The initial chill is occasionally repeated, but rarely more than once; the temperature shows greater remissions, the pulse keeps a lower level, the blood-pressure rises, the patient feels some improvement in her condition, sleeps more, her skin becomes covered with a warm perspiration, the peritoneal symptoms subside or do not even appear, the kidneys act more freely, the bowel movements become normal, and the disease terminates, usually rapidly, by lysis.

If embolic processes are lit up, the symptoms and signs are those peculiar to the organ and location of the new inflammations. One way that acute bacteremias terminate—and this is true of the vascular variety—is by passing over into a subacute or chronic state of pyemia. Some authors call these conditions septicopyemia. The diagnosis, prognosis, and treatment will be discussed later.

Septic Endocarditis.—This usually complicates the severer bacteremias, or septicopyemia, but may occur after a mild local affection, or, rarely, without demonstrable local lesions. The bacteria settle on the valves, oftenest of the left heart, causing ulceration of same. The disease is marked by the presence of miliary embolic abscesses in the brain, liver, kidneys, etc. An endocardium that is already diseased is more prone to infection, and chlorosis seems to favor it, too.

Symptoms.—Severe rigor, high and continuous fever, very rapid pulse, cerebral symptoms, muttering delirium, stupor, or even acute delirious mania, and, later, symptoms of meningitis; retinal hemorrhages in 80 per cent. (Litten); Roth's spots (Doherty); diarrhea; hemorrhages under the skin; scarlatiniform eruptions or blisters. The disease lasts from two to twenty-eight days, and often simulates typhoid, presenting roseola, enlarged spleen, and typhoid tongue. The heart-findings are usually equivocal. Sometimes sudden death occurs.

The *diagnosis* is not easy in the absence of a local cause for the high fever and the rapid pulse. Severe sickness, marked nervous symptoms, retinal hemorrhages, repeated chills without determinable emboli, indicate a severe bacteremia.

The *prognosis* is bad. The *treatment* is symptomatic.

Pyemia, septicopyemia, metastatic bacteremia, are all names for a chronic form of sepsis characterized by repeated chills, high fever with deep remissions and intermissions, and marked tendency to metastatic pus-formation. The essential pathology of this form of infection is a metrophlebitis with extension along the veins of the broad ligaments into the spermatic, the hypogastric, and the iliac veins, even to the vena cava, attended by the formation of thrombi, from which bacteria, bits of fibrin, and droplets of pus are released and carried away in the blood-stream, to find lodgment in distant organs, there setting up purulent processes. The thrombi in these infections are large, and undergo puriform degeneration, while in the acute bacteriemia they are not so extensive and do not break down, but supply myriads of germs to the blood. These thrombi are found mainly in the ovarian vessels if the infection, as is usual, gained entrance at the placental site in the fundus. If the main infection is in the lower part of the uterus, or if the placental site was low (placenta prævia), the uterine veins first, and then the hypogastric and internal iliac or the femoral are involved, causing one form of phlegmasia alba dolens (Fig. 756). There is sometimes a periphlebitis around the veins in the broad ligaments, and from this a peritonitis or a parametritis may develop, which extends upward or down the thigh, the latter causing another form of phlegmasia alba dolens. The uterus will show the changes resulting from the attack of the bacteria—either an endometritis or a phlebitis—and involution will be retarded. Sometimes involution is normal, the disease being located only at the placental site, which shows large and infected thrombi. The bacteria involved are again frequently streptococci of a low grade of virulence or the pyococci, but the others mentioned above may also be causative.

Symptoms.—Often the symptoms of a local infection, especially that of endometritis, precede the development of pyemia, and this process may have subsided and the patient already have been called convalescent when the first chill announces a new complication. Again the puerpera may have had an apparently normal puerperium, only a slight evening temperature or rise of pulse apprising the acute observer that something was brewing, when in the second week a chill and fever declare the disease. I have seen this as late as three weeks after delivery. The initial chill is constant, lasts ten to forty minutes, and is followed by high fever,—even 106° F.,—fast pulse, and defervescence is accompanied by a profuse sweat. Subnormal temperature,—95° F.,—even collapse, may ensue. Another rigor may occur within a few hours or the next day, and these are repeated daily for a variable length of time. One of my cases had more than 100 chills. The severest forms of infection have the fewest number of chills, and the number of rigors cannot be foretold. It is believed that each one indicates that a bit of thrombus has broken off, or at least that the blood has gained a new supply of bacteria or toxins or more bacterial albumins. The bacteria are usually most easily found in the blood during the chill (Warnekros), but may be absent until near death, when the case may assume a more septicemic type. It is impossible to locate the embolism of every chill. The temperature is very irregular; the pulse-curve follows that of the fever, unless an embolism occurs in a vital organ (Fig. 760). Leukocytosis is the rule. The course of the disease is very chronic, lasting from three weeks to three months, or even as long as a year. At first the general condition is little affected, but sooner or later the blood suffers, the strength wanes, and a hectic condition and inanition supervene. The skin becomes waxy-gray, the pulse weak and rapid, bed-sores develop, and the patient may die of exhaustion in four to twelve weeks without metastases occurring. Metastases are the rule, however, and they may protract the course of the disease as long as eight months. The most common metastases are:

(a) *Lungs.*—Emboli here are indicated by pain in the chest, cough, bloody, sometimes purulent, expectoration, dyspnea, and the signs and symptoms of pleurisy, abscess, or pneumonia. Later, gangrene of the lung may occur. If the embolus is large, it may plug one of the larger pulmonary vessels and cause sudden death. If the embolus is exceedingly small, it may pass through the large pulmonary capillaries and lodge in the brain, kidneys, etc. If the foramen ovale is patent, the emboli may pass directly into the greater circulation.

(b) *Joints.*—When the joints are affected, the usual signs of arthritis are present. Suppuration and complete disorganization do not always follow; sometimes a serous effusion is the only finding, and it is reabsorbed, but may leave adhesions, contractures, and partial disability. The knee is most often affected, and the large joints usually, but not one is exempt.

(c) *Subcutaneous tissue* anywhere may be the seat of an abscess, which is shown by the usual signs. Fochier noticed that these abscesses seemed to have a curative effect, and he induced them artificially as a therapeutic measure.

(d) *Kidneys.*—Albuminuria is constant in the bad cases. Emboli here are shown by pain, bloody urine, and the usual course of a pyonephrosis.

(e) *Eyes.*—Two forms occur. Retinal hemorrhages, common with acute endocarditis, and panophthalmitis, with complete disintegration of the eyeball.

(f) *Thyroiditis, Parotitis.*—Metastases of the kidney, eye, and thyroid are of very evil omen, but are not absolutely fatal. Meningitis is always fatal.

If the veins of the pelvis are much involved, edema of the legs is noticed, and the abdominal wall veins enlarge for the collateral circulation. Ascites may be present. On the other hand, all three may be absent, with very extensive thrombosis. Gangrene of the flesh of the calves and posterior aspects of the thighs, leaving deep and eroding bed-sores, occurs in very chronic cases, and the puerpera will be made a bed- or chair-ridden invalid for life.

The *diagnosis* at first may be in doubt, but soon the repeated chills, the sweats,

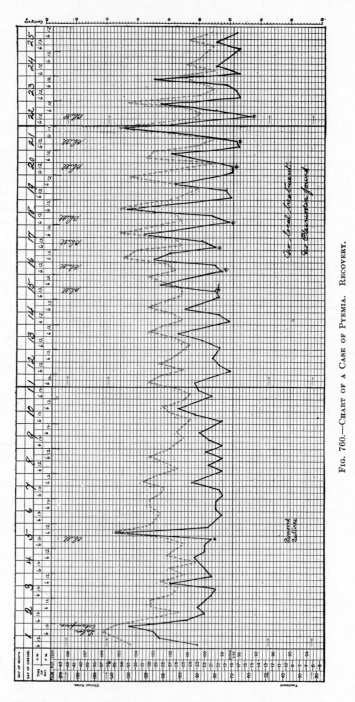

FIG. 760.—CHART OF A CASE OF PYEMIA. RECOVERY.

the zigzag temperature-chart, and the local findings will clear the situation. Vaginally, the uterus may be normal, but usually it is enlarged and slightly tender. At one or both sides the fornices may be found swollen and sensitive; indeed, the thrombosed veins may sometimes be felt as solid, worm-shaped cords. Deep pressure at the sides of the uterus from the belly always elicits tenderness, and the same may be present under Poupart's ligaments. Prognosis and treatment will be considered later.

Phlegmasia Alba Dolens.—This is a term rather loosely applied to several different pathologic conditions. Literally it means a painful white inflammation, and is applied to such occurring in the legs and thighs, although equally applicable to the same condition occurring in the arms. The following forms are observed in practice:

(1) Simple thrombosis of the saphenous and femoral veins or of the iliac, with edema of the extremity beginning at the foot and extending to the trunk, but not onto it, attended by very slight fever, little pain, and, in general, very mild symptoms. The skin is cool, translucent, and mottled, or marbled with distended veins. Puncture would show a thin serum. These cases have been called mechanical thromboses, and have been explained by the stasis of the blood in the pelvic and crural veins during pregnancy and the puerperium, the long rest in the recumbent posture, the anemia, the hyperinosis of pregnancy, marasmus, etc., but the author believes that they are always due to a mild infection, and that it is a rapidly advancing endophlebitis. McLean proved that thrombosis did not occur without infection and Rosenow found a diplostreptococcus in 5 cases of pulmonary embolism. The origin of this infection may be remote from the site of the thrombosis, and may have healed, examples of which, from my own observation, are ulcer of the ankle, mastitis, and infected perineum. At an autopsy in Vienna on a woman who died of pulmonary embolism after a simple perineorrhaphy the pelvic and femoral veins were found filled with clots, and their origin could be traced to the infected wound in the perineum. Many cases of sudden death from embolism are preceded by mild febrile symptoms, rapid pulse, or local symptoms which indicate that disease of some kind exists in the pelvis. Excepting these accidents, the course of the thrombosis is not alarming; the fever keeps a low level, the general health is good, appetite and sleep are but little disturbed, and recovery takes place in from two to six weeks. The disease usually begins after the eighth day of the puerperium, and is caused by an organism of low virulence—either an attenuated streptococcus or the staphylococcus, even sometimes by the bacteria which normally grow as saprophytes in the genitals. This form of phlegmasia occurs not seldom after myoma operations.

(2) Thrombophlebitis of the pelvic and crural veins may be the outward extension of the infected uterine veins, being only a part of a pyemic process, to which reference has already been made, and it may also occur apparently alone. In the former case the symptoms and signs of endometritis or pelvic inflammation precede the pain and swelling of the leg; in the latter case the initial chill is followed at once by the localization in the extremity. Often the intrapelvic symptoms of the early puerperium are overlooked. Usually after the eighth day, and perhaps as late as the twentieth, the puerpera experiences pain in the groin, and at the same time in the calf of the leg. The pain is so great that the leg is immovable. The swelling is noticed first in Scarpa's triangle and in the labium vulvæ of the affected side. The groin is the site of the greatest pain, and sometimes it is possible to feel the thrombosed veins under Poupart's ligament. The upper thigh is sometimes swollen to twice its natural size, has a white, opalescent, or somewhat yellowish tint, feels hot to the touch, is exceedingly sensitive, and pits with difficulty on pressure. Within a few hours or days the whole limb is involved, but sometimes the lower leg and foot seem rather to be edematous, and not infiltrated with lymph. W. A. Freund has differentiated by puncture the lymph of the upper thigh from the serum of the lower leg. The milk-white appearance of the limb gave the disease the popular appellation, "milk-leg"—indeed, the ancients believed it was, in reality, a milk metastasis.

At the beginning a chill may or may not occur, but fever is always present, together with the symptoms of severe illness—i. e., of infection, of a pyemic process. Both limbs may be involved at once or one after the other. The fever pursues an irregular course, with marked remissions; the pulse is usually high, and the course of the disease is very protracted, especially if one limb is involved after the other. Weeks or months may elapse before the signs of inflammation and obstruction of the veins disappear, and the general health may suffer very much. Bed-sores are prone to form over the sacrum and the heels. Even long after the recovery edema of the foot will appear when the patient is much on her feet. In bad bases the inflammation passes over to the arteries; thrombosis occurs here too, and gangrene of the extremity results. If many of the veins of the leg become occluded, the circulation may be stopped, with the same result. Arterial thrombosis may also result from emboli from the valves—endocarditis. Immediate amputation is demanded when the diagnosis of gangrene is made; delay means death, and even amputation may not save. Portions of the calves and thighs may slough off from pressure and poor circulation. Treatment is based on surgical principles. (See Stein, McMalley.)

Pathologically, in these cases one finds the pelvic veins full of firm thrombi, and the inflammation has crept out through the pampiniform plexus to the obturator vein, or even through the hypogastric, to the common iliac, and then backward to the femoral. In addition to the endophlebitis and phlebitis, there is a marked peri-

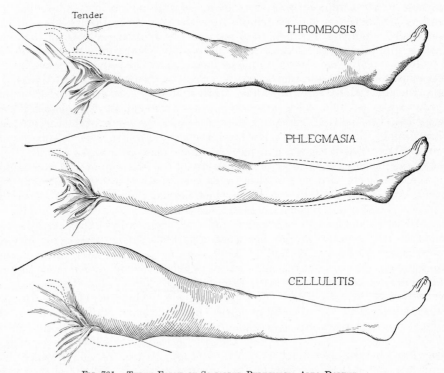

Fig. 761.—Three Forms of So-called Phlegmasia Alba Dolens.

1, Femoral thrombosis with swelling of leg and tenderness over the vein. 2, Phlegmasia alba dolens, with white, tender swelling of whole thigh and later edema of the leg. 3, Crural cellulitis, extension from pelvic cellulitis; red, frequently suppurating, often fatal.

phlebitis with extensive inflammatory edema. The connective tissue around the veins is infiltrated with a gelatinous, mucoid material ("phlegma"), which also fills the lymphatics accompanying the veins. Whether or not there is a lymphangitis or simply a lymphatic stasis with coagulation of the lymph has not been settled— probably both exist. This lymphatic process accompanies the inflammation of the veins as the latter spreads out of the pelvis and down the leg. The large veins are filled with thrombi, partly solid, partly puriform degenerated. The phlebitis may be primary, or secondary to a pelvic cellulitis, and the process may be reversed;

a phlebitis may lead to a cellulitis, and, owing to the proximity of the peritoneum, to a local peritonitis. The clinical picture may then be indistinct, combining symptoms and signs of the three conditions.

(3) *Pelveocrural Cellulitis.*—In this form of phlegmasia the condition is one of extension of a cellulitis from the pelvis. This cellulitis differs from the form described under Parametritis in the rapidity of its spread, its tendency to attack the *subcutaneous cellular tissue*, the lateness of suppuration, if at all, and the severity of its effect on the general system. It resembles the malignant infections of the arm, and is, like them, almost always caused by a virulent strain of streptococci. The infection may leave the pelvis either above or below, and the resulting inflammation of the upper thigh will appear first over Poupart's ligament or in the nates. Swelling, pain, heat, and *redness* characterize this form of phlegmasia, and it often is but part of a general septicemia. Very often, in addition, thrombosis occurs in the crural veins, and then the lower part of the affected extremity swells up with edema, and the picture resembles the ordinary phlegmasia alba dolens more. It may at first be difficult to distinguish between the two forms, but the fact that the inflammation with the swelling began in the upper part of the thigh first and the edema of the foot came a considerable time later,—an observation clearly made by Levret in 1766,—and the demonstration of a pelvic cellulitis, will aid a good deal in the differentiation. Blisters and pustules occur with both forms. Necrosis and abscess are rare with the purely phlebitic phlegmasia, and commoner with the cellulitis. The course of this kind of phlegmasia is rapid and usually fatal, the inflammation involving both limbs, and the bacteremia being pronounced. If healing is to take place, the infection ceases to spread and the general symptoms ameliorate. Abscess formation is a favorable sign unless the whole limb becomes studded with areas of necrosis. Such cases are protracted and serious. The diagnosis is easy, as a rule. Sometimes it may be necessary to shut out neuritis or parametritis, when the thrombosis is deep seated and edema not yet begun.

Treatment.—Prevention. Extreme asepsis in the conduct of all obstetric cases will effectually prevent the vast majority of all the forms of phlegmasia alba dolens. The milder thromboses, phlegmasia of the type first described, may now and again occur with faultless technic, but these are also ascribable to infection, probably endogenous in origin, though many authors believe they are due to stasis of the blood in the veins, prolonged rest in the horizontal position, and alteration of the blood. To forestall such thromboses many authors, especially the Germans, recommend that the puerpera be gotten out of bed as soon as possible after labor— on the second or third day. This is said to improve the circulation and prevent thrombi from forming. I am not strongly in sympathy with such a practice, but give the puerpera much more freedom in bed than formerly, and insist on regular bed exercises. (See Time of Getting Up, p. 354.)

Aside from the general rules applicable to all forms of puerperal infection, which will be discussed later, the treatment of phlebitis and thrombosis requires special precautions. The dangers are embolism and bed-sores. Good nursing is of prime importance. Moving the patient and the affected limb is restricted to a minimum, and is done slowly and with the greatest care to avoid pulmonary embolism. The limb is to be elevated slightly to aid the return circulation, which may be done by means of soft pillows, not rubber covered. For a few hours each day the leg should lie flat, the change being made guardedly. The pad to protect the heel is to be placed under the tendo achillis, and the bed-clothes are to be supported by a cradle of hoops. Drop-foot may be prevented by adjustment of a few soft pillows against the sole. After from ten to twenty days of normal temperature the clot may be considered firm enough, and the patient given a little more freedom, at first tentatively, to see if fever arises—if not, she may carefully get out of bed. When there is great pain in the groin, a light ice-bag or a warm-water bag is applied.

Care is required to avoid freezing and burning, both of which are more likely to occur when the circulation is poor. Morphin may be used for pain. It is important to keep up the nourishment. Later, when the patient gets up, the foot may become edematous. A rubber stocking may sometimes be worn with comfort. Massage of the limb is not permitted for several months after the patient is about. In a subsequent puerperium the thrombosis may recur. For pulmonary embolism see page 862. Homans drained the arteriovenous sheath of the femoral vessels successfully in 2 cases.

Intramural Uterine Abscess.—More commonly than is reported, a uterine lymphangitis or phlebitis results in an abscess within the muscular wall. Such abscesses may be single or multiple, seem to prefer the cornua as sites, and may be the only local cause for the general symptoms, or may be only a part of an extensive local infectious process, as pelvic peritonitis, cellulitis, pyosalpinx, phlebitis. These abscesses may break into neighboring organs—the bladder, the peritoneum, the parametrium, the sigmoid, or the rectum; they may break into the cavity of the uterus, giving rise to a sudden discharge of pus per vaginam, which simulates that of a pyosalpinx, or they may be absorbed or inspissated. The course of the uterine abscess is chronic. The symptoms of the acute stage of the infection subside, and the accoucheur's attention is drawn to this condition by the persistence of the fever, etc. Examination shows the uterus enlarged, and, at some point, a soft, fluctuating tumor is palpable. A soft or suppurating fibroid will give all the symptoms and signs of uterine abscess. Treatment is surgical. If the symptoms persist, the abscess is attacked by laparotomy, but drained if possible from below, otherwise from above, walling off the general peritoneal cavity with gauze and by fixing the omentum to the uterus. A drainage-tube may be inserted into the abscess and led out of the belly, being fastened in place with sutures (Barrows). If the uterus is riddled with abscesses, hysterectomy and free vaginal drainage are indicated. (Lit., Pielsticker.)

Specific Infections.—*Gonorrhea.*—A large number—easily 15 per cent.—of the patients of our public maternities enter with a latent gonorrhea. In private practice the number will perhaps not exceed 10 per cent. Since, with modern aseptic methods, fever is becoming so rare, we conclude that the gonococcus does not play a very important rôle in puerperal infection. Acute gonorrhea is much more likely to spread than the chronic and to become serious, both as regards the mother and also the baby, its eyes, navel, etc. When the disease is latent, the surfaces are usually free from the organisms, the gonococci resting in the crypts of the vulva, the urethra, Skene's tubules, the ducts of Bartholin's glands, and sometimes the cervical glands. If the tubes are already infected, temporary or permanent sterility results. Causes which we do not understand effect an increase of virulence of these cocci; then they spread all over the surface of the parts, even to the uterine cavity, up through and out of the tubes onto the pelvic peritoneum and ovaries, causing pyosalpinx, ovarian abscess, and pelvic peritonitis. This extension on the surface is the rule with gonorrhea, but in exceptional cases the bacteria burrow into the cellular tissue, causing cellulitis, with or without abscess, or into the veins, causing phlebitis, phlegmasia, metastases, gonitis, endocarditis, even general bacteremia—gonococcemia. It is usual to find a mixed infection in these conditions, but there is no doubt but that the gonococcus alone can cause them.

Symptoms.—There is nothing characteristic about gonorrheal infections. Usually the fever begins later in the puerperium than the other infections, because it requires some time for the cocci to attain full virulence and to pass up through the uterus to the tubes and peritoneum. Pelvic peritonitis beginning after the seventh day is almost always gonorrheal. Involvement of a single joint,—the knee or the wrist,—of a very chronic nature, is often gonorrheal; indeed, pregnancy and the puerperium are the most potent predisposing causes of gonorrheal "rheumatism." With the rare exceptions mentioned the symptoms are mild, and apply to the part of the pelvic anatomy which is affected. The course of the cases is usually protracted, which is especially true of pyosalpinges and ovarian abscesses. A collection of pus in the culdesac may be opened when it bulges toward the vagina or the rectum, and healing is then rapid. Deforming scars and adhesions always follow gonococcal infections, and sterility is the usual result. The diagnosis may seldom be made from the clinical course. The finding of the gonococcus in large numbers (rarely in pure culture) in the lochia will indicate the cause of the symptoms, but not positively, because the streptococcus, the pyococcus, or the Bacterium coli in symbiosis may be at the root of the real illness. The prognosis as to life is good, as to health, dubious. The women almost never fully recover if the infection passes beyond the uterus. After many years the tubes may become patulous, and even pregnancy supervene, but, as a rule, the women remain their life long gynecologic invalids and often require capital operations to restore even partial health.

Treatment is based on general principles. Local treatment is absolutely contraindicated in the acute stage. Prolonged rest in bed is imperative. Only after the fever has been absent a week may the puerpera get up. If an internal examination is to be made, it is done very gently. If an abscess is felt in the culdesac, it is to be opened, but not before the surrounding adhesions are very firm. The tubular drain may be removed when the discharge has nearly ceased—usually at the end of ten days; then a bit of gauze is kept in the vaginal opening for a few days. Irrigations of the pus-sac are never made. Pyosalpinges should not be removed, either vaginally or abdominally, for a year at least, and even then only for specially insistent indications. If the pyosalpinx is due to a streptococcous infection, several years may elapse before its removal is positively safe. The sedimentation test should be normal before operation is attempted.

Tetanus.—Nowadays tetanus is the rarest of all infections in the puerperium, but when it does occur, it is of a most virulent type. Pathology, symptoms, diagnosis, and treatment do not differ from those of surgical tetanus. In the differential diagnosis eclampsia must be thought of. Symbiosis is the rule, sometimes apparently favorable to recovery; again, the other bacteria favor the tetanus. Prophylaxis in maternities requires special severity, because, to judge from the experience of one European hospital, when the disease is once introduced, all ordinary means of eradicating it may fail (Pit'ha). If, therefore, one case should occur in a lying-in hospital, the patient had better be removed at once from this institution, and all the rooms she occupied be disinfected in the most thorough manner and left exposed to the elements for at least a week. All instruments and utensils that came in contact with the patient should be doubly sterilized, and all the women exposed to the infection given an immunizing dose of antitoxin. (See Spiegel.)

Diphtheria.—This is rare in the puerperium, and the disease differs in no way, except localization, from that observed in the throat. The membrane, unlike that of the streptococcus, shows a marked tendency to spread all over the parturient canal, and usually leaves no scars. General symptoms of toxinemia are in evidence, and if the streptococcus is associated, a severe septicemia may ensue. Over 42 cases of puerperal diphtheria are on record. I had one. Balard reports an epidemic of 8 cases, started by a puerpera with an innocent sore throat. *Smears* and *cultures* should be taken from every puerperal fever case in order to discover diphtheria. Treatment with antitoxin in maximal doses is indicated, also local treatment. Hospitals are reminded that epidemics of diphtheria occur among the newborn.

LITERATURE

Balard: Arch. Mens. d'Obst. et de Gyn., April–June, 1918, No. 46, p. 136.—*Barrows:* Amer. Jour. Obstet., April, 1911.—*Benthin:* Ref., Amer. Jour. Obstet. and Gyn., October, 1923.—*Cullen:* Surg., Gyn., and Obst., August, 1917, p. 135.—*Curtis:* "Bacteriology and Histology of Endometrium," Surg., Gyn., and Obst., February, 1918, p. 178.—*Doherty:* Jour. Amer. Med. Assoc., August 1, 1931, p. 308.—*Gellhorn:* Amer. Jour. Obstet., July, 1909, p. 31.—*Goodall, J. R.:* Puerperal Infection, Montreal, 1932.—*Homans:* New England Journal of Med., May 14, 1931.—*Kroemer:* "Phlegmasia Alba Dolens," Arch. f. Gyn., 1910, vol. xcii, 2, p. 537.—*Mayer, A.:* Thrombosis from the Standpoint of the Gynecologist, München. med. Wchnschr., January 30, 1931, lxxviii, 179–184.—*McLean:* Chicago Medical Recorder, April, 1923; also *Michaelis:* Zeit. f. Geb. u. Gyn., 1912, Bd. 70, H. 1.—*McNalley, F. P.:* Amer. Jour. Obst. and Gyn., March, 1932, p. 367.—*Pielsticker:* Uterine Abscess, literature, 1916. Zeits. f. Geb. u. Gyn., lxxix, I, p. 74.—*Pit'ha:* Zentb. für Gyn., 1899, No. 29.—*Rosenow:* Jour. of Infect. Dis., Chicago, March, 1927, p. 389.—*Sampson:* Amer. Jour. Obstet., March, 1910. Gives literature on Uterine Abscess.—*Schottmüller:* Zentralbl. f. Gyn., December, 1910, No. 52, p. 1674.—*Spiegel:* Arch. für Gyn., 1914, Bd. 103, H. 2; also Jour. Amer. Med. Assoc., January 2, 1915, p. 90.—*Stein:* Surg., Gyn., and Obst., 1916, vol. xxiii, p. 424.—*Thrombophlebitis:* Arch. Mens. d'Obstet., November, 1912. Literature.—*Thyroiditis:* Ann. de Gyn. et d'Obst., February, 1910. Literature.—*Warnekros:* Arch. f. Gyn., June, 1912, vol. xcvii, H. 1, p. 73.

CHAPTER LXV

DIAGNOSIS OF PUERPERAL INFECTION

Most cases of fever in child-bed are cases of child-bed fever, but this fact must not lead the accoucheur into carelessness in his treatment of feverish puerperæ. Several times I have found the attendant giving intra-uterine douches when the patient was suffering from tonsillitis. In my own experience the following diseases have been mistaken for puerperal infection: typhoid fever, acute miliary tuberculosis, meningitis, acute yellow atrophy of the liver, tonsillitis, pneumonia, la grippe, tuberculous peritonitis, appendicitis, cholecystitis, ureteropyelitis, and mastitis. In practice, therefore, while puerperal infection is the first to be thought of when the puerpera sickens, the patient should be subjected to a complete and careful physical examination, and, by a process of exclusion, the diagnosis reached that the disease has taken its origin in the genitals. It is wise to repeat the general examination at intervals of three or four days to avoid surprises, and early to recognize complications.

After it is certain that the case is one of infection, these questions are to be answered, all being essential to prognosis and treatment: (1) What is the anatomic location of the infection? (2) In what direction is it spreading and how far? (3) Is the infection more general than local, or more local than general? (4) What bacterium is causative? (5) Is there anything in the uterus?

Ad 1: A study of the history of the labor may indicate at once the site of the infection, for example, if the delivery was instrumental, with extensive injury to the cervix, the usual result of infection is a cervicitis followed by parametritis or peritonitis. Perineorrhaphies may suppurate. Manual removal of the placenta is often followed by endometritis and bacteremia, curetage postpartum by bacteremia via the lymphatics, with or without peritonitis, and so on. In addition to the history the site of pain and other local symptoms may point to the anatomic structure involved. Early in the puerperium it is dangerous to make an internal examination, and, further, the information gained is slight. Specular examinations are not recommended. All these manipulations tear open the puerperal wounds, reinoculate the tissues, and carry the infection to parts higher in the parturient canal. Inspection of the vulva, aided by separating the labia to get a good view of the introitus, will give useful information, the condition of the puerperal wounds being a good index of what is going on higher up. (See Endometritis.) Parametritis and pelvic peritonitis are usually easily distinguishable—if not at first, then later in their course.

Ad 2: Ordinarily the spread of the infection can be traced from day to day by the clinical course of the disease. Metastases in various parts of the body give symptoms characteristic to the part affected.

Ad 3: The determination whether the infection is limited to the uterus or has already invaded the blood is not easy—indeed, as was already stated, Schottmüller has proved that in many cases, formerly considered local diseases, that is, toxinemic only, a hemolytic anaërobic streptococcus may be cultivated from the blood. Formerly sterility of the blood was considered evidence that the infectious process was entirely local. Now, unless anaërobic, as well as aërobic, methods and the utmost variety of culture-media are used, sterility of the blood may not be regarded as evidence that the bacteria are restricted to the genitals. In many cases the streptococcus has been found culturally in the blood, the staphylococcus also, as well as other bacteria previously mentioned, and when they are found easily, by the or-

938

dinary methods or in large numbers, one may conclude that a bacteremia exists. For the technic of the bacteriologic study of the blood the reader is referred to appropriate text-books. Clinically, the accoucheur may not be able positively to decide from the symptoms whether he has a purely local infection with toxinemia, or whether the blood is also being disorganized by the bacteria, but in general the severity of the illness is a fair guide. Continuous high temperature, very rapid pulse, severe prostration, etc., point to bacteremia.

Ad 4: It is usually possible to determine what germ is causative—at least the one taking the leading rôle. In order to find out the causative bacteria it is necessary to make exhaustive studies of the blood, as well as of the lochia. A small quantity of the lochia is obtained from the deeper portion of the vagina by means of a simple pipet, and cultures made in all the known bacteriologic media, both anaërobic as well as aërobic. Early tests must be made because the vagina is soon swarming with bacteria. Smears are taken but only the gonococcus may be identified with certainty and this too requires care. Since some strains of streptococci are very virulent and others less so, it is needful to discover which one is active in the particular case. Unfortunately, we are not able to do this. Tests of the virulence of cultures of streptococci on the lower animals are unreliable because the latter do not react as do the humans. Hemolysis in cultures (on blood-agar, for example) has been proved to occur with many kinds of streptococci, and it may betoken a virulent strain. On the other hand, anhemolytic streptococci may be very virulent (Zangemeister). There is some evidence to make us believe that endogenous infections are due to anaërobic streptococci (Schwarz and Dieckmann and Harris.)

The fact that one identifies certain bacteria in the lochia does not permit the deduction that the infection results from that particular organism. If it is found in large numbers, in pure culture, or overshadowing all the others, the conclusion that it is causative may be hazarded, and if, in addition, the same organism is found in the blood, the diagnosis becomes assured. Regarding the streptococcus, Krönig believes that this simple test will enable one to be positive. If a small amount of lochia, inoculated on blood-agar, gives rise to very numerous hemolytic colonies, the puerpera is suffering from puerperal infection. If a finer reagent is used, such as grape-sugar bouillon, streptococci may be grown from 80 per cent. of even normal puerperæ, and the test is less valuable. Occasionally the causative organism may be recovered from the urine.

The gonococcus is easy to recognize in the lochia, and when present in large numbers or pure culture, may be held responsible for the clinical picture. Still, the accoucheur must bear in mind that the gonococcus is frequently associated with the streptococcus and the staphylococcus, and that all, or at least a goodly part of, the disease may be due to the latter. Further, gonococci may appear in the lochia of an apparently healthy puerpera, and their presence may be proved by clinical experience—i. e., gonorrheal ophthalmia neonatorum, the mother remaining well. The discovery of true tetanus bacilli has not yet been made except in tetanus. In one case seen by the writer in consultation diphtheria bacilli were obtained by a competent bacteriologist when neither the appearance of the genitals nor the clinical course suggested diphtheria. In the differential diagnosis of puerperal infections from other diseases accompanied by fever the bacteriologic investigation of the lochia gives only conditional information. For example, if the diagnosis lies between miliary tuberculosis and sepsis, the finding of streptococci in the lochia would not be enough to fix the diagnosis of sepsis. Much more information would be gotten from the blood examination. Here the streptococcus, the finding of the tubercle bacillus, the typhoid bacillus, and the pneumococcus give us dependable information.

Having pursued the investigation of the case along the four lines indicated, the accoucheur may usually make a satisfactory diagnosis. In actual practice other questions arise. One of the most common is—(5) "Is there anything in the uterus?" This has been discussed on p. 895. If the answer cannot be positively made, the case is treated as if there were nothing in the uterus—contrary to older teachings. Another duty of the attendant is the diagnosis of the condition of the vital organs of the body, the state of the liver, of the kidneys, of the lungs, of the heart, of the blood—these must all be watched to discover how they are withstanding the attack of the toxins and bacteria.

If the case becomes chronic, an internal examination is to be made to find any localized suppuration, as pelveocellulitic abscess, perimetritic exudates, pyosalpinx, ovarian abscess, intramural uterine abscess, infected myoma, etc.

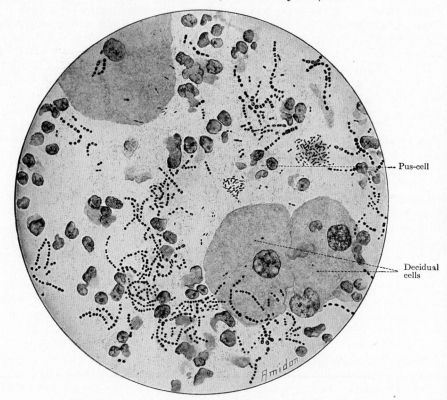

FIG. 763.—LOCHIA IN PUERPERAL SEPTICEMIA. STREPTOCOCCUS INFECTION.
Fuchsin stain. Note the preponderance of streptococci. In acute virulent infections the dominating organism usually does not permit symbiosis.

A word of caution may be permitted here. In all infected cases the utmost gentleness is to be practised in palpating the pelvic structures. Only too easily is the infectious process carried into regions hitherto protected, and also a collection of pus may be broken into the general peritoneal cavity, which usually results fatally, in spite of immediate laparotomy and free drainage above and below.

The differential diagnosis should consider—(1) All the pelvic inflammations, one from the other, and from inflamed tumors (myomata, cysts, etc.); (2) the separation of pelvic infections from those of the urinary system, especially ureteropyelitis; (3) the differentiation from inflammations of other organs in the belly, e. g., the gall-bladder, the appendix; and (4) from all general diseases—typhoid, malaria, tuberculosis, acute uremia, acute leukemia, rheumatism, etc. Obviously, in a treatise of this size a presentment of all these subjects is impossible. Special mention should be made of pneumonia and pleurisy, which may appear as the first symptoms of a uterine infection. Showers of bacteria reach the lungs via the blood.

In considering pyrexia during the puerperium mention must be made of "nervous" temperature. Many accoucheurs and nearly all nurses believe that a puerpera may develop fever from nervous shock or excitement, but such an occurrence has never come under my personal observation. In the dispensary service of the Chicago Lying-in Hospital a woman on the fifth day after delivery, as the result of anger against her husband who drank up their small store of money, and anxiety for her children, who were without food, became intensely wrought up and developed a temperature of 105° F. The nurse brought food for her and her children, and the fever subsided within six hours. No other cause was demonstrable.

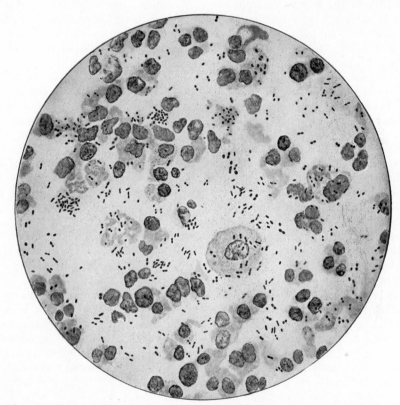

Fig. 764.—Lochia—Saprophytic Infection.

Granting this possibility, it must, however, be emphasized that pyrexia from nervousness is of greatest rarity. Chill and fever after emptying the bladder (catheter fever) occasionally may be noted. Infection is almost always the actual cause.

The Diagnosis of Latent Infection.—Latent or larvated infection means that although the woman has no fever or other signs of illness, bacteria are present in the body, usually at the site of a proposed operation, and are likely to attain virulence or exhibit invasive action if the local barriers are destroyed. This larvated infection is especially to be feared in cases where the vagina is continually supplied with blood, e. g., in protracted abortion, in the stillicidium sanguinis of placenta prævia, or in puerperæ, from placental remnants, the presence of blood seeming to develop the virulence of the streptococci and staphylococci.

Infection may be latent in the parturient canal without bleeding, as we occasionally sadly experience after doing a cesarean section on an apparently clean patient. We can combat practically all the other dangers of abdominal section but this one, which we call the "X quantity" in our deliberations.

In the presence of latent infection all operations are very dangerous, but at the present time we have no certain methods of evaluating the danger. If the course of the case presents those conditions which we know favor infection, *i. e.*, eclampsia and other toxemic states, protracted bleeding, prolonged labor, early rupture of the membranes; if the smears and cultures from the uterus show large numbers of streptococci and staphylococci; if the discharge is unhealthy in appearance; if there are raw places covered with grayish exudates; if there is a slight elevation of temperature—marked leukocytosis or short sedimentation time— one should consider omission or postponement of operative procedure. But usually one will be on the horns of a dilemma, *e. g.*, hemorrhage may command interference, fear of latent infection countermand it. Ruge, Phillips, Koller *et al.* think the laboratory helpful. If there are no streptococci nor staphylococci in the uterus or if those found fail to multiply when cultured on the woman's own blood for three to six hours it is safe to operate.

Prognosis of Puerperal Infection.—Statistics, usually deceptive, are particularly fallacious in puerperal infection. The disease is so protean in its manifestations that it is next to impossible to group cases similar enough to make general deductions from—to say nothing of reducing them to figures. Experience, however, will permit the attendant to give a good or a bad prognosis, and if he has made a complete diagnosis, as outlined in the previous section, much difficulty will be overcome.

Infection varies in gravity with the anatomic part involved, the direction of its spread, the degree of invasion of the blood, and the nature of the infecting organism. Vulvitis and vaginitis are usually not serious—only rarely does the infection break through the natural barriers and get into the blood or travel up to the peritoneum, and this, with the Streptococcus pyogenes. Endometritis is more dangerous, but here, too, the large majority of cases recover, although the streptococcus may be causative, unless improper treatment is instituted. Putrid endometritis, even when there is considerable decaying material, heals rapidly if drainage is good. Lochiometra, responsible for many "one-day fevers," is easily relieved by treatment and almost invariably has a good prognosis. Parametritis, with the exception of the form called erysipelas internum puerperale, which is really but a part of a septicemia, has a good prognosis. Even if the whole connective-tissue framework of the pelvis is involved, the prognosis is good as to life, because if an abscess does not form, nature usually absorbs the exudates, and, further, the bacteria involved are rarely of a virulent type. Perimetritis is more serious, because at the start one cannot say if the disease will remain limited to the pelvis. If the clinical evidence early in the disease seems to indicate such limitation, the prognosis is good and recovery is the rule, since the bacteria are not likely to be virulent (often the gonococcus) and the resistance of the woman is shown to be strong. General peritonitis is almost always fatal. Very few cases of streptococcus peritonitis recover, but even here hope should be by no means abandoned. Bacteremia or general septicemia is, in three-quarters of the cases, fatal. Septicopyemia or metastastic bacteremia is not so dangerous. Bumm complains of a high mortality—80 per cent.—but Schroeder's, Tietze's, Schellenberg's, and mine are more favorable—30 to 50 per cent. These forms of inflammation show that nature is more or less successful in localizing the infection. Indeed, in all cases where the accoucheur detects a tendency at limitation a good prognosis may be given. Spreading infections and invasion of the blood-stream and of the peritoneal cavity are always serious. Phlegmasia alba dolens is usually a favorable outcome of a puerperal infection. The large majority of cases recover unless it be the form of crural cellulitis, which is often fatal.

Much depends on the causative organism. Tetanus is the most fatal of all, hardly any of the women recovering from it. Gonorrhea is the least dangerous of the pus cocci. Saprophytic infections are so varied that we cannot generalize—indeed, some of the bacteria formerly held to be saprophytic have recently been found to possess invasive qualities, for example, the Streptococcus putrificus. Others have long been known to possess them, for example, the Bacterium coli, the gas bacillus, etc. Since the Streptococcus pyogenes causes most of the serious infections, its demonstration in pure culture, or as the dominant organism in the lochia, carries considerable prognostic importance. Unfortunately, it is not easy to determine, as was already shown, whether the streptococcus is of the virulent type, and, further, unless the bacteriologic examination is made early in the puerperium, the organisms may have disappeared from the vagina.

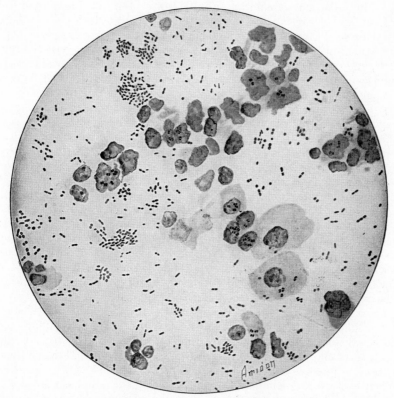

Fig. 765.—Lochia—Gonorrheal Infection.

In judging the severity of any particular case the above information is first considered; next, the apparent severity of the clinical manifestations. If the infection occurs early in labor, develops before it is finished, and does not subside immediately the uterus is emptied—the disease is serious. If the fever begins within thirty-six or forty-eight hours after delivery, the same is true. A single chill at the beginning of the disease is of only moderate significance, but a second chill, or a chill occurring after a preliminary run of fever, indicates graver disease, since these symptoms betoken advancing infection. Repeated chills in pyemia are not a fatal symptom, though very distressing and somewhat ominous. One of my cases had over 100 chills and recovered. Continuous high fever from the start is an unfavorable symptom, as is extreme prostration, both usually indicating a bacteremia. Remittent fever is less serious. Rapid pulse is also bad—a sign of grave toxinemia;

indeed, the pulse is a better indicator of the gravity of the case than the temperature. If the pulse remains around 100, the woman will rarely die. If it goes above 140, the prognosis becomes dubious. A good pulse with volume and force usually means recovery, but if it rapidly increases in rate while diminishing in power, one may decide that the heart muscle is degenerating under the poisoning. A sinking temperature with a running pulse almost always presages death, and since, on the graphic charts, their lines cross, it has been called the cross of death. Restful sleep, a warm, moist skin, and appetite are good symptoms. The advent of septic endocarditis or of septic pneumonia or pleuritis immediately darkens the outlook. Delirium and even the typhoid state are not necessarily bad, but ominous. The general impression on the accoucheur of the severity of the illness, and the feeling of the patient herself, help a great deal in making the decision, but in regard to the latter I must say that sometimes very severe and even fatal cases show remarkable euphoria. This is most common in peritonitis toward the end: the woman feels well, wishes food, and desires to get up, but the Hippocratic facies, the collapse, the thready pulse in a clammy, icy wrist, show that death is not far distant.

Unfortunately, the laborious researches of von Rosthorn, Arneth, Burkhard, von Herff, and others on the morphology of the blood have produced no really useful results so far as prognosis is concerned. Destruction of the red blood-corpuscles and hemoglobin is the rule, which accounts for the pallor of the women and also for the icterus of some cases of infection. In severe toxinemias or bacteremias the reds may sink to less than 1,000,000, the blood-picture being one of acute pernicious anemia. Poikilocytosis and nucleated reds appear in the worst infections. Leukocytosis is the rule, but is of no prognostic significance. There is a physiologic leukocytosis in the puerperium, which may reach 29,000. Absence of leukocytosis shows lessened reaction of the puerpera to the attack of the bacteria, but I have seen recovery take place from severe infection with a leukocytosis that did not exceed 8000. It was hoped that the differential count would give useful data. In health, according to Türck, the relations of the whites are about as follows: Polymorphonuclears, 65 to 75 per cent.; lymphocytes, 20 to 25 per cent.; mononuclears, 3 to 5 per cent.; eosinophiles, 2 to 3 per cent. According to Arneth, increase of the polymorphonuclears indicates an effective reaction against the invaders, because these leukocytes, being older, have strongest phagocytic power. Decrease in the polynuclears and increase in the mononuclears and neutrophiles, with two or three nuclei, show that the bacteria are using up the former, while the blood-making organs are filling the ranks with young leukocytes. The eosinophiles disappear early in the disease. Reappearance of the eosinophiles and increase of the polymorphonuclears may be regarded as a sign of improvement. How far these statements apply in practice is yet to be determined. Agranulocytosis is serious.

When bacteria are demonstrated in the blood, the prognosis is bad, but not necessarily fatal. Lenhartz reports 17 per cent. of recoveries, and Canon 25 per cent. where such were found. If they are numerous and easily discovered by our ordinary cultural methods, and if they are found in all the examinations, the prognosis is worse than if they are few in number and discovered only once in numerous tests. The hemolytic aërobic Streptococcus pyogenes is very fatal, also the staphylococcus (which seems to be exceptionally virulent when it invades the blood), the Bacillus coli, and the Bacillus aërogenes capsulatus.

Albuminuria appearing and increasing is of bad omen, also the presence of granular and epithelial casts. Women exhausted by profuse hemorrhage, by the toxemias of pregnancy, by the shock of severe and contusing operations, debilitated by alcohol, syphilis, tuberculosis, and the acute diseases—all are poor subjects for an added infection.

Finally, in making the prognosis, the state of the previous constitution must be debated. Much depends on the general health of the woman—heart, lungs, and renal and hepatic affections often seriously diminishing her chances of recovery. Normal blood-pressure, or one that rises after being low, with a firm second aortic heart-tone justify a good prognosis, and vice versa (v. Jaschke).

Mortality of Puerperal Infection.—In 1909, in the registered area of the United States, which comprised only 55.3 per cent. of the total population, 7791 women died in childbirth, and of these, 3540 died of "puerperal septicemia." In 1930 in the registered area, which comprised 94.7 per cent. of the total population, 14,836 died in childbirth, and of these, 6087 died from infection. These figures are taken from the mortality statistics of the United States Bureau of the Census. If the same proportion of deaths exists in the non-registered area, it is safe to say that every year there are lost, in the United States, over 7000 mothers from child-bed fever. In reality the numbers are much larger. There is no doubt that women have died from sepsis, and the death reported as due to other causes, either through mistaken diagnosis or deliberate concealment. I do not fear to hazard the statement that 8000 women die annually in the United States from child-bed infections. When one considers that the majority of cases of puerperal infection get well, the conclusion is inevitable that the disease is still—in these modern aseptic and antiseptic times—very prevalent.

In England and Wales, exclusive of Ireland and Scotland, between 1500 and 2000 women die annually from puerperal sepsis, and 2200 to 2900 from the accidents of labor, but Sir. William J. Sinclair asserts that the septic mortality probably varies between 3000 and 5000 per year. Routh believes that the last few years show slight improvement. In Ireland 0.327 per cent. of puerperæ die from infection (Boxall 1903); in Glasgow (1911), 0.57 per cent. In Germany about 6000 women are lost each year from infection, and fully as many more from accidents of childbirth. Von Herff recently called attention to a slight but persistent—and deplorable—rising of the mortality from sepsis, which he ascribes to the lack of aseptic practice *by the physicians* and increase of obstetric operating. Grace L. Meigs points out that puerperal infection has not been decreased in recent years as have tuberculosis, diphtheria, etc., and she shows that childbirth mortality is second only to that of tuberculosis in women of reproductive age.

Without doubt—and to our discredit must it be said—today one woman in 400 giving birth to a child dies from puerperal infection, a humanly preventable disease. In the maternities fatal sepsis has been reduced almost to the vanishing-point. A sharp distinction must be made between the cases delivered in the hospital and treated exclusively by its officers, and those cared for outside, before admission to the institution. With this separation of the figures some maternities show the absence of fatality in successive thousands of cases.

What can be done by the use of an aseptic technic is shown by the results of the obstetric dispensaries—institutions that care for the poor of our large cities in their own homes. Less favorable conditions could hardly be imagined than those in which such obstetric cases are treated, yet the results challenge our admiration. Lea says that in the out-clinic of Queen Charlotte's Lying-in Hospital, London, in 1907–08, 4165 women were delivered without a death from infection. In the first 7000 cases of the Chicago Lying-in Hospital—the dispensary service—one woman died from infection, and there was a series of 3990 cases without death from any cause—that is, of cases handled exclusively by the dispensary staff.

Morbidity of Puerperal Infection.—It is safe to say that for every woman who dies from puerperal infection five others suffer from it, but it is impossible to prove the statement. The morbidity as regards infection is the best available test of the efficiency of a maternity's technic. Statistics from a large number of maternities collected by von Herff and Lea show that 6 to 30 per cent. of puerperæ have fever postpartum, but it is unwise and unjust to make comparisons between these institutions, because—(1) There is no generally accepted standard of what constitutes "fever"; (2) some hospitals take the temperature in the axilla, some in the mouth, and a few in the rectum; (3) some hospitals have trained, intelligent nurses, some midwives, more or less intelligent and conscientious; (4) some hospitals have four-hour temperature readings, others only A. M. and P. M.; (5) many thermometers are inaccurate (I myself have noted inaccuracies of over 1° F.); (6) some authors omit the common initial elevation of temperature to 100° or even 101° F. that follows delivery and subsides within twenty-four hours, while others include it; (7) it is impossible always to separate the cases due to infection from those due to other non-puerperal causes—the statistics, therefore, will always have a subjective or personal bias; (8) some maternities get good material, others the most unfavorable—for example, women debilitated by privation or constitutional disease, heart, pulmonary, or other visceral lesions, gonorrhea, etc.

It is highly desirable that obstetric authorities come to agreement on a standard of puerperal morbidity. Important information could then be obtained as to the relative values of various methods of treatment, of the use and the non-use of rubber gloves, of the vaginal antiseptic douche, of external disinfection, etc. Not until such a standard is adopted may reliable conclusions be drawn from present statistical information, and for this reason the statistics are here omitted. The British Medical Association recommended as standard—"The puerperal morbidity should include all fatal cases and also all cases in which temperature exceeds 100° F. on any two of the bidaily readings from the end of the first to the eighth day after delivery." German authorities adopt 38° C., or 100.4° F., as the normal limit. In my own practice every temperature above 99.5° F. taken with a certificated thermometer, in the mouth, is regarded as morbid; indeed, any rise above 99° F. is viewed with suspicion, and the rise which so often follows labor is also ascribed to an infection and is not held to be a "fibrin ferment fever." In my opinion this postpartum

60

fever is due to the inoculation of the puerperal wounds with the bacteria ever present in the parturient canal; indeed Kulka has found bacteremia in normal labors.

From my own experience in private practice, in practice in the maternity wards of general hospitals, in a special maternity hospital, and in consultation; from my knowledge of the results of my colleagues who treat cases parallel to mine in the same institutions, and from my observation of the work done in maternities at home and abroad; from my studies of the statistical tables of several countries and of a large number of institutions, details of which it is naturally impossible to present here, I have come to the following conclusions: Puerperal infection is still very prevalent—indeed, it is perpetually endemic; it kills 1 in 400 women delivered of full-term children; it leaves as incurable invalids at least ten times this number; although diminished it still occurs in private practice; it is more frequent in maternities that form an integral part of a general hospital than it is in private practice; it is least frequent in the special maternity hospital; it is more frequent in maternities used for the teaching of students than in those not so used, or where only midwives or nurses are taught; it is more frequent in January, February, and March, the time when the general health of the people is below par, when fresh air and sunshine are at the minimum; it is more frequent during the prevalence of la grippe, colds in the head, pneumonia, scarlet fever, erysipelas, bacteremia from other causes (a fact proved by Galabin for England and Wales); it is more common among the delicately bred well-to-do than among the poor, who, through ages of squalor and filth, have developed immunities, which the others in their protected lives do not possess.   Medical practices which are without bad result among the poor would, if applied to the finely bred woman, produce effects horrible to contemplate; it is still carried about on the person of the accoucheur, as a rhinitis or pharyngitis, for example, and, in those times when it seems that an epidemic influence is at work, the cause may be sought in the inefficiency of the means ordinarily practised for its prevention in the presence of numerous alien bacteria.   For example, a certain practitioner, fairly careful and thorough in his aseptic technic, may for years have no infections. Suddenly, when there is a prevalence of streptococcal infections, rhinitis, sinusitis, mastoids, etc., he has a succession of septic cases.   His ordinary methods of prevention are deficient in the presence of extra danger.

It is impossible to learn the number of deaths that occur long after parturition, but indirectly from its action, from operations done to relieve the effects of puerperal infection, or from disease of the heart, lungs, liver, and kidneys, which took its origin in a puerperal process.   Counting such deaths would swell the mortality figures decidedly.   Likewise it is impossible to measure the invalidism suffered by these unfortunate women.   (See Labhardt, Sigwart, Bourne, Bell.)

LITERATURE

Bell, W. Blair: British Med. Jour., May 30, 1931.—Bourne: Recent Advances in Obstetrics, 1926, Blakiston.—Boxall: Puerperal Morbidity, 1903, Sherratt and Hughes, London.—Falls: Jour. Amer. Med. Assoc., November 10, 1923, p. 1590.—Harris: Amer. Jour. Obst. and Gyn., April, 1926.—Ibid., Bull Johns Hopkins Hosp., January, 1929.—Heynemann: "Phagocytosis in the Lochia," Arch. f. Gyn., 1911, vol. xciii, H. 1.—Kulka, Klapsia: Zentb. für Gyn., June 1, 1929.—Labhardt: Halban-Seitz, Biol. und Path. des Weibes, 1927, vol. viii, p. 418. —Lea: Puerperal Infection, Oxford Medical Publications, 1910.—Routh: Jour. Obst. and Gyn., Brit. Empire, October, 1911, p. 165.—Ruge: Abs. Jour. Amer. Med. Assoc., 1923, p. 1657.—Schellenberg: Zentb. für Gyn., 1932, p. 519. Lit.—Schroeder: Deutsche med. Woch., 1930, Nr. 34.—Schwarz and Dieckmann: Amer. Jour. Obst. and Gyn., 1926.—Sigwart: Halban-Seitz, Biol. und Path. des Weibes, 1927, vol. viii, p. 486.—Sinclair, Sir W. J.: The Life of Semmelweis.—Tietze und Plave: Zeitschr. für Geb. u. Gyn., 1932, p. 379.

CHAPTER LXVI

TREATMENT OF PUERPERAL INFECTION

Prophylaxis plays the transcendently important rôle in this disease. So much can be done by prevention and so little by treatment that our efforts should be concentrated on asepsis and on a physiologic conduct of labor.

Much, in a preventive line, can be done during pregnancy to get the woman into perfect condition for the trial of labor. Local diseases, vulvitis, intertrigo, vaginitis, bartholinitis, cervicitis, etc., are to be cured as long as possible before labor supervenes. Zweifel claims that by the use of douches of 0.5 per cent. lactic acid he changed the pathologic vaginal secretion to the acid, flaky, white, or normal, and reduced the incidence of fever in the puerperium by more than half. Coopernail suggested electrocauterization of the diseased cervix during early pregnancy as a prophylactic and H. A. Miller *et al.* report a marked reduction of postpartum infection in more than 2000 cases. It seems to be safe but I have restricted my treatment of diseased cervices to applications of silver nitrate and douches. Appendicitis cases are to be operated on early. The same may be said of salpingitis, but the diagnosis of the latter is harder to make. Suppuration of the ear or of the head sinuses, etc., should all receive appropriate treatment. The patient is to be instructed in the principles of local cleanliness, and coitus and self-examination in the latter months should be expressly forbidden. The gravida should not visit sick puerperæ and should not expose herself to contagious diseases. In the unavoidable presence of one of the above conditions, and during the prevalence of colds in the head, grippal, streptococcal, and other infections, the precautions to be followed during labor are to be redoubled.

Although much experimentation has been done with streptococcal and staphylococcal serums, vaccines, immune bodies, etc., given before and right after labor, no generally convincing results have been published (Lash). In the prevention of tetanus prophylactic injection of antitetanic serum is useful, as was shown by the epidemic in Prague.

Vitamins A and D are said to fortify the gravida against infections.

There are three grand principles in the prevention of puerperal infection: (1) *Preserve the general immunities;* (2) *preserve the local immunities;* (3) *maintain the strictest possible Aseptic Technic.*

The general immunity against infection is strengthened by perfect health, and prenatal care is supposed to provide the parturient with that. During labor the accoucheur is not doing his duty if he does not preserve the woman's forces by getting her sufficient sleep, rest, food, and liquids. Obstetric shock may follow a protracted labor, one in which exhaustion, starvation, and acidosis combine to reduce resistance, and sepsis may be lighted up. Just as important is the prevention of bleeding during labor. "The blood is the life" (Deut. xii : 23), and the woman needs all of hers to fight bacteria, therefore, do not waste a drop. Anemic patients are more liable to thrombosis and embolism.

Credé expressed the second principle: *Limit as far as possible the puerperal wounds.* Every puerpera is a wounded woman. It is good surgery to limit the operative wound and to avoid injuring the tissues, and the same is true of obstetrics. A few concise directions will indicate how this may be done.

947

Limit the number of internal examinations to an irreducible minimum, and make them very gently, so as not to tear the softened mucous membrane. Conduct the labor, so far as possible, by external and rectal examination. The state of the cervix and prolapse of the cord are the only points in labor indeterminable by external examination. In cases of doubt, a vaginal may be necessary, then do not hesitate to make it.

Do not rupture the bag of waters until there is strict indication for it, and let one condition be a completely dilated os. The membranes dilate the cervix with the least trauma, and also mechanically prevent the access of germs to the uterus.

Avoid all measures to shorten the time of normal labor, as manual dilatation of the cervix, of the perineum, or having the woman bear down before the head has slipped through the cervix. Do not give ergot until the placenta has been delivered. Outside of its noxious action on the child, it increases the frequency of operative interference. Do not apply forceps until there is an honest, scientific indication for their use. Do not use douches, especially hot ones or antiseptic ones, in normal labors. These rob the vagina and cervix of their epithelium and their natural protecting secretions. Prevent perineal and vaginal tears, as far as possible, which means a patient conduct of the second stage, but do not allow the other extreme of practice, and permit the head to pound for hours on a rigid perineum until the vitality of the tissues is lost and they are bruised and infiltrated with blood. Early episiotomy and forceps are more scientific procedures.

When a purulent vaginitis complicates labor, antiseptic treatment may be applied with a view to limiting the amount of pus ground into the puerperal wounds by natural and operative processes and it may aid in preventing ophthalmia neonatorum.

The third stage should be conducted as physiologically as possible. Interference should be instituted only on strict indication—above all, manual removal of the placenta should be attempted only when hemorrhage occurs or the organ is pathologically adherent. Great care is to be exerted to obtain the placenta and the membranes complete, as retained portions of either furnish pabulum for the organisms naturally in the vagina, and they retard involution, which, when normally progressing, offers a barrier to infection. The uterus should not be bruised by too early, too frequent, and too strong attempts at Credé expression of the placenta, or too much and too forcible massage.

The placenta and membranes should be carefully inspected, to determine if pieces of the former or shreds of the latter are missing. Such an examination consumes fully five minutes, and should never be neglected. If in doubt, inject milk through the vein of the cord. If a piece of placenta is missing, it must be removed at the time of labor. If a piece of membrane less than one-half of the whole remains in the uterus, I usually do not go in after it. If the uterus balloons out with blood, or if there is external hemorrhage, the cause is frequently found to be such a piece of membrane wrapping up a blood-clot. Removal is then indicated. See that the uterus is free from blood-clots, hard, and firmly contracted before you leave the house. Such a uterus offers resistance to bacterial invasion.

After every operative delivery, and after every breech delivery, and in all cases where there has been a very rapid dilatation of the cervix, examine the whole uterovaginal tract for lacerations. In my own practice I carry out this principle but in cases delivered among the infectious influences of a general hospital and in home service it is best not to invade the parturient channel unless it is positively indicated.

Repair all lacerations of the perineum that are deeper than one-half inch. A large number of cases of infection originate in the perineal wound.

Before introducing the hand into the uterus, in any manipulation, I wash out the introitus and the vagina with bichlorid and lysol solutions wrung out of cotton pledgets, and the hand passes into the vagina under a drenching of lysol solution. This is done to avoid carrying higher, or into the uterus, particles of feces, etc., which may have reached the vagina through the various manipulations connected with an operative delivery.

After the puerpera has been cared for on the lines just indicated, the parturient canal is to be left severely alone. Make no internal examinations, give no douches—practise only external, vulvar antisepsis. Only after the puerperal wounds are well healed may an internal or specular examination be safely made.

The third principle, maintain the strictest possible aseptic technic, was expressed by Credè: "Prevent the infection of the unavoidable puerperal wounds." This comprises the principles and practice of asepsis and antisepsis, and here, after referring to Chapter XX, p. 293, nothing more need be said on this subject. Such a technic should be part of the very body and soul of the accoucheur.

Curative Treatment.—Few subjects in medicine present such diversity of opinion as this one, and, too, owing to the latest discoveries in bacteriology, in the action of bacteria and in immunology, our ideas of treatment have undergone radical changes. In general, it may be said that the polypragmasia of former times has given way to a more physiologic treatment; that we now rely more on aiding and stimulating nature's own methods of combating the disease. The discussion of this subject may be divided into four parts—local, general, specific, and surgical measures—but before considering these, the author wishes to describe the routine treatment he carries out in such cases.

When the careful general medical examination has excluded all other causes for the illness and a diagnosis of puerperal infection is made, the woman is isolated in the lightest, airiest room available, and put at complete physical and mental rest, which means that a good obstetric nurse is put in charge of her. If too poor to obtain proper care at home, she is sent to the best hospital within her means. A laxative is administered; provision is made for a generous semisolid diet, with much fluid; an ice-bag, or, if the patient prefers it, a warm-water bag, is laid over the uterus; the Charles White (1773), commonly called Fowler, position is ordered, and 1 tablet (1 mgm.) t. i. d. or ½ an ampule (0.25 mgm.) of ergotamin tartrate (gynergen) b. i. d. given hypo. for only three or four days. The ergot is given for the purpose of keeping the uterus contracted and hard but with the gynergen one must watch sharply for ergotism (pallor, dizziness, bradycardia, nausea, acrocyanosis, etc.). This prevents the absorption of toxins and bacteria, and expels clots, membrane and lochia, but Louros, from his experiments on mice, believes that ergotamin also helps to cure infection directly, by stimulating the reticuloendothelial system.

If there is any foreign matter in the uterus—clots, secundines, lochiometra— I try to aid its expulsion with medicines: quinin, gr. iij every hour for 5 doses, then one ampoule of pituitary extract every two hours for 3 to 5 doses. Hofbauer believes the latter has a specific curative power in sepsis.

The invasion of an infected puerperal uterus is one of the most dangerous of obstetric operations. (See Köhler, Sigwart.) A little of the lochia is sent to a laboratory for bacteriologic analysis. Sutures in the perineum and cervix are removed at once, to provide free drainage, and the gaping wounds swabbed with pure tincture of iodin, but this is the extent of the local treatment. Developments are then awaited. Even if it is certain that there is something in the uterine cavity, the uterus is not invaded. Curetage, ecouvillonage (brushing out the uterus), douches, packing, etc., are not employed. The sole indication for local treatment is hemorrhage from the uterus. If the woman does not show immediate improvement, the various specific remedies are considered (*vide infra*). When the course of the disease becomes chronic, the patient is carefully watched for signs of localization of the infection, and in a very few cases this point is attacked by operation.

This policy of non-interference—this nihilism with respect to active local and general measures—is the result of my experience in the Dispensary Service of the Chicago Lying-in Hospital. In a series of 25,560 full term deliveries about 10 per cent. had fever over 100° F. In only one case was the uterine cavity invaded and a douche given; in the others we followed the plan above outlined, and only 9 women died of infection, but 5 of these died under questionable treatment in other hands. In none of these cases did the subsequent course show that the event might have been different had a more active policy been followed. With the thoughtful clinician the article of Mermann (Arch. f. Gyn., 1907, vol. iv) carries great weight. Mermann, in 330 cases of fever of all grades of severity, and treated purely expectantly, lost only 7 women. In 30 of the cases the disease was critical, and, even using these only for comparison, the results compare favorably with all other methods of treatment. On the other hand, I can recall numerous cases where, before adopting the above methods, I caused severe illness by active local treatment, and I am not sure but what some of the women died because of the curetage, pelvic drainage, etc., intended for their relief. This has been the experience of my colleagues, working in the same hospitals with me, and whose results I have been able to follow.

Local Treatment.—The local treatment of infection is the attempt to remove the offending bacteria and their toxins, to take away their pabulum—clots, membranes, placental fragments, decidua—and to destroy those bacteria and neutralize those toxins which remain in the genital canal after the mechanical cleansing. The idea is excellent, but experience has shown it is unsuccessful and dangerous. In the hope of accomplishing these purposes the following methods are practised:

(1) Intra-uterine douches of normal salt solution or of antiseptic solutions, such as bichlorid of mercury, lysol, carbolic acid, alcohol, iodin, etc., if the attendant believes that such remedies have real bactericidal action on germs already inside the living tissues. Harvey knew about douches, but Ruleau, in 1704, first used them for fetid lochia. They enjoyed the greatest vogue in the years 1881 to 1900, often being given in normal puerperæ as a routine, but lately have lost, in large part, the confidence of the accoucheurs. The objections to the uterine douche are—(a) It is inefficient, the bacteria being beyond reach within fifteen minutes after they are inoculated; (b) it is painful, sometimes violent uterine action being set up, and if (c), as sometimes happens, part of the liquid escapes through the tubes into the peritoneal cavity, syncope, vomiting, and peritonitis may result; (d) the nervous shock sometimes causes syncope, even convulsions, and coma (Bar); (e) the antiseptic employed may be directly poisonous, over 50 cases of bichlorid and as many more from carbolic acid poisoning being on record, the chemical being absorbed by the uterus, or gaining entrance to the blood through the sinuses (I know of two which have not been recorded); (f) air-embolism; (g) perforation of the uterus; (h) profuse hemorrhage; (i) chill and fever—the infection having been reinoculated by the douche; (j) sudden death, which is usually from air-embolism, but may be due to cardiac paralysis; (k) the infection may be carried up higher in the parturient canal, heretofore unaffected.

Continuous irrigation of the uterus was recommended in 1877 by Schücking. It had some vogue, and until very recently was occasionally practised. The Carrel-Dakin method, continual disinfection with hypochlorite solution, has not qualified.

(2) Swabbing out the uterus with gauze wound around a long dressing forceps, with or without antiseptic or caustic solutions. Alcohol, carbolic acid, iodin, and combinations of these have been used.

(3) Brushing the surface of the endometrium with a round brush, similar to those which are used for cleansing bottles (ecouvillonage). Introduced by Doléris, it was quite popular with French accoucheurs, and is recommended by Lea as safe and efficient. The Germans do not use the brush, nor do American obstetricians. I regard it as dangerous, but perhaps not so much so as the curet.

(4) *Curage*, or digital removal of the contents of the uterus, is recommended by a large number of authorities here and abroad, among whom a few may be mentioned: Hirst, Galabin, Jellett, Sinclair, Bumm, Chrobak, Ahlfeld, Schauta, Bar, Pinard, and Pestalozza.

(5) *Curetage.*—This operation, introduced in 1850 by Recamier, who invented the curet for the purpose, had a very generalized employment, but now is almost passé. It has always had opponents, prominently among the earliest of whom may be mentioned Karl Schröder, and lately many authorities are arrayed against the practice—Walthard, Williams, Noble, Cragin, Edgar, Watkins, Ries, Bumm, Leopold, Fehling, Krönig, Veit, Olshausen, and others, some of whom formerly advised the procedure. The dangers of curetage—and these are present with both blunt and sharp instruments—and of curage with the finger are: (a) The delicate bank of leukocytes, the wall nature throws up to limit the spread of the bacteria, is broken through at innumerable places, and the bacteria literally ground into the lymph-spaces and the venous

lumina—it is a thorough vaccination or inoculation of the uterine tissues, and resembles raking the soil after strewing it with seed; (*b*) curetage, no matter how expertly done, cannot remove all the diseased tissues. The bacteria, within fifteen minutes after inoculation, are already out of its reach, and, further, at autopsy in cases where the curet had been used, invariably parts of the endometrium could be proved never to have been touched by the instrument; indeed, even the whole placenta has been found; (*c*) perforation of the uterus is a common occurrence, and almost always fatal from peritonitis; even the greatest gentleness may not prevent such an accident, because in some cases the muscle is as soft as butter; (*d*) hemorrhage from the reopened placental sinuses, even air-embolism, has been reported; (*e*) the freshly united wounds are torn open and new ones created, into all of which infection is ground; (*f*) a pyosalpinx or other pus-sac may be ruptured by the manipulations. It seems about as reasonable to curet the nose and throat in cases of diphtheria as to curet the uterus for sepsis.

(6) Emptying the uterus with polypus forceps is a very dangerous procedure, because parts of the uterine muscle, even the intestine and omentum, have been pulled out under the impression that ovular remnants were being removed. The forceps may be used to remove pieces floating freely in the uterine cavity or hanging out of the cervix.

(7) Drainage of the uterus with rubber or glass tubes is the practice of some French, Italian, German, and American accoucheurs.

(8) Packing the uterus with gauze, or draining it with the same, may be employed to stop hemorrhage after the operations just considered, and they are employed by some as directly antiseptic measures.

(9) Hobbs of England recommends the injection of sterile glycerin into the infected uterus to promote a flow of bactericidal lymph from the deeper tissues, floating out and killing the bacteria. A soft rubber catheter is left in the uterus and every two or three hours the nurse injects a few cubic centimeters of pure glycerin. I never use the method, but will admit it has promise.

For the last twenty years I have practically dispensed with local treatment in puerperal infection, being convinced that it does much more harm than good. Only if the woman is having uterine hemorrhages do I interfere, and then, by packing the uterus with 2 per cent. iodoform gauze to stop the flow and aid the expulsion of the retained masses causing it. This packing is repeated, if needed, daily for several days. Often the foreign matter comes away when the gauze is removed, and usually the temperature comes down, the patient's general condition improving. Only after the local barriers are considered strong enough and involution of the uterus well advanced is the removal of the retained material attempted. This is safe only after the temperature has been normal two or more weeks. One waits as long as possible. Nature often does wonders. Most authorities do not take this radical position. Bumm, Hirst, the French, and many advise a primary palpation of the uterine cavity with the finger and the immediate removal of its contents, but they all emphasize the danger of the procedure when the infection is streptococcal, urging that it then be omitted. It has already been proved that it is impossible to say—certainly at the first examination—whether a given infection is, or is not, streptococcal, and, further, before the streptococcus can be demonstrated the infection is through the uterine wall and beyond. On the other hand, if the infection is saprophytic, but little danger need be apprehended from it, and it is safe to wait a few days to see what course the disease will take. Winter, of Königsberg, Mermann (*loc. cit.*), Saft, and Baumm, Höhne, Barsony, Traugott, Thorn, Houch, of Cleveland, Watkins and Ries, of Chicago, Davis, Cragin, and Polak, of New York, are opposed to local treatment, and Credé, of Leipsic, shortly before his death, strongly emphasized its dangers, advising its total discontinuance. Vignes reports a complete reversal of the former active local treatment at the Clinique Baudelocque in Paris. It is gratifying to note that one voice after another is being raised against douches, curetage, curage, and other local interferences with the processes of healing adopted by nature, and the author hopes that the curet will soon be recognized as a criminal instrument in simple puerperal infection, and that the other operations will be reduced to the one indication—to stop hemorrhage. (For the treatment of pus collections see Pelvic Peritonitis.)

Local treatment can be summed up in one word—drainage.

General Treatment.—Everything that will improve the woman's general health will help her throw off the disease, and the attendant should count no effort lost that will increase her resisting powers. Fresh air is important, and I have employed the outdoor treatment with good results. Sleep is a prime necessity, and if procuring mental and physical quiet do not bring it, morphin may be used. Aspirin and codein also relieve pain. Pain is depressing and fatiguing. In a maternity the sick woman should be isolated—first, because of the danger, recognized by practically all authorities, of her being the beginning of an epidemic of puerperal infection, and, second, to insure her quiet. Visitors are excluded, and every one about the house should bear a cheerful mien. Nursing the child is stopped, first, because the mother needs all her reserve force to combat the infection; second, the acts of nursing are disturbing and tiring, and, third, the child may be infected. In those cases where, contrary to orders, nursing has been continued, the child often, not always, suffers from the poor quality of the milk.

For the *fever*, as a rule, nothing need be done. If continuously high, cool sponging, cool packs, or the cool bath may be used—rarely the bath, because it involves too much exertion for the patient, and a weak heart may go default; further, in parametritis and perimetritis the patient may not be moved much. Antipyretics are contraindicated. Medicines are very sparingly used. Of tonics, quinin is the best, in two- or three-grain doses. Hexamethylenamin is given if there are signs or fears that the urinary tract may be involved in the infection. Drugging is avoided, so far as possible, first, because it does little good, and, second, because it spoils the stomach, the most important ally of defense. Alcohol, formerly considered almost specific in all kinds of infections, has lost favor. At most the system can utilize ½ ounce a day, and there is no objection to giving this amount in the form of eggnog or a wine to stimulate a flagging appetite.

The Bowels.—In prolonged cases an occasional laxative is ordered, and the bowels usually need enemata. Diarrhea may be one of nature's methods of ridding the system of toxins, and is not interfered with unless pronounced, and when it begins to exhaust the patient. When the diarrhea is too marked, charcoal and salol may be tried, but magnesia usta, in dram doses every three hours, may do better. Opium and starch enemata may be necessary. Vomiting is always a bad symptom, and, if bilious, almost always means a fatal ending. Food by the mouth is withheld for a while and rectal feeding instituted—saline solution with 3 drams of grape-sugar added to each quart, by the drop method. If the vomiting persists, the stomach may be washed out. It is surprising how much greenish-black fluid is removed, and the patient usually feels much relief for several hours. Food is not given by mouth but the body is saturated with fluid by means of Ringer's solution and glucose intravenously, venoclysis. The body needs large amounts of fluid and also the chlorine, sodium, calcium, and potassium ions. To drain the toxins from the upper bowel, enterostomy may be done, or a duodenal tube placed and aspirated frequently.

Meteorism in peritonitis is a troublesome condition. Overfeeding and cathartics are to be avoided and enemata given. Milk and molasses, of each ℥viij, form a very efficient enema in causing flatus to pass, chamomile tea enemata being good also. Physostigmin salicylate, $\frac{1}{60}$ grain, may be given every four hours for four doses, but in my experience it has failed to relieve the distention. Pituitrin may be tried (except after classic cesarean). The rectal tube gives some relief. If the stomach is dilated, the patient is to lie on the abdomen and the foot of the bed is raised, or the stomach is washed out—a sovereign remedy which may be repeated every four hours. The small intestine may be opened through a tiny incision near the navel and drained. The electric vibrator, allowed to play on the belly, may stimulate peristalsis.

For the *chills*, the patient is covered warmly and given a hot drink. If the chill is prolonged, ¼ grain of morphin is given hypodermically.

Attention is given the heart, and all exertion of the patient is forbidden in order to spare its strength. Digitalis, to be useful, must be given prophylactically. To prevent pulmonary stasis the patient's position should be frequently changed, and she should be made to take four or five slow deep breaths several times daily. Deep breathing hurries the circulation of the liver, and Bourcart recommends daily massage of the liver region for this purpose. He believes he can thus enhance the detoxicating action of the organ.

Special attention is directed to the *diet*, and an abundance of sugar and proteins is provided—less of fat. Milk, buttermilk, matzoön, kumiss, eggs, jellies, cereals, sugar, ice-cream, fresh fruits, lettuce, and gelatin in all forms are permissible. The caloric requirements are greater than normal, for reasons readily understood. Small amounts of easily digested food, frequently repeated, daintily served to tempt the appetite, will keep up body weight. Studies in metabolism show that glucose spares protein, and the laboratory has demonstrated that in the presence of glucose many bacteria cannot become virulent. These facts should be made applicable to practice and the patient's desires consulted.

Fluids in quantities to keep the tongue moist must be introduced, and, since acidosis is often present, alkalies may be exhibited.

Latterly I have been experimenting with the infra-red lamp, applied locally, and the ultraviolet for general irradiation. The latter seems to be a good tonic, but not as good as direct sunlight. The infra-red lamp shortens the course of pelvic inflammations by hastening abscess formation and pointing. One must proceed cautiously with these new agents.

Finally, the *mental state* of the patient should be treated. She should be buoyed up with the hope and assurance that she will recover—indeed, speaking from experience, I can say that even the apparently hopeless cases sometimes get well, and I am convinced that the mind of the patient has considerable to do with her struggle with the infection.

A general physical examination is to be made every three or four days—one might discover a medical or surgical complication.

Specific Treatment.—Since the bacteria are beyond the reach of the antiseptic douche and the curet, we try to get at them and to neutralize or remove their poisons by way of the blood. We try to do this in two ways—first, by direct antiseptic or bactericidal action; second, by stimulating the antibacterial and antitoxic power of the blood, as well as we know these forces.

Intravenous injection of mercury, of colloid silver salts (collargol, electrargol, etc.), salvarsan, formaldehyd, gentian violet, mercurochrome, dispargen, yatren, rivanol, etc., deserve only historic notice. We still lack a therapia sterilisans magna.

The hope that bacteriology would supply a remedy for infection has not been borne out as yet. Vaccine therapy is a flat failure. (See Miller, Lit., Teague, and McWilliams, Schottmüller.)

Antistreptococcus sera usually fail, perhaps because there are so many different strains of streptococci. Very rarely one seems to have obtained a good result. Whether this is due to the accident of having matched the causative strain, or to the increase of leukocytosis (Weaver and Tunnicliff), or to the mobilization, through the action of the foreign protein, of other antibacterial agencies, or not to the serum at all, but is a *post hoc* occurrence, we do not know. The antiscarlatinal serum seems to have scored the most successes.

I use it in severe streptococcal infections early in the disease, giving 20 c.c. intravenously and 30 c.c. hypodermically for the first dose. After six hours 50 c.c. more are given, hypodermically, and the next day 100 c.c. at similar intervals. If a good effect is not evident, no more is administered. Beware of anaphylaxis!

Erythema at the site of injection, general urticaria, swelling of the joints simulating pyemic joints, and moderate, temporary increase of fever, may be observed—rarely serious symptoms. It is useless in pyemia, thrombophlebitis, cellulitis, and peritonitis. In early cases of acute streptococcic bacteremia, especially if complicated by erysipelas, one may hope for some effect. As a prophylactic the antistreptococcic serum is useless, but the tetanus serum useful.

Blood and serum of the husband, immunized by killed cultures from the wife's blood, have been tried. Only in several weeks does the blood acquire immune bodies, and by this time it is usually too late. If the serum or blood of a cured patient is available it should be used.

Protein Therapy.—The introduction of a foreign protein (vaccine, serum, milk) into the blood sometimes causes a severe reaction—chill, fever, sweat, prostration, leukocytosis. The foreign protein activates the protoplasm and stimulates all the natural immunizing functions of the body, especially the reticuloendothelial system (Louros). The author would warn to care in the use of such powerful agents, certainly in acute cases. Ehrenfest's review is not encouraging.

Salt and Glucose Solutions.—Whenever the liquid intake is less than normal and sometimes when we wish to "flush the system," saline solution and glucose are prescribed. Saline may be given by the drop method per rectum or by hypodermoclysis, but glucose is best injected intravenously. When vomiting prevents food intake glucose may be introduced by vein—venoclysis, 200 c.c. of a 10 per cent. solution per hour for five to ten hours.

The good effects of salt and glucose solutions lie in the supply of water and food and the stimulation of the circulation and of the skin, kidneys, and intestine. Care must be observed to avoid overloading the heart and causing edema of the lungs.

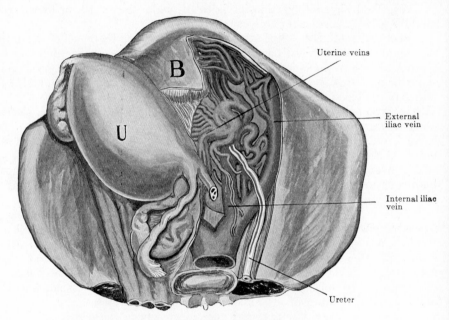

FIG. 766.—VEINS OF THE RIGHT PELVIS (from Kownatski). From a woman who died of eclampsia four days postpartum.

Transfusion.—As an aid to the antitoxic forces of the septic puerpera and to sustain her, especially if she has had severe hemorrhage, blood should be transfused from the husband or other healthy donor. Possibly blood from a pregnant woman or from a puerperal fever convalescent is better. Frequent small transfusions (200 to 300 c.c.) are better than a single large one. Matching and grouping must be meticulously carried out.

The Abscess of Fixation.—It has been known for a long time that if a case of sepsis has a focus of free suppuration, recovery is very probable, and Fochier, in 1892, advised the injection of turpentine into the thigh, with the object of making an abscess and thus inducing leukocytosis. Voiturier, in 1909, reported 120 cases and reviewed the literature. Recently Dunker reports good results.

Surgical Treatment.—Reference has already been made to the treatment of pelvic inflammations by operation, and no real difference of opinion exists regarding the procedures advocated for the treatment of localized suppurations such as pelvic abscesses, pus tubes, ovarian abscess, uterine abscess, necrotic fibroids.

The author believes in a very conservative practice, trusting much to the defensive and reparative processes of nature. Extensive exudates are often absorbed, or, while waiting, become easily accessible for drainage, with the preservation of functionating organs. At least by waiting, the immunities of the patient are developed, and she will not die from acute sepsis the result of the surgical attack.

Two radical operations, however, have been employed in the treatment of severe infections, about which there is still much to be learned. One is extirpation

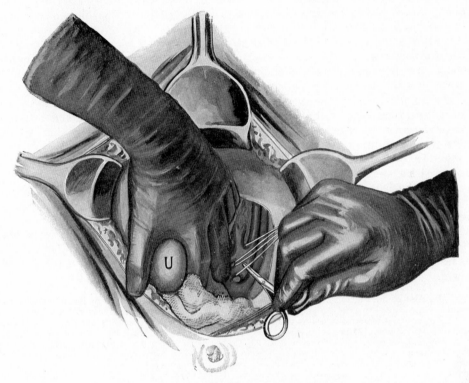

FIG. 767.—LIGATING THE RIGHT MEDIAN AND INTERNAL ILIAC VEINS.
Modified from Kownatski. Martens says the only safe way is extraperitoneally.

of the uterus, the other, ligation of the pelvic veins, with a view to stopping the progress of a thrombophlebitis.

Hysterectomy.—Schultze removed a uterus containing an infected placenta in 1886, and the patient recovered, and since then the operation—total hysterectomy—has been done several hundred times, but with not enough success to give it a firm place in our therapy. At the Congress in Rome in 1902 the subject was one of the main themes, and again in Madrid in 1903. Fehling reported in Rome a mortality of 55.7 per cent., and Cortiguera, in Madrid, 51.8 per cent.; Doléris, 95 per cent.; Mouchotte (all abortion cases), 43.3 per cent. The main difficulty lies in placing the indication. It is generally admitted that in the following conditions—in all of which the local lesion is the predominant factor—hysterectomy is justifiable: (1) Rupture of the uterus or vagina with infection, perforation of the uterus with beginning peritonitis, or perforation of the uterus during the local treatment of an infection within it; (2) infection of a fibroid, or when a fibroid has been much bruised by an operative delivery and infection is feared (a fibroid polypus is often removable from below); (3) cancer of the uterus; (4) infection, with a molar pregnancy; (5) abnormal adherence of the placenta and infection; (6) incarceration of all or of a part of the ovum, for example, missed abortion or labor with infection (in the latter three instances the difficulty of removal of the masses in the usual manner must be also considered); (7) uterine abscess; (8) gangrene of the uterus. (9) Infected inverted or prolapsed uterus. It has been also suggested to remove the uterus in cases of peritonitis, extensive involvement of the tubes and ovaries, and in uterine emphysema (Demelin), but the shock of such operations is very badly borne by these intensely septic patients. The greatest danger is from peritonitis, if such is not already present, and it is impossible, with our present technic, to avoid soiling the peritoneum to some extent when the whole uterus is removed.

Much more uncertainty exists as to the propriety of removing the uterus in cases of bacteremia, or at least in cases of severe endometritis and uterine lymphangitis and phlebitis, when the infection, presumably, is still more or less limited to the uterus. There is the point. If we could tell when the infection is likely to pass the line of safety, we would know when to remove the uterus, and experience has shown that uteri are usually removed too late to do any good, and in those cases, where the courageous operator has done hysterectomy early, he could never be sure that the mutilation of the patient was demanded. The operation may have killed her, or if she got well, may not have contributed to her recovery, but has rendered her sterile. My own experience with the operation is nil—I have never seen a case where I thought it could possibly save life, and in many critical cases recovery ensued without it. If a general bacteremia exists, no one would expect any good from the operation. Weber (1921), Lea, Cragin, Davis, Edgar, and Zangemeister (1927), Walthard and Schottmüller (1930), take the same position. Septic patients are the poorest subjects for operations and anesthetics, and there is no doubt in my mind that many puerperæ annually lose their lives because of them.

Ligation of the Pelvic Veins.—In 1784 J. Hunter cured a case of pyemia by ligating the saphenous vein. Sippel in 1894 proposed it, and in 1897 W. A. Freund ligated thrombotic spermatic veins to cure septicopyemia, but without success. In 1902 Trendelenburg reported 4 failures out of 5 operations. Miller studied the cases reported up to 1917 and figures a corrected mortality of 32.9 per cent. Kauffman collected 174 cases, with 55.1 per cent. deaths. If the ovarian veins alone are involved, the outlook for the operation is more favorable than if the hypogastrics are affected. M. Martens of Berlin has advocated ligation for twenty-two years; he ties both ovarians, both hypogastrics, even the vena cava, if necessary to get beyond the thrombosis and periphlebitic edema. He had 27 cases with 17 recoveries. One must remember that a perivascular lymphangitis usually accompanies the septic thrombosis, and that the collateral veins will readily provide avenues for the infection to travel around the ligatures.

After a positive diagnosis of septicopyemia is made, this operation should be considered. Repeated chills, extreme intermittence of temperature, demonstrated successive showers of bacteria in the blood, thrombocytopenia, hemoglobinemia, and the palpation of hard, worm-like masses in the bases of the broad ligaments justify the diagnosis of thrombophlebitis, and if the attendant feels convinced that only the veins are implicated, it may be justifiable to remove them from the general circulation by ligating them distally from the infection. In subacute and chronic cases of four to six weeks' duration the most success has been attained, but here also are the most spontaneous recoveries. In acute cases the operation is contraindicated. All writers agree on the difficulty of selecting the proper ones for the operation, and that the treatment is still on probation. Three methods of ligation are proposed—the extraperitoneal, the operation being similar to the extraperitoneal ligation of the internal iliac artery; the vaginal route, taught by Taylor of Birmingham; and the transperitoneal, the one that Martens says has the worst mortality. An advantage of the extraperitoneal approach (beside the avoidance of peritonitis) is that one can drain the perivascular infiltrated areas, also a source of bacteremia. Operation may be unilateral when the disease seems thus limited, one can ligate the other side if no improvement follows. Martens tied the cava 4 times safely. (See Koch.) Edema of the pelvic tissues and vulva and, sometimes, permanent varices and venous congestion follow the operation when the majority of the veins are tied, conditions resembling the after-effects of puerperal infections with formation of much fibrous tissue about and in the veins and connective tissue (Sanes, Warnekros, Sigwart, 1927, Lit.). Normal pregnancy and labor following ligation have been reported. Panhysterectomy is sometimes performed at the same time as ligation, but, according to Bumm and Weber, is almost always a fatal injury.

Literature

Baumm: Arch. f. Gyn., vol. lii, iii, p. 579.—*Bourcart:* Ref. Jour. Amer. Med. Assoc., 1922, vol. lxxviii, p. 1008.—*Dunker u. Brandis:* Zentb. für Gyn., February 20, 1932, p. 482.—*Ehrenfest:* Review on Protein Therapy, Amer. Jour. of Obstet. and Gyn., April, 1923.—*Halban and Koehler:* Path. Anat. des Puerp. Prozess, Wien, 1919.—*Hoehne:* Zentb. für Gyn., December, 1914.—*Houch:* Cleveland Med. Jour., March, 1919.—*Huggins:* Amer. Jour. Obst. and Gyn., 1926, 12, 562.—*Hüssy:* Zentb. f. Gyn., 1917, No. 30.—*Koch:* Zentb. f. Gynaek., July 2, 1927, p. 1713.—*Koehler and Ehrenfest:* Therapy of Puerperal Fever, 1925, C. V. Mosby Co.—*Lash, A. F.:* Amer. Jour. Obst. and Gyn., November, 1929.—*Louros:* Klin. Wochenschr., 1928, p. 996.—*Louros and Scheyer:* Zentb. für Gyn., 1927, No. 12, p. 763.—*Martens, M.:* Zeitschr. für Geb. u. Gyn., December 30, 1930, vol. xcix, p. 1.—*Miller:* Surg., Gyn., and Obst., October, 1917, p. 432.—*Sanes:* Amer. Jour. Obst., January, 1913 (full literature).—*Schottmüller:* Zentb. für Gyn., 1931, October 31, p. 3229.—*Sigwart:* Halban-Seitz, Biol. u. Path. des Weibes, 1927, vol. viii, i, p. 716.—*Teague and McWilliams:* Jour. of Immunology, June 11, 1917, p. 376.—*Thorn:* Zentb. f. Gyn., 1912, p. 141.—*Tietze and Plave:* Zeitschr. für Geb. u. Gyn., 1932, p. 379.—*Traugott:* Zeitsch. f. Geb. u. Gyn., Bd. 68.—*Vaccines:* Surg., Gyn., and Obstet., July, 1910.—*Vineberg:* Surg., Gyn., and Obstet., July, 1910. "Ligation of Veins," p. 31.—*Voiturier:* L'Obstetrique, August, 1909.—*von Herff:* v. Winckel's Handbuch der Geburtshilfe.—*Walthard:* Stoeckel's Geburtshilfe, 1930, p. 787.—*Warnekros:* Arch. f. Gyn., June, 1912, vol. xcvii, ii, p. 71.—*Watkins:* Jour. Amer. Med. Assoc., January, 1912; also paper read in June, 1912.—*Weaver and Tunnicliff:* Jour. Infectious Diseases, 1911, vol. ix, p. 130.—*Weber:* Döderlein's Handbuch, 1921, Schlussband, p. 913.

CHAPTER LXVII

DISEASES OF THE BREASTS

FUNCTIONAL DISTURBANCES

THE most common disorder affecting the breasts is **simple engorgement.** The general notion is that with engorgement the breasts are overfilled with milk. This is true only in part. While a small amount of milk forms spontaneously in the breasts, the symptoms are due to lymphatic and venous stasis. One can see this in some cases, even the skin being edematous. The engorgement occurs on the second, third, or fourth day, when the "milk comes in," and it may occur at the time of suddenly weaning the child, when the usual relief produced by nursing is absent.

Symptoms.—The breasts are very heavy, painful, and hot; they feel warm,

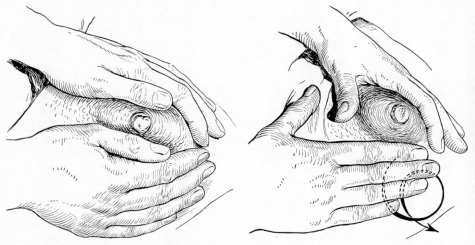

FIG. 768.—MASSAGE OF BREAST. EVEN COMPRESSION OF ENTIRE BREAST. FIRST MOTION.   FIG. 769.—MASSAGE OF BREASTS. SECOND MOTION.

but there is no rise of body temperature. There is no such thing as "milk-fever"— a fever the ancients ascribed to the engorgement of the breasts on the third or fourth day. Fever at such time is usually due to infection. Examination of the breasts shows them to be much enlarged, tender, hard, sometimes edematous, and of a bluish, mottled appearance. The nipple is flattened so that the child cannot grasp it, and the secretion of milk may be suspended—the breasts are choked up with swelling. The part of the gland running up into the axilla enlarges too, and the patient cannot bring her arm to the side.

If let alone, the engorgement gradually disappears, the gland becomes soft, and the milk flows readily when the child nurses. If irritated by too much or too rough massage, by breast pumps, and by too frequent nursing, the engorgement is slower in going down, but it will gradually disappear.

Treatment.—Since the determination of lymph and of blood to the breast is due to hyperactivity, sedative remedies, not stimulation, are needed. A saline cathartic may be given to deplete the system; liquids by mouth are restricted, and the breast is put at rest as far as possible, which means that the periods between nursings are to be lengthened. A tight breast-binder is applied, supplemented by ice-bags if the pain is marked. Some patients prefer warmth—when a warm wet boric dressing may be ordered. Soranus, of Ephesus, A. D. 100, said not to pump the breasts, because it increased their activity. Massage of the breasts is employed in rare cases, and is practised as follows. Massage and the use of the breast-pump are contraindicated if there is the least suspicion of inflammation. See author's Obstetrics for Nurses for details.

The operator sterilizes his hands and anoints the breasts with sterile albolene or oil. The first motion (Fig. 768) is one of even compression of the whole breast. Both hands are spread out as evenly and smoothly as possible over the breast, and firm compression is exerted against the chest. The blood and lymph are thus pressed out and away from the gland. On removing the fingers one may see depressions in the surface. This pressure is not painful, but the contrary. After this even pressure has been practised a few minutes and all the gland covered, gentle circular strokings are made from the nipple toward the periphery (Fig. 769). The four fingers make circles around the nipples, pressing harder as they go away from the nipple. (See diagram, Fig. 770.) The breast is steadied by the other hand.

After circling the breast twice the third motion is instituted (Fig. 771). One hand steadies the breast, while four fingers of the other hand wipe the milk toward the nipple. Any milk formed is thus squeezed out of the nipple. This is the least important of the three motions. The last motion is a repetition of the first motion, and nearly always the patient will feel much relieved by the procedure, even though no milk has been expressed. The breasts are now bandaged smoothly and tightly.

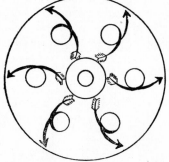

FIG. 770.—DIAGRAM OF OUTWARD STROKINGS.

Polygalactia is the abnormal increase of milk secretion. It occurs mainly in women of sthenic habit, and usually subsides in a few days without treatment or with the measures just considered.

Hyperlactation is a voluntary condition. It means that nursing is prolonged beyond the customary eight or nine months. One case came to my notice where a wet-nurse suckled three successive children in the same family without harm to herself and with benefit to the nurslings. Ploss says that such a practice is common in Spain, and that the Japanese women, the Chinese, Armenian, and more or less civilized tribes nurse their children for several years—some even up to fifteen. There is a popular fallacy among the poor that nursing prevents conception. Hyperlactation is usually bad in its effects on the general health of the woman, causing emaciation, asthenia, oligemia, backache, pain in the breasts, drawing into the shoulders while nursing, anorexia, and general neurasthenic symptoms. Headache, cramps in the shoulder muscles, amaurosis, and lactation psychoses have been observed. More important is the usual hyperinvolution of the uterus,—the so-called lactation atrophy,—which, if the cause is not early removed, may lead to permanent changes in the organ. The uterus is so small sometimes that it can hardly be found. A tuberculous lesion may become active in these conditions. The treatment begins with weaning the child; then tonics, forced feeding, and outdoor living are prescribed.

Galactorrhea.—Continuous flowing of a milk-like secretion from the breasts, irrespective of nursing, and persisting after weaning, is called galactorrhea. It is very rare and rather intractable. The cause is unknown, but the disease is more frequent in neurotic women, and in some cases abnormal practices on the breasts may be suspected if simulation and exaggeration are eliminated. It may be unilateral or bilateral, intermitting for a few days or weeks, to recur again; may follow abortions or full-term labors, may be slight in amount or profuse, as much as several quarts being lost daily.   My case continued for four years, but was free from the flow during two intervening pregnancies, and her milk disagreed with the children, so that they had to be wet-nursed.   Recovery occurred when a small abscess near the nipple was opened.   Perhaps a chronic galactophoritis may explain some of the cases of galactorrhea.   Instances are on record of the flow lasting from eleven to thirty years.   The health usually suffers more or less,—a condition called "tabes lactea,"—but it may not be affected at all.

Treatment.—Compression of the breast by binder is first practised.   Iodid of potash, generally recommended, failed in my own case.   A chronic galactophoritis should be looked for, and, if found, the inflamed portion of the breast excised. Atropin in glycerin (gr. 1/5 ad. ℥j) applied under a binder may be tried.   Duke cured 1 case by desensitizing the patient to her own milk.   Return of the menstruation is usually accompanied by stopping of the flow, and therefore, perhaps, efforts to favor the return of the menses may be useful.   Attention to the general health is advisable, and a little wholesome neglect of the local condition to distract the patient's mind from it may also be useful.   x-Ray treatments, spirits of camphor, ℥ xv t. i. d. theelin, prolan may be tried experimentally.

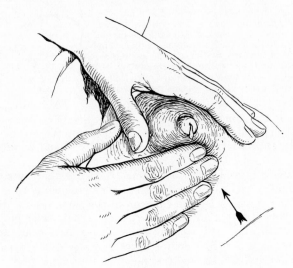

FIG. 771.—MASSAGE OF BREASTS.   THIRD MOTION.

Abnormal Milk.—Remarkable as it may seem, the milk of the mother, although plentiful, may not agree with the child.   The author has seen cases where it seemed to act like an irritant intestinal poison, and fatalities have even been reported. These have all been neurotic mothers, and most of them in the higher classes. Chemic and microscopic examinations have not given satisfactory explanations. Shannon believes that foreign protein from unusual diet of the mother may be responsible.   The condition may or may not recur in subsequent pregnancies.

The child will refuse the breast, in which case the milk may have a foreign taste, or it will vomit the ingested milk or have a diarrhea from it, sometimes with fever.   The milk may appear yellower and thicker in these cases, showing either a persistence of the colostrum or an increase in fat and proteids—that is, it is too rich. Curiously, sometimes a child will refuse one breast and accept the other; in a case of this kind the milk of one breast was said to be salty.

If the milk is believed to disagree with the child, causing green, acrid stools, the nursing should be discontinued for forty-eight hours, the breasts being regularly emptied in the mean time by the breast-pump.   The child is fed on a substitute milk, and at the end of this period another trial is made of the mother's milk. If it again causes intestinal disturbance, the wisest course to pursue is to obtain a wet-nurse for the child.

If the mother's milk is deficient in one or the other ingredient, the physician will instruct the nurse to give an additional feeding of this or that preparation of sugar, cream, barley-water, etc., after each nursing. Not much may be expected from dieting the mother. Illness of the mother affects the quality of the milk, rendering it indigestible, and also diminishing the amount. Bacteria circulating in the maternal blood are excreted in the milk, which is true of tuberculosis, streptococcemia, pyococcemia, and perhaps for malaria. The infant may be infected from the germs thus swallowed, or from the germs contained in pus which comes from a mammary abscess. Exceptions to this statement are not rare. I have seen septic women, even pneumonia cases, nurse their babies with impunity. A woman with diphtheria, given antitoxin, may nurse. That drugs administered to the mother pass over to the fetus is well known.

Strong emotions certainly affect the milk, causing indigestion, diarrhea, green corrosive stools, even convulsions and death of the infant, many authentic cases of which are on record. (Lit., Seiffert.)

Agalactia.—One of the commonest complaints of nursing mothers is scarcity or lack of milk. Total absence of milk is found only when the breasts are absent, a rare anomaly. The causes of deficient milk secretion are general weakness or ill health; malformations or diseases of the nipples, which render nursing impossible or too painful; occlusion of the milk-ducts, or destruction of gland tissue from mastitis; insufficient stimulation of the breast by a puny child; inadequate amount of gland tissue as a congenital anomaly, which might be hereditary, successive generations of women not having nursed their children; disuse of the breast in successive pregnancies; old primiparity—women with the first child after thirty-five seldom being able to nourish the infant; starvation, the wasting diseases, and the effects of febrile affections; emotional states, a quiet, placid disposition contributing to a good supply, worry, fright, pain and anger, reducing or temporarily stopping the flow; lack of love for the child may reduce the amount; menstruation rarely reduces it; obesity—but not invariably; hemorrhage during labor; interruption of lactation for any cause. The milk usually is not so abundant when nursing is resumed. I have seen the milk return five weeks after the child had been removed from the breast, and cases are on record of its return months afterward. Several reports of nursing of the child by its own grandmother are authenticated, and in certain tribes of savages such a custom is common.

Symptoms.—A large breast does not mean a good supply of milk, since it may be made up mainly of fat, with little gland tissue. Small breasts with thin skin and blue veins coursing under the surface usually give plenty of milk.

The symptoms of deficient milk-supply are, first, the distress of the child—its loss in weight; second, pain in the breasts and the absence of secretion. The child is unsatisfied with the nipple; he may suck for a short while, but, finding nothing there, will refuse it and cry. After supplemental feeding he goes to sleep. When there is plenty of milk the mother can feel it leave the breast and see the infant swallow. There are also some drops of "white nourishment" around the mouth. These are all absent in agalactia. Weighing the child before and after nursing proves the lack of milk. If the mother persists in nursing after the supply has diminished, the act comes to be attended with pain in the breasts, radiating around to the back, first only during the nursing, later in the intervals also. Unless nursing is interrupted, serious inroads on the woman's health may result.

Treatment.—If there is not enough milk in the breasts, an attempt may be made to stimulate the secretion by diet, cool baths, and massage of the breasts;

61

but only a few cases are amenable to treatment.   Medicines have very uncertain, if any, action.

By increasing the liquids in the diet the total quantity of milk may sometimes, but not always, be increased.   When the milk supply is not augmented, the patients put on fat.   Milk may be given in large quantities, also water, very weak tea, chocolate, oatmeal and barley gruels, and oyster-stews, in addition to the regular diet.   Cod-liver oil (vitamins A and D) may help.   Alcoholic drinks should be restricted, or, better, avoided, and certainly by a mercenary wet-nurse.   Alcoholics are not good for the infant.

Cool full baths stimulate the skin and the breast also.   They may be taken daily at about 80° to 84° F.   The whole body should be briskly rubbed with a coarse towel, avoiding the mammæ.   Bier's method of producing artificial engorgement has been applied to the breast to stimulate the flow of milk.   The results

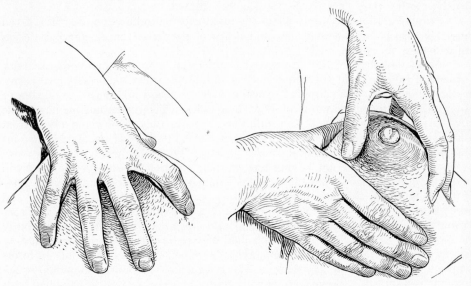

FIG. 772.—STIMULATING MASSAGE.   FIG. 773.—STIMULATING MASSAGE.

thus far have been fair.   Ultra-violet radiation may help and may improve the quality of the milk.

Massage of the breasts stimulates the formation of milk.   When massaging the breast for this purpose, the rules given on p. 959 do not apply.   One wishes here to irritate the gland.   This is done by raising the whole breast from the chest-wall (Fig. 772) and working it gently between the fingers.   Care should be used not to bruise the delicate organ, as an abscess may result.   The gland is then held against one hand, while the tips of the outspread fingers of the other hand make circular movements all around its periphery (Fig. 773).

The best stimulant for the milk secretion is a vigorous infant.   Abt's electric milk pump has proved very useful.

One should not be discouraged too soon, as the establishment of the milk secretion is sometimes slow.   In one case sufficient milk did not come until the fifth month.   Often, after the patient is up and gets outdoors, the milk comes in larger quantities.   One may be misled to believe that this is the action of some special drug or of feeding.   If, however, the measures instituted have no effect, it is wiser to discontinue them as soon as this fact is apparent.   Too great zeal in forcing the breasts to act may result in mastitis.

Drying up the Milk.—Of all the measures recommended for this purpose, the author has found the following the simplest and quickest. Liquids in the diet are reduced, a saline cathartic given on two successive days, a firm breast-binder is applied, and the breasts then left absolutely alone. Pumping and massage only stimulate the gland to further action. Drugs are dangerous or useless. If the engorgement following the weaning is very marked and painful, the treatment described on p. 958 may be employed.

"Caked Breast."—So-called "caked breast" is a local engorgement affecting one or more lobules or lobes. It is sometimes due to occlusion of one or more of the lactiferous ducts, but may be a simple congestion, due to injury, which may have antedated the gestation. A lump made up of hard, convoluted masses of gland tissue is found occupying one or more quadrants of the organ, which is tender to the touch, but presents no signs of real inflammation, nor is there any general reaction. "Caked breast" does not usually lead to mastitis, though it is easy to understand that the bacteria normally present in the tubuli lactiferi could thus more easily attain invasive qualities. If such a breast is roughly handled, as by ill-directed massage, infection is prone to develop. The possibility of carcinoma, although very remote, should always be in the mind, and in doubtful cases a piece of the mass removed for microscopic examination.

Treatment.—Outside of instructing the nurse and the patient to leave the breasts alone, to protect them from injury, not to attempt to massage the lumps away, nothing is done. If the breasts are very painful, an ice-bag or a wet warm dressing may be applied.

DISEASES OF THE NIPPLES

Sore nipples are a frequent complication of the first weeks of nursing. They are worthy the attention of the accoucheur, because they are exceedingly painful, may prevent lactation entirely, thus harming the child, and may lead to infection of the breasts, which may result in abscess or even in death of the puerpera. Over half of nursing mothers suffer from sore nipples; primiparæ more than multiparæ; blonds, particularly red-haired women, more than brunets, who usually have a thicker skin; old primiparæ more than young ones, and they are especially common if the nipple is retracted or deformed (Fig. 774). If the nipple is flat or even inverted, the child will be unable to get hold of it, and if efforts at nursing are too long persisted in, engorgement, cracks, and fissures occur, and, infection being thus introduced, abscess results. The conditions making sore nipples are erosions, blisters, cracks or fissures, and ulcerations. Erosions are caused by the maceration of the thin epithelium and the sucking of the infant, which thus exposes the rete. Sometimes the epithelium is raised up as a blister by the intense suction, and the blister, bursting, leaves the eroded rete. If infection is added, the process may become ulcerative. If the skin cracks, which is especially likely to occur at the bottom of a crevice in the nipple, a little blood is poured out; it hardens to a scab under which a droplet of pus sometimes is found. Nursing breaks off the crust, and if the part is not treated, a deep ulcer may form. Cracks are either circular or vertical. The cracks which run circularly are usually at the base of the nipple, at its junction with the areola, and if the ulceration is deep, the nipple may be partly or wholly amputated. Vertical cracks may split the nipple into two. Bacteria are always present on and in sore nipples, and may cause sickness in the baby. If the cracks bleed, the child may swallow blood, which reappears in the stools or vomit—melæna spuria. Occasionally slight rises of temperature in the mother are due to infected nipples.

The *treatment* of sore nipples begins during pregnancy. (See p. 247.) Of great importance is proper position of mother and baby during nursing, to prevent distorting the nipple. If the woman complains of pain when the child nurses,

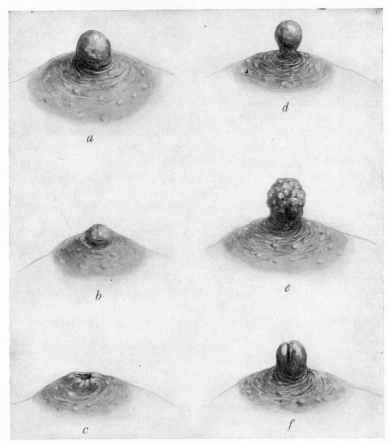

Fig. 774.—Variously Formed Nipples.
a, Normal; b, stunted; c, inverted; d, mushroom; e, mulberry; f, split or bifid.

an inspection of the nipples is to be made—with a magnifying-glass, if necessary. Some neurotic women have pain while nursing, even in the absence of disease of the nipples—sometimes so much that nursing is impossible in spite of sedatives and soothing local applications. This may be due to spasms of the erector papillæ muscles and an ointment of belladonna may help.

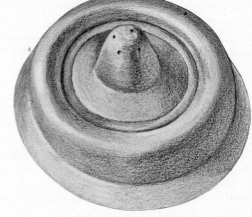

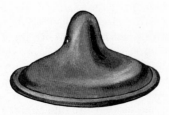

Fig. 775.—Wansbrough's Lead Nipple-shield.

Fig. 776.—"Infantibus." Nipple Shield for Nursing. Adheres to breast on vacuum principle. Helps flat nipples.

A blister is to be opened by a fine sterile needle and the child withheld from the nipple for thirty-six hours. Cracks and ulcerations are first cleansed with hydrogen dioxid, then one of the following measures employed: Leaden nipple-shields (Fig. 775) are worn between nursings; the crack or ulcer is touched with 2 per cent. nitrate of silver solution morning and night, and this is allowed to dry in the sunlight; the whole nipple may be painted with the same; a 50 per cent. alcohol compress is laid on the nipple for an hour thrice daily; the nipple is exposed to the air under a wire tea strainer; glycerol of tannin, glycerin and boric acid applications, a salve of equal parts of castor oil and bismuth, may be applied; compound tincture of benzoin, allowed to dry in; light therapy. A glass nipple-shield is ordered for the nursing or a rubber one (Fig. 776). Sometimes the nipple may be given a respite for healing by milking the breast instead of putting the child to it. The attendant is warned to be scrupulously aseptic in the care of the breasts and nipples, because of the great danger of infection. The breast is not to be touched by the nurse, the nipple being washed with sterile boric solution by means of sterilized cotton wound on toothpicks—the so-called applicators. It may be necessary to stop nursing from the breast until the crack has healed, and if the sore positively refuses to cicatrize, it may be wisest to suspend lactation entirely to prevent a breast abscess. This is especially true of the inverted and deformed nipples, and particularly if the milk is scarce. Such a combination almost inevitably leads to mastitis, which the woman ought to be spared.

MASTITIS

Inflammation of the breast occurs almost exclusively in nursing women. Cases have been found during pregnancy, even in the non-pregnant, and exceedingly rarely in men. The predisposing causes are cracks, fissures, and ulcers, which in turn are caused by deformities of the nipple and occur in primiparæ oftener. While bacteria are the direct cause of mastitis, and while they may often be found in apparently healthy breasts, an exciting agent is usually necessary. Such are bruising of the breast by injury, which may have been remote, by massage, too much pumping of the breast, squeezing it, or efforts to make it secrete milk when it is physically unable to do so. Simple milk stasis or local or general engorgement seldom leads to abscess, if it ever does, alone.

The germs which have been found in mastitis cases are the Staphylococcus albus and aureus, the Streptococcus pyogenes, the Bacillus coli, the pneumococcus, the gonococcus, the Oïdium albicans, and blastomycetes (van de Velde). Symbiosis may be present. These microörganisms are brought to the breasts by the hands of the attendants, the linen, etc., or by the patient herself, the usual source being the lochia. In general hospitals unusual and severe infections may be brought to the breasts. The child may be the source of the infection, having thrush or Bednar's aphthæ (the lesions of which usually contain both the streptococcus and staphylococcus), pharyngitis, ophthalmia, coryza, or pemphigoid or pustular eruptions on the face, etc. Without doubt some of the cases are caused by the attainment of invasive qualities of the bacteria normally inhabiting the outer milk-ducts in the nipple. In 1893 I proved that the staphylococcus existed in the milk of apparently healthy women. When the breast is overstimulated or hurt the bacteria invade it. Finally, it is possible for the germs to get to the breasts via the blood, as is sometimes observed in septicopyemia, but this is very rare.

Forms of Mastitis (Fig. 777).—The infection may be limited to the areola outside the lamina cribrosa, forming an abscess running around the nipple, or in one of the tubercles of Montgomery, or in the milk-glands attached to them; second, the infection creeps along the tubuli lactiferi into the parenchyma of the gland; this is called parenchymatous or glandular mastitis or galactophoritis; third, the bacteria, gaining admission to the connective tissue through a crack or deep fissure, burrow into the fat around the lobes and lobules, causing interstitial or phlegmonous mastitis or lymphangitis; this cellulitis may be superficial or deep;

occasionally the latter two forms are combined; fourth, the infection passes directly through the gland to the areolar tissue under it on the chest-wall, producing here a submammary abscess.

Symptoms.—The parenchymatous form of inflammation is the most common, and begins seldom before the seventh day of the puerperium—most often from the tenth to the twentieth day. Frequently there is a little pain in one portion of the breast, marked while nursing, and occasionally slight fever—99° F.—for a day or two preceding the outbreak. This is manifested by a more or less severe chill and fever. The temperature may reach 106° F. and be accompanied by delirium, but usually does not go over 103° F., and the febrile symptoms are moderate. Pain in the breast is the rule, and over the lobe affected redness and tenderness are found, and usually the nipple will show a fissure, the site of entrance of the infection.

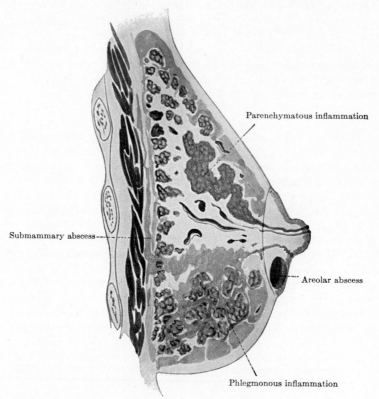

Parenchymatous inflammation

Submammary abscess

Areolar abscess

Phlegmonous inflammation

FIG. 777.—DIAGRAM OF BREAST INFECTIONS.

Often a droplet of pus may be expressed from the sinus lactiferus leading to the affected lobe. Any quadrant of the organ may be inflamed, though usually the outer half, and here one or more large lumps may be palpated. In one case the spot of redness and tenderness was not larger than a nickel, yet the woman's temperature was 105° F. Under appropriate treatment the temperature and pain subside within thirty-six hours unless the other breast is also affected, as in Fig. 779. If the fever continues for more than forty-eight hours, suppuration rarely fails to appear. Then the temperature becomes remittent, chills occur, the portion of the breast affected swells up, containing a large, hard mass. At one spot it softens, and redness of the skin, with a bluish tinge indicates where the pus is coming to the surface. Unless promptly operated, successive lobes are involved until the whole breast is riddled with abscesses. These must all be opened and drained, healing often requiring weeks or even many months. Naturally, in these cases the cellular

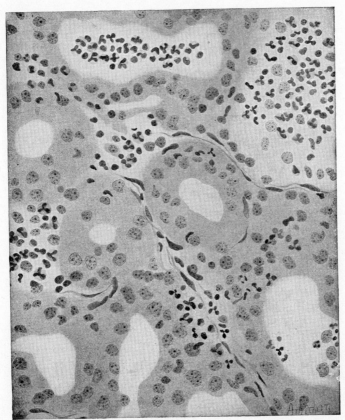

Fig. 778.—Mastitis Purulenta.

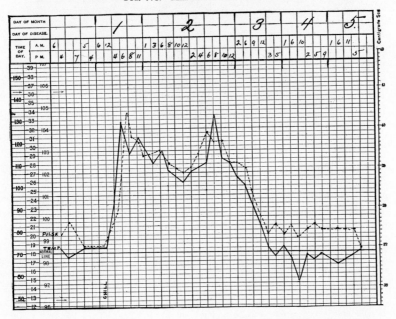

Fig. 779.—Acute Double Mastitis. No Abscess. Right Breast First.

tissue is also involved. Sometimes the acute symptoms subside and the accoucheur believes the process is at an end, but a few weeks later fever begins again and the breast suppurates, or pus is evacuated through the nipple.

In the cellulitic or phlegmonous variety the infection travels into the gland from a fissure and along the connective-tissue septa, and redness, fan-shaped, spreading from the crack, may be seen around the nipple. If the deeper lymphatics are involved, the case resembles one of deep cellulitis anywhere, with brawny swelling of the skin. Usually the streptococcus is here concerned—at least some heterogenous bacterium—and such cases are more frequent in general hospital practice. The fever, though at first less intense, keeps up longer, and the pulse more quickly feels the effect of the toxemia. Erysipelas has been observed, and even a pan-mastitis. Suppuration is much more common in this form of mastitis, but often, too, the breast shows only a firm infiltrate, which may be absorbed in from six to twelve days. After three or four days it is possible to foresee which termination is to occur. The axillary lymphatic glands may be enlarged.

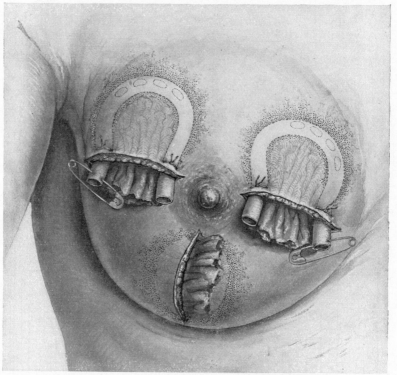

Fig. 779a.—Scheme for Drainage of Multiple Breast Abscesses in a Way that Will Not Leave Ugly Scars.

In the submammary abscesses, which Billroth believed were due to suppuration of deep-seated mammary gland tissue, the pus collects behind the gland, which then seems to float on a cushion, and edema appears at the periphery. The general symptoms are most threatening in this form of infection—indeed, unless promptly evacuated, the pus may burrow far and the patient die of bacteremia.

Treatment.—At the beginning it is not always possible to determine whether the infection is of the parenchymatous or the cellulitic variety, but the treatment is the same for both. The following practice has been found very successful by the author: (1) Remove the infant from the breast, and from both breasts if the symptoms are not very mild; massage and pumping the breast are forbidden; (2) administer a brisk saline cathartic; (3) apply a tight breast-binder; (4) one may use cold or heat in an attempt to allay the inflammation. Both methods have many partisans. If cold is selected put two or three ice-bags on each breast. After gently squeezing the nipple to evacuate a possible pus sac, it is surrounded by a ring of cotton; a layer of the same is laid between the two breasts; a rolled towel is placed to support the organ from the axillary side, and the breasts, lifted up, are tightly bandaged. The ice-bags must keep the breasts cool, but the nurse is instructed to watch the skin for signs of freezing, which, by the way, I have never seen with this treatment. After the temperature has been normal for twelve hours, the bags are removed one by one, and in twenty-four hours the child may be put back to the breast. This treatment is more successful in the parenchymatous forms than the cellulitic. If heat is to be applied we use a therapeutic lamp—sunlight—or put on a 30 per cent. alcohol dressing kept hot with water-bags or a (safe) electric pad.

If an abscess forms, it must be incised as soon as diagnosed. If the attendant is certain that suppuration has begun, the ice is replaced with a hot wet boric dressing. In opening abscesses some respect should be paid to the appearance of the breast. Ugly, visible scarring can be avoided. The incision may be made parallel to the lower or outer margin of the infiltration cutting radially from the nipple, the skin undermined and reflected upward, then the abscess is opened and thoroughly evacuated with the finger, breaking up the septa between the pus pockets. If more than one lobe is involved each one is thus treated. A drainage-tube is inserted into each cavity describing a semicircle, Fig. 779a, the ends fastened at the corners of the wound with a silkgut stitch. The tube has four holes at the vertex of the arch. The wound is washed out with peroxid, then packed with rubber tissue (rubber gloves are excellent), and a large wet dressing applied. This procedure is an extensive operation, and is often followed by chill, fever, and aggravation of the symptoms, sometimes with septic eruptions, but these subside within thirty-six hours, and the patient goes on to recovery. The rubber packing is removed after forty-eight hours, then renewed daily. Healing of the flap is directed to avoid a large scar. The tube is removed when the wound is granulating nicely. A single small abscess might be drained by a simple puncture or aspirated, using a large needle, whereupon the breast is compressed.

Occasionally, especially if the primary operation was not done thoroughly, new portions of the breast break down, forming secondary abscesses which may riddle the breasts, and these may protract the healing for months. I have noticed that if such pockets are not immediately opened, but left for a few days and then incised broadly and the cavity rubbed lightly with the finger (gloved), a sort of auto-inoculation or vaccination is made, which has a good influence on the whole gland. The sinuses drain better under a wet dressing, which is at first renewed thrice daily; later, less often. Attention must be given to building up the general health, which is likely to suffer from the profuse suppuration and prolonged illness. The patient is to be gotten out of bed and out of doors as soon as possible.

I have found that the infra-red lamp hastens recovery of breast abscesses. It is applied at 20 inches for twenty minutes, three or four times daily. General irradiation with the quartz-lamp, and especially out-door sunlight are very helpful, too.

When the sinuses are very persistent and new foci of suppuration constantly appear, vaccine treatment is to be tried. It is best to get the bacterium, usually the Staphylococcus albus, from the patient and make an autogenous vaccine, giving first 5,000,000, then in a few days 25,000,000 or 50,000,000, if necessary.

The author has used the Bier treatment on several cases of mastitis, and does not find that it materially shortens the length of the suppuration, nor does it enable one to dispense with large incisions. In very chronic cases compression of the breast with a rubber bandage hastens the closure of old sinuses.

In the cellulitic variety of mastitis, if diagnosed early, a hot, wet boric dressing covering a large part of the chest would be better than the ice. Incision is to be delayed until definite suppuration is discovered. Surgeons are divided as to the propriety of incising cellulitic infiltrates early. Judging from my experience in treating cellulitis in the pelvis, I would wait for actual pus formation. Submammary abscess is to be opened at once by broad incisions at the periphery of the gland.

The excessively rare carcinoma and adenomata of the breast deserve mention, although in an experience comprising the pathology of over 51,000 obstetric cases carcinoma of the breast was found only once.

SUNDRY COMPLICATIONS OF THE PUERPERIUM

Naturally, a puerpera may suffer from any of the diseases she would contract under other conditions, without any bearing on the puerperal state. A few of these deserve special mention.

Fever from Emotional Influences.—See p. 941.

Fever from Constipation.—Without doubt, overloading of the bowels may cause fever during the puerperium, but such cases must be extremely rare. Almost invariably a temperature that at first was ascribed to stercorrhemia is found later to be due to an infection in the pelvis or the breasts. The diagnosis must be made by exclusion, which is admittedly a precarious method. The therapeutic test—subsidence of the fever following brisk catharsis—is absolutely unreliable, because—(1) Energetic action of the bowels may affect the uterus and stimulate it to contraction, expelling from its cavity clots, lochia, and detritus; (2) the pelvic circulation is hastened by the cathartic, an action most exhibited by aloes, and the relief of an overloaded rectum improves the currents of the blood and lymph in the pelvis; (3) some cathartics produce leukocytosis, which aids in repelling infections; (4) a full rectum may cause lochiometra or stasis of lochia in the vagina—its emptying and the bearing-down efforts of defecation relieve the stasis. Therefore, if the fever subsides after the bowels are emptied, the case may have been one of infection, and not of absorption of toxins from the intestinal tract, as supposed.

Budin, in 1892, called attention to febrile stercorrhemia, and Küstner, Oui, Lavergne, and others have reported typical cases. Fever, headache, anorexia, sometimes nausea and abdominal pain, are the symptoms. The tongue is heavily coated, the breath fetid, the skin muddy or pasty, the belly distended with gas or doughy to the touch over the large bowel, and often tender. The lochia, usually normal, may have a fecal odor (colon bacillus), but the uterus and adnexa are normal. Brisk catharsis and enemata produce copious fetid evacuations, after which the symptoms subside. When the rectum is packed with hardened feces, it may be necessary to inject a softening enema (1 dram inspissated ox-gall triturated in 1 ounce of glycerin, to which are added 2 pints of water). After this has acted for an hour the softened mass may be removed by the gloved fingers, aided by rectal irrigation of saline solution.

Tape-worms have often been expelled during the puerperium. Fever has occasionally been ascribed to them, but in 6 of my cases they existed without causing temperature. The treatment is the usual one, but the child is to be kept away from the breast for the two days required for the action of anthelminthic remedies. During pregnancy treatment might induce abortion.

Tympany and Ileus.—Tympany occurring after delivery seldom becomes obstinate or very marked, and gives no concern if the bowels are moving and the general condition is not affected. If the distention does not quickly subside under the usual treatment (a cathartic, carminative enemata, a 5-grain asafetida pill three times daily, a few doses of pituitary), the possibility of a serious affection should be entertained, and a careful search made for a cause.

Obstruction of the bowels may be due to kinking from adhesions, the sequelæ of former operations or inflammations, and requires the usual treatment. In one case I found that a retroverted puerperal uterus compressed the rectum. After raising this up with one finger in the bowel the obstruction was relieved.

Ileus after cesarean section is the same as that met so often by surgeons, but it may follow operative deliveries from below—hebosteotomy, even natural deliveries. Sometimes an acute dilatation of the stomach is the cause, and, again, paralysis of the small intestine or occlusion of the large bowel. Bruising the bowel when the uterus is massaged, kinking from adhesions, compression of the bowel by the retroverted uterus in the pelvis, thrombosis of one of the celiac or mesenteric arteries, and unrecognized rupture of the uterus, rupture of a pus-sac, rupture of the gut with beginning peritonitis—all these may cause excessive tympany and ileus postpartum. Infection of the peritoneum from some cause must always first be thought of in these cases. The diagnosis is the most important part of the treatment. If it is decided not to open the abdomen, the following measures may be tried: repeated enemata, of which the milk and molasses combination, $\frac{1}{2}$ pint of each, is the best; this may be given with the patient inverted; turning the patient on her stomach; elevation of the head and shoulders; 5-grain asafetida pills thrice daily; washing out of the stomach (very useful); eserin, $\frac{1}{80}$ grain hypodermically every four hours for four doses; pituitrin; puncture of the gut with a fine needle—while said to be safe, to be used only as a last resort. In obstinate cases one should not wait too long to give the patient the benefit of surgery. An intestinal fistula may relieve the intense toxemia resulting from obstruction.

Appendicitis is to be always considered when an "acute abdomen" occurs postpartum. One cannot always differentiate it from puerperal peritonitis and operation may be needed to decide.

Fissures in ano are a not infrequent complication of the late puerperium. Inspection readily reveals them, and stretching of the sphincter with a speculum and a few applications of 10 per cent. silver nitrate solution to the cracks as readily cure them. Oil enemata and free action of the bowels strengthen the cure.

Difficulty of Urination.—This subject has already been touched upon (p. 350), and here need be mentioned only the overfilling of the bladder, with dribbling (incontinentia paradoxa); overfilling with only partial emptying of the bladder (evidenced by pain in the belly, a displaced uterus, a soft tumor above the pubis, sometimes tympany, and lochiostasis and fever); and the dribbling of urine which comes through a vesical fistula or paralysis of the sphincter vesicæ.

Exhaustion psychoses may occur after prolonged and arduous labors in weakened individuals, and I have seen "soldiers' heart" in a few cases. The symptoms are exhaustion, dyspnea, and palpitation of the heart on exertion, precordial oppression, giddiness, tremor, nervous instability. I have observed these symptoms also after serious gynecologic operations.

Gall-stone colic seems to be favored by the conditions in the puerperium, but, as Prochownic says, they may be simulated by disturbances of pancreatic function.

Backache.—Although the subject is immensely important, I can give it only a few lines. The causes: General hypoplasia with overstrain of the pelvic joints and connective tissues; orthostatic backache; sacro-iliac slip; chronic pelvic arthritis; coccygosacral arthritis or fracture; pelvic infections (parametritis postica); granulations in scars of lacerations with consequent periostitis; general destruction of the supports of the pelvic viscera; rarely retroversion itself; these and all other medical and surgical causes.

Literature

Duke, W. W.: Jour. Amer. Med. Assoc., April 23, 1932, p. 1445.—*Prochownic:* Monat. f. Geb. u. Gyn., September, 1916, No. 3.—*Shannon:* Amer. Jour. Dis. of Child., September, 1921, vol. xxii, p. 223.—*Seiffert:* Jour. Amer. Med. Assoc., June 12, 1920. Literature.

PART III

OPERATIVE OBSTETRICS

CHAPTER LXVIII

GENERAL CONSIDERATIONS

DURING pregnancy and labor the accoucheur's duty to his patient is both prophylactic and remedial. After providing for the gravida as described in the Hygiene of Pregnancy, p. 242. his course is one of watchful expectancy. He simply studies the processes of nature and determines when, where, and how he may be of assistance, but he must always bear this in mind, that he never can be of "assistance" unless something in the course of pregnancy, labor, or the puerperium goes wrong. Under such circumstances he makes up his mind that he must interfere. This is the first; second, he studies what he must do, and third, when he should do it. That something in the course of pregnancy, labor, or the puerperium which commands interference, or any mode of treatment, is called an "*indication.*" The many features of each obstetric case are the factors which determine or specify the nature of the procedure to be instituted. We call them "*conditions.*" A condition, therefore, is a prerequisite which must be fulfilled before the procedure demanded by the indication may be carried out. The study of the case, and the determination that there is a reason for the adoption of a particular line of treatment, we call "placing the indication," and this requires very delicate balancing of all the conditions. Speaking broadly, all *indications* for interference lie in the presence of immediate or prospective danger to mother or child. The *conditions* will be found in the state of the mother at the time of the intended treatment. Only when the conditions necessary for carrying out the procedure are present may we act, but the indication may be so strong that we have to "force the condition." For example, a woman has bleeding. The indication is to empty the uterus, but the cervix is tightly closed. A condition for rapid delivery is an open cervix; therefore we must first open the cervix, or choose an operation which has not this binding condition. A condition which absolutely prohibits a given line of treatment we call a "contraindication."

Selection of Operation.—This will depend on the indications and conditions, but often there are other considerations, as the skill of the operator, the environment of the patient, the religion of the family, the desires of the parents. An unskilful practitioner, unless he can obtain competent counsel, should always do that operation which promises the greatest safety to the mother. If the patient is amid bad surroundings, it may be necessary to sacrifice the child, while if she were in a good maternity, cesarean section would save both. A Catholic family does not permit craniotomy on the living child, and a husband may absolutely demand that his wife be subjected to no added risks for the sake of the child.

A clear presentation of the views of the Catholic Church on the propriety of craniotomy, therapeutic abortion, operation for ectopic gestation, cancer with pregnancy, etc., may be found in Rev. E. J. Burke's Acute Cases in Moral Medicine. The general principle here enunciated is that it is never justifiable to perform any operation whose intention is to destroy a living fetus.

971

Diagnosis.—Before every obstetric procedure the accoucheur must have made a careful *general* examination. He must know the exact condition of the kidneys, heart, lungs, thyroid, blood, etc. The "Leit motif" of every case should be sought out (see page 617). Having discovered the basic pathology, the main factor which disturbs the normal progress of the labor, the accoucheur will immediately see his course of conduct clearly, and he will acquire a comforting confidence in his operating. Just before an operative delivery, with the patient on a table and perhaps anesthetized, the examination of the local conditions—presentation, position, attitude of the child, the fetal heart, the cervix, etc.—must be repeated, because things may have changed in the time intervening, or the first diagnosis may have been wrong. If the local findings are different from what was expected, the original plan of procedure must be dropped or altered. Any other course which might be taken to save the accoucheur trouble and mortification usually results in more of each for him, and endangers the patient. It may be wisest to put the woman back in bed and select an entirely different line of treatment.

After the diagnosis is made and proved, the operator may well rehearse the steps of the operation in his mind beforehand, and take cognizance of the various complications which are likely to arise. If he will construct a mental picture of the conditions before him and then do the operation, as it were, "in the air," before the patient, he will be surprised how much the correct procedure is facilitated.

Assistants.—For good surgical operating at least three assistants are required—an anesthetist, a first assistant, and a nurse to hand instruments. Most surgeons demand more help than this, but most accoucheurs are satisfied with less. Why an accoucheur should, voluntarily, deny himself, the patient, and the baby the benefits of sufficient help is incomprehensible. In private practice it is often impossible to obtain more than one assistant to give the anesthetic, and the nurse must do all the rest of the work. Sometimes there is no nurse even, and the accoucheur has himself to give the anesthetic while operating. If the general practitioner would equal the work done in the maternity hospitals, he must educate the public to allow him sufficient help, and it can be done easier than he thinks. Circumstances are very unusual where another physician, one or two medical students, or one or two extra nurses are not obtainable. It is unsafe to trust the husband to help or to hold a light. He may collapse; further, it is cruel.

Prevention of Injuries.—Obstetric operating requires a clear head and a steady hand. Only too easily is the mother injured beyond repair, and the child harmed so seriously that its future is affected. Loss of sleep, the sufferings of the patient and sympathy for her, the importunities of the family, the unfavorable environment, all wear down the nerves. If the accoucheur is then called upon to perform a complicated, forceable, yet delicate operation, one attended with acute emergencies, he may, unless he has a strong will, when suddenly confronted with an unexpected difficulty, get into a frenzy of operating—a *furor operativus*, in which judgment has fled and an acute obsession seizes him—to pull out the child, oblivious of everything. In such a case the baby's head may be torn off its body, its limbs broken, the mother's uterus ruptured, etc. I have seen this operative frenzy many times and in varying degrees from mild nervousness to complete dementia. The older writers sought to combat it by advice and warnings. They insisted the accoucheur should lead a temperate life and avoid alcohol and tobacco. They painted mottoes in the operating-room, *e. g.*,

PRIMUM NON NOCERE

They engraved the words:

NON VI SED ARTE

on the obstetric forceps.

Another frequent and dangerous fault is haste in operating. The operator forgets that there is more danger to the child from traumatism than from asphyxia in slow delivery, and besides, the mother's tissues suffer less. A clock should be placed where the accoucheur can constantly see it, and an assistant should call off the minutes during the delivery. Both have a steadying effect.

Examination of the Patient after Delivery.—I have made it a rule to examine the parturient canal from the fundus to the vulva and the adjacent viscera and pelvis after every operative delivery. The hand is inserted into the uterus, palpates the placental site, removing adherent placental fragments, decidual débris, membranes, and blood-clots, then encircles the lower uterine segment three times, going from right to left, and three times from left to right—this in order to discover a slit-like injury—then the vagina likewise, and then the vulva. Tears of all degrees are carefully searched out. The pubic joint is palpated, the bladder catheterized, and finally, after all repairs have been made and just before applying the vulvar dressing, the finger is passed into the rectum to find out if any stitches have been put through it or if it is otherwise injured. The accoucheur must know and record the location and extent of all the puerperal wounds. It has been objected that such an examination, done by the general practitioner, is more dangerous, from infection, than would be the rare possibility of overlooking a ruptured uterus. Perhaps true, and I would not insist on it where the probability of an intact parturient canal is strong.

After operative deliveries the child, too, requires a careful gentle examination of the head and all its members. It may not be so easy to discover a skull fracture or a broken clavicle as we would like it to be.

Reflection.—A most profitable procedure after it is over is for the accoucheur to review all the details of his case and what he has done, considering the result, and examine himself to see if his judgment has been good and his technic perfect; then to decide what he would do in a similar case or if the same woman became pregnant again. All these impressions should be written on the history card. They will be invaluable for future reference and also for individual improvement.

Anesthetic.—The reader is referred to the chapter on Anesthesia in Normal Labor. For many operations an anesthetic is not necessary, though occasionally it is demanded by a very apprehensive patient. Such are packing the cervix to induce abortion or premature labor, the application of the metreurynter, rupture of the membranes, insertion of bougies, vaginal, even uterine, tamponade. A few sutures may be placed in the perineum without ether, but if the tear is extensive or the patient too nervous, it is necessary. Curetage in abortions with the finger or the curet, and manual removal of the placenta, in a few cases may be done without narcosis, and I have in exceptional instances applied the forceps without it, thus getting the assistance of the labor-pains in the delivery. Occasionally, for a short operation, the patient can be put in a semiconscious condition and kept there by an expert anesthetist; this is the first stage of anesthesia, and precedes the one of excitement, and I have often suggested analgesia to the patient, either by words or by giving whiffs of ether. If there is time for preparation, many operations (perineorrhaphy, curetage) may be done under morphin and scopolamin, complemented by a little ether, if necessary. Increasing experience teaches me to limit general anesthetics wherever possible. Two fatal cases of hepatic cytolysis and 5 cases of icterus after chloroform, 8 fatal ether pneumonias, and several bad bronchitis cases have warned to care, not to mention prolonged nausea and vomiting, and the pain caused by them. These three discomforts often are worse than the pain relieved by the drug. Narcotic drugs also have a bad influence on the child, and I am convinced that many of the deaths ascribed to asphyxia are, in reality, anesthetic deaths.

In cases of marked anemia, in eclampsia, in other toxicoses, with goiter, in Basedow's disease, and in heart, lung, and kidney diseases, in women with marked kyphoscoliosis or great abdominal distention, all anesthetics are dangerous, and may be used only with the greatest circumspection.

Ether, chloroform, nitrous oxid, ethylene—all are good for anesthesia in operative delivery. Chloroform is preferred by many, even today, and perhaps its harmful effects on the liver are balanced by the late deaths from pneumonia, pulmonary abscess and sepsis, that so frequently follow ether. An expert may give nitrous oxid or ethylene with greater safety than attends the usual giving of ether and chloroform.

For general use I recommend ether, and the gases for hospitals where expert anesthetists are available. For version the narcosis must be deep enough to paralyze the uterus which can best be done by chloroform, next by ether, aided by a dose of atropin. For eclamptics, ethylene or ether, no chloroform; for heart cases, ether or ethylene; for anemic women, ether.

Wherever in obstetrics, as in surgery, it is possible to operate under local novocain infiltration or nerve blocking this should be done, since, unquestionably, the dangers are more than halved by the avoidance of general anesthesia. In the Chicago Lying-in Hospital and the home service of the Chicago Maternity Center simple episiotomy and repairs are usually done under "local." We do all varieties of cesarean section under infiltration anesthesia, and over 600 have been successful. With this experience I have no desire to try lumbar or sacral cord anesthesia, because it stands to reason that if the local infiltration method is so easy and practicable, one should not expose the patient to the dangers of invading the central nervous system. These seem to be greater in the pregnant than in the non-pregnant state. Müller and others try to block the pudic nerves. We do it in many cases, but have not yet experimented with extradural sacral anesthesia. For procedure see page 332.

Preparations.—The manner of preparation for operative delivery in a private home will be described as briefly as possible. In maternities the technic is identical with that of major operations plus preparation for the complicities presented by the sudden accidents of delivery and the attention required by the baby. The principles of the practice of asepsis and antisepsis are the same as in the practice of surgery, and have already been considered. If there is no one present capable of resuscitating the child, the head-piece must be arranged to allow the operator to use his mouth for insufflation of air per catheter to the baby. Figure 330 on p. 345 shows the dress of the patient during delivery. When the woman is put on the operating-table, the exposed area of mons, vulva, perineum, to the edges of the leggings, is again disinfected with lysol solution, and 1 : 1500 bichlorid, a pair of sterile leggings put on, and a sterile towel laid over the belly. This towel is frequently changed during the operation, and the skin and vulva are frequently drenched with an antiseptic solution. Even though once sterilized, the leggings are not touched by the operator. If he does so inadvertently, he washes his hands in the solutions. The assistants holding the legs wear gloves. If called upon to hold instruments, etc., they too wash in the antiseptic solutions. One must not trust too much to aseptic drapes. Figure 331, p. 346, teaches what false protection they confer.

In private home practice, although all the sheets, towels, leggings, etc., are sterilized when they have been put on the patient, the accoucheur should touch them as little as possible. *Only the area immediately around the vulva, which has been disinfected and is frequently drenched with antiseptic solutions, and the towel over the abdomen, are to be considered sterile, and may be touched by the accoucheur.* If he will practise this principle as a habit, he will be able to carry out the most complicated obstetric procedures amid the most discouraging surroundings, with greatest safety. Our operating-rooms err in this regard. The sterile field of operation is made too large. The absolute sterility of the immediate site of the operation and of the instruments, sponges, etc., which come into it, is the bacteriologic laboratory idea of asepsis, and, to my mind, the correct one—certainly for private practice. If everything else is considered infected, it is not so hard for the operator and his assistants to preserve the asepsis of the actual field of operation.

During the course of the operation, especially if prolonged, the vulva and thighs are frequently swabbed with antiseptic solutions—1 : 1500 bichlorid and 1 per cent. lysol solution. If feces escape from the anus, they are received with the greatest care in pledgets soaked in bichlorid solution. If the rectum is very full, it may be emptied by pressure from the vagina. To try to keep fecal matter away from the field by holding a towel or swab over the anus is fatuous—the feces are simply smeared all over the perineum by such procedures. It is best to see what becomes of the evacuations, and disinfect the anus continuously, taking extra care during all manipulations not to pass the hands, instruments, or gauze near the source of infection. After delivery, if much use has been made of strong antiseptics, it is a good plan to wash the parts with sterile water to prevent an eczema.

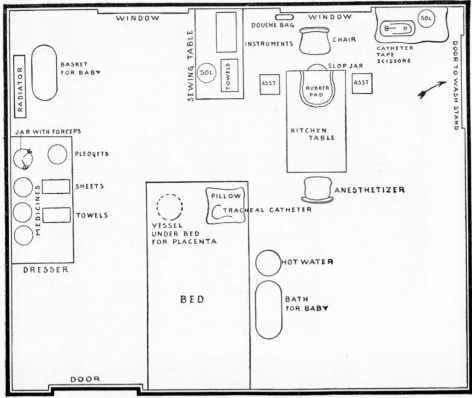

Fig. 781.—Diagram of Room Arranged for Operation.

☞ Aseptic technic is not the final word in the prevention of infection. Good operative technic, the preservation of the woman's immunities, the prevention of shock and hemorrhage, proper selection of operation, etc., contribute certainly as much to success.

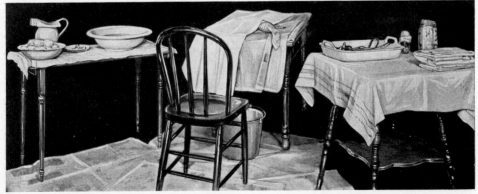

Fig. 782.—Arrangement, Using Kitchen Table for Obstetric Operations at Home.

Sewing table to left carries basin of lysol solution, bowl of bichlorid, saucer with scissors, artery clamp, and tape for cord, and pitcher of hot sterile water. A newspaper is folded into the shape of a Kelly pad and does excellently. Table to right carries pan of instruments, pile of sterile towels, jar of sterile cotton swabs, jar of sterile silkworm-gut and catgut.

Preparation of Patient for Operative Delivery.—If the woman has not been prepared as already described on p. 296, she is gotten ready for operation just before the anesthetic is started. The operator first sterilizes his hands. The vulva

is shaved, scrubbed with soap and water, the smegma under the hood of the clitoris
removed with oil or vaselin, and the parts thoroughly washed with both lysol

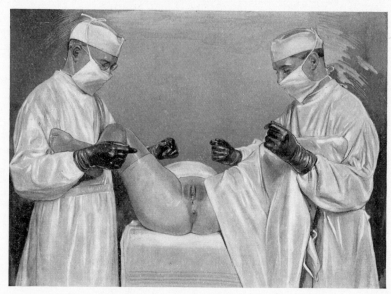

FIG. 783.—PATIENT POSED FOR OPERATIVE DELIVERY. ASSISTANTS HOLDING LEGS.
During passage of head the legs are dropped into half Walcher (Fig. 655). Notice that the sterile assistants do not
touch even the sterile drapes with their hands.

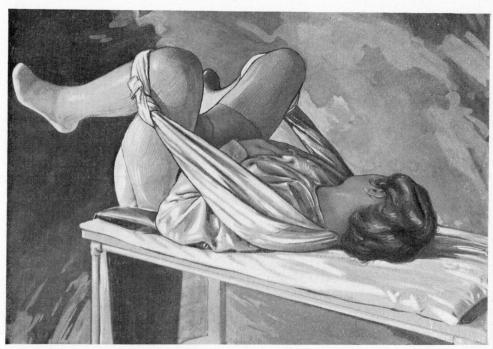

FIG. 784.—PATIENT ARRANGED FOR OPERATIVE DELIVERY WITH SHEET SLING TO HOLD LEGS WHEN SHORT OF HELP.
Note sheet tied below knee and drawn over shoulder.

and bichlorid solutions. The vagina, too, is mopped out with lysol solution, care
being taken to rub lightly and not destroy the epithelium too much. In order to

prevent hairs and wash-water dripping into the vagina during the shaving and washing, a large swab soaked in antiseptic solution is packed into the introitus. After everything else is disinfected, the swab is removed and this part and the vagina are attended to. If the patient had already been prepared for normal labor,

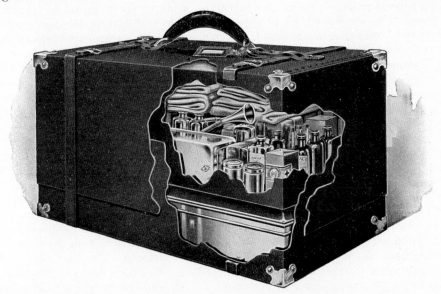

Fig. 785.—Author's Operation Telescope. Portable Sterilizer, Telescoped, at the Bottom.

all that is needful is a thorough washing with the antiseptic solutions. In all cases the accoucheur must be sure that the bladder is empty.

Arrangement of the Room.—Figure 781 is a diagram of a room in a private home, and Fig. 782 shows the arrangement of tables, etc.

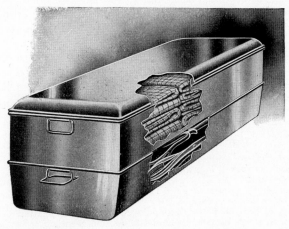

Fig. 786.—Author's Portable Sterilizer, Ready for Stove, with Instruments in Pan, Sheets and Towels in Upper Compartment. The Pan Containing the Instruments is Telescoped in the Tray for Packing.

Provision for good light is essential. An acetylene bicycle lamp or the lamps from an automobile I have many times found useful.

The kitchen or library table makes an excellent operating-table, and should always be used. It is unfair to the woman, the baby, and the doctor to operate on a woman lying across the bed. When the surgeons do appendectomies, and the gynecologists vaginal hysterectomies, with the patients lying in their beds, it may be justifiable to perform obstetric operations in such fashion. I have personal knowledge that many babies have been lost, that several women have been killed, and many more permanently damaged, because the accoucheur did not discard this medieval practice and put his patient on a proper operating-table. It stands to reason that better work can be done on the table, and, further, the dignity of the specialty of obstetrics is concerned. Even the specially constructed obstetric beds do not possess the advantages of a table.

Posture of Patient.—In America and in Continental countries the parturient is always placed on the back for operative delivery or other obstetric operation. England alone uses the side position, but less now than formerly. Kerr uses it only for low forceps operations. Figure 783 shows the most convenient posture. In cases of shoulder presentation, or in breech, when it is desired to get the presenting part away from the inlet, the head of the table may be lowered, as described by Dickinson, a combination of lithotomy and Trendelenburg positions. In some cases it is necessary to turn the woman on her side for a few minutes—for example, to grasp the anterior foot in back-posterior shoulder presentations. The woman's leg then is simply lifted over the head of the operator, and replaced after he has grasped the foot. A few operations—replacement of cord, disentanglement of locked twins—are performed with the patient in the knee-chest position, and I have operated on several women, pulseless from hemorrhage, with the body suspended head down from the shoulders of two assistants. The ease with which version can be done in this posture is surprising. Walcher's position (Fig. 655) is used to aid the passage of the head through the inlet, and the exaggerated lithotomy when it is passing the bony outlet (Fig. 495, p. 623).

Instrumentarium.—In city and town practice it is not required to take to the labor case a complete obstetric outfit. The satchel shown on p. 291 meets all the demands of the usual labor and the operations most commonly performed. If a high forceps or a version, or the care of placenta prævia, eclampsia, etc., is to be attempted, or if the woman lives far from the operator's base of supplies, a complete obstetric armamentarium must be at hand, and such an outfit, if the accoucheur wishes to be abreast of the times and give his patient the benefit of his art, must be an extensive one. Figure 785 shows the author's obstetric bag for operative cases, and Fig. 786, the portable sterilizer. The instruments are packed in the pan of the sterilizer; the other articles are arranged, without any especial order, in the upper compartment of the telescope. I have found it impracticable to have special cases and compartments made for each article—the satchel is complicated enough without them. The instruments may be divided into sets for perineorrhaphy, for forceps, for craniotomy, and wrapped in separate towels.

LIST OF ARTICLES IN TELESCOPE

1 complete operating dress, trousers, sterile gown, head-piece mask.
4 pairs sterile rubber gloves, long and short.
2 sterile hand-brushes.
2 jars sterile antiseptic gauze, one piece 12 yards and one 8 yards long.
4 jars sterile cotton and gauze swabs.
4 ounces French gelatin, or, better, 2 ampules Merck's sterile gelatin.
1 douche-can with sterile rubber tube and salt solution needle.
3 tracheal catheters, 2 rubber catheters.
1 box containing ampules of sterile epinephrin solution, pituitrin, gynergen, ephedrin, digitalis, and 50 per cent. glucose. Tablets for Ringer's solution.
1 glass hypodermic syringe—to be boiled for cesarean section.
1 sac containing a small bottle of fluidextract of ergot; a vial with tapes for the cord (sterile); a vial of bichlorid tablets; 4 ounces of liquor cresolis compound (lysol); a vial of sodium bicarbonate or borax (for boiling instruments); a glass, screw-cap bottle of sterile silk-worm-gut in 1 : 500 bichlorid solution; a bottle of 25 per cent. argyrol solution or 1 per cent. silver nitrate; a baby scale, and a tape-measure.
1 dozen tubes of sterile chromicized catgut, Nos. 1 and 2.
2 cans of ether. A mask. A head stethoscope.
1 set of history sheets for the nurse. Labor cards and birth certificates.

LIST OF INSTRUMENTS

1 pelvimeter.
1 sac containing a set of Voorhees' rubber bags, all sizes, and a syringe for filling.
3 obstetric forceps. One small one for little babies, the ordinary Simpson forceps, and the same with longer shanks for high operations, or an axis-traction instrument.
8 long pedicle clamps; 2 angular clamps.
8 ordinary artery forceps.
3 needle-holders—one long.
1 scalpel.
3 scissors.
4 retractors—various sizes.
3 tissue forceps.
2 ring forceps for cervix.
2 double vulsella for cervix.
1 box needles.
1 uterine packing forceps.
1 embryotomy set, comprising cranioclast, 1 perforator, 1 trephine, 1 heavy scissors, 1 bone forceps, 1 decapitation hook, and 1 blunt hook.
1 hebosteotomy set, comprising 1 special needle, 3 Gigli saws, 2 handles for same, 1 long curved needle, 1 raspatorium, and 1 flat director.

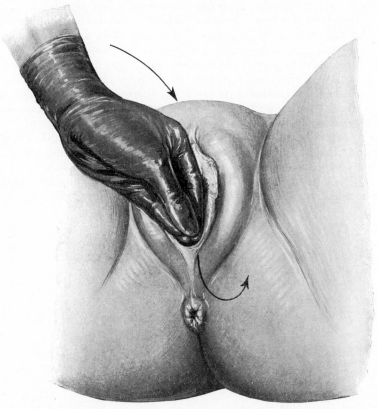

FIG. 787.—METHOD OF INTRODUCING HAND TO AVOID CONTAMINATION FROM FECES.

Previous to operation the instruments required are boiled for thirty minutes in a 1 per cent. soda or borax solution in a covered vessel. This sterilizes them, and the operator serves himself with them from the open trays on the table beside him.

In the author's Obstetrics for Nurses fuller details of the preparation for operations will be found.

Provision for Complications.—It is wise at all times to make preparations to combat postpartum hemorrhage and asphyxia of the child. For the former, the nurse will have the douche-bag sterilized, filled, and covered, ready for instant use, and the accoucheur will have a supply of sterile gauze and instruments for lacerations and for packing. For the child, an appropriate place is provided to lay it, with the tracheal catheters, warm-water bags, towels, and a hot bath close at hand.

Just before the operation the accoucheur surveys the room to see if everything is in readiness—as a general surveys the field of battle.

Care of Feces Issuing from the Anus.—This is a very unwelcome complication of any obstetric operation, because it requires the most constant watchfulness and the greatest dexterity to avoid transporting the infectious material into the genitals. Sometimes the feces contain only saprophytic and harmless organisms—a fact which is proved by the rarity of serious infections, when we know how often fecal matter is brought into the vagina, but occasionally the Streptococcus pyogenes and the gas bacillus in virulent condition exist, and fatalities in considerable number are on record. Measures should have been instituted beforehand to provide for such a contingency, that is, a cathartic administered early in labor, and an enema given to wash the lower bowel clean. If labor lasts several days, these are repeated—taking care that it be not too shortly before delivery.

If the bowels move as the operation is begun, the rectum should be emptied by squeezing out its contents from the vagina, using two fingers. I prefer not to irrigate the rectum with sterile water unless the head is well down in the pelvis and blocks the further downpour of fecal matter. Hard feces are easier to manage than spattering liquids. The anal region must be constantly inspected during the delivery, and, as feces exudes, it is carefully received in wet antiseptic gauze or cotton, the parts then being liberally drenched with 1 : 1500 bichlorid and 1 per cent. lysol solutions. Whenever the hand is inserted into the vagina, it is passed from above under the pubic arch, the possibility of contamination being always kept in mind (Fig. 787). To try to preserve asepsis by fastening a towel or pad over the anus is illusory—the feces being thus simply plastered all over the perineal region from the inside of the cloth, even damming back up into the vulva. Urine may also be infectious, especially if the woman suffers from pyelitis or pharyngitis.

CHAPTER LXIX

PREPARATORY OBSTETRIC OPERATIONS

PREPARATION OF THE SOFT PARTS

Opening the Cervix.—In this chapter only those methods of cervical enlargement will be considered which apply to labors at or near term. For the methods of obtaining access to the uterine cavity in the earlier months of gestation see page 1124, Induction of Premature Labor and of Abortion.

The state of the cervix is a condition which governs the indications of most obstetric operations. In eclampsia, placenta prævia, and all diseases demanding immediate emptying of the uterus the state of the cervix has a guiding influence in the choice of procedure. We have many methods of gaining access to the uterus—some slow, some rapid. The slow ones are those which call the uterus into action to aid in the dilatation, and the process resembles natural labor

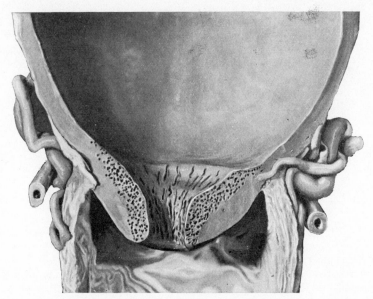

Fig. 788.—Beginning Obliteration of Cervix. Purely Diagrammatic.
A laceration at this time endangers vessels and peritoneum.

more closely. Packing the cervix and metreurysis are slow operations, but in some of the more rapid ones uterine action also aids the process in a marked degree, as in manual dilatation and the employment of the Bossi dilator. The following operations are done to open the cervix: Packing the cervix and lower uterine segment with gauze; manual or digital dilatation; metreurysis; mechanical dilatation with metal instruments; radiating incisions in the cervix; vaginal cesarean section. Which of these methods will be the one selected will depend—(1) On the condition of the cervix, whether it is tightly closed, or already more or less effaced or shortened or drawn up into the body of the uterus; (2) on the urgency of the case and the nature of the complication demanding the interference; (3) on the skill of the operator; (4) on the environment of the patient; (5) the pains.

It is of greatest importance to distinguish between a cervix that is already effaced or obliterated and one that has not been at all taken up, and also to know how far the process has advanced. During the effacement and dilatation of the cervix the pelvic connective tissue is drawn up out of the pelvis; the bladder is drawn up, and its attachment to the cervix loosened and displaced upward, the ureters going with it; the peritoneum is elevated; the broad ligaments unfolded; and the large vessels at the sides of the uterus raised up and retracted, sometimes even above the brim. This means that these important structures are removed from the pelvis, where they are subject to injury from below (Figs. 788 and 789). In primiparæ this unfolding of the cervix may occur to some extent in the last weeks of pregnancy, and is sometimes accompanied by fugitive labor-pains, and this is also true of multiparæ, in whom there is an additional softness of the tissues. Artificial opening of the cervical canal is easiest in the last weeks of pregnancy, but even then there is

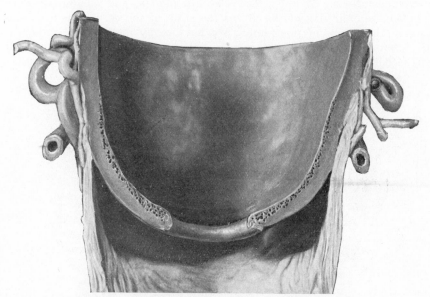

Fig 789.—Cervix Effaced. Diagrammatic. Vessels and Peritoneum Retracted away from Ordinary Danger.

danger of deep lacerations, and the more nature has opened the cervix, the less the accoucheur has to do. Figure 792 will give an accurate idea of the location of the uterine artery, and Fig. 886 on page 1084 shows the development of the uterine veins. The latter are really more important in this connection.

Packing the cervix is shown in Fig. 791. It may be employed to start labor (Hofmeier, 1888), to induce abortion (Wyder, 1888), to soften and dilate the cervix preparatory to the insertion of a colpeurynter, and to stimulate flagging labor-pains in the first stage. Ordinarily, if not already present, pains come on within eight hours, but sometimes not for ten or fifteen, when the first packing is removed and another inserted, if needed, or other methods adopted. This simple operation may be done when the cervix is closed. Anesthesia is rarely required. I have never found it necessary to use a metal dilator after the sixth month to procure enough dilatation to pass the tube, of which there are several sizes, with gauze to fit. It may be done safely at home. It is not useful in urgent cases nor in placenta prævia. The dangers are infection (which can be avoided), rupture of the membranes, which may allow prolapse of the cord, separation of the edge of the placenta if situated near the internal os, and air-embolism. The latter may be avoided by holding the labia spread apart by the fingers and the instrument, by packing slowly,

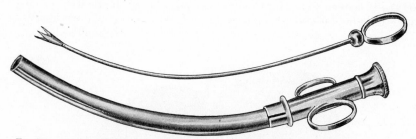

FIG. 790.—MODIFIED GEROTA UTERINE PACKING TUBE FOR USE AFTER THE SIXTH MONTH.
The tube has a lumen ⅜ inch across. Gauze 3 inches wide or a knit bandage is used for packing. It is sterilized and preserved in hermetically sealed bottles. It is served directly from the bottle. Smaller tubes and narrower gauze are used for abortion cases.

and having the shoulders of the patient raised. Separation of the edge of a lowly inserted placenta occurred once in the very many cases in which I have thus packed.

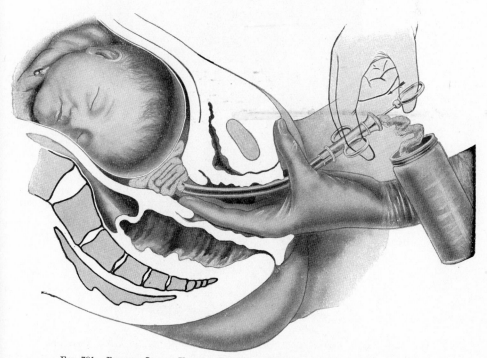

FIG. 791.—PACKING LOWER UTERINE SEGMENT AND CERVIX FOR INDUCTION OF LABOR.
Catching the end of the gauze strip from the bottle, which is held near the vulva, by means of the trident plunger, the gauze is pushed the whole length of the tube. Now, under the guidance of the two fingers, placed in or against the cervix, the tube is inserted into the lower part of the uterus. With short in-and-out strokes of the plunger the gauze is deposited above and in the cervical canal, taking care to distribute it evenly and not to rupture the membranes. This is easily accomplished by moving the end of the tube in circles and retracting it as the cavity fills up. From three to five yards may be inserted. In most cases the vagina need not be plugged. It is occasionally needed in abortions.

It was evidenced by a slight flow of pure blood. I put no more gauze into the uterus, but packed the cervix tightly, and the result was good. Rupture of the membranes occurred several times without bad results—indeed, labor seemed hastened.   In 2 cases the gauze compressed the forelying cord (evidenced by marked slowing of the fetal heart-tones) and had to be immediately removed.   Vaginal tamponade was described under Abortion (*q. v.*).

Manual Dilatation of the Cervix.—This is the oldest method of enlarging the canal, and is spoken of in Hippocrates' writings.   It is the method most naturally adopted, but the ancients also possessed pronged instruments operated by screws. Paré, in the forced operative delivery, which he so much practised, and to which

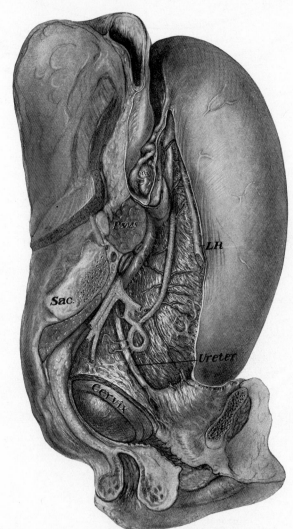

FIG. 792.—UTERINE ARTERY AND URETER.   DILATATION OF THE CERVIX ALMOST COMPLETE.
Adapted from Couvelaire.

his pupil, Guillemeau, gave the name "accouchement forcé," began with digital dilatation of the cervix.   First one and then two fingers are insinuated through the os.   The two fingers may be then spread by one or two fingers of the other hand forced between them like a wedge.   After the tips of four fingers are introduced they are placed back to back, the knuckles acting like a double fulcrum, and the cervical ring is thus expanded.   This is similar to the methods devised by Bonnaire and Edgar.   P. Harris inserts the whole hand into the vagina, and the cervix is dilated by the insinuation into it of, successively, one finger, the thumb and one finger, then two, then three and four, and finally the hand, the thumb being given a motion of extension, the fingers one of flexion. The only advantage this method has over the others is that the hand, being in the vagina, is not so easily contaminated by feces issuing from the anus, but, by raising the hands toward the pubis in the performance of the operation illustrated above, this danger may be avoided.

It is essential to procure complete opening of the canal, otherwise the delivery of the child which follows may be difficult or impossible, and during the fruitless attempts at extraction the undilated uterus may rupture or the child die or be severely injured. The conditions for manual dilatation of the cervix are: The cervix must be effaced, or very nearly so; the pelvis normal; the child normal in size, and the presentation and position favorable or corrigible. The placenta may not be prævia. The vagina, too, must be dilatable, or is to be enlarged by episiotomy. Unless performed under these conditions, the operation is dangerous and may fail of its purpose. It requires from one-half to three hours, and is often painfully tiring

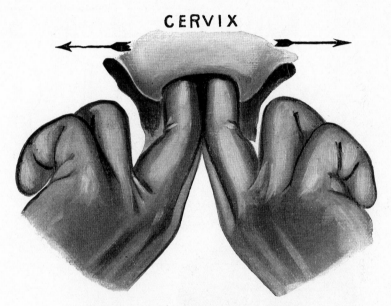

CERVIX

Fig. 793.—Dilating Effaced Cervix with Fingers.
Shows double fulcrum action (90 per cent. of cases have tears).

to the fingers and hands. It is invariably attended by lacerations of the cervix, and these tears are often deep, sometimes even of the importance of a rupture of the uterus, opening the peritoneal cavity, causing death from hemorrhage or from infection. In multiparæ the lacerations are usually somewhat less extensive. In all cases the cervix is bruised and battered, and infection, even in the hands of the cleanest obstetrician, is sometimes unavoidable. In truly exceptional cases the cervix is so soft that it may, within fifteen to thirty minutes, be dilated large enough for safe delivery. Where the cervix needs only a little more enlargement to be complete, manual dilatation is permissible. In other cases we have better means of obtaining access to the uterus. For history see Bauer.

Metreurysis.—*Historic.*—In 1831 Schnakenberg dilated the cervix with a bladder attached to a syringe. In 1851 Carl Braun invented the colpeurynter, a rubber balloon to be distended with fluid after being placed in the vagina. For a long time previously Chiari, Wellenbergh, and others had used pigs' bladders for this purpose, but discarded them because they decomposed. In 1862 Tarnier invented the "dilatateur intrauterin," a soft-rubber bag or condom on the end of a male catheter. Barnes, in 1862, introduced the soft-rubber fiddle-shaped bags, which are not used any more.   In 1888 Champetier de Ribes recommended a large, cone-shaped, inelastic bag, and since then, among the numerous modifications that have been proposed, the

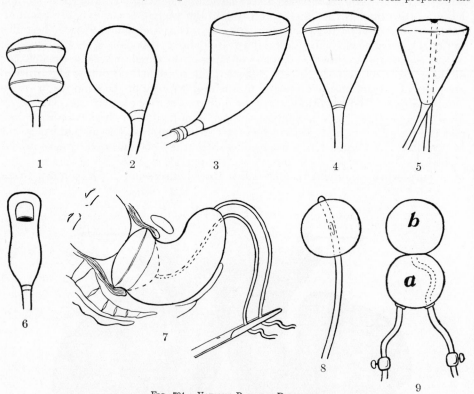

FIG. 794.—VARIOUS BALLOON DILATORS.
1, Hirst's; 2, Braun's; 3, Champetier de Ribes'; 4, Voorhees'; 5, Stowe's; 6, Barnes'; 7, Pomeroy's; 8, Tarnier's; 9, Chassagny's.

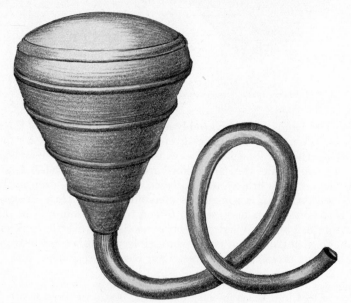

FIG. 795.—MODIFIED VOORHEES' BAG.
Ridges enable one to determine how far the bag has traversed the cervix.

use of cloth bags, rendered impermeable by rubber, has already superseded the old colpeurynter of Braun. Schauta, in 1883, published the use of the bag in the uterus, as practised in Spaeth's clinic. Mäurer, in 1887, introduced constant traction on the bag as a means to hasten its action. In 1907 Stowe invented a bag shaped like the Voorhees bag, but with a tube leading through its center, through which sterile salt solution can be injected into the uterus to replace lost liquor amnii, an idea suggested several years before by Bauer to the Berlin Medical Society. Of all the bags on the market, I have found those of Voorhees, in four sizes, and the large ones of the same shape sold in Europe under the name of Dührssen, the best. Since the bag is usually placed in the uterus, the name hystreurynter or metreurynter is better. The bags are filled with water and boiled in plain water for thirty minutes; paint with ½ per cent. iodin in glycerin, fill with ½ per cent. lysol solution.

The method of application of the hydrostatic bag has been minutely described on p. 502, in the Treatment of Placenta Prævia (*q. v.*). Some operators prefer to pass the bag by sight (Fig. 796), believing that thus it is easier to avoid carrying infection from the vagina into the uterus. The perineum is retracted by a speculum, the cervix is steadied by a ring forceps, and the folded bag is gently insinuated into

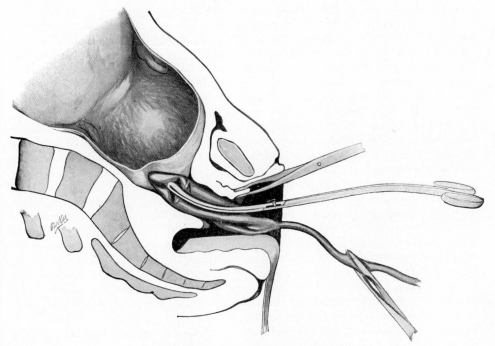

FIG. 796.—PASSING COLPEURYNTER BY SIGHT.

and through the canal, in the direction of one of the sacro-iliac joints, taking due notice of the curves of the canal. Force may not be used, and it is best, in the absence of special indication, to preserve the membranes. Such special indications are eclampsia, in which it has been noticed that the convulsions often cease after the liquor amnii has been let off, polyhydramnion, twins, and other conditions of overfilling of the uterus, and placenta prævia, in order to place the bag on top of the placenta.

If time is no object, traction is not applied, but if the pains are slow in coming, a weight of one or two pounds may be attached to the tube. After the first bag is expelled a larger one may be applied, the membranes punctured, or the labor left to nature, depending on the exigencies of the case.

The action of the metreurynter is three-fold: First, it mechanically dilates the cervix from above downward like a fluid wedge, in which respect it closely resembles the bag of waters; second, by its presence and by the dilatation of the uterus which its increased volume causes, but particularly by pressure on the retrocervical ganglion, the uterus is stimulated to action, and strong pains are usually soon inaugurated. Third, it may be used as a tampon, as in cases of placenta prævia, etc. The selection of the bag will depend on the object sought, and if rapid action is desired, the inelastic bag with traction will more quickly evoke pains and dilate the uterus than the soft-rubber colpeurynter, which, under traction, is likely to pull out into a sausage shape and slip through the poorly dilated cervix. If it is simply desired to evoke pains, as in the induction of labor, either bag may be used without traction, or with a minimum amount of it. As a tampon in the vagina, the soft colpeurynter is preferred; in the treatment of placenta prævia, the Voorhees' conic inelastic bag. Early in pregnancy, and in the late months, just to inaugurate uterine action, a small-sized bag is employed.

Indications.—Metreurysis is very useful for the induction of premature labor where great urgency is not present, though sometimes, if traction is put on the tube and the parts are not too rigid, the pains start up, and they, together with the mechanical dilatation, open the uterus in a few hours. Whenever there is an indication to hasten delivery in the interests of the mother or child, the bags may be used, and to prepare the cervix or the vagina for rapid delivery, as in breech, shoulder, or face presentation, or in the presence of threatening complications, they are often invaluable. In stenosis of the cervix the bags may be useful, but they require the aid of the pains to soften the parts. A sluggish uterus may be stimulated by the metreurynter, but it is wise to find out the cause of the weak pains—rigidity of the cervix, abnormal adherence of the membranes, overdistention of the uterus, pendulous belly, low placenta—all these may require other treatment. In cases of dry labor the bags deserve more general application, since they replace the bag of waters to a considerable extent. In shoulder presentation, to preserve what is left of the liquor amnii and to keep the presenting part from impaction in the pelvis, the metreurynter should be applied and complete dilatation awaited. In contracted pelvis, where spontaneous delivery is to be expected, a bag is to be applied if the membranes rupture prematurely. Generally speaking, metreurysis is useful when the bag of waters ruptures before complete dilatation has been effected. In prolapse of the cord the hystreurynter is of great value. Perhaps the most valuable function of the metreurynter is as a plug in cases of placenta prævia. While properly not belonging here, it may be mentioned that the colpeurynter is useful,—placed in the vagina, to prepare the vagina and pelvic floor for rapid delivery, as in breech presentation, forceps, version, and extraction; to overcome rigidity of the soft parts; to stimulate pains; and, during pregnancy, to lift up a retroflexed uterus, to raise a uterus that may be causing hyperemesis, and in the treatment of pyelo-ureteritis.

Conditions.—The cervix must be open enough to insert the size of bag desired. Rarely is it necessary to use metal dilators first. Packing the cervix with gauze for twelve hours usually suffices to render it soft and dilatable. Cervical carcinoma and threatened uterine rupture contraindicate the operation. In the presence of vaginal infection some other plan should be selected, if possible, such as puncture of membranes, vaginal cesarean section, even the Porro operation.

Dangers and Disadvantages.—In a few cases the uterus does not respond, the bag is not expelled, and traction, within the limits of safety, does not open the cervix. Sometimes traction brings one bag after another through, but the uterine action does not come into play and the cervix closes up again. Several cases are recorded where pregnancy continued. Oftener the repeated manipulations, which in some cases may extend over a period of five or more days, cause fever (infection), and then, unless the pains come on strongly, a formidable condition is presented for treatment. Such torpor of the uterus is rare.

The metreurynter may displace the presenting part, and this may be undesirable, unless version is in contemplation. Prolapse of the cord is a real danger. In spite of close watching and care this happened in 2 of my cases, and in one I lost the infant because of it. The danger of infection is nil—with proper precautions. Three cases, one fatal, of air-embolism from bursting of the bag are reported. A liquid should have been used for filling. Rupture of the uterus has been reported in 11 instances, but in several of them the extraction of the child through an insufficiently dilated passage was probably the real cause. In the others excessive softness of the cervix was a factor—placenta prævia, nephritis. In my case, a primipara aged thirty-eight with placenta prævia, the bag evoked such tumultuous pains that it ruptured the uterus, the woman dying of internal hemorrhage. If too much traction is put on the bag, the uterus acts too violently and such danger is real. If too much fluid is injected into the bag, the uterus is overdistended, as in polyhydramnion, and the uterine action is usually weak, but sometimes the opposite is true. A large experience with the bags, however, together with study of the voluminous literature on the subject, convinces me that most of the disadvantages may be overcome by proper technic and by watching the effects, not leaving the patient to ignorant attendants. They are, indeed, a very valuable, indispensable addition to our obstetric resources. Since the rubber deteriorates with time, the bags are to be kept dry in an ordinary paste-board box, and thus preserved, will last one or two years.

Machine Dilatation.—Tertullian, in the second century after Christ, mentions pronged uterine dilators, and they played a more or less prominent part in gynecology and obstetrics since. Levret (1760) opposed their general use. Goodell's dilator is the type of the instrument used by gyniatrists and in the treatment of early abortions. In 1888 Bossi invented a four-branched dilator for the parturient cervix, which had great vogue in the years 1902 to 1906, but now is almost generally discarded. The principle of the instrument is irrational. Constant elastic distraction of the cervix was invented by Tarnier in his three-branched, glove-stretcher-like "ecarteur uterin," forced apart by elastic bands around the handles. Bossi replaced the bands with a powerful screw and added a scale to show the amount of separation of the blades.

In all the cases in which I have used it, 14 in number, lacerations of greater or less degree resulted, and Bossi's directions were carefully followed. American authorities do not recommend such instruments. Literature and history of all dilating methods are to be found in the articles of Hartz and Lewis and DeLee.

Incisions in the Cervix.—*Hysterostomatomy.*—The first records of cervix incisions to aid delivery are from the eighteenth century, but probably they were made earlier. Baudelocque, about 1790, condemned them; Simpson used them in cases of carcinoma; Godemer (1841), in eclampsia; Skutsch, in 1887, to save the baby; but Dührssen, in 1890, showed their value so conclusively that they are often termed "Dührssen's incisions." The field of usefulness of this operation is very limited, because the incisions are safe only after complete effacement of the cervix. Reference to Figs. 788 and 789 will show that a cut made before the blood-vessels are retracted exposes them to great danger—indeed, several deaths have occurred from hemorrhage, and if the tissues are incised before obliteration of the cervix is complete, the wounds are likely to tear further during the extraction and open up the broad ligaments, even the peritoneal cavity. The ancients made multiple small cuts in stellate fashion, but Dührssen made deep lateral cuts, and if these were not sufficient, posterior and anterior incisions also. Other operators make the cuts in the oblique diameters, two to four as needed, which method is preferable. It is essential that the greatest deliberation be practised in the subsequent extraction of the child to prevent the lacerations from extending—an accident which has happened in the hands of the world's best accoucheurs. The preparations for the operation are the same as for any major obstetric procedure, because sometimes a severe hemorrhage must be faced, and afterward the wounds are to be repaired. The indications are found in those complications bringing danger to mother or child, when the cervix is obliterated, only the thin partition between the dilated lower uterine segment and the vagina being left to overcome. It is a common operation before the application of forceps in occipitoposterior positions in primiparæ, or in other operative deliveries when the cervix is not open enough. Rigid cervix scars, conglutination, etc., are occasional indications. The condition which must be insisted on is *complete effacement of the cervix*. Placenta prævia is a contraindication. Most so-called manual and instrumental dilatations of the cervix are in reality bilateral incisions or tears, but made with blunt instruments.

Accouchement Forcé.—This operation was introduced by Paré, given the name by Guillemeau, his pupil, but, owing to its great maternal (sepsis and hemorrhage) and fetal (asphyxia) mortality, was employed only in the gravest emergencies. Under the protection of asepsis and antisepsis it was revived, but is now rapidly

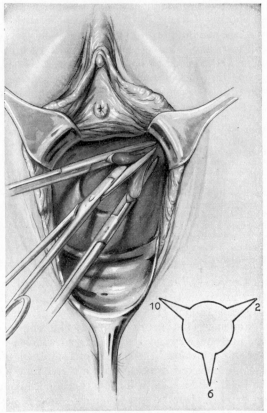

FIG. 797.—DÜHRSSEN'S INCISIONS.
Under wide exposure of the field by broad specula the cervix is grasped and cut between two 8-inch forceps which are left on a few minutes to stop hemorrhage. The author usually makes three incisions corresponding to the 10-2-6 of the clock, and cuts to the fornices vaginæ.

falling into disuse because of the almost invariable severe injuries inflicted on the mother, the frequent hemorrhage and deaths caused, and the paucity of fetal lives saved. The original conception of the operation was rapid dilatation of the cervix by the hands, version, and forced extraction of the child. Recently the term has been used to apply to any one of several methods of rapid delivery from below. While admitting that a few cases occur where it is not extra hazardous to dilate the cervix and extract, according to the original formula, these are so few and the dangers of the others so great that the author would advise dropping both the term and the operation altogether from our obstetric surgery. As a substitute for this brutal and unsurgical operation the metreurynter, in cases of not great urgency, and vaginal or abdominal cesarean section in the others, are suggested.

Delmas, in 1928, sought to revive accouchement forcé, claiming that spinal anesthesia relaxes the cervix and lower uterine segment to such an extent that manual dilatation is easily performed in thirty seconds to six minutes and version and extraction just as readily accomplished in the same length of time. On anatomic and theoretic grounds such a claim is untenable and experience, mainly by the French themselves, has amply proved its fallacy.

Mention may be made, for the sake of condemning the procedure, of the operation of using the body of the child as a dilator of the parturient canal. Unless the infant is dead, and excepting a few cases of placenta prævia, such a method is inadvisable.

Vaginal cesarean section, or colpohysterotomy, is an operation devised by A. Dührssen, of Berlin, April 1, 1895. Acconci, of Italy, devised a similar operation, but Dührssen ("Der vaginale Kaiserschnitt," Berlin, 1904) conclusively proves his priority. The term vaginal cesarean section, used in the eighteenth century for cervical incisions, was considered by Baudelocque unsuitable. Although Dührssen's operation is a formidable one, deserving the name he chose for it, the terms vaginal hysterotomy or colpotrachelotomy might supplant it.

Preparations.—These are the same as for any major obstetric operation. An anesthetist, two assistants, and a nurse are needed if good work is to be done.

A table, the lithotomy position, and good horizontal light are essential. The operation has been successfully done under the exigencies of practice in a home, but with increased technical difficulties. The instruments are those of vaginal hysterectomy plus the forceps, etc.

The Operation.—If the parturient is close to the end of pregnancy and primiparous, it is best to make a deep unilateral episiotomy—on that side to which the occiput points if forceps are to be used; on the opposite side, if version is to be performed. This will prevent laceration of the perineum during the subsequent delivery. If the episiotomy wound bleeds too freely, it may be sewn up temporarily, the line of suture being at a right angle to the line of incision. Dührssen insisted on the necessity, in case the child is at full term, of making both anterior and posterior

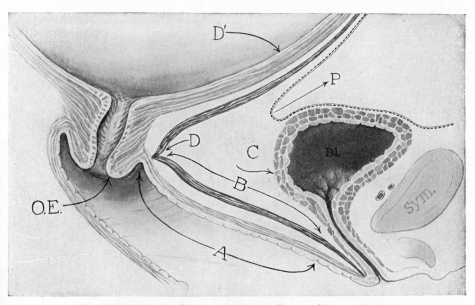

Fig. 798.—Diagram of Surgical Anatomy of Vaginal Cesarean Section.

cervical incisions. Bumm finds the anterior incision, if extended, gives sufficient space. My experience accords with Dührssen's. The cervix must be in the median line. It is often twisted by rotating the presenting part to one or the other side. Figure 799 shows the field exposed by short broad specula, the cervix drawn by vulsellum forceps or by silk traction ligatures, and red lines to indicate the location of the incisions, which go through the mucous membrane of the vagina and the vesicovaginal fascia. After the vagina has been reflected off the base of the bladder, the latter is pushed upward, off the anterior cervical wall (Fig. 800), using the finger

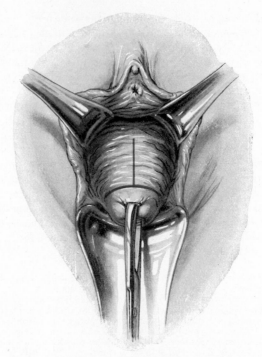

FIG. 799.—VAGINAL CESAREAN SECTION.
Exposure of field and line of incisions.   The anterior cut begins one inch from urethra.

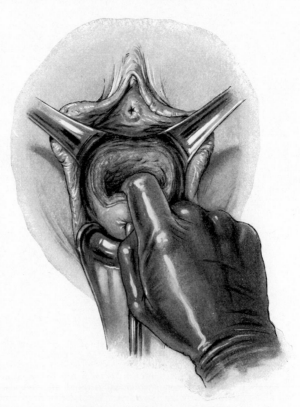

FIG. 800.—PUSHING THE BLADDER OFF THE CERVICAL WALL.
The finger is covered with gauze.

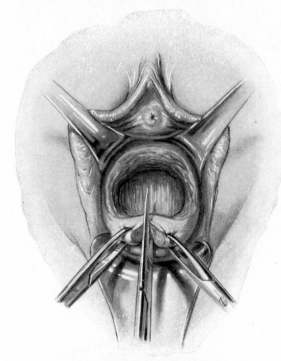

FIG. 801.—SPLITTING THE CERVIX.

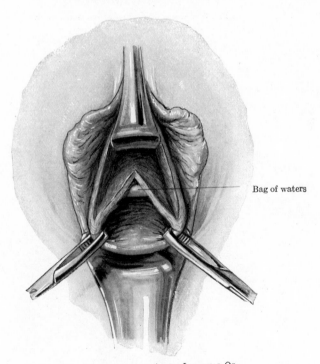

Bag of waters

FIG. 802.—CERVIX SPLIT TO ABOVE INTERNAL OS.

covered with gauze. At the same time the cervix is partly freed from the bases of the broad ligaments at the sides, but care is required here, as large veins may be encountered. Now the cervix is grasped by two vulsellum forceps and split medially (Fig. 801) up to the internal os. Figure 802 shows this section made and the bag of waters pouching in the opening. Operating

63

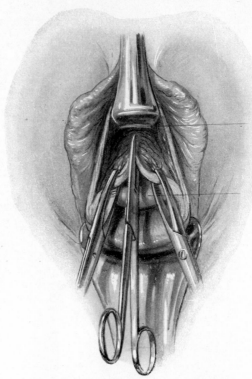

Uterovesical reflection
of peritoneum

Bag of waters

FIG. 803.—INCISING LOWER UTERINE SEGMENT.

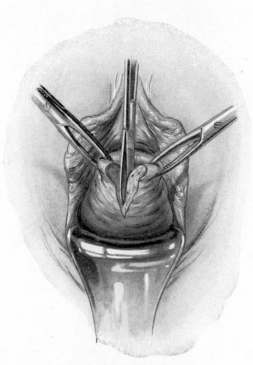

FIG. 804.—INCISING POSTERIOR WALL.

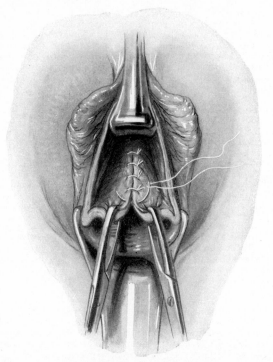

FIG. 805.—SUTURING ANTERIOR INCISION.

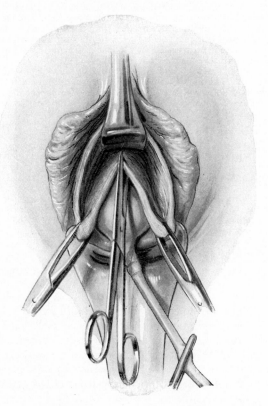

FIG. 806.—VAGINAL CESAREAN SECTION, HAVING FIRST INSERTED A VOORHEES' BAG.
By pulling on the bag the cervix becomes accessible, and as soon as enough room has been obtained the bag comes through.

again as in Fig. 800, the bladder is stripped further off the anterior wall, laying it bare to view, and the uterovesical fold of peritoneum can be seen or felt at the upper end of the wound. A narrow speculum is inserted to expose the field clearly. Now the medial uterine incision is continued upward (Fig. 803), the vulsellum forceps being placed on successively higher portions of the cervix and lower uterine segment, and pulling them down into the bite of the scissors. Care is to be exercised to keep in the median line and to avoid injuring the peritoneum. This is pushed off the fascia covering the lower uterine segment before the advancing scissors by means of the finger, and the uterine muscle and this same fascia are incised just as we do in the laparotrachelotomy.

For a child weighing about 3 or $3\frac{1}{2}$ pounds, an anterior incision 10 cm. in length usually suffices. One may test the size of the opening by passing through it the fist, made about the size of the baby's head, by holding in it a large ball of cotton. If more space is needed, the anterior incision may be extended upward or the posterior wall may be incised also (Fig. 804). Dührssen makes the posterior cut first as routine.

Grasping the cervix with bullet forceps, it is split to the vaginal reflection, then the peritoneum of Douglas' culdesac is pushed upward and loosened at the sides, after which the lower uterine segment is divided as high as needful. Delivery is now accomplished by forceps or by version and extraction, according to preference—I prefer forceps. Solms of Berlin leaves the case to nature.

If labor-pains are present, hemorrhage is not usually profuse, but if it is, manual removal of the placenta and uterine tamponade are rapidly performed, and ergot given hypodermically, or pituitrin injected into the cut edges of the uterine muscle. A careful examination of the parturient tract is made to determine the extent of the wounds. Now the incisions are closed (Fig. 805). By traction on the silk loops or vulsella, placed on the uterine edges, the uppermost angle of the opening is readily drawn into view, which may be aided by a narrow speculum placed so as to retract the bladder. A row of interrupted No. 2 twenty-day catgut sutures, taking part of the muscle, but leaving the mucosa, is rapidly put in, care being observed not to include the uterine packing, and over this a second layer is placed, uniting the outer layer of the muscle of the lower uterine segment and the fascia over it, similarly to the closure in laparotrachelotomy. The vesicovaginal fascia is coapted with the same sutures which unite the vaginal edges—interrupted No. 2 catgut. A strip of gauze may be left to drain the large subperitoneal wound for twenty-four hours. If the posterior wall has been divided, this is sutured first with interrupted through-and-through catgut sutures, tied on the interior of the cervix. Finally, the perineum is repaired. The operation requires from eight to twenty minutes for the delivery of the child, and from twenty to forty minutes to repair the incisions. If, as with cancer, the uterus is to be extirpated, the anterior and posterior incisions are prolonged until the uterus is bisected, and the broad ligaments are clamped and tied, each half being removed after the method of P. Müller.

Dangers.—Injury of the bladder and ureters may be avoided by proper technic, by going slowly without attempts at spectacular operating. In pushing the bladder off the cervix it must be borne in mind that, as labor progresses, the bladder is drawn up, and usually to the right side. In breech and shoulder presentations the bladder is more central. One of my cases whose operation was entirely uncomplicated returned after six years with a displaced and kinked left ureter which causes intermittent hydronephrosis. Hemorrhage is usually not marked if the uterus is divided cleanly in the middle line, if the tissues at the side are spared, and the cuts do not tear further, which they will not do if properly placed at first. In two cases the tissues were so friable that the traction ligatures and vulsella pulled out, and hemorrhage was so profuse that the vaginal route had to be abandoned. After the delivery packing the uterus will stop hemorrhage. Pulling down the uterus strongly also has a good influence. There is no reason why Sehrt's compression may not be applied if needed at this stage. In one case the broad ligaments and pelvic connective tissue were so edematous that the cervix could not be drawn down for incision, and abdominal cesarean section was indicated. To gain access to the cervix when it is high up Dührssen advised a deep paravaginal perineal incision, or deep episiotomy, and also, what seems to be a real improvement in this operation, the metreurynter, by means of which the cervix is pulled down and on which it is incised. When the fully distended colpeurynter can come through the incision, the child can be easily delivered. Should the bladder be opened, it is to be sutured after delivery and a permanent catheter inserted. If the peritoneum is torn, it is sutured at once. In both instances drainage from below is indicated. Rupture of the vagina occurred in two of my cases, threatening hemorrhage from the bases of the broad ligaments in three.

Subsequent pregnancies and labor in five of my cases were entirely uneventful, and many such are reported, so that there need be but little fear that the uterus will rupture, but in several instances the wound did not heal perfectly, leaving an everted eroded cervix.

Indications.—When the cervix is closed and an indication arises for rapid delivery, and, second, when the cervix is diseased and nature is unable to overcome the obstruction, vaginal cesarean section may be done. Under the first caption may be placed eclampsia, abruptio placentæ, hyperemesis gravidarum, uncompensated heart disease, lung disease, œdema pulmonum, asphyxia in utero—in short, all acute complications on the part of the mother or infant. Under the head of obstructions stenosis, antefixatio uteri, scars from old operations, may be mentioned. Cancer is not amenable to this operation.

Conditions.—Delivery from below must be possible, that is, the pelvis must be large enough and presentation and position of the child favorable. Although some authors recommend the operation in placenta prævia, I would consider this a contra-indication, and Bumm recently retracted his recommendation. The child must be living, unless the indication for haste on the part of the mother is imperative. The operation simply overcomes the resistance of the cervix, and it is highly important to determine beforehand if there is an edema of the connective tissue or excessive friability of the tissues. In 60 operations performed by the author many technical difficulties were encountered. It is, therefore, not to be undertaken except by one skilled in pelvic surgery.

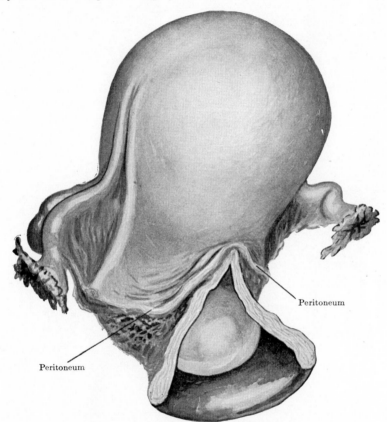

Peritoneum

Peritoneum

FIG. 807.—ANTERIOR VIEW OF OPERATION.

Operations Preparing the Vagina and Pelvic Floor for Delivery.—Episiotomy and the deep paravaginal incisions have already been described, and it has also been said that the colpeurynter may be placed in the vagina to prepare it for the subsequent delivery. This procedure is especially useful in breech and shoulder presentations in primiparæ. Some authors advise manual dilatation of the pelvic floor and vulva preparatory to forceps operation or other rapid operative delivery, and before hebosteotomy. My own experience proves to me that in such cases we do not really stretch the muscle and leave its structure perfect afterward, but we cause innumerable, minute or larger, submucous tears, and afterward the women return, not with torn pelvic floors, but with relaxed pelvic floors, the functional result, however, being the same or worse. I prefer a clean cut to these unsurgical methods, and am convinced that the after-effects are much more favorable. Unfortunately, this ideal practice comes into conflict with the desire to avoid the necessity of "putting in stitches," which carries a certain opprobrium among the women. I know that many children have been lost and much invalidism has resulted from this ill-advised and objectionable sentiment.

LITERATURE

Bauer, A. W.: Wien. klin. Woch., 1928, No. 43, also Zeitschr. für Geb. u. Gyn., xciv; H. iii, p. 720.—*Bürger:* Arch. f. Gyn., 1906, vol. lxxvii, p. 485.—*De Lee:* "The Use of the Colpeurynter," Chicago Medical Recorder, 1900; "The Bossi Dilator," Amer. Jour. Obstet., 1903, vol. xlviii, No. 1.—*Delmas, P.:* Revue Franç. de Gyn. et d'Obstetrique April, 1929. Also Yearbook of Obstetrics, 1930, p. 201–206.—*Hartz:* Monatsschr. f. Geb. u. Gyn., vol. xix.—*Lewis:* Surg., Gyn., and Obstet., December, 1906.—*Schweitzer:* Centralbl. f. Gyn., June 22, 1912.

CHAPTER LXX

PREPARATORY OPERATIONS (CONTINUED).—PREPARATION OF THE BONY PELVIS

Enlarging the Pelvic Canal.—Reference has already been made to the idea of the ancients that the bones of the pelvis soften and separate during delivery. We make use of the softening of the joints and the movability of the bones on each other to produce, by posture, actual enlargement of the diameters of the canal. Thus it is certain that the Walcher position enlarges the conjugata vera, and the exaggerated lithotomy, the bony outlet, particularly in its transverse diameter. The idea of cutting the bony pelvic ring is not recent.

Symphysiotomy and Hebosteotomy.—Pinæus, in 1570, refers to section of the pelvic bones; de la Courvee, in 1655, delivered a child by section of the symphysis pubis after the mother aied in labor; Sigault, in 1768, invented the operation of symphysiotomy, but could not perform it until 1777. The woman, Mme. Souchot, and her child, survived, but she had a permanent vesico-vaginal fistula, fecal incontinence, and difficulty of locomotion. Sigault was given a silver medal. In 1775 Aitken recommended section of the bones on both sides of the joint by means of an articulated saw, but never did it on a live woman; in 1821 Champion de Bar le Duc pointed out the advantages of cutting the bone instead of the symphysis, and in 1830 Stoltz, of Strassburg, perfected the operation of pubiotomy, using a chain-saw, very much as it is done today, but he also operated only on cadavers. In 1832 Galbiati tried Aitken's recommendation, but the mother and babe died from the operation itself, and pubiotomy all but disappeared until Gigli, of Florence, in 1894, drew general attention to the operation and published his saw,—a roughened steel wire,—which he had invented for the express purpose of cutting the pelvic girdle. Bonardi, in 1897, performed the first operation with the saw, Gigli operating in 1902 the first time on the living. Symphysiotomy had a checkered career. In France an acrid polemic was waged about it, and Baudelocque, Caseaux, DuBois, and La Chapelle finally caused its abandonment. In Germany and England the operation never obtained a foothold, but in Italy, in spite of its high mortality and morbidity, it enjoyed a sporadic existence by grace of Galbiati and Morisani. With the improvement in asepsis and instrumentarium of the late eighties and the proper selection of cases naturally the results improved. In 1891 Spinelli, a pupil of Morisani, went to Paris, interested Pinard in the revived operation, and the latter, within a year, performed it 17 times. In 1892 and 1893 it was being done in all countries with the overenthusiasm begotten by every new remedy, and for a time symphysiotomy threatened the firm position held by cesarean section. Toward the end of the last century, however, it lost ground almost entirely. Zweifel, in Leipsic, Kerr, of Glasgow, Jellett, now in New Zealand, and Pinard, in Paris, are among its few fast friends even today.

In 1904, as the result of the publications of Gigli, Van de Velde, and Döderlein, pubiotomy took the center of the stage, and in the subsequent five years hundreds of operations were performed the world over. Now the enthusiasm is waning, because it has been found that the operation has an unavoidable maternal and fetal mortality and a considerable morbidity. While Stoeckel says pubiotomy has about disappeared from Europe, Döderlein, of Munich, Wallich, of Paris, and most American accoucheurs believe it still has a certain but small field of usefulness.

Anatomy.—Figures 808 and 809 show the anatomy of the field of operation. The large venous plexuses are the source of the profuse hemorrhage. It is easily seen how the triangular ligament—the urogenital septum—robbed of its anterior support, is always torn, exposing the urethra, the anguli vaginæ, and the vestibular structures to serious injury.

Symphysiotomy.—There are several methods of opening the pubic joint, some exposing the field, others subcutaneous. Italian operators made a small incision above the pubis, and, under the guidance of the finger, passed a curved, ball-pointed knife around the joint, severing the cartilage from below upward. Farabeuf exposed the field anatomically. Ayres, of New York, did the operation entirely subcutaneously, with a blunt-pointed bistoury, and Zweifel, of Leipsic, does it with a Gigli saw, in a fashion similar to hebosteotomy. Frank has revived Ayres' subcutaneous symphysiotomy and Hüssy holds it superior to other pelvis-enlarging operations. Klee, in lauding Frank's operation emphasizes the importance of cutting the subpubic ligament, but avoiding the pre-urethral fascia (Henle's ligament). This protects the urethra and bulbocavernosi (Fig. 810).

Zarate has devised a subcutaneous partial symphysiotomy which promises to displace all other methods and may, if the future bears out the author's claims,

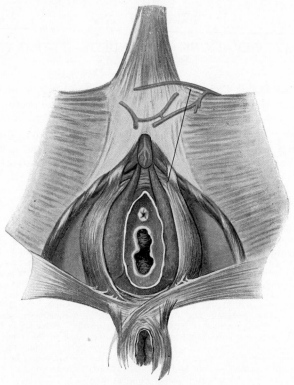

FIG. 808.—SHOWING VEINS AT SITE OF HEBOSTEOTOMY (after Waldeyer).
Line indicates the location of cut.

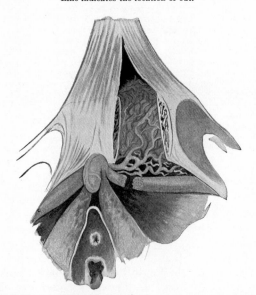

FIG. 809.—AFTER SECTION OF PUBIS. SEMIDIAGRAMMATIC (after Waldeyer).
Note that crus clitoridis is always torn.

rehabilitate the bloody enlargement of the bony pelvis in obstetric esteem. The principle of Zarate's method is to divide the cartilage of the pubis and a part of the arcuate ligament, leaving the superior, the pre-urethral, and as much of the anterior ligament as possible intact. *Technic:* A mark is made on the skin directly over the top of the pubic joint. The patient is put in the exaggerated lithotomy position, with the thighs strongly flexed and abducted. Two fingers of the left hand in the vagina push up the head and deflect the urethra to the right. The sharp-pointed scalpel enters vertically through the mark made at first, to $\frac{1}{2}$ cm. below the upper margin of the cartilage. Figure 810 shows the direction of the movement. The knife is smoothly worked down and up, with the center of oscillation at the point of entry. The handle is bent toward the abdomen, the edge cutting from within outward.

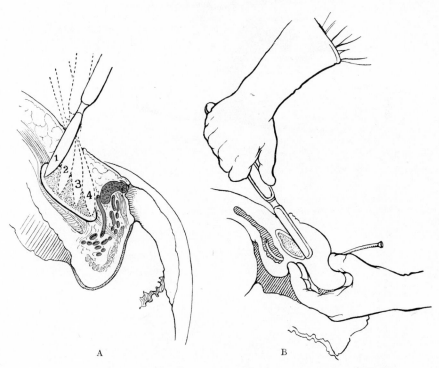

FIG. 810.—A, ZARATE'S PARTIAL SYMPHYSIOTOMY; B, FRANK-HAMMERSCHLAG OPERATION.

At the lower end of the symphysis the tough ligamentum arcuatum offers a little greater resistance, but if the operator finds the bones have already parted, no more of the ligament is cut—but in any event the ligament of Henle should not be cut. If the pubes do not separate, the knife is pushed back to the beginning and the superior pubic ligament is severed. This is all that is expected of the scalpel; the rest of the required enlargement of the pelvis is obtained by stretching the ligaments (strong flexion and abduction of the thighs).

The conditions, indications, details of delivery of the child, and the after-treatment are the same as those for pubiotomy. Zarate and the other advocates of the subcutaneous methods claim that one need not hold the indication so strictly to clean cases, that the element of infection need not be feared so much.

Hebosteotomy.—Gigli's original operation was an open dissection, and the results were no better than with symphysiotomy. Walcher devised a method of operating entirely subcutaneously, which Bumm has simplified. Döderlein, before Walcher, had modified the operation of Gigli, and his is the one usually recommended.

Döderlein's Operation.—Preparations are made for a serious operation. In rare cases hemorrhage and lacerations occur which tax the skill of the most expert. Two trays are to be used—

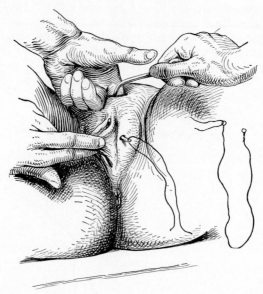

FIG. 812.—HEBOSTEOTOMY. PASSING THE NEEDLE. GIGLI SAW AT RIGHT.

one for instruments for the work on the joint, and the other for the vaginal work. If it is necessary to return to the wound in the joint after the hands have had to do with the parturient canal, the operator should draw on another pair of sterile gloves.

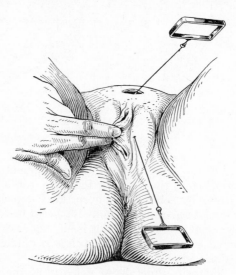

FIG. 813.—HEBOSTEOTOMY. SAW IN POSITION.

The patient is put in the posture for delivery shown in Fig. 783, but the legs are held by the two assistants nearly horizontally. A transverse or longitudinal incision, 1 inch long, is made over the left pubic tubercle, down to the rectus fascia and through it, but the latter cut is always made longitudinally, and only large enough to permit the finger to pass behind the pubis. This finger gently separates the bladder and fat from the bone, until the ligamentum arcuatum is felt.

Now the needle (Fig. 812), armed with a silk ligature, is guided by the finger around the bone, the point of the needle adhering as closely to the bone as possible.   When the point has rounded the ligamentum arcuatum, it is bent sharply forward, while an assistant pulls the labium toward the right side—this to bring the opening in the skin far from the flow of the lochia, and, by the sliding

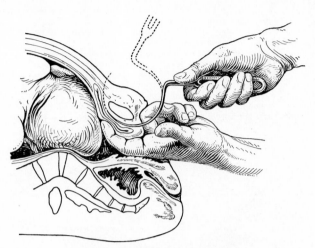

FIG. 814.—HEBOSTEOTOMY (after Bumm).
A catheter in the urethra will help to preserve it from injury.

of the tissues, to close the passage of the needle.   A nick with the knife allows the tip of the dull needle to emerge; the thread is grasped and the needle withdrawn.   The saw is pulled through by means of this thread, and the saw handles attached.   By to-and-fro motions of the saw, the action resembling cutting a bar of soap with a string, and making short strokes, the bone is severed.

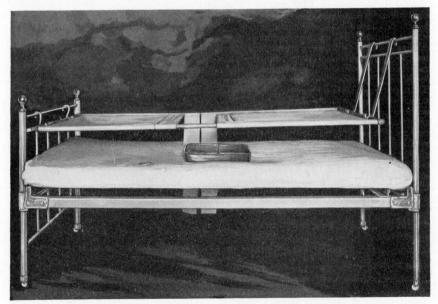

FIG. 815.—HOME-MADE BED FOR SYMPHYSIOTOMY OR FOR HELPLESS PATIENTS.

In this motion the saw may not be sharply bent, but kept in an obtuse arc, and the sawing motion is halted on the instant that the bony resistance is felt to give way.   After the needle has been placed, the bladder is to be catheterized to test its integrity, which, being assured, the sawing is proceeded with.   Mayer advises to place the patient in the Walcher position while sawing the bone, and raise the limbs gradually, to prevent too sudden separation of the two halves of the pelvis and injury to the soft parts between. Costa does the same, and Kerr uses the Walcher for the delivery.

Hemorrhage is usually free from both wounds, during and just after the bone is sawn through. Quickly the upper wound is packed with hot iodoform gauze, a stitch of silkworm-gut closes the lower puncture, and an assistant makes counterpressure from the vaginal surface by means of a large gauze swab. In a few minutes the hemorrhage has usually ceased, the gauze may be removed, and the pubic wound sewed up with three deep silkworm-gut sutures. The bones separate with a dull, crunching sound, which is very unpleasant, at first about 2 cm., and during extraction up to 6 cm. More separation than this endangers the sacro-iliac joints.

Some operators leave the delivery to nature or wait for later indication, especially in primiparæ, but by the majority immediate delivery is practised. In primiparæ I prefer to leave the delivery to nature, as does Stoeckel also. The fetal heart is to be auscultated almost continuously and delivery done at the earliest sign of fetal danger.

Version is generally not advised. The head may be pressed into the inlet from above, or a few pains awaited and then the forceps applied. In primiparæ a deep episiotomy should always

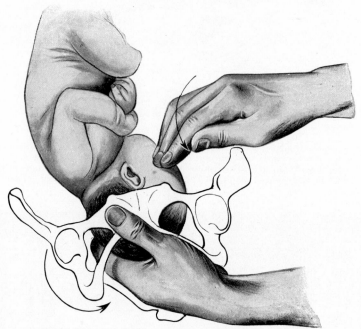

Fig. 816.—Turning Occiput to Front by Combined Manipulation.
The head was engaged, occiput right 135°; it was raised up, mobilized and turned; now it is O.D. 45°. This and similar manipulations are facilitated by lubricating the vagina with sterile liquid soap.

be made before applying the instrument, and in multiparæ also if the introitus is small. The danger now to be avoided is rupture of the anterior vaginal, urethral, and bladder wall, hence the extraction of the child must be very deliberate and the direction of traction be downward, to relax the anterior wall as much as possible. During the delivery the assistants press the pelvis together from the sides, but I believe Kerr's suggestion to use the Walcher position is better. It is highly important that the mechanism of labor be favorable—a posterior occiput or a brow presentation, therefore, should be corrected previous to extraction. It is my practice to remove the placenta very soon, and pack the uterovaginal tract with gauze as a routine. Now all vaginal injuries are repaired, a clean pair of gloves put on, and the pubic wound inspected and treated, if necessary. Catheterization of the bladder now determines if this organ is injured.

Subcutaneous Operation.—Bumm uses a sharp, full-curved needle, and passes it from below upward under the guidance of a finger in the vagina (Fig. 814). It is threaded with the saw, then withdrawn, and the operation completed as above.

Complications.—Hemorrhage is easiest to control in the open symphysiotomy when clamps may be placed on the crura clitoridis and bleeding veins, but in one case I had to pack the vagina tightly and place a sand-bag on the pubis to exert counterpressure. In subcutaneous operations, compression from within and without for five to fifteen minutes almost always stops the hemorrhage, but if it does not, delivery must be effected at once, the uterovaginal tract firmly plugged, and then counterpressure from without provided. If this fails, which is very unusual, a deep suture may be placed on either side of the wound in the bone, but it is better to apply a Sehrt aorta compressor for eight or ten minutes, during which time bimanual compression is kept up, covering the area of separation. If hemorrhage recurs on loosening the compression, the pubic joint must be exposed and the source of the bleeding searched for and quelled. If spontaneous delivery is to be awaited, a vaginal tampon is inserted, firmly compressing the site of bone section, and counterpressure from the outside made with pads and T-binder. These are all removed at the end of thirty or forty minutes, when the cessation of the bleeding is assured.

Hematomata do not develop so long as compression is kept up, but as soon as the woman is placed in bed they may form (one-fifth of the cases reported), and perhaps are favored by rough handling of the patient in transporting her. If they are large and growing, they must be incised and packed—an unlovely operation. If suppuration sets in, which is not unusual, early drainage is indicated.

Lacerations.—Although waiting for spontaneous delivery seems to be the ideal treatment after opening the pelvis, the majority of accoucheurs are not in favor of it, even after proper trial. It is to be reserved for primiparæ, for cases of marked spacial disproportion, when the

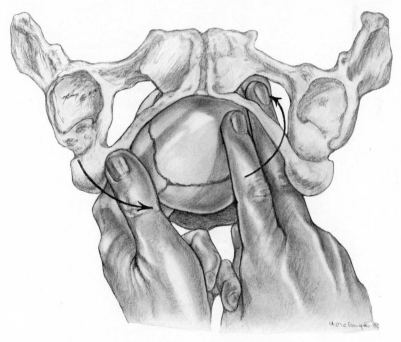

Fig. 816a.—Rotating a Head (O.D.P.) in the Pelvis by Two Fingers of Each Hand.

cervix is not fully dilated, and where no indication for the immediate termination of labor exists. If a vaginal tear communicates with the bone, the immense wound is closed as far as possible, and a gauze drain placed in the prevesical space and led out through the vagina. Injuries to the bladder are usually on its anterior wall, and cannot be repaired at this time. A permanent catheter is placed in the bladder, and 5 grains of hexamethylenamin given four times daily. The catheter is to be removed every six hours and a new one inserted, and the nurse must be instructed to report immediately if the urine ceases to flow—this to avoid urinary infiltration. Lacerations occur from too great or too sudden separation of the bones, from direct injury with the needle, or the soft parts are cut between the head and the sharp edges of the bones.

After-treatment.—After the wound is dressed, a broad adhesive strip is passed three-quarters around the pelvis over the trochanters, and the knees bound together with a towel. This is removed in twenty-four hours, and the adhesive strips in ten days. For the first week great care is required in handling the patient, because the bones are tender and a hematoma may be started. A bed arranged with a frame on which the patient may be raised for catheterization, irrigations, urination, etc., while not absolutely necessary, much facilitates the treatment and increases the puerpera's comfort. For nine days the woman should lie on her back; after this she may move about in bed, and may get out of it at the end of three weeks, and may walk as soon as she feels able to do so, which is usually in the fourth week. Some operators prefer that the woman should move freely in bed, with the intention of favoring fibrous union, and thus facilitating subsequent delivery; others apply a split circular bandage with a weight on each side, as in fracture of the pelvis.

Indications.—Almost the sole indication for hebosteotomy is mechanical disproportion between the head and the pelvis. With a normal-sized fetus the operation is indicated in flat pelves with a conjugata vera of more than 7 cm. and more than $7\frac{1}{2}$ cm. in a generally contracted pelvis. If the child is overgrown, of course, the pelvic diameters must be larger, but with very large children the excessive danger to the soft parts must be considered as contraindicating this opera-

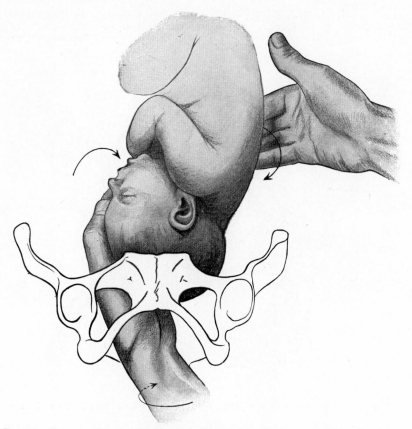

Fig. 817.—Changing Occipitolæva Posterior to Occipitolæva Anterior Before Engagement.
Internal hand obtains purchase on shoulder and pushes it past the promontory. Outside hand pulls body around. Arrows indicate motion of hands. Was O.L. 135°; is now O.L. 90°.

tion. The indication for hebosteotomy really depends on the time the patient is first seen. During pregnancy, if the pelvic contraction is discovered, the induction of premature labor may be preferred, or the patient may be allowed to go to term and some form of cesarean section be performed at the very beginning of labor. The latter is my choice. If the labor test shows that the head will not go through one chooses between the bone operation and laparotrachelotomy. I prefer the latter. A head deeply engaged in a funnel pelvis may, forceps failing, be delivered after pubiotomy, this in my opinion being one of the very few indications for the operation. If the woman is already infected, or presumably so; if prolonged attempts with forceps have been made and the maternal parts much bruised; if the child is injured or not in good condition—hebosteotomy becomes a dangerous and unsatisfactory operation and unless extraperitoneal cesarean section proves feasible, craniotomy must be substituted. With a dead or dying child embryotomy is the only operation. It will be seen that hebosteotomy is useful only in border-line cases, where the attendant, believing the child would be delivered, has waited until labor has advanced so far that cesarean section would be too dangerous, or has even attempted delivery with the usual methods. The selection of the operation now is one of judgment of the condition of the mother and babe and of the probable outlook for both. It is, therefore, largely subjective. In shoulder and breech presentations, where, of course, we cannot await the test of labor, placing the indication

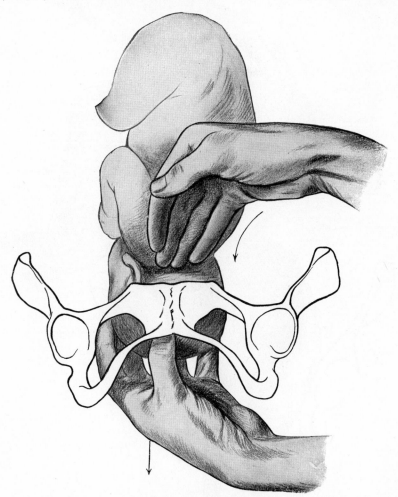

Fig. 818.—Leading Head into Pelvis by Combined Pressure and Traction.

becomes still more subjective and will be aided by knowledge of previous deliveries, pelvic and fetal mensuration, the state of the soft parts, etc. I feel that pubiotomy should be restricted in favor of abdominal delivery in good cases, and the older methods should be preferred in unfavorable ones. In persistent occipitoposterior, and in face presentation with the chin immovably posterior, an occasional indication for section of the pelvis may arise. Lewis and Montgomery did symphysiotomy for such conditions, but there are only 8 others reported (Morse, Titus, Hoppe).

Conditions.—(1) The pelvis may not be too small, that is, less than 7 cm. in the flat, and $7\frac{1}{2}$ cm. in generally contracted, with a child of 7 pounds. It may not be ankylosed, as by tuberculous disease, advanced age, etc. (2) The child may not be too large, especially in primiparæ; (3) the child must be in good condition and not deformed, for example, hydrocephalus, anencephalus; (4) the maternal soft parts may not be infantile or rigid, hence hebosteotomy should seldom be attempted in primiparæ, especially if very young or old; (5) there may not be too

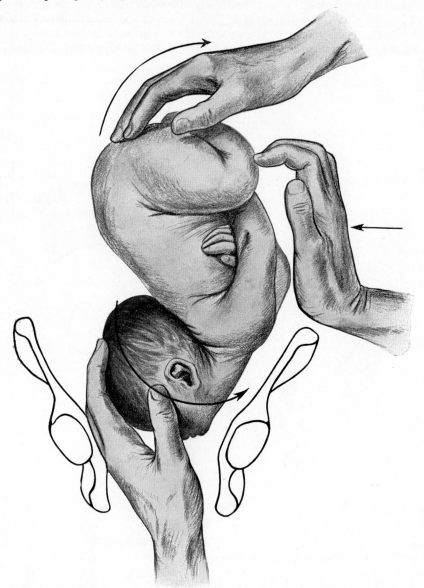

Fig. 819.—Thorn's Method of Changing Face to Occipital.
Operator's inside hand pulls occiput down, while his outside hand pushes the chest over. At the same time an assistant draws the breech to the opposite side.

many varicose veins; (6) the mother must be in good condition and not infected, that is, no fever, slow pulse, clean conduct of labor; (7) the cervix must be effaced and dilated; (8) the woman must be in a well-equipped obstetric operating-room, with plenty of assistants, since the operation is not one to be done in the home.

Prognosis.—The reader is referred to p. 774. After symphysiotomy there is often a slight permanent enlargement of the pelvis, so that subsequent deliveries may be spontaneous, but after hebosteotomy it is not so marked. This is one of the advantages of the operation over cesarean, and should have weight when the two come in close competition. Union of the bones by a strong fibrous callus is the rule, but in many cases, especially after eight months, it is bony, and dystocia from too big a callus has been reported. Subsequent labors may not be treated by a second symphysiotomy because of the immense scar which involves the bones, the bladder, the urethra, etc., but pubiotomy has on several occasions been performed twice. I have performed cesarean section in these cases on principle, and in one case because of the enormous varicosities of the vulva and pelvis which followed the previous (infected) pubiotomy.

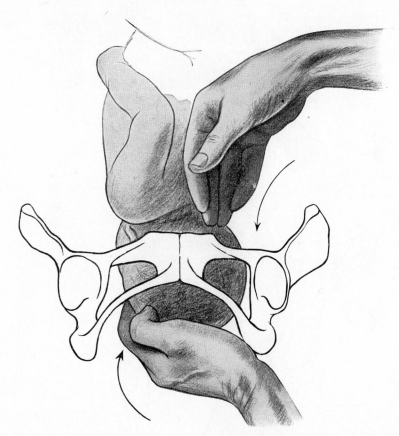

Fig. 820.—Changing Face to Occipital. Second Movement.
The fingers of the inside hand push up the face, the thumb trying to push down the occiput, while the outside hand forces the occiput down too.

Osteoplastic operations on the pelvis, with the object of permanently enlarging its cavity and thus rendering spontaneous labor possible have been invented by Olliver, 1850 (prophylactic symphysiotomy); Credé, 1879; Frank, 1894; Füth, 1907 (pelveoplastics on the rami); Rotter, 1912 (removal of the promontory of the sacrum); Costa, 1921 (superior symphysiectomy). They are all irrational, and what little experience has been published shows them to be impractical.

Improving Occiput Posterior Positions.—Occipitoposterior positions occasionally require correction, and the indications will be found on p. 636. The simple manœuvre of Hodge, pressing up on the sinciput during the pains, may increase flexion and thus assist rotation, or Tarnier's plan may be preferred. The position may have to be corrected during the progress of labor or precedent to delivery by forceps. In the former case after the correction is made the woman is allowed to finish her labor or is assisted by art should a new indication arise. In the second instance, having decided on forceps, one seeks to rotate the occiput to the front before applying the blades. The manipulation must vary with the station of the head. First, occiput deep in pelvis; after lubricating the vagina with liquid soap, and raising and mobilizing the head a very little, two fingers of one hand obtain a purchase on the skull behind the baby's ear, and seek to pull the occiput downward and forward, while the other hand, outside, pushes the forehead toward the

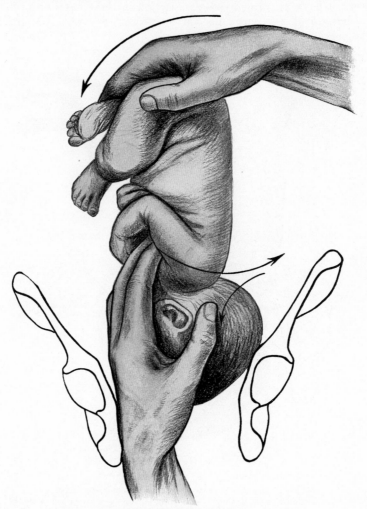

FIG. 821.—CHANGING FACE TO OCCIPITAL. THIRD MOVEMENT.
The fingers now push the child's chest toward the side, the thumb at the same time forcing the occiput down, the other hand presses the breech over, to flex the trunk.

back part of the pelvis (Fig. 816), or we may aid the inside hand by pressure with two fingers on the malar bone from behind the pubis (Fig. 816a). In a large pelvis the whole hand inserted may pull the occiput forward with the fingers behind the ear, while the thumb pushes the forehead backward. When the head is in proper position, an assistant, working from the outside, holds the forehead at the point to which the operator pushed it, while the latter uses his free hand to insert one blade of the forceps. The other hand, which has been kept inside to prevent the occiput from rolling backward again, guides the forceps blade into place. In many cases

I have retained the occiput in its new position by means of a vulsellum forceps affixed to the scalp while the forceps were being adjusted.

If it appears desirable to rectify an occiput posterior position before the head is engaged, two operations claim the preference—manual correction and podalic version. The conditions for manual correction are: (1) The pelvis may not be too contracted for the subsequent delivery; (2) the child must be living; (3) the cervix must be dilated to admit the hand; (4) the bag of waters ruptured; (5) the uterus

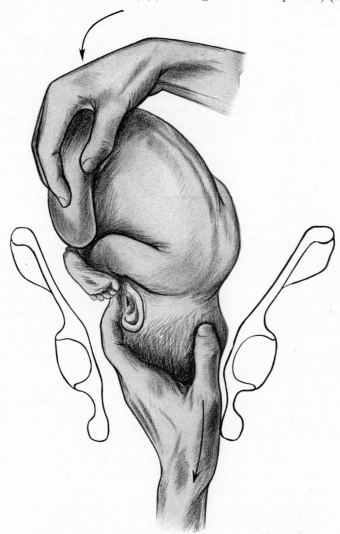

FIG. 822.—CHANGING FACE TO OCCIPITAL. FOURTH MOVEMENT.
Leading the child downward into engagement.

may not be in tetanic contraction or on the point of rupturing; (6) placenta prævia and prolapse of the cord may not exist.

Excepting the sixth these conditions also govern podalic version, and, therefore, when they are thus evenly balanced, individual skill or preference will decide which method is chosen.

Manual correction as shown in Fig. 817, p. 1006, has been practised by the author for many years. Eden and Kerr publish similar methods. Success in obtaining and maintaining an anterior position depends on getting the fetal dorsum to the front, otherwise the head will turn back as soon as the pressure is relieved.

Under deep anesthesia the whole hand is passed into the uterus, pushing the head up, but out of the pelvis only if necessary. That hand is selected which will have its palm directed toward the face of the infant. The posterior shoulder of the child is sought, and with the tips of the fingers is swung around to the front, past the promontory of the sacrum. The head fitting into the hollow of the hand goes with the trunk. The other hand, working in the flank outside, aids this motion by pulling the shoulder toward the front. When the inside hand is leading the head into the pelvis in its new position, the outside hand forces the head down by pressure on the occiput, which is now over the pubic ramus (Fig. 818, p. 1007). It may be advisable to draw the head down deep into the pelvis with forceps, await four to six labor-pains, remove the forceps, and leave the case to nature, or to follow a later indication. This is the two-stage operation. The indication for correction of the malposition having been satisfied and no new indication for delivery being present, one may rest. The latter plan is especially successful in primiparæ when recession of the pericervical tissues and dilation of the cervix are not yet complete, because the molding of the head, the retraction of the tissues produced by a few hours' labor, and the progress of the head toward the outlet immensely facilitate and disendanger the subsequent delivery.

During the manipulations a little dilatation of the cervix is permissible, but usually it is best not to attempt the correction until the cervix is fully dilated, because sometimes an unexpected indication for rapid delivery arises during the operation—e. g., prolapse of the cord, abruptio placentæ.

In rare instances the manipulation fails, or must be given up because the force required is too much to be safely applied. Now the forceps alone will be able to effect delivery, but the operator must be aware that they are very difficult to apply under such conditions and invariably cause superficial and deep injuries to the maternal parts. If the operation is forced, a still-birth frequently results.

Improving the Attitude of the Child.—Faulty attitudes, face, brow, and other malpresentations, prolapse of extremities and of the cord, with indications for treatment, have already been considered (p. 688). It remains to show how face and brow presentations may be corrected.

Baudelocque recommended to push up the chin and face, and then slide the fingers over the occiput and pull this down into the pelvis—all being done by the inside hand. Schatz (1872) sought to alter the posture of the head by changing the extension of the trunk to flexion. In face presentation the usual C shape of the child's spinal column is changed to resemble the letter S, and Schatz, operating from the outside, by pulling the shoulder in one direction while he pushed the breech over in the opposite, in favorable cases could alter the attitude of the trunk so that the head went over from a condition of extension into one of flexion. Thorn (1893) combined both methods, and was more successful than Schatz in breaking the curves of the fetal body and producing the C shape (Fig. 819, p. 1008).

My own method, which has failed only twice in 25 cases of face presentation, and once in 3 cases of brow presentation where it was attempted, is similar to Thorn's, but more is done by the inside hand.

Author's Method.—A good table, the obstetric position, with the nates well over the edge to allow the operator to sink his elbow, and deep anesthesia are indispensable. The operation consists of four acts: first, raising and releasing the head and shoulder from the grasp of the uterus, so that the baby floats free above the inlet; second, flexion of the chin and forcing down the occiput; third, pushing in the prominent convexity of the chest to a concavity; fourth, leading the now flexed head into the pelvis.

1. The hand, whose palm will lie against the child's face (for example, in M.D.P., the left), is introduced into the lower uterine segment, and with the fingers widely apart the head is grasped, and with a circular motion is loosened from its fixed position in the inlet. It may be necessary to raise the whole head above the inlet into the false pelvis. The fingers then slide by the head

and disengage the shoulders from the uterine walls. The child is thus rendered movable, being freed from the grasp of the lower uterine segment. Information is also gained of the condition of the uterus as to rigidity, thinning, etc.

2. With the same hand the chin and then the face are pushed up, the tips of the fingers being applied in the nasal fossæ (Fig. 820), while the outside hand presses the occiput down.

3. The same internal hand now continues farther past the face, either in front of the promontory or behind the pubis, until the finger-tips reach the chest and shoulder of the child. Obtaining purchase on the shoulder, the fingers are flexed, which throws the chest first into a straight line and then into a concavity, and at the same time the thumb makes downward traction on the occiput, bringing the latter into the palm of the hand (Fig. 821, p. 1010). The outside hand meanwhile pushes the breech to the side on which the chin lay.

4. The inside hand, holding the head in the now flexed attitude, with the fingers over the face and the thumb hooked into the suboccipital region, gently leads the head into the pelvis, the outside hand forcing the child into extreme flexion and down toward the inlet (Fig. 822, p. 1011). An assistant now places his one hand on the breech, the finger-tips of the other being over the occiput, while the operator uses his free hand to insert the blades of the forceps. A few slight tractions bring the head down into the pelvis, and engagement having been obtained, recurrence of the face presentation is impossible. Sometimes the first attempt at correction fails, or the head, having been flexed, extends again as soon as the pressure of the hand is removed. To avoid this the above advice is given. In addition, the assistant, from the outside, should maintain the flexion of the trunk by firm pressure on the breech, and the operator, by holding the child in its new posture for five minutes, perhaps aided by a few pains, may make the conversion permanent. Should the head show a tendency to slip back, it may be held in its new attitude by means of a vulsellum attached firmly to the scalp until the forceps are applied. One may wait for natural delivery or apply forceps, depending upon conditions. The tiny wounds are dressed antiseptically afterward.

Indications.—The sole indication for this operation is the mentoposterior position, where, from close observation of the course of labor, the accoucheur is convinced that the case is not likely to terminate with anterior rotation of the chin. It is not the routine treatment of face presentation.

Conditions.—(1) The cervix must be fully dilated because the hand must be introduced, and it may be necessary to deliver at once; (2) the bag of waters is to be ruptured; (3) the child may not be too large or the pelvis too small (very important); (4) the uterus must not be too much thinned or on the point of rupturing; (5) the head may not be deeply engaged in the pelvis; (6) placenta prævia may not be present; (7) the child must be living and viable.

If an indication for immediate delivery on the part of the mother or child exists, it may be better to perform version and extraction, and the same may be said of minor degrees of pelvic contraction. In placenta prævia and prolapse of the cord version is the operation of choice, unless—and one must always remember this—other conditions exist which require cesarean section.

VERSION

Version, or "turning," is an operation which changes the polarity of the fetus with reference to the mother, the object being to change an abnormal, or relatively abnormal, relation into a normal, or relatively normal, one. Thus version may change a transverse presentation to a longitudinal one, or a head presentation to one of breech.

Version is also very useful as a preparatory operation before rapid delivery, when the latter is indicated by the condition of the mother or child. Version is only a preparatory operation. When it is completed, the indication for it is satisfied. A new indication must be present for the extraction, which may not follow without such indication.

Version, bringing down the head, is called "cephalic," and when the breech is brought down, "podalic." Version may be done by purely external, by internal, and by combined manipulation—sometimes called "bipolar." Nowadays the purely internal version is not done, the external hand being used to aid the internal one.

Historic.—Internal cephalic version was done even before Hippocrates' time, and was generally preferred to podalic because of the belief that the child could best be born if it came head first. Celsus, about the time of Christ, Soranus, one hundred years after, and Aëtius (sixth century A.D.) performed podalic version, but this knowledge was lost in the dark ages, until Ambroise Paré, in 1550, described and very successfully performed the operation. Wiegand, in 1807, introduced external version, but the procedure had been previously used in Japan and Mexico as an empiric measure during pregnancy to favor labor, and by Pechey, in England, as early as 1698. Baudelocque, in 1780, Hohl, in 1845, Wright, of Cincinnati, in 1854, and Braxton Hicks, in 1860, perfected the combined methods of version.

At the present writing there appears in Buffalo an interesting figure, modeled after the famous Scotchman, Mr. Figg, of Simpson's time—Dr. Irving W. Potter. He has reduced the science and art of obstetrics to a very simple formula. Excepting those few cases where the baby is born before he arrives, he delivers all women by cesarean section or podalic version and immediate extraction. The author has kept careful account of his work and has thoughtfully considered his published opinions and the results of his practice. There is little if anything new, either in the idea of doing version in normal cases or in his technic of turning and of the extraction which always follows. However, Potter has recalled to attention the advantages of version, which operation was being fast relegated to undeserved desuetude by the other methods of delivery. With this exception his principles of practice are condemnable in every way, being, in my opinion, unscientific and misleading and dangerous to both mothers and babies.

Version in Transverse Presentation.—If recognized during pregnancy, the transverse position of the child may be changed by the woman assuming, when in

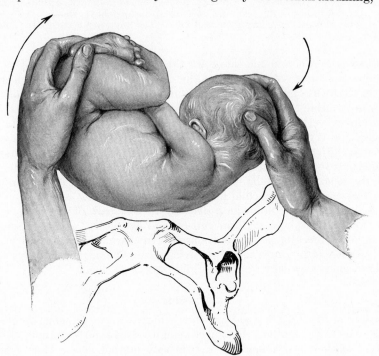

FIG. 823.—WIEGAND'S EXTERNAL VERSION.

bed, a posture which favors descent of the head—that is, she should lie on that side on which the head lies. The breech then falls over to the side, the head sliding over the inlet. In spite of a snugly fitting binder the child may not remain in the new relation. Even during the first stage of labor postural treatment is to be tried, but here external cephalic version is the operation of choice if operation is needed. Unquestionably, cephalic presentation is the most favorable for mother and child, and we should try to bring the head into the inlet by external cephalic version, governed, however, by the following conditions: (1) There should be no contraction of the pelvis unless pubiotomy is in anticipation, and the child may not be too large; (2) there should be no immediate or prospective indication for the rapid termination of labor, because if, under such circumstances, the head did not at once engage, another operation—podalic version—would of necessity have to follow; (3) the fetus must be very movable, which means that the bag of waters must be intact and the pains absent or weak. Placenta prævia, prolapse of the cord, and monstrosities are contraindications, and a fat or tender abdomen may make the manœuver impossible.

Cephalic version has very limited application, but I am convinced it is used less often than it should be. Most accoucheurs prefer to wait for complete dilatation and then do podalic version and extraction.

Wiegand's Method.—Anesthesia is rarely needed, but the patient must learn to relax the belly-wall. By using a partial Trendelenburg posture the child falls away from the inlet and becomes more movable. One hand is placed over the breech, the other over the head, and by alternate stroking and pushing movements the head is brought over the inlet. Operating between pains one holds, during the time the uterus is contracting, what has been gained. Time is no object, and force may not be used. Now the foot of the table is lowered, and the head forced down into the inlet, where it is held for five minutes or until the pains fix it there. If the cervix is completely dilated, and if the cord or the extremities have not prolapsed, the bag of waters may be ruptured, still holding the head firmly in the inlet. If the cervix is not dilated, or if the cord lies over the os, the membranes may not be ruptured. Combined internal and external version to bring the head over the inlet is almost never practised nowadays, though it should be.

Wright's Method of Combined Cephalic Version.—In Sc. L. A. the right hand grasps the shoulder girdle and presses the child's body in a curvilinear direction to the right, while the left hand, operating on the abdomen, forces the breech in a curvilinear direction upward and inward toward the left. The shoulder is not pushed upward more than is sufficient to dislodge it from the inlet, and no direct action on the head is made, but after the head has come down it is received in the hollow of the right hand and led into the pelvis in a manner similar to that shown on page 1011, Fig. 822. Gentleness and patience are required for success. Dilatation should be complete or nearly so, an indication for immediate delivery absent, and the child living.

Podalic Version.—When version or turning is mentioned, it is usually the podalic one that is meant, and it is preferred, because—(1) As a rule, cephalic version is too difficult or impossible; (2) there is an immediate or prospective indication, either on the part of the mother or the child, for rapid delivery; and (3) there is often slight pelvic contraction. Lately the latter indication is being much restricted in favor of pubiotomy and cesarean section. If a case of transverse presentation occurs in a contracted pelvis, the pelvis and not the presentation of the child decides the course to pursue, i. e., the pelvis is the "Leit motif."

Very few operators try to turn by the breech with external manipulations alone, but I have several times succeeded in doing so, and it is almost always possible if the case is simply one of deflected breech presentation. There are two methods of combined or bipolar version which are employed, according as the cervix is open enough to admit the hand or only enough for one or two fingers. The name of Braxton Hicks is most often associated with the last method, because he did so much to popularize it. The other method might, with propriety, be called "bimanual" version.

Which of these methods is used depends on the condition of the cervix and the mobility of the fetus. If the cervix is completely dilated, bimanual version, rupturing the bag of waters, is performed. If the cervix is not dilated and the bag of waters is intact, it is best to wait. One may not go away, but should stay by the patient so as to interfere when needed. If the cervix will admit only two fingers, but the bag of waters is ruptured, Braxton Hicks' version is indicated. It is dangerous to wait after the bag of waters is ruptured for the cervix to dilate to a size sufficient to allow the hand to pass through. Braxton Hicks' version should be considered, and if not thought feasible, a metreurynter should be put into the lower uterine segment to preserve the balance of the liquor amnii, to keep the shoulder away from the inlet, and to prevent prolapse of the cord and extremities, a plan preferred by the author. When the cervix is well dilated the time is ripe for the bimanual version. Should an indication on the part of the child for rapid delivery arise before full dilatation is accomplished, the various methods of opening the cervix must be taken up as additional preparatory measures. Version, followed by extraction through an only partly opened cervix, is a dangerous and often fruitless operation.

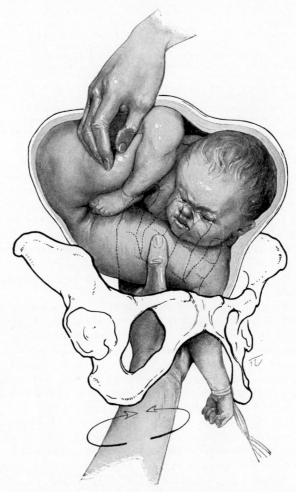

Fig. 824.—Version. First Motion. Hand Inside Pushes up the Shoulder and Frees it from Grasp of the Uterus by Smoothing Away the Uterine Wall.

In passing the hand through the vulva the labia are to be widely parted; the direction is at first downward toward the sacral hollow, then upward in the axis of the inlet, sinking the elbow downward, and the motion should be spiral, from left to right. The hand is well lubricated with lysol solution. While the outside hand steadies the uterus, the inner one gently pushes up the shoulder, and, by stroking the uterine wall, frees it from its grasp on the child, at the same time noting its thinness, or perhaps any present break in its surface.

Bimanual Version in Transverse Presentation.—Few operations are so satisfactory as version, but none is more dangerous if performed without due consideration of the conditions.

Conditions.—(1) The cervix must be dilated enough to allow the hand to pass, and, if the version is done in the presence of an indication for extraction also, it must be fully dilated; (2) the pelvis may not be too much contracted—this in view of the extraction to follow; (3) the uterus may not be in tetanus or retracted over the fetus—that is, the case may not be one of neglected transverse presentation with the uterus on the point of rupture; (4) the child must be mobile, that is, not engaged, or in the process of spontaneous evolution; (5) unless the version promises to be exceptionally easy, the child must be living.

The third and fourth conditions require most careful thought; indeed, it is at this point that the art of the accoucheur comes into play. To know when it is safe to turn and when the risks of rupture of the uterus are too great requires much experience and delicate judgment. Only too easy is it to rupture a thinned lower uterine segment, and the inexperienced accoucheur would do better to err on the

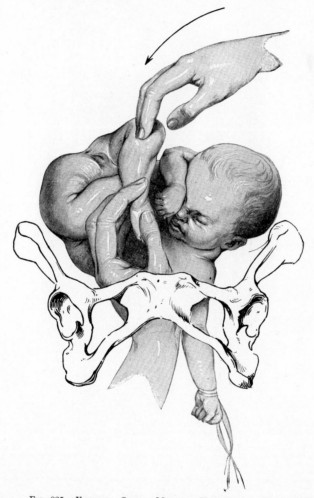

FIG. 825.—VERSION. SECOND MOTION. HAND SEIZING FOOT.

Passing the hand directly along the belly or side of the fetus, taking care to avoid the cord, the fingers touch, successively, thigh, knee, and ankle. Aided by the outside hand, the upper foot is pressed into the grasp of the thumb and the two first fingers, which seize it, without making the hand into a knobby fist. This is avoided because the uterus might tear over the sharp knuckles, and, further, the fist and the body of the child make too wide a mass for the safety of the lower uterine segment.

side of safety to the mother. It is impossible to lay down a set rule as to how long after the rupture of the membranes a version is still permissible. All depends on the degree of retraction and contraction of the uterus. The longer the time, the more difficult and dangerous the operation. I have done a turning three days after the membranes ruptured, and again have found it impossible two hours afterward.

The preparations are the same as for all obstetric operations. The instruments required are those for the operation chosen for the delivery of the child—as forceps or breech extraction. For the version several slings are to be provided, smooth tape a yard or more long and $\frac{1}{2}$ inch wide, and some sort of sling-carrier.   Profound narcosis is needed for the actual turning, but later a lighter sleep is preferable. Most often the dorsal posture is sufficient, but in back-posterior positions and pendulous belly the lateral (the one on which the child's feet are) may be required. A modified Trendelenburg may be used instead.   One is here governed by surrounding conditions.   Long gantlet gloves and lubrication are essential.

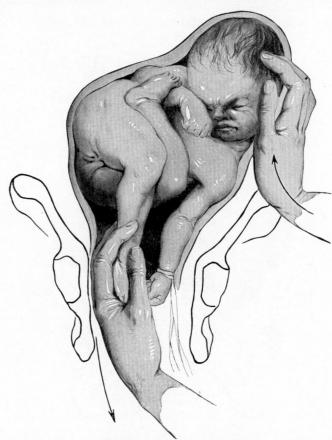

FIG. 826.—VERSION. THIRD MOTION.

Gently the foot is drawn into the pelvis, sliding it down the wall of the uterus behind the pubis.   In back-anterior presentations the foot is led down posteriorly near the sacro-iliac joint, where there is more room.   The outside hand aids the turning by pressing the head toward the midline and upward. *During the uterine contraction no motion may be made:* the hands are to lie absolutely quiet.   Between pains the operation is resumed.   At all stages the back of the internal hand should feel the wall of the uterus and discover a separation of its fibers, or a beginning abruptio placentæ. When the knee has passed the vulva, the version is complete; the head will now be found in the fundus.

If there is difficulty in performing this act—the actual turning—see that the narcosis is deep enough to paralyze the uterus; pass the hand around the child to find if the shoulder is caught on the pelvic brim; then, if necessary, bring down the other leg too.

If, during the operation, the hand instead of the foot be brought down, no harm is done—a sling is put on it.   It is rare not to be able to reach the feet—then the knee may be pulled down.   If the cord prolapses, the version must be hurried.   Such an accident is to be avoided, if possible, and shows the wisdom of procuring complete dilatation before turning.   Should, during the operation, a beginning rupture of the uterus be discovered, further attempts to turn are too dangerous—cesarean section is considered, and, if this is contraindicated, embryotomy is required.

Which hand shall be introduced?   That hand whose palm will lie against the breech when in the uterus—when the breech is to the left, the right, when to the right, the left, hand.   The bag of waters is usually ruptured; if not, the membranes are to be opened just as the hand passes the cervix; the forearm then will fill the vulva and prevent the escape of all the liquor amnii.   Peu, in 1694, recommended that the membranes be stripped up until the feet were reached, but this is bad practice because vaginal bacteria are thus rubbed into the uterine wall and there is danger of abruptio placentæ.

through a slightly contracted pelvis easier coming last than going first? Experience and experiment on the cadaver prove that it does, but it has to come through quicker, and as a result many babies die. Wolff and Leopold showed that the results were about the same. The amount of damage done the children and the mother is about equal; it remains, therefore, a matter of personal choice. British accoucheurs, prominently Kerr, have given up prophylactic version in favor of prolonged expectancy and forceps, which is the position I take in the matter because, if a gentle attempt with the forceps fails, pubiotomy is in reserve.

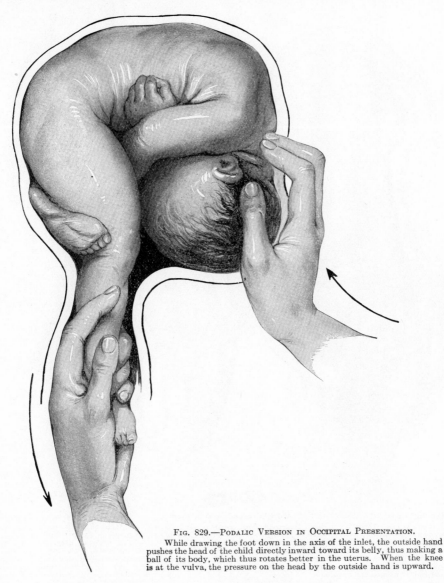

Fig. 829.—Podalic Version in Occipital Presentation.
While drawing the foot down in the axis of the inlet, the outside hand pushes the head of the child directly inward toward its belly, thus making a ball of its body, which thus rotates better in the uterus. When the knee is at the vulva, the pressure on the head by the outside hand is upward.

Conditions.—(1) The cervix must be dilated enough for the method of version chosen, and if the operation is done to save the child, it must always be fully effaced and dilated; (2) the head must be movable, not engaged, but under profound anesthesia an apparently fixed head may often be easily pushed up into the false pelvis; (3) the pelvis must be roomy enough for the extraction to follow; (4) the soft parts may not be too rigid—in primiparæ version is to be restricted to the minimum possible; with some accoucheurs primiparity contraindicates version; (5) the uterus may not be in tetanus or on the point of rupturing.

Methods.—Of these there are three: Wiegand's external version, the bimanual, or combined internal and external, using the whole hand in the uterus, and Braxton Hicks', inserting only one or two fingers through the cervix. What was said about

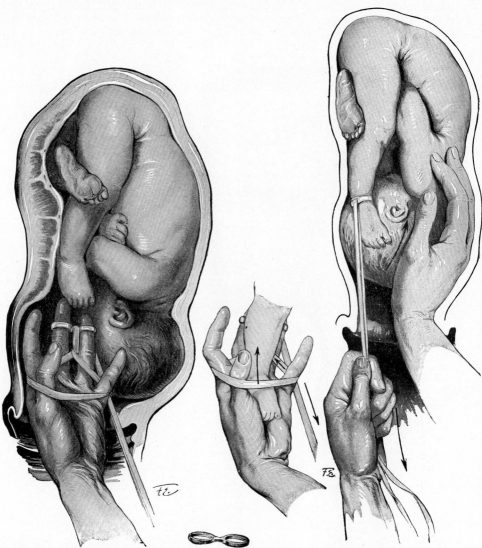

FIG. 830.—APPLYING A SLING TO FOOT WITH MORALES' SLING-CARRIER.

If the foot cannot be readily grasped or does not give purchase enough for traction, a sling may be put on it. The ringed bar of Morales is mounted on the middle and fourth fingers, a tape adjusted over it like a pulley, and the loop spread out by the little finger and thumb. When the loop has been adjusted around the part to be grasped (the foot or hand), pulling on the tape draws the loop upward and tightly around the member.

FIG. 831.—SHOE-HORN MANŒUVER.

If the head is arrested by the contraction ring catching in the nape of the child's neck, one hand may be used, after the manner of a shoe-horn, while the other pulls on a sling attached to the foot. It is rarely advisable to bring down the two legs, but this and Sigmundine's manœuver may often be found useful.

version in shoulder presentation regarding preparations, posture, hand to choose, bag of waters, bringing down one or both legs, prolapse of the cord, and rupture of the uterus applies here. The anterior foot is the one to seize because it brings the back to the pubis. In face cases it is necessary to pass the hand far up into the fundus, but it is also wise first to bend in the child's chest curve and force the breech down on to the internal hand, making the child more of a ball than of long cylinder shape. The "double manual," a procedure invented by Justine Sigmundine, consisting of pulling on a sling attached to the leg while pushing the head up

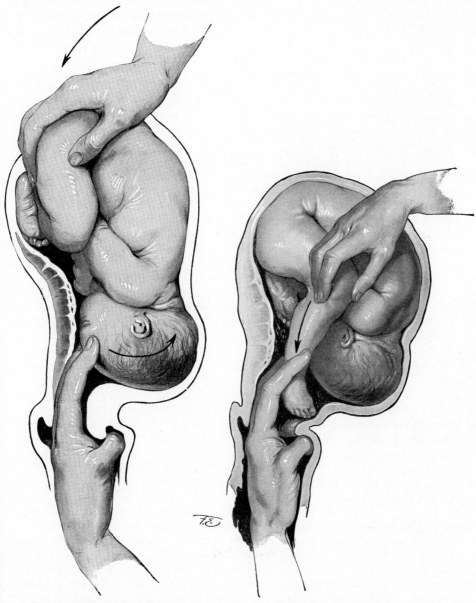

FIG. 832.—BRAXTON HICKS' VERSION.

While the whole hand lies in the vagina, only one or two fingers pass through the cervix. The head is pushed away from the inlet and upward, while the outside hand presses the breech in the opposite direction—that is, downward toward the inside fingers.

FIG. 833.—BRAXTON HICKS' VERSION.

Forcing foot into grasp of two fingers. Seizing the foot is not always easy, since it may slip from between the fingers, and a blunt ring forceps (Fig. 690) or long polypus forceps may be then used. After the foot is down in the vagina the head is pushed up as usual.

with the hand from the inside, and the manœuver illustrated in Fig. 831, are often needed.

Version in Face and Brow Presentation.—The general principles of turning are applicable here, but owing to the extension of the child's body difficulties are likely to be met, first in grasping the foot, and second in overcoming the retraction of the uterus, which has adapted itself to a long fetal ellipse. Version is hard, and if forced may rupture the uterus. These difficulties are met as follows: (1) Secure complete uterine relaxation by deep anesthesia and a dose of atropin; (2) using the hand whose palm will lie over the chest push up the head and flex it partially; (3) fold the arms over the chest and press the latter toward the baby's back—this manœuver flexes the trunk a little and brings the legs nearer; (4) pass the hand further and grasp the anterior foot; (5) draw gently on the foot, aiding the turning by upward pressure on the head from the outside.

This method may fail when the over-extension of the body is extreme, the child being in a contortionist's attitude, with the feet near the occiput, and, in addition, sometimes with the spine twisted or lateroflexed. The condition is recognized at once because the hand does not find the arms and feet where they are expected. The tense uterus in these neglected cases does not permit flexion of the baby's trunk as above described. Here one must change hands, push the face up and to the side and search for the feet over the baby's back just above the occiput. During the version the child is made to turn a complete back-somersault.

Braxton Hicks' version has a limited application because, in cases where version is indicated, it is almost always desirable to be in a position to extract the child when the turning is complete, and, too, as we have seen, often an accident happens during operation which demands immediate extraction. Therefore the author recommends, in all cases where possible, to procure complete dilatation of the cervix before attempting to turn the child.

The main indication for Braxton Hicks' version is placenta prævia. It is sometimes done for prolapse of the cord, occasionally in shoulder presentations, and very exceptionally to turn the head down in breech presentation. The conditions are the same as for the operation last described, but the mobility of the fetus must be absolutely free.

Cephalic Version in Breech Presentation.—This is the oldest kind of version, and is only recently being revived. It was done by the ancients because they considered all other than cephalic presentations pathologic and insuperable. During labor in a primipara with breech presentation, with or without a contracted pelvis, it may be desirable, though seldom possible, to bring the head down. Cephalic version might also be a preparatory operation before pubiotomy. The dangers of the operation are detachment of the placenta, coiling and prolapse of the cord, and recurrence of the breech presentation. The usual conditions for version must be insisted on, especially full mobility of the child, but the presence of a contracted pelvis may not cancel the indication if a pelviotomy or laparotrachelotomy is to be performed after a test of labor. A primipara with contracted pelvis and breech presentation may present the indication for laparotrachelotomy.

Version may be accomplished by external manipulations, by inserting the whole hand, and by the Braxton Hicks' method. The breech is pushed upward and to one side, while the hand outside strokes the head along the inner wall of the abdomen toward the inlet. When it has been brought over the brim, it is grasped as in Fig. 818, p. 1007, and forced down into the pelvis, or pulled in by the forceps. In these cases, also, it is wise to procure full enlargement of the cervical canal before operating, so as to be able to care for all possible accidents—for example, prolapse of the cord or abruptio placentæ—by immediate delivery.

External Cephalic Version in Breech Presentation.—When, during the prenatal examinations in the twenty-eighth week of pregnancy, a breech presentation is discovered one should try to change it to a head, because the mortality of breech deliveries is 6 to 10 per cent.

The patient is instructed to lie in the knee chest posture for fifteen minutes four times daily, and to sleep on her side—the left, if the baby's back is on the right, and vice versa. If at the end of two weeks the breech persists, external version is attempted. This maneuver does not always succeed at first nor does the baby always remain in its new presentation. Then the operation is to be repeated.

Technic.—First the location of the placenta is determined, and the fetal heartbeat counted. The placenta can sometimes be located by sight, a bulging of one part of the uterus, or felt as a soft spongy area. If the bell of the stethoscope is pressed against it hard, a loud souffle is heard (equivocal) and often the fetal heart is slowed for the moment. The direction of the round ligaments may also give a little aid (see page 305). If the placenta is on the anterior wall, only the gentlest attempt at version may be permitted—perhaps it had better be given up entirely.

The patient (bladder and rectum empty) is placed in a moderate Trendelenburg position, and asked to relax the belly. The child is mobilized by gentle manipulation, then with one hand the breech is drawn out of the inlet into one iliac fossa, while with the other hand the head is pressed down into the opposite flank. We first try to turn the baby in the sense of flexion of the trunk, the short route, by operating on its two poles synchronously. If the resistance met is more than expected—try to turn the child in the opposite direction. Hold the fetus in its new position for five minutes. Listen to the fetal heart after each step. The baby may suffer so much that the effort must be suspended, and the child returned to its original position. One may not cause any pain, nor may the operation be forced if difficulties are encountered. It is not without danger. (See Lit.)

The **prognosis of version** may never be lightly estimated. It depends largely on the skill of the operator. The operation may be directly fatal to the mother from rupture of the uterus, of the cervix, or from abruptio placentæ. The danger of rupture of the uterus during version cannot be too strongly emphasized. For the child, the conditions requiring the interference usually determine the outlook. The turning itself, unless unduly prolonged by complications, by abruptio placentæ, or by prolapse of the cord, affects the infant but little.

LITERATURE

Bartholomew: "Cephalic Version in Breech Pres.," Transactions, Amer. Gyn. Soc., 1927.—*Costa, Loschi:* Zentralbl. für Gyn., October 22, 1921, p. 1524. Literature.—*Hoppe:* Zentb. f. Gynäk., 1927, May 21, No. 21, 1329.—*Hüssy:* Arch. f. Gyn., Bd. 104, H. 3, p. 572, 1915.—*Kerr:* Operative Midwifery.—*Klee:* Zeitschr. f. Geb. u. Gyn., 1925, vol. 88, H. 3, p. 574.—*Morse:* Surg., Gyn., and Obstet., February, 1912.—*Stoeckel:* Praktische Ergebnisse, Geb. u. Gyn., 1911, Heft 1; also Zentrb. für Gyn., 1915, p. 56.—*Titus:* Surg., Gyn., and Obstet., December, 1916, p. 734. Literature.—*Zarate:* Gynécologie et Obstét., 1926, Tome xiv, p. 289. Also Archiv. für Gynaek., 1931, vol. 147, H. 3, p. 759.

65

CHAPTER LXXI

OPERATIONS OF DELIVERY

UNDER this heading will be considered those operations which remove the child from the parturient canal—breech delivery, forceps, craniotomy, and cesarean section. The technical term "extraction" would apply to all such manœuvers, but usage has limited it to the removal of the unmutilated child through the natural passages.

The differences between spontaneous and artificial delivery must always be borne in mind. In spontaneous delivery the fetal body is compressed into a smoothly rounded cylinder and the uterus contracts upon it evenly from all directions propelling it downward.

In artificial delivery, whether by the head or the breech, we put traction on the child and the fetal cylinder is broken at several places,—for example, at the neck, the shoulders being held back by the soft parts,—or at the shoulder-girdle in breech presentation.

In addition, the uterus is not smoothly applied to the fetus, but may be caught and folded on any prominence of its body. Further, the impingement of a sharp point of the fetus may cause anomalous contraction rings. It is wise, therefore, to make our tractions synchronous with the uterine contractions, or, if the uterus is in spasm, relax it completely by narcosis.

The baby may suffer cerebral concussion and shock from trauma.

EXTRACTION

General Indications.—Why should we desire to deliver the woman? Why must we extract the child? Here is the broad indication in a few words. We deliver the child because the mother is unable to do so. The indication for extraction, therefore, is insufficiency of the powers of labor, and, as Schauta did, this general indication may be subdivided into, first, absolute weakness of the powers; second, relative insufficiency; third, insufficiency of the powers in relation to the necessary rapid termination of labor. Under the first head, actual weakness of the forces of labor, may be mentioned weak pains from maldevelopment of the uterus, fibroids, overdistention, poor innervation, tetanus uteri, hour-glass contraction, infantilism, rupture of the uterus, generally poor muscular development, diastasis recti, inflammatory conditions in the abdominal cavity which weaken the abdominal muscles, etc.

Relative insufficiency of the powers may be due to increase of the resistances offered—(a) on the part of the mother, such as rigidity of the cervix, vagina, perineum; contracted pelvis; tumors of the passage; and (b) on the part of the child, such as overgrowth, hydrocephalus, malpresentations, malpositions, etc. The pains may be strong or even stronger than usual, yet unable to complete delivery.

Insufficiency of the powers in relation to the desired rapidity of the delivery is a very common indication for extraction. The powers may be sufficient and efficient, the resistances may be normal or even less than normal, and the woman could complete the labor unaided, but a complication has arisen demanding immediate delivery. A few may be cited—on the part of the mother, eclampsia, acute and chronic pulmonary and heart diseases, hernia, appendicitis, hemorrhage from the genitals or from the lungs, etc., and, on the part of the child, asphyxia threatening from any cause, or severe compression of the brain, etc.

General Conditions.—(1) The pelvis may not be too severely contracted. A flat pelvis with a conjugata vera of less than 8 cm. will very rarely permit a normal-sized child to pass, and if the pelvis is a justominor one, a conjugata vera of nearly 9 cm. is necessary. If the child is estimated to weigh over 8 pounds, the conjugata vera must be over 9 cm. In short, an absolute prerequisite for extraction is that there be no insuperable disproportion between the babe and the pelvis. If pubiotomy or embryotomy is in reserve, the degree of contraction may not go below $7\frac{1}{2}$ cm. and $6\frac{1}{2}$ cm. respectively.

(2) The cervix must be effaced and the os dilated. This condition is impor-

tant in relation to the ease of the extraction, the integrity of the maternal tissues, and the life and safety of the child. If it is necessary, in the interests of the infant or the mother, to deliver before this prerequisite is fulfilled, the cervix must be opened by one of the preparatory operations—metreurysis, incisions, etc. The

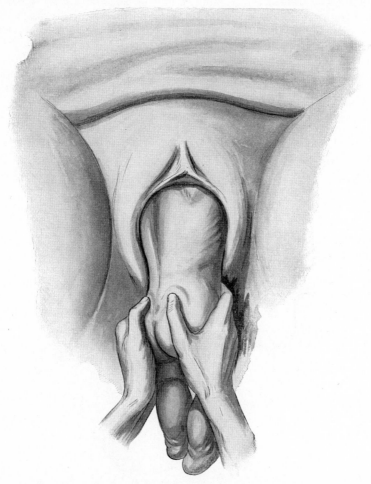

FIG. 834.—SECOND ACT OF EXTRACTION. DELIVERY OF BREECH TO SHOULDERS.

An assistant makes continuous even pressure over the whole uterus with both hands. The accoucheur takes the breech in two hands, with the thumbs over the back of the sacrum, the index-fingers resting on the anterior superior spines, the others evenly distributed over the pelvis and thighs, Gentle, even traction is made downward in the direction of the axis of the inlet *until the anterior shoulder-blade comes well under the pubis.* Now the fingers are gently insinuated into the vagina along the chest of the child to discover the location of the arms. If they are in the normal attitude, crossed over the chest, it is easy to pull them down by hooking a finger in the elbow-flexure, and simply drawing the arms out, first one, then the other. If they have been stripped up, out of easy reach, proceed as in Fig. 834a.

evils of extraction before dilatation is complete have been referred to, and will bear reiteration.

(3) Before delivery the bag of waters must be ruptured.

(4) With few exceptions one must insist that the child be living.

If the child is dead, embryotomy is, as a rule, a preferable operation. If in doubt, the child gets the benefit, within a reasonable limit.

(5) In cephalic presentations the head must be engaged in the pelvis, or so nearly engaged that it is almost certain that a slight pull from below will complete the engagement. (*Vide* Forceps.)

Extraction by the Breech.—The reader is referred to p. 660 for the details of the treatment of breech presentation.

Manual Aid.—Even though the majority of breech labors end without the necessity of aid by the accoucheur, it is wise to have the woman on a proper table and to have all the instruments for forceps delivery and for the repair of lacerations ready, with the room cleared for operation. When the breech has been delivered, the woman is urged to bear down, failing which an assistant exerts strong pressure on the child from the abdomen, and if this does not make rapid progress, the indication for "manual aid" is present. In multiparæ manual aid is seldom required. An anesthetic is used only if the woman is unruly or if the soft parts are very rigid. In primiparæ I make a deep unilateral episiotomy—on the side on which the occiput will come down—as a routine measure. It facilitates all the manipulations of the delivery, preserves the child from injury due to the application of force, saves time,

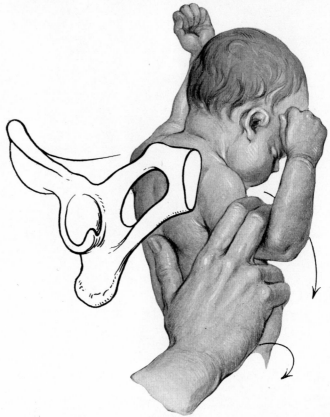

Fig. 834a.

Two fingers slip upward under the pubis over the child's back, and down to its elbow flexure. By flexing the two fingers and twisting his wrist, the operator sweeps the baby's arm over its chest and down and out. If the anterior arm proves inaccessible or requires too much force for its liberation, bring down the posterior arm first, as in Fig. 835.

which lessens the danger of asphyxia, and safeguards the sphincter ani from laceration. If the child is astride the cord, the latter is gently loosened and stripped over one thigh, failing which it is cut between two ligatures and the delivery rapidly ended. The bladder is to be empty. Feces issuing from the anus must be carefully removed, and this part watched with great solicitude, because in the hurry of the successive maneuvers it is only too easy to soil the operating hand and carry infection into the uterus. Lubricate the passages with green soap. Figures 834, 835, 836, and 837 describe the operation of "manual aid."

Complete Extraction.—When in breech cases an indication arises for delivery, preparations are identical with those for version. The operation itself is divided into four acts: First, bringing out the breech and legs; second, delivery to the shoulders; third, disengaging the shoulder-girdle; and fourth, the birth of the head. Complete extraction is manual aid preceded by one act, *i. e.*, bringing down the foot or feet.

First Act.—How to deliver the breech will depend on its station or location and upon the attitude of the child. If the breech is deeply engaged in the pelvis, a little traction with the finger in one groin may suffice; if one or both feet are down, traction is made on the extremity. The following methods have been employed to deliver the breech: (*a*) Bringing down one leg; (*b*) the finger in the groin; (*c*) the use of a fillet or sling placed over the groin; (*d*) a blunt hook, or two hooks, one in each groin, or specially constructed forceps, shaped like hooks; (*e*) use of the obstetric forceps on the breech.

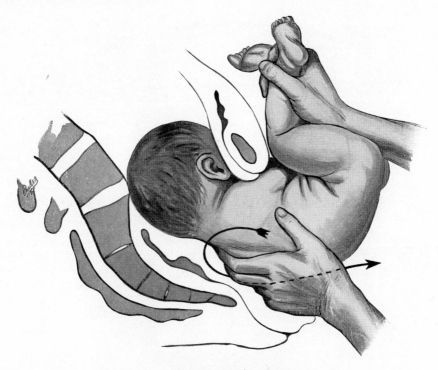

FIG. 835.—DELIVERY OF POSTERIOR ARM AND SHOULDER.

The posterior shoulder and arm are being disengaged, using the hand, whose palm will apply flat to the child's back. The other hand seizes the two feet of the infant and swings the body through an arc toward the mother's groin, which motion draws the shoulder down into the hollow of the sacrum, bends the child around the ramus pubis, and gives more room for the insertion of the hand. Leaving the thumb outside, two fingers are passed over the back, over the shoulder, down the arm, *to* the elbow, and wipe the arm over the face and chest, down and out of the vulva. During this act there should be no pressure by the assistant from the abdomen.

Of all these methods, extraction on one or both legs is by far the best, and I have not yet met a case where it was impossible to get a foot down. Deep anesthesia and the Trendelenburg posture have always enabled me to reach the extremity, no matter how firmly the breech seemed wedged into the pelvis at the start. In cases of contracted pelvis, unless cephalic version is to be performed, it is advisable to bring down the foot, and in pendulous abdomen it is also desirable, the leg straightening out the child in the axis of the inlet, which permits the uterus to work to good advantage. In single breech presentations the manœuver is the hardest to carry out; in double breech, two fingers may be able to grasp the ankle, which lies near the internal os. The anterior limb is to be selected whenever possible, because this brings the back to the pubis, but if too much trouble is experienced, the posterior one is seized, and in the subsequent extraction due notice is taken of the mechanism intended by nature.

Delivery by the finger in the groin is the least harmful of all the other methods mentioned, which possess real dangers of injuring the skin, vessels, and nerves in the groin and of fracturing the neck of the femur. The blunt hook, the fillet, the breech forceps, and the head forceps, in my opinion, should be used only on a dead fetus. But very few authorities recommend them, and in my practice so far they have been entirely dispensable. Robert Barnes, in his immense experience, never failed to bring down a leg. (See Figs. 838–841.)

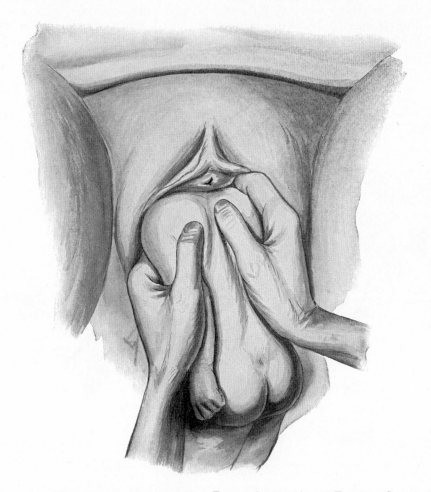

Fig. 836.—Delivery of Anterior Arm. Turning Anterior Arm to Hollow of Sacrum.

Having brought out the posterior arm there is more room to reach the anterior one. It may be visible behind the pubis and easily got out. If not, the child is allowed to fall onto the hand which delivered the arm, the arm is laid as a splint alongside the chest, the operator grasps the chest of the child with both hands, the index-finger of the second hand obtaining a purchase on the anterior scapula, and the other fingers being evenly distributed over the thorax. Then, with gentle rotation, the anterior arm is turned to the back, following the direction of the child's belly, and the now-posterior second arm and shoulder are delivered, reversing the action shown in Fig. 835, p. 1029. Don't crush the child!

The second, third, and fourth acts of extraction have been fully described under Manual Aid (q. v. p. 1028 and Figs. 834–837).

Complications.—It remains to discuss the difficulties that are likely to arise during the extraction. Two facts require emphasis at the very start. One is that the mechanism of breech labor may be pathologic throughout its whole course, or may rectify itself at any point, and a normal mechanism may become pathologic at any point. The other is that when an extraction is done to save the child, the conditions for delivery must be insisted upon, especially the one relating to the complete dilatation of the cervix. To force the delivery through an ill-prepared cervix is to expose the mother to the greatest danger of rupture of the uterus, and for so much hazard, in all probability, lose the child. The rigid cervix delays the extraction so long that the child succumbs, unless the accoucheur is prepared to make deep incisions into the constricting structures.

Complications During the First Act.—If the posterior leg is brought down, the anterior hip may catch on the pubic ramus. Sometimes the operator brings one leg down so that it crosses the other which lies athwart the inlet. Treatment: A sling is put on the ankle delivered and the other extremity brought out. Occasionally the foot drags out the cord, and this demands rapid delivery if the conditions are fulfilled.

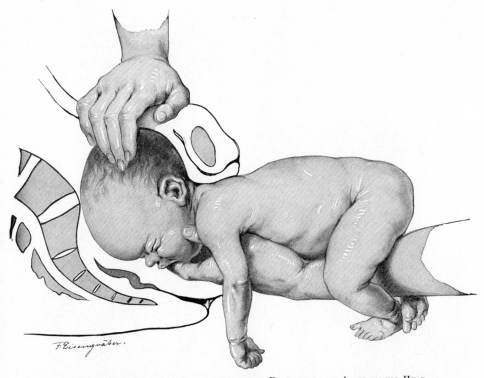

FIG. 837.—CELSUS-WIEGAND-MARTIN METHOD OF DELIVERING THE AFTER-COMING HEAD.

Remembering the mechanism of breech labor, the accoucheur will know on which side of the pelvis the mouth will be. The hand whose palm applies to the belly searches for the child's mouth, and two fingers are passed into it until they come to rest at the posterior angles of the jaw, the child lying on the forearm. Standing to the patient's side, the accoucheur places the other hand on the head from the outside (having carefully pushed the intestines out of the way), and, by combined pressure from above, with very light traction from below, the head is brought down into the pelvis, rotated, and delivered, following the mechanism usually adopted by nature. The chin is kept well flexed, and when the nape of the neck stems behind the pubis, the chin, face, forehead, and vertex are brought slowly over the perineum. In primiparæ episiotomy is usually performed. Gentleness! Deliberation!

Complications, Second Act.—Large or very fat babies or a contracted pelvis may render the delivery from the breech to the shoulders difficult. Care must be exercised in applying pressure to avoid injuring the abdominal viscera. If more than ordinary resistance is met, pass the fingers alongside the child to find if a distended abdomen exists (for example, ascites, cystic kidneys, liver tumor, etc.). With large and fat babies it is wise to deliver the arms before the shoulders have become wedged into the pelvis, therefore, not to draw the trunk down until the scapula is palpable under the pubis, but to begin the third act a little sooner. Moderate pressure from above, lubrication of the vagina with sterile, liquid soap, slow traction from below, the fingers being evenly spread over the lower trunk, with a minimum of squeezing of the baby, will almost always succeed in bringing the shoulder girdle within reach.

Complications, Third Act.—Normally, the arms lie crossed over the chest, and if nothing interferes are delivered in this position. If traction is made on the body

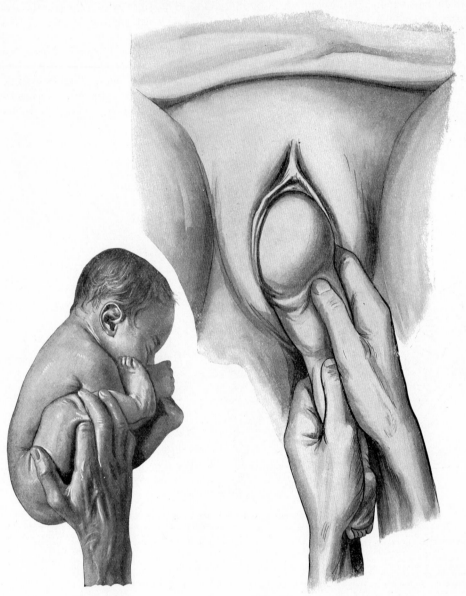

FIG. 838.—BRINGING DOWN FOOT. PINARD'S MANŒUVER.

Passing the hand high up into the uterus, avoiding the cord, which is kept on the back of the hand, the index-finger is pressed into the popliteal space. This shortens the hamstring muscles and flexes the leg, upon which the three fingers slip over the knee to the ankle, the foot now being wiped along the other thigh posteriorly into the pelvis and out. During the pains no move may be made—the hand should lie passive until the uterus relaxes.

FIG. 839.—DELIVERY OF ANTERIOR HIP.

Laying the thumbs parallel to the long bones and distributing the fingers evenly over the rest of the limb, traction is made downward in the axis of the inlet until the crest of the ilium has passed the ligamentum arcuatum, the hands being adjusted higher and higher as the limb appears. No bending nor twisting motions are allowable, and the action must be smooth, not jerky. The vagina should be well lubricated with sterile liquid soap. The slippery leg is held with a dry towel.

too soon; if the pelvis is small; if the cervix is not sufficiently dilated—the arms may be arrested and stripped up above the child's head (Fig. 842). In such cases it is necessary to pass the four fingers high into the pelvic inlet, leaving the thumb outside, and, as usual, gliding over back, shoulder, humerus, elbow, to the forearm; this latter is pushed to the side of the pelvis, wiping across the face and then down and out. The posterior arm is first delivered. Episiotomy is the rule in primiparæ, because the thickness of the hand added to that of the chest is usually too much for the perineum. It may be well to push the child back a little to loosen the arms from the wedge-like action of the head. If it is too hard to get the posterior arm, one tries to bring down the anterior arm from behind the pubis. Failing this, the child may be rotated ventrally so as to bring the anterior arm to the hollow of the sacrum, and this arm is liberated first, then the trunk is rotated back for the

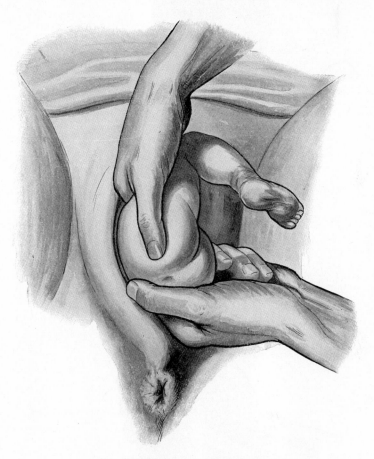

Fig. 840.—Delivery of Posterior Hip.

As soon as possible the index-finger—only one finger—of the other hand is passed over the back, along the crest of the ilium, into the posterior groin, and with combined traction the whole pelvis is brought out, following the usual mechanism. The second leg is allowed to drop out.

other arm. If the operator's fingers are short, or if the arm is very high up, the whole hand should be passed in to get the arms. Then the thumb should lie parallel to, never opposed to, the fingers, and it may not be used to grasp the arm. During these manœuvers the assistant should not exert pressure on the fundus uteri, since this renders internal manipulation difficult, but the operator himself can sometimes assist the inner hand to reach the arms by gently pressing them down into the pelvis from the outside.

In version cases one usually puts a sling, prophylactically, on one arm. When the extraction is begun, an even, gentle pull is made upon the sling, so as to bring the hand down over the baby's chest, and the delivery of the arm occurs together with the trunk.

A second and a bad complication occurs in the third act, when the arms are thrown back into the nape of the neck and cross the pelvis under the head. This is usually caused by anomalous rotation of the child's trunk, and is commoner after version and improper efforts at extraction (Fig. 843). This condition is recognized only when the fingers are passed in to liberate the posterior arm. Without delay

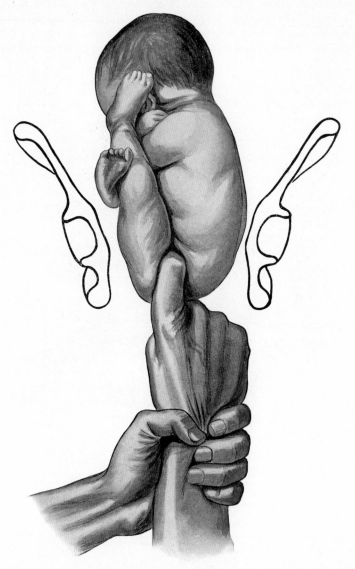

FIG. 841.—DELIVERY OF BREECH WITH FINGER IN GROIN. OTHER HAND SUPPORTS WRIST.

In extracting the breech with one finger in the anterior groin the whole hand is placed in the vagina, the finger passes from in front, while the thumb seeks to aid a better grasp on the pelvis. Traction is to be made downward, but the pull must be toward the belly of the child, to avoid injury to the structures in the inguinal region and fracture of the femur. This operation is very tiring, hence the hands may be changed and the wrist supported as shown. Episiotomy and patience are required. As soon as the posterior groin is accessible, the index-finger of the other hand is placed in it, and delivery of the breech accomplished easier. Aid by Kristeller expression.

the body of the child is pushed back, or stuffed in a few inches, to release the arms from their imprisonment by the head, and the half hand inserted directly up the child's back to the forearm. This, then, is pushed up, the fingers wiping the baby's elbow and forearm over its face, past the sacral promontory to the other half of the pelvis, down and out. If this does not succeed the first time, the child should be pushed back a little further and the manœuver tried once more, failing which the anterior arm should be liberated. Grasping the chest as indicated in Fig. 836, p. 1030, the child is rotated ventrally so as to bring the anterior arm behind; then, with four fingers deeply inserted, or even the whole hand, the just mentioned motion with the child's forearm is carried out. Rotation of the trunk much facilitates the release of the arm, but beware of causing Erb's paralysis!

It is not allowable to pull down on the shoulder to make the arm and elbow more accessible. Fracture of the clavicle is the certain result. Nor may the arm be brought down over the back, obviously, for the same reason. If the accoucheur will go at his work deliberately, it will not be needful to exert brute force and break the clavicle or humerus. To try to deliver the head without previous liberation of the arms (Deventer) is not good practice.

Complications, Fourth Act.—Arrest of the head may occur at the pelvic inlet, and after it is in the excavation or at the outlet. If the child is large or the pelvis

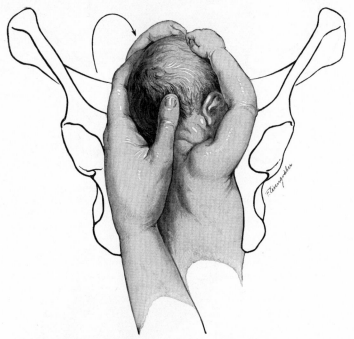

Fig. 842.—Arms Stripped Up. Whole Hand Required to Bring Them Down.
The thumb may not be used to grasp the arm.

small, the head wedges into the inlet with the sagittal suture in the transverse diameter. Extension occurs and the mouth is thrown up high—sometimes above the brim. Treatment: Wiegand-Martin's method, remembering that the chin is high up and to the side, that the head must be brought through the inlet in the transverse diameter, that it should not be strongly flexed, and that it may not be rotated to bring the occiput forward until it is deep in the excavation. The pull must be downward in the axis of the inlet, hence the patient is best on a high table, but most of the work is to be done by pressure with the outside hand. Where this method fails, the Mauriceau-Smellie-Veit method is tried (Fig. 844). One hand searches the mouth, and two fingers are placed, as before, on the lower insertions of the pterygomaxillary ligaments. The other hand is placed fork-like over the shoulders, *with the finger-tips resting on the sternum,* not on the sides of the neck. The knuckles rest against the mastoid processes. While an assistant presses the head forcibly downward from without, the operator pulls gently, but firmly, downward from within, observing the mechanism just described. In particularly difficult cases the Walcher position may be used, and the operator, by pushing the head to one or the other side of the promontory, may gain more room for the large biparietal diameter to pass, or, by tilting the head upward or downward, may seek to bring the biparietal plane through the inlet on a slant. *Non vi, sed arte* applies with double force in this operation.

If the head will not come into the pelvis under the exhibition of moderate force applied above and below, unless the accoucheur is expert with the forceps, it is best to desist, because the end sought, a living child, will be defeated by the at-

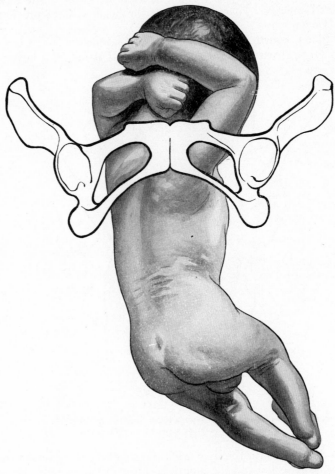

Fig. 843.—Arms in Nape of Neck.
These arms can be made more accessible by manipulation from the outside.

tempt itself, and the mother will suffer irreparable injury. Now there is no occasion for hurry. Craniotomy should be performed. In practice there is usually no compunction about such a course, since the child has almost always died by this time.

When the head is arrested in the excavation, a quick examination determines if the delay is caused by the cervix or by the bony pelvis. A tight cervix must be stripped back or cut, which is not always a simple matter. If the methods of delivery just mentioned do not show immediate results, the forceps should be applied to the after-coming head. My practice for years has been to apply forceps

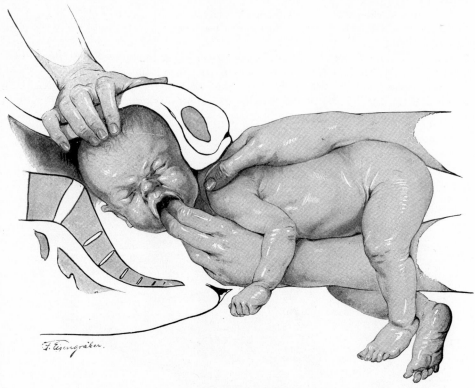

FIG. 844.—GUILLEMEAU-MAURICEAU-SMELLIE-VEIT METHOD, AIDED BY OUTSIDE HAND.
(Klein proves this method should be called simply Guillemeau's.)

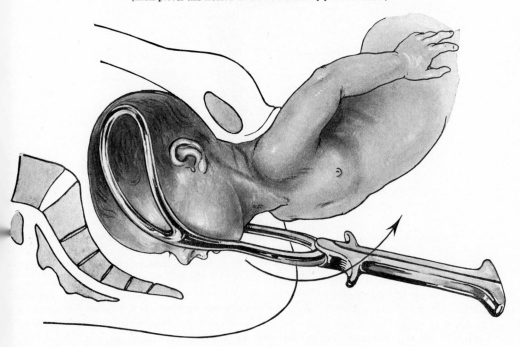

FIG. 845.—FORCEPS ON THE AFTER-COMING HEAD.

An assistant holds the child up and out of the way with its arms behind the back, and the blades are applied in the usual manner. In his hurry the operator may not forget the usual precautions to safeguard the cervix, pelvic floor, and the child. This head is engaged; only an expert with the forceps may be allowed to try them when the head is arrested at the inlet. They are then dangerous to the mother and usually barren of results.

to the after-coming head if it does not quickly follow moderate traction, and Kerr recommends it very highly, quoting also Smellie, Barnes, and Hermann in its favor. Williams opposes the practice, as do some of the German authorities, though several —Nagel, Klein, Nürnberger (Lit.), and others, and French operators, Bar and Tarnier—employ the instrument in some cases. I am convinced that many children will be saved, that fracture of the clavicle, hematoma of the sternomastoid, dislocation of the vertebræ, Erb's paralysis, and many lesser injuries could be avoided if the application of the forceps to the after-coming head were taught in

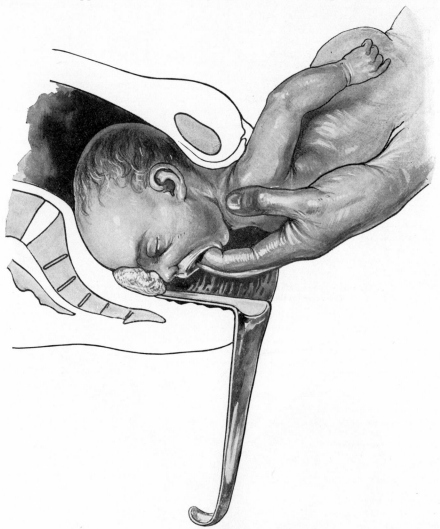

Fig. 846.—Letting Air to Child's Lungs when Head is Arrested in Breech Delivery.

the schools and more generally practised. It is a more humane way of delivering the head in cases of moderate difficulty than the Mauriceau-Smellie-Veit method. At least in all breech cases the forceps should be ready for use. Piper of Philadelphia invented a special forceps for the delivery of the after-coming head.

A very valuable manœuver, practised for many centuries, is the retraction of the perineum by the hands or by broad specula, wiping the vagina dry and allowing the child to breathe with its head still in the pelvis (Fig. 846). A stiff rubber tube may also be inserted into the child's pharynx. Stowe, in one case, did tracheotomy and saved the infant.

Abnormal Rotation in Breech Cases.—Thus far we have considered the operation of delivery when the mechanism of labor has been the usual one—that is, with the back anterior. Just as in vertex presentations, we have errors in the mechanism due to abnormal rotation. In some breech deliveries the child's back turns to the mother's back, and the belly lies forward, behind the pubis. This complication occurs oftener in footling presentations when the posterior leg has come down, after version when the operator has seized the posterior leg, and, rarely, during an otherwise natural breech labor when improper attempts at rotation had been made. As was said in discussing breech presentation, nature almost always rectifies the abnormal start of the mechanism by turning the back three-fourths of a circle, making it rotate the "long route," past the promontory, through the other half of the pelvis to the front. The back rotates in the direction opposite from that which one would expect. An acute observer will notice this tendency of the breech to swing around in front of the sacrum. By not appreciating this point and resisting the mechanism sought by nature, the accoucheur may cause the back to remain directed behind. During the first and second acts this is of little moment. Watching the rotation intended by nature, the operator seeks to aid it by pulling harder on that groin which tends to turn forward. In a few cases, even when the posterior limb is down, the back takes the "short route," through one-fourth of a circle, to the pubis.

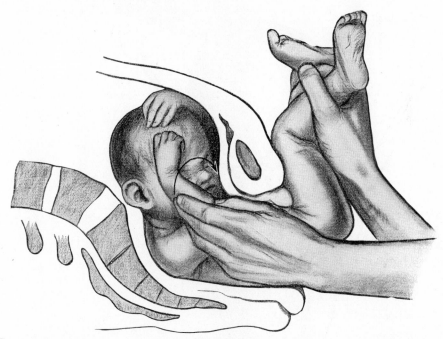

Fig. 847.—Bringing Down Arms in Back to Back Position.   Arrow Indicates Direction of Movement.

Abnormal Rotation During the Third Act.—The arms may lie folded across the chest, may be stripped up alongside the head, or may be crossed in the nape of the neck. In the first case the matter is very simple. The child is supported a little above the horizontal with one hand, while two fingers of the other go in over the back, over the shoulder, down the arm to the elbow, and wipe the forearm over the chest, out from behind the pubis, the usual manœuver being reversed. It may also be possible, sinking the trunk toward the floor, to go directly to the forearm from behind the pubis, and, indeed, this may be the only way if the child is large or the pelvis small—there may be no room behind. When the arms are stripped up above the head, great difficulties are usually met, and if they are in the nucha, it may be impossible to liberate them without fracture. Under no conditions may the arms be brought down over the child's back. In the first place, if the accoucheur sees that the child's back remains persistently posterior, he will bring the arms down as early as possible. It is sometimes necessary to pass the whole hand into the parturient canal in order to reach the arms—especially if the accoucheur has short fingers. This overdistends the vagina and perineal floor, hence a deep episiotomy is made, as a rule. Some authors recommend that the arms be brought down after sinking the child's trunk and entering and operating behind the pubis. I prefer, with Fritsch and the majority, to raise the body of the child somewhat (one cannot pull it up so far as when the back is anterior), and pass the four fingers from behind up to the head and push the forearm forward and to the opposite anterior quadrant of the pelvis, then down over the chest, as in Fig. 847. If the first attempt does not succeed, the trunk of the child is rotated, at the same time stuffing it back somewhat to free the arms above the inlet, and the anterior arm is delivered first. The child is now turned back for the other arm to come behind. Pulling on the shoulder to make the arm more accessible fractures the clavicle. In a few cases I was able to aid the internal hand by letting an assistant support the body of the child, while I pushed the arms into proper position from the outside. External manipulation is not used enough in our obstetric operations. In only one case from a very large number was I constrained deliberately to break the arm in order to preserve the life of the child, which was jeopardized by the delays in the delivery. It is wise to announce this necessity beforehand. A. Müller's procedure, delivery of the shoulder-girdle without previous liberation of the arms, succeeds only in easy cases. When force is used there is danger of breaking the spine.

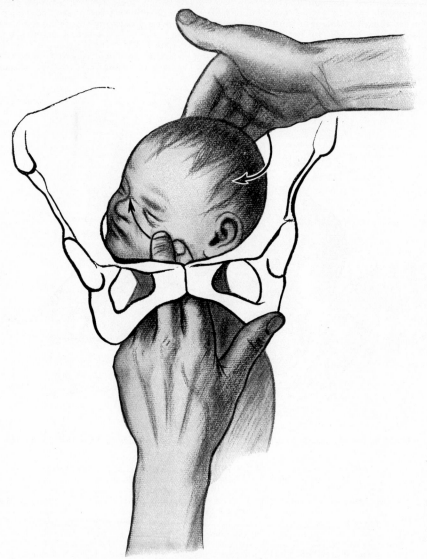

FIG. 848.—ROTATING HEAD BY CONJOINED MANIPULATION.

During the Fourth Act.—Referring to the chapter on Abnormal Mechanisms with Breech, it will be found that the head may be arrested at the inlet with the chin caught over the ramus pubis, or the head may engage in the pelvis with the chin to the front, and that nature may terminate these cases in two ways—one is by flexion: the body depends, the chin remains applied to the sternum, and the face, forehead, and vertex roll out from behind the pubis, the nape of the neck resting on the perineum; the other is by extension: the chin leaves the sternum, and if the child is lifted up to the belly of the mother, the occiput, vertex, and face come over the perineum, the neck resting behind the pubis, and the face issuing the very last.

In the first case the accoucheur may attempt to turn the head so as to bring the occiput to the front, the chin to the rear or to the side, if the pelvis is a flat contracted one. LaChapelle passed the hand in on the side opposite that on which the chin lay and tried to pull the face around. Zweifel recommended pressure with four fingers on the upper jaw. In four cases the following manœuver succeeded quickly: Two fingers behind the pubis obtained a purchase on the malar bone, and, while pushing this to the rear, the outside hand pulled the occiput to the front (Fig. 848). Now the mouth was readily accessible, and the usual mechanism could be carried out. In another case I pulled the chin to the side with the outside hand, while the inside hand pulled the occiput to the front.

If rotation of the head does not quickly take place, it may be better, since seconds are very valuable, to try to deliver the head without turning the chin behind. Van Hoorn's method is used if the occiput has not engaged in the pelvis, combined with pressure on the forehead from the outside (Fig. 849). This pressure should do most of the work. The child is lifted up over the pubis, to which its chest applies, and thus the occiput rolls past the promontory into the hollow of the sacrum. Too much force exerted now will break the child's neck. When the occiput comes into the hollow of the sacrum, the accoucheur quickly determines if the mouth of the infant is accessible behind the pubis—that is, if extension or flexion is present. If the finger can be inserted into the mouth, the Guillemeau-Mauriceau-Smellie-Veit method upside down is performed; if extension has occurred, the chin lying above the pubis, a modified Van Hoorn's method is practised. The forceps are preferable to either of these manœuvers. Indeed, the necessity for them is of the greatest rarity, since it is almost always possible to bring the head down in proper rotation.

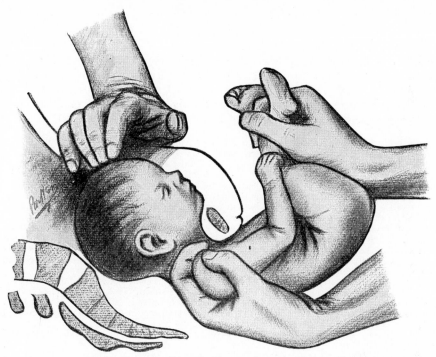

FIG. 849.—VAN HOORN'S METHOD, AIDED BY OUTSIDE HAND.

A complete extraction by the breech, if properly executed, is one of the most brilliant operations, and, if the complications are successfully mastered without injury to the mother or child, it takes rank with the technically most difficult of all surgery. Every motion is the result of centuries of study and practice by the world's best accoucheurs, and the movements must follow each other with deliberation, exactness, and speed. Four minutes are allowed for the arms and four for the head. More time consumed endangers the child. It is a good plan for an assistant to count aloud the minutes. While a child may live five minutes after its placental circulation is cut off, it is greatly endangered, and may die later of atelectasis, pneumonia, sepsis, or the results of profound asphyxia.

Finally, attention should be drawn to complications offered by the soft parts. If extraction is undertaken before the cervix is fully dilated, dangers of no mean order are incurred for both mother and child. For the mother there is risk of tears

66

of the lower uterine segment and cervix, which in placenta prævia are particularly fatal from hemorrhage. Sepsis is a later result. For the child the risk lies in the delay incident to the stripping up of the arms by the tight ring of the cervix, and, too, even after liberation of the arms the cervix may close down around the neck or face, at the root of the nose, buttonholing the head in the uterus. Traction in such cases brings the constricting cervix into view as a thick purplish and white band. This ring may be carefully stripped back, or if too tight, may be incised. It may be possible to admit air to the child's mouth by means of specula and wait for the head to come through (Fig. 846, p. 1038).

Deep lacerations of the perineum, even to the third degree, are very common in breech deliveries. They occur when the hand is inserted alongside the trunk or during the rapid delivery of the head. I make an extensive episiotomy in most breech cases not alone to preserve the sphincter ani but also to facilitate all the required manipulations, which save the child from asphyxia and from injury.

Lack of space prevents reference to the many accoucheurs who perfected each of the various manœuvers above detailed. (See Lit. p. 1077.)

FORCEPS

Definition.—The forceps of obstetrics is an instrument designed to extract the fetus by the head from the maternal passages, without injury to it or to the mother. As soon as the right of either is encroached upon, the instrument ceases to be the forceps of obstetrics, but becomes simply an instrument of extraction, similar to the craniotomy forceps, and not so good.

History.—Hippocrates advised pulling on the head with the hands, but probably used the manœuver only for small heads; the Arabians used a three- or four-bladed hooked tractor for dead fetuses; in 1554 Rueff, of Zürich, published a jointed forceps similar to that used in lithotomy; in 1561 Pierre Franco advised a three-bladed duckbill speculum, obviously impractical; the Japanese for centuries used whalebone loops and silk nets brought over the head by means of strips of whalebone; Smellie tried to draw fillets over the occiput and chin. It is remarkable that the idea of the obstetric forceps was so long in coming. As Schröder says, this was probably because men were not allowed at the confinement-bed except in the most difficult cases And here, for lack of experience in normal cases, they knew little except to mutilate the child and extract it, and often the viscera of the mother, with sharp hooks. Unless the child presented by the breech or shoulder, so that the accoucheur could grasp a leg on which to pull, he was powerless, except as stated. Small wonder the women took alarm when a "man-midwife" had to be called, because they had observed, says Smellie, that "either the mother or the child or both were lost."

In 1720 Palfyn, of Courtrai, near Ghent, laid before the Academy of Medicine in Paris his forceps (Fig. 850, c) for the extraction of the child without mutilation. This rough, clumsy instrument was modified by others. Dussè crossed the blades and lengthened them, and Levret, 1746, added the pelvic curve, also the French lock, still used, though modified. The forceps depicted on Palfyn's memorial plaque in the cathedral in Ghent shows a pelvic curve.

The first forceps were invented probably in 1580 by Peter Chamberlen, the elder, the son of a Huguenot, William Chamberlen, who fled from Paris in 1569 and settled in Southampton. In 1670 Hugh, one of the large family, went to Paris and tried to sell the instrument for $7500. Mauriceau, to test the value of Chamberlen's pretenses, suggested that the latter attempt the delivery of a woman with extreme contraction of the pelvis, upon whom he had decided to perform cesarean section. Chamberlen declared that nothing could be easier, and at once, in a private room, set about the task. After three hours of vain effort he was obliged to acknowledge his defeat. The woman died from injury to the uterus, the negotiations for the sale were dropped, and Chamberlen returned with his secret unrevealed to England. Later, after wrecking a bank, he fled to Holland, where he sold the secret to a Roonhuysen, in Amsterdam, who sold it in turn to any doctor having the necessary large amount of money, but sold only half the forceps,—the vectis,—adding fraud to infamy.

In 1753 Vischer and van de Poll purchased the secret and made it public, but by this time, through Palfyn, Drinkwater, and others, the forceps had become common property. Palfyn, at the time seventy years of age, had walked to Paris to show his invention. It was not well received and he died poor and neglected, but in 1784 his resting-place in Ghent was marked by a statue of a weeping woman. The original forceps of the Chamberlens were found in 1815 in a hidden attic of a house in Essex, England, occupied by several generations of the family (Ingraham). Numberless alterations and modifications have been made on the forceps. Figure 850 shows a few of them, the only radical changes from the original Chamberlen and Dussè models being the addition of axis-traction by Tarnier in 1877. For history of forceps see Schroeder, Das.

Description.—The forceps consists of two blades, which are named right and left, according to the side of the mother's pelvis in which they lie when applied. Each blade has a handle and a hook-like projection, added by Busch. Gregoire (1740) put the fenestrum in the blade, but the Chamberlen forceps also had it. Some of the latest forceps are unfenestrated, for example, the McLane-Tucker.

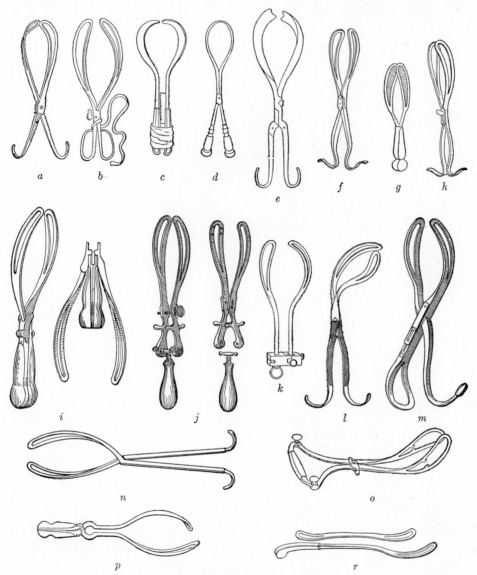

FIG. 850.—A FEW OF THE HUNDREDS OF FORCEPS MODELS.

a, Chamberlen No. 1; *b,* Chamberlen No. 2; *c,* Palfyn; *d,* Palfyn, 1721; *e,* Dussè, 1733; *f,* Gregoire, 1746; *g,* Smellie, 1752; *h,* Levret, 1747; *i,* Mathias Saxtorph, 1791; *j,* Coutouly; *k,* Hamon, 1867; *l,* Baumers of Lyon, 1849; *m,* Santarelli, 1794; *n,* Japanese forceps; *o,* Chassagny; *p,* Rudford's asymmetric; *r,* Pean's vectis.

The blades are curved on the flat to fit the head,—the "cephalic curve,"—and on the edge to fit the concavity of the sacrum—the "pelvic curve." The two blades are fitted together by a lock, which in the English forceps consists of opposing shoulders with a flange; in the French forceps, a screw or pin; and in the German instrument, a sort of combination of both principles. Smellie and the English used a very short forceps, because the operation was practised only after the head was well down in the pelvis. The French used long forceps, since they often extracted the head before engagement had occurred. The German forceps are rather long, and resemble the French in having a small cephalic curve and a marked pelvic curve.

Over six hundred kinds of forceps have been invented and reinvented (Das). I recommend for general use the Simpson or Vienna School forceps. I lengthened

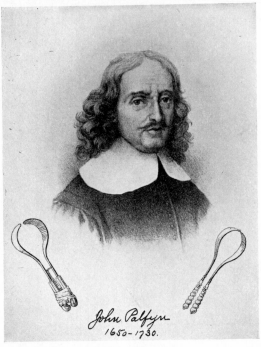

John Palfyn
1650-1730.

FIG. 850a.

the shanks so as to keep the handle away from the anus, made the hooks larger and flatter so as not to hurt the hand and modified the handles a little to secure lightness and ease of cleansing.

The Function of the Forceps.—Levret, in 1746, said that the forceps should be a tractor and nothing else, to supply from below the force that was lacking

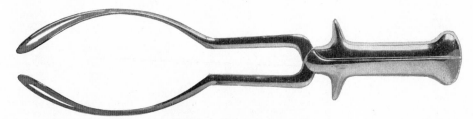

FIG. 851.—SIMPSON'S FORCEPS.
Made longer and handle modified by the author.

from above. Smellie in 1752, used his short, straight forceps as a rotator, Scanzoni, in 1865, developed an operation in which instrumental rotation was the main feature. Tarnier, in 1881, demonstrated the principle on which the forceps may be used to correct the position of the head in the pelvis. He pointed out that, owing to the pelvic curve of the instrument, if one twists the handles, the blades, with the head in their grasp, do not turn on the axis of the shanks, but tend to describe part of a circle within the pelvis (Fig. 862). In order, therefore, to make the head rotate around an axis it is necessary to sweep the handles of the forceps through a large circle outside the pelvis. The apex of the forceps blades then will act as a center and the head will turn around on it. Bill has improved on Tarnier's maneuver by first raising the head out of the pelvic floor gutter, and then sweeping the handles around to impart the movement of rotation to the head within the pelvis. Kielland, in 1915, devised a forceps without pelvic curve, and with the blades bent

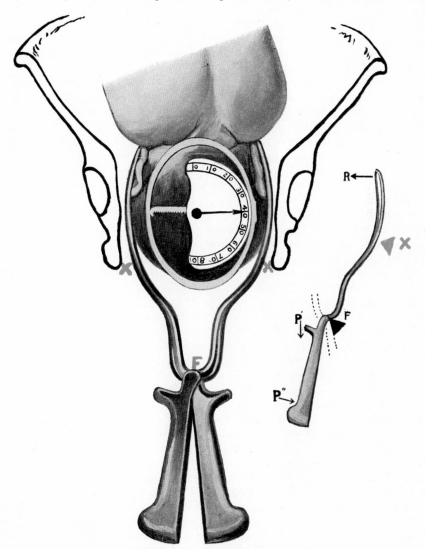

FIG. 852.—EXPERIMENT TO SHOW COMPRESSION EFFECT OF TRACTION.

a little downward. With this instrument a head may be grasped biparietally, no matter in which diameter it lies in the pelvis and it may, according to Kielland, be twisted safely to any position desired (*vide infra*).

The forceps has been used as a lever. Baudelocque, Osiander, Tarnier, Farabeuf, et al. applied the blades anteroposteriorly to the head lying above the inlet, and by up and down leverage movements canted it past the promontory. They also made large pendulum motions from side to side. The maternal soft parts, being the fulcrum, are usually bruised and torn.   Rudford, Fig. 850, page 1043, and Farabeuf constructed special instruments for grasping the head above the inlet.   These are now obsolete but Barton has reinvented Farabeuf's "prehenseur," and added an axis-traction device.   Kielland's forceps are said to be a good lever, but only in skilled hands.   The forceps should never be used as a dilator of the cervix.

Compression of the head is inevitable, but we seek to reduce it to the minimum. Experiments have proved what a little reflection would show, that we can reduce the volume of the fetal head but a few cubic millimeters by means of outside force, and even this is attended by great danger to the child.   If one applies forceps to the head of a still-born child in mannikin practice, it will be observed that closing the blades causes the head to bulge out in the diameter at right angles to the direction of compression, but only slightly.   What is more noticeable is the lengthening of the head in its long diameter, a point which Levret, Baudelocque, Budin, and Milne-Murray refer to.   Much depends on the softness of the head and the shape of the canal through which it is to pass.   Reference to Fig. 852 will show how the head suffers compression in two ways.   By squeezing the handles of the forceps together at P'', the action is that of a lever of the first class, the lock being the fulcrum, F, the resistance being the head, R.   Traction downward at P', with the fulcrum at X (the maternal parts), also produces a lever of the first class, resulting in additional compression of the head.   The compression at P'' we can regulate ourselves, but the amount exerted at P' depends entirely on the amount of pull exerted to deliver the head and increases with the resistances met.   The power is applied at P', or, as is advised in practice, at F, but the fulcrum is at X, and the power is applied to the long arm of the lever, obviously the most dangerous circumstance for the fetal head.   Taking these facts into consideration, I must disagree with Barnes, believing that the compression is not one-half of the power of the traction, but probably greater than the traction.   Farabeuf says it is ten times greater.   By eliminating resistance (e. g., by episiotomy) we reduce compression to a minimum.   Compression of the head has very noxious influences on the brain. If suddenly applied, the child suffers from concussion.   If slower in action, the circulation is hindered, the pneumogastric is stimulated, the pulse being slowed, and asphyxia resulting, or smaller or larger hemorrhages occur—all these outside of direct injury to structure or fracture of the bones.   Children vary very much in their ability to stand compression.   Some seem to have charmed lives.

While traction is the dominant function of the forceps, strength is giving way to art, and an artistic operator can use the forceps also as a rotator and, though rarely, as a lever, without serious damage to mother or child.   How much traction may safely be applied is hard to say.   Attempts to measure it with dynamometers have failed.   It is rarely necessary to pull with more than the strength of the biceps, as in Fig. 859.   To brace the feet against the table and pull with all the strength of the back and shoulders is brutal, unscientific, and murderous.   Craniotomy is more humane.   The accoucheur should always remember, when working with the forceps, that he has a child's brain in the grasp of a powerful vise, and that only the greatest care and gentleness will save its wonderfully delicate structure from injury.

Indications for Forceps.—These are the same as for extraction in general, comprising those conditions which threaten the life of the mother or child.   The accoucheur should not allow the woman to remain many hours in the second stage, waiting for signs of actual danger to the mother or child, when it is apparent that she will not be able to deliver herself.   As Barnes said, we should wait to see what the woman is able to accomplish, not what she can endure.   Then, too, when the signs of danger to the mother or the child are present, often real damage has been done—it were wiser if the accoucheur had anticipated the dangers.   In America 75 per cent. of the forceps operations are done because of *insufficiency of the powers* of labor when the head has come on to the perineum, or even is visible during a pain. Either the head is a little too large, or the perineum a little too resistant, or the woman's nerves have given out. In either case labor has come to a standstill, the pains weaken, the woman bears down less and less strongly, and, if not relieved, may get into a highly nervous, even delirious condition, which is not without after-effects on her constitution. The child suffers, too, the heart-tones are slowed, then grow faster and irregular, and a caput succedaneum forms and soon attains large dimensions and hardness.

It is not easy to select just the right time to interfere in these cases. Needless to say, the conditions must all be fulfilled. In general, it is wise to operate long before the exhaustion is marked, before the signs and symptoms of threatened rupture of the uterus are present, and before the child presents evidences of asphyxia. It is impossible to assign an arbitrary limit. As a general rule one should not wait more than one or one and a half hours after the head has reached the perineum and progress has ceased. If the perineum seems to be too resistant, a deep episiotomy may allow the head to go through—a procedure which is much preferable to forceps. If episiotomy does not give exit to the head, nothing has been lost, because the perineum would probably have been incised for the succeeding delivery anyway. (Compress bleeding areas; save blood!)

Arrest of the rotation of the head is another frequent indication for forceps. Occipitoposterior positions are most often here concerned, the occiput not turning completely to the front, but stopping usually in the transverse diameter of the pelvis—the so-called *deep transverse arrest*. It is not uncommon to find the child in the "military attitude," that is, one of slight deflexion, with the head set squarely on the shoulders. The sagittal suture runs across the pelvis, the two fontanels being about on one level.

Third in frequency may be grouped a large number of *complications* which affect the mother, but secondarily, the child also, a few of which may be mentioned. Eclampsia, fever, or infection during labor, with or without tympania uteri; acute diseases, as pneumonia, typhoid; chronic diseases, tuberculosis, heart disease, with the possibility of hemoptysis, heart-failure, or edema of the lungs; hernia, appendicitis, and other intra-abdominal conditions; placenta prævia, abruptio placentæ, prolapse of the cord, etc.

Face and brow presentations per se do not indicate forceps or any interference, but the accoucheur is more often called upon to intervene.

Contracted pelvis of itself is really a contraindication for forceps. Schröder says they fit the contracted pelvis like the fist on one's eye. After the head is molded so that it is almost ready to come down into the excavation, and in cases of generally contracted pelvis, where the powers give out after the head has engaged, it is justifiable to use the forceps as an instrument of trial, but the accoucheur must be constantly aware of their murderous possibilities.

Finally may be mentioned the use of forceps on the *after-coming head,* a practice which should, in my opinion, supersede many of the difficult Smellie-Veit extractions.

Prophylactic Forceps.—In 1920 the author created much comment in the profession by publishing a method of delivery to which he applied the name "prophylactic forceps." Briefly the procedure is as follows: Morphin and scopolamin are given in the first stage and perfect spontaneous dilatation of the cervix secured. When the head has come well down on to the pelvic floor, in complete anterior rotation, and has begun to part the levator ani pillars (and not before), the perineum and the fascia over the levator pillar are incised and the child delivered by forceps. Sometimes the pains are so good that the forceps are unnecessary after the episiotomy. Upon the birth of the child pituitrin is given, and after the placenta, ergot also. Another smaller dose of morphin and scopolamin is given to reduce the amount of ether needful for repair.

The objects of this interference with nature are: (1) To reduce the muscular and nervous strain of the second stage of labor; (2) to save the pelvic floor and adjacent fascia from overstretching; (3) to save the woman's blood; (4) to save the baby's brain from the evil results of prolonged compression and congestion *ex vacuo.*

The author strongly warned against the wide adoption of this procedure, believing that this would result in a high maternal and fetal mortality, which would defeat the very purposes intended. "Watchful expectancy" should still be the guide for the general practitioner and he should interfere only in the presence of immediate or prospective danger to mother or baby. On the other hand, the obstetric specialist, in his exquisitely equipped maternity, must do something to reduce the morbidity of the women and the mortality and morbidity of the babies. He must, where he can, improve on faulty nature. Many accoucheurs have practised this principle for years without applying any particular name to their forceps operations. The author is keenly aware that all operations can be abused, but he presented this mode of delivery to the profession confidently trusting each man to do honestly with his patients.

Conditions for Forceps.—These are the same as for extraction in general. (1) The pelvis must be large enough to permit delivery of the unmutilated child. If this point cannot be settled beforehand, the forceps, if used, is only an instrument of trial—of diagnosis. Forceps may not be used on a hydrocephalus, since the blades will usually slip off. If the child is very small, a diminutive pair of forceps is to be employed. (2) The cervix must be effaced and dilated, or sufficient enlargement must be easily procurable. Dilatation of the cervix by means of the head pulled down by forceps is a dangerous—really unjustifiable—procedure. (3) The membranes must be ruptured and out of the way, because of the danger of dislocation of the placenta. (4) The head must be engaged, or so nearly so that a cautious trial of the forceps may be permissible. (5) The child must be living. If the fetus is dead, craniotomy should be performed to reduce the damage to the pelvic floor; if in doubt, the forceps.

Technic.—We speak of "high," "low," and "medium" forceps, but there is no uniformity of teaching as to what these terms mean. It would be better to designate the operation by the name of the plane in which the biparietal diameter is found, for example, *outlet* (for low), *midplane* (for medium or mid), when the parietal bosses lie in the bispinous line, and *inlet* forceps (for the term high) when the head lies in the plane of the inlet, but has not yet completely engaged. To apply the forceps on the floating head is usually a lapsus artis.

Greater scientific accuracy may be obtained by using the plan shown on page 310. One will say, the forceps were applied to the head at 0 or at +1 or +2, as the case may be.

A few commonly used expressions require explanation. The "front" of the forceps is the side of the concavity, the side on which the lock opens, and to which the tips of the blades point. The tips are called the apex. The forceps may lie in the pelvis in any of its diameters. The forceps is said "to lie in this or that diameter" when a line drawn through the centers of the fenestra lies in the diameter specified. The front of the forceps, therefore, would look in the diameter at right angles to the one the forceps lies in. The best diameter for the forceps to take is the transverse, because then their pelvic curve corresponds to the mother's pelvic curve. The child's head is said "to lie in this or that diameter" of the pelvis when the sagittal suture lies in that diameter. When the head lies in the anteroposterior diameter and the forceps lies in the transverse, the head will be grasped in the most favorable manner, and the delivery of the child will be attended with the least difficulty (Fig. 853). When the head lies in an oblique diameter of the pelvis, the forceps should be applied in the opposite diameter, the front of the forceps pointing in the direction in which the point of direction lies (Fig. 854). Some operators still place the blades in the sides of the pelvis, that is, in the transverse diameter, letting them grasp the head whichever way they will. Most operators try to apply the blades to the sides of the head, the original method taught by the pioneers. This might be called the "ideal," or normal prehension. When the child's head lies with its long diameter transversely in the pelvis, the only way the forceps can get a good hold on it is when they lie in the anteroposterior diameter, but then one blade would rest on the promontory while the anterior one would cut into the bladder, the curves of the forceps and of pelvis antagonizing each other. I prefer to first bring the occiput to the front by combined manipulation and then apply the forceps. Rotation failing, a compromise must be made, and the blades are laid in one oblique of the pelvis, and grasp the child's head over one malar bone and the opposite

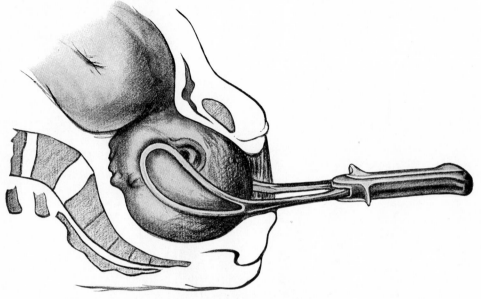

Fig. 853.—The Forceps Lying in Their Most Favorable Position (O. 0°). ("Ideal")
The head is on the perineum and rotation is complete.

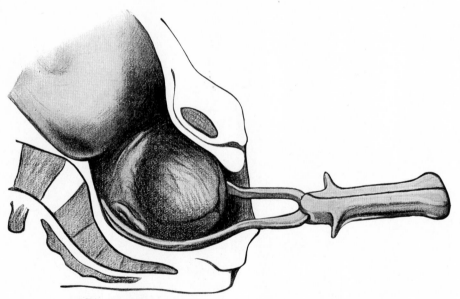

Fig. 854.—Forceps in O.D.A. (O.D. 45°). ("Ideal Prehension")
The forceps lie in the right oblique diameter of pelvis.

parietal (Fig. 856). This is better than to place the blades one over the face and the other over the occiput, the instrument lying in the transverse, as in Fig. 855. If the head is excessively flexed, this last is not so objectionable.

A rule of the forceps operation, to which there are no exceptions, is that the front of the forceps should point in the direction of the point of direction. If the occiput lies on the right side of the pelvis, the front of the forceps points to the right, and as the occiput rotates to the front, the front of the forceps looks more and more forward.

Of the two blades, the left is, with rare exceptions, passed first; it is grasped in the left hand and laid in the left side of the mother. The right blade is held by the right hand, and comes to lie in the right side of the pelvis.

Every forceps operation consists of four acts: Application of the blades; adaptation or locking; extraction of the head; removal of the instrument.

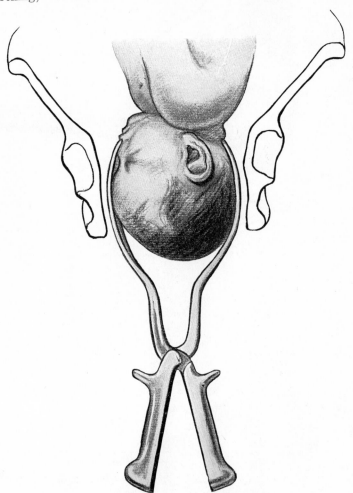

FIG. 855.—FORCEPS GRASPING HEAD IN AN UNFAVORABLE DIAMETER.
There is a strong tendency to slip. This application is to be avoided. Causes tentorium tears.

FIRST ACT.—*Application of Blades to Head.*—Having reassured himself that his diagnosis is correct by a careful bimanual examination after the patient is asleep and quiet, paying particular attention to the station of the fetal head, the accoucheur seats himself on a chair of convenient height and rehearses the intended operation in the air before the patient. Two fingers of the right hand are passed into the vulva, vagina, and, if the cervix can be reached, inside the cervix and within the membranes. Nothing may lie between the forceps and the head, and, to be certain of this, the fingers must feel the head all the way and be passed up as high as possible, guarding the tip of the forceps until it goes beyond reach. In higher forceps operations the half-hand should be inserted. Now the left blade of the forceps is taken in the left hand, poised vertically in the introitus vaginæ, being held like a pen (Fig. 857), and passed with the delicacy of a urethral sound. As the blade glides along the fingers in the vagina the tip is held closely to the head, so as to get under the cord or the membranes if they should fall in the way. The thumb of the right hand is used to guide and press the blade into place. As the fenestrum disappears inside the vulva, the time is come to sink the handle, and when the lock rests near the perineum, the first half of this act is completed. In most forceps operations the blades, if properly applied, will fall into the right position of their own weight. As the handle sinks down, the operating hand glides over the top and now grasps it like a scalpel (Fig. 858). It is not good to hold the forceps like a catlin, in the whole fist. Lubrication of the blade facilitates its passage.

The right blade is passed in like manner, the two fingers of the left hand being inserted and acting as guide and protectors of the maternal tissues. The lock being

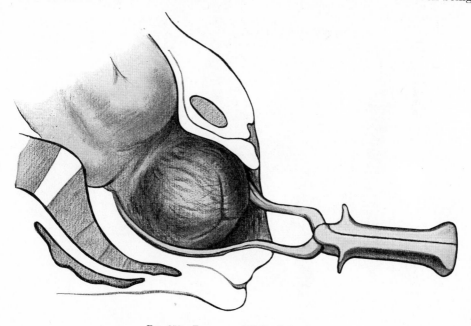

FIG. 856.—FORCEPS IN O.D.T. (O.D. 90°).
The head lies in the transverse, the forceps lies in the right oblique. The front of the forceps points to the right anterior.

on the top of the left blade, this one must be passed first, otherwise the handles would have to be recrossed outside the vulva, after the application, which would subject the maternal tissues and the child to injury by the tips of the instrument and allow the cord to fall into the grasp of the blades.

SECOND ACT.—*Adaptation or Locking; Grasping the Head.*—The technic of this movement will depend on the presentation and position of the head, since the blades must be applied so as to fit it in the best way.

In the usual operation of forceps the head is low down, and the small fontanel has rotated all the way or nearly all the way to the front, and the blades, after being inserted, fit naturally to the sides of the head. Often, however, they need a little adjusting before it is possible to fit the lock neatly. The simplest method to bring the blades into position is to press the handles gently downward on to the perineum. If this is not successful, they are depressed, and at the same time twisted lightly by means of the hooks on the handles, and if this does not do, a triplex motion is given the instrument. The handles are pressed downward, pushed upward into the pelvis, and twisted slightly, all in one movement, but *without the exhibition of much force*. If it does not succeed easily, the forceps must be removed and re-applied, because there is some obstacle to locking, which must be recognized and

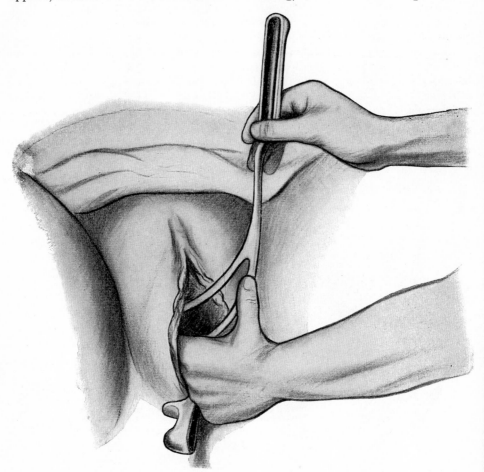

Fig. 857.—Grasping Blade Like a Pen, First Motion. Insertion of Second (Right) Blade.

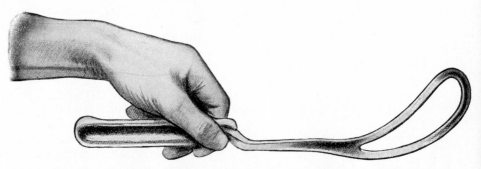

Fig. 858.—Grasping Forceps Blade Like a Scalpel. Second Motion of Insertion.

relieved. To force the locking is bad practice, and always results in fetal or maternal injury. Usually, the accoucheur will find he has made an error in diagnosis of position, or that the child has a hydrocephalus. As a rule the occiput, if not fully rotated already, turns forward while the forceps are being locked. Should this not occur, one must adjust the blades smoothly to the sides of the head by making one blade "wander" a little anteriorly, the other a little posteriorly (Fig. 867). The forceps will now lie as in Fig. 854 or Fig. 856.

After locking, the heart-tones should be auscultated. First listen and note their frequency and strength, then close the blades and listen again. If the tones at once become faint or slow, the cord is in the grasp of the forceps; if the slowing occurs only when the handles are kept tightly closed, it is due to cerebral compression. By pushing one or two fingers up along the back of the child's neck, behind the pubis, it is possible to feel the cord if it encircles the neck. Should there be a suspicion that the tip of the forceps squeezes the cord, the instrument must be removed and reapplied. If compression of the cord is unavoidable, the delivery must be quickly effected. An internal examination is also made, to find if the cord or cervix or an arm is caught in the grasp of the instrument.

THIRD ACT.—*Extraction.*—After locking the forceps one gentle pull is made on them to see if the blades lie properly and fit well, also to give the accoucheur an idea of the amount of resistance likely to be met. This is called the trial traction, and after it is done the heart-tones should again be listened to. Four points must be borne in mind with each traction: (1) Each traction is made with the uterine pains, and if these are absent, the pain is imitated, that is, the pull is gradual at first, slowly reaches an acme, is held for a moment, and then slowly relaxed; (2) as little power is exhibited as possible, regulating the amount by the advance of the head. With the elbows at the side and the arms flexed the strength of the biceps alone should suffice, and more than 60 pounds will almost never be required—usually much less. Time should be disregarded, but the fetal heart-tones carefully watched; (3) with the few exceptions soon to be considered the traction should be simple, not combined with pendulum, corkscrew, nor twisting motions; (4) the line of traction should correspond to the axis of the parturient canal (Fig. 876a).

After the trial traction the forceps are grasped, as shown in Fig. 859, the right hand on one shank with the index-finger in the crotch, the thumb underneath the handle. The left hand steadies the forceps, keeps the blades applied to the head, but does not make traction unless great force is necessary, in which event the fingers are applied to the hooks from above. One slow, even pull is made, at first in the horizontal plane or downward, or somewhat upward, depending on the station of the head and the curve of the parturient canal at that particular point. Carefully note the amount of progress of the head, and allow the head to recede very slowly; then listen to the heart-tones, loosening the forceps after each traction, but not separating the handles too far, because the cord might slip under the blades. After one or two full minutes by a clock placed directly in front of the operator, another traction is made—if necessary, a little stronger than the first. The descent and rotation of the head are determined by frequent examinations, the fingers searching for the location of the small fontanel. As the head bulges the perineum traction is more upward, and the usual precautions to save the pelvic floor are to be observed, such as slow delivery, bringing the head through with its most favorable diameters, and episiotomy. In my own practice I seldom deliver a primipara with forceps without first doing an episiotomy. This saves the child's head from prolonged compression, shortens the time of operation, forestalls fetal asphyxia, and prevents a ragged laceration, which is almost inevitable. After every traction listen to the fetal heart-tones. When the head is well engaged in the vulvar outlet, the forceps may, if preferred, be removed, and the delivery completed by pressure on the head from behind the anus—Ritgen's manœuvre. If the operator is right handed, he stands off at the left side of the patient, and if he uses his left hand, to her right (Fig. 860). He grasps the forceps at the lock with the right (or left) hand, with the little finger between the shanks, and gently, slowly, advancing line by line, he turns the head out, the handles of the forceps pointing toward the abdomen. At the same time the head is pulled up vertically somewhat, to keep the nucha applied snugly to the subpubic ligament. From fifteen to thirty minutes are required for an ordinary forceps delivery, most of which time is spent in bringing the head to the perineum. If the operator wishes to deliver without episiotomy and tries to "save the perineum," he must bring the head through the pelvic floor very slowly, taking as much time as a natural

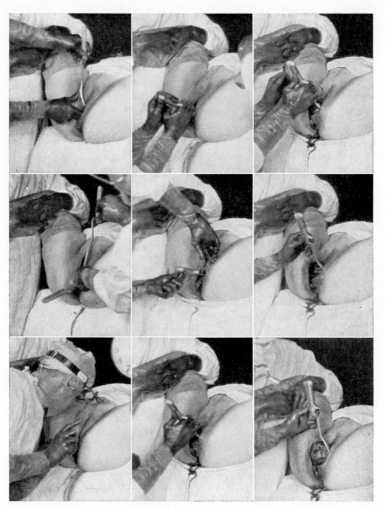

Fig. 859.—Strips from the Author's Motion Picture of the Forceps Operation.

delivery would take. My experience with this method was not encouraging, and Kerr found the same—the children got asphyxiated—and now I perform episiotomy (Fig. 876a).

FOURTH ACT.—*Removal.*—When the head is about ready to pass the vulvar ring I usually remove the forceps, as the slight lessening of the circumference ($\frac{1}{2}$ to $\frac{3}{4}$ cm.) may be just enough to save the sphincter from damage.

The action is the reverse of that of the application, taking care not to tear the scalp, the ear, or the soft parts of the mother. A few points in technic: Watch for feces issuing from the anus; wipe from above downward; do not let baby's chin glide over the perineal region; cleanse baby's mouth and throat before it makes the first gasp; have assistant "follow down" uterus as child escapes and apprise you at once if it balloons out or does not contract firmly; after head is born give 1 c.c. pituitary extract into deltoid, and after placenta is out, 1 c.c. aseptic ergot or gynergen into gluteus; while tying the cord, keep a watchful eye on the blood escaping from the vulva—save blood!; drench the externalia and introitus with

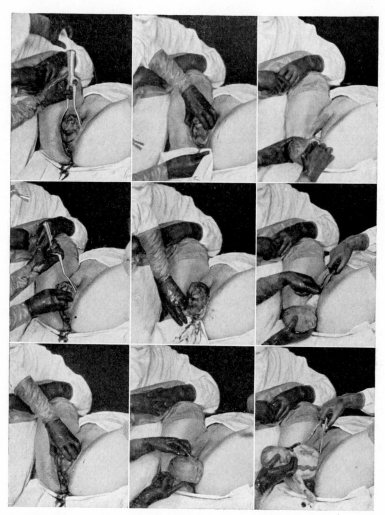

Fig. 860.—Note Light Traction without Compression, and Blades Removed to Save Perineum.

antiseptic solution, and resterilize gloves before entering parturient canal; always prepare to treat postpartum hemorrhage and asphyxia of the newborn.

Low or Outlet Forceps.—Here rotation is complete or nearly so, the head is most easily seized by the instrument, and the blades lie on the sides of the head, over the ear. Applying the blades to the sides of the pelvis allows them to grasp the head properly. This is the commonest forceps operation, also the least dangerous. The general description just given is all that need be said about it.

FORCEPS IN THE UNUSUAL MECHANISMS OF OCCIPITAL PRESENTATION

The occiput, when an indication arises for forceps, may be found at any point of the pelvic circle. We have just described the operation when anterior rotation has been completed or nearly so. This is the easiest of forceps deliveries—the hardest is that which finds the occiput in or near the hollow of the sacrum, occiput R. or L. 180° (Fig. 869, p. 1063, and Fig. 230, p. 213.) These are tersely called "occiput posteriors," and are the bane of the obstetrician. While they cause the majority of operative stillbirths, under proper management they can be successfully dealt with.

The small fontanel seldom lies directly in the median line, i. e., O. 180°, being usually to the right or left depending on the location of the back, i. e., the original position before labor began, nature thus giving the operator a useful hint. In the subsequent maneuvers he should follow the proper mechanism of labor, and not turn the head away from the direction the back must take.

Without question it is best for both patients if the child is delivered with the occiput anterior, i. e., after rotation has been effected—providing this can be done without the exhibition of too much force. Art and patience will triumph here when raw strength fails. Only rarely will it be necessary to pull the head out with the small fontanel over the perineum (Fig. 869), i. e., unrotated. Therefore, the accoucheur should learn the methods and acquire the skill wherewith to improve the position of the head before extracting it, and this is not difficult. Since the arrest of rotation of the occiput may occur in any sector of the pelvic circle, the operator, in order to bring the small fontanel to the front, under the pubis, may have to turn it from 1° to 180°. Naturally the more nature has accomplished, the less he will have to do, but the principles of the operation are the same at all points in which the occiput happens to be. First let us take the complete occipito-sacral, O. 180°, then O.D.P., O.D. 135°, then O.D.T., O.D. 90°, or "deep transverse arrest."

Forceps in Occipito Sacral Position and O.D.P., O.L.P.—The reader will find the details of the treatment of unrotated occiput positions on page 636, under the title "Persistent Occiput Posteriors." Nature usually does not fail to bring the occiput to the front—at least it usually is found well out of the hollow of the sacrum. If progress in labor ceases at this point three courses are open—correction and expectancy, podalic version, and forceps. To avoid repetition, the reader is referred to page 1009 for a discussion of the first two. Having failed with them our only alternative is forceps. Cesarean section for the single indication, occiput posterior, alone, is not permissible (Fig. 861).

Technic.—Four objects must be accomplished to complete the operation, flexion, synclitization, rotation, extraction. Disregard of the first two may render the others difficult or impossible. It is understood that the cervix is retracted and out of the way, the pelvic floor prepared by manual stretching and, later, episiotomy, and the uterus relaxed by an anesthetic. First a perfect diagnosis must be made. It would be fatal to try to turn the head in a direction opposite to that intended by nature. It will help a great deal if the diagnosis of position had been settled early in labor. In back-right positions the small fontanel must sweep around the right side of the pelvis, in back left, around the left. If, when coming to operate, the caput succedaneum is large, obliterating the usual landmarks, *locate the ear*—the tragus points to the face. Study the degree of synclitism and of the flexion of the head, and finally reassure yourself by bimanual examination that you have not made a mistake in judging the size of the pelvis and the baby's head, and the degree of engagement. Do not be ashamed to change your mind.

Now lubricate the vagina and the baby's head with liquid soap, raise the head up out of its embedment, i. e., mobilize it freely, flex it by pressing lightly on the forehead, and reduce asynclytism if necessary by pushing up one side of the head

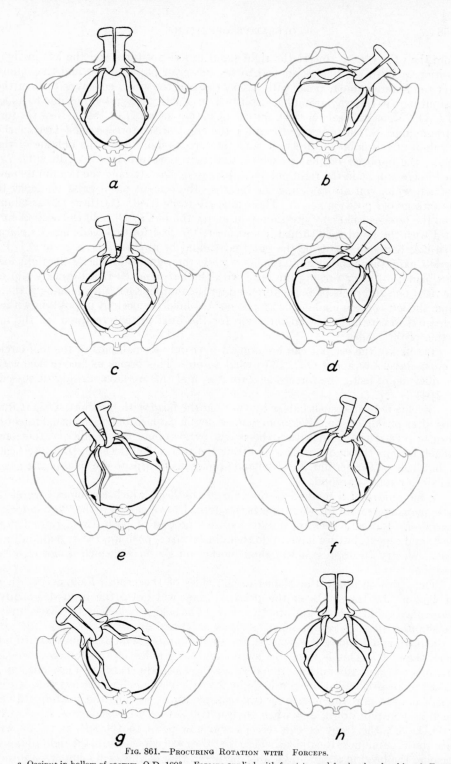

FIG. 861.—PROCURING ROTATION WITH FORCEPS.

a, Occiput in hollow of sacrum, O.D. 180°. Forceps applied with front toward forehead and pubis. *b*, Forceps are locked, pushed up in axis of pelvis and handles swept over an arc of 45°, in sectors of 5°, *not all at once;* now O.D. 135°. *c*, Holding what was gained, the forceps are readjusted, in the transverse; head grasped obliquely; repeat key in lock manœuver; push up, sweep handles through an arc of 45°, in sectors of 5° each, bringing occiput to position *d*, *i. e.*, O.D. 90°. *e*, Preventing the head from twisting back, with the fingers, the forceps are made to "wander" into the left oblique, front to the occiput. Repeat, push up, sweep handles through arc of 45°, in sectors of 5°, *i. e.*, coax the occiput around to *f*, taking time and avoiding brusque motions. Now O.D. 45°. At the beginning of this stage an expert operator may apply the forceps in the anteroposterior diameter of the pelvis, in the ideal prehension and proceed as usual (Fig. 865). *g*, Holding the head as O.D. 45°, with a vulsella, if it persists in rotating back, the forceps are reapplied, at last in the normal or ideal prehension and the rest of the rotation is accomplished by the push up, twist, and pull method, remembering that extreme gentleness will accomplish more with less damage than force. NON VI, SED ARTE; not with force but with skill.

more than the other. Insert the right hand in left positions and the left in right positions. With the fingers applied to the posterior parietal boss and the thumb over the anterior malar bone, with a slow twist of the wrist, endeavor to turn the occiput part of the way around as described on p. 991. It is often possible to make an O.D. 75°, or at least an O.D. 90° (O.D.T.) out of an O.D. 180°. Now the forceps are applied, remembering the rules, the front of the forceps must face in the direction of the point of direction, and the forceps must lie in the oblique of the pelvis, the opposite of that in which the sagittal suture lies, i. e., in O.D. 75° the forceps will lie in the right oblique. It may be hard to hold the head in its new position while you are applying the forceps—the occiput has a great tendency to slip into its old position again. These aids are to be tried: (1) Have the assistant keep the forehead back by pressing on it above the pubis; (2) hold the occiput forward with the hand that turned it and insert the first forceps blade into its place, even if it happens not to be the one that should be applied first, e. g., in O.D.P., the left hand turns the head and holds it while the right hand inserts the right forceps blade; (3) after turning the head with the left hand (O.D.P.) quickly slip in the right one and press back the forehead on the mother's left side, holding it there while the left forceps blade is being put on; (4) hold the occiput in position with a vulsellum forceps attached to the scalp for the brief instant required for the insertion of the blades.

Let us say the occiput can be brought over only a small part of the half-circle it must travel—to about O.D. 135—what to do? This brings us face to face with the question of using the forceps as a rotator, and this we have already discussed, (p. 1044).

Smellie delivered such babies by twisting the head with his short straight forceps after pushing it up. Scanzoni made a double application of the usual forceps, Tarnier turned the head within the pelvis by sweeping the handles of the long French forceps through a wide arc outside the pelvis, Bill does not push the head up but does as Tarnier did, and Kielland applies his forceps to the sides of the head and simply rolls it around.

I have devised a method of rotation of the head which combines several of these maneuvers, and for want of a better term I have named it the "key in lock" operation. It really tries to imitate nature's process of push, twist, retract, untwist, and repeat, but we have to do them in reverse—push up, twist, pull, and repeat. We try to impress a wriggling motion on the head, which is not easy to describe.

One tries to apply the blades to the sides of the head. Failing this, they are laid in the transverse of the pelvis. They will grasp the head diagonally, in an unfavorable manner, and are, therefore, to be held very delicately. Now, under the slightest possible compression, the head is pushed up about 2 c.m. in the axis of the birth canal and gently twisted, the small fontanel being brought forward not more than 5°. This is done by sweeping the handles of the forceps through an arc of about 10° outside the pelvis á la methode Tarnier, Figs. 862, 863. Then the head is pulled down a little in the axis of the pelvis, *but less than it was pushed up*. Repeat this maneuver two or three times, pushing the head up only as much as you pull down, and when the sagittal suture is transverse, i. e., O.D.T. or O.D. 90°, the front of the forceps will now point to the left, and they will lie in the left oblique. Readjust them so that they will come to lie in the right oblique, grasping the head in a more favorable diameter, that is, the ideal manner. Indeed, sometimes the head slips around the rest of the way itself within the blades. By pushing up a little, twisting a little, and levering a very little (to overcome asynclitism), imparting a wriggling motion to the head not unlike fitting a key to a stubborn lock, one can usually coax the occiput to the front, whereupon the rest of the operation—the extraction, is completed without trouble. One should not

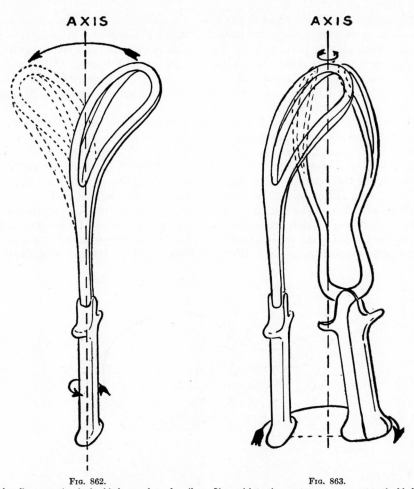

FIG. 862.

If handles are twisted, the blades tend to describe an arc in the pelvis, tearing the vagina from its attachments.

FIG. 863.

If we wish to give a rotatory movement to the blades, the handles should be made to describe an arc.

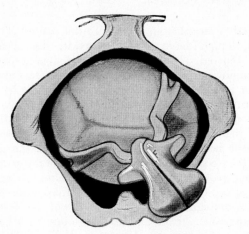

FIG. 864.—DIAGRAM OF FORCEPS IN O.D.T. (O.D. 90°). USUAL APPLICATION.
F indicates front of forceps.

hurry nor do too much turning at once, not more than 5°; it is like taking mincing steps. Readjust the forceps pari passu as the rotation is effected.

The prehension of the head at the beginning of this operation need not always be made as described. Variants must be recognized, but the principle does not change. Sometimes it is possible to lay the blades to the head anteroposteriorly in the pelvis with their front directed toward the small fontanel. Again one may apply the forceps with the front toward the forehead (like Scanzoni), and when the occiput is brought into the anterior quadrant of the pelvis, remove them and re-apply as for an anterior position.

In rare cases it is impossible to turn the occiput to the front either by manual effort, or the forceps, or by a combination of the hands with the forceps. To force the issue would entail great damage to the mother and probably kill the baby, therefore we must observe and discover the mechanism intended by nature and then aid it. If the occipito-sacral mechanism is inevitable it is best to deliver the head in extreme flexion as will be learned if you refer to page 632.

The application of the blades is made as usual, but the front of the forceps looks toward the forehead, which, from now on, becomes the point of direction (Fig. 869). Locking the blades is the same as usual, but after they are locked the handles are raised a little toward the pubis—this to increase flexion. Traction is made on the

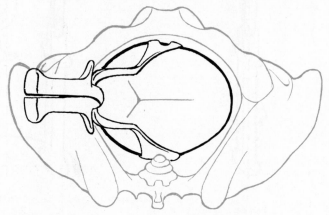

FIG. 865.—FORCEPS IN O.D.T.; O.D. 90°.

Application by expert in anteroposterior diameter of pelvis. Ideal prehension but danger to soft parts because pelvic curve of forceps does not correspond to pelvic axis.

parietal bosses, a little upward from the horizontal plane. This increases flexion, and it has happened, though I have never observed it, that, even as late as this, anterior rotation has occurred. The occiput is first delivered over the perineum, the forehead resting behind the pubis; then the brow and face come from under the pubis. Much power is often necessary, and it is advisable to perform episiotomy in primiparæ, as a rule, and almost always in multiparæ, to avoid extensive lacerations of the pelvic floor and sphincter. If conditions are favorable one might deflex the head and deliver as a face presentation. These cases are claimed by the Kielland forceps enthusiasts. Some accoucheurs prefer the axis-traction forceps since the mobility they confer on the head allows the latter to adapt itself somewhat to the parturient passage, but for the man who knows the mechanism of labor and is willing to be guided by the action of the natural powers they are unnecessary, and in the hands of a man ignorant of the principles of the science of obstetrics the instrument is too dangerous. (See page 1073, "Failure with Forceps.")

Forceps in Deep Transverse Arrest.—O.D.T., O.D. 90°, and O.L.T., O.L. 90°. In some cases where a delay in labor has been manifest for some time, an examination reveals the head well down in the pelvis, the sagittal suture in the transverse diameter, the small fontanel to one side, generally the right, the large fontanel to the other side, and both on the same level. This condition is called "deep transverse arrest"—sometimes "impaction," the head being wedged in between the ischial tuberosities. (See Deflexion Attitudes, p. 637). Lack of flexion and weak pains are usually causative, but often we find persistent asynclitism as well. The principles of treatment are similar to those of occiput posteriors in general, we must favor flexion, complete the rotation and extract. Manual correction having failed the forceps must be relied upon.

It is obvious that, in transverse arrest, if the forceps were applied to the sides of the head, the blades would have to lie in the conjugate diameter of the pelvis,

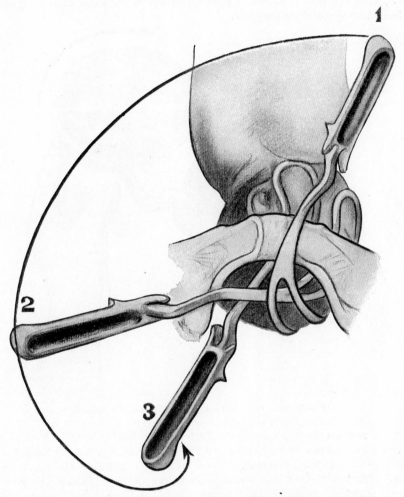

FIG. 866.—ROTATING LEFT BLADE AROUND HEAD IN O.D.T. (O.D. 90°). "WANDERING."

which is mechanically a bad principle, the pelvic curve of the forceps being then directly opposed to the curve of the pelvis, and there being danger of injury to the bladder by the anterior blade. If the instrument were laid transversely, it would seize the head over the face and occiput (Fig. 855), injuring the eyes, deflexing the head, and inviting a tendency to slipping. When, therefore, the operator cannot rotate the occiput to the front manually, he will have to grasp the head obliquely (Fig. 864), one blade lying on the parietal bone, the other on the malar. The forceps then will lie in an oblique diameter of the pelvis. In O.D. Transverse, the forceps will lie in the right oblique, in O.L. Transverse, in the left.

Technic for O.D. 90°.—Since the front of the forceps must point in the direction of the point of direction, in this case the occiput, the blades must be brought to lie in the right oblique diameter of the pelvis, one anteriorly behind the iliopubic tubercle, lying over the anterior malar bone, the other posteriorly, opposite the right sacro-iliac joint, lying on the posterior parietal bone. The left blade, therefore, has to be guided around the side of the pelvis over the child's face, to come into position (Figs. 866 and 867), while the right blade does not have to "wander" at all, but may be laid directly opposite the sacro-iliac joint. While the blade is being pushed in by the outside hand, the fingers inside pull it around the pelvis. Locking is not easy in these cases, but is done as before described, and the operator, knowing that the head is grasped in one of its long diameters, will not bring the handles too close together.

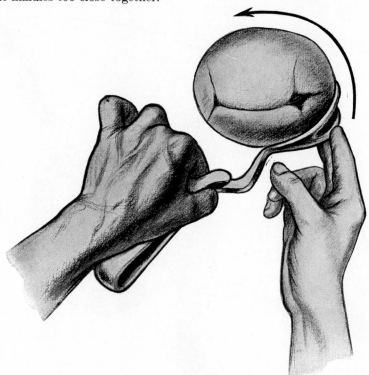

Fig. 867.—Showing How to Turn Forceps Blade. "Wandering."

A good way for the accoucheur to assure himself that the child's head does not suffer injurious pressure is for him to put the index-finger of his left hand between the handles while making traction. The details of the rotation and extraction are identical with those given for occipito-sacral position—in fact delivery in deep transverse is the latter half of this maneuver, and the "key in lock" method is very successful. A clever operator might lay the forceps blades in the anteroposterior diameter of the pelvis, i. e., on the sides of the head, obtaining at once the normal or ideal grasp (Fig. 866), and thus when the small fontanel has been brought to 0° he will have the forceps in position for extraction without adjustments.

Many authors recommend the turbinal movement for deep transverse arrest, i. e., the downward pull is accompanied by a slight and gentle rotation, the two motions being absolutely synchronous, thus effecting spiral progress of the head, rotating 5° and advancing 5 mm. with each traction (Fig. 868). There is danger in this method—danger of abrupting the vagina and bladder from their attachments, and for this reason, the new method is preferred, and the turbinal operation reserved for the exceptional case.

After rotation is complete the forceps may be removed and the birth left to nature—*i. e.*, if the heart-tones are good. This may be desirable in primiparæ with contracted outlet or large babies. In a few hours the pains will have molded the head so as to permit spontaneous delivery after episiotomy or a very easy low forceps operation. The benefits may outweigh the manifest objections to such a two-stage procedure.

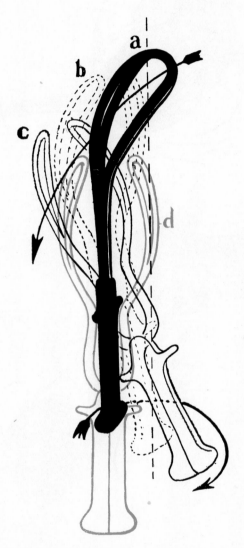

FIG. 868.—TURBINAL MOTION OF THE FORCEPS.
This is as applied to a head in O.L.T. (O.L. 90°).

Scanzoni-Fritsch Operation.—This is a method of turning the head by means of the forceps. It is entirely dispensable, and, in my opinion, is fraught with too great dangers to the maternal soft parts, and with too much risk of Erb's paralysis to be practised by any but experts. The forceps are applied with the front looking toward the forehead. By rotating the instrument the forehead is brought to the rear, which, of course, inverts the forceps. They are removed and reapplied, with the front toward the occiput, which has come to the pubis, and the operation is completed as usual after rotation has occurred. We have better means for correcting occiput posterior positions.

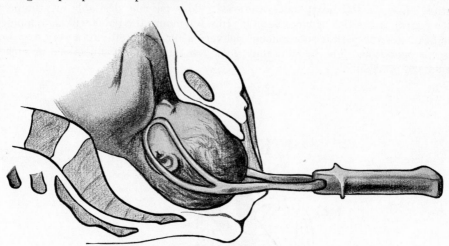

FIG. 869.—FORCEPS IN OCCIPUT POSTERIOR POSITION ON PELVIC FLOOR (O.D. 180°).

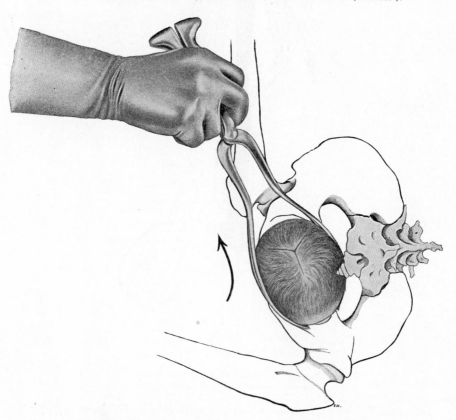

FIG. 869a.—DELIVERY OF THE HEAD OVER THE UPPER RAMUS PUBIS.
This method is used in cases of anchylosis of one hip and rarely when rotation is impossible.

Forceps in Face Presentations.—*Per se* face presentation is no indication for forceps, but labor is often delayed and help often required with all the deflexion attitudes. In face presentation, to the conditions demanded for forceps in general one new one must be added—the chin may not be behind the transverse diameter of the pelvis—that is, anterior rotation of the chin, at least to the transverse diameter, must have occurred.

Application of the blades after the chin has rotated is very easy, although care is required not to injure the baby's eyes. Adaptation or locking is different. Instead of depressing the handles, it is best to raise them well. This sinks the blades toward the hollow of the sacrum, and thus they obtain a firmer hold over the parietal bosses. If the blades are placed and locked in the usual manner, they will slip off the narrow brow and face—they are, therefore, locked with the handles raised, and the latter are lowered, which manœuver increases extension (Fig. 870). Traction is first downward, to increase deflexion, then in the horizontal plane, until the chin is well out from under the pubis, then upward, but not so acutely as with the occiput, because the delicate larynx is between the spine of the child and the bone. Episiotomy is the rule in primiparæ.

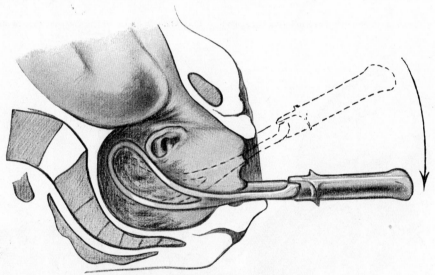

Fig. 870.—Forceps in Face Presentation.
Dotted line shows forceps as first applied. Traction is applied after handles are lowered.

Forceps in Arrested Rotation of the Chin.—To deliver with forceps when the chin is directed toward the hollow of the sacrum is possible only when the child is small, and then only at the expense of extensive lacerations. To try to rotate the chin anteriorly by means of forceps from a posterior quadrant of the pelvis is equivalent to a craniotomy, and much more damaging to the mother's tissues. It is, however, possible safely to deliver a face presentation arrested in rotation after the chin has reached or passed the transverse diameter, but the operation is very delicate, very difficult, usually causes deep tears, and often costs the child's life. The reason for the last is obvious. One blade compresses the neck and always injures the structures exposed by the extreme extension of the cervical spine. The forceps lies in an oblique, the front pointing in the direction of the point of direction. In M.D.T. the forceps lie in the right, in M.L.T. in the left, oblique. Extraction must be most carefully done, loosening the forceps frequently and readapting them at the earliest possible moment to the sides of the head. Rotation is effected by giving the forceps a slight turbinal movement, but much may also be accomplished by manipulation with the fingers aided by the hand outside.

Forceps in Brow Presentation.—What was said under Face Presentation applies here. The brow, instead of the chin, must come to the pubis and appear in the

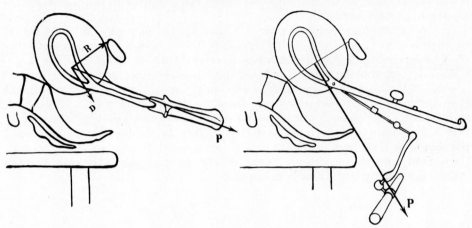

FIG. 871.—DIAGRAM SHOWING TRACTION WITH USUAL FORCEPS.

FIG. 872.—DIAGRAM OF ACTION OF AXIS-TRACTION FORCEPS.

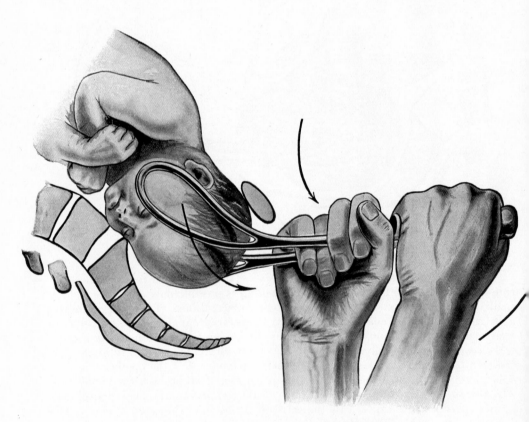

FIG. 873.—PAJOT'S (OSIANDER'S) MANEUVER WITH FORCEPS.
By this method axis-traction is obtained. First practised by Saxtorph in 1772.

vulva, the face resting behind the symphysis until the occiput can be brought over the perineum, after which the face comes down from behind the pubis. Episiotomy is the rule in primiparæ and in multiparæ, too, if the child is large.

Inlet Forceps Operations—"High Forceps."—In most of the cases of forceps just described the head occupies the excavation of the pelvis, and we might speak of "midplane forceps," as was already mentioned. The term "high forceps" is

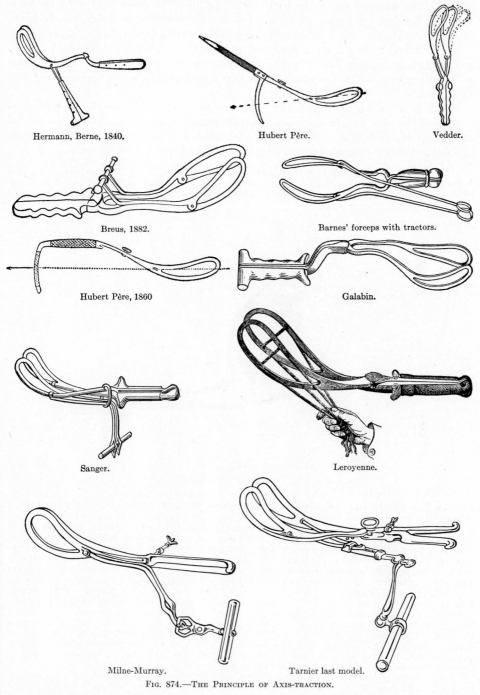

Hermann, Berne, 1840.

Hubert Père.

Vedder.

Breus, 1882.

Barnes' forceps with tractors.

Hubert Père, 1860

Galabin.

Sanger.

Leroyenne.

Milne-Murray.

Tarnier last model.

FIG. 874.—THE PRINCIPLE OF AXIS-TRACTION.

best limited to those cases where the biparietal diameter is in the region of the superior strait, but has not yet passed lower, or has not even as yet entered the inlet, but is arrested just above it. Some operators permit the use of forceps on the "floating head." Version is preferable. In some cases the head is so well fixed that it may be impossible to move it away to do version, and yet it is not quite engaged so as to fulfil the condition for forceps. Under these circumstances the forceps is an instrument of trial, or, as Carl Braun said, "an instrument of diagnosis." We want to see if the head will come into the pelvis. If, after suitable trial, the head will not come in, we must do a craniotomy, even if the child be alive, or, if both patients are in prime condition, pelviotomy or section. (See p. 1001.)

For deliveries begun when the head is above the level of the spines of the ischia many authors recommend a special instrument—the axis-traction forceps—that is, an instrument which will enable us to apply force to the head parallel to the axis of the pelvis.

The head, when high up, has a curve to traverse. Owing to the forward projection of the sacrum and perineum, traction cannot easily be applied in the axis of the inlet. If applied in any other line, the problem is like trying to pull an object around a corner—both the corner and the object suffer.

Figure 871 shows the effect of the ordinary forceps when applied on the high head; if traction is made in the usual way, a large part, estimated by Tarnier as almost half, of the force will be exerted against the symphysis. The older obstetricians appreciated the fact that the head would

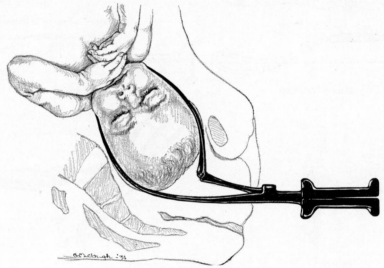

FIG. 875.—BARTON'S FORCEPS.

thus impinge on the anterior pelvis wall, and Levret (1750) recommended that tapes be put through the fenestra of the forceps, and, while pulling in the usual manner, also to pull downward on the tapes, thus making the head follow the curve of the parturient canal. Saxtorph (1772) advised to pull downward toward the floor with one hand over the lock, while the other pulled the forceps straight out—a maneuver which is generally known as Pajot's (Fig. 873). In 1840 Hermann, of Berne, instead of the tapes, attached a straight hook to the blade near the head, and the Huberts, in 1860, bent the handles down so that when traction was made on the lowest parts the force was transmitted through the bent lever to the head in the axis of the inlet. Finally, in 1877, Tarnier invented a forceps which he believed possessed these advantages—(1) It allowed traction to be made in the axis of the inlet; (2) while the head was fixed in the forceps proper the traction apparatus was so jointed that the head was given free mobility and could follow the impulses of the mechanism of labor; (3) the handles of the forceps could be used as indicators of the lines the head was following. Tarnier constructed over 100 models before he considered the instrument perfect (Fig. 876). Simpson, Murray, Lusk, Breus, Felsenreich, and many others sought to improve on Tarnier's instrument, but of all axis-traction instruments, in my opinion, those of Tarnier and Simpson are the best.

Axis-traction forceps are not universally recommended by obstetric authorities. In England Kerr, Milne-Murray, Eden, and others recommend them; in Germany opinion is nearly evenly divided, the balance being slightly in their favor; in France Pajot, Depaul, and others opposed Tarnier, but the large majority was with him; in America nearly all writers are in favor of them. Vienna is lukewarm, and Bossi, in Genoa, says they are entirely dispensable. For my part I cannot share the enthusiasm of Williams, Kerr, Murray, and others. By means of Pajot's maneuver I can give the head a direction which a knowledge of the mechanism of labor will indicate; by careful observance of the tendencies of movement which the forces of nature give the head I can determine in which way to apply traction, and I can aid one or the other, as required. With the axis-traction device there are so many joints between the operating hand and the head that it is impossible to impress on the latter any specific motion. All the knowledge one has accumulated regarding normal and abnormal labor mechanisms goes for naught, and all one can do is to pull blindly on the cross-bar. In this respect the axis-traction forceps are not artistic. In actual practice, where I have applied both instruments on the same case, I have been better satisfied with the simple Simpson forceps and seldom use any other. Deep injuries to the maternal tissues are just as frequent with the new forceps, a fact which W. A. Freund proved. The Tarnier instrument has a murderous cephalic curve, cognizance of which should be taken when screwing together the handles, otherwise a large number of dead and injured children will be the result. In all axis-traction instruments there is the possibility of the curved arms or the joints bending or breaking under the powerful force applied, having witnessed three such accidents myself.

Indications for High Forceps.—These are the same as usual—danger to the mother or child, but in this case, occurring at a time when the head has not yet passed through the inlet. Let it be well emphasized that the indication for forceps here must be unusually strict.

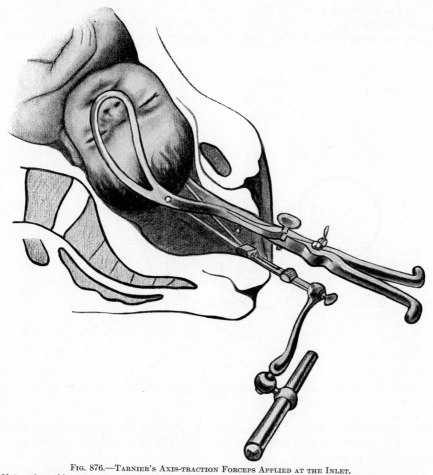

FIG. 876.—TARNIER'S AXIS-TRACTION FORCEPS APPLIED AT THE INLET.
Note unfavorable prehension. Fortunately, the head is often more flexed, and there is some slight anterior rotation, wherefore the blade does not injure the face as much as would occur in the case illustrated. Traction should be made, according to Tarnier, in the direction indicated by the handles, the traction rods lying 1 cm. away from the shanks.

Conditions.—These also are as usual, and to be strictly insisted on. Engagement of the head must be so nearly accomplished that the accoucheur feels certain that a little pull from below will help the head into the pelvis, which means that molding of the head be well advanced. The alternatives, if he fails, are craniotomy, pelviotomy, laparotrachelotomy, Porro. The pelvis may not be too contracted—not less than $8\frac{1}{2}$ cm. in flat, and 9 cm. in the justo-minor types. Dilatation of the cervix and retraction of the pelvic organs above the inlet must be positively complete.

The high forceps operation has always been and still is a controversial subject. Aside from the question of the propriety of the use of the forceps at all upon the high head, and of the employment of axis-traction, the difference of opinion has been upon the prehension of the head. Smellie, Baudelocque, Burns, Dewees, Farabeuf, *et al* grasp the head in its biparietal diameter, the blades lying in the anteroposterior diameter of the pelvis, the front of the forceps pointing to the occiput. Massini reverses the forceps, the front pointing to the face. Kielland claims his straight forceps is especially fitted for anteroposterior application. (Fig. 877.)

Most accoucheurs, however, place the blades in the sides of the pelvis and let them seize the head in any way they will. Thus, since the head usually enters the pelvis in the transverse, they will lie over the occiput and forehead—or, if the head is deflexed, over the face, as shown in Fig. 876. Frequently the head is slightly oblique, in which case the forceps grasp it in a more favorable manner. Indeed, an attempt should be made, even when the head is high, to follow the

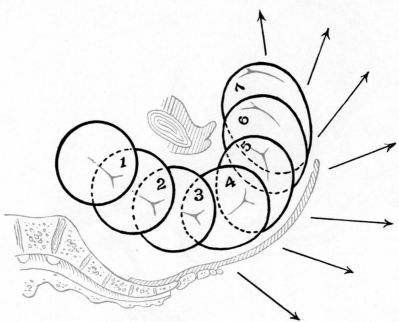

Fig. 876a.—Diagram to show descent, flexion, and rotation of head and direction for forceps traction at different stations.

general rules of forceps application, either by turning the occiput into a good position by combined manipulation, or by adjusting the blades to the sides of the head as far as possible.

In all events the first grasp of the forceps is continued only until the head is engaged in the pelvis. Then the operation follows nature's mechanisms.

In applying the blades the half or even the whole hand should be inserted as a guide, as the operation is much more complicated than usual. Locking the instrument is also attended with more difficulty. To prevent serious injury to the head the handles may not be tightly screwed nor forced together. Adaptation of the blades may be helped by the hand outside, since one can see and feel the tip of the instrument through the lower abdomen.

It is wise to approach a high forceps operation without preconceived inten-

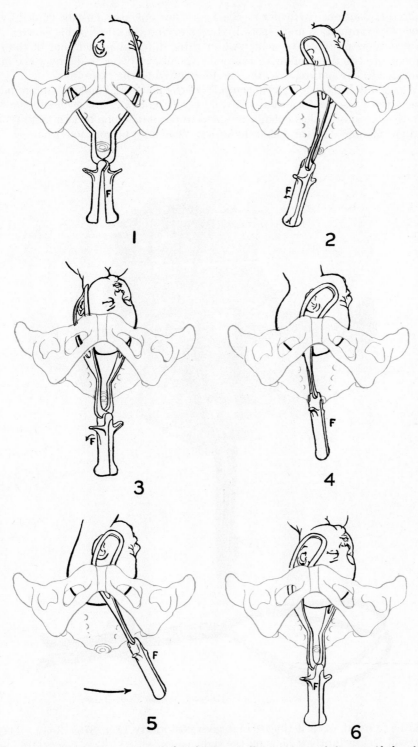

Fig. 876b.—1, Forceps in transverse, bad prehension. 2, Forceps in sagittal diameter, ideal prehension. 3, Occiput shows tendency to turn posteriorly; not to be antagonized. 4, Massini's manœuver, first step. 5, Ditto, flexion of head. 6, Ditto, posterior rotation before engagement.

tions to carry out one particular mechanism. The operator must be guided by the findings on examination and especially by observing the effect of his efforts. It is allowable, indeed proper, to make two or three different prehensions of the head and moderate tractions following each one, the object being to discover the mechanism intended by nature, *i. e.*, the one best suited to the case.

We usually lay the forceps in the sides of the pelvis and make an unprejudiced traction using the Saxtorph-Pajot manœuver (Fig. 873). Occasionally the head enters the pelvis or makes enough progress to encourage one or two more pulls in the same manner. If the head shows any tendency of rotation whatever, this

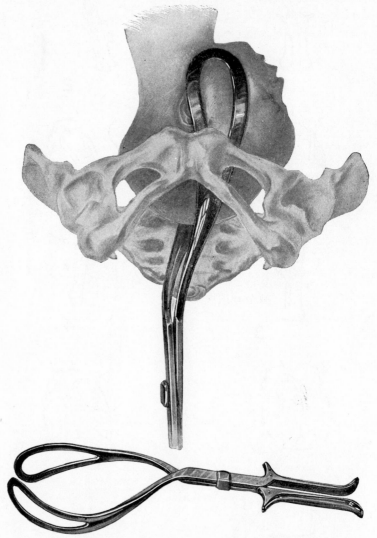

Fig. 877.—Kielland's Forceps. Applied at the Inlet.

should be favored, even if the occiput goes posteriorly (Fig. 876b, 2–3). The operator will feel instantly if he is on the right track.

If not, a second application of the forceps should be made, grasping the head anteroposteriorly, front of forceps pointing to the occiput (Fig. 876b, 2). In a flat pelvis the head is to be brought through the inlet with the sagittal suture in its transverse diameter. In a normal pelvis one may try to bring it down in one of the obliques, following nature's guidance as to whether the occiput is to go anteriorly or posteriorly, and it is necessary to take into account the degree of flexion and asynclitism and act accordingly. One tries to impart first one, then the other movement, following that which seems more favorable. The manœuver might be likened to one's trying to pull his clenched first through a knot-hole in a board.

Massini reverses the blades of the forceps, directing their front to the face, flexes the head by sweeping the handles to the corresponding side, mobilizes the head a little, rotates it so as to bring the occiput posteriorly into a diagonal of the inlet and then draws it down into the pelvis (Fig. 876b, 4, 5, 6).

In extracting, it is to be remembered that the high forceps is an operation of trial—of diagnosis. If six, or at most eight, powerful, well-directed tractions make no impression—do not bring the head lower—the instrument must be removed. Two or three of the tractions should be made with the patient in the Walcher position. Craniotomy now must be done, or if the mother and babe are in prime condition and the environment is favorable, hebosteotomy or low, cervical cesarean section. If the head does move a little with each traction, the operation should be gently completed, taking plenty of time. After the head has entered the pelvis it may rotate within the forceps, which should be opened to permit this, or it may be turned by combined manipulation, the case now being simply one of arrest at the midplane. Now remove the axis-traction apparatus and deliver as in ordinary forceps, or it may be best to leave the delivery to nature, or to follow a subsequent indication.

The Kielland Forceps.—In 1915 Chr. Kielland, of Christiana, Norway, introduced a new forceps to the profession. It bears slight resemblances to several ancient models, and its principles are not new. Kielland asserts that by discarding the pelvic curve of the forceps one can apply the instrument in the sagittal diameter of the pelvis, thus adapting the blades to the sides of the head when it lies with its long diameter in the transverse of the pelvis. He also uses his forceps as a simple rotator after the head is engaged in the excavation, claiming to master both high transverse arrest and occiput posteriors with ease and safety. For mentoposterior positions and brow presentations the forceps are said to be particularly successful. Several cherished practices are unseated by Kielland—the high application of the forceps always in the transverse diameter of the pelvis; the ban on the use of the forceps as a rotator; the method of application of the blades (Kielland puts the anterior blade in place upside down and then twists it into position).

Lack of space forbids a fuller consideration of the new forceps. I have used it sufficiently often to believe that it should have a place in the specialist's armamentarium, but I cannot join the chorus of German laudators. It is the man behind the forceps more than the instrument itself that accomplishes the results. In low operations the Simpson forceps cannot be superseded; in deep transverse arrest and engaged occiput posteriors almost always sufficient anterior rotation can be effected manually without the necessity of using the forceps as a rotator; in high arrest, version is usually the operation of choice if cesarean section is not selected—otherwise one makes a trial with the forceps. Here the Kielland instrument should score its greatest success, but in my hands the long Simpson forceps has been equally as efficient. In unfavorable face and brow presentations conversion and podalic version are preferable to any forceps operation. Complete Literature, Greenhill.

Failure of the Forceps.—The instrument has been applied and several tractions made, but the head does not advance. What to do? In the olden time another pattern of forceps would be sent for, and another doctor would try to deliver with them. Cases are on record where five or six such trials were made, and with awful results. Fortunately this day is past.

When unexpected difficulty appears, the forceps are to be removed and the cause of the failure investigated. Errors in position (an unrecognized occiput posterior), insufficient preparation of the soft parts, and a greater disproportion between the head and the pelvis than was expected, will be found the usual causes of the unsuccess. To mention the last first; if the pelvis is found too small or the head too large, two operations demand consideration, laparotrachelotomy and pubiotomy. If the baby has not suffered from overzealous attempts at delivery, and if the chances of infection are slight, one of them may be performed, otherwise, embryotomy is the horrible alternative. Unprepared soft parts occasionally defeat a forceps operation, and if their resistance is overcome by force, frightful lacerations are the result and the baby is usually lost too. Therefore, the operation had better be suspended and a large colpeurynter inserted into the constricting zone. Unrecognized abnormal position of the head is the most frequent cause of failure with the forceps. When this is corrected the delivery is usually surprisingly easy.

Curiously, and in contravention to all classic obstetric rules of conduct in such cases, one may sometimes perform podalic version and extraction, even after the head is engaged, and after attempts with the forceps have failed. Version and forceps are not complementary operations; rather, where version is indicated, the forceps are contraindicated (see the conditions for these two operations on pages 1015 and 1048). Yet occasionally a case will occur where the circumstances detailed above exist, or a mistake in judgment has been made, or the cord prolapses, and one may depart from accepted dogma and secure a happy result by an unorthodox procedure.

Prognosis of the Forceps Operation.—For the mother the dangers are injury, hemorrhage, and infection. Some tearing of the pelvic organs is inevitable, and the number and severity increase the higher up the forceps operation is done. High forceps show the most and the worst injuries, which may be atrocious if the condition relating to the dilatation had not been fulfilled. If rotary motions with the forceps are made, the vagina may be twisted from its connective-tissue attachments, or the cervix may be caught in the grasp of the forceps and be bruised or torn off bodily; or the operator, thinking the blade is inside the cervix, may use force, and as the tip of the instrument is in the fornix, he may punch through this up, under, or through the peritoneum.

The vagina itself may be torn or cut by the blades of the forceps and the vulva also, especially when the blades are bent upward in the delivery of the head. The edges may cut the crura of the clitoris and cause severe hemorrhage, or pressure necrosis which may go to the bone. In severe forceps operations the symphysis pubis has been ruptured, also the sacro-iliac articulations, and the woman will have a pain in the lower spine and back, with more or less invalidism all the rest of her life. Injury to the sacro-iliac joints is a frequently overlooked cause of backache, leukorrhea, and many gynecologic conditions. The bladder may be torn into, or may be pulled off its pelvic attachments and be permanently prolapsed. Scars in the vaginal wall may distort the bladder sphincter, causing incontinence and cystitis. Injury to the levator ani and pelvic floor is a constant sequel to forceps delivery. At autopsy one is astonished at the extent and number of the tears and bruises. Postpartum hemorrhage results from the tears and from atonia uteri. Infection is common from lapses of asepsis and from the ease with which contused wounds are successfully attacked by the bacteria.

Most dangerous to both mother and child is the slipping of the forceps. This happens in two ways, according to Mme. La Chapelle: in the vertical sense, that is, the forceps slide off in the direction of the line of traction; and in the horizontal sense, that is, the forceps slip off in a line perpendicular to the line of traction, *the patient being imagined erect* (Figs. 878 and 879). I believe the terms "axial" and "exaxial" slipping would more clearly express the conditions.

The causes of slipping of the forceps are: Grasping the head too low, the forceps not being inserted high enough, under a mistaken idea of the degree of engagement; the blades feather too much—a poor instrument; the head may be too small or too large—hydrocephalus; the head is not grasped right; the handles are bent up too soon as the head nears the outlet.

The sensation of slipping of the forceps is unmistakable. The handles tend to separate, and if the direction is to the front or back of the pelvis, the blades seem to jump off the head with a snapping noise, and they are usually disarticulated. If the forceps slip off in the line of traction, *i. e.*, axially, one can feel the instrument advance while the head seems not to follow. Slipping of the forceps is commonest at the inlet, because here the walls of the pelvis do not hold the blades to the sides of the head. It is highly essential to discover the tendency to slip early, because the lacerations caused by it are frightful. Removal of the blades and reapplication are the treatment. If the head is small, a small forceps must be secured. If there is a hydrocephalus, puncture is required.

Dangers to the Child.—(1) Compression of the brain, slowing of the heart, asphyxia. (2) Fracture of the skull, with or without subdural hemorrhage. (3) Hemorrhage from rupture of the sinuses at the base or from rupture of the tentorium cerebelli. (4) Concussion of the brain. (5) Crushing of the orbital plates, with retrobulbar hematoma and injury to nerves and muscles, causing squint, ptosis, etc. (6) Injury to the eyes, traumatic cataract, abruption of the choroid, corneal opacity, retinal hemorrhage, enucleation of the eye. (7) Facial paralysis, from compression of the nerve as it comes out in front of the mastoid. Usually good prognosis.

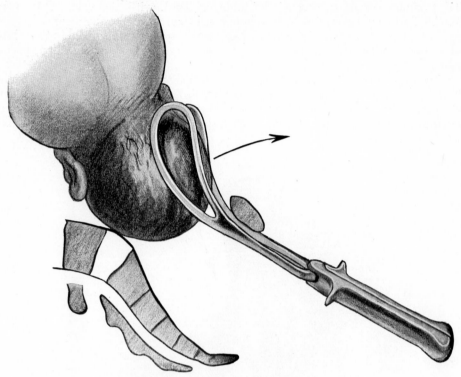

FIG. 878.—SLIPPING OF FORCEPS. HORIZONTAL SENSE. EXAXIAL.

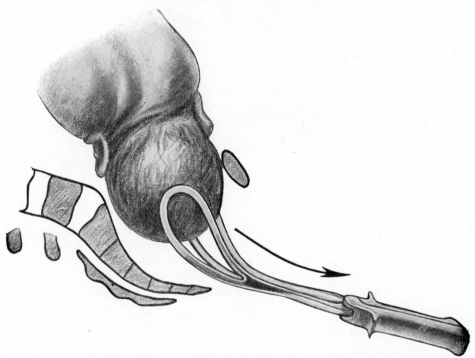

FIG. 879.—SLIPPING OF FORCEPS. VERTICAL SENSE. AXIAL.

(8) Pressure necrosis of the scalp, perhaps to the bone. (9) It is said that idiocy is more frequent after forceps. (10) Cephalhematoma—usually good prognosis.

(11) Compression or cutting of the umbilical cord, with asphyxia. (12) It is possible that deafness may be due to injury or hemorrhage into the organs of hearing, etc. (13) Erb's paralysis. (14) Indeed, nearly every imaginable injury has been observed, and, in general, forceps babies are more liable to infection, pneumonia, atelectasis, meningitis, hemophilia, etc.

Dystocia Due to the Shoulders.—If, after delivery of the head, the shoulders do not immediately follow gentle traction, applied as indicated under the conduct of normal labor, the accoucheur should make an examination with four fingers to determine the cause of delay. One or the other of the following conditions will be

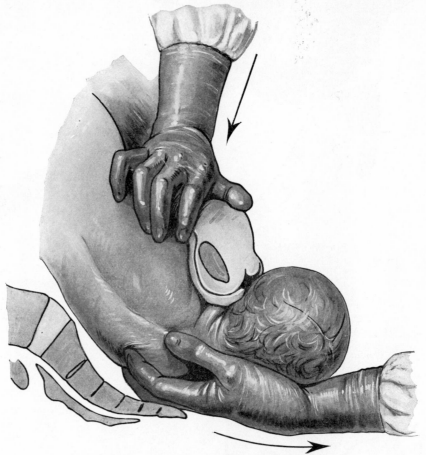

Fig. 880.—Bringing Down Posterior Arm in Head Presentation.

found: (1) The shoulders are broad and firm or the pelvis contracted; (2) they have followed an unfavorable mechanism, the anterior shoulder being caught on the ramus pubis, or having over-rotated, and, the accoucheur not observing this, he tries to bring the shoulder-girdle down in the wrong diameter; (3) the cord is too short; (4) the chest of the child is too large (anasarca); (5) locked twins or a monster exists.

The head springs backward against the perineum, pressing this well up into the pelvis, and traction serves only to stretch the neck. Not a few children have been lost at this stage of delivery.

Treatment.—If the woman is conscious, she should be exhorted to bear down strongly, her legs are firmly pressed against her belly and the assistant aids with a light Kristeller expression. Now, by means of the fingers inside and the hand outside, the shoulder-girdle is rotated into the most favorable pelvic diameter—one of the obliques and the anterior shoulder tucked down behind the pubis. Next, the accoucheur inserts two fingers behind the pubis gaining a purchase on the scapula. By gentle pressure and slight traction in the axilla, the anterior shoulder is pushed to one side (ventrally) and drawn down, the pressure imparting a slight twist to the body, as you would coax the finger out of a tight ring. We call this "tight ring maneuver No. 1." If this fails we try to dislodge the posterior shoulder from the promontory and lead it down into the excavation by tight ring maneuver No. 2. Four fingers pass high up the vagina over the baby's back, the index is insinuated into the posterior axilla. Aided by pressure from the outside (Fig. 880) the shoulder-girdle is turned into a favorable oblique and at the same time drawn down into the pelvis, the torso being given a turbinal motion, which may, if necessary, carry the back over into the opposite side of the pelvis. Excessive caution is here required because only too easily is the clavicle fractured or the cervical plexus torn or pulled out of the spinal cord, the baby's neck broken or a hemorrhage made into the spinal canal.

Failing these plans, next to do is to deliver the posterior arm, it being necessary to insert the whole hand in order to reach it, and it is wiped down over the face —not over the back. Now extraction is always possible unless there is some monstrosity. This will at once be discovered by the hand which has been introduced, and, of course, the treatment will be guided by what is found. Exenteration, cleidotomy, or other cutting operation will usually be advisable under such circumstances.

Since these manipulations take much time, during which the child may die, a few moments should be spared to insert a catheter into the child's trachea and to blow sufficient air into its lungs to prevent asphyxia. Time to effect the disengagement of the shoulders is thus obtained, the operator may work deliberately, and more certainly avoid damage to the child and the mother.

LITERATURE

Das, K.: The History of Forceps, Calcutta, 1929. Enormous work, a classic.—*Davis:* Amer. Jour. Obstet., December, 1910, p. 978.—*Greenhill:* Amer. Jour. Obstet. and Gyn., March, 1924, p. 349.—*Ingraham:* "History of Forceps," Amer. Jour. Obstet., 1911, vol. ii, p. 830.—*Klein:* History of Breech Extraction, Münch. med. Woch., 1902, No. 31.—*Massini:* Gynéc. et Obstét., Paris, 1926, No. 6, p. 369.—*Nürnberger:* Monatsschr. für Geb. u. Gyn., May, 1922, p. 305.—*Reynolds and Newell:* Amer. Jour. Obstet., January, 1910.—*Schroeder:* Münch. med. Woch., 1923, No. 48; "Cephalic Version in Breech Pres.," Trans. Amer. Gyn. Soc., 1927.—*Winckel-Edgar Text-book:* History of Breech Extraction.

CHAPTER LXXII

CESAREAN SECTION

CESAREAN section is the removal of the child from the uterus through an incision made in the abdominal wall. The term may not be applied to the removal of the child from the belly after rupture of the uterus, nor to operations for ectopic pregnancy.

The term probably is derived from the Latin, *partus cæsareus*, from *cædere*, to cut. The term cesarean section, therefore, is really a redundancy. There is no evidence to show that Julius Cæsar was thus delivered. Cæsones (children delivered by section from their dead mothers) were known long before Cæsar's time, and the operation was not performed on the living in Rome. Cæsar's mother was alive at the time of his wars, as is proved by his letters to her.

Cesarean section on the dead woman has been done for ages, possibly even by the early Egyptians, and the operation is referred to in the myths and folklore of European races. Dionysus was cut from the dead Semele. The Lex Regia of Numa Pompilius, 715 B. C., Buddha and the ancient Jews expressly commanded the removal of the child before the burial of its mother.

Cesarean section on the living is of more recent date, though it is more than possible that it was performed by earlier peoples. That the Jews did the operation successfully is shown by their laws. In the Mischnejoth (before 140 B. C.), the rights of twins delivered by section are gravely considered and in the Talmud (400 A. D.) the law reads, a woman need not observe the usual days of purification after abdominal delivery (Rigby). "Jotze Dofan" was the name they applied to operation through the flanks of their mothers and "Kariyath Habbeten" to the classic cesarean. In the heart of Uganda in 1879 Felkin witnessed a cesarean section performed by a native. The operator—a specialist—washed his hands and the operative field with banana wine (antisepsis!), the patient being drunk with the same (anesthesia!). A quick incision opened the uterus. After cutting the cord and removing the placenta the cervix was dilated from above, the uterus massaged and compressed, the peritoneal cavity cleansed by raising the woman up, then the abdomen closed by pin and figure-of-8 sutures, the wound being dressed with a paste of crushed herbs. The temperature remained below 101° F. and the wound healed in eleven days. For how many centuries must these savages have been doing this operation to have developed so good a technic?

The first authenticated report of cesarean section was made by J. Trautman, of Wittenberg, in 1610, on a case of hernia uteri gravidi, although Bishop Paulus of Meirada, Spain, is said to have done one in the thirteenth century, and Christ. Bein reported one in 1540. Estienne, 1539, performed section on a moribund woman, saving the baby (Gail). About 1500 J. Nufer, a swine-gelder in Switzerland, had successfully delivered his own wife after a dozen midwives and several barbers had failed, and in 1581 F. Rousset had published 15 cases, which probably were not all extra-uterine pregnancies, as has been suggested. Rousset's monograph established the operation, and in spite of its own frightful mortality and the resultant opposition by many of Europe's best accoucheurs, it very slowly became an acceptable resource in those forlorn cases where the parturient almost to a certainty would have died without it. The Catholic Church had much to do with the habilitation of the operation, since it enabled the rite of baptism to be given to the child. Sigault's symphysiotomy for a few years only was a competitor of cesarean section.

Kayser (Copenhagen, 1844) found a mortality of 62 per cent. for the previous eighty years, but Tarnier said that up to his time there had not been a successful case in Paris during the nineteenth century, and Spaeth said the same thing of Vienna in 1877. Harris collected 80 cases in the United States, with a mortality of 52 per cent. The causes of death were hemorrhage and infection. In cesarean sections, sutures were not put in the uterine wound because the ends could not be left long for the subsequent removal, as was the custom in olden days. As a result the women often died of hemorrhage into the peritoneal cavity. For the same reason lochia escaped into the belly and usually set up peritonitis. Further, aseptic technic was unknown, and all laparotomies were fearfully dangerous. In 1769 Lebas put three stitches in the uterine wound and left the ends long, by which they were subsequently removed, with success, but a true efficient uterine suture was not made until Kehrer and Sänger recommended it in 1882. In 1877 Porro, of Pavia, to avoid the dangers of hemorrhage and of infection from the leaking of the lochia, advised the supravaginal amputation of the uterus after the child was delivered, and for a short time this operation bid fair to replace the old conservative cesarean section. Sänger's operation in 1882 showed such good results that Porro's was soon relegated to its proper place—as an operation where there is some special indication for sacrificing the uterus. The essentials of Sänger's operation are: median abdominal incision; median uterine incision, with or without eventration of the uterus; use of rubber ligature around cervix to stop hemorrhage; resection of a strip of uterine muscle under the peritoneum; interrupted silver-wire seromuscular sutures, avoiding the decidua—8 or 10; interrupted fine silk seroserous (Lembert) sutures, 20 to 25; extreme antisepsis.

Previous to Sänger the abdominal incision had been made in all possible locations, the uterus

1078

opened in many different places and ways, drainage of the uterus, of the abdominal cavity, above and below, and many other devices had been practised. Osiander, in 1805, thought out, performed, and recommended the low or cervical cesarean almost as it is done today. Joerg came on the same idea in 1806. Others sought to empty the uterus without opening the peritoneal cavity. The operation consisted of making an incision above and parallel to Poupart's ligament, blunt dissection under the peritoneum to the cervix and vagina, followed by a flank delivery—a "Jotze Dofan" or "Buddha Birth." Ritgen did it in 1821, and Physick, of Philadelphia, recommended it to Dewees in 1824, but he did not do it. Baudelocque named it "gastro-elytrotomy" in 1823, and T. Gaillard Thomas in 1870 revived the defunct operation, but it was soon discarded for the Porro operation, introduced in 1877, just as the latter was displaced by the improved cesarean of Sänger. The object of all these measures was to avoid hemorrhage, seepage of lochia with peritonitis, adhesions of the uterus to the abdominal wall, to the omentum, and the danger of rupture of the scar in subsequent pregnancies. With the general improvement of our aseptic technic the results of Sänger's operation got better, and it was found possible to dispense with many things he considered necessary. Many varieties of suture have been recommended—through-and-through interrupted or continuous, buried muscular, seromuscular, decidual, three layers, four layers, silkworm-gut, wire, silk, catgut, etc.

In spite of all improvements and a refined aseptic technic the classic cesarean left much to be desired, especially when it was measured with modern requirements. In the first place, it is not safe where infection is present or even suspected, therefore it cannot always be used to obviate craniotomy on the living child; second, postoperative intestinal complications are frequent, and, while seldom fatal, are always disturbing; third, peritoneal adhesions are often left, causing suffering and trouble later; fourth, the uterine scar may rupture in a subsequent labor; fifth, there is still a mortality of 1 to 10 per cent. and higher in just those cases where one would like to adopt this method of delivery.

To obviate these faults Frank, of Bonn, in 1906 recalled attention to the operation of Joerg. Frank, however, opened the peritoneal cavity just above the pubis, and united the parietal to the peritoneum of the lower uterine segment, thus shutting off the peritoneal cavity, after which delivery was effected. Sellheim clarified the surgical anatomy of the parts, demonstrated the advantages of delivering the child through the zone of dilatation or exit passage rather than through the contracting portion of the uterus, and devised several methods of approach to the lower uterine segment. His work is fundamental to all later modifications. Latzko pushed the bladder to one side and the peritoneum upward from off the lower uterine segment, gaining access to the uterus entirely extraperitoneally. More than twenty different varieties of the low operation have been proposed. All have the object in common, to avoid manipulation in the general peritoneal cavity as much as possible, and to place the incision in the uterus entirely in the lower uterine segment. The idea is that the greatest dangers of immediate and remote complications come from the uterine opening into the peritoneal cavity, and that an incision in the lower uterine segment will obviate peritonitis and rupture of the uterus in subsequent labor. The reader is referred to Nicholson, Küstner, Vogt, and DeLee for the history of the twenty or more modifications of the low operation. Schilling gives complete literature.

The latest addition to the abdominal delivery is the operation suggested by Gottschalk of Berlin, in 1909 and 1911, and performed, independently, by Portes of Paris in 1924 for frankly septic cases—temporary exteriorization of the cesareanized uterus for four weeks, or until the infection has cleared away, then return of the organ to its proper place. It is gaining but little ground.

At the present time there are five methods of abdominal delivery. The old, the classic or conservative cesarean section now rapidly passing into discard. The incision is made in the fundus uteri—in the corpus—and thus the operation could be called corporeal section. In two other methods the incision is made in the cervix, and they are called low, or cervical cesareans. All the low operations invented may be divided into two groups—those where access is gained to the cervix through the peritoneal cavity, i. e., trans- or per-peritoneally, or better, intraperitoneally, and those where the cervix is reached purely extraperitoneally—in a manner similar to the ligation of the external iliac artery.

Then there is the Porro, supravaginal amputation of the uterus, which may follow either of the above and lastly the Gottschalk-Portes operation.

Indications for Abdominal Delivery in General.—There is hardly an obstetric complication that has not been treated by cesarean section. Indeed, many surgeons know of but one way out of a difficult obstetric situation, i. e., suprapubic delivery. Older writers, having to do mainly with contracted pelves, divided the indications into absolute and relative.

The absolute indication for cesarean section exists when the parturient canal is narrowed so much that the child, even reduced by mutilating operations, cannot be gotten through with safety to the mother. Contracted pelvis with a conjugata vera of 6 or $6\frac{1}{2}$ cm. or an immense child will give the absolute indication, but the narrowing of the passage may be produced by exostoses, irremovable tumors, stenosis of the cervix and vagina, and neoplasms of the uterus and adnexa, prolapsed before the child. If these conditions are discovered early in pregnancy, some may be removed before labor. During labor there is no choice.

The relative indication, speaking broadly, will exist when the accoucheur decides that the abdominal delivery offers better chances for both mother and child than delivery from below. It is largely subjective.

In contracted pelvis, excepting the absolutely contracted, cesarean section is considered only with a view to saving the life of the child, because we can, by means of embryotomy, very safely deliver from below. The field claimed for cesarean section from the relative indication is in pelves with a conjugata vera of from $6\frac{1}{2}$ to 9 cm., depending on the size of the child. This is also the field claimed by pubiotomy, prophylactic version, forceps, and expectancy. This brings us again to the treatment of contracted pelvis. (See pp. 764–778.)

Another indication on the part of the child is prolapse of the cord. Nowadays so much value attaches to the life of the fetus, and the abdominal delivery has such a small mortality that this is a just indication when the cervix is closed and the conditions favorable. A soft, open cervix or one easily dilatable will permit delivery from below.

Habitual death of the fetus in or just before labor, and habitual abruptio placentæ in or before the second stage—a distinct clinical entity—may give the indication for section.

Abnormal presentation of the child (*e. g.*, breech, face), *per se*, does not offer an indication, but will do so if there are adjuvant factors which make dystocia, *e. g.*, aged primiparity, contracted pelvis, rigid soft parts. A mammoth child puts its case in the class of contracted pelvis.

All the other indications consider the benefits to both mother and child, and they are relative in this sense, that, in the opinion of the accoucheur, abdominal delivery will be less dangerous and less damaging, to both parent and fetus, than delivery from below, which, however, could be done. These indications are almost wholly subjective, leaving a wide field for the play of individual preference, the influence of isolated experience, and the clash of contending statistics. Therefore the operation is much abused, and even by men whose intentions are honest.

The following is an incomplete list of other conditions for which cesarean section is done: Eclampsia; placenta prævia; abruptio placentæ; old primiparity (women of difficult and delayed conception); stenosis of cervix; vaginal stenosis, congenital and acquired; antefixed uteri; ovarian cyst; fibroids; healed vesicovaginal fistulæ and extensive repair operations; dystrophia dystocia syndrome; heart disease; tuberculosis; pulmonary edema; combinations of these with contracted pelvis. For details the reader is referred to the appropriate chapters.

The decision for abdominal delivery must depend largely on the choice of method. The numbers of the low or cervical operations performed the world over are large enough now for us to say positively that it is safer than the classic. Therefore, we are enabled to spread the indication for abdominal delivery over a wider field, and also give the baby better chances for life and health. The terrific mortality still attending the classic cesarean in the United States is an opprobrium. The indications for the old method should be as restricted as they were twenty-five years ago.

Should the dictum "once a cesarean always a cesarean" hold? Much disagreement exists on this point, and a decision cannot be reached until we know how many cesarean uteri rupture in subsequent labors. Findley, Spalding *et al.* find numerous reports of such fatalities. Holland found the frequency of rupture was 4 per cent., with a maternal mortality of 30 per cent. and fetal, 70 per cent. Without doubt the uterus after section is weakened in the scar, and this is especially marked if the muscle was sewed improperly or if its healing was disturbed by infection, or if glandular tissue has formed in the scar, but in the majority of instances it stands the strain of subsequent labor well. The healing of the uterine incision is usually a complete muscular restitution, but the thickness of the uterine wall has suffered, and, therefore, it is more or less weak at this site. Sometimes part or all of the union is by scar tissue and in rare instances only the peritoneum and mucosa have united. This makes rupture in subsequent pregnancy and labor almost inevitable. In all cases, if the placenta is implanted over the scar, it impairs the uterine wall still more, and bursting of the uterus is more frequent and more dangerous. Since it is impossible here to discuss the subject fully, I will state my position: Subsequent cesarean is necessary—(*a*) when the reason for the first one still exists, *e. g.*, contracted pelvis; (*b*) when infection occurred after the first; (*c*) when it is known to have deen done imperfectly; (*d*) when other conditions make it desirable to reopen the abdomen, *e. g.*, a hernia in the scar, the advisability to tie off the tubes, appendicitis, fibroids.

When it is decided to allow vaginal delivery after a previous cesarean section or myomectomy, the birth-room should be set up all ready for laparotomy. Should the uterus show signs of thinning or rupture, labor should be terminated by forceps, and in all cases when the cervix is fully dilated. The scar in the low cervical cesarean is much less likely to part than the fundal. Only 23 cases of rupture are on record.

Conditions.—For the absolute indication there are no governing conditions— the child must be removed abdominally whether or not it is alive, and regardless of the condition of the patient. If she is infected, extirpation of the uterus should follow, or extraperitoneal cesarean section is performed, or, if it qualifies, the Gottschalk-Portes operation.

For the relative indication to hold, the mother and babe should be in prime condition. It is very important to make sure that the child is not a monstrosity, as an acephalus, which is not easy. One may now get an *x*-ray picture of the child. In the presence of kidney, lung, heart, or general diseases the questions of risk of anesthetic, of shock, and of infection must receive careful consideration with a medical consultant. After prolonged labor, with or without rupture of the membranes and in the presence of infection the classic cesarean section is contraindicated. Gonorrhea comes in this class. When infection is only suspected, one may do the low operation. In cases of abruptio and placenta prævia we do not insist that the child be alive.

The cervix must be patulous for the escape of the lochia; if there is cicatricial stenosis, the uterus must be removed. Barnes (1876) advised to operate just before labor began in order to avoid the disadvantages of emergency. Everything can be gotten ready without hurry, as for ordinary laparotomy, which means much for the assistants and nurses; operation by daylight; the accoucheur can usually have had some rest; the bag of waters is still intact; the cord or extremities will not have prolapsed; accidents and delays in transportation, etc., are avoided. The disadvantages of early operating are readily overcome.

By the prophylactic administration of ergot, the injection of pituitrin, by packing the uterus, brisk massage, and, if needed, by compression of the aorta the hemorrhage is controllable; nature usually provides for lochial drainage, but if the cervix seems too tight it may be dilated a little; and by careful study of the case the approximate date of term may be decided and non-viability avoided.

When a Porro is to be performed, the element of danger from hemorrhage and lochial seepage is eliminated, and, therefore, the operation may be undertaken at any time. The cervical cesareans should also, if possible, be performed before labor begins, although they are much easier if the pains have fully developed the lower uterine segment.

Classic Cesarean Technic.—It is important to get the patient into the best possible general health beforehand. Regulated outdoor exercise, care of the bowels, and much sleep are provided. The skin of the belly should be cured of eczematous and other eruptions. As a routine may be recommended daily washing of the belly with tincture of green soap. Douches, without special indication, are forbidden, and the patient is impressed with the importance of local cleanliness and the *abstinence from intercourse or self-examination*. If possible, she should be in the maternity a week or more in advance of the date set, especially if she has had a previous section. General diseases—for example, nephritis, hemophilia—are treated as thoroughly as we know how. Gentle laxatives are used a few days before, and an enema the day of the operation.

The Operation.—Preparations for reviving the child should never be forgotten. Four assistants are needed—one for the anesthetic, one, especially trained, to resuscitate the child, one to help on the other side, and one to hand instruments, thread needles, supply sponges—duties which in most modern hospitals fall to the nurse. Another sterile assistant may be needed if the case is complicated or requires extirpation of the uterus.

Local anesthesia is the best anesthetic. We have done 600 laparotrachelotomies with it, and find it reduces the general mortality and morbidity. Next in order but far away comes ethylene, then ether.

For the preparation of the abdomen, shaving, washing thoroughly with tincture of green soap and hot water, with bichlorid 1 : 1000, with 65 per cent. alcohol; just before adjusting the laparotomy sheet a wash with 40 per cent. of tr. iodi in alcohol, which is washed off with 65 per cent. alcohol immediately prior to the incision.

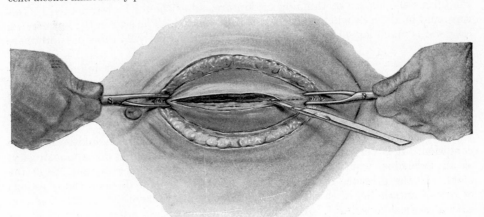

FIG. 881.—CLASSIC CESAREAN SECTION.
Steadying uterus with vulsella.   (Keeps spill out of abdomen.)

Just before starting the anesthetic a hypodermic of aseptic ergot is given and the patient catheterized. The incision is made in the linea alba, should be about 5 inches long, with its upper end just below the navel. As the belly wall is sometimes very thin, one may not cut too deeply. It is best to make a small opening and cut the balance with scissors on two fingers inserted into the peritoneal cavity. Now the uterus is brought to the middle line and steadied by the assistant. A long narrow sponge is packed around the fundus in horseshoe shape to prevent spreading of the "spill." By means of volsella or a stitch at either end of the intended incision the assistant holds the uterus up against the abdominal opening. With another knife a longitudinal incision, 4½ inches long, corresponding to the abdominal one, is made half through the thickness of the uterine wall, and with lessening strokes the cavity of the egg is opened; then, cutting between two fingers with scissors, the opening is enlarged both ways to the size of the first uterine cut. Liquor amnii gushes out while the operator searches for one foot, on which he makes the breech extraction, following minutely the classic operation, with Smellie-Veit on the after-coming head. Now a full cubic centimeter of pituitary extract is given intramuscularly (deltoid). The assistant presses the sides of the belly against the retracting uterus to keep liquor amnii and blood out of the peritoneal cavity. Clamping the cord in two places and cutting between requires only an instant, the operator handing the child to an assistant who stands at his elbow bearing a large tray covered with an aseptic blanket. The placenta usually falls free into the hollow of the uterus, but the membranes must be pulled off gently and slowly to get them all. After the secundines are out, with a gauze pad the interior of the uterus is wiped perfectly smooth, all shreds of placenta and membranes being removed, and a clean pad is stuffed into the gaping cavity, which rapidly closes as the organ retracts and contracts. This is aided by gentle kneading and firm compression. The pack is removed just before finishing the first row of stitches. The most important part of the operation is the uterine suture. Beginning at the upper end of the incision a row of sutures is inserted just beneath the endometrium, taking care this is not turned into the wound. Four rows of sutures are put in, mostly interrupted. Number 2 twenty-day catgut is used. Care should be used to get accurate coaptation in the angles and to avoid too much constriction of the tissues for fear of necrosis when the uterus contracts and tightens the sutures. The knots must be firmly tied. It is usually possible to determine three layers of muscle—one, the thickest, internal, next to the decidua, and darker in color, probably because the fibers are cut across; another, a little thinner—the middle coat; and a third, very thin, to which is attached the peritoneum. Time taken to apply an accurate uterine suture and make a thorough abdominal closure is well spent. Too rapid and spectacular operating is responsible for many bad results.

Complications.—*Adhesions* are seldom met in primary operations, but, nevertheless, it is wise not to cut too boldly into the belly. After previous sections adhesions are the rule. The most common are of the omentum, or of the uterus to the abdominal wall, or the omentum to the uterus. Rarely a coil of gut is attached to the uterus under the line of the incision, and still more rarely the cecum, appendix, or sigmoid may be adherent behind and tear when the uterus is eventrated. Where adhesions are known or suspected, the belly should be opened at a spot free from them, and two fingers inserted to determine their location and extent. A clear space on the uterus should be quickly made, and the child and placenta delivered, after which the adhesions are dealt with according to general surgical principles. It is best not to deliver the uterus if there are adhesions. Adherent gut must be very tenderly handled. If the omentum can be tied off the uterus or abdominal wall without denuding it much, this should be done—large rough areas, however,

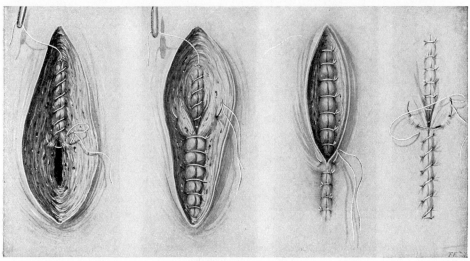

FIG. 882.—UTERINE SUTURE, FIRST ROW.

Takes in thin layer of muscle and goes to edge of, but not through the mucosa. If a dry field use interrupted.

FIG. 883.—SECOND ROW.

Buried, takes a good part of muscle. Interrupted.

FIG. 884.—THIRD ROW.

Edge of peritoneum and 8 mm. of muscle. Interrupted.

FIG. 885.—FOURTH ROW. ON PERITONEAL SURFACE (LEMBERT).

Takes in part of muscle. Upper portion of wound may not be coverable by Lembert. Then a few extra sutures.

only invite new adhesions. If the uterus is intimately bound to the abdominal fascia, it may be best not to attempt its separation unless extirpation of the organ is to be performed or the tubes exsected. In the latter instance a segment of the uterus, together with the abdominal scar, may be excised. In a second cesarean section the uterine incision should be parallel to and close to the scar of the first one, and weak portions of the muscle exsected.

If a hernia of the old scar is present, the sac is to be exsected and the edges of the fascia brought together anew.

The Placenta.—In 42 of 67 cases where the site of the placenta was noted the organ was situated on the anterior wall and had to be cut to gain access to the infant. It is not possible to be sure of the location of the placenta beforehand. The course of the round ligaments (converging anteriorly) and the prominence of the veins in the violaceous surface of the uterus give some indication of it. If the first cut into the muscle causes profuse hemorrhage, anterior insertion may be suspected, but the operation does not differ from the usual one, except that the movements must be hastened. I usually cut right through the placenta.

Hemorrhage.—Nowadays severe bleeding is rare, because we use local anesthesia and give a hypodermic of ergot before the anesthetic is started and one of pituitary extract immediately after the delivery of the child, but if the placenta has been cut or torn or the section made before labor, more blood may be lost than is permissible (*e. g.*, in an anemic woman), and the flow must be

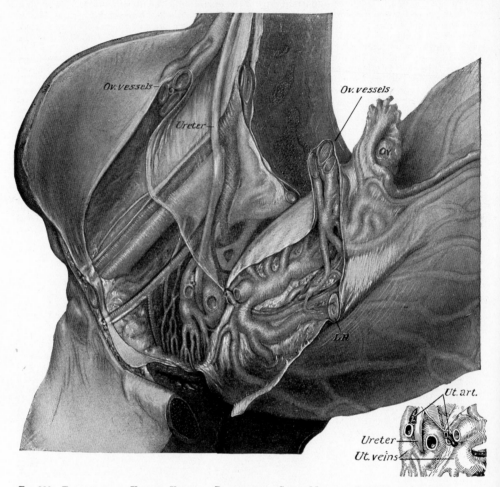

FIG. 886.—TOPOGRAPHY OF UTERINE VESSELS.   PREGNANCY OF SEVEN MONTHS.   *L. R.*, LIGAMENTUM ROTUNDUM.
Adapted from Couvelaire.

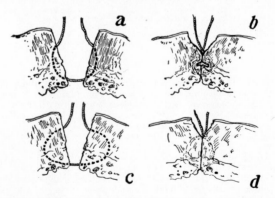

FIG. 887.—WRONG WAY (*a* AND *b*) AND RIGHT WAY (*c* AND *d*) TO PASS NEEDLE IN UTERINE SUTURE.

very quickly stanched.   In such cases another injection of pituitrin is made directly into the uterine wall and the cavity of uterus packed with a hot wet laparotomy sponge.   The uterus is then massaged and squeezed together until it contracts well.   The quickest way to stop the bleeding is by closing the uterine wound, which should be done with the utmost despatch, consistent with thoroughness. Then the massage is repeated. While these maneuvers are being carried out, an assistant compresses the aorta as shown in Fig. 713. If these measures do not quickly cause uterine contraction and cessation of the bleeding, extirpation of the uterus must be considered. The operator must not forget that the blood may escape per vaginam also and in large quantities. If it is desirable to preserve the uterus and the hemorrhage persists, uterine tamponade may be resorted to. Since the wound has been closed, packing is inserted from below in the usual manner. On three occasions I deemed it best to tampon. Recovery.

Infection.—If the case is known to be infected, the conservative cesarean section is contraindicated, and if delivery must be made abdominally, either the Porro operation or complete extirpation must be practised. In cases of gonorrhea conservative section is very dangerous, a point Leopold emphasizes, and it is best to consider these, too, infected. There is no way of determining beforehand that the parturient canal is aseptic. Fever, fetid discharge, tympania

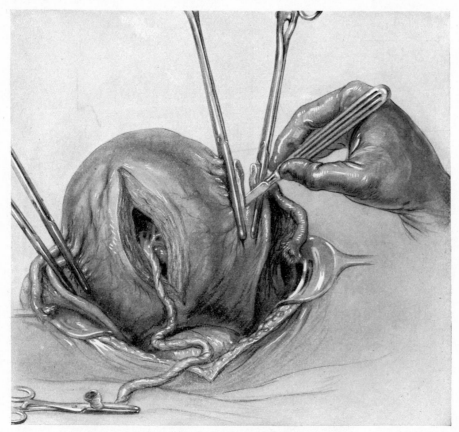

FIG. 888.—PORRO CESAREAN SECTION.
Both broad ligaments are clamped, taking in the round ligaments because of the varicosities.

uteri, and unhealthy wounds at the introitus are evidences of infection of the uterus—at least, are danger signals. In borderline cases the technic must be modified. (See Extraperitoneal Cesarean Section.) If during an ordinary cesarean section a septic focus is unexpectedly opened, for example, an infected dermoid, the intestine, an appendical abscess, it is best to remove the uterus and provide free pelvic drainage.

Uterine Drainage.—While rubbing the interior of the uterus smooth, it is a good plan to pass the finger down into the cervix, but *not* through it into the vagina, to see if it is patulous, unless examination beforehand has shown that the os is open. If the cervix is closed by scars so that a crow's quill cannot pass, the uterus is to be amputated. A normal cervix will open spontaneously under the influence of the after-pains. If the accoucheur fears that there is not enough drainage, he may pass gauze or a tube through the cervix into the vagina. It is highly important not to catch the gauze in the uterine stitches. One fatality from this cause is on record.

After-treatment.—This does not differ from that after the usual laparotomy. Cathartics are usually not administered until the fifth to the eighth day, and then not unless required, the bowels being unloaded by enemata. Milk and molasses, ½ pint of each, make a very efficient clyster, which may be repeated. Sometimes a camomile tea enema produces free evacuation of feces and flatus. The baby is put to the breast at the end of twelve to twenty-four hours.

Of the various postoperative complications, peritonitis, ileus, and uterine abscess only will be mentioned. If a beginning peritonitis is diagnosed, the patient must be constantly watched, that is, hourly observations must be made, and if the pulse grows steadily faster, the nausea increases to emesis, the temperature rises higher, the abdominal rigidity increasing, with or without leukocytosis, Fahraeus positive, in short, if sure—and the time required to know seldom need exceed eight hours—that the infection is progressing, the belly is to be reopened and drained. Ileus and acute dilatation of the stomach occur, it seems to me, oftener after the classic cesarean

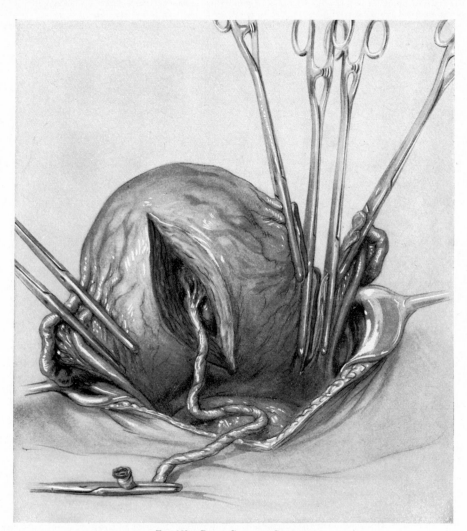

Fig. 889.—Porro Cesarean Section.
After cutting one side, two clamps are placed, reaching to about the level of the uterine artery.

section than after other celiotomies. For ileus the usual methods of treatment are practised. One that is serviceable after cesarean section is to hang the woman, inverted, from the shoulders of assistants, and with the finger in the rectum push the heavy uterus up out of the pelvis and give a high colonic flushing of milk and molasses, with the patient depending. In one case an electric vibrator applied to the distended bowel seemed to help. Eserin had failed. Pituitrin is not recommended, because the grinding contraction of the uterus may tear the sutures apart. Wyss reports 14 cases of bursting of the line of suture by the uterine contractions, and some had been sewn with silk and silver wire! Pituitrin is serviceable after the low cesarean. In obstinate cases of ileus permanent drainage of the stomach by nasal tube and aspiration, failing which enterostomy and drainage of the upper bowel to relieve toxic absorption is to be done before the patient is *in extremis*.

These measures have been successful in my practice in the treatment of gastric dilatation: having the woman lie on the stomach, the foot of the bed being elevated 18 to 24 inches; the knee-chest position; gastric lavage, repeated every four to six hours; massage of the stomach; rectal feeding. Dehydration, which is very rapid in these patients, must be prevented. Hypodermoclysis by the continuous axillary drip, salt and glucose solutions intravenously and by rectum should be kept up until the stomach is settled. Duodenal drainage is worth a trial. Both ileus and dilatation may be caused by a too tight abdominal binder, a point that I would emphasize strongly. In all probability a mild peritoneal infection is responsible for most of the cases, and bursting of the fascial suture for a few others. Uterine abscess is to be suspected if there is a mild fever, with signs of local peritonitis or partial ileus. Usually the abscess breaks on the surface, the wound opening. With good drainage the patient quickly recovers, but the uterus is permanently ventrofixed and the scar may give way in a subsequent pregnancy.

The lochial discharge is scanty after cesareans, rarely retention. Usual treatment.

Massive collapse of the lung occasionally imposes as a partial ileus. The findings and the x-ray will make the diagnosis, and turning the patient on the unaffected side will cure (Sante).

Prognosis.—By rigid examination of the cases, and the exclusion of all that present even a suspicion of infection, the mortality of the conservative cesarean delivery can be reduced to about

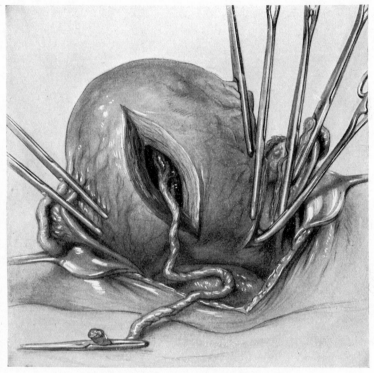

FIG. 890.—PORRO CESAREAN SECTION.
A clamp is put on the uterine artery, taking care that it grasps the tissue at the side of the uterus, not toward the pelvis, to avoid the ureter.

2 per cent. Routh in 1910 collected with great labor the statistics of Great Britain, comprising 1282 cases, and these may be taken as a type for all civilized countries. He shows that there has been a steady decrease in mortality until now; in favorable cases it is from 2 to 4 per cent. In cases where labor had been prolonged or even attempts made with the forceps, the death-rate was 34 per cent. and over. After labor had been in progress some time with the membranes ruptured he found 10.8 per cent. mortality, the best showing being made in those cases where labor had just begun, the bag of waters being intact—2.2 per cent. Eardly Holland collected 1954 sections done for contracted pelvis in Britain, 1910–20, and found mortalities ranging from 1.6 per cent. for elective cases to 27 per cent. for cases with previous attempts at delivery. The average was 4.3 per cent., which is about the same as those of Winter (4.2 per cent.) and Hornung (4.3 per cent.) for Germany in 1929. It is generally admitted that the dangers of cesarean section increase with every hour the woman labors, especially if the membranes are opened, the vaginal bacteria rapidly invading the uterine cavity. The exhaustion of active labor diminishes the woman's vital resistance to infection. Newell makes the startling statement that in several of the towns near Boston the recovery of a patient from cesarean section is a rarity. There were 30 cesarean deaths in Chicago in 1927, and in Massachusetts in 1922 the classic cesarean section stood second to puerperal infection as a cause of death!

If the low, cervical section were generally practiced, this mortality would be cut in half.

The operation as generally performed has a high morbidity. Fever is present in about 40 per cent. of the cases, while postoperative bronchitis and pneumonia, uterine abscess, ileus or gastric dilatation of some degree, infected catgut with hernia, may too often complicate the recovery. Taken all in all, it is not an operation to be lightly advised. The mortality of the children should be zero if the infant was well at the start.

Repeated cesarean sections have been done in large numbers, Nancrede in 1875 having done the sixth operation on the same woman. In such cases the uterus is so broadly adherent to the belly wall that it may be opened without entering the general peritoneal cavity. I do not recommend to try this, because intestines may be adherent to the scar.

Sterilization with Section.—Should the woman be sterilized to prevent future pregnancies? Authorities differ between wide extremes, and in deciding one must consider the dangers of subsequent pregnancies and labors and the necessity for consecutive cesarean sections.

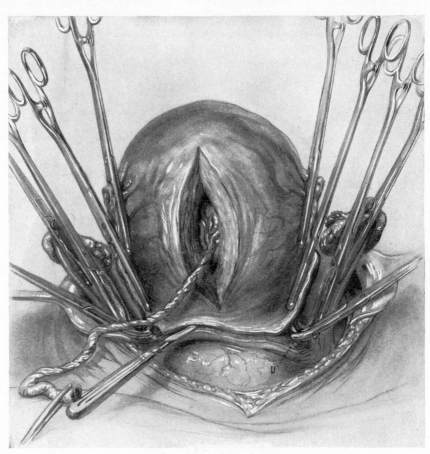

FIG. 891.—PORRO CESAREAN SECTION.

After the process has been repeated on the right side, the peritoneum is severed half an inch above its reflection on to the bladder. The ureter does not come into view, and lies a short distance farther away from the forceps than is indicated in the drawing. The location of the uterine artery may be determined by touch.

If the woman has tuberculosis, chronic nephritis, osteomalacia, or any disease which in itself is a contraindication to pregnancy, she should be sterilized. Any one who admits the propriety of inducing abortion for such conditions must admit the above postulate.

The danger of rupture of the uterine cicatrix in subsequent labor is no indication by itself, but may strengthen other reasons.

If the first section is done for eclampsia, placenta prævia, abruptio placentæ, prolapse of the cord, faulty mechanism of labor, pelvic tumors, in the absence of other indications the woman should not be sterilized. If the woman has a large family, the question is discussable, but if there is only one child, and that one weak or deformed, it is better not to sterilize her.

If the cesarean operation is done for contracted pelvis, I earnestly dissuade the patient from such a procedure at the first section, pointing out the fact of the safety of subsequent operations, the possibility of the death of the only child, and the unhappiness of a one-child family. At the second cesarean I willingly sterilize, if requested, although lately, since the mortality has been so much reduced, I often suggest a third operation. At operation one may reverse the intention to sterilize if the child is not of the desired sex, or if it is asphyxiated and of doubtful recovery.

For many years the ethics of sterilization have been debated. Green created an extensive discussion of it at the 1903 meeting of the American Gynecologic Association, taking an extreme negative position. In Catholic families the priest's advice is to be sought, and, in certain cases, a lawyer's. Some states have strict laws (Miller). Most American, English, and Continental authors concede the right of decision to the mother and her family, after they have been given

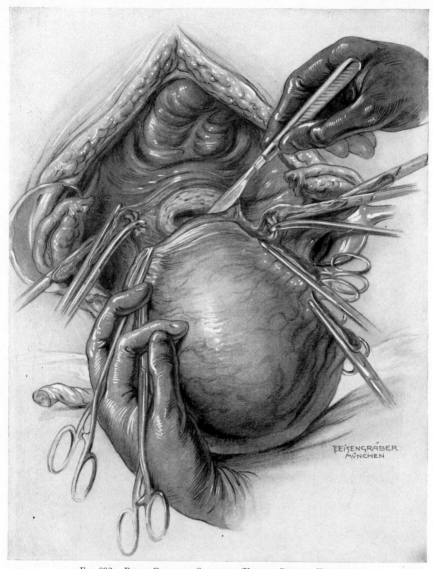

FIG. 892.—PORRO CESAREAN SECTION. (VIEW OF BACK OF UTERUS.)

The large uterus now hangs only at the cervix. It is pulled sharply over the pubis and cut off half an inch above the cervicovaginal junction, beginning from behind. When cutting the anterior cervical wall the relation of the knife to the bladder must be watched. There is usually little hemorrhage.

a fair presentation of all the facts. By following the Golden Rule I have had no difficulty in arranging a satisfactory course in these matters.

Methods.—Ligation, simple section or exsection of a portion of the tube, as recommended by Blundell in 1819, have proved insufficient, pregnancy having occurred in spite of them. Salpingectomy and exsection of the uterine cornua are safe. Madlener's method, simply crushing a loop of the tube and ligating with silk has given good results so far. Extirpation of the uterus as a means of simple sterilization is hardly to be recommended, certainly not in young women. The desire to have all the functions of a woman is strong, and seldom do the patients not regret the loss of the menses. The operation can be done in the same time as removal of the tubes, and

69

the postoperative recovery is prompter and more satisfactory than in the conservative cesarean section, but the technical difficulties are greater with amputation of the uterus, and premature menopause is not rare, even if one or both ovaries are preserved.

The Porro Cesarean Section.—In 1877 Porro, of Pavia, to avoid the dangers of hemorrhage and of infection from the large uterus, which was poorly sewn up, advised the amputation of the body of the uterus and the adnexa above an elastic ligature placed about the cervix, and the anchoring of the stump in the lower angle of the abdominal wound—an operation similar to supravaginal hysterectomy for

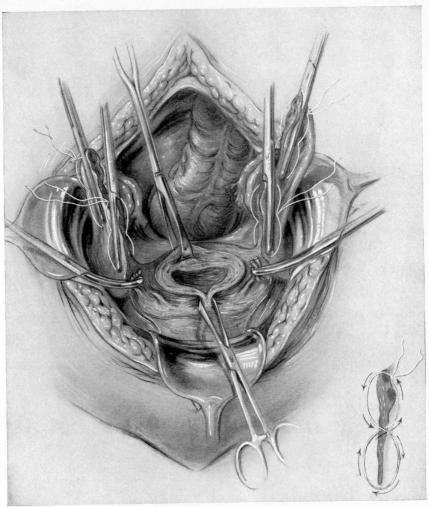

FIG. 893.—PORRO CESAREAN SECTION.

After raising the stump with vulsellum forceps, ligatures replace the artery clamps. The uterines are secured by special ligatures. Sketch below shows how the ligature is applied to prevent slipping. Most troublesome oozing would result from the immense veins. (See Fig. 886, p. 1084.)

fibroid, with extraperitoneal treatment of the stump. The operation had been suggested by Cavallini in 1768, and performed successfully on rabbits by Blundell in 1823. Storer, of Boston, did it for fibroids in 1869. Later, when Schröder dropped the sutured hysterectomy stump back into the pelvis, Isaac E. Taylor did the same for the stump after Porro's operation. Porro's radical operation did reduce the mortality of cesarean section, and gained some vogue, but was soon replaced by the improved conservative operation of Sänger. This was called "conservative" because the uterus was not sacrificed.

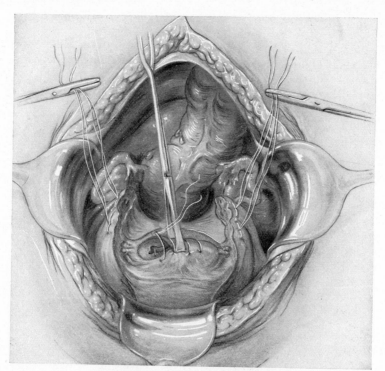

FIG. 894.—PORRO CESAREAN SECTION.

A few interrupted sutures, not taking in the mucosa, close the stump. In suspected septic cases this may be omitted to favor drainage, just the peritoneum being closed, or the cervix may be anchored extraperitoneally in the lower corner of the abdominal wound (original Porro).

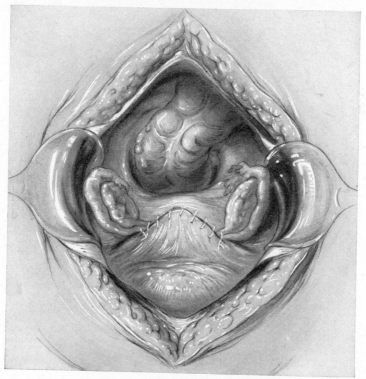

FIG. 895.—PORRO CESAREAN SECTION.

The peritoneum is sewed over the stump after uniting to it, with one suture, the severed ends of the round ligaments, the tubes and of the ovaries. If the tubes and ovaries have been removed, the round ligaments are to be united to the stump.

Indications.—It may be necessary to remove the uterus when myomata are present, especially if large or if they block the pelvis. Myomectomy may be performed in favorable cases if the woman desires more children. Sepsis in labor, when vaginal delivery is undesirable, is the most common indication. In abruptio placentæ, especially if one encounters a "Couvelaire" uterus and in placenta prævia it may be the quickest and most bloodless way of effecting delivery and stopping hemorrhage. Carcinoma cervicis, osteomalacia, placenta accreta,

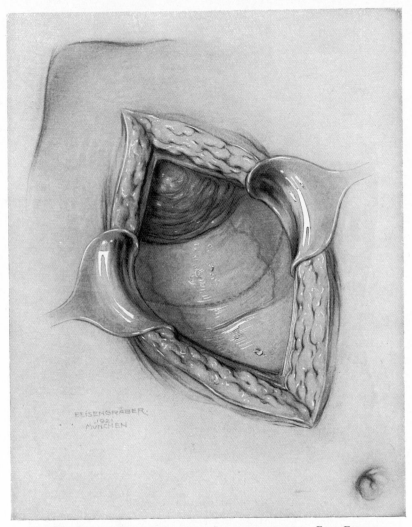

FIG. 896.—CERVICAL CESAREAN SECTION OR LAPAROTRACHELOTOMY. FIELD EXPOSED.

Trendelenburg position. Bladder empty—leave catheter in. Hypo. of ergot. Median incision from pubis to about 2 inches below navel (6½ inches). Watch for bladder when opening belly. Now a long narrow lap. sponge is tucked in horseshoe shape around the inside of the opening. Dotted line shows intended cut which is 2 cm. below firm attachment of peritoneum to uterus. This incision varies with the height of the bladder on the uterus.

intractable postpartum bleeding, rupture of the uterus are rarer indications for hysterectomy.

There are no conditions. The best time to operate is before labor begins.

The technic is a slightly modified, supravaginal hysterectomy. If the plan of operation is known beforehand, the abdominal incision should be nearer the pubis. After the child is delivered, two clamps are put on each broad ligament close to the uterus. Unless diseased, both tubes and ovaries are left. Both round ligaments are also clamped separately, or, if they are near the tubes, or if the broad ligaments are full of varicose veins, they are included in the first clamp.

After cutting to the tip of the clamps, two more are put on the broad ligaments, reaching below the level of the uterine arteries, keeping close to the uterus to avoid the ureters, and the tissue is cut between. Now a curvilinear incision is made through the peritoneum across the face of the uterus, just above the bladder, extending from the cut edge of the peritoneum around one round ligament to the other, and the bladder is pushed down by the finger covered with a piece of gauze. Owing to the usual immense development of the veins of the broad ligament, the varicosities making it sometimes as large as one's wrist, it is impractical always to open up the connective tissue to isolate the uterine arteries, as is done in gynecologic hysterectomies. After both broad ligaments are clamped and the uterus freed, the latter is pulled sharply forward over the pubis and cut off, beginning from behind, just above the vaginal insertion, the point being determined by palpation. It

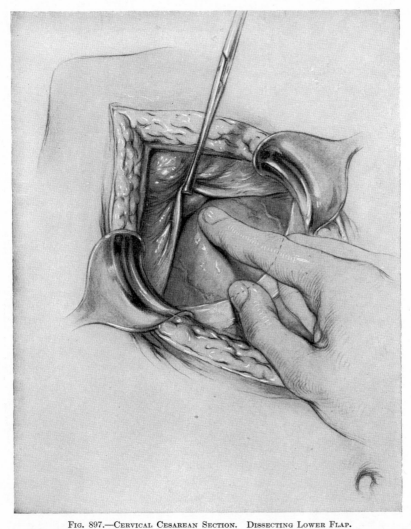

FIG. 897.—CERVICAL CESAREAN SECTION. DISSECTING LOWER FLAP.
After incising the peritoneum, it is gently stripped toward the pubis together with the bladder, using the finger. Large bleeding veins are tied with fine catgut (rarely needed). The point of raised peritoneum shown in illustration is sewed with one suture to the skin of the pubic end of incision, or held with Allis forceps.

is wise to cut carefully because of the softness of the uterine tissue and its thinness near the bladder. I usually cut from the right behind, to the left in front, then strip the uterus from the bladder, if need be, forming a new pedicle of the base of the right broad ligament, which is clamped and severed last. The ligaments are tied off under the clamps, using No. 2 hardened catgut. Then the large vessels are secured by separate individual ligatures. Before removing the clamps it is wise to secure perfect hemostasis, because oozing from the veins in the soft tissues may be exceedingly troublesome. A few through-and-through sutures in the stump may be required, but I usually apply them in such a manner as to turn the cut edges of the cervix against each other, leaving the cervical canal open for drainage. Now the peritoneum is sewed together after turning the ligated stumps in underneath it and uniting them to the cervical stump with a few sutures.

Michaëlis in 1809 recommended the removal of the whole uterus, and Bischoff in 1880 first practised it—a case of cancer. The operation is much more formidable than the amputation of the fundus. The hemorrhage from the cut vagina and bases of the broad ligaments is less easily controlled.

Cesarean section, with amputation of the uterus in clean cases, and with an expert operator, has the same mortality as the conservative operation, and the morbidity is decidedly less. Recovery is prompter, less painful, and less complicated than after the ordinary cesarean operation. The reason for this is the elimination of the large, involuting, really necrosing uterus, the clearing out of the pelvis (less absorption), and the covering in of all raw surfaces by peritoneum. In septic cases the mortality is still high—probably near 20 per cent. It is a question if total hyster-

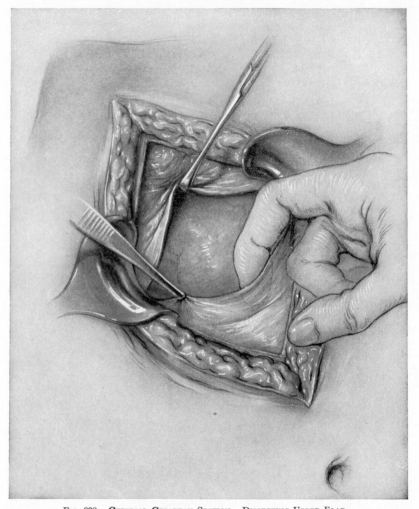

Fig. 898.—Cervical Cesarean Section. Dissecting Upper Flap.

The upper flap of peritoneum is made in the same way, being pushed up toward the navel to a point which delimits the upper end of the uterine incision. Be sure the bladder is pushed down far enough to expose an area of lower uterine segment sufficient for the exit of the child.

ectomy would improve the results. In septic cases the *unopened* uterus is to be brought out, the abdomen partly closed behind it, and walled off by large dry sponges. If the child is dead, one proceeds deliberately with the amputation of the unopened septic container. When the child is alive this may also be done—but speedily. If the field is carefully insulated (rubber dam, thick towels) the usual Porro suffices and is safer for the child.

Suprasymphyseal Cervical Cesarean Section.—Since the greatest dangers of the classic section arise from opening the peritoneal cavity, the old accoucheurs sought to avoid this by delivery of the child through a flank incision, gaining access to the cervix without incising the peritoneum. Owing to imperfect technic and more imperfect asepsis their patients died, and the operations were forgotten. Frank in 1906 disinterred the idea, and since then more than 20 low cervical operations have been devised. In some the peritoneum is not opened at all, but is peeled up off the lower uterine segment after displacing the bladder to one side and then delivery effected. In others the peritoneal cavity is opened above the pubis, the general peritoneum walled off by sponges, or the parietal and visceral layers of peritoneum temporarily united, and then the child delivered. Various kinds of incisions are made—too many for a text-book to discuss.

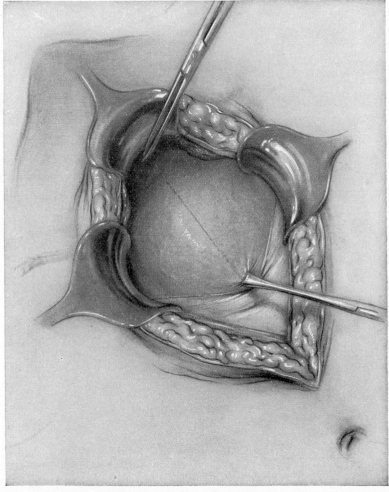

Fig. 899.—Cervical Cesarean Section. Intended Incision in L.U.S.
The bladder is held by a well-rounded retractor. With two Allis forceps (or two catgut sutures, if preferred) the upper and lower ends of the intended incision are delimited and the uterus steadied. Select a line midway between the two round ligaments. Now be ready for the "spill" either by a supply of large laparotomy sponges or the vacuum pump. Some operators prefer the transverse incision,

All the methods depend on certain anatomic changes which occur in the lower uterine segment and the overlying peritoneum and bladder during pregnancy. Owing to the softening and the loosening of the peritoneum and pelvic connective tissues, and to the development of the lower uterine segment in the latter months of pregnancy, and particularly during labor, the cervix is dilated and drawn away from the pelvis and from its relations to the vagina and the bladder. The vesico-uterine culdesac is usually obliterated. The peritoneum is easily moved on the subjacent structures. It is, therefore, possible to elevate this portion of the peritoneum and to push the bladder off its cervical attachments with great ease, thus exposing an area of the cervix and lower uterine segment large enough for the delivery of the child without encroaching on that portion of the peritoneum which is opened in the classic cesarean section.

In general, these operations fall in two classes, the true extraperitoneal and the intraperitoneal. The author recommends Latzko's method for the first, and as the intraperitoneal type the laparotrachelotomy to be now described.

Laparotrachelotomy.—This term is applied to the operation of abdominal delivery through an incision in the neck of the womb—trachelotomy. The tech-

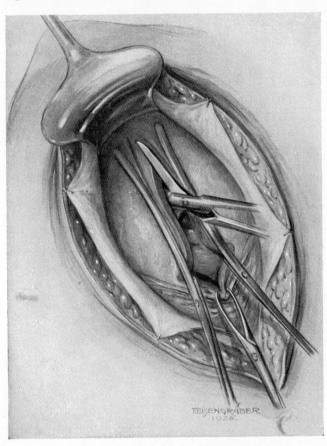

FIG. 900.—CERVICAL CESAREAN SECTION.

A small opening is made in the uterus close to the upper reflected peritoneum, the index finger inserted to push away the cord, if nearby, and to plug a possibly bleeding vessel. Take good care of the spill. Two ordinary, light, intestinal clamps are applied to the sides of the proposed incision to stop bleeding from the sometimes large, uterine sinuses and more superficial varicose veins. Having care not to clamp or cut the cord, the opening is extended down to the bladder with scissors. One can see the cut sinuses, and they should be closed temporarily with Allis forceps as the intestinal clamps are removed.

nic is based on Sellheim's third method and we have added several features which strengthen the scar and guarantee against seepage of the lochia. To avoid repetition the reader is referred for the details to the legends under the illustrations, Figs. 896–907.

The operation is much simpler if the patient has been in strong labor for some time. Uterine action stretches the lower uterine segment and draws the cervix away from the bladder. While technically more difficult, laparotrachelotomy may be done before labor, even in the eighth month of pregnancy.

Complications.—Adhesions are very rare, even in second operations. After previous abdominal uterine fixation one may have to work through a broad field of adhesions. Hemorrhage has already been discussed (see page 1083). Only in placenta prævia need it be feared. The woman is already anemic and the slogan "save blood," already emphasized when we studied the treatment of placenta prævia, applies with the same force. One quart of salt solution is given per rectum just before the anesthetic is started or the axillary drip begun. Remember transfusion. The pituitrin is administered earlier, a second dose is injected directly

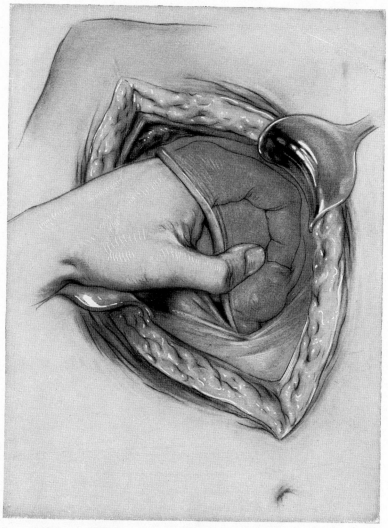

FIG. 901.—CERVICAL CESAREAN SECTION. BRINGING FACE TO FRONT.
The face of the child is now pulled into the wound by means of a finger introduced into its mouth. Do not hurry, do not use force. Clear the throat with sponges or the vacuum pump. If the occiput comes more readily into the wound, steady it with an Allis, grasping the scalp, and apply forceps as usual (Fig. 902a).

into the uterus or into a vein the instant the head has been delivered, the edges of the incision are to be clamped at once with broad tongue forceps, the placenta is to be removed if hemorrhage begins, then the fundus is tamponed. The rough bed of the placenta is momentarily compressed to determine if it has a tendency to bleed—if so, the bleeding area is lifted up with a vulsellum forceps and the ridge thus created is to be whipped over with a continuous suture of No. 1 plain catgut. Then the uterine packing is completed and the end of the gauze led into the vagina.

It is removed in twenty-four hours. Right after the patient is put to bed 3 quarts of saline solution are given by the rapid drip method per rectum.

The *after-treatment* is incomparably simpler than that after the classic cesarean section, to which the reader is referred. Vomiting, tympany, and gas-pains are often absent, seldom annoying, and almost never threatening. Fever may come from absorption, from suppuration in the wound, from lochiostasis, from pyelo-

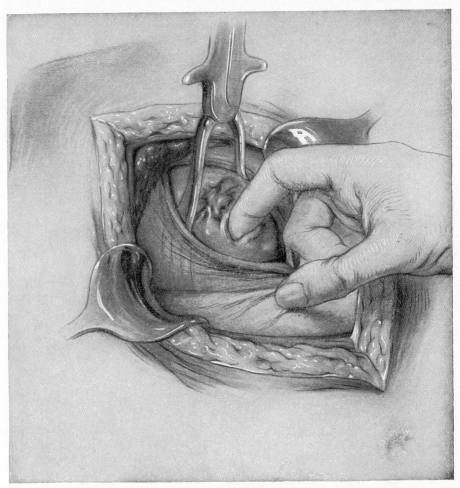

FIG. 902.—CERVICAL CESAREAN SECTION.

The assistant holds the head steady with his finger. The forceps are applied with the concavity of the blades toward the pubis. (In the illustration straight forceps are being used.) Remove all retractors. Sometimes the head may be expressed by Kristeller, or squeezed out from the flanks. Deliver the chin first over the upper (navel end) edge of the wound and the rest of the head by flexion. Do not hurry. Deliver shoulders slowly and carefully, giving time for the uterus to contract. Child may breathe freely now. Nurse gives a full cubic centimeter of pituitrin into deltoid muscle. The cord is severed, the child handed to an assistant, then the edges of the wound are grasped with Allis or tongue forceps, using as many as are needed to stop bleeding. The separation of the placenta is now observed. Manual removal is not done at once—rather wait a few minutes, but do not permit bleeding. Credé expression of the placenta is sometimes feasible. Wipe out the uterus carefully and pack temporarily with a long laparotomy sponge. We usually pack the uterus with gauze and lead the end down into the vagina, as a routine. It is necessary if there is too much bleeding and when the cervix is not open enough. If the uterus is sluggish, inject 1 c.c. strong pituitrin directly into it and compress aorta.

ureteritis, from a bronchitis, most rarely from peritonitis. At the first sign of the last the wound is to be reopened and drained. If suppuration is suspected, a careful combined examination will determine where the pus is. If in the abdominal wound or in the cavity of Retzius, removal of the stitches will give access to it; if under the bladder, it may easily be reached by anterior colpotomy or by reopening the uterine suture via the gaping cervix. In only 13 of 264 cases did we need to drain the abdominal wound, and in only 1 did we have to reopen the uterine suture from below. Lochiostasis is cured by giving ergot and pituitrin, the Fowler position, and raising the uterus with a finger in the rectum. It is rarely necessary to dilate the cervix.

Indications for Cervical Cesarean Section.—(See page 1079.) The old classic cesarean is rapidly giving way the world over, to the new cervical method. In

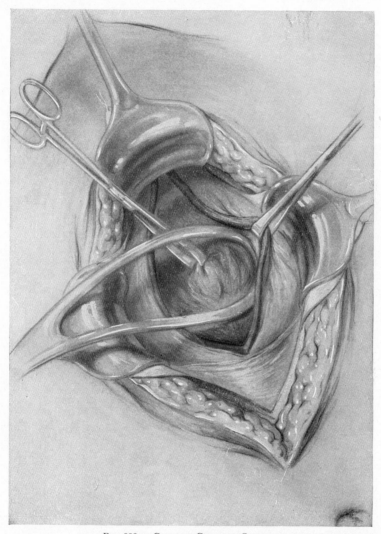

Fig. 902a.—Cervical Cesarean Section.

If it seems easier to bring the occiput out first, one searches rapidly for the small fontanel and fastens an Allis forceps to the scalp near it. The head is now gently turned to bring the small fontanel to the midline, and, lifting up the edge of the cervix with an Allis, the forceps blade is slipped underneath. It glides easily around the head and the prehension is the ideal or normal one.

Germany laparotrachelotomy is the accepted cesarean, in Britain, Kerr and Holland laud it, in America, Hirst, Adair, Beck, Lynch, Watson, Falls, Harris, Plass, and many others have adopted it. Williams acknowledged it in his later years. Indeed, I believe that laparotrachelotomy should replace the old classic cesarean in all but a few exceptional cases, such as inaccessibility to the parts from pendulous belly, kyphoscoliosis, etc., and where instant delivery is required to save the child and even here a very low classic should be done.

The advantages of the cervical incision are both immediate and remote. At the operation, the spill is limited to the lowest portion of the abdomen; the hemorrhage is less, and more easily controlled, being directly under the eye and finger; the omentum and intestines do not come into view; there is less peritoneal shock. True, the operation requires greater technical skill, but this should be possessed by a man who considers himself capable of deciding whether an abdominal delivery is or is not necessary.

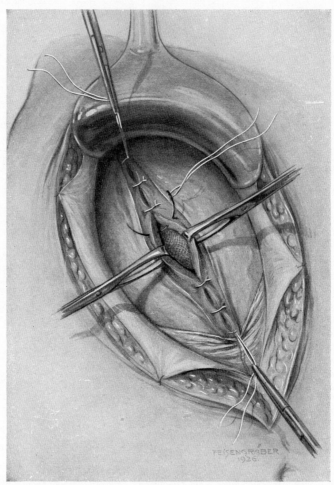

FIG. 903.—CERVICAL CESAREAN SECTION. SUTURE OF WOUND.

While waiting for the placenta, bleeding sinuses in the wound are clamped with Allis or tongue forceps (Fig. 418a, p. 508). A few stitches may also be applied, but not tied. After the uterus is packed, the sides of the wound are raised up with Allis forceps. In the picture only two are shown—six or ten may be necessary to clamp vessels. The corner retractor (Fig. 686) provides good exposure. Interrupted sutures, No. 2 twenty-day catgut, 1 cm. apart or closer if needful to stop bleeding, going down to, but not through the mucosa, and not taking in the fascia. Exceptionally where haste is required a continuous suture is used.

Postoperative complications are much rarer than after the corporeal section. Particularly are ileus, gastric dilatation, and peritonitis conspicuously absent. This is because the spill is so well controlled, because there was so little exposure and manipulation of the peritoneum, and none of the gut or omentum; because the uterine closure is in the cervix, accurately coapted, *at rest during the healing process*, and thickly covered by fascia and peritoneum—almost absolutely preventing seepage of lochia. Visualize the fundus uteri, heavy, contracting and relaxing, making excursions all over the abdomen, and imagine a leaky wound in it!

Adhesions are very seldom left, for the same reasons, and rupture of the uterus in subsequent labor is much rarer than after the classical operation, there being only 23 cases reported up to date. This is because the cervix heals better than the fundus, being undisturbed by the uterine contractions.

The maternal mortality of the cervical operations is less than the classic. We have done 1100 at the Chicago Lying-in Hospital, with only 15 deaths, and many of these cases were unfavorable ones. Eight of the deaths were not due to the operation—eclampsia, tuberculous meningitis, abruptio placentæ, diabetes, etc.

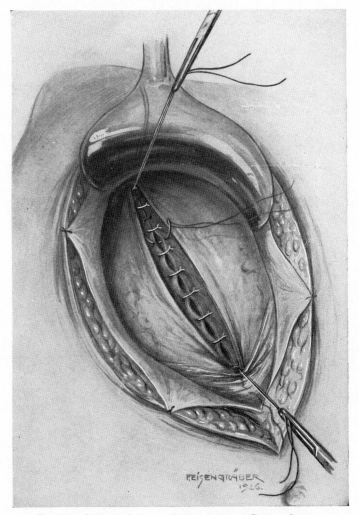

Fig. 904.—Cervical Cesarean Section. Second Row of Suture.
A second row of apposition sutures is now applied; No. 1 twenty-day catgut. Careful not to catch the gauze in any stitch!

One of the greatest advantages of laparotrachelotomy is that it may be performed after the woman has had a real test of labor. The mortality of the classic section increases with every hour the woman has had pains, and especially if the membranes are ruptured (Routh). Being able, safely, to give the woman a good test of labor, many operations will be avoided, since nature often surprises with a normal delivery when dystocia was predicted. We are doing laparotrachelotomy in cases where the classic would not be considered, e. g., after a few attempts with forceps have been made, after several vaginal examinations, and even when there is a slight possibility of infection.

Extraperitoneal Cesarean Section.—Access to the lower uterine segment is gained by a dissection similar to that for ligation of the external iliac artery, and a knowledge of the anatomy of the spaces of Retzius and of Bogros is essential.

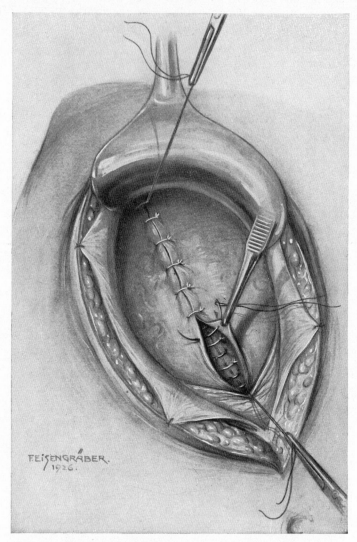

FIG. 905.—CERVICAL CESAREAN SECTION. THE IMPORTANT FASCIAL SUTURE.

Now the fascia over the lower uterine segment is reunited with a special interrupted suture so placed that the edge of one side overlaps that on the other ½ cm. Occasionally a superficial vein bleeds and requires a mattress-suture (No. 0 plain catgut). The bladder end of the suture is kept as a tractor to lift the tissues out of the depths of the wound until all oozing has been perfectly stanched.

Of true extraperitoneal operations that devised by Latzko is the best. The reader is referred to the illustrations (Figs. 908–912).

Contrary to the transperitoneal method, the true extraperitoneal is not an easy operation, since the pushing of the bladder off the uterus and raising the peritoneum from its attachments are sometimes very difficult. The longer the pains have acted, the more the uterus has pulled itself off the bladder, and the easier becomes the separation. It is just the cases of prolonged labor where the operation is most useful. Küstner injured the bladder in 7 per cent. of his cases; ureteral fistula,

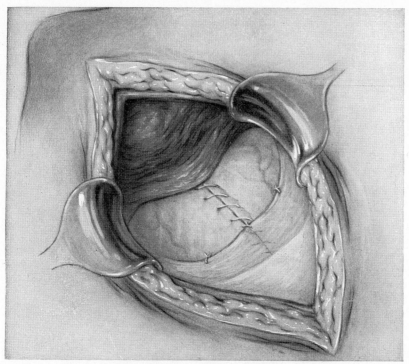

FIG. 906.—CERVICAL CESAREAN SECTION. ANCHORING THE UPPER FLAP.

Now the upper flap of peritoneum is pulled down over the fascia and fastened with a few small single stitches.

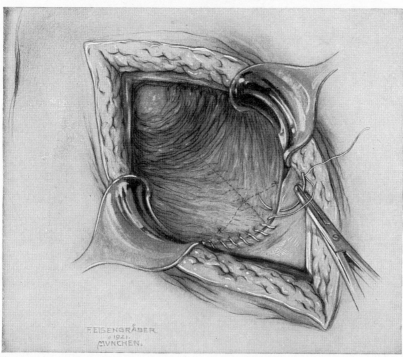

FIG. 907.—CERVICAL CESAREAN SECTION.

Finally the bladder flap is raised up and sewed with a continuous No. 1 twenty-day catgut, burying the knot under the peritoneum, leaving a hardly visible line of suture which the bladder, when filled, completely hides. In clean cases the two peritoneal flaps are not overlapped but reunited where cut. The peritoneal toilet is very simple. Usually intestines and omentum have not been seen. Drainage is not needed.

hemorrhage from the large vessels in the broad ligaments, thrombosis, and a high fetal mortality have been reported. Bumm tore the peritoneum in one-third of his operations. Nevertheless, Küstner and Bumm together report 226 cases, with 4 maternal deaths, less than 2 per cent., again a marvelous showing, because many of Küstner's cases were frankly septic and half were suspicious.

At present the adherents of the cervical operations are divided in opinion as to which method, the extra- or the intraperitoneal, is the best, with the honors of discussion about even. Does the pelvic peritoneum care for an infectious spill as well as or better than the pelvic connective tissue? Are the results in extraperitoneal operating in suspect and infected cases (the only ones where it is considered) really better than laparotrachelotomy? We cannot enter the controversy here. Only years of experience can decide. My opinion is firm—laparotrachelotomy for all but those where infection is suspected, then Latzko's operation, Porro, or craniotomy.

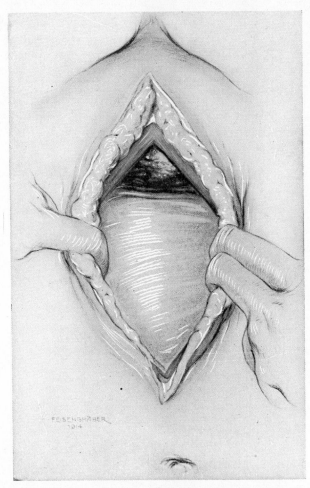

FIG. 908.—LATZKO EXTRAPERITONEAL CESAREAN SECTION.

Trendelenburg position. Bladder filled with 150 c.c. sterile water, the catheter, clamped, remaining in place. Bladder appears at top of wound; after thorough orientation the water is let out, the catheter left in place. Incision beginning at the pubis to about 2 inches from navel, a fingerbreadth left of the median line, down *to* the peritoneum. Great care not to puncture the latter. Space of Retzius exposed. By deeper and more lateral dissection the spatium Bogrosi is opened.

The strongest appeal the new operations make is their claim that through them craniotomy on the living child may be abolished. Unfortunately this is not true. Parturients are sent to our hospitals, lacerated and infected, with the child dying or so injured that it dies soon after birth. In the frankly infected case and where many attempts at delivery have been made, no cesarean is safe, though Küstner says that the extraperitoneal method may still be used. Where the infection is apparently mild or only suspected, Latzko's operation competes with the Porro cesarean, and in young women it may be done unless the conditions demand craniotomy; in older mothers of many children a Porro is preferable. Unfortunately there is no scientific means of telling if there are dangerously infective organisms in the parturient canal.

Cesarean Section on the Dying or Dead Woman.—A fetus will live from five to twenty minutes after the death of its mother. Reported cases of longer periods are not authenticated. The length of time of survival depends on the suddenness of the mother's death, the child living longer if she dies of apoplexy, accident, hemorrhage, eclampsia, or very acute affection than if the agony is prolonged, as in tuberculosis, heart disease, etc., though in some of the latter cases the vitality

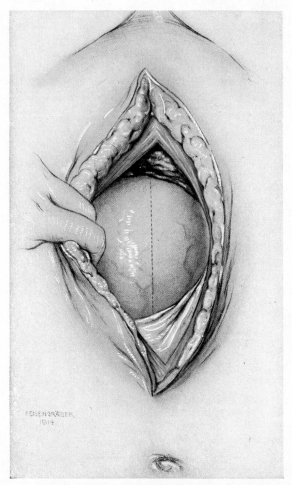

Fig. 909.—Latzko Extraperitoneal Cesarean Section.

Vesico-uterine plica is gently pushed upward and medially, while the bladder is worked downward and to the right of the lower uterine segment. Be sure you have the deepest part of the vesico-uterine fold. The first whitish fold is not it. After the lower uterine segment is freed for a small space the rest of the denudation is easy—careful at the top. Separate at the side as little as possible to avoid the large vessels and ureter, in the space of Bogros.

of the child is remarkable. Since the mother uses up the child's oxygen, the latter usually dies first. Even before Numa Pompilius, attempts to save the child by cesarean section after the death of its mother were made, but the results were so poor that most men discountenanced the procedure. In recent times the operation has often been done, and the results are more encouraging. If the pregnancy has advanced beyond the twenty-sixth week, no delay is to be allowed after life is positively extinct, but the belly opened at once. It is not even necessary, legally

70

to obtain the consent of the husband or the family, though for his own protection the accoucheur should get it if possible. Bacon, of Chicago, in 1911 proved this. Nor should precious minutes be lost trying to hear the heart-tones, because several children have been saved when they were inaudible. (See Remy, Fallon and Wyder, Lit., Neumann.)

The Talmudists and the Catholic law demand that cesarean section be performed on the dying woman to save the child, but this operation, painful to all concerned, has rarely been done. If the woman's death is only a matter of a few

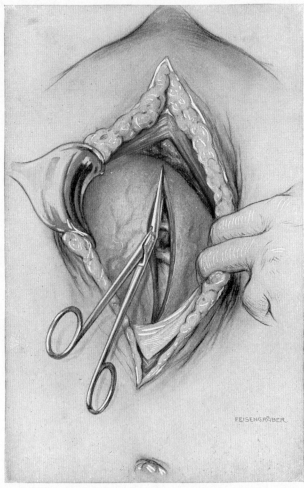

FIG. 910.—LATZKO EXTRAPERITONEAL CESAREAN SECTION.
Guided by the fingers, the thin lower uterine segment is incised. Avoid sharp retractors and too violent lateral pulling.

hours, this being the opinion of a consultation of physicians, and the child is living and viable, the operation is indicated, but here, legally, it is needful to get the written consent of the husband or the next of kin. In practice it may be required to prepare for the operation, and, awaiting the woman's death, to watch the heart-tones, operating before death only if the child shows signs of distress. Naturally, if conditions are right for a quick delivery from below, this is preferable. In Strassburg a woman with mitral disease was operated on, supposedly in agony, but it was only catalepsy, and she recovered. Operate aseptically!

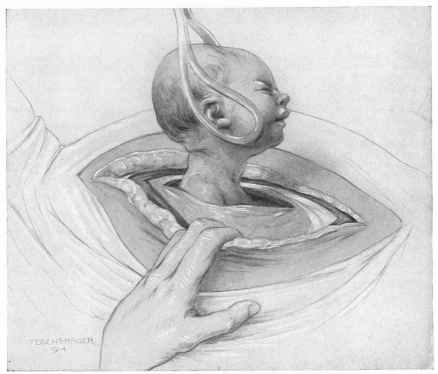

FIG. 911.—LATZKO EXTRAPERITONEAL CESAREAN SECTION.

Table horizontal. The head is pulled into position for forceps either by means of a finger in the mouth and the child delivered as in face presentation, or a vulsellum is fastened to the occiput and thus the head steadied for the application of the blades. Deliver slowly. If necessary to enlarge the uterine incision, do it under the eye. A tear would extend toward the side where are the ureter, large veins, and the uterine artery. The placenta may be removed manually or expressed by Credé. If needed, an injection of pituitrin may be given into the uterine muscle.

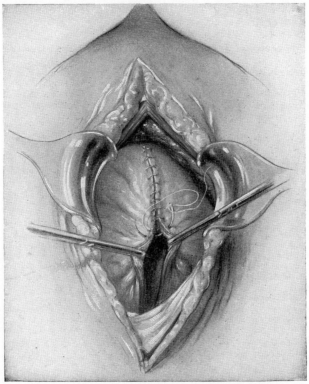

FIG. 912.—LATZKO EXTRAPERITONEAL CESAREAN SECTION.

Uterine suture. I always put in three rows. Now draw the peritoneum down, bring the bladder into position, and fasten it with a few sutures. Leave a rubber drain in the lowest corner of wound. Abdominal closure.

THE GOTTSCHALK-PORTES OPERATION

In 1909, and again in 1911, Gottschalk of Berlin recommended a two-stage cesarean with the object of preserving the uterus when the woman is infected. Independently, in 1924, Portes of Paris, thought out and performed an identical operation. It is very simple. The unopened uterus is delivered, the abdomen closed, watertight, around the cervix, the child and placenta are removed, the aperture sutured, and the mass, covered by moist dressings, is exteriorized for four or more weeks, *i. e.*, until the infection is gone. Now the belly is reopened and the clean, involuted uterus is replaced (Fig. 912a).

About 100 cases are on record up to date with a mortality of 11 per cent. Four women have since had live babies by cesarean section. I have had no personal experience with this innovation as yet, and I think some of the reported cases were thus treated, experimenti causa, but the idea is attractive and soon its worth will be demonstrated. I would be inclined to leave the uterus un-

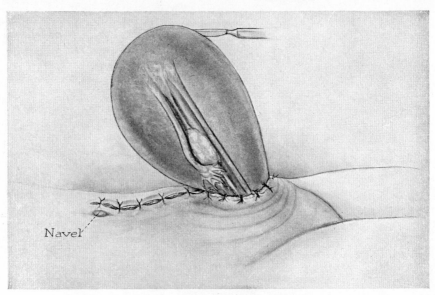

FIG. 912a.—GOTTSCHALK-PORTES OPERATION.
Side view. Abdomen is protected from the spill by towels and large rubber dam.

sutured (if there is no bleeding) to get the advantage of free drainage of the infected uterine wall —an idea Chaput suggested for the treatment of puerperal infection.

If Gottschalk-Portes' procedure proves successful we shall have to rewrite the indications for treatment of infected labors. It will restrict Porro's operation to multiparæ and give us another alternative to craniotomy on the living child. (Lit. Phaneuf, Latzko.)

LITERATURE

Bacon: Trans. Chic. Gyn. Soc., 1911.—*Chaput:* Presse méd., Paris, February 15, 1917, p. 94.—*Cholmogoroff:* Zent. f. Gyn., 1911, p. 743, and Arch. f. Gyn., 1911, vol. cxv, Heft 1, p. 23. Gives literature of rupture of cesarean section scars.—*DeLee:* Amer. Jour. Obst. and Gyn., October, 1925, vol. x, No. 4.—*Fallon:* Boston Med. and Surg. Jour., November 11, 1926, p. 929.—*Gall:* Gyn. et Obst., Paris, 1925, No. 1, p. 24.—*Gottschalk:* Verhand. d. Deutsch. Gesell. für Gyn., 1911, Bd. xiv, p. 651.—*Holland:* London Lancet, September 18, 1920.—*Küstner:* Zentb. für Gyn., 1914, No. 10.—*Ibid.:* Der Abdominale Kaiserschnitt, Zentb. für Gyn., 1915, No. 31. Complete literature.—*Ibid.:* July 4, 1932, p. 882.—*Latzko:* Zeitschr. für Gyn., November 28, 1931, p. 3470.—*Lewis:* Amer. Jour. Obst., October, 1909, p. 587.—*Madlener:* Zentb. für Gyn., 1926, p. 219.—*Miller, Justin:* American Bar Ass'n. Jour., March, 1930, p. 158.—*Neumann:* Zeitschr. für Geb. u. Gyn., 1929, xciv, Heft 3, p. 749.—*Nicholson:* Surg., Gyn., and Obst., February, 1914, p. 245.—*Phaneuf:* Surg., Gyn., and Obst., June, 1927, p. 788.—*Portes:* Bull. de Soc., de Gyn. et Obst., Paris, 1924, No. 3.—*Remy:* Arch. de Tocologie, vol. xxi, p. 819.—*Rigby:* System of Midwifery, 1841, p. 249.—*Routh:* "Cesarean Section," Jour. Obstet. and Gyn., British Empire, January, 1911.—*Sante:* Jour. Amer. Med. Assoc., May 14, 1927, p. 1539.—*Schilling:* Iowa State Med. Jour., November, 1923.—*Spalding:* "Cesarean Section Scars," Jour. Amer. Med. Assoc., December 1, 1917, p. 1850. See also Amer. Jour. Obstet., December, 1916. Literature.—*Stoeckel:* Jahreskurse für Ärtzl. Fortbildung, July, 1916, p. 27.—*Winckel:* "Cesarean Section on the Dead and Dying," Artliche Rundschau, 1892, No. 5.—*Wyder:* Arch. f. Gyn., vol. lxxxii, pp. 725 and 771.—*Wyss:* Quoted by Wolff, Zeitschr. f. Geb. u. Gyn., 1914, p. 742.

CHAPTER LXXIII

MUTILATING OPERATIONS ON THE CHILD

UNDER this caption will be considered the operations which reduce the bulk of the child. Lessened in size, it can be easier gotten through the parturient canal. Embryotomy would be a good general term for all the procedures, but it has been given a particular significance.

Craniotomy is an operation which consists in opening the fetal head, the evacuation of the brain, and extraction by means of a large bone forceps or a sharp hook.

Perforation is the first step in craniotomy, but is sometimes applied to the whole operation.

Cranioclasis is the third step in the operation, and is also sometimes applied to the whole operation. The instrument, which is nothing more nor less than a large, strong, especially constructed bone forceps, is called a cranioclast.

Cephalotrypsis is an operation in which the head is crushed by means of a powerful forceps supplied with a compression screw, no perforation of the head being made. The instrument is called a cephalotryptor, and was invented by Baudelocque, the nephew. It is an obsolete operation.

Decapitation means what it says,—amputation of the head,—and is accomplished either by means of a blunt hook or a sickle-knife, the écraseur, or scissors.

Embryotomy is applied to decapitation, to the section of the fetal trunk, or to the opening of the body cavities.

Exenteration means disemboweling the fetus to diminish the size of the trunk. It is the same as evisceration.

Brachiotomy means section of an arm.

Cleidotomy is an operation done by Ferondi in 1877 and introduced by Herbert Spencer in 1895. It consists of section of the clavicles, and is used when the shoulders are too broad to pass, the head being delivered and the child dead.

Spondylotomy is section of the spinal column.

Before forceps and version were known, removal of the child piecemeal was the only means the ancients had of accomplishing delivery in cases of mechanical obstruction. Fig. 913 shows some of their crude instruments. Until 1830 the sharp hook was mostly used for extraction, and it tore through the bladder and rectum as often as it safely delivered the head.

Craniotomy.—*Indications*—(A) *On the Dead Child.*—No accoucheur should have any compunctions about mutilating a dead child, yet I have seen the most atrocious operations carried out by physicians in order to avoid the necessity of perforating a piece of lifeless clay. Either they fear opprobrium, or they overrate the dangers of craniotomy. Craniotomy is chosen, the fetus being dead, when an indication arises for the immediate termination of labor. Craniotomy is less dangerous than the forceps, especially if the child is large, the pelvis small, or the soft parts unprepared. It is the rule for hydrocephalus. Sentimental reasons advanced by the family should not stand in the way of the accoucheur's doing the best for the mother.

When the child is surely dead, even if there is no indication for the immediate termination of labor, perforation of the cranium and reduction of its size may be desirable. This is true of primiparæ—we wish to save the levator ani and pelvic outlet from overstretching, and, further, it is thus possible to shorten the time of labor. It would perhaps be best in such cases to perforate the cranium, evacuate

1109

a large part of the brain, and leave the expulsion to nature. In private practice, unless the family is intelligent, objections will be raised to the disfigurement of the child, or even its death may be ascribed to the attendant. In delivery of the after-coming head, the fetus having died, hurry should cease, and the head be perforated. It is not wise to delay too long, since much blood may accumulate behind the head.

(B) *When the child is living*, the indication for craniotomy is dreadfully hard

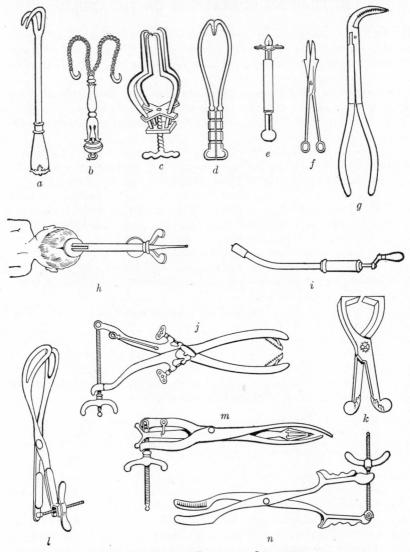

FIG. 913.—TYPES OF DESTRUCTIVE INSTRUMENTS.

a, Ambroise Paré; *b*, Andre de la Croix; *c*, Ambroise Paré; *d*, Levret; *e*, Burton's perforator; *f*, Smellie's scissors; *g*, Meigs; *h*, Mauriceau; *i*, trephine of Braun; *j*, Pajot; *k*, Ambroise Paré; *l*, Lusk's cephalotribe; *m*, Tarnier's basiotribe (recommendable); *n*, C. Braun's cranioclast.

to place. Nowhere in all medicine does so heavy a responsibility rest on the medical attendant. He is judge, jury, and, perhaps, executioner of an innocent baby, and he can hardly be blamed if he shrinks from the painful task. It is imperative to have consultation whenever the question of craniotomy on the living fetus arises. The decision will rest not alone on scientific grounds, as we shall show directly.

In practice, craniotomy will come up for consideration in cases of moderately contracted pelves, in incorrigible occipitoposterior positions, face and brow presentations, when the child has suffered much from injudicious operating and tumors blocking the passage. Regarding the course of conduct of contracted pelves, the reader is referred to the appropriate chapter. The conditions almost always met are these: The woman has been in labor many hours or even days, unclean hands have frequently examined her, attempts at delivery with the forceps have failed, the vulva is torn and bruised, the cervix hangs in shreds, the urine is bloody, the child is injured or perhaps dying. Here there is only one course—craniotomy. The responsibility for the death of the child rests on those who conducted the labor up to this point. On the other hand, if the woman is not injured, not infected, and the child is in perfect condition one is not justified, at least from a scientific point of view, in doing craniotomy.

Pinard and a few Catholic authors demand the abolition of craniotomy on the living child, but the overwhelming majority of obstetric authorities declares this extreme position untenable. All, however, agree that the necessity for destroying the child is less and less frequent as the diagnosis of spacial disproportion is earlier discovered, giving a chance for cesarean section and pubiotomy. It follows, therefore, that craniotomy will be more frequently performed in home practice. In a good maternity the necessity for sacrificing the babe will be of the rarest occurrence. For centuries craniotomy was the opprobrium of obstetric science. It is this no longer in the science, but remains such in obstetric practice. The newer methods of cesarean section bid fair to bring the necessity for craniotomy on the living child almost to the vanishing point.

Legally, the mother has a right to demand that she be exposed to no unusual danger for the sake of her child, and she may refuse to do so even at the request of her husband. Also, she has the right, even if opposed by her husband, to run added risk for its sake if she wishes. The legal status of the unborn child is still unsettled (Kiernan). At present it is part of its mother, and has no legal existence until the cord is cut. The mother may recover damages for its loss by wilful or negligent means, though itself it has no redress if it survives the injury. The moral and ethical aspects of the question are too broad to be more than mentioned here. The stand of the Catholic Church has been alluded to,—"Non Occides!"—and in such families the attendant is guided by the word of the priest, who is always to be summoned. If the accoucheur is convinced that the cesarean section demanded would kill the mother, he may retire from the case. On the other hand, if the family insists on the sacrifice of the child, when the accoucheur feels that there are good chances for a successful cesarean section, he should likewise decline, but, legally, he must stay by the patient until another qualified practitioner has assumed charge.

Is consent of the patient or next of kin necessary? Legally, yes—indeed, the attendant could be held for malpractice if the mother suffered injury from an operation less safe than a craniotomy, performed without her consent. The facts of the particular case are to be laid, unvarnished, before the family for decision, which is their right. Here much depends on the ability of the accoucheur in prognosis, for he has to evaluate the condition of the mother and of the babe and to foretell their probable chances of life and health, admittedly a very difficult and delicate task. After all, the family will usually rely on the accoucheur's judgment, and he will be immensely aided and comforted by adherence to the Golden Rule.

After craniotomy it is the accoucheur's bounden duty to warn the family that the next labor should be so conducted that a child-life saving operation may be done. A second craniotomy is criminal.

In posterior occiput positions not amenable to the usual treatment, and where the forceps fail, craniotomy may be necessary, if the patient is at home far from competent help. Forced forceps deliveries here, as well as in face and brow presentations with the chin posterior, are equivalent to craniotomies as far as the child is concerned, but have not the saving grace of the latter in sparing the woman from serious, often fatal, mutilations. Let no man pride himself on having accomplished a hard operative delivery with a whole but dead child. Let him ask himself if craniotomy had not been more humane. In the well-equipped maternity laparotrachelotomy will usually help out such a distressful situation.

Craniotomy is not a good operation when a tumor is impacted in the pelvis. Necrosis of the tumor often ensues.

Conditions.—The pelvis may not be too contracted. Barnes believed it possible to deliver a mutilated fetus through a conjugata vera of less than 2 inches, but most authors place the limit at 6.2 cm. for flat and 6.5 cm. for generally contracted pelves. Naturally, these figures must be raised if the child is of unusual size or hardness. The cervix must be well dilated or easily dilatable—the more, the better.

Technic.—In addition to the special instruments for craniotomy, all those used in a forceps operation should be boiled. Naegelè's perforator (Fig. 914) is one of the best, but the trephine makes a larger opening in the skull, and the vagina is less likely to be injured by spiculæ of bone, which is also true of the rubber gloves of the accoucheur (Fig. 915). For crushing the perforated head the best instrument is Zweifel's cranioclast (Fig. 916). It has three blades, and while more difficult to apply than the generally recommended Carl Braun instrument, it does better work.

The head is steadied by an assistant from the outside, or seized by means of a

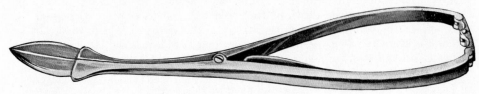

FIG. 914.—NAEGELÈ'S PERFORATOR.

strong vulsellum forceps sunk into the scalp. In some cases I hold it with the obstetric forceps. Under cover of the whole hand the perforator is introduced and applied to the most accessible portion of the head, care being taken that it does not glance off, which advice is to be specially heeded when the cutting perforator is

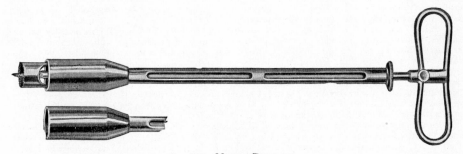

FIG. 915.—MARTIN TREPHINE.
Made more easily cleansable by the author.

used (Fig. 918). It is also possible to expose the head by specula and do the operation by sight. After the opening is made, one finger is hooked into it, then the brain matter is thoroughly broken up by means of a long forceps, taking special care to tear the tentorium and destroy the medulla, this to avoid the painful experience of seeing the child gasp after delivery. Two cases are recorded where the child lived a while in spite of the mutilation. Now the cranium is washed out with a stream of sterilized water, an operation facilitated by the cannula shown in Fig. 917. The third step of the operation is crushing the empty skull. The middle blade of the cranioclast is introduced through the opening in the cranial vault and bored into the base of the skull, until it is solidly fixed here, with its convexity, indicated by a little sign on the handle, directed toward the face. In order to insert this blade properly one must depress the perineum strongly, and one obtains the securest hold by screwing it into the foramen magnum. The head being thus steadied the first outer blade is laid over the face, in a manner similar to the application of forceps. By means of the compression screw the two are brought slowly together, *but after they are locked and before they are tightened the accoucheur should assure himself that nothing is caught in the grasp of the jaws.* When the handles are in contact, the two are locked with the hasp, then the third blade applied and also screwed down tight. The fourth act—extraction—is done with the same care and gentleness as the forceps operation, and the proper mechanism of labor should be followed. There is no occasion for hurry. Frequent examinations are made to determine if the head is following, to preserve the parts from injury by spiculæ of bone, which may be sharp and piercing, and to aid in stripping the cervix back over the head. If the instrument is well applied, it will not slip off. Spiculæ or sharp edges of bone are removed by means of the Mesnard-Stein forceps (Fig. 919). The perineum is to be preserved by slow delivery—at least, the woman should be spared the injury of this structure.

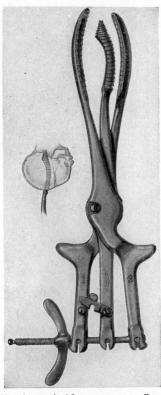

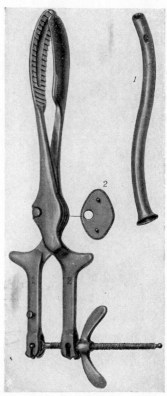

FIG. 916.—AUTHOR'S MODIFICATION OF ZWEIFEL'S CRANIOCLAST.

Little sketch shows how the center blade is bored into base of skull to hold the head, while the outside, crushing blades of the cranioclast, are applied and screwed together.

FIG. 917.—AUTHOR'S MODIFICATION OF ZWEIFEL'S CRANIOCLAST.

The same instrument as Fig. 916, used as a cephalotribe after being assembled by means of the little plate, 2. The cannula at the side is for breaking up and evacuating the brain. A rubber catheter is pushed through it and the cavity irrigated with a forcible stream of sterile water.

In many cases, after the head is delivered, the shoulders are arrested. It is not prudent to use force. The size of the shoulder-girdle is reduced by the operation of **cleidotomy.** One hand searches for the more accessible of the two clavicles, and under the guidance of this hand the tip of the decapitation scissors is passed to a point on the neck of the child adjacent to it. With tiny snipping motions the points of the scissors are pushed under the skin of the neck, and, guided by the fingers, a clavicle is reached and cut. The other is treated the same way. It is now possible to deliver the trunk of the child. In very exceptional cases the sternum must be bisected and the chest emptied—this in cases of monsters or anasarca. If delivery of the trunk still causes difficulty, one arm may be brought down and traction made on it, or, better, the blunt hook is passed into the axilla and combined traction made on it and the head.

If the craniotomy is performed in face presentation, the perforation is made through the glabella or through one eye, using the Naegelè instrument.

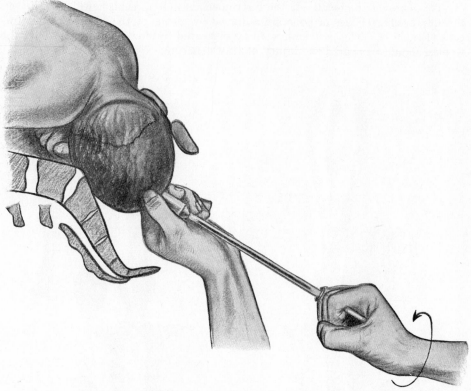

FIG. 918.—PERFORATION WITH TREPHINE.

In all cases, as soon as the mouth of the child is accessible, the throat is to be stuffed full of wet cotton, because sometimes the elasticity of the chest causes the

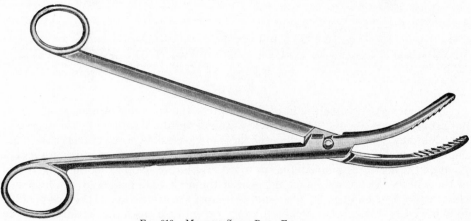

FIG. 919.—MESNARD-STEIN BONE FORCEPS.

child to make a sort of inspiration which the bystanders mistake for a gasp and evidence of life.

Craniotomy on Aftercoming Head.—One may puncture the skull through either the roof of the mouth or the occipital plate. I prefer the former as it helps break up the massive base of the skull, and does not disfigure the head. The jaw is pulled down, and the Naegelè perforator is slowly bored through the hard palate; by spreading the instrument and twisting it around in all directions a large hole is reamed out. After breaking up the brain with a long forceps it is easy to wash

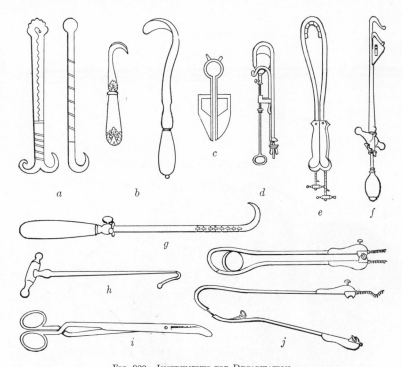

FIG. 920.—INSTRUMENTS FOR DECAPITATION.

a, Arabian; b, Ambroise Paré; c, Abulcasis; d, Baudelocque; e, Van der Ecken; f, Tarnier's embryotome; g, Jacquemier; h, Braun's hook; i, Dubois scissors; j, Ribemont Dessaignes' chain saw.

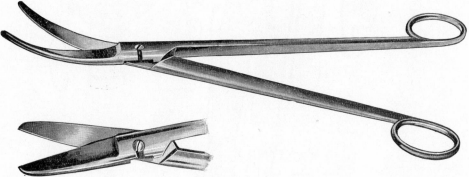

FIG. 921.—DECAPITATION SCISSORS.

it out with a douche. A few tractions are made to see if the collapsed head will follow. Perhaps it is too hard to collapse.

The solid blade of the cranioclast is inserted through the opening in the skull, and another laid over the face. While desirable it is not usually possible to put on the third blade. If extraction fails with two blades (rare), the body of the child must be got out of the way to provide room for the insertion of the third blade. First the skin of the neck is cut all around to make a cuff for the protection of the mother's soft parts in all subsequent manipulations; this cuff is pushed up and the spine severed near the head by means of heavy Siebold scissors. The head is now readily accessible.

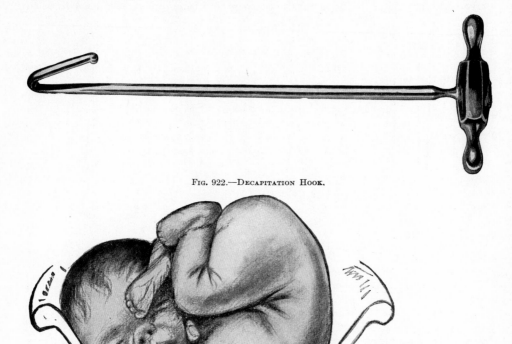

FIG. 922.—DECAPITATION HOOK.

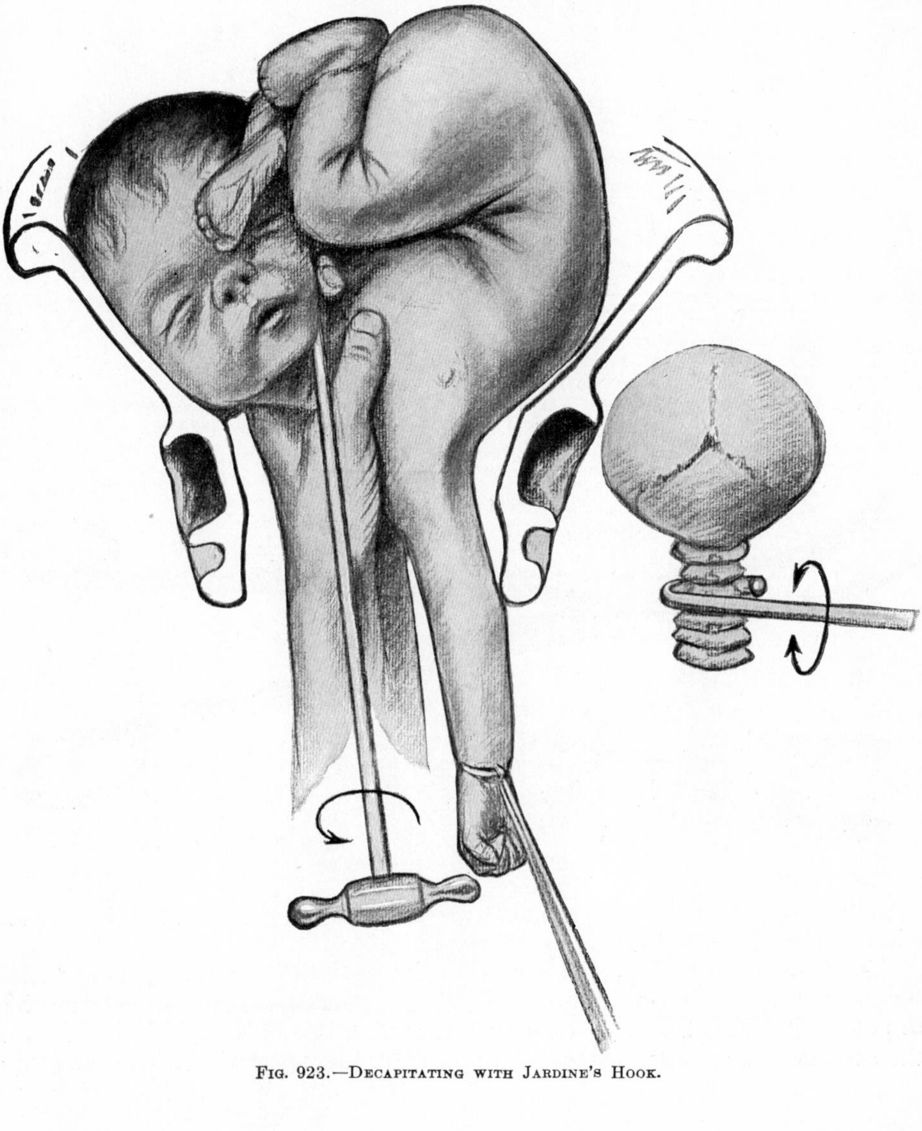

FIG. 923.—DECAPITATING WITH JARDINE'S HOOK.

It has been advised to decapitate the child as routine, after perforation, then to seize the stump with powerful vulsellæ and with the head thus securely held, to apply the cranioclast or cephalothryptor. It is good to know an alternative procedure, since this operation is occasionally very laborious.

Decapitation.—Hippocrates did decapitations, using a curved knife. It is the rarest of all operations, nowadays, owing to the general improvement of obstetric practice. Neglected transverse presentation is the usual indication, but sometimes it is needed to decapitate the first of interlocked twins, and, still more rarely, in the treatment of double monsters. The conditions for the operation are the same as for craniotomy, and the same question will arise as to the propriety of performing it when the child lives. In neglected transverse presentations, however, it is most exceptional for the child to be found alive. Of prime importance in these cases is an accurate knowledge of the state of the uterus. If the lower uterine segment is excessively thinned, indeed, on the point of rupturing, decapitation should be superseded by evisceration, because this operation will not increase the distention—rather the opposite. If the shoulder is wedged deeply into the excavation, the neck being stretched almost parallel with the long axis of the fetal body, evisceration is a better procedure and requires no special instruments. If the neck is readily accessible and the uterus not dangerously thinned, decapitation is a very satisfactory operation. Figure 920 shows some of the instruments used for severing the neck. Carl Braun's hook has been modified by Jardine by making the inside somewhat sharp—an improvement. I have usually performed the operation as here described, all under the guidance of the hand, but I can see advantages in doing it with the aid of sight, the field being exposed by broad specula and the neck being pulled down with the hook or powerful vulsella.

Decapitation with the saw, illustrated in Fig. 920, *j*, is a more surgical and a safer procedure (the thinned out lower uterine segment is not endangered by twisting the head), but the instrument is available only in large maternities.

First Act.—To make the neck more readily reached, traction is put on the arm. Passing the whole hand into the vagina, the neck is encircled by two fingers and the thumb. Guided by the latter, the hook is passed over the neck, where it is firmly pulled into the soft parts. No attempt to twist should be made until the hook is well placed and the fingers are apposed to the thumb, thus encircling the neck and guarding the mother's tissues from injury. Now the handle is twisted, slowly pulling at the same time, turning the knob in the direction of the head. The first half-turn breaks the cervical spine, after which the hook takes a deeper hold on the muscles, and a full turn severs these. The skin now remains, and this is packed into the hook by means of the fingers, and a few complete turns cut it with the cleanness of a knife. Sometimes a few tough shreds must be severed with the scissors (Fig. 921).

Second Act.—Extraction of the trunk is made on the prolapsed arm; only rarely is it necessary to open the chest or apply the hook to the trunk. The neck must be covered by the fingers during delivery to protect the vagina from being pierced by spiculæ of bone.

Third Act.—Delivery of the head is accomplished by expression from above, traction on the jaw from below, or, if need be, by forceps or even craniotomy. In the latter instance the head must be firmly fixed either by the forceps or by strong vulsella. Sharp projections of bone may do much damage if unobserved.

Evisceration.—In cases of arrested delivery of the child, in conduplicatio corpore (see p. 664) the neck is inaccessible to the hook or the scissors. Exenteration is the best operation. A large hole is made in the chest with the scissors, several ribs being resected. With the fingers the entrails are pulled out—first out of the chest, then, after boring through the diaphragm, out of the abdomen. Usually the body collapses, and the child can be easily extracted, but if there is the least resistance, the spinal column should be cut through with the scissors (spondylotomy), a perfectly safe procedure, since the instrument operates inside the body of the child, the maternal soft parts being protected. Now the extraction may be made by pulling on the arm or pulling down the feet of the child, or by hooking the blunt hook over the spinal column.

Bi-sectio Feti.—Very difficult, and fortunately very rarely needed is embryotomy in breech labors.   The delivery of a large fetus can tax the ingenuity and strength of a most capable accoucheur.   Naturally a mammoth child would require section, a Porro.   Aimless hacking at the mass will accomplish nothing and probably force the attendant to the conviction that cesarean section is the only way out, but there is a safer and better one.

Disarticulate one leg at the hip; draw down firmly on the other, split the pelvis along the spinal column delivering the small half; pulling on the spine via the leg, bring the liver into reach, exenterate abdomen; perforate the diaphragm; eviscerate chest; bisect chest; bring down one arm and amputate, if necessary taking part of the chest; bring down other arm; craniotomy.   During this long operation the maternal soft parts are protected by broad flat specula and by cutting inside a cuff made of the skin of the fetus.

In concluding the author cannot refrain from sounding a warning.   Every hospital should have a complete set of destructive instruments.   They are, in effect, constructive.   Often, for the want of them, or a man skilful enough to use them, cesarean section is performed.   As these cases are always the protracted, the neglected, the botched, the infected labors, the mortality of the mothers is frightful.

LITERATURE

Ferondi: Zentralb. für Gyn., 1912, p. 599.—*Kerr:* Operative Midwifery.—*Kiernan:* The Alienist and Neurologist, May, 1911.—*Spencer:* Personal communication, 1913.—*Stratz:* Zeitschr. für Geb. u. Gyn., 1915, p. 724.

CHAPTER LXXIV

INDUCTION OF PREMATURE LABOR

THIS means the artificial interruption of pregnancy, after the child has become viable, but before term. Louise Bourgoise, midwife to Mary of Medici, in 1608 introduced the operation of inducing labor prematurely as a therapeutic measure. Smellie did it in 1756, and in 1793 Denman reported 20 cases of induced premature labor for contracted pelvis. In all probability, according to Kleinwächter, the ancient Greeks performed abortion for the same reason. Soranus, of Ephesus, in the second century, mentions it.

Indications.—There is hardly any condition affecting the pregnant woman that may not give the indication for emptying the uterus. The most common are—first, contracted pelvis, the idea being that a small fetus will pass through easily; and, second, diseases which affect the health of the woman so deeply that it is feared she will not survive until term, or that the inroads on her constitution will be such as materially to shorten her life. The indications may be grouped under five headings: 1. Contracted pelvis. 2. Diseases which are incidental to pregnancy. 3. Diseases accidental to pregnancy. 4. Habitual death of the fetus after viability, but before term. 5. Prolonged pregnancy and overgrowth of the child.

For contracted pelvis see p. 769. Under diseases incidental to pregnancy see the chapters on Eclampsia, Toxemia, Chorea, Pernicious Vomiting, Pernicious Anemia, Placenta Prævia, Abruptio Placentæ, Psychoses, Multiple Neuritis, Impetigo Herpetiformis, Polyhydramnion, Hydatidiform Mole, etc. The keynote of the treatment is to stop the gestation at a point before either mother or child, or both, are in danger, either to life or to health.

Under diseases accidental to pregnancy see the chapters on Bright's Disease, Tuberculosis, especially of larynx, Heart Disease, Diabetes, Retinitis, Psychoses.

A very interesting condition is the habitual death of the child after viability, but before term. In apparently healthy women successive children die, either just before labor or directly after. Sometimes the boys die, the girls live. The causes are mostly unknown. Syphilis is the most common, and my practise is, even if no history of the same is forthcoming, and even if the seroreaction of both parents is negative, to submit both to a mild mercurial treatment. An occasional success has encouraged me to continue this plan. During pregnancy this pill is administered three times daily: Hydrargyri iodidi rubri, gr. $\frac{1}{20}$; Ferri carbonatis, gr. iij; Acidi arseniosi, gr. $\frac{1}{50}$. Bright's disease in a latent form explains a few cases; anemia and constitutional disorders, diabetes, avitaminosis, and hypothyroidism a few more. Smith says hypothyroidism causes still-births in sows. Infection of the decidua and ovum from a distant focus (e. g., tonsil, teeth), without doubt, may kill the fetus and thus terminate successive pregnancies, as I pointed out many years ago (See Lit.). Often enough no cause can be found. Without doubt, the husband is sometimes to blame, and I am convinced that some men cannot produce a spermatozoid capable of giving the normal ovum sufficient life impetus to carry it through a full gestation. This has been observed in alcoholism, lead-poisoning, in tobacco-workers, x-ray operators, and even without apparent reason. The rôle of bacteria issuing from pus pockets in the male urethra and reaching per coitum the ovum has not yet been studied. The treatment of such cases is causal, and

1119

in addition to this good results have been observed in a complete reversal of the usual mode of life. For example, a man overloaded with business cares may be sent, with his wife, to spend six months in camp on the plains or in the mountains.

If the exact time when the children usually die is known, labor may be brought on a few weeks before this. In some of these cases every alternate child dies, or the habit is broken up from some cause or other. It will be noticed that this indication is precarious, but most authors allow it.

Prolonged Pregnancy and Overgrowth of the Child.—Some women habitually go over the usual period of pregnancy, and not seldom the child dies or suffers so much during delivery that it succumbs shortly after. In these cases the cranium is usually hard and angular, the bones stiff and unmoldable, the flesh firm and unpliable, and the body-length increased. In some instances the child as a whole is of greater size than ordinarily, and the mechanical labor difficulties are pronounced. I have already (p. 690) discussed this subject, and stated that my practice is not to allow the women to go too far beyond term. Some women come to the accoucheur giving a history of difficult labors with immense children. It is wise to accept the story with much reservation, because often, for various reasons, the previous attendant will exaggerate the size of the child, and again the patient herself will do the same, sometimes forgetting. Nevertheless, such a pregnancy requires watching, and if the child actually does grow too large, it is best to interrupt it.

Conditions.—The child must be living and viable in all cases where the pregnancy is terminated in its interests. It may not be deformed. A child delivered before the thirtieth week of gestation has but little chance of survival. Speaking broadly, with every week of gestation after this period the child's chances improve 10 per cent. In determining the size of the child by palpation the possibility of twins is to be borne in mind.

The pelvis may not be too markedly contracted, it being generally conceded that in pelves below 7 and 7½ cm. the outlook for an infant, even at the thirty-second week, is dubious.

The condition of the mother must be such that she will probably live through the operation. Although several cases are on record of the operation being done on a moribund woman, actual practice seldom justifies it. The consent of the mother or next of kin must be obtained, and in all cases a consultation is essential, first, because human judgment is fallible, and, second, to avoid legal entanglements later. A written statement is desirable.

The Prognosis.—In a collection of 2200 cases Sarwey found a maternal mortality of 1.4 per cent.—0.6 per cent. due to infection, but part of this may have been due to causes not inherent in the operation itself. Nowadays, with our perfected technic, the induction of labor should be without mortality ascribable to infection carried in by the accoucheur, but it is not possible always to avoid infecting the woman with virulent bacteria already present in the genitalia, for example, in gonorrhea, in the urine from a ureteropyelitis, even those of the ordinary vaginal flora. If, as not seldom happens, the operation requires repeated internal manipulations extending over several days, the streptococci in the vagina, given blood, bruised tissue, and a depressed woman, acquire invasive virulence; therefore it is not uncommon in prolonged cases, in spite of the most painstaking aseptic technic, for the patient to have fever, and in a few cases fatal sepsis may arise.

The morbidity is not small. Dilatation of the cervix is usually imperfect and lacerations are common, which is also true of the pelvic floor to a less degree. Operative termination of the labor is oftener required, which carries with it the dangers so often referred to. If the uterus is very sluggish, the various operations have to be repeated day after day. Such cases act badly on the nervous system of the patient. In a few cases on record the attempt to get the uterus to act had to be abandoned, and the pregnancy went to term. Some of the methods employed are not without danger—the insertion of a bougie, for instance, may detach the placenta.

For the child, the general mortality is from 30 to 60 per cent., depending on the period of pregnancy and the indication which demanded the interference. Ahlfeld collected the authentic cases of very premature children, and found 19 of weights ranging from 500 to 1000 grams that survived. Ylppoe made a most exhaustive study of the early life of premature infants. The child of a sickly mother will have less chance of survival than one from a healthy parent. The dangers besetting the child in passing a narrowed pelvis are to be carefully weighed. Nowadays specialized obstetric nursing and the scientific incubator have done much for the premature infant. The presentation of the child has much to do with the prognosis, that of the breech being particularly unfavorable. It is best to secure cephalic presentation before operating—at least, perfect dilatation of the parturient canal—to make the exit of the tender child the easiest possible.

Technic.—Of the 20 or more methods that have been recommended, only a few are practised, and the selection will depend on the urgency of the case, the rapidity with which it is necessary to empty the uterus, and individual preference.

Puncture of the Bag of Waters.—This is the oldest method, mentioned by Denman in 1793, as the generally known, probably only, one. Any long-pointed instrument may be used, as scissors, but where obtainable, a thin trocar is better. By forcing the head down into the cervix, by allowing the water to trickle away, not to rush out in a stream, better, using the Sims' position, prolapse of the cord may be prevented. If the head is movable and prolapse of the cord likely, it is wiser to substitute another method. In primiparæ, with a closed cervix, the disadvantages of a dry labor are to be borne in mind. Puncture of the membranes is the most certain of all methods, and may be used when other, milder means fail. An overdistended uterus is to be handled gently—a slight increase in its hydraulic pressure may burst it. Feel for pulsating fetal vessels, velamentous cord.

Bougies.—Krause in 1855 introduced one or two elastic solid bougies into the uterus between the membranes and the wall. In 2 cases of my own the placenta was encroached on, with severe but controllable hemorrhage. The bag of waters may be punctured, and I think the danger of infection is higher than with other methods. In a case seen in Berlin, necrosis of the track of the bougies was found postmortem.

By the light of broad specula the cervix is exposed, and two No. 24 French size, soft-rubber bougies are passed into the uterus, going to either side, behind, in the direction of the least resistance. If the least blood appears, both are to be removed and the vagina packed. Next day another method of induction, usually puncture of the membranes, is to be practised.

Dilatation of the Cervix.—Hydrostatic dilatation of the cervix is often used to hasten labor and in the treatment of placenta prævia. A bag in the cervix both dilates it and stimulates the pains. For details see p. 502. When the bags are used simply to start labor-pains, the small sized ones are selected. Pains usually come on within six hours, but often subside immediately the bag is expelled, requiring the insertion of another. Sometimes the pains do not come on for several days, even if larger and larger bags are put in every twenty-four hours. It cannot be denied that sometimes the bag displaces the head and allows malpresentations and prolapse of the cord to occur, killing the baby.

Packing the cervix and lower uterine segment with gauze is a favorite method of the author. It is illustrated in Fig. 791. Under the guidance of the fingers, or in the view provided by broad specula, and with the cervix drawn down by vulsellum forceps, a strip of gauze 3 to 5 yards long and 3 inches wide is snugly and evenly placed in the lower part of the uterus and the cervical canal.

Sometimes the separation of the membranes, by swinging the finger around the

71

lower pole of the uterus, is enough to bring on contractions (Hamilton). I have used this method at term with labor imminent.

Medicines.—The old combination, quinin and castor oil, will bring on labor (if the woman is at or over term) in about 30 per cent. of cases. In rare instances the pains are tetanic and jeopardize the child. (See Williamson.) Occasionally quinin can cause the death of the fetus in utero (Gellhorn).

Pituitary extracts are dangerous when used as they are at present. I know of one rupture of the uterus, and, therefore, proceed warily (*vide infra*).

Author's Practice.—Where there is no great hurry, my practice is as follows: One trial of quinin and castor oil is made. The oil is given at 8 A. M., and quinin, gr. iii, as soon as the bowels begin to act. At the end of twenty-four hours, if there is no result, the patient is prepared as for any major obstetric operation. Under the strictest aseptic precautions the cervix is dilated with the finger-tip and straightened, then the region just above the internal os is loosely, and the cervical canal tightly packed with gauze, as described on p. 983, leaving no ends hanging out the vulva. I usually do this about 9 A. M. Pains usually come on by 3 or 5 o'clock the same day, and as soon as they are well established the gauze may be removed. If pains do not come on by 9 A. M. the next day, a medium-sized Voorhees bag is inserted. While the uterus may not have gotten into regular action some pains always have occurred, and they have softened the cervix and produced some effacement. If, within fifteen hours, regular pains have not set in, the membranes are ruptured, and now, with very few exceptions, the labor goes on quickly.

In a few cases I combine minute doses of pituitary extract with the quinin and oil, as follows: One hour after the quinin, $\frac{1}{2}$ unit of a standard pituitary preparation is given, hypodermically; fifteen minutes later, exactly 1 unit, in twenty minutes, 2 units, and if there is no effect, in twenty minutes, 3 units. The medicine must be given by an accoucheur, who listens to the fetal heart almost constantly and notes the uterine response. He has by him a can of ether wherewith to check untoward action of the uterus.

Since Hofbauer has shown that pituitary extract applied on cotton in the nose is absorbed, and that too strong effects can be controlled by quick removal of the tampon, I have tried thus to induce labor. I prefer the minute hypo doses as being more scientific.

In cases where emptying the uterus is urgently needed—edema pulmonum, cardiac decompensation, eclampsia and preëclampsia, and in hemorrhagic disease, pulmonary tuberculosis, thyrotoxicoses, etc., abdominal delivery is preferred—laparotrachelotomy under local anesthesia. In the exceptional multipara with relaxed cervix—vaginal hysterotomy.

Where the urgency is less acute, especially in multiparæ, puncture of the membranes and insertion of a balloon dilator will usually suffice to induct pains.

Irregular uterine action, abnormal contraction rings, malpresentations and malpositions of the fetus, insufficient dilatation of the cervix, nervous exhaustion, sleeplessness, prolonged anxiety of the patient, fever, prolapse of the cord, lacerations of the soft parts, operative interference, postpartum hemorrhage, and many other grave and less grave complications must be expected when you induce labor.

Premature children suffer severely from the traumatism of labor. Breech deliveries are especially fatal to them, therefore version, as a rule, is contraindicated. They are prone to fracture of the bones, cerebral hemorrhage, and atelectasis pulmonum. For these reasons I often do laparotrachelotomy to guarantee the life of the baby, especially if this is to be the mother's only one.

If delivery is effected by forceps, episiotomy is desirable to spare the head the perineal pressure. After delivery it is essential that the lungs be well inflated, that the infant be kept warm, and that it be placed in a properly ventilated and disinfected incubator. Mother's milk and good nursing, however, are more important than the incubator. The best results are obtained by combining the three.

For the sake of completion a few obsolete and dangerous methods may be named: Puncture of the membranes high up in the uterus with a trocar; intrauterine injection of water, hot and cold, of glycerin, milk, etc.; the Kiwisch douche —a stream of hot water against the cervix; carbon dioxid water irrigations of the vagina; vaginal tamponade; colpeurysis; electricity; the x-ray; irritation of the nipples; medicines, as cimicifuga, ergot, cathartics, etc. (Literature in Williamson).

Induction of Abortion.—This operation has been done since remotest antiquity, and in savage as well as civilized lands. By some it was done to prevent overpopulation, and was a recognized procedure; by others to avoid the discomforts and dangers of the function of reproduction, or even the disfigurement of the person wrought by gestation, as in decadent Rome. The child was considered to be without a soul—only a growth on its mother. As a therapeutic measure, abortion was done long before Christ; indeed, the production of abortion by a physician for other reasons was considered unethical, as witness the oath of Hippocrates. The ancient Jews considered abortion a great sin, but admitted it as a means of cure of disease affecting the mother. The promulgation of Christian principles did much to stop the practice, at least openly, and soon the law made it a punishable offense. (See Lecky, History of European Morals.)

One of the saddest commentaries on our modern "civilization," in a so-called religious and ethical era, is the prevalence of criminal abortion. A young physician is not long in practice before he is approached with the request, in a hundred ways, open or concealed, to perform a criminal abortion. Not alone the single woman, but the married, will come. All arguments will be brought to bear— that of friendship for a stricken family, the disgrace of a child under untoward circumstances, the impossibility of caring for a large number of children, ill health, even gold will be offered. The physician should allow none of these things to influence him to do an abortion, because, first, it is murder, and conscience will make his later days miserable; second, it is a criminal offense, and, performed in the way most of such operations have to be done, infection will likely follow, and perhaps death of the patient, with a prison term for the perpetrator, in the perspective; third, accidents, like perforation of the uterus and anesthetic deaths, are not uncommon; fourth, if he does it once he is a lost man,—the woman, no matter how firmly she has been bound to secrecy, will tell her friends, and soon his reputation as an abortionist will be established. There are other reasons, but the conscientious physician will not need any at all. A word of warning: Let the inexperienced physician beware of simulated disease. A woman will read up on some disease which she knows sometimes gives the indication for abortion, and will try to impress the doctor that she is deathly ill. We cannot discuss here the many legal points involved in cases of rape and in abortion in general. See Hartman, Olshausen, and Peterson, Haines, and Webster. The position held by the Catholic Church is clearly set forth by Rev. E. J. Burke.

Therapeutic abortion is rarely indicated, and lately our general therapy has improved so much that few affections justify its performance. (1) Contracted pelvis with a conjugata vera below 6 cm., mentioned by Soranus of Ephesus in the second century A.D., and by Cooper in 1772, to avoid the terrific mortality of cesarean section. Nowadays, with the safety of cesarean section, the accoucheur should refuse to perform abortion for this indication unless there are other, scientific reasons, *e. g.*, heart, lung, or kidney disease. (2) Hyperemesis gravidarum and other forms of toxemia (Gestoses). Without doubt, here is a real indication for abortion, but a restricted one. In cases of toxemic vomiting, with the evidences of real involvement of the structure of the liver and kidneys, one should not wait too long before emptying the uterus. (3) Incarceration of the retroflexed, gravid uterus is usually better treated by laparotomy. (4) Advancing tuberculosis, as shown by loss of weight, evening fever, hemoptysis, etc., unresponsive to treatment. Opinion is divided as to whether pregnancy aggravates tuberculosis or not. (See Hill.) A combination of hyperemesis gravidarum and tuberculosis is a positive indication for abortion, as is also tuberculous laryngitis. (5) Heart disease is only an indication when the muscle is badly inefficient, as advanced myocarditis and decompensation. (6) Diabetes and other constitutional diseases, as under induced labor. In preparing for operations on diabetics, and in the acidosis and coma which may follow them, insulin is invaluable. (Cf. Reveno.) (7) Diseases of the kidneys, especially if complicated by retinitis. (8) Other diseases which seriously jeopardize the mother, as Basedow's disease, leukemia, pernicious anemia, chorea, otosclerosis, etc. (see Lit.). (9) Nervous and mental diseases (multiple sclerosis, epilepsia, amentia, etc.) seldom indicate abortion (Herschman, Lit.). (10) Diseases of the ovum—polyhydramnion, hydatidiform mole, death. In the last mentioned, hemorrhage from the uterus usually indicates interference, and then the procedure cannot be called true abortion; rather we are simply completing a process nature has begun. Hemorrhage during the early months of pregnancy may come from placenta prævia, placenta marginata, cornual placenta, and chronic abortion, and may require interference. Repeated bleedings are almost always followed by complete abortion. Sometimes the pregnancy continues to term, and trouble arises in the placental stage from placenta accreta and postpartum hemorrhage. Again, a placenta prævia will show itself in the seventh or eighth month. While a few of my cases have gone to term, as a rule I find frequent hemorrhages in the early months sufficient indication for interference. (See Winter's Monograph on this subject, also Fairbairn.)

In one case, a neurotic, highly bred, "overcivilized" (Reynolds) woman, the psychic shock of the pregnancy was so great that the question of therapeutic abortion was seriously considered. I refused to do it, advising mental treatment, and the woman disappeared, but had she not, in my hands, quickly recovered from the continuous nervous excitement, the sleeplessness, the almost maniacal fear of pregnancy, which reminded me very much of the overwhelming terror some people have of thunder-storms, I am sure that abortion would have been justified. Tokophobia, the exaggerated fear of labor, is advanced by many women as a reason for requesting an abortion.

The conditions for the operation are about the same as for induced labor. The moral and religous aspects of the case must be considered, never forgetting that in those cases where disease in pregnancy threatens the life of the mother, the induction of abortion is a conservative operation, "saving the mother," not "sacrificing the child," because, as Pinard says, the mother would otherwise become the "coffin" of the child. (See p. 1111.) Always insist on a consultation, draw up a written statement of the facts in the case, and have it signed by the woman, her next kin, and all the physicians in charge. In Catholic families advise with the priest. Every appearance of mystery and secrecy must be sedulously avoided. It is best to perform the operation in a hospital.

Technic.—The operations may be divided into those done during the first eight weeks, those done from the eighth to the sixteenth week, and those from this time until the child is viable.

In the first eight weeks the uterus usually can be emptied all at one sitting. An anesthetic is not always required, but the accoucheur must be able to do everything with the greatest deliberation and comfort. A careful bimanual examination is made to discover an ectopic pregnancy or a retroflexion. The cervix is dilated with Goodell dilators of increasing sizes, this part requiring from fifteen to twenty-five minutes. Then the contents of the uterus are removed with the curet and polypus forceps, after which the cavity is lightly filled with a strip of gauze. This stops the bleeding, and when, next day, it is removed, it brings with it shreads of decidua which may have been overlooked. In rare cases the cervix is so hard that it is impossible or unsafe forcibly to dilate it. Here the cervix may be packed with iodoform gauze for twenty-four hours, when it will be found softened and dilatable. Perhaps a tent may be put in, but I do not recommend them, since I consider them dangerous. When haste is not demanded, the two-stage method may be chosen.

During the third and fourth month the abortion is done in two stages. On the first day the os is opened a little with a Goodell dilator, then with a curet the ovum is broken up, making certain that the amnion has been punctured; then the cavity of the uterus is lightly, the cervix and vagina tightly, packed with gauze by means of the tubular packer shown on p. 983. Pains almost always start up within twelve hours, and if the packing is not expelled, at least the cervix is opened enough to put in one finger. If it is not, the packing may be repeated—this time I usually use a piece of weak iodin gauze. At the end of another twenty-four hours the uterus may be emptied, as described under Abortion. If the uterus must be emptied quickly, this may be done by anterior vaginal hysterotomy, but I do not advise the cutting operation as routine.

If sterilization of the patient is to be combined with therapeutic abortion, the best way is to make a short, low abdominal incision (preferably Pfannenstiel), empty the uterus, and exsect the tubes or amputate the fundus—*i. e.*, to do a miniature cesarean section or Porro. These operations are usually possible under morphin, scopolamin, and local anesthesia.

During the fifth and sixth months the process resembles the induction of premature labor more. The bag of waters should be ruptured, and a small-sized Voorhees bag inserted. In cases of great urgency vaginal cesarean section should be performed. Let me warn the accoucheur against the removal of a small fetus piecemeal through a long, narrow cervical canal. It will tax his skill to the utmost, especially if, as so frequently happens, the body is torn off the head, which bobs around in the blood in the uterine cavity. If he attempts this operation, every bit of the body of the fetus should be laid out on a clean towel, and he may not call the work complete until all the parts of the fetus are accounted for. After the placenta is removed, the whole interior of the uterus is lightly cureted, and finally the cavity is filled with gauze, which is removed the next day. *Wherever possible, the fingers are to be used instead of the curet or ovum forceps.*

There is no medicine which will safely bring on abortion, though many are vaunted for the purpose. Other methods of inducing abortion have been named under Induced Labor.

After-treatment.—Ergot and hydrastis, of each 10 minims, are administered thrice daily for a week. Douches are not used—only external washings with a weak antiseptic solution. The woman should lie abed for one week and only gradually assume her duties.

Prognosis.—The induction of abortion is attended by a certain, though in proper hands small, mortality. The dangers are infection, which is not always avoidable, since the woman may have it within her, and perforation of the uterus. I consider the operation of induced abortion one of the most dangerous in obstetrics, a view confirmed by Albert in recent statistics. The most painstaking asepsis does not always guarantee an afebrile convalescence. Perforation of the uterus by the curet is sometimes very easy. It has happened to every accoucheur of experience—either the cervix tears into the broad ligaments or peritoneal cavity, or the curet, even the finger, goes through the wall of the uterus. In one recorded case the uterine muscle was so soft that the weight of the curet held vertically on the extirpated uterus sufficed to make it go through to the table underneath. I confess I use the curet only with the greatest distrust, and dispense with it entirely if the finger can gain access to the uterus. The ovum forceps, too, are dangerous, and many cases are reported annually of the drawing out of coils of gut and omentum through perforations in the uterus. Spiculæ of bone from a dismembered fetus may also puncture the uterine wall, and the lower uterine segment may be torn during forced attempts to draw the fetus through it. In view of all this the operation is not to be lightly undertaken, and is to be performed with the greatest gentleness and circumspection.

LITERATURE

Albert: Zentralb. für Gyn., September 19, 1931.—*Browne:* Fetal Death from Strep. Hemolyt., Jour. Amer. Med. Assoc., September 11, 1926.—*Burke, Rev. E. J.:* Acute Cases in Moral Medicine, McMillan, 1922.—*DeLee:* "A Study of the Causes of Some Stillbirths," Jour. Amer. Med. Assoc., July 29, 1916; also "Fetal Infection as a Cause of Stillbirth," Bulletin New York Lying-in Hospital, January, 1917.—*Fairbairn:* London Lancet, January 29, 1927.—*Gellhorn:* Amer. Jour. Obst. and Gyn., June, 1927.—*Hartman:* Annales de Gyn. et d'Obst., April, 1915, p. 466.—*Henkel:* Halban and Seitz, Biol. und Path. des Wiebes, 1924, Band ii, p. 545.—*Herschmann, H.:* Zentb. für Gynaek., August 22, 1931, p. 2576. Report of Symposium.—*Hill, Alice M.:* American Review of Tuberculosis, Fall, 1927.—*Le Count:* "Embolic Decidual Endometritis," Transactions Chicago Gyn. Soc., February, 1918.—*Olshausen:* Medizinische Klinik, 1915, No. 48.—*Otosclerosis:* Zentb. für Gyn., February 26, 1927, and Zeitschr. für Geb. u. Gyn., 1927, xci, p. 194.—*Peterson, Haines, and Webster:* Toxicology and Legal Medicine.—*Reveno:* "Insulin in Diabetic Coma Complicating Pregnancy," Jour. Amer. Med. Assoc., December 22, 1923.—*Smith:* Jour. Amer. Med. Assoc., July 7, 1917, p. 43.—*Temesvary:* Zentb. für Gyn., 1927.—*Thalheimer:* "Insulin in Hyperemesis," Transactions of the Chicago Gyn. Soc., April, 1924.—*Williamson:* Surg., Gyn., and Obst., June, 1922, p. 812; *Idem,* Jour. Obst. and Gyn., Brit. Empire, August, 1905, p. 254.—*Winter:* Der Künstliche Abort, Stuttgart, Enke, 1926.—*Ylppoe:* Zeitsch. f. Kinderheilk., 1919, Band 24.

A BRIEF OBSTETRIC CHRONOLOGY

Reproduced (with additions by the author) from Ottow's chapter in Stoeckel's Lehrbuch der Geburtshilfe, with the kind permission of the two authors and the publisher, G. Fischer, Jena.

Prehistoric Times. Primitive methods of giving help in all early peoples, carried on by women aided by priests and transmitted to modern times in the cults and practices of savage tribes.

3500 B. C. Egyptians had maternities.

1500 B. C. India—Brahmanism, Jews. Isolation of puerperæ (Ayur Veda of Susruta). Egyptians, Jews preach extreme cleanliness in obstetric practice. Eight presentations of fetus distinguished. Podalic version. Later separation of priests from medical practice. Cesarean section after sudden death obligatory. Embryotomy.

Circa 400 B. C. Zenith of empiric medicine among the Greeks. The time of Hippocrates. Dawn of anatomic basis for medicine. Midwives. Physicians knew theory only, learned mostly from sacrificial animals. They performed destructive operations, knew fetal positions, believing cephalic only the normal, and advised internal cephalic version. Believed pelvis spread during labor. Intra-uterine injections.

Circa 300 B. C. Greek—Alexandrian period. Human anatomy studied. Herophilus discovers the ovaries.

200 B. C. Greek—Alexandrian medicine in Rome. Midwives care for births, slave physicians begin to learn obstetrics. Lex regia (of mythical origin) habilitated in practice. Jewish Talmud (Babylon) mentions cesarean section on the living and for twins.

A. D. Celsus about Christ's time, Roman Encyklopedist, mentions version in transverse position of a dead fetus.

100 A. D. Soranus of Ephesus wrote a good book for midwives. Positions of child, describes version, bringing down arms. Induces labor. Treats dystocia in modern fashion. Protects perineum.

150 A. D. Galen reconstructs medicine of the past. No influence on obstetrics.

400 A. D. Cesarean section done by Jews.

Middle Ages. The gloomy period of medicine; previous acquisitions preserved in monasteries (not used); Arabian and Jewish physicians kept alive Grecian medicine. (Avicenna, et al.) Medical school in Salerno, 850–1200. Greco-Arabic science. Scholastic Medicine. Nadir of obstetrics. Midwives rule; version forgotten; surgeons craniotomize and extract. Puerperal infection rife.

14th Century. Maternity wards in hospitals. Nuremberg 1339. Paris 1378 et al.

1452. Attempt to regulate midwifery practice and establish the guild. Regensburg, Germany.

1513. First German text-book for midwives, by Eucharius Roesslin, later one by Walther Rüff, in 1545.

16th Century. Renaissance. Reëstablishment of medicine based on ancient principles but soon followed by disbelief in their authority resulting from the anatomical discoveries of Vesalius, Falloppio, Eustachi et al. Wound surgery flourishes.

1550. Ambroise Paré resurrected podalic version. Founds (although a surgeon) school of obstetrics in France. Son-in-law Guillemeau treats placenta prævia by version and extraction. Marks beginning of scientific era in obstetrics.

1589. First German school for midwives; Munich.

1595. Mercurio, Italy; obstetric anatomist; invents Walcher position; says contracted pelvis requires cesarean.

1609. Louise Bourgeois, Parisian midwife, describes face presentation; introduces induction of premature labor.

1610. Trautmann, Wittenberg, first report of cesarean section.

1620. The obstetric forceps. Kept a secret by the French family Chamberlen.

1630. Midwife school in Paris, Hotel Dieu. Men excluded.

1650. Ph. Legoust discovers the fetal heart tones.

1651. William Harvey declares, "Omne vivum ex ovo." Postulates the fetal circulation. (Later, 1786, studied anatomically by John Hunter.)

17th Century. Men succeed in gaining entrance to obstetric practice in France and Spain. One permitted to study in the Hotel Dieu; learn normal labor.

1668. François Mauriceau. Elevates French obstetrics. Describes eclampsia, mentions ectopic gestation, calls lochia a wound secretion and suspects the epidemic nature of puerperal infection. Invents a method of extraction of after-coming head. (Mauriceau-Levret-Smellie-Veit maneuver.)

1670. Hugh Chamberlen tries his forceps on a patient given him by Mauriceau;—fails, patient dies of injury.

1670. Regnerus de Graaf describes the Graafian Follicle and Corpus Luteum.

1685. Paul Portal (Paris) educated in the Hotel Dieu, recognizes true nature of placenta prævia —Paré thought it a prolapsed placenta.

1690. Justine Sigmundine, Brandenburg midwife, writes a book for midwives, classifies positions of head according to occiput and invents the tape-on-leg maneuver for versions.
1701. Hendrik van Deventer founds the science of contracted pelves, and begins the study of the mechanism of labor.
1720. Jean Palfyn of Ghent, Belgium, presents his obstetric forceps to the Paris Academy of Medicine.
1722. De la Motte develops internal version (he had a very small hand); emphasizes the inlet as important in contracted pelvis.
1725. Frederik Ruysch recommends expectant treatment of third stage, advising against pulling on cord, squeezing uterus, etc.
1738. Johann Jakob Fried extends the Strasbourg midwife school to teach doctors.
1742. Sir Fielding Ould exalts obstetrics in Ireland, develops knowledge of mechanism of labor, invents episiotomy.
1747. André Levret (Paris) invents French obstetric forceps with a pelvic curve.
1751. Johann Georg Roederer establishes clinical obstetrics in Germany. Teaches the head enters pelvis in oblique attitude.
1752. William Smellie of London teaches advanced obstetrics; emphasizes natural labor; invents short and long (curved) forceps; describes forceps in occiput posterior positions; publishes obstetric atlas, measures conjugata diagonalis.
1772. William Cooper advises therapeutic abortion for contracted pelvis.
1774. William Hunter publishes Anatomy of Pregnant Uterus.
1775. Jean Louis Baudelocque develops obstetrics in Paris; improves pelvic mensuration.
1777. Jean Réné Sigault performs first symphysiotomy on living.
1780. Charles White, England, recommends position later named "Fowler" for uterine drainage.
1784. Aitken of Edinburgh recommends pelviotomy with chain saw.
1788. Thomas Denman, London, advises artificial premature labor, for contracted pelvis.
1791. Lucas Johann Boër founds Vienna Obstetric School. Extreme conservatism; only 0.47 per cent. forceps deliveries.
1796. Friedrich Benjamin Osiander in Goettingen recommends much interference in labor; 45 per cent. forceps. In 1799 writes first history of obstetrics.
1799. Franz Anton Mai recommends puncture of membranes to induce labor.
1805. Osiander invents and performs low, cervical cesarean section.
1806. Wendelstaedt invented uterine tamponade.
1807. Joerg (Leipzig) describes low, cervical section.
1808. John Stearns of Massachusetts uses Ergot.
1812. Franz Carl Naegelè (Heidelberg) established his rule for computation of length of pregnancy. Describes entry of fetal head in pelvis. "N's obliquity."
1818. Fr. Isaac Mayor, Geneva, re-discovers fetal heart tones. Philip Legoust had heard them in 1650.
1818. W. J. Schmitt (Vienna) and J. H. Wigand (Hamburg) develop abdominal diagnosis of presentation and position. Baudelocque.
1821. F. Ritgen attempts extraperitoneal cesarean section.
1822. Lejumeau de Kergaredec establishes clinical importance of fetal heart tones.
1827. Carl Ernst von Baer (Königsberg) discovers the human ovum.
1829. A. Baudelocque (nephew) invents cephalotripsy.
1831. J. Berschins (Stockholm) studies liquor amnii chemically.
1832. Gennaro Galbiati (Italy) performs pelviotomy.
1833. First clinic for students of medicine opened in Paris.
1833. James Blundell (London) did Porro operation on rabbits. S. Storer of Boston did it for fibroids in 1869.
1839-45. E. C. Jak. v. Siebold writes classic history of obstetrics.
1839. Franz Carl Naegelè describes pelvis named after him. Others follow.
1842. Carl Rokitansky describes pregnancy in uterine horn, also acute yellow atrophy of liver.
1843. Oliver Wendell Holmes (Boston) proves puerperal fever a contagious disease carried by physicians and midwives, but misses the point of exactly how it is transmitted. Dropped the fight for his theory after two efforts.
1843. John C. W. Lever of London discovers albuminuria in eclampsia.
1847. Sir James Young Simpson introduces ether and chloroform in obstetrics.
1846. James Marion Sims invents vaginal speculum.
1847. Ignaz Philipp Semmelweis (Budapesth) recognizes the true nature of puerperal infection and teaches a good method of prevention.
1850. Sir James Young Simpson introduces prophylactic version.
1851. Carl v. F. Braun (Vienna) invents rubber colpeurynter, replacing the pig's bladder.
1851. Gustav Adolf Michaëlis (Kiel) founds our modern knowledge of contracted pelves. Aided by Litzmann (Kiel).
1853. Carl Siegmund Credé (Leipzig) introduces his method of expelling the placenta; also the use of AgNo₃ to prevent gonorrheal ophthalmia (Eisenmann in 1830 had recommended chlorine water).
1854. Marmaduke Burr Wright of Ohio introduces combined cephalic version.
1855. Steinau recommends rubber gloves to prevent puerperal infection.
1863. John Braxton Hicks (London) describes his method of combined podalic version.
1862. Robert Barnes (London) invents the fiddle-shaped bag for dilating cervix.
1864. Hugh Lennox Hodge, Philadelphia, publishes work on mechanism of labor giving the parallel pelvic planes.

1867. Joseph Lister (Edinburgh) promulgates theory of infection of wounds by the air and introduces antisepsis.

1872. Christian Wilhelm Braune (Leipzig) makes frozen sections of pregnant women for anatomic study.

1875. Oscar Hertwig (Jena) discovers the process of conception.

1875. Ludwig Bandl (Vienna) describes uterine action in rupture and the formation of Bandl's ring.

1876. Eduardo Porro (Milan) performs supravaginal amputation of uterus following cesarean with exteriorization of stump.

1877. Stéphene Tarnier (Paris) begins his work on axis-traction forceps.

1879. Albert Neisser (Breslau) discovers the gonococcus.

1881. Stéphene Tarnier (Paris) introduces carbolic acid antisepsis in obstetrics.

1882. Max Saenger (Leipzig) introduces improved and practical cesarean section.

1882. Ferdinand Adolph Kehrer (Heidelberg) suggests low transverse incision in cesarean section.

1883. Robert Lawson Tait (England) does first successful operation for ectopic pregnancy.

1886. O. Morisani (Italy) publishes indications and technic of symphysiotomy. Tarnier replaces carbolic acid by HgCl₂.

1887. Alfred Duehrssen (Berlin) establishes value of deep episiotomy.

1892. Albert Doederlein (Leipzig) founds modern bacteriology of the lochia, advancing bacteriology of the parturient canal.

1893. E. Ries (now Chicago) and Krönig (then Leipzig) introduce rectal examination.

1894. Leonardo Gigli (Italy) reintroduces pubiotomy, inventing the wire saw.

1895. Wilhelm Konrad Roentgen (Würzburg) discovers x-ray.

1896. Alfred Duehrssen (Berlin) introduces vaginal cesarean section, upon which the "surgical era" in obstetrics begins.

1902. Richard von Steinbüchel (Graz) recommends morphin-scopolamin, "twilight sleep," for obstetrics; later developed by Krönig and Gauss.

1905. Fritz Schaudinn and Erich Hoffmann (Berlin) discover the cause of syphilis, the Spirochæta pallida.

1906. H. Dale (Edinburgh) discovers the oxytocic action of pituitary extract; beginning of the hormonal treatment of labor pains.

1907. Fritz Frank (Bonn) resurrects the low cervical cesarean section.

1908. Hugo Sellheim (Tubingen) places anatomic foundation under low cervical cesarean section.

1913. Hugo Sellheim (Tubingen) establishes principles of mechanism of labor.

1916. Christian Kielland (Oslo) invents a new obstetric forceps.

1927. S. Aschheim and B. Zondek invented first successful hormonal test for pregnancy.

1931. J. Whitridge Williams describes uterine involution.

INDEX

72

Date Due

'47